Biofunctional Cosmetics for Health

Biofunctional Cosmetics for Health

Exploring Nature's Ingredients for Safety, Efficacy, and Sustainability

Edited by

Alexandros Tsoupras
Hephaestus Laboratory,
School of Chemistry, Faculty of Sciences,
Democritus University of Thrace,
Kavala University Campus, Kavala, Greece

George Z. Kyzas
Hephaestus Laboratory,
School of Chemistry, Faculty of Sciences,
Democritus University of Thrace,
Kavala University Campus, Kavala, Greece

ELSEVIER

ACADEMIC PRESS
An imprint of Elsevier

Academic Press is an imprint of Elsevier
125 London Wall, London EC2Y 5AS, United Kingdom
50 Hampshire Street, 5th Floor, Cambridge, MA 02139, United States

ISBN: 978-0-443-27500-5

For information on all Academic Press publications visit our website at https://www.elsevier.com/books-and-journals

Publisher: Mara Conner
Acquisitions Editor: Nicole Denis
Editorial Project Manager: Kritika Sharma
Production Project Manager: M. Balakrishnan
Cover Designer: Mark Rogers

Printed in England by CPI Group (UK) Ltd
Croydon CR0 4YY
United Kingdom

Typeset by Integra Software Services

Alexandros's dedications

To my wife, Maria, and to the rest of my family, colleagues, and students for their love and continuous support, and especially to the memory of my Mother, Georgia (Γεωργία), my Father, Vasileios (Βασίλειος), and my two brothers, George (Γεώργιος) and Nestor (Νέστωρ), who, due to their kind hearts and their deep knowledge in both chess and history/philosophy/psychology and theology, all managed to inspire me during our short co-presence on how to be innovative by using all pieces on the chessboard, and always after thorough studying/evaluating everything that has been done/found so far and after viewing/re-viewing things from all possible angles, in a way that will benefit all and without losing one's self/soul.

(«Τι γαρ ωφελείται άνθρωπος εάν τον κόσμον όλον κερδίσει, την δε ψυχήν αυτού ζημιωθεί;»)/"What good will it be for someone to gain the whole world, yet forfeit their soul?" (Matthew Gospel 16:26).

"Thank you all for Everything!"

Contents

Section II
Health benefits of bioactive ingredients from sustainable plant-based sources and their by-products

Contributors

Rony Aad Politecnico di Milano, Department of Electronics, Information, and Bioengineering, Milan, Italy

Theodora Adamantidi Hephaestus Laboratory, School of Chemistry, Faculty of Sciences, Democritus University of Thrace, Kavala University Campus, Kavala, Greece

Chryssa Anastasiadou Fisheries Research Institute, Hellenic Agricultural Organization-DIMITRA (ELGO-DIMITRA), Nea Peramos, Kavala, Greece

Sotirria Anastasiou Hephaestus Laboratory, School of Chemistry, Faculty of Sciences, Democritus University of Thrace, Kavala University Campus, Kavala, Greece

Dimitrios Argyropoulos d-Lab: Digital Agriculture and Bioresources, School of Biosystems and Food Engineering, University College Dublin, Dublin, Ireland

Evangelia Baltzi Department of Food Science & Technology, School of Agricultural Sciences, University of Patras, Agrinio, Greece

Apostolos Beloukas Department of Biomedical Sciences, School of Health and Care Sciences, University of West Attica, Athens, Greece

Ida Bogdani Hephaestus Laboratory, School of Chemistry, Faculty of Sciences, Democritus University of Thrace, Kavala, Greece

Antigoni Bourgani Hephaestus Laboratory, School of Chemistry, Faculty of Sciences, Democritus University of Thrace, Kavala University Campus, Kavala, Greece

Michail Chalaris Hephaestus Laboratory, School of Chemistry, Faculty of Sciences, Democritus University of Thrace, Kavala University Campus, Kavala, Greece

Vassiliki Chrysikopoulou Hephaestus Laboratory, School of Chemistry, Faculty of Sciences, Democritus University of Thrace, Kavala University Campus, Kavala, Greece

Sunil Kumar Deshmukh Research and Development, Greenvention Biotech Pvt. Ltd., Pune, Maharashtra, India

Gkentsidis Georgios Hephaestus Laboratory, School of Chemistry, Faculty of Sciences, Democritus University of Thrace, Kavala University Campus, Kavala, Greece

Pol Gimenez-Gil Laboratory of Food Chemistry, Department of Chemistry, National and Kapodistrian University of Athens, Athens, Greece

Despina A. Gkika Hephaestus Laboratory, School of Chemistry, Faculty of Sciences, Democritus University of Thrace, Kavala University Campus, Kavala, Greece

Mayurika Goel Sustainable Agriculture Program, The Energy and Resources Institute, TERI-Gual Pahari, Gurugram, Haryana, India

Ronald Halim UCD Algae Group, School of Biosystems and Food Engineering, University College Dublin, Dublin, Ireland

Maria-Chrysanthi Kafentzi Hephaestus Laboratory, School of Chemistry, Faculty of Sciences, Democritus University of Thrace, Kavala, Greece

Haralabos C. Karantonis Laboratory of Food Chemistry – Technology and Quality of Food of Animal Origin, Department of Food Science and Nutrition, School of Environment, University of the Aegean, Lemnos, Greece

Mehak Kaur Sustainable Agriculture Program, The Energy and Resources Institute, TERI-Gual Pahari, Gurugram, Haryana; Department of Botany, University of Delhi, Delhi, India

Maria Kioiloglou Hephaestus Laboratory, School of Chemistry, Faculty of Sciences, Democritus University of Thrace, Kavala University Campus, Kavala, Greece

Eleftherios Kotos Laboratory of Food Chemistry, Department of Chemistry, National and Kapodistrian University of Athens, Athens, Greece

Ioanna Koumentakou Hephaestus Laboratory, School of Chemistry, Faculty of Sciences, Democritus University of Thrace, Kavala University Campus, Kavala, Greece

Eleni Kourmazou Hephaestus Laboratory, School of Chemistry, Faculty of Sciences, Democritus University of Thrace, Kavala University Campus, Kavala, Greece

Kusum Kumari Sustainable Agriculture Program, The Energy and Resources Institute, TERI-Gual Pahari, Gurugram, Haryana, India

Konstantina Kyprou Hephaestus Laboratory, School of Chemistry, Faculty of Sciences, Democritus University of Thrace, Kavala University Campus, Kavala, Greece

George Z. Kyzas Hephaestus Laboratory, School of Chemistry, Faculty of Sciences, Democritus University of Thrace, Kavala University Campus, Kavala, Greece
Kalliopi Ladomenou Hephaestus Laboratory, School of Chemistry, Faculty of Sciences, Democritus University of Thrace, Kavala, Greece
Maria-Parthena Lafara Hephaestus Laboratory, School of Chemistry, Faculty of Sciences, Democritus University of Thrace, Kavala University Campus, Kavala, Greece
Kassiani Lalexou Laboratory of Biochemistry, Department of Chemistry, University of Ioannina, Ioannina, Greece
Evgenia Lamprianidou Hephaestus Laboratory, School of Chemistry, Faculty of Sciences, Democritus University of Thrace, Kavala University Campus, Kavala, Greece
Sophia Letsiou Department of Biomedical Sciences, School of Health and Care Sciences; Department of Food Science and Technology, Faculty of Food Sciences, University of West Attica, Athens, Greece
Maria Nektaria Magkoulia Laboratory of Biochemistry, Department of Chemistry, University of Ioannina, Ioannina, Greece
Elpida Mantzakopoulou Laboratory of Food Chemistry, Department of Chemistry, National and Kapodistrian University of Athens, Athens, Greece
Margarida Matias Centre for Applied Bioscience Research, Technological University of the Shannon, Limerick, Ireland
Stefanos Michailidis Hephaestus Laboratory, School of Chemistry, Faculty of Sciences, Democritus University of Thrace, Kavala University Campus, Kavala, Greece
Patrick Murray Centre for Applied Bioscience Research, Technological University of the Shannon, Limerick, Ireland
Constantina Nasopoulou Laboratory of Food Chemistry – Technology and Quality of Food of Animal Origin, Department of Food Science and Nutrition, School of Environment, University of the Aegean, Lemnos, Greece
Anna Ofrydopoulou Hephaestus Laboratory, School of Chemistry, Faculty of Sciences, Democritus University of Thrace, Kavala University Campus, Kavala, Greece
Despoina Pantazi Laboratory of Biochemistry, Department of Chemistry, University of Ioannina, Ioannina, Greece
Konstantinos Pavlidis Hephaestus Laboratory, School of Chemistry, Faculty of Sciences, Democritus University of Thrace, Kavala University Campus, Kavala, Greece
Anastasia Pilakouri Hephaestus Laboratory, School of Chemistry, Faculty of Sciences, Democritus University of Thrace, Kavala University Campus, Kavala, Greece
Charalambos Proestos Laboratory of Food Chemistry, Department of Chemistry, National and Kapodistrian University of Athens, Athens, Greece
Sushanta Kumar Saha Centre for Applied Bioscience Research, Technological University of the Shannon, Limerick, Ireland
Marina Seferli Hephaestus Laboratory, School of Chemistry, Faculty of Sciences, Democritus University of Thrace, Kavala University Campus, Kavala, Greece
Katie Shiels Centre for Applied Bioscience Research, Technological University of the Shannon, Limerick, Ireland
Nikolaos Stasinopoulos Hephaestus Laboratory, School of Chemistry, Faculty of Sciences, Democritus University of Thrace, Kavala University Campus, Kavala, Greece
Eleana Toma Department of Biomedical Sciences, School of Health and Care Sciences, University of West Attica, Athens, Greece
Nikolaos Toulis Department of Biomedical Sciences, School of Health and Care Sciences, University of West Attica, Athens, Greece
Theodora-Evelina Traga Hephaestus Laboratory, School of Chemistry, Faculty of Sciences, Democritus University of Thrace, Kavala University Campus, Kavala, Greece
Evangelia Tsikopoulou Hephaestus Laboratory, School of Chemistry, Faculty of Sciences, Democritus University of Thrace, Kavala University Campus, Kavala, Greece
Konstantina Tsikrika Laboratory of Food Chemistry, Department of Chemistry, National and Kapodistrian University of Athens, Athens, Greece
Alexandros Tsoupras Hephaestus Laboratory, School of Chemistry, Faculty of Sciences, Democritus University of Thrace, Kavala University Campus, Kavala, Greece
Athina Velissaridou Hephaestus Laboratory, School of Chemistry, Faculty of Sciences, Democritus University of Thrace, Kavala University Campus, Kavala, Greece
Athena Venieri Hephaestus Laboratory, School of Chemistry, Faculty of Sciences, Democritus University of Thrace, Kavala University Campus, Kavala, Greece
Simone Vesentini Politecnico di Milano, Department of Electronics, Information, and Bioengineering, Milan, Italy
Jessica Walshe Centre for Applied Bioscience Research, Technological University of the Shannon, Limerick, Ireland

Editors' short biographies

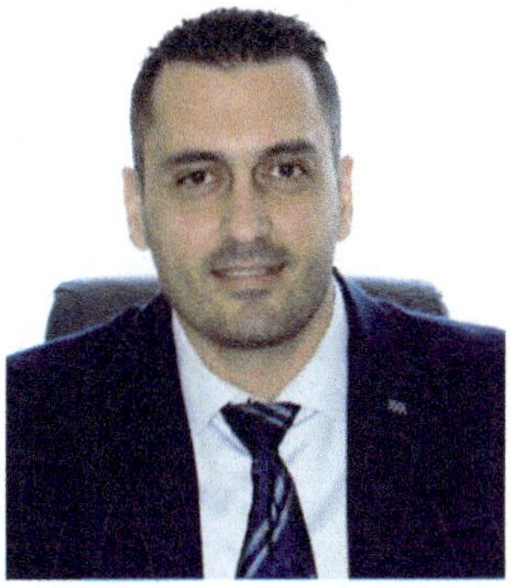

Dr. George Z. Kyzas is a Chemist and Full Professor at the Department of Chemistry, Democritus University of Thrace (DUTh). He was born in Drama (Greece) and studied Chemistry at the Department of Chemistry, Aristotle University of Thessaloniki (AUTh). He obtained his B.Sc., M.Sc., and Ph.D. degrees from the same department specializing in Chemical Technology. He is currently working at the Department of Chemistry (Democritus University of Thrace, Kavala, Greece), where he has been the Head of the Department (since 2019). He is also the Head of the Hephaestus Laboratory of the Faculty of Sciences (since 2023) and the Head of the M.Sc. in Cosmetic Chemistry (since 2021). His research interests include the synthesis and characterization of various (majorly adsorbent) materials (inorganic, aluminates, polymers, graphene, activated carbons, agrofood residues, nanomaterials, CNTs, etc.) for environmental applications (adsorption/photocatalysis and wastewater treatment). His scientific work has been published in more than 360 papers in international journals with high impact factors, while he has published 8 books and 42 chapters in scientific books and holds 5 patents. He has also served 11 times as a Guest Editor for Special issues of journals and has delivered more than 240 invited announcements at international conferences. His work is widely recognized with 26,000 citations (h-index: 89). He is the Editor of the journal *Environmental Science and Pollution Research* (Springer, IF 5.8). At the age of 42 years, he was included in the list of Highly Cited Researchers for 2022 (Thomson Reuters - Clarivate WoS) (0.1% most impactful scientists in the world). His name is also included in the list of the World's Top 2% Scientists for 2019–2024, which is compiled by the Stanford University (United States) based on standardized citation indicators. He has been awarded scholarships from the Research Committee of the Aristotle University of Thessaloniki (2009, 2013), the Greek State Scholarship Foundation (2013), and the Stavros Niarchos Foundation (2016). He has also participated in about 25 research projects. He is a reviewer for more than 200 scientific journals (ACS, Elsevier, Springer, Wiley, Taylor & Francis, etc.) and participates as Chair of Expert Panelists and as an Assessor/Evaluator/Reviewer in national, European, and international research proposals/calls/projects.

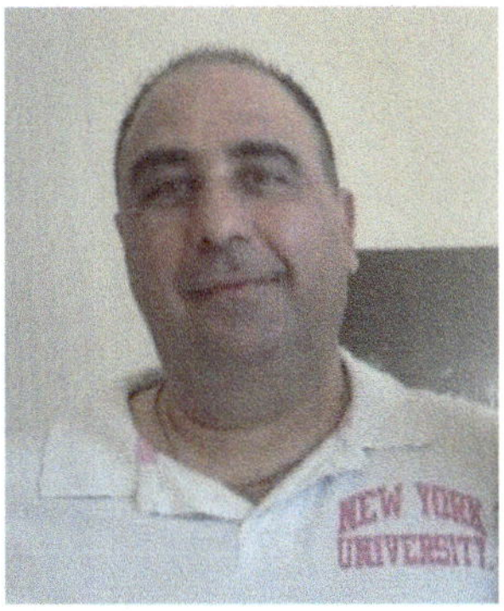

Dr. Tsoupras Alexandros is an Assistant Professor of Biochemistry at the Department of Chemistry, Democritus University of Thrace (DUTh). He holds a bachelor's degree in Chemistry and a master's degree and a Ph.D. in Chemistry–Biochemistry from the Department of Chemistry, the National and Kapodistrian University of Athens (NKUA), with scholarships from the "State Scholarship Foundation (IKY)" (first throughout Greece). During his studies, he worked as a Postgraduate Research and Teaching Assistant (2002–2008) and after graduating as a Postdoctoral Research and Teaching Associate both at NKUA (2008–2011) and at other Greek and international academic institutions, including "Albany Medical College," NY, United States (2011), and the "University of Limerick," Ireland (2017–2019). He also worked as a Lecturer at several higher education institutions and colleges (2012–2013), as a Public Servant (Chemist–Biochemist, 2023–2027), and finally as an Assistant Professor at the Department of Chemistry of NKUA (fixed-term contract at 2008), at the University of Limerick in Ireland (2019–2022), and currently at the Department of Chemistry of DUTh (2023–present).

Throughout his academic experience, Alexandros has participated in research studies investigating the implications of inflammation, thrombosis, and oxidative stress in chronic diseases and the evaluation of the antiinflammatory, antioxidant, and antithrombotic potential of several pharmaceuticals, synthetic compounds, and natural bioactives from sustainable natural sources, as active ingredients for the development of new biofunctional products (e.g., functional foods, dietary supplements, nutraceuticals, nutricosmetics, cosmeceuticals, cosmetics, and drugs–pharmaceuticals) to reduce the risk of inflammation-related chronic diseases in the context of sustainable development and circular economy.

He has also participated in several funded research programs, with relevant patents, and has contributed as a main author and/or corresponding author to more than 180 scientific publications in high-impact journals (Q1), with more than 3500 citations (h-index: 33, Scopus). He has also participated in more than 50 Panhellenic and international scientific conferences with several presentations and/or published announcements–posters having received awards. Finally, he is an evaluator of research proposals and a reviewer, a Guest Editor, and a permanent member of the Editorial Team in a multitude of journals and serves as a Main Author–Editor of scientific books and book chapters for major publishers (e.g., Elsevier, Springer, Wiley, Taylor & Francis, MDPI, etc.) within these scientific fields.

Alexandros's acknowledgements

First, I would like to thank my coeditor, Prof. George Kyzas, for the fruitful collaboration and his continuous support, not only throughout this excellent and innovative project, but also throughout all my research and teaching journey at my current Institution (School of Chemistry, Faculty of Science, Democritus University of Thrace, Kavala University Campus, Greece).

I am also grateful to all my colleagues both here in my current Institution and especially to my PostDoc Researcher, Dr. Anna Ofrydopoulou, for all her valuable support in this project, but also to those from my previous Institutions (Biochemistry and Food Chemistry Lab, Chemistry Department, University of Athens, the Department of Biological Sciences, University of Limerick, Ireland, the Region of Attica, etc.), and many others for believing in me and for giving me the opportunity to travel with them and continue my research/teaching trip.

A special thank you to all my undergraduate and postgraduate students (M.Sc. in Cosmetics Chemistry, in Biochemistry, etc., and Ph.D.s), who keep inspiring me throughout this journey toward creating a brighter, more innovative future, through lifelong learning and personal growth for becoming a better educator and human being that can shape the next generation of leaders.

I wish also to express my gratitude to my parents Vasilios and Georgia (Βασίλειος and Γεωργία), my big brothers Nestor (Νέστωρ) and George (Γεώργιος), who passed away too early, to my wife Maria (Μαρία), and to the remaining members of my family, Ioanna (Ιωάννα), Christos (Χρήστος), and Makrina (Μακρίνα) and their children, for their constant love, support, and encouragement.

I also feel gratitude to *The Three Hierarchs*—Saint Basil the Great, Saint Gregory the Theologian, and Saint John Chrysostom—who, as patrons of education with deep knowledge of medicine at the time, also taught that the human body should not be neglected, but instead it should appropriately be taken care of, especially by utilizing natural products, but also to view our body as a creation of God that works in harmony with nature and the soul, rather than a prison to be despised.

I also feel eternal gratitude to *Holy Trinity (Αγία Τριάδα—"Agia Triada")*, and especially to *"Logos" (Λόγος—"The Word")*, for always lighting the fire within me for Science and Research, for the good of all, based on the saying:

"ἐρευνᾶτε τὰς γραφάς, ὅτι ὑμεῖς δοκεῖτε ἐν αὐταῖς ζωὴν αἰώνιον ἔχειν" (Research and investigate the Scriptures diligently, because you believe and hope that within them you will find eternal life); St. John's Gospel 5:39.

Section I

Exploring biofunctional cosmetics and health properties

Chapter 1

Prologue: An introduction to sustainable natural sources of bioactive compounds for biofunctional cosmetics

Alexandros Tsoupras
Hephaestus Laboratory, School of Chemistry, Faculty of Sciences, Democritus University of Thrace, Kavala University Campus, Kavala, Greece

1 Introduction

Our modern way of life has evolved in such a way that, on the one hand, it provides us with several benefits, while on the other hand, it forces us to face several traditional and emerging challenges. Among these, one of the most important is the continuously evolving exposome, meaning the factors that we encounter each day and that can epigenetically affect the expression of important genes necessary for our daily biological function. Some factors of the exposome are not modifiable (i.e., sex, origin, age, and genetic background), while others are modifiable [i.e., dietary habits, physical activity or inactivity, smoking, alcohol consumption or abuse, and environmental conditions such as pollution and ultraviolet (UV) radiation]. Due to the presence of harmful epigenetic exposome factors, the human body reacts by activating intrinsic biochemical mechanisms in an effort to eliminate the threats it faces. Characteristic examples include the inflammatory activation of several biological mechanisms responsible for removing either the threat itself or its consequences, such as dead cells produced following exposure to UV radiation. However, when such responses become continuous or excessive, they may evolve into systemic inflammatory stimuli and the expression of genes that favor thromboinflammatory manifestations and oxidative stress. These processes can damage both cells and the extracellular matrix of connective tissues, eventually leading to unfavorable conditions that threaten human health and well-being (Tsoupras et al., 2018, 2024a).

Particularly with regard to the skin, the skin exposome refers to the cumulative environmental exposures experienced throughout a person's lifetime that may influence or alter skin health and contribute to the development of skin diseases. Key external and internal factors include solar radiation, air pollution, hormonal activity, nutrition, and psychological stress. Chronic exposure to UV radiation is strongly associated with photoaging, photocarcinogenesis, and pigmentation changes. In addition, pollutants related to traffic emissions contribute significantly to skin aging; particulate matter and nitrogen dioxide have been linked to increased pigmentation and the appearance of lentigines, while ozone exposure has been associated with wrinkle formation and the exacerbation of dermatological conditions such as atopic eczema. Hormones also play a significant role in skin physiology, regulating numerous biological processes, although their levels decline with age and contribute to age-related skin changes.

Nutrition influences essential biochemical pathways, including oxidative stress, inflammation, and glycation, which can affect the progression of skin aging and photoaging. Furthermore, psychological stress and sleep deprivation promote a proinflammatory state that may weaken extracellular matrix components, particularly collagen. Combined factors such as hormonal imbalance, inadequate nutrition, and chronic stress may therefore contribute to the development or exacerbation of inflammatory skin conditions, including atopic dermatitis, psoriasis, acne, and rosacea (Passeron et al., 2020). By considering the paradigm of the benefits derived from the Mediterranean Diet, which has been recognized by UNESCO as part of the Intangible Cultural Heritage of Humanity (Decision 5.COM 6.41), it becomes evident that this dietary pattern represents not only a nutritional practice but also a comprehensive way of living characterized by specific lifestyle choices. Recent research has demonstrated that adherence to the Mediterranean Diet provides substantial health benefits, including positive effects on skin health (Annunziata et al., 2025). Although research has investigated the role of nutrition and specific nutrients and phytonutrients in maintaining skin health, there is still a lack of clear dietary recommendations specifically aimed at achieving healthy skin. Despite the evident link between nutrition and skin health, often referred to as

Biofunctional Cosmetics for Health. https://doi.org/10.1016/B978-0-443-27500-5.00013-7

nutritional dermatology, further research is required to identify the intersection between these two disciplines (Assaf and Kelly, 2024).

Consequently, several studies have focused on how lifestyle-related factors can contribute to improved skin health and the prevention of skin aging. Lifestyle medicine is increasingly recognized as an evidence-based approach, demonstrating how daily habits and behaviors influence disease prevention and overall well-being. Even small and gradual lifestyle modifications can produce meaningful improvements in general health and may also benefit skin condition and appearance. Nevertheless, the role of lifestyle factors in maintaining skin health has received relatively limited attention in the scientific literature. Current findings suggest that four key lifestyle components can significantly support dermal health: proper nutrition and diet, adequate rest and sleep, regular physical activity, and positive social or community interactions. Overall, these lifestyle factors may contribute to healthier skin and improved well-being during aging (Knaggs and Lephart, 2023). Nevertheless, as previously mentioned, when individuals are continuously exposed to an unfavorable exposome that negatively affects skin health, lifestyle choices alone may not be sufficient, and additional protective measures may be required to overcome such threats. An important aspect of modern lifestyle choices is the increasing recommendation to incorporate natural products into everyday life, including their use in daily skincare products and general skin protection practices. The use of natural products in daily routines, particularly in skincare, represents a growing wellness trend focused on the use of raw, minimally processed, and nontoxic ingredients derived from natural sources to support long-term skin health, reduce exposure to synthetic chemicals, and promote environmental sustainability.

This shift toward the concept of "clean beauty" involves the use of several natural bioactive compounds, botanicals, essential oils, and mineral-based ingredients obtained from sustainable natural sources. These ingredients are intended to work in harmony with the skin's natural physiological functions rather than relying primarily on synthetic chemicals. Traditionally, when referring to natural materials used in cosmetics, botanical sources—particularly aromatic and medicinal plants—are the most widely recognized. However, the range of natural sources has expanded significantly in recent years and now includes additional plant-based materials such as spices, as well as marine and aquatic plants. Of particular interest in recent years are natural bioactive compounds derived from agrifood by-products, which represent a healthier and more cost-effective sustainable solution for sourcing ingredients used in biofunctional cosmetics (Fig. 1.1) (Adamantidi et al., 2025; Kontaxi et al., 2024; Letsiou et al., 2025; Marra et al., 2024; Moysidou et al., 2024; Papadopoulou et al.,

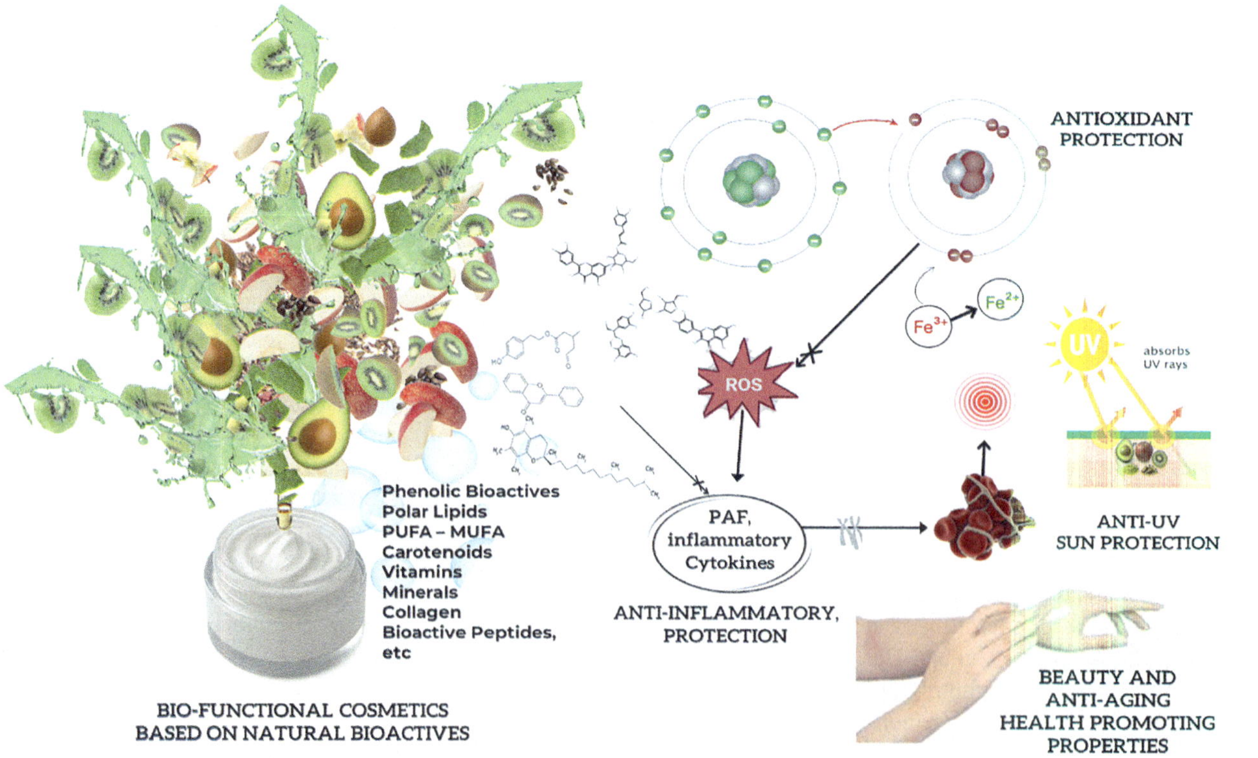

FIG. 1.1 Utilizing bioactives from sustainable natural sources for biofunctional cosmetics with health-promoting properties and benefits for skin health. Abbreviations: MUFA, monounsaturated fatty acids; PAF, platelet-activating factor; PUFA, polyunsaturated fatty acids; ROS, reactive oxygen species; UV, ultraviolet.

TABLE 1.1 Sections of the book on natural biofunctional cosmetics.

Section I	Exploring biofunctional cosmetics and health properties
Section II	Health benefits of bioactive ingredients from sustainable plant-based sources and their by-products
Section III	Sustainable bioactive ingredients from microorganisms
Section IV	Health benefits of bioactive ingredients from sustainable animal-based sources
Section V	Sustainable inorganic bioactive ingredients from natural resources
Section VI	Natural bioactives for environmentally friendly cosmetic and nutricosmetic packaging
Section VII	Epilogue

2025a, 2025b; Tsiapali et al., 2025a, 2025b; Tsoupras et al., 2024b, 2024c; Papadopoulou et al., 2024; Seferli et al., 2024; Vandorou et al., 2024; Venetikidou et al., 2025).

Within this conceptual framework, the present book explores in depth the rapidly emerging and highly promising scientific field of biofunctional cosmetics derived from natural products. Biofunctional cosmetics are advanced topical products designed to produce measurable biological effects on the skin, hair, or body, extending beyond traditional cosmetic functions that primarily focus on appearance. These products interact with physiological processes such as skin barrier repair, oxidative balance, inflammation, pigmentation, and the regulation of the skin microbiome.

Several examples of cosmetics based on natural ingredients already exist and demonstrate promising outcomes, with numerous products currently available on the market, indicating significant growth potential for natural biofunctional cosmetics. Major categories include barrier repair formulations, antiaging and longevity products, microbiome-modulating cosmetics, antioxidant and antiinflammatory formulations, pigmentation modulators, marine-derived ingredient formulations, and delivery-enhanced systems utilizing nanotechnology. These products typically contain bioactive compounds such as ceramides, peptides, antioxidants, botanical extracts, and vitamins that target specific biological pathways.

Advances in biotechnology and formulation technologies have improved ingredient stability, penetration, and efficacy, enabling biofunctional cosmetics to positively influence skin health while remaining within the regulatory domain of cosmetic products rather than medical treatments. Nevertheless, several limitations still exist, particularly those related to safety and regulatory considerations concerning the use of natural materials, as well as sustainability challenges regarding the sources utilized within a circular economy framework, which is increasingly encouraged and supported by both the European Union and the United Nations.

Within this context, this book incorporates several thematic sections aimed at introducing readers to the diverse types of natural bioactive compounds derived from sustainable sources that can be successfully incorporated into biofunctional cosmetic products to provide health-promoting properties and support overall skin health. These sections are presented in Table 1.1.

Overall, within the present chapter, a brief overview and the major key points of the chapters included in these sections are provided as a prologue, facilitating readers' first encounter with these concepts before they delve deeper into the more detailed analyses presented in the subsequent chapters.

2 Section I: Exploring biofunctional cosmetics and health properties

This section refers to an introduction of the book through a prologue (Chapter 1), which explains why it is important to incorporate biofunctional cosmetics with natural products as one of our healthy lifestyle choices, along with regulatory (Chapter 2), market-related concepts (Chapter 3), and safety issues (Chapter 4) associated with such innovative natural products of the cosmetics industry.

More specifically, within Chapter 2, the regulatory framework for biofunctional cosmetics is thoroughly reviewed, which primarily follows general cosmetic legislation but requires stronger scientific substantiation due to their biological activity. In the European Union, Regulation (EC) No. 1223/2009 governs product safety, manufacturing standards, ingredient restrictions, and documentation requirements such as the Product Information File and Cosmetic Product Safety Report. Functional claims must comply with Regulation (EU) No. 655/2013, meaning that they must be truthful, evidence-based, and not imply therapeutic effects. Additional frameworks, such as Good Manufacturing Practice (ISO 22716), the REACH chemical regulation, and nanospecific rules, ensure ingredient safety, quality control, and transparency. Safety assessments rely on toxicological data, exposure analysis, and nonanimal testing methods, while efficacy must be supported by laboratory and human studies. Overall, biofunctional cosmetics represent a scientifically evolving sector that requires rigorous safety evaluation, responsible claims, and compliance with international regulatory standards.

Moreover, Chapter 3 introduces the reader to a market-wise analysis of biofunctional cosmetic natural products. The cosmetics industry is a rapidly growing global sector, increasingly influenced by consumer demand for sustainable, natural, and biofunctional products. Biobased cosmetics are formulated with ingredients derived from plants, marine resources, and other natural materials that provide biological benefits such as antioxidant, antiinflammatory, antimicrobial, and antiaging effects. Advances in biotechnology, green chemistry, and nanotechnology have supported the development of these ingredients, while patented actives—such as peptides, UV filters, vitamins, and microbial ferments—play a key role in innovation and product differentiation. Major multinational companies, including L'Oréal, Estée Lauder, Unilever, and Shiseido, dominate the market through strong research and development, strategic marketing, and global distribution networks. Market growth is further driven by increasing consumer awareness of environmental and health issues, as well as trends such as clean beauty, multifunctional ingredients, artificial intelligence–based product development, and circular economy practices like ingredient upcycling and sustainable packaging. Despite its strong growth, the biofunctional cosmetics market faces several challenges that may limit its expansion. Biobased ingredients often involve higher production costs, complex extraction processes, and expensive safety and performance testing before commercialization. Additional barriers include regulatory restrictions, environmental concerns related to large-scale natural resource use, misinformation about natural versus synthetic ingredients, and difficulties in replacing conventional synthetic compounds while maintaining product performance and stability. However, the adoption of sustainable production methods, renewable raw materials, and eco-friendly packaging solutions is expected to strengthen the sector in the long term. Overall, the cosmetics industry is gradually transitioning toward more sustainable and innovative formulations, with biofunctional products positioned as a key component of future market development.

Importantly, Chapter 4 analyzes safety issues and concerns in the cosmetic industry for natural products. Real-world experiences in cosmetic laboratories demonstrate that effective safety management evolves through the analysis of incidents, successful interventions, benchmarking practices, and technological innovation. Case studies reveal how accidents, near-misses, and operational errors—such as improper solvent handling, poor chemical labeling, or misuse of personal protective equipment—highlight weaknesses in safety systems and provide opportunities for improvement. Conversely, proactive safety initiatives, including advanced training programs, strong leadership engagement, quality control monitoring, and health surveillance, have proven effective in reducing incidents and strengthening organizational safety culture. Industry leaders such as L'Oréal and Beiersdorf set benchmarks by integrating safety management systems, digital monitoring tools, and structured risk assessment frameworks into their operations, demonstrating how safety can be embedded within corporate strategy, innovation pipelines, and sustainability goals. Technological advancements are increasingly transforming laboratory safety by enabling real-time hazard monitoring, digital documentation, and predictive risk analysis. Tools such as digital safety data sheet platforms, wearable exposure sensors, smart laboratory equipment, and cloud-based safety management systems improve hazard communication, emergency response, and exposure tracking. At the same time, broader safety challenges—including raw material contamination, preservative reformulation risks, and laboratory accidents—highlight the importance of rigorous supply chain control, robust quality testing, and strong safety culture. The future of cosmetic safety management lies in integrating toxicological research, green chemistry, computational modeling, and new approach methodologies, such as in vitro and in silico tools, which aim to enhance risk assessment while reducing reliance on animal testing. Together, continuous learning, technological integration, and regulatory compliance form the foundation of a resilient safety framework that protects workers, consumers, and the credibility of the cosmetics industry.

3 Section II: Health benefits of bioactive ingredients from sustainable plant-based sources and their by-products

This section delves deeper into the health-promoting properties of biofunctional cosmetics containing natural bioactives from sustainable plant-based sources or their by-products, in a circular economy design, as mandated by the EU and UN.

More specifically, Chapters 5–9 refer to the more traditional plant-derived sources of bioactives for the cosmetic industry, including medicinal and aromatic plants, spices, and freshwater and marine photosynthetic organisms and plants. These chapters provide paradigms of biofunctional cosmetics that leverage bioactive compounds from medicinal plants, spices, and photosynthetic aquatic organisms to deliver therapeutic and preventive skin benefits beyond superficial esthetics. Bioactive compounds derived from such cosmetic and pharmaceutical plants—like polyphenols, flavonoids, carotenoids, vitamins, saponins, and essential oils—exhibit antioxidant, antiaging, antiinflammatory, antimicrobial, and photoprotective activities. These bioactives regulate cellular pathways, including collagen synthesis, sebum production, pigmentation, and oxidative stress, supporting skin rejuvenation, barrier repair, and overall dermal health. Spices contribute complementary phytochemicals, like curcumin, thymoquinone, and eugenol, offering antioxidant, antiinflammatory, antimicrobial, and regenerative effects. Similarly, freshwater and marine algae provide metabolites such as carotenoids, fucoidans, phlorotannins, and peptides that enhance hydration, UV protection, collagen synthesis, and antiaging responses, positioning these natural sources as multifunctional ingredients for modern cosmetic and cosmeceutical formulations.

Advances in green extraction and innovative delivery systems have increased the potential of these bioactives for industrial application. Techniques such as ultrasound-, microwave-, enzyme-assisted, supercritical fluid, and pulsed electric field extraction improve yield, selectivity, and environmental sustainability, while nanoemulsions, liposomes, phytosomes, and solid lipid nanoparticles enhance stability, bioavailability, and targeted skin delivery. Despite this progress, challenges remain, including species- or cultivar-specific variability, compound instability, standardization, regulatory compliance, and production scalability. Future research should focus on sustainable cultivation, extraction optimization, formulation strategies, and clinical validation to fully exploit plant-, spice-, and aquatic-derived bioactives for next-generation cosmetics that integrate efficacy, safety, and environmental responsibility.

Moreover, Chapters 10–15 refer to plant-derived sources of bioactives that were traditionally used in more agrifood sector applications rather than cosmetics, while recent research has shown that several of them, and especially their by-products, can be valorized for added-value biofunctional cosmetic products. For example, vegetables and fruits are rich sources of bioactive compounds—including polyphenols, polar lipids and unsaturated fats, carotenoids, glucosinolates, betalains, vitamins, and minerals—that provide antioxidant, antiinflammatory, photoprotective, and regenerative effects for skin health. Vegetables such as broccoli, carrots, tomatoes, and sweet potatoes supply sulforaphane, lycopene, luteolin, and anthocyanins, enhancing hydration, elasticity, and protection against UV and oxidative stress. Fruits and fruit-processing by-products, like apple pomace, grape pomace, and citrus peels, deliver polyphenols, flavonoids, enzymes, and vitamins that support moisturizing, antiaging, skin renewal, and enzymatic exfoliation, aligning with circular economy principles by valorizing agroindustrial residues. Advanced green extraction methods—such as ultrasound-, microwave-, enzyme-assisted, supercritical fluid, and subcritical water extraction—maximize yield and preserve bioactive stability, while nano-encapsulation, liposomes, and solid lipid nanoparticles improve bioavailability, transdermal absorption, and formulation compatibility.

Edible plant oils—including palm, soybean, rapeseed, sunflower, and olive—and their by-products provide fatty acids, phenolics, tocopherols, carotenoids, phytosterols, proteins, and squalene, delivering hydration, antioxidation, antiaging, antiinflammatory, photoprotective, and regenerative effects. Similarly, cereals and their by-products (bran, germ) supply β-glucans, ceramides, and polyphenols like ferulic acid, supporting barrier function, collagen preservation, wound healing, and antioxidant protection. These compounds also serve technological roles in formulations, such as thickeners, stabilizers, and water-binding agents. Despite promising bioactivities, challenges in raw material variability, stability, solubility, and regulatory compliance necessitate innovations in green extraction, encapsulation, and advanced delivery systems. Integrating these plant-, fruit-, oil-, and cereal-derived bioactives with sustainable processing and circular economy practices offers multifunctional, safe, and environmentally responsible solutions for next-generation biofunctional cosmetics and cosmeceuticals.

4 Section III: Sustainable bioactive ingredients from microorganisms

In this section, Chapters 16–19 focus on the roles of several microorganisms as powerful biotechnological tools and sustainable biofactories for the production of functional ingredients used in next-generation biofunctional cosmetics. Bacteria, fungi, protozoans, and microalgae can generate a wide range of valuable metabolites—including probiotics, prebiotics, postbiotics, polysaccharides, lipids, peptides, enzymes, pigments, and antioxidants—that support skin health and cosmetic performance. Bacterial lysates, fermentation products, and postbiotics can help regulate the skin microbiome, strengthen the skin barrier, and provide antiinflammatory, antioxidant, and antiaging benefits. Similarly, fungal metabolites such as mycosporines, chitosan, polysaccharides, and organic acids contribute to skin repair, hydration, photoprotection, pigmentation control, and antimicrobial activity. Through advanced fermentation technologies, strain optimization, and controlled cultivation systems, microorganisms can be harnessed to sustainably produce high-value cosmetic ingredients while reducing environmental impact compared to traditional synthetic or plant-based sources.

Beyond bacteria and fungi, protozoans and marine microalgae further expand the microbial reservoir of bioactive compounds for cosmetic innovation. Protozoans produce diverse biomolecules—including exopolysaccharides, sterols, sphingolipids, peptides, and enzymes—that support hydration, wound healing, UV protection, microbiome balance, and antioxidant defense. Meanwhile, marine microalgae function as renewable biofactories capable of synthesizing carotenoids, polyunsaturated fatty acids, vitamins, phenolics, and UV-absorbing mycosporine-like amino acids, which contribute to photoprotection, skin barrier maintenance, and antiaging effects. Biotechnological strategies such as controlled fermentation, photobioreactor cultivation, and advanced encapsulation technologies enable the stable delivery of microbial probiotics, prebiotics, and bioactive metabolites into cosmetic formulations. With appropriate safety assessments, regulatory compliance, and transparent production practices, microorganisms represent a versatile and environmentally sustainable platform for developing innovative biofunctional cosmetics aligned with modern consumer demand for natural, effective, and eco-conscious skincare solutions.

5 Section IV: Health benefits of bioactive ingredients from sustainable animal-based sources

Within this section, Chapters 20–22 review the utilization of marine animals—including mollusks, crustaceans, and fish—and their processing by-products as a vast and sustainable reservoir of bioactive compounds with remarkable potential for the development of biofunctional cosmetics. Tissues, shells, exoskeletons, skin, mucus, ink, and processing residues from these marine organisms are rich in valuable biomolecules such as proteins, peptides, polysaccharides, lipids, pigments, minerals, vitamins, and enzymes. These compounds—including collagen, gelatin, chitin, chitosan, glycosaminoglycans, carotenoids, omega-3 fatty acids, and marine phenolics—exhibit a wide range of beneficial biological activities, such as antioxidant, antiinflammatory, antimicrobial, moisturizing, photoprotective, wound healing, and antiaging effects. Bioactives derived from marine animals can promote skin regeneration, enhance hydration and elasticity, stimulate collagen synthesis, protect against oxidative stress and UV damage, and improve skin barrier function, making them highly valuable ingredients for skincare, haircare, oral care, and other cosmetic formulations. Importantly, the valorization of marine animal by-products—such as fish skin, bones, scales, crustacean shells, and molluskan shells or ink—aligns strongly with circular economy principles and sustainable biotechnology strategies. Through environmentally friendly extraction technologies, enzymatic hydrolysis, and marine biorefinery approaches, seafood processing residues can be transformed into high-value functional ingredients such as marine collagen, bioactive peptides, chitosan derivatives, astaxanthin, polar lipids, and mineral complexes. These compounds not only enhance the performance and multifunctionality of cosmetic formulations but also contribute to reducing marine waste and improving resource efficiency. Consequently, marine animals and their by-products represent an environmentally responsible and innovative platform for developing next-generation biofunctional cosmetics and cosmeceutical products.

Within the same section, Chapters 23–24 review other alternative animal sources as sustainable ones for bioactive ingredients in biofunctional cosmetics, such as insects and their products and by-products. In addition, dairy products from other animals in the agrifood sector, especially fermented dairy products, are also reviewed. Such alternative animal-derived resources—including insects and dairy products—are increasingly recognized as sustainable and innovative sources of bioactive compounds for the development of biofunctional cosmetics. Insects represent a highly sustainable and efficient biological resource due to their rapid growth, low environmental footprint, and ability to convert organic side streams into valuable biomass. Insect-derived compounds—including chitin, chitosan, antimicrobial peptides, proteins, lipids, and fatty acids—demonstrate antioxidant, moisturizing, wound healing, and microbiome-regulating properties, making them promising natural ingredients for innovative cosmetic and cosmeceutical formulations. Dairy-derived materials further contribute to this group of alternative bioresources by providing proteins, peptides, lipids, and other bioactive molecules capable of enhancing skin hydration, barrier repair, antioxidant defense, and antiinflammatory responses. The valorization of dairy by-products, particularly whey from cheese production, offers significant sustainability benefits by converting agricultural residues into high-value cosmetic ingredients. In particular, fermented dairy products represent a promising future direction, as microbial fermentation can generate a wide range of bioactive metabolites, including peptides, organic acids, exopolysaccharides, vitamins, and postbiotic compounds. These fermentation-derived molecules may improve skin hydration, support microbiome balance, enhance bioavailability, and reduce allergenicity compared with nonfermented dairy ingredients. Together, alternative animal-based sources for bioactives, like insects and fermented dairy, offer environmentally responsible and biotechnologically versatile platforms for producing multifunctional bioactive ingredients that can support the development of next-generation sustainable biofunctional cosmetic products.

6 Section V: Sustainable inorganic bioactive ingredients from natural resources

Within this section, Chapters 25 and 26 review inorganic matter like natural minerals, metal ions, and carbon-based materials as functional ingredients in cosmetic formulations. More specifically, Chapter 25 reviews the use of natural minerals, metal ions, and plant-derived complexes in biofunctional cosmetics for their multifunctional benefits, including UV protection, antimicrobial defense, wound healing, antioxidant activity, and skin regeneration. Key ingredients—clays, silicates, zeolites, volcanic and marine minerals, and metal oxides such as zinc, copper, and titanium—provide structural, sensory, and therapeutic effects, while plant-derived compounds enhance bioactivity through metal chelation and phyto-mediated nanoparticles. Sustainable sourcing strategies, including responsible mining, phytomining, bioleaching, marine and geothermal resource utilization, and waste valorization, ensure environmental and social responsibility. Emerging innovations such as hybrid mineral–polymer systems, nanocosmetics, smart delivery technologies, and personalized mineral supplementation integrate efficacy with eco-consciousness, positioning inorganic bioactives at the forefront of next-generation, safe, and sustainable cosmetic formulations.

Chapter 26 explores the role of natural and synthetic carbon-based materials in biofunctional cosmetics, emphasizing their unique properties, applications, and sustainability potential. Materials such as activated carbon, carbon nanotubes, graphene derivatives, fullerenes, and carbon dots exhibit exceptional adsorption, antioxidant, antimicrobial, and photoprotective capabilities. These characteristics allow them to enhance the performance, stability, and longevity of cosmetic formulations for skin, hair, eyes, lips, and oral care. Biomass-derived carbon materials, obtained from agricultural and forestry residues, offer a sustainable and eco-friendly alternative to conventional sources, aligning with circular economy and green chemistry principles. By enabling controlled release of active ingredients and multifunctional effects, carbon-based nanomaterials contribute to innovative, high-performing cosmetic products while supporting environmental responsibility. Despite their advantages, the chapter underscores the importance of rigorous safety evaluation and regulatory oversight. While dermal exposure to carbon nanomaterials is generally safe, inhalation and environmental release present potential risks, particularly for nanoscale particles. The chapter calls for standardized toxicological testing, careful synthesis, and green production methods to ensure consistency, biocompatibility, and minimal ecological impact. Future directions include combining carbon nanomaterials with natural bioactives and adopting plant-based or biodegradable systems to create synergistic, multifunctional cosmetic products. Overall, carbon-based materials are positioned as pivotal agents in shaping the next generation of biofunctional cosmetics that integrate efficacy, safety, and sustainability.

7 Section VI: Natural bioactives for environmentally friendly cosmetic and nutricosmetic packaging

Within this section, Chapter 27 discusses the urgent need for sustainable and eco-friendly packaging in the cosmetics industry, which traditionally relies heavily on plastic due to its low cost, durability, and protective properties. However, plastic waste has severe environmental consequences, prompting a shift toward biodegradable and biobased materials such as polylactic acid (PLA), polyhydroxyalkanoates (PHAs), cellulose, starch, and chitosan. These materials, derived from renewable resources, can offer comparable mechanical and barrier performance while reducing carbon footprints and supporting a circular economy. The chapter reviews the specific characteristics required for cosmetic packaging, emphasizing stability, safety, barrier performance, and esthetic appeal. It also highlights the challenges of reusability, microbial contamination, and chemical interactions between packaging materials and complex cosmetic formulations. The text further examines advances in biopolymer-based packaging, detailing modifications and nanocomposite strategies that enhance mechanical strength, thermal stability, barrier performance, and antimicrobial properties. PLA, PHAs, and polysaccharides are explored in depth, showing how reinforcement with nanoclays, cellulose fibers, lignin, or metal oxide nanoparticles can address inherent limitations like brittleness, moisture sensitivity, and poor gas or UV barrier properties. Despite progress, long-term stability, microbial safety, and formulation–material compatibility remain critical research gaps. Future efforts should focus on systematic testing of biodegradation, chemical interactions, and mechanical performance under real-world conditions, requiring interdisciplinary collaboration across material science, microbiology, and cosmetic chemistry to achieve reliable "green" packaging solutions for the cosmetics industry.

8 Section VII: Epilogue

Finally, within this section, Chapter 28 explores the growth and evolution of cosmetic and cosmeceutical products formulated with natural ingredients and bioactives, highlighting key milestones in research and development, global market growth, regulatory frameworks, and technological innovations within the field. The cosmetics and cosmeceuticals industry represents one of the fastest-growing sectors of the global consumer market, driven by technological innovation, changing lifestyles, and increasing consumer awareness regarding ingredient safety, sustainability, and product efficacy. In recent years, demand for formulations containing natural ingredients and bioactive compounds has expanded considerably, shaping the development of green cosmetics, dermatocosmetics, and clean-label products. Natural cosmetics now constitute a rapidly growing market segment worldwide, particularly in skincare and haircare, supported by consumer preference for safer, environmentally responsible, and functionally effective products. Historically, natural substances derived from plants, animals, and minerals were widely used in traditional cosmetic practices. Over time, advances in analytical chemistry, biotechnology, and formulation science have transformed these empirical practices into evidence-based cosmetic research, enabling the identification, extraction, and utilization of bioactive molecules such as polyphenols, carotenoids, peptides, vitamins, and polysaccharides. These compounds provide diverse cosmetic benefits, including antioxidant protection, skin hydration, antiaging activity, pigmentation regulation, antiinflammatory effects, and antimicrobial preservation.

Modern cosmetic research increasingly integrates green extraction technologies, biotechnology, and advanced delivery systems to enhance the stability, bioavailability, and skin penetration of natural bioactives. Encapsulation platforms such as liposomes, nanoemulsions, and lipid nanoparticles allow controlled release and improved performance of sensitive ingredients, while sustainable sourcing strategies, fermentation technologies, and circular economy principles support environmentally responsible product development. At the same time, regulatory frameworks, safety assessments, and transparent labeling remain critical for ensuring product efficacy and consumer protection. Despite rapid progress, challenges related to ingredient variability, stability, clinical validation, and sustainability persist. Future research directions emphasize interdisciplinary collaboration, advanced omics technologies, artificial intelligence-assisted discovery, and responsible innovation to develop next-generation cosmetic and cosmeceutical products that combine scientific validation, environmental sustainability, and personalized skincare solutions.

AI disclosure

During the preparation of this work, the author(s) used ChatGPT to recheck putative grammatical and syntax errors. After using this tool/service, the author(s) reviewed and edited the content as needed and take(s) full responsibility for the content of the publication.

References

Adamantidi, T., Lafara, M.-P., Venetikidou, M., Likartsi, E., Toganidou, I., Tsoupras, A., 2025. Utilization and bio-efficacy of carotenoids, vitamin A and its vitaminoids in nutricosmetics, cosmeceuticals, and cosmetics' applications with skin-health-promoting properties. Appl. Sci. 15, 1657. doi:10.3390/app15031657.

Annunziata, G., Verde, L., Zink, A., Muscogiuri, G., Albanesi, C., Paganelli, A., Barrea, L., Scala, E., 2025. Plant-based foods for chronic skin diseases: a focus on the Mediterranean diet. Curr. Nutr. Rep. 14 (1), 42. doi:10.1007/s13668-025-00632-5. PMID: 40048018; PMCID: PMC11885338.

Assaf, S., Kelly, O., 2024. Nutritional dermatology: optimizing dietary choices for skin health. Nutrients 17 (1), 60. doi:10.3390/nu17010060. PMID: 39796494; PMCID: PMC11723311.

Knaggs, H., Lephart, E.D., 2023. Enhancing skin anti-aging through healthy lifestyle factors. Cosmetics 10, 142. doi:10.3390/cosmetics10050142.

Kontaxi, N.-I., Panoutsopoulou, E., Ofrydopolou, A., Tsoupras, A., 2024. Anti-inflammatory benefits of grape pomace and tomato bioactives as ingredients in sun oils against UV radiation for skin protection. Appl. Sci. 14, 6236. doi:10.3390/app14146236.

Letsiou, S., Tsakni, A., Antonopoulos, D., Tsoupras, A., Houhoula, D., 2025. Unveiling the biological properties of *Rosa rubiginosa* L. leaf extract as a bio-functional ingredient based on 2D cell-based models and in vitro assessments. Cosmetics 12, 62. doi:10.3390/cosmetics12020062.

Marra, A., Manousakis, V., Zervas, G.P., Koutis, N., Finos, M.A., Adamantidi, T., Panoutsopoulou, E., Ofrydopoulou, A., Tsoupras, A., 2024. Avocado and its by-products as natural sources of valuable anti-inflammatory and antioxidant bioactives for functional foods and cosmetics with health-promoting properties. Appl. Sci. 14, 5978. doi:10.3390/app14145978.

Moysidou, A.M., Cheimpeloglou, K., Koutra, S.I., Finos, M.A., Ofrydopoulou, A., Tsoupras, A., 2024. A comprehensive review on the antioxidant and anti-inflammatory bioactives of kiwi and its by-products for functional foods and cosmetics with health-promoting properties. Appl. Sci. 14, 5990. doi:10.3390/app14145990.

Papadopoulou, D., Chrysikopoulou, V., Rampaouni, A., Tsoupras, A., 2024. Antioxidant and anti-inflammatory properties of water kefir microbiota and its bioactive metabolites for health promoting bio-functional products and applications. AIMS Microbiol. 10 (4), 756–811. doi:10.3934/microbiol.2024034.

Papadopoulou, S.N.A., Adamantidi, T., Kranas, D., Cholidis, P., Anastasiadou, C., Tsoupras, A., 2025a. A comprehensive review on the valorization of bioactives from marine animal by-products for health-promoting, biofunctional cosmetics. Mar. Drugs 23, 299. doi:10.3390/md23080299.

Papadopoulou, S.N.A., Anastasiou, E.A., Adamantidi, T., Ofrydopoulou, A., Letsiou, S., Tsoupras, A., 2025b. A comprehensive review on the beneficial roles of vitamin D in skin health as a bio-functional ingredient in nutricosmetic, cosmeceutical, and cosmetic applications. Appl. Sci. (15), 796. doi:10.3390/app15020796.

Passeron, T., Krutmann, J., Andersen, M.L., Katta, R., Zouboulis, C.C., 2020. Clinical and biological impact of the exposome on the skin. J. Eur. Acad. Dermatol. Venereol. 34 (Suppl 4), 4–25. doi:10.1111/jdv.16614.

Seferli, M., Kotanidou, C., Lefkaki, M., Adamantidi, T., Panoutsopoulou, E., Finos, M.A., Krey, G., Kamidis, N., Stamatis, N., Anastasiadou, C., Tsoupras, A., 2024. Bioactives of the freshwater aquatic plants, *Nelumbo nucifera* and *Lemna minor*, for functional foods, cosmetics and pharmaceutical applications, with antioxidant, anti-inflammatory and antithrombotic health promoting properties. Appl. Sci. 14, 6634. doi:10.3390/app14156634.

Tsiapali, O.I., Ayfantopoulou, E., Tzourouni, A., Ofrydopoulou, A., Letsiou, S., Tsoupras, A., 2025a. Unveiling the utilization of grape and winery by-products in cosmetics with health promoting properties. Appl. Sci. 15, 1007. doi:10.3390/app15031007.

Tsiapali, O.I., Kontaxi, N.-I., Pavlidis, K., Ofrydopoulou, A., Prokopiou, V., Letsiou, S., Kosheleva, R.I., Mitropoulos, A., Tsoupras, A., 2025b. Anti-inflammatory and antioxidant properties of anti-UV creams enriched with natural extracts from avocado, apple, and kiwi by-products, with and without nanobubbles. Cosmetics 12, 231. doi:10.3390/cosmetics12050231.

Tsoupras, A., Lordan, R., Zabetakis, I., 2018. Inflammation, not cholesterol, is a cause of chronic disease. Nutrients 10 (5), 604. doi:10.3390/nu10050604. PMID: 29757226; PMCID: PMC5986484.

Tsoupras, A., Adamantidi, T., Finos, M.A., Philippopoulos, A., Detopoulou, P., Tsopoki, I., Kynatidou, M., Demopoulos, C.A., 2024a. Re-assessing the role of platelet activating factor and its inflammatory signaling and inhibitors in cancer and anti-cancer strategies. Front. Biosci. (Landmark Ed) 29 (10), 345. doi:10.31083/j.fbl2910345. PMID: 39473406.

Tsoupras, A., Panagopoulou, E.A., Kyzas, G.Z., 2024b. Anti-inflammatory, antithrombotic and anti-oxidant bioactives of beer and brewery by-products, as ingredients of bio-functional foods, nutraceuticals, cosmetics, cosmeceuticals and pharmaceuticals with health promoting properties. AIMS Agric. Food 9 (2), 568–606. doi:10.3934/agrfood.2024032.

Tsoupras, A., Panagopoulou, E.A., Kyzas, G.Z., 2024c. Olive pomace bioactives for functional foods and cosmetics. AIMS Agric. Food 9 (3), 743–766. doi:10.3934/agrfood.2024040.

Vandorou, M., Plakidis, C., Tsompanidou, I.M., Adamantidi, T., Panagopoulou, E.A., Tsoupras, A., 2024. A review on apple pomace bioactives for natural functional food and cosmetic products with therapeutic health-promoting properties. Int. J. Mol. Sci. 25 (19), 10856. doi:10.3390/ijms251910856. PMID: 39409182; PMCID: PMC11476848.

Venetikidou, M., Lykartsi, E., Adamantidi, T., Prokopiou, V., Ofrydopoulou, A., Letsiou, S., Tsoupras, A., 2025. Proteolytic enzyme activities of bromelain, ficin, and papain from fruit by-products and potential applications in sustainable and functional cosmetics for skincare. Appl. Sci. 15, 2637. doi:10.3390/app15052637.

Chapter 2

Current rules and regulations

Constantina Nasopoulou
Department of Food Science and Nutrition, School of the Environment, University of the Aegean, Myrina, Lemnos, Greece

1 Categories of biofunctional cosmetics

1.1 Introduction

Biofunctional cosmetics are topical formulations developed to exert biologically measurable effects on the skin, hair, or body, extending beyond traditional esthetic functions. These products act on skin barrier integrity, cellular signaling, oxidative balance, inflammatory pathways, pigmentation mechanisms, and the skin microbiome, thereby occupying a scientific space between conventional cosmetics and dermatological therapeutics (Draelos, 2019; Badilli and Inal, 2025). Advances in molecular biology, microbiology, and delivery technologies have significantly contributed to the emergence of this category, supporting efficacy claims through mechanistic and clinical studies (Kim and Lee, 2024).

1.2 Overview of biofunctional cosmetic categories

Biofunctional cosmetics may be broadly classified according to their primary biological targets and mechanisms of action, as summarized in Table 2.1.

1.3 Skin barrier and repair biofunctional cosmetics

The epidermal barrier plays a crucial role in preventing water loss and protecting against environmental stressors. Disruption of this barrier is associated with increased transepidermal water loss (TEWL), inflammation, and susceptibility to irritation (Elias, 2005). Biofunctional cosmetics targeting barrier repair typically incorporate ceramides, cholesterol, fatty acids, and humectants, which mimic the natural lipid organization of the stratum corneum (Elias and Wakefield, 2014).

Recent studies demonstrate that topical supplementation with physiological lipids significantly improves barrier recovery and hydration, while also influencing microbial colonization patterns on the skin surface (Danby et al., 2025). Moreover, niacinamide has been shown to enhance ceramide synthesis and improve barrier resilience through the modulation of keratinocyte differentiation (Tanno et al., 2000).

1.4 Antiaging and skin longevity biofunctional cosmetics

Skin aging is driven by intrinsic factors such as cellular senescence and extrinsic factors, including ultraviolet (UV) radiation and pollution, which induce oxidative stress and extracellular matrix degradation (Fisher et al., 2002). Antiaging biofunctional cosmetics target these mechanisms using retinoids, bioactive peptides, antioxidants, and growth-factor-like molecules.

Signal peptides and carrier peptides have been reported to stimulate collagen synthesis and improve dermal density, while antioxidants such as vitamin C and polyphenols reduce oxidative damage and matrix metalloproteinase activity (Schagen, 2017; Kim and Lee, 2024). Advances in lipid-based nanocarriers further enhance the penetration and stability of these actives, increasing clinical efficacy (Badilli and Inal, 2025).

Biofunctional Cosmetics for Health. https://doi.org/10.1016/B978-0-443-27500-5.00002-2

TABLE 2.1 Major categories of biofunctional cosmetics and their biological targets.

Category	Biological target	Mechanism
Barrier and repair	Stratum corneum lipids	Lipid replenishment, TEWL reduction
Antiaging and longevity	Dermal matrix, oxidative pathways	Collagen stimulation, ROS reduction
Microbiome modulation	Skin microbial ecosystem	Restoration of microbial balance
Antioxidant and "antiinflammatory"	ROS and inflammatory mediators	Free radical scavenging, cytokine modulation
Pigmentation modulation	Melanocytes	Regulation of melanogenesis
Delivery-enhanced systems	Epidermal penetration	Improved bioavailability
Marine-derived and bioderived actives	Multifunctional targets	Hydration, antiaging, photoprotection

1.5 Microbiome-modulating biofunctional cosmetics

The skin microbiome is increasingly recognized as a key regulator of skin homeostasis, immunity, and barrier function. Dysbiosis has been linked to acne, atopic dermatitis, rosacea, and accelerated skin aging (Byrd et al., 2018; Hong et al., 2025).

Biofunctional cosmetics in this category employ prebiotics, probiotics (or bacterial lysates), and postbiotics to selectively support beneficial microorganisms while suppressing pathogenic strains (Theodorou et al., 2024). Both clinical and in vitro studies suggest that microbiome-targeted formulations can reduce inflammation, enhance barrier integrity, and improve hydration (Knackstedt et al., 2020; Hong et al., 2025).

1.6 Antioxidant and "antiinflammatory" biofunctional cosmetics

Oxidative stress is a central driver of inflammation, premature aging, and pigmentary disorders. Biofunctional antioxidant cosmetics incorporate plant-derived polyphenols, vitamins C and E, carotenoids, and enzymatic antioxidants to neutralize reactive oxygen species (ROS) (Pandel et al., 2013).

In addition to antioxidant activity, many botanical and marine-derived compounds exhibit "antiinflammatory" effects by downregulating proinflammatory cytokines such as IL-1α and TNF-α (Kim and Lee, 2024). These dual-function activities are particularly valuable in products designed for sensitive, photoexposed, or aging skin.

1.7 Pigmentation-modulating biofunctional cosmetics

Hyperpigmentation results from dysregulated melanogenesis involving tyrosinase activity, melanosome transport, and inflammatory signaling. Biofunctional cosmetics targeting pigmentation commonly use alpha-arbutin, kojic acid, tranexamic acid, and vitamin C derivatives to inhibit melanin synthesis or transfer (Briganti et al., 2003).

Clinical studies indicate that tranexamic acid not only suppresses melanocyte activation but also reduces inflammation-induced pigmentation, supporting its classification as a biofunctional cosmetic active rather than a purely esthetic agent (Cho et al., 2016).

1.8 Marine-derived and bioderived functional ingredients

Marine organisms are a rich source of polysaccharides, peptides, proteins, and pigments with proven bioactivity. Marine polysaccharides, such as alginates and fucoidans, exhibit moisturizing, antioxidant, and "antiinflammatory" properties, while marine peptides demonstrate antiaging and antimicrobial effects (Wang et al., 2025).

These ingredients are increasingly incorporated into biofunctional cosmetic formulations due to their multifunctionality and favorable biocompatibility profiles (Badilli and Inal, 2025).

1.9 Delivery-enhanced biofunctional systems

Effective delivery remains a major challenge in biofunctional cosmetics. Nanotechnology-based systems, such as liposomes, nanoemulsions, and solid lipid nanoparticles, have been shown to improve penetration, stability, and controlled release of active compounds (Prow et al., 2011). Such systems enable lower active concentrations while maintaining biological efficacy, reducing irritation risk, and improving consumer safety (Badilli and Inal, 2025).

1.10 Conclusion

Biofunctional cosmetics represent an evidence-based evolution of cosmetic science, integrating biological mechanisms with advanced formulation technologies. Research increasingly supports the efficacy of these products in modulating skin physiology, although further long-term clinical trials and standardized evaluation methods are required to substantiate claims and support regulatory clarity (Draelos, 2019; Theodorou et al., 2024).

2 Regulatory framework

2.1 Introduction

Biofunctional cosmetics are a subclass of cosmetic products formulated with bioactive ingredients that claim specific biological functions beyond basic esthetic effects, for example, antioxidant activity, modulation of the skin microbiome, cellular repair processes, or targeted biosignaling effects. These products often bridge the traditional boundaries between cosmetics and cosmeceuticals, a term commonly used in scientific and commercial literature to denote cosmetic products with purported therapeutic or functional biological effects. However, no regulatory authority formally defines "cosmeceuticals" as a separate category; rather, products must be classified based on their intended use and claims.

Regulatory objectives for all cosmetics, including biofunctional cosmetics, are to protect human health, ensure safe use, prevent misleading claims, and provide transparency in labeling and consumer information. These objectives are reflected across global regulatory frameworks but vary in how they treat functional or biologically active cosmetics, especially in the European Union (EU) (Table 2.2).

2.2 EU regulatory framework

2.2.1 *Regulation (EC) No. 1223/2009 on cosmetic products*

The cornerstone of EU cosmetic regulation is Regulation (EC) No. 1223/2009, which sets *binding requirements* for cosmetic products placed on the EU market. Its main goals are to protect human health and ensure a functioning internal market for cosmetics. The key requirements include:

- Definition of a *cosmetic product* and ingredient safety standards
- Obligations for the *responsible person* to ensure compliance
- Creation of a comprehensive *product information file*
- Prior notification via the *cosmetic product notification portal*

TABLE 2.2 Major biofunctional cosmetic categories and regulatory considerations in the EU.

Biofunctional category	Typical active ingredients	Intended cosmetic function	Key regulatory concern
Antioxidant cosmetics	Vitamin C, vitamin E, polyphenols, resveratrol	Protection against oxidative stress	Claim substantiation; concentration–effect relationship
Antiaging/cellular renewal	Retinoids, peptides, alpha hydroxy acids (AHAs)	Reduction of wrinkles, skin renewal	Borderline medicinal claims
Skin barrier repair	Ceramides, cholesterol, fatty acids	Restoration of barrier function	Evidence of functional effect
Microbiome-targeted cosmetics	Prebiotics, probiotics, postbiotics	Balance of skin microbiota	Biological mechanism claims
"Antiinflammatory" /soothing	Niacinamide, bisabolol, botanical extracts	Reduction of irritation or redness	Disease-related claim avoidance
Skin lightening/tone correction	Niacinamide, arbutin, vitamin C	Reduction of hyperpigmentation	Safety, discrimination concerns

A cosmetic product must be safe under foreseeable conditions of use before market placement, and its safety must be supported by documented evidence. Manufacturers are required to compile a Cosmetic Product Safety Report (CPSR), which shall include comprehensive toxicological profiles for all constituent ingredients, microbiological quality specifications, and the results of relevant physicochemical testing. In addition, the report must provide a clear rationale for the intended use of the product, together with an assessment of consumer exposure.

Scientific literature highlights that the EU adopts a *risk-based and claim-driven approach* when evaluating advanced cosmetic formulations, especially those bordering on medicinal functions (Dreno et al., 2014; Nohynek and Antignac, 2017).

Scientific reviews emphasize that these categories remain legally cosmetic only when claims do not imply treatment, prevention, or modification of pathological conditions (Nohynek et al., 2010; European Commission, 2016).

Regulation (EC) No. 1223/2009 includes positive and negative lists (Annexes II–VI) controlling ingredient use. Biofunctional ingredients may be:

- Prohibited (Annex II),
- Restricted (Annex III),
- Authorized preservatives, UV filters, or colorants (Annexes IV–VI).

Scientific literature highlights that bioactive potency does not exempt ingredients from cosmetic use, provided safety is demonstrated at intended concentrations (Nohynek et al., 2010).

Nanomaterials require explicit notification and labeling, reflecting EU precautionary principles regarding novel delivery systems (European Commission, 2021).

2.2.2 Regulation (EU) No. 655/2013 on cosmetic claims

For biofunctional cosmetics, claim substantiation is the most critical regulatory challenge. Regulation (EU) No. 655/2013 requires that all claims suggesting biological or functional effects (e.g., "skin barrier repair," "microbiome balance") must be supported by adequate scientific justification, avoiding misleading language (European Commission, 2013).

Peer-reviewed research highlights that mechanistic plausibility alone is insufficient; instead, human-relevant data are strongly preferred for functional cosmetic claims (Korting and Schäfer-Korting et al., 2011; Lodén and Maibach, 2017).

According to industry–academia consensus, human clinical data using validated noninvasive methods (e.g., TEWL, corneometry, profilometry) represent the gold standard for substantiating biofunctional cosmetic claims in the EU (Pinnagoda et al., 2016).

3 Good Manufacturing Practice (EN ISO 22716)

Good Manufacturing Practice (GMP) represents a fundamental component of quality assurance in cosmetic manufacturing, ensuring that products are consistently produced and controlled according to appropriate quality standards. Within the EU, compliance with GMP is a legal requirement under Regulation (EC) No. 1223/2009 on cosmetic products, which stipulates that cosmetic products must be manufactured in accordance with GMP to ensure consumer safety (European Parliament and Council of the European Union, 2009). Although EN ISO 22716:2008 is formally a voluntary international standard, it is widely recognized as the *de facto* reference framework for demonstrating GMP compliance in the cosmetic sector across the EU.

EN ISO 22716:2008 provides comprehensive guidelines covering all critical aspects of cosmetic product manufacturing, including personnel qualifications and hygiene, premises and equipment, raw material control, production operations, in-process and finished product controls, storage, distribution, and handling of deviations, complaints, and recalls (International Organization for Standardization (ISO), 2008). The standard also emphasizes the implementation of robust quality management systems and appropriate documentation practices to ensure traceability, consistency, and accountability throughout the product lifecycle. By adopting ISO 22716, manufacturers can systematically minimize risks related to contamination, mix-ups, and quality defects during production and distribution.

In addition to ISO 22716, several complementary ISO standards support best practices in cosmetic manufacturing and quality assurance. ISO 22715 provides guidance on packaging and labeling, helping ensure that cosmetic products are presented in a manner that preserves product integrity and complies with regulatory and consumer information requirements. ISO 16128 establishes guidelines for defining and calculating the natural and organic content of cosmetic ingredients and finished products, thereby promoting transparency and harmonization in marketing claims related to natural and organic cosmetics (International Organization for Standardization (ISO), 2016).

Collectively, these ISO standards contribute to the global harmonization of cosmetic manufacturing practices and quality expectations. However, it is important to note that ISO standards do not supersede or replace legally binding regulatory requirements. Rather, they function as technical tools that support manufacturers in achieving and demonstrating compliance with applicable cosmetic legislation, particularly within the EU regulatory framework (European Commission, 2013).

4 Regulation of bioactive and functional ingredients

The incorporation of bioactive ingredients and nanomaterials into cosmetic formulations has expanded rapidly due to advances in biotechnology, nanoscience, and skin biology. Bioactive cosmetic ingredients—such as peptides, antioxidants, botanical polyphenols, and vitamins—are designed to interact with the biological pathways of the skin, while nanomaterials are employed to enhance stability, penetration, and controlled release of active substances. However, the same properties that improve performance may also alter toxicokinetics and biological interactions, raising concerns regarding skin penetration, systemic exposure, and long-term safety (Bowman et al., 2010; Nohynek and Dufour, 2012).

These concerns have prompted regulatory authorities to refine cosmetic safety frameworks, with the EU adopting nano-specific provisions, while other regions rely primarily on general safety principles and postmarket surveillance (Magnusson and Wilkinson, 2019).

4.1 Regulatory challenges associated with bioactive cosmetic ingredients

Bioactive cosmetic ingredients are frequently described as "cosmeceuticals," although this term lacks legal recognition in most regulatory systems. The regulatory challenge arises from the biological activity of these ingredients, which may influence cellular signaling, collagen synthesis, pigmentation, or inflammatory pathways while remaining legally classified as cosmetics (Draelos, 2005).

Several studies highlight that bioactive ingredients can exhibit dose-dependent effects, necessitating robust safety evaluation despite their cosmetic classification (Sivamani et al., 2014). Botanical extracts, for example, often contain complex mixtures of secondary metabolites, some of which may be sensitizers or endocrine-active compounds (Bilia et al., 2018). Consequently, regulatory toxicology increasingly emphasizes full ingredient characterization, margin-of-safety (MoS) calculations, and exposure-based risk assessment for bioactive substances (Basketter et al., 2014a).

Importantly, claims associated with bioactive ingredients are closely monitored, as therapeutic or disease-related claims may trigger reclassification as medicinal products or drugs, particularly in the EU (Rastogi et al., 2018).

4.2 Regulation of nanomaterials in cosmetics

The EU represents the most advanced regulatory environment for nanomaterials in cosmetics. Regulation (EC) No. 1223/2009 introduced a definition of nanomaterials—defined based on particle size (typically 1–100 nm in at least one dimension)—and established mandatory premarket notification and labeling requirements. This regulatory approach reflects growing scientific evidence that nanoscale materials may display toxicological profiles distinct from their bulk counterparts (Nohynek et al., 2007; Fadeel et al., 2018).

Safety assessment of nanomaterials in EU cosmetics is supported by scientific opinions issued by the Scientific Committee on Consumer Safety (SCCS), which evaluates data on particle size distribution, solubility, surface reactivity, dermal penetration, genotoxicity, and systemic toxicity (Scientific Committee on Consumer Safety (SCCS), 2018). Peer-reviewed studies emphasize that insoluble or biopersistent nanomaterials, such as metal and metal–oxide nanoparticles, warrant regulatory attention due to their potential for accumulation and cellular uptake (Labouta and Schneider, 2013; George et al., 2019).

Recent regulatory actions restricting or prohibiting certain nanoforms of metals and polymers demonstrate the EU's application of the precautionary principle, whereby regulatory intervention may occur in the presence of scientific uncertainty (Bowman et al., 2014).

5 Role of Registration, Evaluation, Authorization and Restriction of Chemicals (EC No. 1907/2006) in the regulation of biofunctional cosmetics

The Registration, Evaluation, Authorization and Restriction of Chemicals (REACH) Regulation (EC No. 1907/2006) constitutes the overarching chemical safety framework in the EU. Although cosmetic products, as finished formulations, are exempt from REACH registration, substances used as cosmetic ingredients are subject to REACH obligations when manufactured or imported into the EU at quantities of ≥ 1 ton per year (European Parliament and Council of the European Union, 2006; Nohynek et al., 2010).

For biofunctional cosmetics, which incorporate ingredients with targeted biological activity such as peptides, botanical extracts, enzymes, and advanced delivery systems, REACH plays a critical upstream role by ensuring that ingredient-level hazard and risk data are generated prior to cosmetic use.

5.1 Interaction between REACH and the EU cosmetics regulation

REACH operates in parallel with Regulation (EC) No. 1223/2009 on cosmetic products, and the two frameworks are legally complementary. While the Cosmetics Regulation governs product safety, exposure assessment, and consumer protection, REACH focuses on intrinsic substance hazards, including carcinogenicity, mutagenicity, reproductive toxicity (CMR), persistence, bioaccumulation, and endocrine-disrupting properties (Basketter et al., 2014b).

Importantly, REACH does not require the duplication of animal testing for cosmetic purposes. Data generated under REACH—particularly toxicological endpoints such as repeated-dose toxicity, genotoxicity, and reproductive toxicity—are usually used in the CPSR, supporting the safety assessment of biofunctional ingredients (Nohynek and Dufour, 2012).

5.2 REACH requirements relevant to biofunctional ingredients

Biofunctional cosmetic ingredients, including novel peptides, fermentation-derived actives, and botanical isolates, must be registered under REACH when used above the tonnage threshold. Registration requires comprehensive physicochemical, toxicological, and ecotoxicological data, scaled according to production volume (European Parliament and Council of the European Union, 2006).

Complex substances of biological origin, such as botanical extracts, may be registered as substances of unknown or variable composition, complex reaction products, and biological materials (UVCBs). This presents regulatory challenges due to compositional variability, but REACH nevertheless requires sufficient characterization to enable hazard assessment (Bilia et al., 2018).

REACH identifies Substances of Very High Concern (SVHCs) based on properties such as CMR toxicity, endocrine disruption, or environmental persistence. Ingredients classified as SVHCs may be placed on the Candidate List, triggering communication obligations and potential future restrictions (Magnusson and Wilkinson, 2019).

For biofunctional cosmetics, this mechanism has significant implications:

- Certain bioactive compounds may be restricted or prohibited regardless of cosmetic exposure scenarios.
- SVHC classification can lead to reformulation or ingredient substitution, even where cosmetic-specific risk assessment suggests low consumer risk.

REACH restrictions under Annex XVII may limit or prohibit the use of substances in cosmetic ingredients, irrespective of their functional benefits. In contrast to cosmetic regulation, which considers route-specific exposure, REACH restrictions are often hazard-driven, reflecting a precautionary approach (Bowman et al., 2014).

Biofunctional ingredients intended to modulate biological pathways—such as hormone-like plant compounds—are particularly scrutinized under REACH due to concerns about endocrine activity and systemic effects (Sivamani et al., 2014).

5.3 REACH and innovation in biofunctional cosmetics

While REACH has been criticized for its regulatory burden, several studies suggest that it has contributed to improved ingredient transparency, data availability, and safer-by-design innovation in cosmetics (Basketter et al., 2014b). For developers of biofunctional cosmetics, early alignment with REACH data requirements can facilitate faster cosmetic safety assessment under Regulation (EC) No. 1223/2009, reduce regulatory risk during ingredient commercialization, and improve acceptance of novel bioactive substances by regulators and consumers.

5.4 Limitations of REACH in cosmetic risk assessment

Despite its strengths, REACH has limitations when applied to cosmetics. The regulation does not account for cosmetic-specific exposure patterns, such as repeated low-dose dermal application or vulnerable populations (e.g., infants). Consequently, hazard-based REACH decisions may not always align with cosmetic risk assessment outcomes (Nohynek et al., 2010).

For biofunctional cosmetics, this divergence highlights the need for integrated risk assessment approaches that combine REACH hazard data with cosmetic exposure modeling.

6 Safety and efficacy assessment for biofunctional products

Safety assessment of biofunctional cosmetics is a mandatory regulatory requirement and is primarily focused on ensuring that products do not cause adverse effects under normal or reasonably foreseeable conditions of use. The process begins with detailed ingredient characterization, including chemical identity, source, purity, concentration, and potential impurities or degradation products (Scientific Committee on Consumer Safety (SCCS), 2021).

Toxicological evaluation of cosmetic ingredients relies on a weight-of-evidence approach that integrates existing toxicological data, in vitro testing, in silico modeling, and exposure assessment. Key toxicological endpoints include skin irritation, skin sensitization, phototoxicity, genotoxicity, and systemic toxicity, depending on the ingredient's physicochemical properties and dermal penetration potential (Basketter et al., 2014b). In the EU, animal testing for cosmetic ingredients is prohibited, necessitating the use of validated alternative methods and computational toxicology tools (Adler et al., 2011).

Dermal exposure assessment is central to cosmetic safety evaluation, as it considers product type, frequency of application, duration of contact, and the body surface area exposed. These parameters are used to calculate the MoS, which compares the systemic exposure dose with toxicological reference values, such as the No Observed Adverse Effect Level (Api et al., 2018). Special consideration is given to vulnerable populations, including individuals with compromised skin barriers, children, and pregnant consumers.

Postmarket safety monitoring, including cosmetovigilance systems and adverse event reporting, provides real-world data that support continuous safety evaluation and regulatory compliance (Vigan et al., 2014).

Efficacy assessment aims to substantiate the claimed biological or functional benefits of biofunctional cosmetics using scientifically robust methods. A clear definition of the product's mechanism of action is essential, particularly when claims relate to skin physiology, such as collagen synthesis, antioxidant activity, or inflammation modulation (Lodén and Maibach, 2012).

Preclinical evaluation often involves in vitro skin models, reconstructed human epidermis, and ex vivo human skin to assess biological activity, penetration, and target engagement of active ingredients (Ponec et al., 2014). These models support early screening and help identify relevant biomarkers linked to cosmetic claims.

Human studies are the cornerstone of cosmetic efficacy substantiation. Clinical and instrumental evaluations may include noninvasive biophysical measurements (e.g., TEWL, skin elasticity, wrinkle depth), dermatologist assessments, and consumer perception studies (Farris, 2014). Study design should be appropriate to the claim, incorporating adequate sample size, control products, blinding, and statistical analysis to ensure validity and reproducibility.

The bioavailability and stability of active ingredients within the cosmetic formulation are critical determinants of efficacy. Factors such as the formulation matrix, delivery systems (e.g., liposomes, nanoparticles), and skin penetration behavior significantly influence clinical outcomes (Benson and Watkinson, 2012).

Risk–benefit evaluation integrates safety and efficacy data to determine whether the demonstrated benefits of a biofunctional cosmetic justify any identified risks. Regulatory authorities require that cosmetic claims be truthful, substantiated, and not misleading, as outlined in frameworks such as EU Regulation (EC) No. 1223/2009 and international ISO standards for cosmetic claims substantiation, e.g., ISO standards for microbial limits (ISO 17516) (European Commission, 2013; International Organization for Standardization (ISO), 2017).

Ethical considerations, including informed consent, data protection, and transparency in consumer communication, are integral to responsible product development and market authorization.

7 Labeling and packaging requirements

7.1 Labeling requirements

Cosmetic labeling serves as a critical communication tool between manufacturers and consumers and must be clear, truthful, and not misleading. Mandatory labeling elements include:

- Product name and function, unless the function is obvious from presentation
- Name and address of the manufacturer
- Country of origin, for imported products
- Nominal content at the time of packaging
- Date of minimum durability or period after opening
- Precautions for use and warnings, particularly for products containing bioactive ingredients
- Batch number or reference for traceability
- Ingredient list (International Nomenclature of Cosmetic Ingredients, INCI), listed in descending order of concentration (European Parliament and Council of the European Union, 2009)

For biofunctional cosmetics, particular attention must be paid to claims related to biological activity, such as "stimulates collagen synthesis" or "restores skin barrier function." According to Commission Regulation (EU) No. 655/2013, cosmetic claims must be supported by adequate and verifiable evidence and comply with the principles of legal compliance, truthfulness, evidential support, honesty, fairness, and informed decision-making (European Commission, 2013). Claims suggesting pharmacological or therapeutic action are prohibited.

7.2 Packaging requirements

Packaging plays a dual role in biofunctional cosmetics by ensuring product protection and consumer safety, while also supporting sustainability goals. Packaging materials must be compatible with the formulation and must not release substances that could compromise product safety or stability. This is particularly relevant for biofunctional cosmetics containing sensitive ingredients such as peptides, probiotics, antioxidants, or plant-derived actives (Dreno et al., 2014).

Primary packaging must protect against microbial contamination, oxidation, light degradation, moisture, and air exposure.

Airless systems, opaque containers, and single-dose packaging are frequently used to preserve bioactivity. In addition, packaging must comply with GMPs (ISO 22716:2007), which emphasize hygiene, traceability, and quality control throughout the product lifecycle (International Organization for Standardization (ISO), 2007).

8 Conclusions

The regulatory landscape for biofunctional cosmetics is built on the same frameworks as regular cosmetics but with additional complexity in claim substantiation and ingredient safety evaluation. Regulatory compliance requires robust scientific evidence, comprehensive documentation, and adherence to international standards.

References

Adler, S., Basketter, D., Creton, S., Pelkonen, O., van Benthem, J., Zuang, V., et al., 2011. Alternative (non-animal) methods for cosmetics testing: current status and future prospects. Arch. Toxicol. 85 (5), 367–485.

Api, A.M., Basketter, D.A., Cadby, P.A., Cano, M.F., Ellis, G., Gerberick, G.F., et al., 2018. Dermal sensitization quantitative risk assessment (QRA) for fragrance ingredients. Regul. Toxicol. Pharmacol. 97, 1–12.

Badilli, U., Inal, O., 2025. Current approaches in cosmeceuticals: peptides, biotics and marine biopolymers. Polymers 17, 1123.

Basketter, D.A., Alépée, N., Ashikaga, T., Barroso, J., Gilmour, N., Goebel, C., et al., 2014a. Categorization of chemicals according to their relative human skin sensitizing potency. Dermatitis 25 (1), 11–21.

Basketter, D.A., Gerberick, G.F., Kimber, I., Loveless, S.E., 2014b. The identification, classification, and risk assessment of skin sensitizers: regulatory considerations. Regul. Toxicol. Pharmacol. 69 (2), 142–156.

Benson, H.A.E., Watkinson, A.C., 2012. Topical and Transdermal Drug Delivery: Principles and Practice, Wiley.

Bilia, A.R., Guccione, C., Isacchi, B., Righeschi, C., Firenzuoli, F., Bergonzi, M.C., 2018. Essential oils loaded in nanosystems: a developing strategy for a successful therapeutic approach. Evid. Based Complement. Alternat. Med. 2018, 6468593, 1–20.

Bowman, D.M., Schulte, P.A., Barone, S., 2014. Nanotechnology and cosmetics: regulatory and safety challenges. J. Toxicol. Environ. Health, Part A 77 (13), 737–745.

Bowman, D.M., van Calster, G., Friedrichs, S., 2010. Nanomaterials and regulation of cosmetics. Nat. Nanotechnol. 5 (2), 92–95.

Briganti, S., Camera, E., Picardo, M., 2003. Chemical and instrumental approaches to treat hyperpigmentation. Pigment Cell Res. 16, 101–110.

Byrd, A.L., Belkaid, Y., Segre, J.A., 2018. The human skin microbiome. Nat. Rev. Microbiol. 16, 143–155.

Cho, H.H., et al., 2016. Tranexamic acid in melasma. J. Dermatol. Treat. 27, 1–6.

Danby, S.G., et al., 2025. Topical supplementation with physiological lipids rebalances the stratum corneum ceramide profile and strengthens skin barrier function in adults predisposed to atopic dermatitis. Br. J. Dermatol. 193 (4), 729–742. doi:10.1093/bjd/ljaf200.

Draelos, Z.D., 2005. Cosmeceuticals: definitions and regulatory considerations. Clin. Dermatol. 23 (5), 457–460. doi:10.1016/j.clindermatol.2005.01.001.

Draelos, Z.D., 2019. Cosmeceuticals: efficacy and safety. Dermatol. Clin. 37 (1), 55–62.

Dreno, B., Araviiskaia, E., Berardesca, E., et al., 2014. The science of dermocosmetics and its role in dermatology. J. Eur. Acad. Dermatol. Venereol. 28 (11), 1409–1417. doi:10.1111/jdv.12496.

Elias, P.M., 2005. Stratum corneum defensive functions. J. Invest. Dermatol. 125, 183–200.

Elias, P.M., Wakefield, J.S., 2014. Mechanisms of abnormal lamellar body secretion and the dysfunctional skin barrier in patients with atopic dermatitis. J. Allergy Clin. Immunol. 134 (4), 781–791. doi:10.1016/j.jaci.2014.05.048.

European Commission, 2013. Commission Regulation (EU) No 655/2013 laying down common criteria for the justification of claims used in relation to cosmetic products. Off. J. Eur. Union L190, 31–34.

European Commission, 2016. Manual on the Scope of Application of the Cosmetics Regulation (EC) No 1223/2009 (Borderline Products), European Commission, Brussels.

European Commission, 2021. Nanomaterials in Cosmetic Products: Guidance for Safety Assessment. Publications Office of the European Union.

European Parliament and Council of the European Union, 2006. Regulation (EC) No 1907/2006 of the European Parliament and of the Council of 18 December 2006 concerning the Registration, Evaluation, Authorisation and Restriction of Chemicals (REACH), establishing a European Chemicals Agency. Offic. J. Eur. Union L396, 1–849.

European Parliament and Council of the European Union, 2009. Regulation (EC) No 1223/2009 of the European Parliament and of the Council on cosmetic products. Off. J. Eur. Union L342, 59–209.

Fadeel, B., Farcal, L., Hardy, B., Vázquez-Campos, S., Hristozov, D., Marcomini, A., Lynch, I., Valsami-Jones, E., Alenius, H., Savolainen, K., 2018. Advanced tools for the safety assessment of nanomaterials. Nat. Nanotechnol. 13 (7), 537–543. doi:10.1038/s41565-018-0185-0.

Farris, P.K., 2014. Cosmeceuticals: a review of ingredients and efficacy. Dermatol. Surg. 40 (6), 652–659.

Fisher, G.J., et al., 2002. Mechanisms of photoaging. Arch. Dermatol. 138, 1462–1470.

George, S., Lin, S., Ji, Z., Thomas, C.R., Li, L., Mecklenburg, M., Meng, H., Wang, X., Zhang, H., Xia, T., Hohman, J.N., Nel, A.E., 2019. Engineered nanomaterials for health and safety: from toxicological screening to mechanism-based risk assessment. Acc. Chem. Res. 52 (7), 1631–1640.

Hong, J.Y., et al., 2025. Microbiome-based interventions for skin aging. Ann. Dermatol. 37, 101–112.

International Organization for Standardization (ISO), 2007. ISO 22716:2007 – Cosmetics — Good Manufacturing Practices (GMP): Guidelines on good manufacturing practices. International Organization for Standardization (ISO).

International Organization for Standardization (ISO), 2008. ISO 22716:2008—Cosmetics—Good Manufacturing Practices (GMP)—Guidelines on good manufacturing practices. International Organization for Standardization (ISO).

International Organization for Standardization (ISO), 2016. ISO 16128-1:2016—Guidelines on technical definitions and criteria for natural and organic cosmetic ingredients and products—Part 1: Definitions for ingredients. International Organization for Standardization (ISO).

International Organization for Standardization (ISO), 2017. ISO 16128-2:2017—Guidelines on technical definitions and criteria for natural and organic cosmetic ingredients and products—Part 2: Criteria for ingredients and products. International Organization for Standardization (ISO).

Kim, C.M., Lee, Y.M., 2024. Revolutionizing cosmetic ingredients. Cosmetics 11, 157.

Knackstedt, R., et al., 2020. The role of topical probiotics in skin conditions. J. Drugs Dermatol. 19, 827–832.

Korting, H.C., Schäfer-Korting, M., et al., 2011. The benefit–risk ratio of topical corticosteroids: evidence-based approach. Clin. Dermatol. 29 (1), 103–112.

Labouta, H.I., Schneider, M., 2013. Interaction of inorganic nanoparticles with the skin barrier: current status and critical review. Nanomed.: Nanotechnol. Biol. Med. 9 (1), 39–54. doi:10.1016/j.nano.2012.02.003.

Lodén, M., Maibach, H.I., 2012. Dry Skin and Moisturizers: Chemistry and Function, second ed., CRC Press.

Lodén, M., Maibach, H.I., 2017. Treatment of Dry Skin Syndrome: The Art and Science of Moisturizers, second ed. Springer International Publishing. doi:10.1007/978-3-319-29352-7.

Magnusson, B., Wilkinson, S.C., 2019. Global cosmetic regulation: a comparative overview. Toxicol. Appl. Pharmacol. 377, 114626.

Nohynek, G.J., Antignac, E., 2017. Safety assessment of personal care products/cosmetics and their ingredients. Toxicol. Appl. Pharmacol. 243 (2), 239–259.

Nohynek, G.J., Antignac, E., Re, T., Toutain, H., 2010. Safety assessment of personal care products/cosmetics and their ingredients. Toxicol. Appl. Pharmacol. 243 (2), 239–259.

Nohynek, G.J., Dufour, E.K., 2012. Nano-sized cosmetic formulations or solid nanoparticles in sunscreens: a risk to human health? Arch. Toxicol. 86 (7), 1063–1075.

Nohynek, G.J., Lademann, J., Ribaud, C., Roberts, M.S., 2007. Grey goo on the skin? Nanotechnology, cosmetic and sunscreen safety. Crit. Rev. Toxicol. 37 (3), 251–277.

Pandel, R., et al., 2013. Skin photoaging and antioxidants. J. Dermatol. Sci. 69, 1–11.

Pinnagoda, J., Tupker, R.A., Coenraads, P.J., Nater, J.P., 2016. Prediction of susceptibility to irritation by skin barrier measurements. Contact Derm. 22 (3), 164–168.

Ponec, M., Boelsma, E., Gibbs, S., Mommaas, M., 2014. Skin models for dermatological research. J. Dermatol. Sci. 75 (3), 205–214.

Prow, T.W., Grice, J.E., Lin, L.L., Faye, R., Butler, M., Becker, W., Wurm, E.M.T., Yoong, C., Robertson, T.A., Soyer, H. P., Roberts, M.S., 2011. Nanoparticles and microparticles for skin drug delivery. Adv. Drug Deliv. Rev. 63 (6), 470–491. doi:10.1016/j.addr.2011.01.012.

Rastogi, S., Patel, K.R., Singam, V., Silverberg, J.I., 2018. Allergic contact dermatitis to personal care products and topical medications in adults with atopic dermatitis. J. Am. Acad. Dermatol. 79 (6), 1028–1033.e6. doi:10.1016/j.jaad.2018.07.017.

Schagen, S.K., 2017. Topical peptide treatments with effective anti-aging results. Cosmetics 4 (2), 16. doi:10.3390/cosmetics4020016.

Scientific Committee on Consumer Safety (SCCS), 2018. Notes of Guidance for the Testing of Cosmetic Ingredients and Their Safety Evaluation (10th Revision). European Commission.

Scientific Committee on Consumer Safety (SCCS), 2021. Notes of Guidance for the Testing of Cosmetic Ingredients and Their Safety Evaluation (11th Revision). European Commission.

Sivamani, R.K., Goodman, J., Gitis, N.V., Maibach, H.I., 2014. Clinical and biological effects of commonly used cosmetic ingredients. J. Drugs Dermatol. 13 (2), 234–241.

Tanno, O., Ota, Y., Kitamura, N., Katsube, T., Inoue, S., 2000. Nicotinamide increases biosynthesis of ceramides as well as other stratum corneum lipids to improve the epidermal permeability barrier. Br. J. Dermatol. 143 (3), 524–531. doi:10.1046/j.1365-2133.2000.03705.x.

Theodorou, I.M., et al., 2024. Clinical evidence of probiotics and postbiotics in cosmeceuticals. Nutrients 16, 2184.

Vigan, M., Castelain, F., Le Coz, C.J., 2014. Cosmetovigilance: definition, regulation and use in practice. Eur. J. Dermatol. 24 (5), 555–560.

Wang, H., et al., 2025. Marine bioactives in functional cosmetics. Mar. Drugs 23, 205.

Chapter 3

Exploring marketability

Despina A. Gkika, Alexandros Tsoupras, and George Z. Kyzas
Hephaestus Laboratory, School of Chemistry, Faculty of Sciences, Democritus University of Thrace, Kavala University Campus, Kavala, Greece

1 Introduction

The cosmetic industry is among the most significant and rapidly expanding sectors of the global economy, generating revenues of 100.49 billion USD worldwide (Mondello et al., 2024). Within the European Economic Area, approximately 2320 thousand tons of cosmetic products are sold annually (van Dijk et al., 2023). The cosmetics market is divided into several key categories, including skincare, haircare, makeup, perfumes, toiletries and deodorants, and oral cosmetics (Mondello et al., 2024). These products serve to rejuvenate and enhance the appearance of skin, hair, and scent (Babich et al., 2025). The leading companies in the sector are primarily multinational corporations, with L'Oréal standing out as the top manufacturer worldwide in 2021, reporting revenues of about 35 billion USD (Statista Research Department, 2026). The cosmetic industry continues to grow on a global scale. In 2017 the European cosmetic market alone was valued at €77.6 billion (Bom et al., 2019). The global cosmetics market was valued at about USD 296 billion in 2023 and is forecast to reach USD 446 billion by 2030, growing at a 6.1% compound annual growth rate (CAGR) (Grand View Research, 2025). To remain competitive, companies within this industry aim to either mass-produce specific ingredients or enhance existing methods to maximize product yield while minimizing costs (Heath et al., 2022). Cosmetic ingredients fulfill a wide range of functions depending on their intended purpose. They can enhance sensory qualities such as color, texture, and brightness, stabilize the formulation against physical, chemical, or microbial changes, or provide protective effects for the skin, such as shielding against UV radiation, signs of aging, and inflammation (Rischard et al., 2025). When combined in formulations, multiple ingredients may result in synergistic or, conversely, antisynergistic effects (Senthilkumar et al., 2024).

Conventional skincare formulations often rely on petroleum- or mineral oil-derived ingredients, which are nonbiodegradable and environmentally harmful (Goyal and Jerold, 2021). Contemporary society faces growing challenges, including the exhaustion of natural resources, waste accumulation, climate change, and the contamination of air and water (Heath et al., 2022; Lin et al., 2022). These challenges have prompted changes in both consumer behavior (Liobikienė and Bernatonienė, 2017) and industrial practices, especially in the creation of environmentally-friendly products (L'Haridon et al., 2018). To achieve circular economy (CE) objectives, address environmental concerns, and satisfy consumer demand for sustainable cosmetics, many leading companies are shifting from fossil-based to biobased ingredients (Goyal and Jerold, 2021). The industry is increasingly adopting green chemistry, biotechnology, and extraction methods to reduce environmental impact.

Consumer preference has become a decisive factor in shaping the market, with growing demand for organic cosmetic products considered safer alternatives to conventional formulations. Growing awareness of the risks of synthetic compounds has boosted interest in natural solutions across research and industry (Sianipar et al., 2023). Biocosmetics, based on natural resources like plants, minerals, and marine materials, have emerged as an alternative to synthetic products due to concerns over health, environmental impact, and animal testing (Minocha et al., 2025). From an industrial perspective, conventional processing methods also pose challenges, as they often require long processing times and high heat, both of which increase energy demands and significantly raise manufacturing costs (Bhatia et al., 2021).

The emergence of biocosmetics marked the introduction of natural, eco-friendly, and biodegradable constituents into the cosmetics market. This transition seeks to reduce reliance on synthetic chemicals and aggressive ingredients, offering healthier and more sustainable options for personal care products (Minocha et al., 2025). Natural ingredients contain active compounds with valuable bioactive properties, including antioxidant, photoprotective, antiaging, antimicrobial, wound

Biofunctional Cosmetics for Health. https://doi.org/10.1016/B978-0-443-27500-5.00012-5

healing, and antiinflammatory effects, which benefit skin, hair, and dental care. Unlike synthetic ingredients, they stimulate the skin's natural regeneration processes, enabling recovery and the self-resolution of various conditions (Yang et al., 2023). Biobased ingredient production aims for minimal modification, simpler processes, and lower environmental impact, following green chemistry principles (Cao et al., 2025). The use of natural products in cosmetics has a long history, with archeological and historical records showing that plant extracts and vegetable oils have been employed for therapeutic and esthetic purposes for millennia (Christaki et al., 2019). Today, the demand for sustainable, natural, and greener cosmetics is immense, as such products gain consumer trust by respecting and preserving nature (Goyal and Jerold, 2021). The biobased cosmetics and personal care ingredients market was valued at USD 5.54 billion in 2024 and is projected to grow to USD 9.14 billion by 2033 at a 5.72% CAGR (Bothare, 2026).

Nevertheless, the biocosmetics sector faces challenges that require further exploration. High product costs remain a barrier (Goyal and Jerold, 2021). For instance, biosurfactants hold significant promise as alternatives to conventional surfactants (Manga et al., 2021), but production expenses must be reduced to compete effectively with synthetic counterparts. In hair care formulations, product developers must choose between widely used, low-cost surfactants and more specialized options that deliver unique benefits (Cornwell, 2018). This highlights the need for standardized, cost-effective, and environmentally sustainable protocols for biobased ingredient production. With growing commercial interest and scaling of production, it is expected that costs will gradually decline, improving competitiveness with traditional products (Baccile et al., 2021).

By analyzing market segmentation and product positioning, this review identifies the dominant trends shaping the biofunctional cosmetics market. Its novelty lies in consolidating fragmented literature to provide updated, comparable insights into current trends and market developments. The following sections address key aspects: Section 2 reviews the current status of biofunctional ingredients in cosmetics and patented innovations, Section 3 examines the economics of cosmetic formulation and market analysis results, Section 4 outlines the main drivers and inhibitors of market growth, Section 5 discusses strategic marketing approaches for prevailing trends, and Section 6 presents the conclusions derived from the findings.

2 Status quo of biofunctional ingredients in cosmetics

Drawing inspiration from natural adaptation mechanisms, the cosmetics industry applies bioinspired and biomimetic strategies for eco-design, while emphasizing responsible sourcing and fair trade (Luengo et al., 2023).

An average cosmetic product includes about 15–20 ingredients, and since people typically use at least five products each day, they may apply roughly 75–100 different chemicals to their skin. While formulations vary, the main ingredients generally include water, emulsifiers, preservatives, thickeners, colorants, emollients, and fragrances (Goyal and Jerold, 2021). Cosmetic ingredients serve multiple purposes, such as ensuring safety, maintaining efficacy, enhancing sensory qualities, and stabilizing physicochemical properties. In practice, a single product may contain between 15 and 50 components, ranging from water, emollients, surfactants, solvents, preservatives, polymers, and UV filters to antioxidants, chelators, and fragrances (Bom et al., 2019).

Bioingredients are defined as substances used in the preparation of a product that remain present in the final formulation, possibly in a modified form, while retaining biological activity for consumers (Premkumar and Vasudevan, 2018). The term "active ingredient" in cosmetics differs from its pharmaceutical use. In cosmetics, it is primarily a marketing concept, referring to compounds that claim to address specific skin concerns. Such ingredients are often supported by scientific evidence and may be classified into antioxidants, astringents, exfoliants, humectants, skin conditioners, and surfactants. Adjuvants, on the contrary, are formulation-supporting ingredients that enhance the delivery of actives. Examples include emulsifiers, buffers, thickeners, preservatives, fragrances, emollients, occlusives, penetration enhancers, and humectants (Goyal and Jerold, 2021). Biocosmetic materials, whether active or adjuvant, are typically derived from animal or vegetable sources. Common natural ingredients in cosmetics include fats, oils, waxes, extracts, and colorants, with shea butter, coconut oil, mango butter, frankincense, patchouli, and licorice extract among the most used in Europe (Goyal and Jerold, 2021).

Until recently, ingredient selection in cosmetics has largely prioritized maximizing performance while reducing costs (Luengo et al., 2023). However, an increasing range of biobased alternatives is now available as substitutes for petrochemical-derived ingredients. These materials offer significant advantages, including improved safety profiles, better biodegradability, and environmentally friendly characteristics, which are becoming central to the industry's future development (Joondan et al., 2018). Despite these benefits, certain challenges remain, such as stability, compatibility with existing formulations, and the complexity of natural mixtures. Fermentation-derived compounds, for instance, can vary subtly in chemical structure, yet these small differences may result in significantly different functional behaviors and hinder batch-to-batch reproducibility (Fernández-Peña et al., 2020). Table 3.1 summarizes a selection of biofunctional ingredients, highlighting key findings from studies and their associated health-related properties.

TABLE 3.1 Biofunctional ingredients and health functional properties.

Biofunctional Ingredients	Key finding	Health functional properties
Peptides	Peptides play a vital role in stimulating collagen synthesis, reducing fine lines and wrinkles, and improving skin firmness. In one study, the administration of a formulation containing collagen peptides, acerola fruit extract, vitamin C, zinc, biotin, and a vitamin E complex led to enhanced skin hydration, greater elasticity, a reduction in wrinkles, and increased skin density (Bolke et al., 2019).	ACE inhibitor/antihypertensive (Løkra et al., 2008). Anticancer, antitumor, antiproliferative (Negi et al., 2017). Antioxidant (Shih and Cherng, 2012). Cryoprotectant (Nikoo et al., 2015). Emulsifier (Løkra et al., 2008).
Marine resources (sea grasses, seaweeds, sea cucumbers, DSW, microalgae, and so on)	Marine organisms are also valuable sources of structurally diverse bioactive compounds with a wide range of biological properties (Fan et al., 2014). Since marine species represent nearly half of the world's total biodiversity, they provide an extensive reservoir for the discovery of novel bioactive compounds (Kim et al., 2014).	Antibacterial, anticoagulant, antiinflammatory, antifungal, anthelmintic, antiplatelet, antiprotozoal, and antiviral activities, along with effects on the cardiovascular, endocrine, immune, and nervous systems, have been reported (Mayer et al., 2010).
Fruits and vegetables (pomace, skin, extracts)	Fruit pomace, a by-product of fruit juice or concentrate processing, is another promising resource. It contains significant amounts of dietary fiber and phenolic compounds, making it a valuable ingredient for cosmetic applications (Gouw et al., 2017).	Bioactive compounds, such as dietary fibers and phenolics, demonstrate antibacterial properties and can act as preservatives, acidifiers, and flavoring agents. They are also associated with lipid-lowering effects, antihypertensive activity, and protection against atherosclerosis (Öncül and Karabıyıklı, 2016). Colorant, mucilage, and α-tocopherol content (Melgar et al., 2017).
Spices and spice extracts, essential oils	Spices contain active components that can serve as natural bioingredients, with potential applications in the treatment of a wide range of conditions, including cancer, aging-related disorders, metabolic, neurological, cardiovascular, and inflammatory diseases (Tajkarimi et al., 2010).	Antioxidant (Stoilova et al., 2007). Antimicrobial, antibacterial, antifungal (Alves-Silva et al., 2013). Antiinflammatory, antiatherogenic (Kim et al., 2014).

Marine-derived compounds play a leading role in the bioingredients market, with academic–industry collaboration essential for developing and commercializing new actives. The food industry serves as a major contributor to bioingredient innovation, with many new compounds being identified from by-products of food processing. However, preclinical trials remain essential to determine the safe usage limits of these compounds. Bioactive compounds obtained in this way hold therapeutic potential for managing chronic diseases and their associated complications (Premkumar and Vasudevan, 2018). Nanotechnology enables safer, more effective cosmetics by enhancing ingredient delivery and reducing harmful chemicals, with nano-encapsulated sunscreens using zinc oxide or titanium dioxide providing broad UV protection without systemic toxicity (Ghosh et al., 2025).

2.1 Patented biofunctional ingredients in cosmetics: From discovery to market adoption

The biofunctional cosmetics market has become increasingly shaped by patented actives. Cosmetic ingredients are increasingly moving beyond traditional beautification to provide functional skin health benefits, including photoprotection, repair, antiaging effects, and barrier enhancement. Table 3.2 presents representative patented biofunctional cosmetic actives, outlining their molecular identity, regulatory approval status, and global market presence. Sunscreen agents such as Ecamsule (Mexoryl SX), Drometrizole Trisiloxane (Mexoryl XL), and BASF's Uvinul A Plus or Tinosorb filters exemplify the evolution of patented actives designed to meet contemporary photoprotection requirements. These molecules, protected across the United States, Europe, and Asia, have been engineered to ensure broad-spectrum ultraviolet A (UVA) and ultraviolet B (UVB) coverage while simultaneously meeting strict regulatory and safety standards. Consequently, product launches often occur in a staggered regional sequence, with intellectual property strategy and regulatory clearance serving as decisive factors for market entry.

Alongside UV filters, biofunctional peptides form a key class of patented actives in the domains of antiaging and skin repair. Examples include acetyl hexapeptide-8 (Argireline), copper tripeptide-1 (GHK-Cu), and Sederma's Matrixyl complex, which employ biomimetic or signal peptide mechanisms to stimulate collagen synthesis, modulate neurotransmission,

TABLE 3.2 Key patented biofunctional cosmetic actives: ingredients, market, and commercialization landscape.

Patent/publication	Biofunctional material/active/INCI	Product	Assignee/applicant	Commercial product	Regions in market/approval	Key reference URLs	Patent office(s)
US4,585,597A	Terephthalylidene Dicamphor Sulfonic Acid (Ecamsule, Mexoryl SX)	UV filter	L'Oréal	La Roche-Posay Anthelios SX (US NDA), Anthelios line (EU/CA/AU/JP)	United States (via NDA), EU, Canada, Australia, Japan, others	https://patents.google.com/patent/US4585597A/en; https://www.federalregister.gov/documents/2003/06/20/03-15692/grant-of-interim-extension-of-the-term-of-us-patent-no-4585597-anthlios-sp-topical-cream-mexoryl-sx; https://inside-our-products.loreal.com/ingredients/mexorylr-sx	USPTO (United States)
Patented by L'Oréal (see formulations: US9138395B2 mentions MX XL)	Drometrizole Trisiloxane (Mexoryl XL)	UV filter	L'Oréal	Anthelios (EU/CA/AU/JP formulas using Mexoryl XL)	EU, Canada, Australia, Japan (not OTC in the United States)	https://inside-our-products.loreal.com/ingredients/mexorylr-xl; https://patentimages.storage.googleapis.com/ae/08/d8/54ee79c13373a2/US9138395.pdf	USPTO (United States)
US20070031352A1	Diethylamino Hydroxybenzoyl Hexyl Benzoate (DHHB, Uvinul A Plus)	UV filter	BASF	Multiple EU/JP sunscreens (e.g., Eucerin, Nivea, La Roche-Posay EU formulas)	EU, Japan, Australia, many others (not US OTC)	https://patents.google.com/patent/US20070031352A1/en; https://carecreations.basf.com/product-formulation/products/uv-filters/uvasorb-a-plus-granular	USPTO (United States)
EP3229766B1; US20210161793A1	Methylene Bis-Benzo-triazolyl Tetramethylbu-tylphenol (Bisoctrizole, Tinosorb M)	UV filter (particulate organic)	BASF/others	Eucerin Oil Control, La Roche-Posay Anthelios (EU)	EU, Australia, Japan (not US OTC)	https://patentimages.storage.googleapis.com/12/f8/d1/c1bab105623170/EP3229766B1.pdf; https://patentimages.storage.googleapis.com/2d/41/b2/9ed2819802b4c6/US20210161793A1.pdf; https://go.drugbank.com/drugs/DB11262	EPO (European Patent Office); USPTO (United States)
US20130336908A1; EP3463259B1	Bis-Ethylhexyloxyphenol Methoxyphenyl Triazine (Bemotrizinol, Tinosorb S)	UV filter	BASF/others	Many high-SPF EU/JP sunscreens	EU, Australia, Japan (not US OTC)	https://patents.google.com/patent/US20130336908A1/en; https://patentimages.storage.googleapis.com/47/da/d2/a0cd796a10977b/EP3463259B1.pdf	USPTO (United States); EPO (European Patent Office)
EP4054727B1; US20240041736A1	Ethylhexyl Triazone (Uvinul T 150)	UV filter (UVB)	BASF/others	La Roche-Posay (EU), Nivea (EU), many others	EU, Australia, Japan, Korea (not US OTC)	https://patentimages.storage.googleapis.com/25/fd/51/5edbcab966964c/EP4054727B1.pdf; https://patents.justia.com/patent/20240041736	EPO (European Patent Office); USPTO (United States)
EP2838886A1; US20240041735A1	Diethylhexyl Butamido Triazone (Isocotrizinol, Uvasorb HEB)	UV filter (UVB/UVA II)	3V Sigma/others	Various EU/JP sunscreens (HEB)	EU, Japan, others (not US OTC)	https://patents.google.com/patent/EP2838886A1/en; https://patents.google.com/patent/US20240041735A1/en	EPO (European Patent Office); USPTO (United States)
WO2000/064932	Acetyl Hexapeptide-8 (Argireline)	Peptide (neu-rotransmission-modulating)	Lipotec (now Lubrizol)	The Ordinary Argireline Solution 10%; various creams and serums	Global (cosmetic)	https://www.ncbi.nlm.nih.gov/pmc/articles/PMC3510654/; https://hairlc.com/lipotec-argireline-acetyl-hexapeptide-3/	WIPO (International)
US5135913A	Copper Tripeptide-1 (GHK-Cu)	Peptide (signal/repair)	Pickart/ProCyte	NIOD Copper Amino Isolate Serum; Skin Biology products	Global (cosmetic)	https://patents.google.com/patent/US5135913A/en	USPTO (United States)

EP3233210B1; EP4141877A1 (solubility/processing)	Palmitoyl Pentapeptide-4 (Matrixyl)/palmitoyl Tripeptide-1 + Palmitoyl Tetrapeptide-7 (Matrixyl 3000)	Peptides (matrikines)	Sederma (Croda)	The Ordinary Matrixyl 10% + HA; many antiaging serums	Global (cosmetic)	https://data.epo.org/publication-server/rest/v1.0/publication-dates/20200205/patents/EP3233210NWB1/document.pdf; https://patentimages.storage.googleapis.com/61/d0/52/6b4cb3e04710c8/EP4141877A1.pdf; https://eyzhnelen.gr/wp-content/uploads/2018/05/ProductInformationFile_MATRIXYL-3000.pdf	EPO (European Patent Office); EPO (European Patent Office)
EP1345919A1/A2	Hydroxypropyl Tetrahydropyrantriol (Pro-Xylane)	Sugar-derived skin matrix booster	L'Oréal	Lancôme Rénergie/Absolue; L'Oréal Paris Revitalift lines	Global (cosmetic)	https://patents.google.com/patent/EP1345919A1/en; https://patents.google.com/patent/EP1345919A2/en	EPO (European Patent Office)
EP1974720A1	*Vitreoscilla filiformis* Lysate (Aqua Posae Filiformis/Life Plankton)	Postbiotic/lysate	L'Oréal	La Roche-Posay Lipikar Baume AP + M; other L'Oréal brands	EU, United States, JP (cosmetic)	https://patents.google.com/patent/EP1974720A1/en; https://www.laroche-posay.com/en_US/aqua-posae-filiformis-ingredients.html	EPO (European Patent Office)
US5939082A; WO2000/071093	Niacinamide (vitamin B3), topical cosmetic use	Vitamin/barrier & tone	Procter & Gamble	Olay Regenerist, Olay Super Serum, and many P&G products	Global (cosmetic)	https://patents.google.com/patent/US5939082A/en; https://patents.google.com/patent/WO2000071093A1/en; https://us.pg.com/blogs/olay-launches-super-serum/	USPTO (United States); WIPO (International)
CN103822976A (analytical method; Shiseido ingredient)	Potassium Methoxysalicylate (4-MSK)	Brightening agent	Shiseido/CN inventors	Shiseido White Lucent line; Anessa whitening products (JP)	Japan, China (ingredient allowed per local regulations)	https://patents.google.com/patent/CN103822976A/en	CNIPA (China)
FR2947449B1; EP2448549B1	Tetrahydrojasmonic Acid derivative (LR2412)	Jasmonate derivative (anti-aging)	L'Oréal	Lancôme Visionnaire LR2412-Cx	Global (cosmetic)	https://patents.google.com/patent/FR2947449B1/en; https://pubmed.ncbi.nlm.nih.gov/26885790/; https://www.loreal.com/en/articles/science-and-technology/the-major-active-ingredients-developed-by-l-oreal-research/	INPI (France); EPO (European Patent Office)
Referenced in EP2066291A2 (as SK-II PITERA)	Galactomyces Ferment Filtrate (PITERA™)	Ferment/postbiotic	Procter & Gamble (SK-II brand)	SK-II Facial Treatment Essence	Japan; Global cosmetic markets	https://patents.google.com/patent/EP2066291A2/en; https://www.sk-ii.com/product/essence/facial-treatment-essence; https://www.mdpi.com/2077-0383/12/3/1168	
US6756045B1; US8685391B2	Idebenone (topical)	Antioxidant	S. Kerscher et al./Allergan & Elizabeth Arden (related filings)	Elizabeth Arden PREVAGE line (including PREVAGE MD)	Global (cosmetic; MD physician line in the United States)	https://patents.google.com/patent/US6756045B1/en; https://patentimages.storage.googleapis.com/a8/e6/d6/0d24e03d0803f2/US8685391.pdf; https://www.happi.com/breaking-news/elizabeth-arden-and-allergan-enter-into-co-ma/	USPTO (United States); USPTO (United States)
EP2934430B1	Combinations incl. Avobenzone + BEMT + Uvinul T150 + Mexoryl SX/XL	UV filter system	L'Oréal	High-SPF Anthelios (EU) using multifilter systems	EU, other RoW	https://data.epo.org/publication-server/rest/v1.2/publication-dates/20191106/patents/EP2934430NWB1/document.pdf	EPO (European Patent Office)
EP0952836B1	Sulphoquinovosyldiacylglycerols (SQDG)	Antiinflammatory skin actives	Scotia LipidTeknik AB	(none widely commercialized)	Europe (patent expired)	https://www.google.com/url?q=https://patents.google.com/patent/EP0952836B1/nl&source=gmail&ust=1757405760222000&usg=AOvVaw1iHyzUOIi-KAPXKdBwZVfA	EPO (expired)

or accelerate tissue regeneration. Their widespread incorporation across prestige, mass market, and dermocosmetic lines demonstrates how proprietary peptide technologies create brand differentiation within a highly competitive marketplace. Patent protection further secures exclusivity for developers such as Lubrizol, Croda, and L'Oréal, while branded ingredient identities linked to clinically demonstrated efficacy enhance consumer trust and recognition.

Beyond UV filters and peptides, new categories of biofunctional actives highlight the convergence of biotechnology and cosmetic innovation. Sugar-derived matrix enhancers such as Pro-Xylane, microbial lysates, including *Vitreoscilla filiformis* (Life Plankton), and postbiotic ferments such as Galactomyces Ferment Filtrate (PITERA) illustrate the expanding diversity of functional materials. Widely adopted vitamins and small molecules, including niacinamide, idebenone, and LR2412, further support this trend, combining well-established biochemical activity with either strong patent protection or proprietary positioning. Collectively, these developments underscore how innovation in biofunctional actives is closely tied to intellectual property management, where patents not only protect discoveries but also foster consumer confidence, market premiumization, and effective navigation of complex regulatory environments.

The present landscape compels the cosmetics industry to adopt sustainable production and consumption practices (Kolling et al., 2022). To meet emerging sustainability requirements and regulatory standards, companies must update and adapt their operational strategies. Examples include the introduction of fair-trade certifications and sustainability indexes, often aligned with Corporate Social Responsibility frameworks. These tools are designed to strengthen relationships with diverse stakeholders, particularly end users, by clearly communicating the sustainability-oriented attributes of products and encouraging broader stakeholder engagement in supporting the core pillars of sustainability (Acerbi et al., 2023).

3 The economics of cosmetic formulation

From an economic perspective, sustainable practices in the cosmetics industry represent a necessity for long-term success and viability. Enhancing sustainability does not always require large investments and can generate multiple benefits, including cost savings, increased sales, and improved corporate reputation (Bom et al., 2019). Until recently, ingredient selection in cosmetics has primarily focused on maximizing performance while minimizing costs, often overlooking the environmental impact of production processes, by-products, and residues. This underscores the importance of adopting green approaches in both the sourcing of raw materials and production methods.

In broader terms, sustainability is grounded in three fundamental principles (Luengo et al., 2021). According to Bom et al., cosmetics sustainability is a multidimensional concept that must be evaluated holistically across environmental, social, economic, and product performance factors (Bom et al., 2019). Cosmetic companies often pursue sustainability primarily for its economic benefits, such as creating higher-value products and reaching more consumers (Civancik-Uslu et al., 2019).

3.1 Global cosmetic industry transformation and market trends

3.1.1 Regional analysis

In 2021 biobased cosmetics and personal care ingredients accounted for approximately 45% of the market in North America, making the region the leader in this sector (Bothare, 2026). High per capita income has supported strong demand for skincare and haircare products, thereby driving the use of biobased ingredients. The presence of both major industry players and innovative startups has further fueled market growth by continually introducing new and effective biobased products. Regulatory oversight from authorities such as the Food and Drug Administration (FDA) has also encouraged manufacturers to prioritize safer, natural formulations.

North America's well-developed retail infrastructure, encompassing specialty stores and online platforms, provides consumers with broad access to biobased cosmetics. In addition, social media and beauty influencers play a decisive role in shaping consumer preferences and raising awareness about natural and sustainable beauty options. High disposable incomes and strong economies support North America's leading role in the global biobased cosmetics market (Omkar, 2023).

3.1.2 Segmentation analysis

Fig. 3.1 Projected global market segmentation for cosmetics, toiletries, and fragrances to 2025 (Grand View Research, 2025; Presendence Research, 2025; Mordor Intelligence, 2026; Fortune Business Insights, 2025).

Europe's cosmetics market continues to expand across multiple segments, supported by sustainability, innovation, and evolving consumer preferences. Forecasts differ in scope (Fig. 3.1), with CAGR estimates ranging from 4.90%–6.07% in conservative scenarios to 6.50%–7.20% in more optimistic projections. Fig. 3.2 presents projected market values (USD

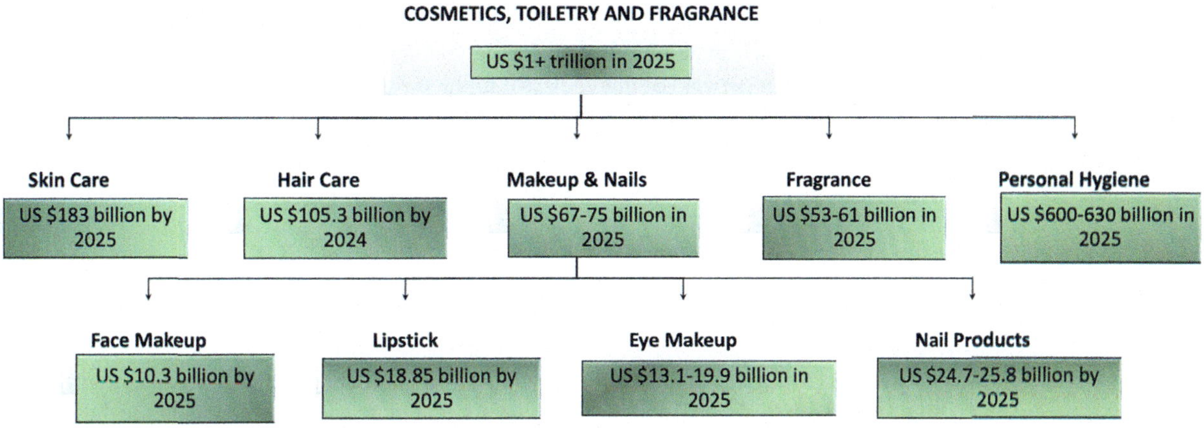

FIG. 3.1 The structure of the cosmetics industry, showing product classification and global market size by category in 2001. Projections for 2025 reveal significant differences across cosmetics and personal care segments. Personal hygiene is expected to dominate, with a market size estimated at US $600–630 billion, nearly three times larger than skincare, the second-leading segment, valued at US $183 billion. Hair care maintains a stable yet smaller share, projected at US $105.3 billion by 2024. Makeup and nail products together account for US $67–75 billion, though the segment remains fragmented: nail products (US $24.7–25.8 billion) and lipsticks (US $18.85 billion) surpass face makeup (US $10.3 billion) and eye makeup (US $13.1–19.9 billion). Fragrances occupy an intermediate position, with a projected market of US $53–61 billion, which is less than one-third the size of the skincare category. Overall, these comparisons emphasize the dominant role of personal hygiene and skincare in global revenues, while also highlighting the intense competition and product diversification that define the color cosmetics and fragrance segments.

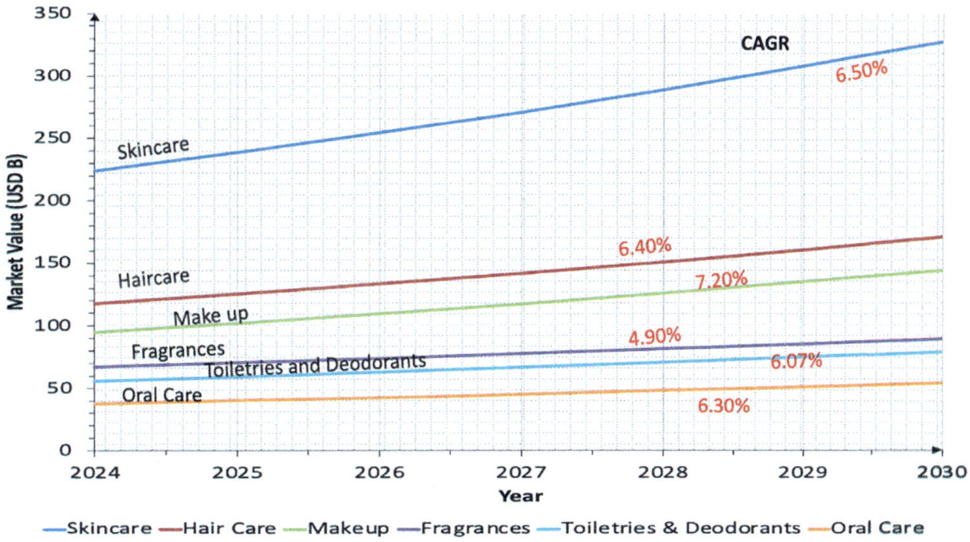

FIG. 3.2 Projected global market growth of major cosmetic categories (2024–2030) (Grand View Research, 2025; Presendence Research, 2025; Teerasumran et al., 2023; L'oreal Finance, 2025).

billions) and CAGR across key cosmetic categories. Skincare is expected to remain the leading sector, surpassing USD 330 billion by 2030 with a CAGR of 6.5%. Makeup, although smaller in overall value, shows the strongest momentum with a CAGR of 7.2%, reflecting dynamic consumer demand. Hair care is projected to grow steadily (CAGR 6.4%), while toiletries and deodorants (CAGR 6.07%) and oral care (CAGR 6.3%) maintain consistent performance. Fragrances, despite representing a smaller segment, continue to contribute to the positive overall trajectory with a CAGR of 4.9%.

3.1.3 Market restraint/high cost of biobased cosmetic products

The expansion of the biomaterials industry in developing and emerging countries is significantly constrained by the high cost of products manufactured from these materials (Bothare, 2026). In the cosmetics sector, biobased formulations typically rely on high-quality natural and organic ingredients, which tend to be more expensive than synthetic alternatives (Omkar, 2023).

Competitive landscape

Table 3.3 highlights the leading industrial beauty corporations, including L'Oréal, Estée Lauder, Unilever, and Shiseido, which dominate the global market through extensive brand portfolios, advanced research and development, and well-established distribution networks. L'Oréal, for example, accounted for about 11.5% of the global beauty and personal care market in 2023 and reported revenues of €43.5 billion in 2024, supported by substantial investment in innovation and international research centers (Statista Research Department, 2026). These conglomerates capitalize on economies of scale, implement strategic marketing across both traditional and digital channels, and increasingly adopt beauty technologies such as artificial intelligence (AI) and augmented reality to deliver personalized products and immersive consumer experiences (Statista Research Department, 2026).

3.1.4 Key industry developments

July 2024 (Partnership): Debut partnered with L'Oréal to develop bioidentical ingredients as sustainable alternatives for use across skincare, haircare, cosmetics, and fragrances.

April 2024 (Launch): Roquette Beauté introduced its latest innovation, Beauté by Roquette ST 730 (INCI: Hydroxypropyl Starch), to the cosmetics market. This novel ingredient responds to the rising consumer demand for plant-based formulations, combining sustainability with clinically validated efficacy for use in both skincare and makeup products (Omkar, 2023).

TABLE 3.3 Key cosmetic industry players.

Company	Origin	Short description	Flagship brands
L'Oréal Group	France	The world's largest cosmetics company; a leader in skincare, makeup, haircare, and luxury beauty.	L'Oréal Paris, Lancôme, Maybelline, Garnier, Kiehl's, La Roche-Posay, Yves Saint Laurent Beauty
Estée Lauder Companies	United States	Prestige beauty giant with a portfolio of high-end brands.	Estée Lauder, Clinique, MAC, Bobbi Brown, La Mer, Jo Malone, Aveda, Tom Ford Beauty
Procter & Gamble (P&G) Beauty	United States	Mass-market beauty leader; strong in skincare and haircare.	Olay, Pantene, Head & Shoulders, Herbal Essences, SK-II
Unilever	UK/Netherlands	Consumer goods leader with a strong beauty portfolio.	Dove, TRESemmé, Vaseline, Lux, Pond's, Simple, Dermalogica
Shiseido	Japan	Premium skincare powerhouse expanding globally.	Shiseido, Clé de Peau Beauté, NARS, bareMinerals, Drunk Elephant
Beiersdorf AG	Germany	Skincare specialist with a strong mass and luxury presence.	Nivea, Eucerin, La Prairie, Labello
Coty Inc.	United States	Global fragrance and cosmetics leader.	CoverGirl, Max Factor, Rimmel, Philosophy; Licensed: Gucci, Burberry, Hugo Boss, Calvin Klein
LVMH (Moët Hennessy Louis Vuitton)	France	Luxury conglomerate with a strong perfume and cosmetics division.	Dior Beauty, Guerlain, Fenty Beauty, Benefit Cosmetics, Make Up For Ever
Kao Corporation	Japan	Major beauty and personal care player.	Kanebo, Bioré, Molton Brown, Jergens, John Frieda
Amorepacific	South Korea	K-Beauty leader known for innovation and natural formulations.	Sulwhasoo, Laneige, Innisfree, Etude House

4 Factors that inhibit and enable the marketability of biocosmetic products

Within this evolving landscape, the cosmetics industry encounters both significant challenges and promising opportunities. Researchers have examined the factors influencing consumer decisions to purchase biofunctional cosmetics. Fig. 3.3 illustrates the key drivers that stimulate growth, as well as the inhibitors that constrain the expansion of the biofunctional cosmetics market.

4.1 Market drivers facing cosmetic product marketability

4.1.1 Scientific evidence

Kumar et al. (2021) demonstrated that consumer health consciousness and environmental concerns are key factors driving the intention to purchase green cosmetics.

4.1.2 Market trends

Cosmetic ingredients are shifting toward natural, organic, and ethically sourced options as consumers demand cleaner and greener products. This trend reflects a fundamental change in formulation, development, and marketing strategies (Alnuqaydan, 2024). Beyond ingredients and packaging, manufacturers are reducing their carbon footprint through energy efficiency and renewable energy adoption (Chel and Kaushik, 2018). Ethical considerations play a central role in the movement toward green and sustainable beauty. Companies are prioritizing cruelty-free practices and striving to establish transparent, ethical supply chains. As a result, consumers can place greater trust in sustainable beauty (Suphasomboon and Vassanadumrongdee, 2022).

4.1.3 Consumer's attitude

Lavuri et al. (2022) and Shimul et al. (2022) emphasized that consumer attitudes, specifically a positive predisposition toward green products, are among the strongest predictors of purchase intentions for green cosmetics. Similarly, Zollo et al. (2021) found that product knowledge, understood as consumers' self-perceived awareness of product characteristics and their health and environmental implications, serves as a key antecedent of purchase intention.

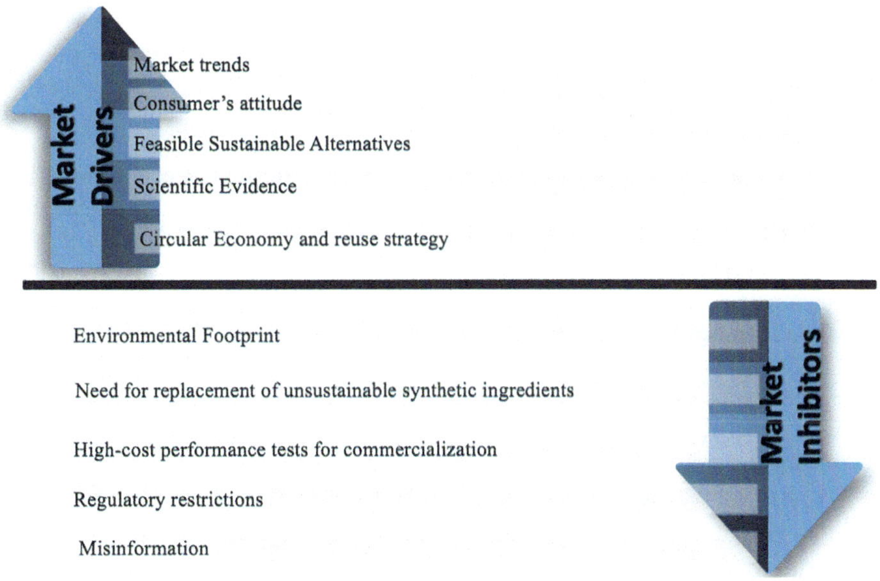

FIG. 3.3 Market drivers and market inhibitors that propel and hinder biofunctional cosmetics market growth.

Feasible sustainable alternatives

The structural diversity of natural ingredients enables tailored cosmetic functions, especially in hair care, where greener alternatives are needed to replace cationic polyelectrolytes and silicones (Luengo et al., 2023). Sustainable ingredients must meet environmental, social, ethical, and economic criteria, requiring companies to balance affordability with quality through technology and supply chain optimization (Omkar, 2023). One effective strategy is the upcycling of industrial waste and by-products, particularly from the agrofood sector, such as spent coffee grounds, olive oil residues, and grape or fruit skins. These materials can be repurposed into high-value, sustainable ingredients for cosmetic formulations (Martins and Marto, 2023). Another innovative approach is the development of waterless products. Originally introduced to increase the concentration and efficacy of active compounds, these formulations also carry significant environmental and economic benefits. Their reduced water content results in smaller product sizes, requiring less packaging and lowering transportation costs, while also decreasing the environmental burden associated with packaging waste (Aguiar et al., 2022).

4.1.4 Adoption of CE and reuse strategy

Improving both economic and environmental performance often goes hand in hand, as demonstrated by the application of CE principles (Acerbi et al., 2021). Interest in CE within the cosmetics sector has grown considerably, particularly in relation to input valorization for product formulation (Mondello et al., 2024). COVID-19 highlighted the urgency of CE models in cosmetics, prompting many companies to replace fossil-based ingredients with biofunctional alternatives, as discussed at the 2020 Sustainable Cosmetics Summit (Goyal and Jerold, 2021).

Bom et al. introduced the concept of "Cosmetic product life cycle with a sustainable approach, life cycle thinking (LCT)," outlining how green cosmetics can be developed through sustainable cultivation, raw material extraction, energy and water efficiency, and effective waste management. Within this context, upcycling has become a transformative approach that improves industrial processes while supporting CE goals. Upcycling, or creative reuse, converts waste streams into higher-value products, thereby reducing environmental impacts and generating new market opportunities. By-products from the fruit and vegetable processing sector, such as spent coffee grounds, olive oil residues, and grape skins, are rich in bioactive compounds like vitamins and phenolics. Repurposing these materials as cosmetic ingredients offers functional and environmental benefits (Martins and Marto, 2023), supporting CE principles of reducing waste, conserving resources, and limiting virgin material use (Martins et al., 2025).

Packaging represents another critical area for CE adoption, as plastics remain the dominant material used in cosmetics. To support eco-friendly packaging, the development of bioplastics derived from biomass has become a priority. Key technologies are focused on maximizing efficiency and sustainability (Khalil et al., 2016). However, scaling biobased plastics to commercial production has proven challenging. Algae, both micro- and macroalgae, have gained attention as a promising biomass source since they do not compete with food production, require minimal water and chemicals, and contain high levels of polysaccharides, lipids, and proteins. These characteristics make algae a sustainable option for bioplastics, supporting both the circular and bioeconomy (Cinar et al., 2020). Emerging materials such as polyhydroxyalkanoates are also expected to play a pivotal role in sustainable packaging (Gómez-Gast et al., 2022), while cellulose-based materials have been shown to improve protection, shelf life, and overall marketability of containers (Iversen et al., 2022).

Reducing manufacturing waste is another pressing concern due to the high costs associated with its disposal. Ancuța and Sonia (202) demonstrated that recovering bioactive compounds allows waste reuse, reduces disposal costs, and minimizes related risks. From an economic standpoint, valorizing by-products through CE practices benefits both waste producers and processing industries by decreasing costs tied to disposal and providing alternatives to conventional materials (Panwar et al., 2021). Conventional waste treatment carries annual costs of up to USD 1 trillion, plus significant social and environmental expenses, while a circular bioeconomy could yield EUR 1.8 trillion in benefits and create 3 million EU jobs by 2030 (Machado et al., 2024).

Reusable packaging represents yet another efficient strategy to reduce the carbon footprint in the postuse phase. Several brands now offer refillable packaging systems, which not only decrease packaging and transportation impacts but also strengthen customer loyalty. According to the Ellen MacArthur Foundation, if all beauty and personal care product bottles were refillable, greenhouse gas emissions could be reduced by 80%–85% (Martins and Marto, 2023).

4.2 Inhibitors facing cosmetic product marketability

Despite the rapid expansion of the green cosmetics sector, it still represents only around 15% of the global cosmetics industry (Sadiq et al., 2021). Scholars have noted that barriers, such as high product prices and consumer skepticism regarding the authenticity of natural claims, significantly influence purchasing decisions (Siddiqui et al., 2023).

4.2.1 Environmental footprint

As the global beauty and personal care market grows, so too does its environmental footprint (Omira et al., 2025). The rising demand for natural alternatives may generate considerable ecological pressures, including deforestation and the unsustainable exploitation of natural resources. For instance, the large-scale cultivation of essential oils and plant extracts can drive the conversion of forests into farmland, leading to biodiversity loss and soil degradation (Couceiro et al., 2025).

4.2.2 Strong investment in innovative, green, and sustainable chemistry

There are still various occurrences where the production of biobased ingredients relies on chemical processes that are not entirely green. It is, therefore, essential not only to derive ingredients from renewable sources but also to ensure their production follows eco-responsible methods with minimal environmental impact. At the same time, biobased ingredients must demonstrate performance equal to or greater than that of petroleum-based components. There is a need for research and investment in sustainable chemistry to design and modify biobased substances into functional cosmetic ingredients (Luengo et al., 2023).

4.2.3 Need for replacement of unsustainable synthetic ingredients

Substituting unsustainable synthetic ingredients with greener options remains a challenge, as it demands a thorough evaluation of their functionality, safety, stability, and performance, along with comparative studies against conventional counterparts (Bom et al., 2019).

4.2.4 High-cost performance tests for commercialization

From an economic standpoint, the use of natural extracts provides important sustainability benefits but also entails higher costs due to the complexity of extraction, the need for stabilization methods, and the addition of compounds to mask unwanted colors. These factors increase formulation expenses and make it difficult to maintain batch-to-batch consistency. However, the rising interest in eco-friendly cosmetic products may help to overcome these barriers, particularly with increased investment in research and innovation aimed at delivering effective and appealing formulations (Adeel et al., 2022). The high cost of isolating plant essential oils has also led to the availability of synthetic substitutes in the market (Başer and Buchbauer, 2023). Although synthetic antioxidants remain dominant, demand for natural antioxidants has been growing in recent years and is expected to continue increasing (Kim et al., 2018). Similarly, the demand for perfumes containing natural plant-derived aromatic components remains strong, as essential oils offer unique and persistent aromas that cannot always be replicated synthetically (Başer and Buchbauer, 2023).

In addition to cost challenges, cosmetic products must undergo extensive preclinical and clinical testing to ensure human safety before reaching the market. These assessments often begin with animal testing, typically in rodents, before progressing to higher-order animals to identify adverse reactions and evaluate formulation safety. Analytical evaluations are then followed by clinical and dermatological studies to assess compatibility and toxicity in humans. Such testing ensures compliance with regulatory requirements prior to commercialization. Conventional approaches to safety testing include cell culture assays, patch testing, cutometric and corneometric evaluations, as well as toxicity analysis in live animal models. This phase is resource-intensive, time-consuming, and represents one of the most challenging stages of product development (Pai et al., 2025). The extraction and preservation of natural ingredients are complex and costly (Pai et al., 2025), leading to higher retail prices that limit the accessibility of biobased cosmetics (Omkar, 2023).

4.2.5 Misinformation

Another important consideration is the prevalence of misinformation in the marketplace, particularly the widespread assumption that all synthetic ingredients are harmful while all natural ones are beneficial. This perception is not always accurate. In addition, many ingredients listed under a single name may originate from animal, plant, or synthetic sources, leaving consumers uncertain about their actual origin. Current EU legislation does not mandate disclosure of ingredient origin, which limits transparency. Requiring full disclosure would enable consumers to make more informed and conscious choices when purchasing cosmetic products (Bom et al., 2019).

4.2.6 Regulatory restrictions

Developing innovative cosmetic ingredients requires strategic regulation, yet stricter global safety standards, driven by concerns over toxicity, environmental impact, and health risks, pose significant challenges (Ghosh et al., 2025).

In the European Union, particular emphasis is placed on sourcing environmentally friendly alternatives for raw materials used in cosmetic formulations. These alternatives must also comply with the requirements of the Registration, Evaluation, Authorization and Restriction of Chemicals (REACH). Under REACH, the list of substances permitted for production, commercialization, and use is established with environmental safety considerations in mind. Substances are evaluated by the European Chemicals Agency, which applies a cross-sectoral assessment framework to ensure environmental and consumer safety. In this context, the demand for natural and organic cosmetic products is increasing, reflecting both consumer preferences and regulatory restrictions on many synthetic ingredients. Nevertheless, challenges remain, as natural ingredients often do not perform as effectively as conventional ones, and all new ingredients must comply with safety requirements outlined in the Annexes of the EU Cosmetics Regulation (Mondello et al., 2024). Europe is a leading exporter and global hub of the cosmetics industry, with the EU playing a key role in regulation and international trade. To support these functions, the EU has developed the CosIng database, which provides transparent access to information on cosmetic substances. Cosmetics legislation requires that all products be registered in the Cosmetic Products Notification Portal before entering the EU market. Further provisions include the prohibition of animal testing for cosmetic safety evaluation, national-level market surveillance by EU member states, and stricter monitoring of products considered to pose higher risks to consumer health. EU cosmetics are regulated under Regulation (EC) No. 1223/2009, which bans most carcinogenic, mutagenic, reprotoxic (CMR) substances (categories 1A, 1B, and 2), with limited exceptions allowed under strict conditions (Alnuqaydan, 2024). In the United States, cosmetic safety is regulated by the Environmental Protection Agency (EPA) and FDA, while in Asia, stricter measures apply, including Japan's Chemical Substances Control Law (CSCL) and Ministry of Health, Labour and Welfare (MHLW) standards for chemical substances (Ghosh et al., 2025).

Such regulatory frameworks must be taken into account before placing novel ingredients on the market, since authorization to claim all assessed functions for a single ingredient can take several years. Companies also aim to commercialize products globally, yet conflicting regulations complicate this process. For example, animal testing is still required for certain products in China, whereas it is prohibited in the European Union. These contradictions create obstacles for market access and highlight the importance of strategic navigation of regulatory landscapes, as compliance directly affects both entry to market and the ability to substantiate functional claims (Rischard et al., 2025). Cosmetic regulation faces challenges as rapid product innovation can outpace oversight, leaving supervision gaps and delaying responses to emerging safety concerns (Alnuqaydan, 2024).

Packaging is another critical aspect of cosmetic regulation and sustainability. Before commercialization, packaging undergoes rigorous testing to ensure functionality, safety, and durability. These assessments include barrier performance (gas and moisture protection), impact resistance, sealing efficiency (to prevent leaks), as well as evaluations of thickness, tear strength, friction coefficient, and solvent residue. Such measures are vital to guarantee consumer safety, preserve product quality, and maintain integrity during storage and distribution (Omira et al., 2025). However, sustainability challenges extend beyond raw materials to encompass formulations and packaging (Luengo et al., 2023).

Plastics dominate the cosmetics packaging sector due to their affordability, light weight, versatility, and durability. Yet, their nonbiodegradable nature poses major environmental concerns, as plastic waste accumulates in landfills and oceans. Alternatives such as glass and metal are increasingly adopted by natural cosmetics brands, but they are more expensive, heavier, and energy-intensive to transport, which increases emissions (Srivastava et al., 2022). Packaging sustainability also depends on minimizing product residues left in empty containers, as these contribute to consumer losses, environmental waste, and reduced recyclability. Klein et al. (2025) stress the importance of choosing packaging optimized for different products to prevent waste, protect recyclate quality, and improve sustainability outcomes. Among promising alternatives, cellulose-based polymers represent versatile and renewable substitutes for conventional plastics, offering broad applicability in cosmetic packaging.

5 Strategic marketing approaches for dominant trends in the cosmetics sector

5.1 Multifunctional ingredients

The deliberate use of multifunctional ingredients (Fig. 3.4) enhances product performance while addressing consumer expectations for effective and efficient skincare solutions (Rischard et al., 2025). These ingredients are defined by their ability to deliver multiple benefits within a single formulation, often combining protective, stabilizing, and sensory functions to target several skin concerns while ensuring formulation stability. The industry has increasingly prioritized the identification of such multipurpose components, particularly from natural and biobased sources, in response to rising demand for eco-friendly solutions. Their advantages are wide-ranging and explain their growing popularity in cosmetic

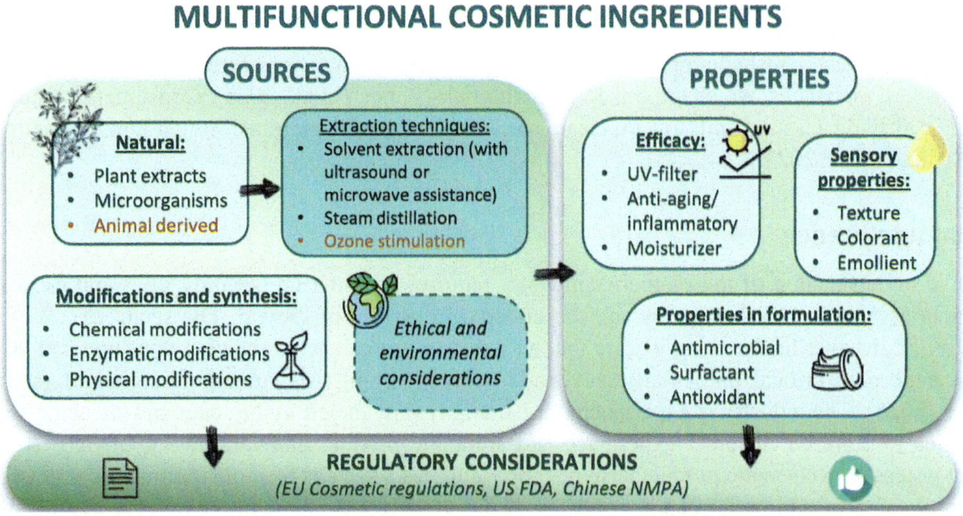

FIG. 3.4 Multifunctional cosmetic ingredients. *(Reproduced with perimssion from Rischard, F., Gore, E., Flourat, A., Savary, G., 2025. The challenges faced by multifunctional ingredients: a critical review from sourcing to cosmetic applications. Adv. Colloid Interface Sci. 00018686. 340, 103463. doi:10.1016/j.cis.2025.103463.); Reproduced with perimssion from (Third Party Material Rightsholder WebReproduced with perimssion from Link: https://www.sciencedirect.com/science/article/pii/S0001868625000740#f0020. Mode of Contact: Rightslink.)*

TABLE 3.4 Synergistic effect of ingredients.

Synergistic effect of ingredients	Key finding
Probiotics with peptides	Strengthen the skin's barrier and reduce inflammation (De Luca et al., 2016).
Marine collagen peptides and plant-derived antioxidants, such as coenzyme Q10, grape-skin extract, luteolin, and selenium	Improved skin properties without increasing oxidative stress (De Luca et al., 2016).
Antioxidants and vitamins	Protects against environmental stressors and promotes healthy cell regeneration (Woodby et al., 2020).
Topical antioxidants, such as vitamins C and E, carotenoids, resveratrol, and pycnogenol, can be complemented with dietary supplementation	Topical antioxidants, such as vitamins C and E, carotenoids, resveratrol, and pycnogenol, may be used in combination with dietary supplements (Woodby et al., 2020).
Probiotics and plant extracts	Probiotics and plant extracts offer a promising approach for delivering active compounds more effectively and enhancing their bioavailability and activity (Holkem et al., 2023).
Lactobacillus acidophilus and *Curcuma longa* rhizome extract	The combined use of *Lactobacillus acidophilus* and *Curcuma longa* rhizome extract has demonstrated synergistic antibacterial effects against C. acnes. This suggests that this synbiotic pairing holds promise for therapeutic applications in cosmetics or medical treatments targeting C. acnes (Kim et al., 2020).

applications. A major benefit lies in their higher efficacy, as multifunctional ingredients can perform several roles at once, reducing the number of components required in a formulation. This simplification not only strengthens overall product performance but also lowers the risk of adverse interactions that could compromise stability or effectiveness. In addition, many bioactive multifunctional ingredients with surface-active or emulsifying properties, such as lignin, biopolymers, and biosurfactants, contribute to physical stabilization while offering further functional benefits (Rischard et al., 2025).

Table 3.4 presents the synergistic effect of key ingredients.

Eco-design in cosmetics is challenging, requiring ingredients that balance cosmetic performance, environmental impact, and economic viability. Guided by green chemistry, the industry invests in new formulations and product redesigns while weighing consumer expectations, feasibility, and sustainability across the product lifecycle (Luengo et al., 2023).

5.2 Clean beauty

The clean beauty movement is reshaping personal care, driving innovation toward formulations free from harmful chemicals like parabens and phthalates, which are linked to health risks (Ghosh et al., 2025). Consumer demand for natural and ethical materials is driving a lasting shift toward clean, sustainable ingredients, transforming how cosmetics are developed and marketed (Alnuqaydan, 2024).

5.3 Artificial intelligence

A comprehensive understanding of the cosmetics industry requires considering not only sales and esthetics but also the complex interactions between market agents and the underlying drivers of growth. The sector exerts a broad influence across all stages of consumer life, making it "rare that an industry is so closely related to consumers at all stages of life." Consumer trust is therefore critical, particularly as AI and machine learning (ML) transform digital interactions (O'Higgins and Fatorachian, 2025). The industry is experiencing a paradigm shift fueled by big data and AI, with brands leveraging these technologies to enhance customer experience and stimulate product innovation (Ustymenko, 2023). AI and ML hold significant potential in cosmetic product design, supporting tasks such as formula optimization, ingredient screening, structure–property analysis, and performance evaluation. For gel scientists, some of the most pressing challenges include formula screening, process optimization, and high-throughput property measurements. AI and ML offer practical solutions in these areas, including predicting swelling and rheological properties, optimizing conditions for 3D printing, and refining formulations (Xin et al., 2024). AI and ML are driving personalization, efficiency, and innovation in cosmetics, enabling smaller brands to compete with global leaders while reshaping marketing, customer engagement, and supply chains (O'Higgins and Fatorachian, 2025).

5.4 Commitment to sustainability

The growing demand for natural and eco-friendly products has intensified concerns regarding sustainability. True sustainability is multidimensional, requiring the integration of economic, environmental, and social considerations. Fig. 3.5 illustrates these three core dimensions of sustainability (Luengo et al., 2023).

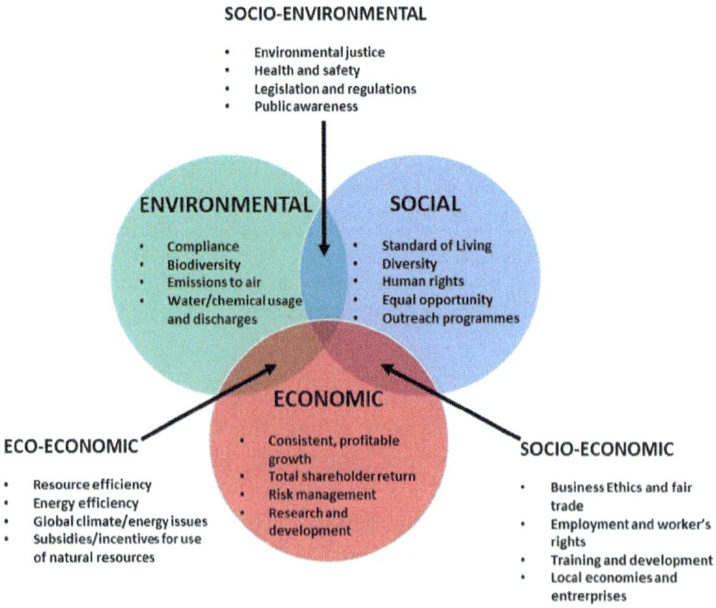

FIG. 3.5 The facets of sustainability. *(Reproduced with permission from Luengo, G.S., Leonforte, F., Greaves, A., Rubio, R.G., Guzman, E., 2023. Physico-chemical challenges on the self-assembly of natural and bio-based ingredients on hair surfaces: towards sustainable haircare formulations. Green Chem. 14639270. 25 (20), 7863–7882. Available from: https://pubs.rsc.org/en/journals/journal/gc. doi:10.1039/d3gc02763e.); Reproduced with permission from (Third Party Material, Rightsholder Web Link: https://pubs.rsc.org/en/content/articlelanding/2023/gc/d3gc02763e. Mode of Contact: Rightslink.)*

Sustainability in cosmetics spans the full value chain, from design and sourcing to postuse management. Ingredient selection follows three key principles: use of renewable resources, eco-friendly manufacturing, and minimized environmental impact, aligning the industry with the UN Sustainable Development Goals (Luengo et al., 2023).

5.5 Economic sustainability paradigm in the cosmetic industry

The cosmetics sector is one of the key industries requiring a long-term vision to effectively manage sustainability. The transition toward greener practices is driven by an increasing emphasis on enhancing both the environmental and social sustainability of activities and products (Bom et al., 2019). Companies are gradually integrating environmental and social objectives into their economic strategies, reflecting a shift toward holistic sustainable practices (Rocca et al., 2022). Economic sustainability remains a fundamental objective, and in many cases, the economic and environmental dimensions are closely linked, particularly through efforts to reduce costs associated with waste removal, storage, and disposal (Clodoveo et al., 2022). For most companies, the initial decision to adopt sustainability commitments is primarily motivated by the potential for economic benefits, whether through the development of higher-value products or the attraction of a broader customer base (Civancik-Uslu et al., 2019).

6 Conclusions

In recent years, the cosmetics industry has made substantial investments in addressing environmental, social, and economic challenges. This study has examined multiple dimensions of market analysis, highlighting key trends, challenges, and opportunities shaping the current landscape. The cosmetics industry, defined by its innovation and dynamism, is continually advancing through research often influenced by market trends. A clear shift can be observed toward the development of products that are less harmful to both the environment and human health. Cosmetics formulated with natural ingredients or those designed to minimize environmental impact have become particularly popular among consumers, a trend that is also reflected in the increasing number of patent applications. These dynamics have strongly shaped the development of biofunctional products, which hold the potential to transform the sector by offering sustainable and eco-friendly alternatives to conventional chemical-based formulations. In Europe, the cosmetics market continues to expand across multiple segments, with momentum driven by sustainability, innovation, and changing consumer values. Growth forecasts vary, ranging from conservative estimates of 4.90%–6.07% CAGR to more optimistic projections of 6.50%–7.20% CAGR. Projections for 2025 highlight significant variation among categories: personal hygiene is expected to dominate with a market size of USD 600–630 billion, nearly three times larger than skincare, the next leading category at USD 183 billion. Global leadership in the sector is maintained by major players such as L'Oréal, Estée Lauder, Unilever, and Shiseido, which leverage extensive brand portfolios, advanced research and development, and well-established distribution networks. However, despite strong growth prospects, the market faces important barriers. These include the environmental footprint of production, regulatory constraints, high costs of performance testing for commercialization, and the pressing need to replace unsustainable synthetic ingredients. Researchers now have access to diverse experimental and computational tools that facilitate the shift from traditional to biobased ingredients. Considerable progress has been made by pioneers in the field, and the molecular diversity of biobased compounds presents vast opportunities for innovation. Nonetheless, advancing sustainable cosmetics requires ensuring that these ingredients deliver key functional benefits while addressing cost and performance challenges.

References

Acerbi, F., Rocca, R., Fumagalli, L., Taisch, M., 2023. Enhancing the cosmetics industry sustainability through a renewed sustainable supplier selection model. Prod. Manuf. Res. 21693277. 11 (1). Available from: https://www.tandfonline.com/tpmr. doi:10.1080/21693277.2022.2161021.

Acerbi, F., Sassanelli, C., Terzi, S., Taisch, M., 2021. A systematic literature review on data and information required for circular manufacturing strategies adoption. Sustainability. 2071-1050. 13 (4), 2047. doi:10.3390/su13042047.

Adeel, S., Habiba, M., Kiran, S., Iqbal, S., Abrar, S., Hassan, C.M., 2022. Utilization of colored extracts for the formulation of ecological friendly plant-based green products. Sustainability. 2071-1050. 14 (18), 11758. doi:10.3390/su141811758.

Aguiar, J.B., Martins, A.M., Almeida, C., Ribeiro, H.M., Marto, J., 2022. Water sustainability: a waterless life cycle for cosmetic products. Sustain. Prod. Consum. 23525509. 32, 35–51. Available from: http://www.journals.elsevier.com/sustainable-production-and-consumption/. doi:10.1016/j.spc.2022.04.008.

Alnuqaydan, A.M., 2024. The dark side of beauty: an in-depth analysis of the health hazards and toxicological impact of synthetic cosmetics and personal care products. Front. Public Health 22962565. 12. Available from: http://journal.frontiersin.org/journal/public-health/section/public-health-education-and-promotion#archive. doi:10.3389/fpubh.2024.1439027.

Alves-Silva, J.M., Dos Santos, S.M.D., Pintado, M.E., Pérez-álvarez, J.A., Fernández-López, J., Viuda-Martos, M., 2013. Chemical composition and in vitro antimicrobial, antifungal and antioxidant properties of essential oils obtained from some herbs widely used in Portugal. Food Control. 09567135. 32 (2), 371–378. doi:10.1016/j.foodcont.2012.12.022.

Ancuța, P., Sonia, A., 2020. Oil press-cakes and meals valorization through circular economy approaches: a review. Appl. Sci. 2076-3417. 10 (21), 7432. doi:10.3390/app10217432.

Babich, O., Ivanova, S., Bakhtiyarova, A., Kalashnikova, O., Sukhikh, S., 2025. Medicinal plants are the basis of natural cosmetics. Federation Process Biochem. 13595113. 154, 35–51. Available from: https://www.sciencedirect.com/science/journal/13595113. doi:10.1016/j.procbio.2025.04.009.

Baccile, N., Seyrig, C., Poirier, A., Alonso-De Castro, S., Roelants, S.L.K.W., Abel, S., 2021. Self-assembly, interfacial properties, interactions with macromolecules and molecular modelling and simulation of microbial bio-based amphiphiles (biosurfactants). A tutorial review. Green Chem. 14639270. 23 (11), 3842–3944. Available from: http://pubs.rsc.org/en/journals/journal/gc. doi:10.1039/d1gc00097g.

Başer, K.H.C., Buchbauer, G., 2023. Handbook of Essential Oils: Science, Technology, and Applications. CRC Press, Taylor & Francis Group. ISBN: 978-1-4200-6315-8.

Bhatia, S.K., Bhatia, R.K., Jeon, J.-M., Pugazhendhi, A., Awasthi, M.K., Kumar, D., Kumar, G., Yoon, J.-J., Yang, Y.-H., 2021. An overview on advancements in biobased transesterification methods for biodiesel production: oil resources, extraction, biocatalysts, and process intensification technologies. Fuel. 00162361. 285, 119117. doi:10.1016/j.fuel.2020.119117.

Bolke, L., Schlippe, G., Gerß, J., Voss, W., 2019. A collagen supplement improves skin hydration, elasticity, roughness, and density: results of a randomized, placebo-controlled, blind study. Nutrients 20726643. 11 (10). Available from: https://www.mdpi.com/2072-6643/11/10/2494/pdf. doi:10.3390/nu11102494.

Bom, S., Jorge, J., Ribeiro, H.M., Marto, J., 2019. A step forward on sustainability in the cosmetics industry: a review. J. Clean. Prod. 09596526. 225, 270–290. doi:10.1016/j.jclepro.2019.03.255.

Bothare, V., 2026. Bio-Based Cosmetics and Personal Care Ingredients Market Size, Share & Trends Analysis Report Based on Active Ingredient (Vitamins and Derivatives, Ceramides, Peptides, Resveratrol, Potassium Sorbate, Bio-Succinic Acid, Hyaluronic Acid, Glycerin, Creatine, Alpha Hydroxy Acids), Based on Application (Skin and Sun Care, Hair Care, Make-up and Color Cosmetics, Fragrances) and By Region (North America, Europe, APAC, Middle East and Africa, LATAM) Forecasts, 2025-2033. Straits Research, SRCP1910DR. [Online]. Available from: https://straitsresearch.com/report/bio-based-cosmetics-and-personal-care-ingredients-market (Accessed 14 Sepetember 2025).

Cao, X., Luo, X., Barros, S.M., Xing, W., MacGregor, M., Delcheva, I., Campbell, J.A., He, S., Kirk, B.P., Tang, Y., Raston, C.L., 2025. Vortex fluidic-mediated transesterification enhancement of mongongo fatty acid ethyl ester production for haircare applications. RSC Sustain. 27538125. 3 (4), 1909–1922. Available from: https://www.rsc.org/journals-books-databases/about-journals/rsc-sustainability/#scope. doi:10.1039/d4su00763h.

Chel, A., Kaushik, G., 2018. Renewable energy technologies for sustainable development of energy efficient building. Alexandria Eng. J. 11100168. 57 (2), 655–669. Available from: http://www.elsevier.com/wps/find/journaldescription.cws_home/724292/description#description. doi:10.1016/j.aej.2017.02.027.

Christaki, E., Giannenas, I., Bonos, E., Florou-Paneri, P., 2019. Innovative uses of aromatic plants as natural supplements in nutrition. In: Florou-Paneri, P., Christaki, E., Giannenas, I. (Eds.), Feed Additives: Aromatic Plants and Herbs in Animal Nutrition and Health. Elsevier, Greece, pp. 19–34. Available from: https://www.sciencedirect.com/book/9780128147009. doi:10.1016/B978-0-12-814700-9.00002-9.

Cinar, S.O., Chong, Z.K., Kucuker, M.A., Wieczorek, N., Cengiz, U., Kuchta, K., 2020. Bioplastic production from microalgae: a review. Int. J. Environ. Res. Public Health. 16604601. 17 (11). doi:10.3390/ijerph17113842.

Civancik-Uslu, D., Puig, R., Voigt, S., Walter, D., Fullana-i-Palmer, P., 2019. Improving the production chain with LCA and eco-design: application to cosmetic packaging. Resour. Conserv. Recycl.. 09213449. 151, 104475. doi:10.1016/j.resconrec.2019.104475.

Clodoveo, M.L., Crupi, P., Annunziato, A., Corbo, F., 2022. Innovative extraction technologies for development of functional ingredients based on polyphenols from olive leaves. Foods 23048158. 11 (1). Available from: https://www.mdpi.com/2304-8158/11/1/103/pdf. doi:10.3390/foods11010103.

Cornwell, P.A., 2018. A review of shampoo surfactant technology: consumer benefits, raw materials and recent developments. Int. J. Cosmet. Sci. 14682494. 40 (1), 16–30. Available from: http://onlinelibrary.wiley.com/journal/10.1111/(ISSN)1468-2494. doi:10.1111/ics.12439.

Couceiro, B., Hameed, H., Vieira, A.C.F., Singh, S.K., Dua, K., Veiga, F., Pires, P.C., Ferreira, L., Paiva-Santos, A.C., 2025. Promoting health and sustainability: exploring safer alternatives in cosmetics and regulatory perspectives. Sustain. Chem. Pharm. 23525541. 43, 101901. doi:10.1016/j.scp.2024.101901.

De Luca, C., Mikhal'Chik, E.V., Suprun, M.V., Papacharalambous, M., Truhanov, A.I., Korkina, L.G., 2016. Skin antiageing and systemic Redox effects of supplementation with marine collagen peptides and plant-derived antioxidants: a single-blind case-control clinical study. Oxid. Med. Cell. Longev. 19420994. 2016. Available from: http://www.hindawi.com/journals/oximed/. doi:10.1155/2016/4389410.

Fan, X., Bai, L., Zhu, L., Yang, L., Zhang, X., 2014. Marine algae-derived bioactive peptides for human nutrition and health. J. Agric. Food Chem. 15205118. 62 (38), 9211–9222. Available from: http://pubs.acs.org/journal/jafcau. doi:10.1021/jf502420h.

Fernández-Peña, L., Guzmán, E., Leonforte, F., Serrano-Pueyo, A., Regulski, K., Tournier-Couturier, L., Ortega, F., Rubio, R.G., Luengo, G.S., 2020. Effect of molecular structure of eco-friendly glycolipid biosurfactants on the adsorption of hair-care conditioning polymers. Colloids Surf. B Biointerfaces. 09277765. 185, 110578. doi:10.1016/j.colsurfb.2019.110578.

Fortune Business Insights, 2025. Makeup Market Size, Share & Industry Analysis, By Product (Powders, Gels, Lotions, and Others), By Application Area (Lips, Eyes, Face, and Nails), By Distribution Channel (Supermarkets & Hypermarkets, Exclusive Brand Stores, Online/E-Commerce, and Others), and Regional Forecast, 2025-2032. FBI102587. Accessed: Sept. 14, 2025 AD. [Online]. Available from: https://www.fortunebusinessinsights.com/makeup-market-102587?utm_source=chatgpt.com.

Ghosh, J., Rupanty, N.S., Noor, T., Asif, T.R., Islam, T., Reukov, V., 2025. Functional coatings for textiles: advancements in flame resistance, antimicrobial defense, and self-cleaning performance. RSC Adv. 20462069. 15 (14), 10984–11022. Available from: http://pubs.rsc.org/en/journals/journal/ra. doi:10.1039/d5ra01429h.

Gómez-Gast, N., Cuellar, M.D.R.L., Vergara-Porras, B., Vieyra, H., 2022. Biopackaging potential alternatives: bioplastic composites of polyhydroxyalkanoates and vegetal fibers. Polymers 20734360. 14 (6). Available from: https://www.mdpi.com/2073-4360/14/6/1114/pdf. doi:10.3390/polym14061114.

Gouw, V.P., Jung, J., Zhao, Y., 2017. Functional properties, bioactive compounds, and in vitro gastrointestinal digestion study of dried fruit pomace powders as functional food ingredients. LWT 00236438. 80, 136–144. Available from: https://www.journals.elsevier.com/lwt. doi:10.1016/j.lwt.2017.02.015.

Goyal, N., Jerold, F., 2021. Biocosmetics: technological advances and future outlook. Environ. Sci. Pollut. Res. 30 (10), 25148–25169. doi:10.1007/s11356-021-17567-3.

Grand View Research, 2025. Cosmetics Market Size, Share & Trends Analysis Report By Product (Skin Care, Hair Care), By End-user (Men, Women), By Distribution Channel (Offline, Online), By Region (North America, Europe), and Segment Forecasts, 2024–2030. Market Report GVR-4-68039-924-6. [Online]. Available from: https://www.grandviewresearch.com/industry-analysis/cosmetics-market (Accessed 14 September 2025).

Heath, R.S., Ruscoe, R.E., Turner, N.J., 2022. The beauty of biocatalysis: sustainable synthesis of ingredients in cosmetics. Nat. Prod. Rep. 14604752. 39 (2), 335–388. Available from: http://pubs.rsc.org/en/journals/journal/np. doi:10.1039/d1np00027f.

Holkem, A.T., Silva, M.P.D., Favaro-Trindade, C.S., 2023. Probiotics and plant extracts: a promising synergy and delivery systems. Crit. Rev. Food Sci. Nutr. 15497852. 63 (28), 9561–9579. Available from: https://www.tandfonline.com/loi/bfsn20. doi:10.1080/10408398.2022.2066623.

Iversen, L.J.L., Rovina, K., Vonnie, J.M., Matanjun, P., Erna, K.H., 'Aqilah, N.M.N., Felicia, W.X.L., Funk, A.A., 2022. The emergence of edible and food-application coatings for food packaging: a review. Molecules 14203049. 27 (17). Available from: http://www.mdpi.com/journal/molecules. doi:10.3390/molecules27175604.

Joondan, N., Laulloo, S.J., Caumul, P., 2018. Amino acids: building blocks for the synthesis of greener amphiphiles. J. Dispersion Sci. Technol. 15322351. 39 (11), 1550–1564. Available from: https://www.tandf.co.uk/journals/titles/01932691.asp. doi:10.1080/01932691.2017.1421085.

Khalil, H.P.S.A., Davoudpour, Y., Saurabh, C.K., Hossain, M.S., Adnan, A.S., Dungani, R., Paridah, M.T., Mohamed, Z.I.S., Fazita, M.R.N., Syakir, M.I., Haafiz, M.K.M., 2016. A review on nanocellulosic fibres as new material for sustainable packaging: process and applications. Renew. Sustain. Energy Rev. 18790690. 64, 823–836. Available from: https://www.journals.elsevier.com/renewable-and-sustainable-energy-reviews. doi:10.1016/j.rser.2016.06.072.

Kim, J.J., Kim, K.S., Yu, B.J., 2018. Optimization of antioxidant and skin-whitening compounds extraction condition from tenebrio molitor larvae (Mealworm). Molecules 14203049. 23 (9). Available from: http://www.mdpi.com/1420-3049/23/9/2340/pdf. doi:10.3390/molecules23092340.

Kim, J., Kim, H., Jeon, S., Jo, J., Kim, Y., Kim, H., 2020. Synergistic antibacterial effects of probiotic lactic acid bacteria with curcuma longa rhizome extract as synbiotic against cutibacterium acnes. Appl. Sci. 20763417. 10 (24), 1–6. Available from: https://www.mdpi.com/2076-3417/10/24/8955/pdf. doi:10.3390/app10248955.

Kim, N.H., Jung, S.H., Kim, J., Kim, S.H., Ahn, H.J., Song, K.B., 2014. Purification of an iron-chelating peptide from spirulina protein hydrolysates. J. Korean Soc. Appl. Biol. Chem. 2234344X. 57 (1), 91–95. doi:10.1007/s13765-013-4211-5.

Klein, M., Tacker, M., Apprich, S., 2025. Product Waste resulting from insufficient emptiability of cosmetic packaging and its economic and environmental implications. Sustainability. 2071-1050. 17 (3), 1056. doi:10.3390/su17031056.

Kolling, C., Ribeiro, J.L.D., de Medeiros, J.F., 2022. Performance of the cosmetics industry from the perspective of Corporate Social Responsibility and Design for Sustainability. Sustain. Prod. Consum. 23525509. 30, 171–185. Available from: http://www.journals.elsevier.com/sustainable-production-and-consumption/. doi:10.1016/j.spc.2021.12.002.

Kumar, S., Dhir, A., Talwar, S., Chakraborty, D., Kaur, P., 2021. What drives brand love for natural products? The moderating role of household size. J. Retail. Consum. Serv. 09696989. 58, 102329. doi:10.1016/j.jretconser.2020.102329.

L'Haridon, J., Martz, P., Chenéble, J.-.C., Campion, J.-.F., Colombe, L., 2018. Ecodesign of cosmetic formulae: methodology and application. Int. J. Cosmet. Sci. 0142-5463. 40 (2), 165–177. doi:10.1111/ics.12448.

L'oreal Finance, 2025. Annual report. [Online]. Available from: https://www.loreal-finance.com/eng/annual-report (Accessed 14 September 2025).

Lavuri, R., Jabbour, C.J.C., Grebinevych, O., Roubaud, D., 2022. Green factors stimulating the purchase intention of innovative luxury organic beauty products: implications for sustainable development. J. Environ. Manag. 10958630. 301. Available from: https://www.sciencedirect.com/journal/journal-of-environmental-management. doi:10.1016/j.jenvman.2021.113899.

Lin, Y., Yang, T., Shen, L., Zhang, J., Liu, L., 2022. Study on the properties of Dendrobiumofficinale fermentation broth as functional raw material of cosmetics. J. Cosmet. Dermatol. 14732165. 21 (3), 1216–1223. Available from: http://onlinelibrary.wiley.com/journal/10.1111/(ISSN)1473-2165. doi:10.1111/jocd.14197.

Liobikienė, G., Bernatonienė, J., 2017. Why determinants of green purchase cannot be treated equally? The case of green cosmetics: literature review. J. Clean. Prod. 09596526. 162, 109–120. doi:10.1016/j.jclepro.2017.05.204.

Løkra, S., Helland, M.H., Claussen, I.C., Strætkvern, K.O., Egelandsdal, B., 2008. Chemical characterization and functional properties of a potato protein concentrate prepared by large-scale expanded bed adsorption chromatography. LWT 00236438. 41 (6), 1089–1099. Available from: https://www.journals.elsevier.com/lwt. doi:10.1016/j.lwt.2007.07.006.

Luengo, G.S., Fameau, A.L., Léonforte, F., Greaves, A.J., 2021. Surface science of cosmetic substrates, cleansing actives and formulations. Adv. Colloid Interface Sci. 00018686. 290. Available from: https://www.journals.elsevier.com/advances-in-colloid-and-interface-science. doi:10.1016/j.cis.2021.102383.

Luengo, G.S., Leonforte, F., Greaves, A., Rubio, R.G., Guzman, E., 2023. Physico-chemical challenges on the self-assembly of natural and bio-based ingredients on hair surfaces: towards sustainable haircare formulations. Green Chem. 14639270. 25 (20), 7863–7882. Available from: https://pubs.rsc.org/en/journals/journal/gc. doi:10.1039/d3gc02763e.

Machado, M., Silva, S., Costa, E.M., 2024. Byproducts as a sustainable source of cosmetic ingredients. Appl. Sci. 20763417. 14 (22). Available from: https://www.mdpi.com/journal/applsci/. doi:10.3390/app142210241.

Manga, E.B., Celik, P.A., Cabuk, A., Banat, I.M., 2021. Biosurfactants: opportunities for the development of a sustainable future. Curr. Opin. Colloid Interface Sci. 18790399. 56. Available from: https://www.elsevier.com/inca/publications/store/6/2/0/0/5/3. doi:10.1016/j.cocis.2021.101514.

Martins, A.M., Marto, J.M., 2023. A sustainable life cycle for cosmetics: from design and development to post-use phase. Sustain. Chem. Pharm. 23525541. 35, 101178. doi:10.1016/j.scp.2023.101178.

Martins, A.M., Silva, A.T., Marto, J.M., 2025. Advancing cosmetic sustainability: upcycling for a circular product life cycle. Sustainability. 2071-1050. 17 (13), 5738. doi:10.3390/su17135738.

Mayer, A.M.S., Glaser, K.B., Cuevas, C., Jacobs, R.S., Kem, W., Little, R.D., McIntosh, J.M., Newman, D.J., Potts, B.C., Shuster, D.E., 2010. The odyssey of marine pharmaceuticals: a current pipeline perspective. Trends Pharmacol. Sci. 01656147. 31 (6), 255–265. doi:10.1016/j.tips.2010.02.005.

Melgar, B., Pereira, E., Oliveira, M.B.P.P., Garcia-Castello, E.M., Rodriguez-Lopez, A.D., Sokovic, M., Barros, L., Ferreira, I.C.F.R., 2017. Extensive profiling of three varieties of *Opuntia* spp. fruit for innovative food ingredients. Food Res. Int. 18737145. 101, 259–265. Available from: https://www.elsevier.com/inca/publications/store/4/2/2/9/7/0. doi:10.1016/j.foodres.2017.09.024.

Minocha, S., Lal, N., Parveen, R., 2025. Biocosmetics: an era of natural friendly constituents in the cosmetic market. Curr. Cosmet. Sci. 26667797. 04. doi:10.2174/0126667797336316250212100308.

Mondello, A., Salomone, R., Mondello, G., 2024. Exploring circular economy in the cosmetic industry: insights from a literature review. Environ. Impact Assess. Rev. 01959255. 105. Available from: https://www.sciencedirect.com/science/journal/01959255. doi:10.1016/j.eiar.2024.107443.

Mordor Intelligence, 2026. Toiletries Market Size & Share Analysis - Growth Trends and Forecast (2025 - 2030). [Online]. Available from: https://www.mordorintelligence.com/industry-reports/global-toiletries-market?utm_source=chatgpt.com (Accessed 14 September 2025).

Negi, B., Kumar, D., Rawat, D.S., 2017. Marine peptides as anticancer agents: a remedy to mankind by nature. Curr. Protein Pept. Sci. 18755550. 18 (2). Available from: http://benthamscience.com/contents-JCode-CPPS-Vol-00000013-Iss-00000001.htm. doi:10.2174/1389203717666160724200849.

Nikoo, M., Regenstein, J.M., Ghomi, M.R., Benjakul, S., Yang, N., Xu, X., 2015. Study of the combined effects of a gelatin-derived cryoprotective peptide and a non-peptide antioxidant in a fish mince model system. LWT 00236438. 60 (1), 358–364. Available from: https://www.journals.elsevier.com/lwt. doi:10.1016/j.lwt.2014.07.051.

O'Higgins, B., Fatorachian, H., 2025. Consumer trust in artificial intelligence in the UK and Ireland's personal care and cosmetics sector. Cogent Bus. Manag. 23311975. 12 (1). Available from: https://cogentoa.tandfonline.com/journal/oabm20. doi:10.1080/23311975.2025.2469765.

Omira, A., Grira, S., Mourad, A.H.I., Alkhedher, M., 2025. The new generation of cosmetics packaging: a paradigm shift. Glob. Transit. 25897918. 7, 223–246. Available from: https://www.sciencedirect.com/science/journal/25897918. doi:10.1016/j.glt.2025.04.004.

Omkar, R., 2023. Bio-based cosmetics market. Kings Res. Accessed: Sept. 14, 2025. [Online]. Available from: https://www.kingsresearch.com/bio-based-cosmetics-market-377.

Öncül, N., Karabıyıklı, Ş., 2016. Survival of foodborne pathogens in unripe grape products. LWT 00236438. 74, 168–175. Available from: https://www.journals.elsevier.com/lwt. doi:10.1016/j.lwt.2016.07.043.

Pai, S., Binu, A., Lavanya, G.S., Harikumar, M., Herga, S.K., Citartan, M., Mani, N.K., 2025. Advancements of paper-based microfluidics and organ-on-a-chip models in cosmetics hazards. RSC Adv. 20462069. 15 (13), 10319–10335. Available from: http://pubs.rsc.org/en/journals/journal/ra. doi:10.1039/d4ra07336c.

Panwar, D., Saini, A., Panesar, P.S., Chopra, H.K., 2021. Unraveling the scientific perspectives of citrus by-products utilization: progress towards circular economy. Trends Food Sci. Technol. 09242244. 111, 549–562. Available from: http://www.elsevier.com/wps/find/journaldescription.cws_home/601278/description#description. doi:10.1016/j.tifs.2021.03.018.

Premkumar, J., Vasudevan, R.T., 2018. Bioingredients: functional properties and health impacts. Curr. Opin. Food Sci. 22147993. 19, 120–128. Available from: http://www.journals.elsevier.com/current-opinion-in-food-science/. doi:10.1016/j.cofs.2018.03.016.

Presendence Research, 2025. Perfume market growth drivers and competitive landscape, 4401. Accessed: Sept. 14, 2025. [Online]. Available from: https://www.precedenceresearch.com/perfume-market?utm_source=chatgpt.com.

Rischard, F., Gore, E., Flourat, A., Savary, G., 2025. The challenges faced by multifunctional ingredients: a critical review from sourcing to cosmetic applications. Adv. Colloid Interface Sci. 00018686. 340, 103463. doi:10.1016/j.cis.2025.103463.

Rocca, R., Acerbi, F., Fumagalli, L., Taisch, M., 2022. Sustainability paradigm in the cosmetics industry: state of the art. Cleaner Waste Syst. 27729125. 3, 100057. doi:10.1016/j.clwas.2022.100057.

Sadiq, M., Adil, M., Paul, J., 2021. An innovation resistance theory perspective on purchase of eco-friendly cosmetics. J. Retail. Consum. Serv. 09696989. 59, 102369. doi:10.1016/j.jretconser.2020.102369.

Senthilkumar, K., Vijayalakshmi, A., Jagadeesan, M., Somasundaram, A., Pitchiah, S., Alharbi, S.A., Ansari, M.J., Ramasamy, P., 2024. Preparation of self-preserving personal care cosmetic products using multifunctional ingredients and other cosmetic ingredients. Sci. Rep. 2045-2322. 14 (1). doi:10.1038/s41598-024-57782-9.

Shih, M.F., Cherng, J.Y., 2012. Protective effects of Chlorella-derived peptide against UVC-induced cytotoxicity through inhibition of caspase-3 activity and reduction of the expression of phosphorylated FADD and cleaved PARP-1 in skin fibroblasts. Molecules 14203049. 17 (8), 9116–9128. Available from: http://www.mdpi.com/1420-3049/17/8/9116/pdf. doi:10.3390/molecules17089116Taiwan.

Shimul, A.S., Cheah, I., Khan, B.B., 2022. Investigating female shoppers' attitude and purchase intention toward green cosmetics in south africa. J. Glob. Mark. 15286975. 35 (1), 37–56. Available from: http://www.tandfonline.com/toc/wglo20/current. doi:10.1080/08911762.2021.1934770.

Sianipar, R.N.R., Suryanegara, L., Fatriasari, W., Arung, E.T., Kusuma, I.W., Achmadi, S.S., Azelee, N.I.W., Hamid, Z.A.A., 2023. The role of selected flavonoids from bajakah tampala (*Spatholobus littoralis* Hassk.) stem on cosmetic properties: a review. Saudi Pharm. J. 13190164. 31 (3), 382–400. Available from: http://www.sciencedirect.com/science/journal/13190164. doi:10.1016/j.jsps.2023.01.006.

Siddiqui, M., Chakraborty, D., Siddiqui, A., 2023. Consumers buying behaviour towards agri-food products: a mixed-method approach. J. Retail. Consum. Serv. 09696989. 73, 103349. doi:10.1016/j.jretconser.2023.103349.

Srivastava, P., Ramakanth, D., Akhila, K., Gaikwad, K.K., 2022. Package design as a branding tool in the cosmetic industry: consumers' perception vs. reality. SN Bus. Econ. 26629399. 2 (6). Available from: https://link.springer.com/journal/43546. doi:10.1007/s43546-022-00222-5.

Statista Research Department, 2026. Cosmetics industry - statistics & facts. Available from: https://www.statista.com/topics/3137/cosmetics-industry/ (Accessed 14 September 2025).

Stoilova, I., Krastanov, A., Stoyanova, A., Denev, P., Gargova, S., 2007. Antioxidant activity of a ginger extract (*Zingiber officinale*). Food Chem. 03088146. 102 (3), 764–770. doi:10.1016/j.foodchem.2006.06.023.

Suphasomboon, T., Vassanadumrongdee, S., 2022. Toward sustainable consumption of green cosmetics and personal care products: the role of perceived value and ethical concern. Sustain. Prod. Consum. 23525509. 33, 230–243. Available from: http://www.journals.elsevier.com/sustainable-production-and-consumption/. doi:10.1016/j.spc.2022.07.004.

Tajkarimi, M.M., Ibrahim, S.A., Cliver, D.O., 2010. Antimicrobial herb and spice compounds in food. Food Control. 09567135. 21 (9), 1199–1218. doi:10.1016/j.foodcont.2010.02.003.

Teerasumran, P., Velliou, E., Bai, S., Cai, Q., 2023. Deodorants and antiperspirants: new trends in their active agents and testing methods. Int. J. Cosmet. Sci. 14682494. 45 (4), 426–443. Available from: http://onlinelibrary.wiley.com/journal/10.1111/(ISSN)1468-2494. doi:10.1111/ics.12852.

Ustymenko, R., 2023. Trends and innovations in cosmetic marketing. Econ. Educ. 2592-8236. 8 (3), 12–17. doi:10.30525/2500-946x/2023-3-2.

van Dijk, J., Figuière, R., Dekker, S.C., van Wezel, A.P., Cousins, I.T., 2023. Managing PMT/vPvM substances in consumer products through the concepts of essential-use and functional substitution: a case-study for cosmetics. Environ. Sci. Process. Impacts 20507895. 25 (6), 1067–1081. Available from: http://pubs.rsc.org/en/journals/journal/em. doi:10.1039/d3em00025g.

Woodby, B., Penta, K., Pecorelli, A., Lila, M.A., Valacchi, G., 2020. Skin health from the inside out. Annu. Rev. Food Sci. Technol. 19411421. 11, 235–254. Available from: http://www.annualreviews.org/journal/food. doi:10.1146/annurev-food-032519-051722.

Xin, H., Virk, A.S., Virk, S.S., Akin-Ige, F., Amin, S., 2024. Applications of artificial intelligence and machine learning on critical materials used in cosmetics and personal care formulation design. Curr. Opin. Colloid Interface Sci. 18790399. 73. Available from: https://www.sciencedirect.com/science/journal/13590294. doi:10.1016/j.cocis.2024.101847.

Yang, Y., Li, B., Wang, M., Pan, S., Wang, Y., Gu, J., 2023. Effect of natural polymer materials on skin healing based on internal wound microenvironment: a review. Front. Chem. 22962646. 11. Available from: http://journal.frontiersin.org/journal/chemistry. doi:10.3389/fchem.2023.1257915.

Zollo, L., Carranza, R., Faraoni, M., Díaz, E., Martín-Consuegra, D., 2021. What influences consumers' intention to purchase organic personal care products? The role of social reassurance. J. Retail. Consum. Serv. 09696989. 60, 102432. doi:10.1016/j.jretconser.2020.102432.

Chapter 4

Exploring safety issues

Michail Chalaris, Sotirria Anastasiou, and Nikolaos Stasinopoulos
Hephaestus Laboratory, School of Chemistry, Faculty of Sciences, Democritus University of Thrace, Kavala University Campus, Kavala, Greece

Learning objectives

After completing this chapter, the reader should be able to:

1. Understand the global regulatory frameworks governing cosmetic safety, including European Union Regulation (EC) No. 1223/2009, Modernization of Cosmetics Regulation Act, and Cosmetic Supervision and Administration Regulation.
2. Identify major classes of cosmetic ingredients and their toxicological concerns.
3. Apply core risk assessment principles, including exposure evaluation and the margin-of-safety approach.
4. Recognize the role of new approach methodologies and next-generation risk assessment in modern safety evaluation.
5. Discuss emerging challenges such as microplastics, endocrine disruptors, and fragrance allergens, and the importance of cosmetovigilance.

1 Introduction

Cosmetics have long served purposes beyond beautification, carrying religious, social, and symbolic significance (Schaffer, 2006; Adkins and Adkins, 1998). Early records show that Ancient Sumerians (c. 5000 BC) ground semiprecious stones into powders for facial use (Schaffer, 2006). Ancient Egypt advanced cosmetic use and production, embedding it into daily life and ritual, though some pigments proved toxic, such as iodine- and bromine-based mixtures dubbed "the kiss of death" (Riesmeier et al., 2022). Ancient Greece emphasized grooming and ceremonial applications, establishing early workshops (myreseia) for systematic production (Adkins and Adkins, 1998).

The Industrial Revolution transformed cosmetics into mass-produced consumer goods through mechanization, chemical advances, and packaging innovations (Jones, 2008). By the 20th century, global corporations and media helped make cosmetics daily essentials, while scientific, ethical, and environmental concerns reshaped the sector. Consumer demand for natural and eco-conscious products surged, alongside innovations in nanotechnology, biotechnology, and skin microbiome research, which introduced both opportunities and new safety challenges (Atallah et al., 2025). Regulatory frameworks tightened in response to risks posed by parabens, phthalates, and formaldehyde-releasing agents (Kaushik et al., 2023; Environmental Working Group (EWG), 2023).

Today, the industry is shaped by advanced research, digital diagnostics, and personalized skincare technologies such as artificial intelligence (AI) and wearable sensors (Alnuqaydan, 2024). Yet, the core concerns remain safety, efficacy, and trust. Modern laboratories handle surfactants, solvents, preservatives, fragrances, colorants, and ultraviolet (UV) filters daily, exposing workers to physical, chemical, and biological hazards that require strict occupational safety protocols (Panico et al., 2019). Proactive toxicological assessments are essential, from formulation to production and postmarket surveillance.

The shift away from animal testing has accelerated the use of *in vitro* methods, quantitative structure–activity relationship (QSAR), and in silico tools (Barthe et al., 2021; Tcheremenskaia et al., 2019; SCCS—Scientific Committee on Consumer Safety, 2009). Laboratories must embed these approaches into routine operations to protect both workers and end users. Because interns and students often lack training, comprehensive onboarding, regular refreshers, and accessible emergency procedures are critical.

Chemical hazards in laboratories include volatile organic compounds (VOCs), allergens, reactive agents, and nanomaterials, posing risks via dermal, inhalation, and ocular routes (Lv et al., 2015). Control measures rely on structured risk assessments, Good Laboratory Practice (GLP) adherence, and up-to-date Safety Data Sheets (SDSs). Within the European Union (EU), Registration, Evaluation, Authorization and Restriction of Chemicals (REACH), Classification, Labeling and

Biofunctional Cosmetics for Health. https://doi.org/10.1016/B978-0-443-27500-5.00005-8

Packaging (CLP), and Cosmetics Regulation (EC No. 1223/2009) form the legal foundation for chemical safety, supported globally by standards like ISO 22716 (EC Regulation No. 1223/2009).

Despite their ubiquity, cosmetics have complex formulations with varying concentrations, application methods, and exposure durations, all influencing toxicological outcomes (Barthe et al., 2021; SCCS—Scientific Committee on Consumer Safety, 2021). Novel ingredients, especially natural compounds, are often introduced without complete toxicological validation, increasing the need for advanced risk assessment (OECD, 2023a). Public health concerns, such as allergic reactions, endocrine disruption, and carcinogenicity, have already driven regulatory reforms, including mandatory premarket safety assessments and cosmetovigilance requirements in the EU (EC Regulation 1223/2009).

Good Manufacturing Practices (GMPs) complement occupational health and safety by addressing hygiene, sanitation, quality control (QC), and recalls. Each production stage—from chemical handling to packaging—carries risks, including chemical exposure, ergonomic strain, and psychosocial stress, all mitigated by a strong safety infrastructure.

Ultimately, toxicology underpins both product innovation and worker protection. As cosmetics evolve, science-based risk assessment, regulatory compliance, and a culture of safety remain central to sustainable and ethical industry growth.

2 Regulatory framework

The regulatory framework for laboratory safety and toxicology in the cosmetics industry is built upon a robust structure of European legislation and international standards, aiming to protect both consumers and workers. At the core of this framework are three key EU regulations: REACH (EC 1907/2006), CLP (EC 1272/2008), and the EU Cosmetics Regulation (EC 1223/2009) (European Parliament and Council, 2009; ECHA (European Chemicals Agency), 2024a). These collectively govern the registration, classification, labeling, and safe use of chemicals across the EU. In the context of cosmetic laboratories, they provide clear guidance on raw material selection, chemical handling and disposal, and the responsibilities of manufacturers and researchers.

REACH obliges companies producing or importing substances over one ton per year to identify and manage associated risks. Detailed toxicological and ecotoxicological data must be submitted to enable proper hazard evaluation (ECHA (European Chemicals Agency), 2024a). Cosmetic laboratories must therefore ensure that only substances with validated safety profiles are used and that supporting documentation is up to date.

CLP, which complements REACH, mandates the classification and labeling of substances and mixtures based on health and physical hazards. Through standardized pictograms, hazard statements, and precautionary language, it enables laboratory personnel to recognize and respond to risks effectively (ECHA (European Chemicals Agency), 2024a).

The EU Cosmetics Regulation (EC 1223/2009) governs cosmetic product safety, explicitly banning animal testing for both ingredients and final products. This has spurred the development and regulatory acceptance of validated alternatives, such as *in vitro* assays and QSAR models. Toxicological evaluations conducted in cosmetic laboratories must integrate these alternative approaches and support the development of the Cosmetic Product Safety Report (CPSR), a mandatory component of the product information file (European Parliament and Council, 2009).

SDSs are another cornerstone of chemical safety, required under both REACH and CLP. These documents provide vital information on substance properties, handling, storage, personal protective equipment (PPE), and emergency procedures. Given that cosmetic products may contain dozens of ingredients, effective SDS management—often via digital systems—is essential for ensuring compliance and safety (ECHA (European Chemicals Agency), 2024a). In addition to EU regulations, member states apply national occupational health and safety laws.

SDS: A standardized document that provides detailed information about a chemical's properties, hazards, safe handling, storage, protective equipment, and emergency measures.

Cosmetic laboratories must also comply with GLP and GMP standards. ISO 22716 outlines GMP guidelines specific to cosmetics, covering raw material handling, personnel hygiene, documentation, and traceability. GLP ensures the reliability of nonclinical safety studies, reinforcing data integrity and regulatory acceptance (ISO, 22716:2007).

The definition of a cosmetic product, according to Regulation (EC) No. 1223/2009, includes any substance or mixture intended for external use on the body (e.g., skin, hair, nails, lips, or external genital organs) or the oral cavity, for the purpose of cleansing, perfuming, changing appearance, protecting, or correcting body odors. This external-use criterion distinguishes cosmetics from pharmaceuticals, which are more stringently regulated (European Parliament and Council, 2009).

In contrast, the US Food and Drug Administration (FDA) defines cosmetics more broadly, including any article applied to the human body for beautifying or altering appearance, even allowing dual-function products (e.g., antiacne creams) depending on labeling claims (U.S. Food and Drug Administration, 1938/2011).

Asian regulations often align closely with the EU model. Notably, China lifted its mandatory animal testing requirement for general cosmetics in 2021, provided specific criteria—such as GMP certification—are met. Nonetheless, animal testing remains mandatory for certain product categories or special claims.

2.1 Importance of regulation in cosmetics

In an industry as dynamic and globally integrated as cosmetics, regulation serves as both a safeguard and a driver of innovation. The application of regulatory controls is essential to maintaining public health, ensuring the integrity of products, promoting environmental responsibility, and preserving consumer trust through transparent marketing. Regulatory frameworks exist at national, regional, and international levels to ensure that cosmetic products placed on the market meet rigorous standards of safety, quality, and ethical responsibility. The following sections delve into the multidimensional role of regulation in shaping the modern cosmetics industry.

2.1.1 Protection of human health

The foremost priority of cosmetic regulation is the protection of human health. Consumers routinely apply cosmetic products to sensitive and permeable parts of the body, such as the face, lips, and eyes. Given the frequency and duration of exposure, the potential for adverse effects—including allergic reactions, dermal toxicity, microbial contamination, endocrine disruption, and even systemic toxicity—necessitates a comprehensive risk management framework (Alnuqaydan, 2024; Kalofiri et al., 2023; Altıokka, 2022).

Regulations such as Regulation (EC) No. 1223/2009 in the EU impose strict requirements for ingredient safety, including the prohibition or restriction of substances known to cause harm. For example, Annex II of this Regulation contains a list of over 1300 substances that are explicitly banned from use in cosmetic products due to their toxic, carcinogenic, mutagenic, or sensitizing properties (Foley, 2019). The Regulation also mandates the submission of a CPSR for each product, comprising toxicological profiles, exposure scenarios, and margin-of-safety (MoS) calculations for all ingredients (Cosmedesk, 2024a).

Moreover, regulations require companies to monitor postmarket safety through mechanisms such as cosmetovigilance, where adverse reactions reported by consumers or healthcare professionals are investigated and addressed (Altıokka, 2022). This lifecycle approach—from premarket safety assessment to postmarket surveillance—ensures that the health of consumers remains the central concern at every stage of cosmetic development and commercialization.

2.1.2 Assurance of product quality

Quality assurance (QA) is a foundational principle of cosmetic regulation, closely linked to both consumer satisfaction and product safety. A product's efficacy, shelf-life, and safety can be compromised by microbial contamination, instability of formulations, or inconsistent manufacturing practices (Detmer, 2010; Lyapina et al., 2023). Regulations address these risks by requiring adherence to GMPs, standardized procedures that encompass all aspects of production, from raw material sourcing and handling to packaging, labeling, and storage.

In the EU, ISO 22716:2007 provides detailed guidance on GMP specific to cosmetic products. This standard ensures that each batch of product is manufactured under controlled conditions, with appropriate QC checks and traceability systems in place (International Organization for Standardization (ISO), 2007). Hygiene protocols, personnel training, equipment maintenance, and contamination control are critical aspects of these requirements.

In addition, QA extends to the physical and chemical properties of the product itself. Parameters such as pH stability, viscosity, and emulsion integrity must be tested to confirm that the product remains effective and safe throughout its intended shelf life. Regulatory authorities may also require validation of claims such as "hypoallergenic," "dermatologically tested," or "noncomedogenic" through scientific evidence. In this way, regulation ensures that cosmetic products not only meet consumer expectations but also maintain consistency, reproducibility, and integrity across production cycles.

2.1.3 Environmental protection

In recent years, the cosmetics industry has faced increasing scrutiny over its environmental footprint. From unsustainable sourcing of raw materials to the ecological impact of synthetic compounds and packaging waste, the environmental implications of cosmetics are now a major concern for regulators, companies, and consumers alike (Ecovia, 2024; Martins and Marto, 2023).

Regulations have begun to address these concerns by placing restrictions on ingredients that pose ecological risks, such as microplastics, persistent organic pollutants, and nonbiodegradable UV filters. For example, the EU has moved to ban or phase out certain microbeads in rinse-off products due to their accumulation in aquatic ecosystems (ECHA (European Chemicals Agency), 2023b).

Furthermore, regulatory frameworks increasingly encourage or require life-cycle assessments and eco-label certifications to evaluate the environmental sustainability of products. Regulatory affairs professionals play a critical role in ensuring that companies adhere to these emerging standards and that environmental claims—such as "biodegradable," "eco-friendly," or "carbon neutral"—are substantiated by verifiable data. This helps prevent greenwashing, a deceptive marketing practice where companies misrepresent the environmental benefits of their products (European Commission, 2023; Evans, 2024). Beyond ingredient safety, packaging regulations are evolving to address issues such as recyclability, plastic reduction, and the use of renewable materials. The alignment of environmental goals with regulatory policy is expected to expand further in the coming years, driven by both policy shifts and consumer demand for sustainable practices.

Greenwashing: A misleading marketing practice in which a company exaggerates or falsely claims the environmental benefits of its products or practices.

2.1.4 Accurate labeling and marketing

Product labeling is the primary interface between a cosmetic company and its consumers, serving not only as a source of information but also as a tool of accountability. Regulatory requirements ensure that labels provide accurate, clear, and accessible information that allows consumers to make informed choices about the products they use.

Under frameworks such as EU Regulation No. 1223/2009, cosmetic labels must include:

- The name and function of the product
- The name and address of the responsible person (RP)
- Nominal content
- Expiry date or Period After Opening (PAO) symbol
- Usage instructions and safety warnings
- Batch number
- A full list of ingredients, using the International Nomenclature of Cosmetic Ingredients (INCI)
- Text presented in the official language(s) of the country of sale (CIRS Group, 2024)

In the United States, labeling is governed by the Fair Packaging and Labeling Act (FP&L Act) and the Federal Food, Drug, and Cosmetic Act (FD&C Act). These require not only accurate ingredient disclosure but also prohibit false or misleading statements. Claims related to performance, safety, and even sensory attributes must be backed by reliable scientific data to avoid legal consequences under "misbranding" regulations (Beauty Labelling Guide, 2022).

With the rise of digital marketing and global e-commerce, regulators are also expanding their oversight of online claims. This includes product websites, social media campaigns, and influencer endorsements. Regulatory affairs teams are now tasked with monitoring all advertising and promotional content to ensure compliance with both domestic and international laws (Federal Trade Commission (FTC), 2025).

Ultimately, truthful labeling and marketing protect consumers from misinformation, reduce the risk of adverse reactions (e.g., due to allergens), and foster trust in brands. They also enable traceability in case of product recalls or regulatory investigations.

2.2 Key regulatory bodies and frameworks

The global nature of the cosmetics industry necessitates a diverse yet harmonized regulatory landscape. While each country or region has its own legal and institutional framework for ensuring cosmetic safety, there are significant overlaps in their core principles: consumer protection, ingredient transparency, QA, and ethical production practices (Martins and Marto, 2023). This section outlines the major regulatory bodies and legal instruments that govern cosmetic products in key jurisdictions and at the international level.

2.2.1 EU: Regulation (EC) No. 1223/2009

The EU has established one of the most comprehensive and progressive regulatory frameworks for cosmetic products globally. Regulation (EC) No. 1223/2009, which came into full effect in July 2013, replaced the earlier Cosmetics Directive (76/768/EEC) and consolidated cosmetic regulation under a directly applicable regulation across all EU Member States (European Parliament and Council, 2009).

This Regulation introduces several pivotal requirements:

- Mandatory GMP: Manufacturers must adhere to GMP protocols to ensure product quality and hygiene (International Organization for Standardization (ISO), 2007; GOV.UK, 2023).

- Ban on Animal Testing: The EU is the first and only major jurisdiction to impose a full ban on animal testing for both cosmetic products and their individual ingredients, setting a global precedent for cruelty-free practices.
- CPSR: Every product placed on the EU market must be supported by a comprehensive CPSR that evaluates ingredient safety, toxicological profiles, exposure levels, and MoS (EC Regulation 1223, 2009).
- RP: A designated individual or legal entity within the EU is legally responsible for the compliance of the cosmetic product (EcoSistant, 2024).

Crucially, the Regulation is grounded in the precautionary principle, which emphasizes preventive action in the face of potential risk. This framework reflects a commitment not only to consumer safety but also to ethical standards and environmental responsibility.

Precautionary principle: Preventive measures are taken to protect health or the environment, even if full scientific certainty about the risks is lacking.

2.2.2 United States: FDA and Modernization of Cosmetics Regulation Act

In the United States, the regulation of cosmetics is governed primarily by the FDA under the authority of the Federal FD&C Act. For decades, the FDA's oversight of cosmetics was relatively limited compared to pharmaceuticals or medical devices (Brooks and Tassonyi, 2023). However, this changed significantly with the passage of the Modernization of Cosmetics Regulation Act (MoCRA) in 2022 (Axios, 2024).

Key provisions under MoCRA include:

- Mandatory Facility and Product Registration: Cosmetic manufacturing and packaging facilities must now register with the FDA, and all marketed products must be listed in the agency's electronic system (U.S. Food and Drug Administration, 2025).
- Adverse Event Reporting: Companies are required to report serious adverse events related to cosmetic use within specified timelines (U.S. Food and Drug Administration, 2025).
- GMP Compliance: The FDA will establish standardized GMP requirements, bringing US practices more in line with international norms (Burdock, 2024).
- Fragrance Allergen Disclosure: MoCRA introduces a requirement to disclose allergens from fragrance components, an area previously exempt from detailed labeling (U.S. Food and Drug Administration, 2024).

Unlike the EU, the United States still allows certain dual-purpose products to be classified as both cosmetics and drugs, depending on their intended use and claims (e.g., antidandruff shampoo, sunscreen). Premarket approval is not required for most cosmetics, except for color additives, but MoCRA represents a significant shift toward stronger postmarket surveillance and consumer protection (Brooks and Tassonyi, 2023).

2.2.3 China: Cosmetic Supervision and Administration Regulation

China, one of the world's largest and fastest-growing cosmetics markets, restructured its regulatory approach with the implementation of the Cosmetic Supervision and Administration Regulation (CSAR) in 2021 (Chemlinked, 2025). CSAR replaced outdated frameworks and introduced a clearer, tiered structure differentiating between general and special cosmetics. Special cosmetics include products such as hair dyes, sunscreens, and cosmetics with functional claims, which require more rigorous evaluation and registration (Su et al., 2020).

Functional claims: Product claims suggesting a physiological or corrective effect, such as whitening or antihair loss.

Notable features of CSAR include:

- Partial Ban on Animal Testing: As of May 1, 2021, China no longer mandates animal testing for general cosmetics imported into the country, provided they meet specific conditions (e.g., GMP certification and safety assessment documentation) (Chemlinked, 2021a; Intertek, 2021).
- Digital Registration Systems: A streamlined online platform for submitting product dossiers enhances transparency and regulatory efficiency (Su et al., 2020).
- Ingredient and Efficacy Disclosure: Enhanced scrutiny on functional claims and the scientific evidence backing them (EU SME Centre, 2021).

CSAR reflects China's broader effort to harmonize its regulatory landscape with global standards, while still retaining stricter controls over high-risk or functional products (Chemlinked, 2025).

2.2.4 International regulatory frameworks

Several international organizations play a crucial role in fostering global consistency in cosmetic regulation. These frameworks are not legally binding but serve as benchmarks and references for national authorities and multinational companies.

- **ISO 22716:2007—Cosmetics—GMPs:** This standard provides comprehensive guidelines for the production, control, storage, and shipment of cosmetic products. It is widely adopted by cosmetic manufacturers and forms the basis of GMP compliance in many jurisdictions (International Organization for Standardization (ISO), 2007).
- **International Cooperation on Cosmetics Regulation (ICCR):** A voluntary group of regulatory authorities from major economies—including the United States, EU, Canada, Brazil, Japan, South Korea, Israel, and China—ICCR promotes the alignment of safety standards, the avoidance of animal testing, and the mutual recognition of assessments.
- **International Fragrance Association (IFRA):** IFRA issues standards that regulate the use of fragrance ingredients to ensure consumer safety. Compliance with IFRA standards is considered essential for companies involved in fragrance formulation (International Fragrance Association (IFRA), 2023).
- **World Health Organization (WHO):** While not directly involved in regulation, the WHO provides scientific guidance on chemical safety, toxicological risk, and public health aspects of cosmetic ingredients (World Health Organization, 2023a).

Together, these bodies contribute to the harmonization of cosmetic safety standards and foster international cooperation on emerging issues such as nanomaterials, allergenic compounds, and environmental impact.

2.3 Labeling regulations

Labeling regulations are fundamental to ensuring transparency, product traceability, and consumer protection in the cosmetics sector. Labels serve as the primary communication tool between manufacturers and end-users, offering essential information for safe and informed product use (Lionetti and Rigano, 2018).

2.3.1 EU labeling requirements: Regulation (EC) No. 1223/2009

According to Article 19 of Regulation (EC) No. 1223/2009, cosmetic product labels must include a specific set of mandatory information to be legally sold in the EU:

- Product name and intended function
- Name and address of the RP
- Nominal content at the time of packaging
- Expiry date or the PAO), denoted by the jar symbol and the number of months or years
- Batch number or reference for traceability (European Parliament and Council, 2009)
- Usage instructions and safety precautions, particularly for professional-use products or those listed in Annexes III and VI (CEPRASRL, 2024)
- Full ingredient list in descending order by weight, using INCI nomenclature
- Language compliance: All information must be provided in the official language(s) of the country where the product is marketed.

These requirements are designed to ensure safety, facilitate product recalls if necessary, and support informed consumer choices (Lionetti and Rigano, 2018).

2.3.2 US labeling requirements: FDA (FD&C Act and FP&L Act)

In the United States, cosmetic labeling is governed by both the Federal FD&C Act and the FP&L Act. These statutes require that all label information be truthful, not misleading, and clearly visible to the average consumer (U.S. Food and Drug Administration, 2022c; Federal Trade Commission (FTC), 2023).

Mandatory labeling elements include:

- Net quantity of contents, expressed in US customary units (Federal Trade Commission (FTC), 2023)
- List of ingredients, ordered by predominance of weight (ECFR (Electronic Code of Federal Regulations), 2022)
- Warnings or cautionary statements, as required by regulation (e.g., 21 CFR 740 for products with specific safety concerns) (U.S. Food and Drug Administration, 2022c)
- Manufacturer's or distributor's name and address (U.S. Food and Drug Administration, 2022c) Failure to comply with these requirements constitutes misbranding, which is a violation of federal law and may result in enforcement actions, including product recalls or fines (U.S. Food and Drug Administration, 2022c; ECFR (Electronic Code of Federal Regulations), 2022).

In both jurisdictions, accurate labeling not only ensures consumer safety but also plays a key role in preventing allergic reactions, enabling responsible use, and ensuring regulatory compliance during inspections and audits.

2.4 Regulatory portals

In the context of modern regulatory compliance, digital notification and registration platforms serve as essential tools for enforcing cosmetic legislation. These portals facilitate the secure submission of regulatory data, enhance transparency, and streamline communication between cosmetic companies and regulatory authorities. They also contribute to public health by supporting traceability, surveillance, and emergency response systems, such as poison control centers. Each major cosmetics market has developed its own digital infrastructure to accommodate the regulatory needs of manufacturers, importers, and distributors.

2.4.1 *EU: Cosmetic Product Notification Portal*

The Cosmetic Product Notification Portal (CPNP) is a centralized, EU-wide online system created under Regulation (EC) No. 1223/2009 to simplify compliance with product notification requirements (Cosmedesk, 2024a). This free digital platform allows companies to submit essential information about cosmetic products, including formulations, packaging, RPs, and toxicological data, before the product is placed on the EU market.

Key features of the CPNP include:

- Single notification: Once a cosmetic product is registered via CPNP, no additional national registrations are needed in individual EU member states (European Commission, n.d.a; Health Products Regulatory Authority (HPRA), 2024).
- Realtime accessibility: Competent authorities across the EU can instantly access submitted data for market surveillance and regulatory oversight (Cosmedesk, 2024a).
- Poison center support: Poison control centers use CPNP data to provide timely and accurate treatment advice in cases of accidental exposure or misuse.
- Compliance monitoring: National authorities can analyze submissions for compliance with labeling, safety, and ingredient restrictions (CMA ComplianceGate, 2024).

By eliminating redundant paperwork and providing a unified platform, CPNP enhances regulatory efficiency and supports the EU's objectives of safety, harmonization, and transparency.

2.4.2 *United States: FDA electronic systems*

While the US FDA does not operate a dedicated cosmetics portal equivalent to the CPNP, it has developed integrated digital systems for oversight as part of its broader regulatory infrastructure. With the enactment of the MoCRA, electronic registration of cosmetic facilities and products became mandatory (Crowell, 2023; U.S. Food and Drug Administration, 2025).

FDA's digital systems support:

- Facility Registration and Product Listing: Required for all domestic and foreign manufacturers, these registrations help the FDA monitor compliance and identify the sources of adverse events.
- Adverse Event Reporting: MoCRA mandates the electronic submission of serious adverse events through FDA portals, helping the agency track product-related health risks in real time.
- Recall Coordination: FDA's electronic systems support the management of voluntary or mandatory product recalls to minimize consumer harm (Brooks and Tassonyi, 2023; U.S. Food and Drug Administration, 2025).

Although less centralized than the EU's CPNP, the FDA's evolving digital ecosystem reflects a significant shift toward transparency, risk mitigation, and realtime regulatory interaction (Crowell, 2023).

2.4.3 *China: National Medical Products Administration Registration Systems*

China's National Medical Products Administration (NMPA) administers regulatory oversight of cosmetics through a set of digital registration and filing platforms, aligned with the CSAR. These systems are particularly robust, given China's large and complex cosmetics market (Chemlinked, 2021a; National Medical Products Administration (NMPA), 2022).

Key functions of the NMPA portals include:

- Premarket registration for special-use cosmetics, such as sunscreens, hair dyes, and whitening products.
- Postmarket surveillance through mandatory safety reporting and inspection mechanisms

- Ingredient transparency by requiring detailed information about raw materials, including their origin, concentration, and function.
- Digital Dossier management, streamlining the review of efficacy claims and safety documentation (Chemlinked, 2024; Zhu, 2023).

These platforms are critical for companies seeking to enter the Chinese market, and they form an integral part of China's strategy to align with global best practices in cosmetic regulation (Chemlinked, 2024).

2.5 Challenges in the regulation of "natural" cosmetics

The increasing consumer demand for natural, organic, and eco-friendly cosmetics has outpaced the development of corresponding regulatory frameworks. Despite growing market share, "natural" cosmetics remain poorly defined and inconsistently regulated, resulting in a host of safety, ethical, and commercial concerns. Both the EU and the United States lack dedicated regulatory categories or legally binding definitions for what constitutes a "natural" cosmetic product (U.S. Food and Drug Administration, 2022c; CTPA (Cosmetic, Toiletry and Perfumery Association), 2023).

Key challenges include:

Health risks: There is a widespread misconception that natural equals safe. However, scientific research has shown that many so-called natural products contain toxic compounds, including allergens, sensitizers, or substances that may interact with other chemicals in the formulation. A review found that naturally derived ingredients may carry microbial contaminants, phenolics, heavy metals, and allergenic compounds, underscoring the need for rigorous safety evaluations (Manful et al., 2024).

Heavy metals such as lead, arsenic, or mercury can occur in natural raw materials and may accumulate to toxic levels if not controlled.

Marketing misuse and greenwashing: The unregulated use of vague or misleading claims, such as "100% natural" or "eco-certified," enables companies to engage in greenwashing, a practice that falsely suggests environmental or health benefits. Such marketing misleads consumers and erodes trust in genuinely safe and sustainable products. Regulatory bodies often lack the mechanisms to verify such claims unless specific standards or certifications are invoked (Environmental Working Group (EWG), 2017).

Ecocertified typically refers to products verified by third-party environmental certification schemes, though criteria vary widely between programs.

Regulatory gaps: In the United States, the absence of federal-level guidelines for natural cosmetics has led to a patchwork of state-level laws, causing inconsistency and legal confusion. This lack of uniformity not only complicates compliance for manufacturers but also exposes consumers to potentially unsafe or mislabeled products, increasing the risk of litigation and enforcement actions (NatLaw Review, 2019).

Validated analytical methods are standardized laboratory procedures tested to reliably detect and measure substances in cosmetic formulations.

Lack of scientific validation: Many natural ingredients, while traditional, have limited clinical or toxicological data supporting their safety and efficacy. This lack of research leaves consumers vulnerable to adverse reactions, especially when formulations are based on untested ingredient combinations. Furthermore, the absence of validated analytical methods for identifying and quantifying natural constituents complicates product standardization (Manful et al., 2024; Klaschka, 2015).

To ensure public health and commercial integrity, it is essential that regulatory agencies develop a consistent definition for "natural" cosmetics, alongside science-based safety assessment protocols and labeling standards.

3 Chemical substances in the cosmetics industry

The cosmetics industry has experienced substantial growth in recent decades, driven by advances in formulation science, biotechnology, and consumer demand for multifunctional, high-performance products. This growth has brought with it an increased reliance on a wide range of chemical substances, both natural and synthetic. Each chemical ingredient included in a cosmetic formulation must meet strict safety criteria: it must be nontoxic, nonirritating, effective, and stable under specified conditions. Moreover, the functionality of these substances—whether as preservatives, pigments, emollients, or active agents—is closely tied to their chemical structure and physicochemical properties. Understanding the chemical composition of cosmetics is essential not only for regulatory compliance and product innovation but also for the protection of consumers and professionals working in laboratories or manufacturing environments (SpecialChem, 2025; U.S. Food and Drug Administration, 2022c).

3.1 Preservatives

Cosmetic products often contain a high percentage of water or water-based ingredients, which create a favorable environment for microbial growth. Without proper preservation, these products can become breeding grounds for bacteria, yeasts, and molds, potentially compromising product stability and posing health risks to users. The inclusion of preservatives in cosmetic formulations is, therefore, a fundamental aspect of product safety (SpecialChem, 2025; Pinto et al., 2021). Preservatives inhibit microbial growth, extending the shelf life of cosmetics and maintaining their safety and efficacy throughout the product's intended use. Commonly used preservatives include both traditional and multifunctional ingredients such as sodium benzoate, benzyl alcohol, phenoxyethanol, ethylhexylglycerin, and caprylyl glycol. In addition, newer options like gluconolactone, tropolone, and sodium levulinate are favored in "clean" or "green" cosmetic formulations for their milder profiles and broader acceptance in natural product lines (SpecialChem, 2025). While preservatives are indispensable, their use is subject to strict regulation. Each must be evaluated for safety, permissible concentration, and potential allergenicity, especially when used in leaveon products or around sensitive areas like the eyes and lips.

3.2 Pigments

Pigments are vital to the sensory and esthetic appeal of many cosmetic products, particularly in color cosmetics such as lipsticks, foundations, blushes, and eyeshadows, as well as in hair dyes and skin tints. They provide the visual identity of the product and help create a wide range of shades and effects. Pigments can be derived from natural sources, such as iron oxides, anthocyanins, or mica, or they may be synthetically produced, including aniline dyes and lipophilic colorants. Synthetic pigments are often preferred in modern formulations due to their higher color intensity, greater photostability, cost efficiency, and better resistance to external conditions such as light, pH variations, and heat (NYSCC, 2023). However, the use of pigments also raises important safety and regulatory issues. Some synthetic colorants have been linked to allergic reactions or systemic toxicity if used improperly. As a result, most countries require that pigments be specifically approved for cosmetic use and must meet purity criteria set by regulatory authorities such as the European Commission (Annex IV, Regulation EC No. 1223/2009) or the US FDA (21 CFR parts 70 and 74).

3.3 Fragrances

Fragrances are among the most complex and variable components in cosmetic products. They can be either synthetic compounds or derived from natural essential oils, such as those from lavender, citrus, rose, and other botanicals. A single fragrance compound may consist of hundreds of individual molecules, each with different volatility, solubility, and interaction profiles. One major concern associated with fragrances is their potential to cause sensitization or allergic reactions, particularly when components oxidize in the air or interact with skin enzymes. Some molecules become allergens only after undergoing metabolic transformation on the skin. Consequently, many regulations require the labeling of known fragrance allergens when they exceed specific thresholds (e.g., 0.001% in leaveon products under EU Regulation 1223/2009). As fragrance compositions are often considered proprietary, striking a balance between trade secrecy and consumer transparency remains a persistent challenge in regulatory policy.

3.4 Emollients, humectants, and surfactants

Emollients are substances that soften, condition, and moisturize the skin and hair. By forming an occlusive layer on the skin, they help reduce transepidermal water loss, thereby improving skin hydration and smoothness (Franco-Gil et al., 2024). Emollients can be derived from natural sources—such as shea butter, jojoba oil, and coconut oil—or may be synthetically produced, such as dimethicone or glyceryl stearate. Hydrocarbon-based emollients, like mineral oil and petrolatum, are also widely used for their barrier-forming properties (Barnes et al., 2021). Closely related are humectants, which draw moisture from the atmosphere into the skin. Examples include glycerin, sorbitol, and hyaluronic acid, ingredients that are widely used in moisturizers and antiaging products for their hydrating and plumping effects (Mawazi et al., 2022). Surfactants are another essential group of functional ingredients, particularly in cleansing products. They reduce the surface tension between water and oils or dirt, allowing them to be rinsed away. Surfactants are categorized by their charge:

- Anionic surfactants (e.g., sodium lauryl sulfate): Excellent cleansers, used in shampoos and facial cleansers.
- Cationic surfactants (e.g., cetrimonium chloride): Common in hair conditioners for their antistatic properties.

- Nonionic surfactants (e.g., polysorbate 20): Mild and compatible with sensitive skin, often used in baby care products.
- Amphoteric surfactants (e.g., cocamidopropyl betaine): Mild surfactants suitable for products designed for sensitive skin or mucous membranes (AOCS, 2024; Verywell Health, 2025).

3.5 Antioxidants

Antioxidants play a crucial role in both the stability of the product and the protection of the skin. They neutralize free radicals, which are unstable molecules generated by UV exposure, pollution, and natural metabolic processes, and which contribute to oxidative stress and skin aging (Vinardell and Mitjans, 2017). Common antioxidants include:

- Vitamin C (ascorbic acid): Water-soluble; promotes collagen synthesis and reduces pigmentation.
- Vitamin E (tocopherol): Fat-soluble; stabilizes cell membranes and helps maintain skin barrier function (Subroto et al., 2023).
- Vitamin A derivatives (retinoids): Regulate keratinization and improve skin cell turnover (Franco-Gil et al., 2024).

Innovations in delivery systems, such as solid lipid nanoparticles, have enhanced the stability and bioavailability of antioxidants in cosmetic formulations (Oehlke et al., 2017; Subroto et al., 2023). Clinical studies indicate that products containing vitamin C and botanical extracts improve hydration and skin radiance without increasing sebum production (Pareek et al., 2025).

3.6 UV filters

UV filters are among the most scientifically scrutinized ingredients in cosmetics. They protect the skin from UV-A and UV-B radiation, which are major contributors to photoaging, hyperpigmentation, and skin cancer (Chatzigianni et al., 2022). UV filters are categorized into:

- Inorganic (physical) filters, such as zinc oxide and titanium dioxide, which reflect and scatter UV rays (Carve et al., 2021).
- Organic (chemical) filters, such as avobenzone, which absorb UV radiation and dissipate it as heat (Sabzevari et al., 2021).

The concentration of UV filters in a product determines its sun protection factor. While essential, some filters have been associated with allergic reactions, endocrine disruption, or environmental harm, especially when used in high concentrations or in aerosol formulations (Santander Ballestín and Luesma Bartolomé, 2023). Regulatory agencies worldwide continuously reassess the safety profiles of UV filters to balance efficacy and consumer protection (Bergeson and Hutton, 2022).

3.7 Nanomaterials

Nanotechnology represents one of the most transformative innovations in the cosmetics industry. Defined by the EU as intentionally engineered insoluble materials sized between 1 and 100 nm, nanomaterials are now found in a broad range of personal care products (European Commission, 2023). Their appeal lies in:

- Enhanced penetration into the stratum corneum for better delivery of active ingredients (Vinardell and Mitjans, 2015).
- Improved product stability and texture (Subroto et al., 2023).
- Increased transparency in sunscreens using nanosized titanium dioxide or zinc oxide (Sabzevari et al., 2021).
- Controlled release mechanisms, ideal for perfumes and antiaging serums (Oehlke et al., 2017).

Despite these advantages, concerns remain regarding the safety of nanomaterials, particularly regarding penetration beyond the epidermis and potential systemic effects. Aerosolized nanoparticles pose inhalation risks for workers (SCCS—Scientific Committee on Consumer Safety, 2023). Studies have investigated the cytotoxic and genotoxic effects of commonly used nanomaterials (Hansen and Baun, 2012). Consequently, Regulation (EC) No. 1223/2009 mandates explicit labeling of nanomaterials and rigorous premarket safety assessments (EC Regulation No. 1223/2009).

3.8 Ongoing safety concerns and research needs

The trend toward plant-based, "clean," or minimalist cosmetic formulations has raised complex challenges for regulatory and toxicological science. While reducing synthetic ingredients is often perceived as a safer option, this shift can lead to increased exposure to untested or insufficiently researched substances. Studies have shown that the average woman uses

8–30 cosmetic products per day, resulting in cumulative exposure to a broad range of chemicals, many of which may interact synergistically or antagonistically (MacKendrick, 2015; Ficheux et al., 2019).

Long-term exposure to certain ingredients—such as phthalates, parabens, and formaldehyde-releasing agents—has been associated with adverse outcomes (AOs), including:

- Endocrine disruption
- Neurodevelopmental delays in children
- Reproductive toxicity
- Increased cancer risk (Wang and Qian, 2021; Johnson et al., 2022; Kohli et al., 2024)

Given these concerns, there is a critical need for:

- Expanded toxicological research on ingredient interactions and chronic exposure.
- Stricter regulatory oversight of ingredient claims and labeling.
- Workplace protections for cosmetic industry professionals exposed to hazardous substances during manufacturing.

Protecting both consumer health and occupational safety in the cosmetics sector depends on the continuous evolution of safety standards, transparent communication, and the integration of cutting-edge science into policy and practice (Kohli et al., 2024; Wang and Qian, 2021).

4 Integrated approaches to chemical safety and toxicological assessment in the cosmetic industry

The cosmetic industry operates within a highly regulated framework that prioritizes consumer safety, product efficacy, and ethical responsibility. This evolving landscape has driven the development and adoption of alternative safety evaluation strategies, including *in vitro* assays, computational modeling, and the use of validated biochemical methods (Filaire et al., 2022). At the same time, occupational safety in cosmetic laboratories has become increasingly relevant, as researchers and technicians are frequently exposed to a wide array of chemical substances, some of which carry health risks if not properly managed (Cosmetic Chemist Safety, 2019; OSHA, 2021). The convergence of product safety and workplace safety has led to the need for integrated approaches that address both consumer and worker protection.

This chapter presents a unified view of the key elements involved in chemical safety and toxicological evaluation within the cosmetic sector. It explores the assessment of raw materials and finished products, the identification and management of chemical hazards in laboratory environments (University of North Carolina, Laboratory Safety Manual, 2019; Cornell University EHS, 2020), and the application of modern biochemical and computational methods in safety testing (Raies and Bajic, 2016).

4.1 Toxicological assessment of cosmetic substances

The toxicological evaluation of cosmetic substances forms the scientific backbone of product safety assurance, ensuring that ingredients and formulations do not pose risks to human health under normal or foreseeable conditions of use. This process begins with the comprehensive assessment of raw materials—including surfactants, preservatives, fragrances, colorants, and emollients—each of which must be supported by a well-documented toxicological profile. These profiles are essential for identifying potential health effects, such as acute toxicity (typically expressed via LD_{50} values), chronic toxicity from repeated exposure, systemic effects, and organ-specific damage (Nohynek et al., 2010).

LD_{50} (lethal dose, 50%): The dose of a substance that causes death in 50% of test organisms; traditionally used as a measure of acute toxicity.

Beyond systemic toxicity, safety assessments focus heavily on local effects such as skin and eye irritation, corrosion, and sensitization. Given the high incidence of allergic reactions linked to fragrances and preservatives, sensitization testing is especially critical. Standardized assays are used to evaluate whether substances may trigger immune responses after repeated exposure (Api et al., 2008; Lyapina et al., 2023). Phototoxicity and genotoxicity represent additional endpoints of concern. The former relates to the potential for substances to cause skin damage upon exposure to light (Ford et al., 2000), while the latter assesses the likelihood of DNA damage, mutations, or carcinogenic effects (Barthe et al., 2021). Equally important is the evaluation of the final cosmetic formulation, which may exhibit interactive effects not evident in the analysis of individual ingredients. In this context, the Human Repeat Insult Patch Test (HRIPT) is frequently used to determine cumulative irritation and sensitization potential under *in vivo* conditions, while *in vitro* methods—such as ocular and dermal tolerance tests using reconstructed human tissue models—support ethical and regulatory demands for nonanimal testing (Barthe et al., 2021; Goebel et al., 2012).

To enhance and complement experimental testing, alternative approaches such as read-across (RAX) and QSAR models are increasingly employed. These in silico tools allow safety assessors to infer toxicological properties based on data from structurally similar compounds or from molecular descriptors and physicochemical characteristics (Mishra and Petry, 2025; Kroes et al., 2007). When appropriately validated, such methods are recognized under EU regulations and are particularly valuable when empirical data are unavailable or when conventional testing raises ethical, technical, or financial concerns.

RAX infers the properties of an untested substance by comparing it with data from structurally or mechanistically similar chemicals.

Another critical aspect of toxicological assessment involves identifying and evaluating impurities, either inherent in raw materials or formed during manufacturing and storage. These may include residual solvents, unreacted monomers, or degradation products. Even trace concentrations of such substances can present safety concerns, particularly if they are classified as carcinogenic, mutagenic, or toxic to reproduction (CMR). The toxicological relevance of these impurities is typically evaluated using exposure-based thresholds, such as the threshold of toxicological concern, to determine whether additional testing or reformulation is necessary (Bury et al., 2021; Kroes et al., 2007).

4.2 Chemical hazards in cosmetic laboratories

Cosmetic laboratories serve as critical environments for product development, testing, and QC, yet they also represent occupational settings where personnel are routinely exposed to a diverse range of chemical substances. Each class of substances carries distinct physicochemical properties that can pose risks to human health if not adequately controlled (Kaushik et al., 2023).

Routes of exposure in the laboratory environment are diverse and depend on the form of the substance and the procedures employed. Dermal contact is the most common, given the manual nature of sample handling, weighing, and preparation. Inhalation exposure can occur during processes that involve heating, mixing, or working with volatile compounds or aerosols, particularly when engineering controls, such as fume hoods, are lacking. Accidental splashes pose a risk for ocular exposure, especially during pipetting or dilution of concentrated solutions. These scenarios necessitate a detailed risk assessment and the implementation of appropriate PPE, engineering controls, and hygiene practices (Occupational Safety and Health Administration, 2011).

The emergence of nanomaterials, such as titanium dioxide, zinc oxide, and silica nanoparticles, has introduced new challenges to chemical safety in cosmetic laboratories. These materials offer performance benefits—such as enhanced UV protection or improved product texture—but their nanoscale dimensions allow for deeper biological penetration and unique interactions with cellular components. Due to their high surface area-to-volume ratio and potential for oxidative stress induction, nanomaterials demand specialized toxicological assessment and stringent exposure control measures (SCCS—Scientific Committee on Consumer Safety, 2019).

To address the broad spectrum of chemical hazards, cosmetic laboratories are required to comply with international standards for chemical classification, labeling, and communication. The Globally Harmonized System (GHS) provides a standardized framework for identifying and conveying hazards through pictograms, signal words (e.g., Warning, Danger), and hazard statements. All containers, reagent bottles, and formulated products must be clearly labeled according to GHS criteria. Moreover, personnel must be trained not only in the use of PPE and emergency procedures but also in the interpretation of labels and SDSs (OSHA, 2012).

4.3 Biochemical and alternative testing methods

In response to regulatory, ethical, and scientific demands, the cosmetic industry has progressively shifted toward nonanimal testing strategies that rely on biochemical, cellular, and computational approaches. These methods not only align with the principles of the 3Rs (Replacement, Reduction, and Refinement) but also provide high-throughput, mechanistically informative, and cost-effective tools for toxicological evaluation. Their integration into safety assessment frameworks has become essential for ensuring compliance with each country's Cosmetics Regulation, which prohibits animal testing for both finished products and their individual ingredients (Filaire et al., 2022). Biochemical assays offer valuable insights into the cellular and molecular mechanisms underlying toxicity. Enzyme-based assays, for instance, are commonly used to assess tissue damage and viability. Models such as reconstructed human epidermis (RhE) (e.g., EpiDerm, SkinEthic) simulate skin architecture and serve as platforms for irritation and corrosion testing. The European Center for the Validation of Alternative Methods (ECVAM) international validation of these models resulted in their acceptance under OECD Test Guideline 439 (Spielmann et al., 2007; OECD, 2019a). Lactate dehydrogenase release assays measure cell membrane integrity by quantifying enzyme leakage upon chemical exposure, providing a quantitative alternative to animal skin irritation tests (Eskes et al., 2003).

The **3Rs** are ethical principles in animal research: Replacement (use nonanimal methods), Reduction (minimize animal use), and Refinement (reduce suffering).

Similarly, specific enzymatic pathways may be targeted to evaluate endocrine-disrupting activity or interference with metabolic functions. Cytotoxicity assays form the cornerstone of *in vitro* toxicology in cosmetics. The MTT(Repetto et al., 2008) assay, which detects mitochondrial dehydrogenase activity, and the neutral red uptake assay, which assesses lysosomal function, are standard techniques used to evaluate cellular viability following exposure to cosmetic ingredients or formulations (Rodrigues et al., 2023). These methods provide dose-response data that inform safe concentration ranges, helping formulators to optimize ingredient selection and regulatory dossiers.

Beyond direct cell viability, biochemical methods can elucidate sublethal effects that signal longer-term or systemic risks. Oxidative stress assays, such as those measuring reactive oxygen species generation or glutathione depletion, are used to assess whether compounds may promote free radical formation or disrupt cellular redox balance. In parallel, inflammatory responses can be detected through cytokine profiling—for instance, measuring interleukins (IL-1α, IL-8) and tumor necrosis factor-alpha (TNF-α)—which are indicators of immunological activation, skin irritation, or sensitization potential (Filaire et al., 2022).

To supplement *in vitro* methods, computational approaches are increasingly adopted in toxicological assessments. RAX allows the inference of toxicological properties for a given compound based on structurally similar substances, while QSAR models predict biological activity or toxicity based on molecular descriptors. These techniques are particularly valuable in early formulation stages, where empirical data may be scarce, and are accepted under regulatory frameworks when justified by appropriate structural, mechanistic, and metabolic analogies (Mishra and Petry, 2025). These alternative methods are not only scientific advancements but also regulatory necessities. Organizations such as the ECVAM and the OECD maintain lists of validated test guidelines, many of which are mandated for use in the preparation of the CPSR (OECD, 2019a; Spielmann et al., 2007). The integration of biochemical and computational techniques ensures the robustness of safety evaluations while supporting ethical imperatives and public expectations for cruelty-free testing.

5 Toxicological risk assessment

As cosmetic products comprise a wide array of chemical substances—many of which are applied directly to the skin or inhaled—systematic evaluation of their toxicological profiles is essential throughout the product lifecycle. Case studies drawn from historical incidents and current literature underscore the evolving nature of toxicological challenges in cosmetic formulation and occupational environments. By integrating empirical evidence with modern predictive approaches, toxicological risk assessment plays a dual role in safeguarding public health and promoting responsible innovation in cosmetic science (Ebmeyer et al., 2024).

5.1 Toxicological evidence, predictive tools, and historical lessons in cosmetic safety

At the core of toxicological risk assessment is the understanding of toxicokinetics, how a substance is absorption, distribution, metabolism, and excretion (ADME) in the human body. This framework helps predict systemic exposure and internal dose following dermal application or accidental inhalation or ingestion. In cosmetics, the dermal route is the primary exposure pathway, but inhalation (e.g., aerosols, powders) and ocular exposure (e.g., splashes) must also be considered. Differences in absorption rates, metabolic capacity, and excretion patterns across populations, such as children or individuals with compromised skin barriers, further emphasize the need for precise risk characterizations (OECD, 2011; Tcheremenskaia et al., 2019). Quantitative benchmarks are used to assess the toxicological acceptability of substances. The No Observed Adverse Effect Level (NOAEL) represents the highest dose at which no harmful effects are observed in toxicological studies. From this, the Derived No-Effect Level is calculated, accounting for uncertainty factors such as interspecies differences and individual sensitivity. These values are then compared to the estimated systemic exposure dose (SED) to calculate the MoS. A MoS greater than 100 is generally required under the EU Cosmetics Regulation to consider a substance safe for use. This calculation underpins the toxicological section of the CPSR and informs regulatory decisions (Cronin et al., 2026; CosmeDesk, 2023; ChemSafetyPro, 2018).

The final element of a toxicological risk assessment involves the critical review and interpretation of the toxicological sections of SDSs. Section 11 of the SDS typically includes data on acute toxicity, irritation, sensitization, carcinogenicity, and other relevant endpoints. Safety assessors must evaluate this information alongside lab-specific exposure conditions and population-specific risks. Importantly, toxicological risk assessment serves both consumer safety by determining the acceptability of ingredients in end-use products, and occupational health by informing risk controls for laboratory personnel and production staff who may encounter higher concentrations or more frequent exposure (Westerholm and Schenk, 2014).

When empirical data are incomplete or unavailable—particularly for novel substances or complex mixtures—a weight-of-evidence (WoE) approach is employed. This strategy integrates multiple sources of information, including *in vitro* data, RAX from structurally similar substances, historical usage, and mechanistic insights, to form a scientifically justified conclusion. WoE assessments are critical for ingredients with limited toxicological testing, allowing risk assessors to draw meaningful conclusions without compromising safety standards. Transparency in the justification and limitations of this method is essential for regulatory acceptance (Suter and Lizarraga, 2022).

Advancements in computational toxicology have further enhanced risk assessment methodologies. Tools such as QSARs, the OECD QSAR Toolbox, and the US EPA's ToxCast database offer powerful predictive capabilities for estimating toxicological endpoints based on molecular structure and known biological activity. These tools are especially valuable for screening large ingredient libraries, prioritizing substances for further testing, and supporting RAX arguments in the absence of animal data. Their integration into modern safety assessments aligns with both scientific innovation and the EU's commitment to reducing animal experimentation (Suter and Lizarraga, 2022; European Food Safety Authority Scientific Committee, 2025).

As was indicated in the preceding section, workers in the cosmetics sector may be exposed to dangerous substances included in products, defying the popular assumption that consumers are the most vulnerable group. In order to enhance the health and safety of workers in the cosmetics sector, it is imperative to secure healthier workplaces in the future and to develop long-term legislative solutions (Datta et al., 2017; Vitoux et al., 2020).

5.2 New approach methodologies

Animal testing was the main method used to evaluate the safety of substances for many years. This methodology is facing growing opposition, not only because of ethical issues that make it unacceptable to significant sectors of society, but also because it causes delays in regulatory decisions and raises questions about the applicability of the findings to human beings. As per the Cosmetics Regulation (EC) No. 1223/2009, the full use of conventional methods to produce toxicological data in animals for the purpose of assisting the safety assessment of cosmetics was prohibited on March 11, 2013.

At this moment, methodologies for evaluating chemical risks are introduced under the umbrella of new approach methodologies (NAMs), including *in vitro* (laboratory-based), in chemico (in a chemical/artificial environment), and in silico (computer-based). Any technique, methodology, approach, or combination that can provide information on the risk and hazard assessment of chemicals without using animals is referred to as a nonanimal model (NAM). NAMs include high-throughput data, *in vitro* bioactivity testing, toxicogenomics-based tests, ex vivo systems, RAX and grouping methods, microphysiological systems, *in vitro* to*in vivo* extrapolation (IVIVE), in silico and modeling tools, AI, and machine learning systems. Because they can replicate human biology and provide mechanistic knowledge on how a chemical may cause toxicity in people, they are a superior option when conducting safety evaluations (Stucki et al., 2022; Haber et al., 2024). By addressing important biological pathways or targets, they employ more compassionate approaches and help to shift the paradigm away from animal research.

AI and **machine learning systems** analyze large toxicological datasets to identify patterns, predict chemical hazards, and support decision-making.

The next-generation risk assessment (NGRA) incorporates data from NAMs from multiple sources, allowing it to participate in the decision-making process. Mechanistic data can be organized into adverse outcome pathway (AOP) networks and AOPs. Through causal linkages, the AOP paradigm connects an initial exposure event to a sequence of mechanistic and measurable key events (KEs) and, eventually, to a clinically relevant illness outcome. AOPs can be transformed into fully quantitative toxicity models by enriching them with dose-response information for each of the many KEs in the pathway. AOPs have already been developed for a variety of harmful effects. However, by measuring molecular or cellular events *in vitro* at lower levels of biological organization without testing on whole animals, it may become possible to predict AOs and their safe doses in an ever-expanding toxicological space as more AOPs and quantitative AOPs (qAOPs) are developed for more key endpoints (Paini et al., 2022; Vinken et al., 2020).

Physiologically based kinetic (PBK) modeling is a potent approach for converting a qualitative AOP into a qAOP that can determine human-relevant guideline values. To estimate time-dependent concentrations in plasma and tissues, PBK models integrate data on exposure, physiology, and chemical characteristics that describe the processes of absorption, distribution, metabolism, and excretion (ADME) of a chemical. For risk evaluation utilizing PBK models, No Observed Effect Concentrations obtained from *in vitro* studies assessing lower KEs in a qAOP can be converted into *in vivo* NOAELs (Vinken et al., 2020; Najjar et al., 2022).

Table 4.1 provides a consolidated overview of the toxicological assessment methodologies discussed in Sections 5.1 and 5.2. It highlights the main advantages and limitations of traditional approaches, predictive tools, and new approach methodologies (NAMs), offering a comparative perspective on their applicability in cosmetic safety evaluation. By presenting both established and emerging strategies, the table underscores the complementary role of these methods in ensuring consumer protection, regulatory compliance, and ethical advancement in toxicological science.

TABLE 4.1 Comparison of toxicological assessment methodologies (integrated Sections 5.1 and 5.2).

Methodology	Strengths	Limitations
Empirical toxicological studies (*in vivo*, historical data)	Provide systemic data (ADME, chronic effects)—long history of regulatory acceptance—benchmark for thresholds (e.g., NOAEL)	Ethical concerns (animal use)—expensive and time-consuming—limited human relevance for some endpoints
In vitro assays (cell/tissue models, reconstructed skin/eye)	Nonanimal, ethically acceptable—mechanistic, human-relevant endpoints—high-throughput possible—Accepted by OECD (e.g., TG 439)	Mostly local endpoints (irritation, sensitization)—cannot fully capture systemic/long-term effects—requires extrapolation to the whole body
In chemico assays	Directly assess chemical reactivity (e.g., skin sensitization)—quick, inexpensive—some OECD-standardized methods	Narrow scope—no metabolic context—cannot predict systemic toxicity
In silico tools (QSAR, read-across, AI/ML, ToxCast, QSAR Toolbox)	Very rapid, low-cost—useful for early screening and prioritization—Accepted under EU regulations if validated—leverages large datasets	Reliability depends on input data and structural similarity—limited for novel chemistries—requires strong justification for regulatory acceptance
Weight-of-evidence (WoE)	Integrates *in vitro*, in silico, and historical data—flexible for data-poor compounds—promotes transparency in decision-making	Requires expert judgment—evidence quality may vary—regulatory acceptance depends on the robustness of justification
Safety Data Sheets (SDS, Section 11)	Readily available—provide standardized data (acute toxicity, irritation, CMR)—essential for occupational safety	Often incomplete or generic—may lack cosmetic-relevant endpoints—quality varies by supplier
Microphysiological systems (organs-on-chips, ex vivo models)	Mimic human organ-level responses—capture complex interactions (barrier, metabolism)—bridge between *in vitro* and *in vivo*	Expensive, technically complex—still under validation—limited scalability for routine use
PBK (physiologically based kinetic) modeling	Converts *in vitro/in silico* data into human-relevant doses—supports quantitative NGRA—valuable for exposure extrapolation	Requires high-quality ADME input data—demands modeling expertise—regulatory acceptance still limited
NGRA/AOP-based frameworks	Integrates multiple NAMs + exposure science—human-centric and mechanistic—internationally supported (OECD, ICCR)	Still evolving—many pathways have data gaps—requires interdisciplinary expertise and transparency

5.3 A 10-step framework for NAMs

Under the auspices of the ICCR, a working group met in 2018 and established a set of guidelines that may facilitate the use of NAMs in cosmetic risk assessments. This new method of evaluating cosmetics is predicated on potential damage reduction and is human-centric. A tiered 10-step strategy was devised to demonstrate how these ideas and NAM data creation could be used in conjunction with the next-generation RAX concept (Vaillancourt et al., 2025; Paini et al., 2022) (Table 4.2).

Determining and characterizing the exposure scenario is the first stage. The Scientific Committee on Consumer Safety (SCCS) (SCCS—Scientific Committee on Consumer Safety, 2021, Europe) guiding notes establish basic assumptions on how much of each product type a consumer uses each day (SCCS—Scientific Committee on Consumer Safety, 2021). The second tier uses more practical methods to determine a suitable exposure measurement. This involves utilizing product presence data to account for the probability of a customer using the element in various product types on a daily basis. A NAM for exposure can be created using the outputs from all tiers of this particular exposure modeling, and the internal dose can be estimated using PBK modeling. Internal systemic exposure concentrations in human blood, plasma, and target organs are compared with concentrations based on cell assays as points of departure for bioactivity New Approach Methodologies–derived Point of Departure (PODNAM) when NAM data are used to perform an ab initio (use of exclusively *in vitro* and in silico data) NGRA instead of the RAX principle (Najjar et al., 2022).

Parabens and caffeine, at levels observed in cosmetic items, were evaluated in two case studies released by the OECD as a means of demonstrating the actual implementation of the 10-step NAM/RAX framework in NGRA. The "target substance" (parabens or caffeine) in these case studies is intended to be unknown but is assumed to be a member of a family of compounds for which historical toxicological data and comparable points of departure already exist (OECD, 2023a). It is crucial that there is sufficient evidence to support the similarity hypothesis in order for it to be accepted and deemed suitable for the intended use. For the compounds, sufficient, high-quality historical toxicological data are crucial. Toxicochemical data, *in vitro* cytotoxicity test data, and toxicogenomic data can all be utilized to identify similarities between the test material and analogs. Consequently, in the case of caffeine, the decision was made to use the primary metabolites of caffeine

TABLE 4.2 Ten-step framework for NAMs in cosmetic risk assessment.

Step	Description
1. Define exposure scenario	Establish product type, frequency, amount, and route of exposure based on SCCS guidance.
2. Refine exposure estimation	Use realistic consumer-use and product-presence data to model actual exposure.
3. Characterize internal dose	Apply physiologically based kinetic (PBK) modeling, supported by *in vitro–in vivo* extrapolation (IVIVE), to translate external exposure into internal concentration metrics (e.g., C_max, C_ss) in relevant human tissues.
4. Identify relevant endpoints	Determine which toxicological endpoints (e.g., irritation, sensitization, endocrine activity) need evaluation.
5. Select NAMs	Choose appropriate *in vitro*, in chemico, or in silico methods aligned with the identified endpoints.
6. Generate NAM data	Conduct laboratory or computational studies to generate mechanistic and quantitative toxicity data.
7. Establish Points of Departure (PODNAM)	Derive points of departure from NAM data (e.g., benchmark dose, AC50, EC10) using concentration–response modeling, and apply IVIVE together with PBK modeling to compare bioactivity thresholds against predicted internal exposure.
8. Integrate with read-across (RAX)	Use data from structurally similar substances to strengthen conclusions where direct data are limited.
9. Perform NGRA	Combine exposure, NAM outputs, PBK modeling, and RAX evidence into a next-generation risk assessment.
10. Regulatory interpretation & decision-making	Present results transparently, highlight uncertainties, and justify conclusions for regulatory acceptance.

as source substances for the target caffeine after looking for chemically related compounds and taking into account what is currently known about its metabolism. Regarding parabens, a number of short-chain n-alkyl parabens were the focus of the search for compounds with comparable chemical properties. The limits of similarity were also defined with the help of physicochemical parameters (Paini et al., 2022; OECD, 2023a).

5.4 Limitations and future challenges for NAMs

NAMs are a good substitute for conventional animal testing in the safety evaluation of chemicals used in the cosmetics industry and elsewhere, but their broad adoption is hampered by a number of issues. *In vivo* animal testing is a major component of chemical safety assessment, especially for higher-tier hazardous endpoints, including repeated-dose toxicity and reproductive toxicity. Furthermore, efforts to replace animal testing with NAMs based on independent, stand-alone investigations are being made as of right now. This approach is not likely to work for complicated dangers, at least not right now (Nicola et al., 2023).

The rate of advancement in chemical safety assessment is being hindered by notable constraints and impediments. These include institutionalized, stringent criteria for animal-based evidence for a variety of substances. Furthermore, a significant number of NAMs have not been updated by the OECD, which makes regulatory adoption difficult in many jurisdictions. In addition, there is a dearth of expertise in handling and analyzing fresh data sets derived from cutting-edge technology. There are also major limitations in comprehending complicated risks. There is a widespread worry that the toxicological domain covered by whole-animal testing is not entirely covered by emerging technologies (Stucki et al., 2022; van der Zalm et al., 2022). Integrated methods, however, may be a component of the solution, as certain NAMs are thought to be more promising than others. It is more likely that NAMs will be employed initially for screening and prioritization, and that tiered techniques will need to be explored first (Rovida et al., 2015). However, as understanding grows, safer approaches—where assessments are created using a blend of conventional methods and NAMs—might boost trust in the use of NAMs.

6 Safety management and risk applications in the cosmetics industry: A holistic approach to laboratory and production environments

The cosmetics industry encompasses a range of laboratory and production environments where chemical handling, formulation, testing, and packaging occur. Ensuring the safety of employees, consumers, and the environment requires a comprehensive and integrated approach to occupational safety. This chapter consolidates key components of safety management in cosmetic laboratories and production facilities, offering a unified framework that spans regulatory compliance, preventive controls, personal protection, training, and sustainability (SCCS—Scientific Committee on Consumer Safety, 2021).

6.1 Safety management systems and safer-by-design approaches in cosmetic laboratories

The implementation of a structured safety management system (SMS) is essential in cosmetic laboratories to safeguard personnel and maintain compliance with regulatory frameworks. A well-functioning SMS integrates organizational policies, operational procedures, and technical controls into a cohesive framework that systematically addresses occupational risks (International Organization for Standardization (ISO), 2018a). Hazard identification and risk assessment form the foundation of this framework, ensuring that incidents are prevented, emergencies are managed effectively, and a culture of continuous improvement is fostered. This approach not only meets regulatory requirements but also represents a commitment to ethical and responsible laboratory operations (OECD, 2019a).

Hazard identification involves systematically recognizing chemical, physical, and biological risks present in the laboratory. For formulation work, this includes reviewing toxicological data on ingredients such as acute and chronic toxicity, sensitization potential, genotoxicity, reproductive effects, and bioaccumulation. Data are sourced from SDSs, regulatory databases such as ECHA and CosIng, scientific monographs from SCCS or CIR, and historical adverse event reports (ECHA (European Chemicals Agency), 2022a, 2024a; CIR (Cosmetic Ingredient Review), 2023). Risks are then evaluated for likelihood and severity, with control measures applied according to the hierarchy of controls: elimination, substitution, engineering controls, administrative procedures, and PPE (National Institute for Occupational Safety and Health (NIOSH), 2023). Applying toxicological screening at this stage supports proactive risk management and aligns with the precautionary principle (Patlewicz et al., 2014; United Nations Environment Programme (UNEP), 2021b).

Safer-by-design strategies, integrated into SMS frameworks, aim to eliminate or reduce hazards at the source. These strategies prioritize substituting higher-risk substances with safer alternatives, while balancing toxicological profiles with formulation compatibility, stability, cost, and consumer expectations.

The operationalization of safety and design principles requires robust standard operating procedures (SOPs). These protocols govern formulation, testing, equipment cleaning, and spill response, ensuring consistency and accountability (OSHA, 2023a). Training ensures that all staff, including students and interns, are competent in SOP use (International Organization for Standardization (ISO), 2018a). Chemical inventory control further strengthens SMS implementation, with centralized systems tracking chemical identities, hazard classifications, and storage locations. Such systems facilitate risk assessments, regulatory compliance under frameworks like REACH, and rapid access to SDS. High-risk reagents must be stored according to compatibility guidelines, segregated to minimize accidental reactions or exposures (OECD, 2019a; National Institutes of Health (NIH), 2019).

To maintain and improve safety performance, laboratories must implement internal audits, incident reporting, and corrective and preventive actions (CAPA). Incident reporting systems encourage the documentation of near-misses for root cause analysis (International Organization for Standardization (ISO), 2018a; OSHA, 2015; International Atomic Energy Agency, 2016). Compliance with international standards—including ISO 45001 for occupational health and safety and GLP for data integrity—reinforces both operational reliability and stakeholder trust (International Organization for Standardization (ISO), 2018a; OECD, 2023a; European Parliament and Council, 2009).

Through this integrated approach, cosmetic laboratories not only protect their workforce but also innovate responsibly, ensuring products are safe, effective, and aligned with consumer and regulatory expectations.

6.2 Laboratory-level safety and QC measures

In cosmetic industry laboratories, safety relies on a combination of PPE, engineering controls, toxicological testing, and GLPs. QC laboratories serve as critical checkpoints, assessing raw materials and finished products to confirm compliance with health, stability, and regulatory standards before market release (ECHA (European Chemicals Agency), 2024a; SCCS—Scientific Committee on Consumer Safety, 2021). By embedding toxicological controls into analytical testing, QC laboratories act as a safeguard against unsafe products.

The correct selection and use of PPE are fundamental to protecting laboratory personnel from chemical, physical, and biological risks. PPE requirements are guided by SDSs, risk assessments, and institutional policies, ensuring appropriate protection for different tasks (National Institute for Occupational Safety and Health (NIOSH), 2023). Training is essential to ensure PPE is used correctly and consistently and must include donning, doffing, inspection, and maintenance (OSHA, 2011).

Engineering controls serve as essential complements to PPE, providing ventilation, containment, and protection against exposure. Examples include fume hoods, biosafety cabinets, laminar flow systems, and dedicated storage infrastructure that comply with international safety standards (European Committee for Standardization, 2004; National Institute for Occupational Safety and Health (NIOSH), 2023). Emergency preparedness requires the presence and regular maintenance of spill kits, eyewash stations, and safety showers.

QC laboratories apply standardized analytical and toxicological tests, such as microbiological controls, physicochemical characterization, heavy metal analysis, and allergen screening, to ensure product safety (International Organization for Standardization (ISO), 2017b; SCCS—Scientific Committee on Consumer Safety, 2021; European Food Safety Authority, 2012; European Parliament and Council, 2009). These processes are reinforced by GLPs and SOPs, which standardize safety-critical laboratory operations and are regularly assessed through audits, inspections, and interlaboratory proficiency testing (OECD, 2023a; International Organization for Standardization (ISO), 2007; ISO/IEC, 2017).

Interlaboratory proficiency testing is a QA process in which multiple laboratories analyze the same samples to compare performance and ensure accuracy.

Together, these measures safeguard personnel, ensure reliable product safety outcomes, and strengthen compliance with regulatory frameworks.

6.3 Production-level controls and safety report compilation in cosmetic manufacturing

In the cosmetics industry, product safety and consistency are ensured by process control measures and systematic documentation that extend from manufacturing to regulatory approval. Production processes must operate under defined parameters to prevent contamination, preserve stability, and ensure compliance with standards (SCCS—Scientific Committee on Consumer Safety, 2021). In parallel, manufacturers are required to compile a CPSR, mandated under Annex I of the EU Cosmetics Regulation (EC No. 1223/2009), which provides the scientific and legal foundation for market authorization (European Parliament and Council, 2009).

Production-level controls focus on identifying and monitoring critical control points—parameters such as temperature, mixing time, and pH—that directly affect product quality. These are complemented by inline monitoring, endproduct testing, and traceability systems that link finished products with raw material records, operator logs, and cleaning histories (U.S. Food and Drug Administration, 2022c; International Organization for Standardization (ISO), 2017b). QA and QC functions ensure system integrity, supplier reliability, and compliance with microbiological and chemical safety requirements (ISO, 2016; U.S. Food and Drug Administration, 2022c).

The CPSR provides a structured assessment of product safety, compiling toxicological and exposure data, physicochemical and microbiological parameters, and relevant regulatory references (European Parliament and Council, 2009; Gądarowska et al., 2022; European Chemicals Agency (ECHA), 2020). Central to the assessment is the calculation of the MoS, which compares the NOAEL with the SED. Exposure assessments must consider all relevant routes and vulnerable populations (European Parliament and Council, 2009; SCCS—Scientific Committee on Consumer Safety, 2021). Predictive toxicology tools may supplement incomplete data, supporting safety decisions in line with international best practices (OECD, 2021a).

Both production controls and CPSR compilation emphasize traceability, transparency, and scientific rigor. By integrating process monitoring, toxicological evaluation, and structured documentation, the cosmetics industry ensures product safety and reinforces consumer and regulatory confidence.

6.4 Exposure monitoring and health surveillance

In cosmetic industry laboratories, exposure monitoring and health surveillance are essential for safeguarding personnel. Monitoring airborne contaminants such as VOCs, particulate matter, and biological agents helps evaluate the effectiveness of control measures and ensures exposures remain below occupational limits (National Institute for Occupational Safety and Health (NIOSH), 2023).

PPE, guided by SDSs and risk assessments, is required for high-risk tasks. Engineering controls, such as fume hoods, laminar flow cabinets, and localized extraction systems, provide additional protection (National Institute for Occupational Safety and Health (NIOSH), 2023; American Conference of Governmental Industrial Hygienists, 2021).

Health surveillance programs address occupational illnesses most relevant to cosmetic laboratories, including respiratory conditions, contact dermatitis, and sensitization reactions. These programs may involve medical examinations, questionnaires, and targeted assessments, depending on institutional or regulatory requirements (European Agency for Safety and Health at Work (EU-OSHA), 2020).

A critical component of exposure monitoring is the documentation and analysis of near-miss incidents, which highlight weaknesses in protective systems and training. Establishing a transparent, nonpunitive reporting culture encourages early identification of risks and supports continuous improvement (OSHA, 2015; Jones et al., 1999).

Comprehensive reporting and follow-up after exposure incidents reinforce accountability and support CAPA. These processes align with international safety standards and GLP, ensuring consistency and compliance through audits and inspections (OECD, 2023a; International Organization for Standardization (ISO), 2007; ISO/IEC, 2017).

6.5 Culture training, auditing, and safety culture in cosmetic laboratories

The establishment of structured training programs and a proactive safety culture is fundamental for occupational health and safety in cosmetic laboratories. Given the diverse backgrounds of laboratory personnel—including chemists, technicians, interns, students, and contractors—training must be tailored to each individual's role, experience level, and exposure risks. Onboarding programs include safety orientation sessions covering general hazards, chemical handling, emergency protocols, and the use of PPE. Introducing safety concepts early fosters responsible work habits and improves risk perception (Zohar and Polachek, 2014; National Institute for Occupational Safety and Health (NIOSH), 2016; Reason, 1997).

Hazard communication standards are regulations requiring employers to inform workers about chemical hazards through labels, training, and SDSs.

Blended training approaches should combine theoretical knowledge with supervised laboratory instruction to reinforce hazard communication standards, chemical classification systems, and emergency procedures. Refresher courses are scheduled regularly, often incorporating findings from near-miss events or audit outcomes (Wu et al., 2008). Advanced modules for supervisors may cover regulatory compliance, incident investigation, and risk assessment methods.

Auditing complements training by verifying compliance and identifying gaps. Audits may be internal, external, or thematic, depending on the scope and objectives. Findings are documented in reports that assign risk ratings and corrective actions, which are reviewed in management meetings to maintain accountability (International Organization for Standardization (ISO), 2007, 2018a; OECD, 2018; International Labour Office, 2009). Linking audit outcomes to training updates ensures a cycle of continuous improvement.

A proactive safety culture extends beyond compliance to emphasize behavioral engagement. Promoting near-miss reporting encourages early hazard detection and prevents escalation into serious incidents. Cultivating an environment where reporting hazards, halting unsafe procedures, and suggesting improvements are actively supported is essential. Supervisors and senior staff play a decisive role by demonstrating commitment to safety and mentoring junior personnel (Geller, 2005).

Tracking performance requires quantitative and qualitative indicators, such as training completion rates, near-miss frequency, corrective action closure time, and employee survey results. Leading indicators are preferred over lagging injury counts, as they identify trends and enable proactive intervention (Schulman et al., 2004). Through this integrated system of training, auditing, behavioral safety, and leadership, laboratories can strengthen resilience and build a robust safety culture.

6.6 Emergency preparedness, response, and digital innovation

In cosmetic laboratories, the frequent use of flammable solvents, sensitizing agents, and reactive chemicals necessitates structured emergency preparedness and response planning. Effective planning protects personnel, limits property damage, and ensures compliance with regulatory standards (OSHA, 2015; National Fire Protection Association (NFPA), 2022). Preparedness must be hazard-specific, addressing scenarios such as chemical spills, fires, burns, or inhalation of toxic vapors. This requires clear procedures, trained personnel, and immediate access to appropriate resources (Centers for Disease Control and Prevention, 2023).

Digital innovation in emergency response refers to the use of electronic tools such as safety apps, QR-coded SDS access, or digital training simulations to improve readiness and response time.

SDSs are essential tools in emergency response, providing guidance on first aid, fire-fighting, and accidental release management (European Commission, 2020). Personnel must be trained to interpret SDS rapidly, apply appropriate extinguishing methods, and use protective equipment during incidents (European Agency for Safety and Health at Work (EU-OSHA), 2020).

Laboratories must maintain specialized first aid kits, eyewash stations, and safety showers, which should be strategically located and regularly maintained (ANSI/ISEA, 2014). Staff training emphasizes first aid for chemical exposures, burns, and inhalation incidents (American Red Cross, 2021). Preparedness drills—such as fire evacuations and spill simulations—are essential for testing readiness and refining protocols (OSHA, 2015; National Fire Protection Association (NFPA), 2022). Clear exit signage, accessible fire extinguishers, and posted emergency contacts further support rapid response. Collaboration with external responders, including fire departments and hospitals, ensures that site-specific hazards are addressed in advance (American Industrial Hygiene Association, 2020).

Integrating emergency preparedness into overall safety management requires coordination, documentation, and continuous improvement. Regular review of protocols, combined with training and external collaboration, fosters a proactive safety culture, strengthens incident response, and supports product integrity in an industry handling complex chemical formulations.

6.7 Psychosocial and ergonomic aspects

While laboratory safety often emphasizes chemical and physical hazards, psychosocial and ergonomic factors are equally important to the wellbeing and performance of personnel (Duffy et al., 2021; World Health Organization, 2023b). In highpaced cosmetic laboratories, employees and students face tight schedules, overlapping tasks, and complex analytical procedures. These pressures contribute to fatigue, cognitive overload, and mental stress. Prolonged strain can impair concentration, increase risk-taking, and heighten error rates when handling hazardous materials or operating advanced instrumentation (ISO, 2021; National Institute for Occupational Safety and Health (NIOSH), 2018).

Workload imbalance is a key psychosocial risk. Staff may juggle formulation development, testing, compliance, and documentation simultaneously, often under strict deadlines. This multitasking environment fosters burnout, dissatisfaction, and long-term health issues if not addressed (European Agency for Safety and Health at Work (EU-OSHA), 2022). For students, a lack of confidence and limited exposure to an established safety culture can intensify stress. Equitable workload distribution, respect for breaks, and task assignments that match training levels are essential in reducing these pressures.

Ergonomic concerns are another critical dimension. Laboratory work typically involves repetitive and posture-intensive activities such as pipetting, weighing samples, or microscope use. These actions increase the risk of repetitive strain injuries, musculoskeletal disorders, and trauma to the neck, shoulders, and wrists (Baker and Chaffin, 2021). Risks escalate when benches, chairs, or instruments are poorly adjusted to user needs, making workstation design a fundamental element of prevention.

Practical interventions can ease ergonomic stress. Adjustable benches and chairs, ergonomic pipettes, task lighting, and antifatigue mats support neutral working postures (OSHA, 2023; Santos et al., 2025). Complementary measures, such as job rotation, task alternation, and scheduled microbreaks, help reduce cumulative strain and improve focus (National Institute for Occupational Safety and Health (NIOSH), 2018).

Equally important is the promotion of mental health and work-life balance. Access to counseling services, wellness programs, and resources like yoga or mindfulness sessions supports coping strategies for laboratory staff (World Health Organization, 2023b). Creating open communication channels, offering feedback, and cultivating a culture that values rest and recovery further mitigate the risks of chronic stress and emotional exhaustion (European Agency for Safety and Health at Work (EU-OSHA), 2022).

In conclusion, addressing psychosocial and ergonomic risks in cosmetic laboratories is essential to both worker health and scientific quality. Beyond managing chemicals and equipment, a holistic safety strategy must safeguard mental resilience, reduce workload stressors, and ensure ergonomic support. By embedding these elements into organizational practice, laboratories foster environments where safety, wellbeing, and performance thrive together.

6.8 Ethical and sustainability considerations

As the cosmetics industry evolves, ethical responsibility and sustainability have become central to laboratory operations. Laboratories are expected not only to ensure product safety and efficacy but also to reduce ecological harm and reflect consumer values. This shift has driven the adoption of green chemistry principles, which promote safer processes, renewable feedstocks, and solvents with lower environmental impact, while maintaining product performance (OECD, 2021a).

A key element of sustainable formulation is the **"safer-by-design"** approach, which replaces known irritants, sensitizers, and toxicants with safer alternatives at the early stages of development. This strategy supports toxicological safety, enhances consumer confidence, and facilitates regulatory acceptance (Schug et al., 2013). For instance, substituting formaldehyde-releasing preservatives with naturally derived ingredients can reduce allergenic risks while improving sustainability. Predictive toxicology tools further strengthen this approach by allowing early hazard screening (Kavlock et al., 2018).

Ecolabeled suppliers are vendors certified to meet environmental standards, ensuring materials are sourced with a lower ecological impact.

Operational practices also contribute to sustainability. Laboratories can reduce their footprint by recycling solvents, minimizing single-use plastics, and adopting energy-efficient equipment such as low-consumption fume hoods and LED lighting (Khan et al., 2024). Process optimization to lower reagent use and environmentally responsible procurement—such as selecting eco-labeled suppliers—further improve resource efficiency and compliance with sustainable procurement standards (United Nations Environment Programme (UNEP), 2023).

Ethical responsibility extends beyond laboratory practice to labeling and transparency. Consumers increasingly seek vegan, cruelty-free, and ethically sourced products, requiring laboratories to substantiate claims with verifiable data, including animal-free testing, the absence of animal-derived ingredients, and adherence to regulatory frameworks (Hartlieb and Jones, 2009; SCCS—Scientific Committee on Consumer Safety, 2021). Third-party certifications, such as Leaping Bunny, PETA, and Ecocert, reinforce brand credibility and demonstrate genuine commitment to ethical values.

These efforts also align with broader sustainability agendas. The United Nations Sustainable Development Goals (SDGs) highlight this connection: SDG 3 (Good Health and Wellbeing) supports the creation of safe, nontoxic products, while SDG 12 (Responsible Consumption and Production) emphasizes reducing waste and environmental impacts (United Nations, 2015). By embedding ethics and sustainability into daily laboratory practices, organizations demonstrate alignment with global goals and reinforce their license to operate in an increasingly conscious market (United Nations Environment Programme (UNEP), 2023).

7 A synthesis of real-world safety performance, drawing on field-tested practices, organizational benchmarks, and emerging technologies

While theoretical frameworks and regulatory guidelines provide the foundation for laboratory safety, it is through the analysis of practical experiences—both adverse incidents and successful interventions—that laboratories truly evolve. In the cosmetics industry, where the manipulation of complex chemical substances intersects with rapid product development cycles, real-world safety applications offer critical insight into what works, what fails, and why. This chapter presents a series of case-based lessons, success stories, and benchmarking practices from across the sector. It highlights how laboratories have responded to emergencies, adopted technology-driven solutions, and cultivated safety cultures that promote resilience and continuous improvement. By examining these examples, readers can gain a nuanced understanding of how best practices are formed, tested, and adapted in everyday laboratory operations (Veltri and Pagell, 2007; Zohar, 2003).

Benchmarking practices are systematic comparisons of an organization's safety performance against industry peers or established standards to identify gaps and improvements.

7.1 Incident-based lessons learned

Real-world incidents provide critical insight into the strengths and weaknesses of laboratory safety systems. Unlike theoretical models, actual events reveal the interplay between human behavior, environmental conditions, equipment use, and procedural adequacy, forming a feedback loop for continuous improvement in protocols, risk communication, and organizational preparedness (Reason, 2000; Hughes et al., 2020).

One example occurred in a cosmetic formulation laboratory where a fire broke out during ethanol handling near an unshielded heating plate. While no injuries occurred, equipment damage and halted production triggered an internal investigation. Contributing factors included a lack of localized ventilation, insufficient training on flammable liquid storage, failure to enforce SOPs near ignition sources, and inadequate emergency preparedness. The case highlighted the need for multilayered risk assessments and showed how complacency in routine operations can mask the risks of common solvents (Dunn et al., 2023).

Corrective measures included mandatory fume hoods or explosion-proof enclosures, revised training modules on flammable liquid risks, stricter SOPs, and tailored fire drills (Wang et al., 2020). Another lesson comes from audits that revealed expired chemicals and poor labeling. These issues, though often dismissed as administrative lapses, pose hazards such as chemical instability, misuse, or delayed emergency response. Robust inventory systems, regular audits, and corrective documentation are critical (International Organization for Standardization (ISO), 2018a; OSHA, 2015; International Atomic Energy Agency, 2016).

Human error in PPE use also contributes to risk. Common mistakes—wearing contaminated gloves outside laboratory areas or reusing single-use equipment—undermine protection and increase crosscontamination. Addressing these requires rigorous training and reinforcement of best practices (Princeton University Environmental Health & Safety, 2025; University of Minnesota, Environmental Health & Safety, 2025). Similarly, near-miss incidents (VOC exceedances, splashes, equipment malfunctions) are vital early warnings. Their documentation strengthens protective measures and training programs, especially when supported by a nonpunitive reporting culture (OSHA, 2015; Jones et al., 1999). Engagement improves further with anonymous reporting via mobile forms or QR kiosks, linked to recognition programs such as "Safety Champion" awards (Geller, 2001; European Agency for Safety and Health at Work (EU-OSHA), 2021; Wei et al., 2023).

Technology-driven adjustments also demonstrate impact. A French cosmetics laboratory achieved a 30% reduction in overexposure incidents by introducing wearable sensors and relocating fume extraction units based on heatmap data, showing how targeted interventions can mitigate risks (Tsow et al., 2009).

Together, these cases emphasize the importance of comprehensive hazard evaluations beyond initial setup or inspections. Equipment placement, procedural discipline, and team awareness must be reassessed as staff, formulations, and processes evolve (Xu et al., 2026). Transparent analysis of incidents and near-misses, when shared across departments or externally, reinforces organizational learning and proactive safety behaviors (Guldenmund, 2010).

In conclusion, incident-based reviews should be institutionalized as learning opportunities rather than reactive audits. They help laboratories move beyond minimum compliance toward a culture of anticipation, accountability, and vigilance, essential for managing the complex risks inherent in cosmetic product development.

7.2 Success stories in safety implementation

While incidents expose vulnerabilities, success stories highlight the benefits of proactive, integrated safety strategies. These examples show how forward-thinking laboratories embed safety into operations, culture, and innovation pipelines (Xu et al., 2026).

A notable case is a European cosmetics manufacturer that restructured its chemical safety program to achieve ISO 45001 certification (Alshreef, 2025; International Organization for Standardization (ISO), 2018a). Changes included digital compatibility charts that flagged storage conflicts (Straut and Nelson, 2020), automated storage systems with access controls, and the substitution of parabens and formaldehyde releasers with safer agents such as phenoxyethanol and ethylhexylglycerin (Darbre and Harvey, 2008). Together, these initiatives exceeded regulatory compliance while reducing occupational risks.

Laboratories also reported improvements through PPE training aligned with hazard-specific risks, addressing errors such as contaminated glove use or reusing disposable equipment. Embedding PPE protocols in onboarding and refresher modules reduced exposure incidents (Princeton University Environmental Health & Safety, 2025; University of Minnesota, Environmental Health & Safety, 2025; National Institute for Occupational Safety and Health (NIOSH), 2023). Blended training approaches combined digital modules and simulations with drills such as spill responses and fire exercises, while refresher courses linked to audit results further reinforced learning (Hale et al., 2015; Veltri and Pagell, 2007; Wu et al., 2008; Wei et al., 2023). Incentives such as "Safety Champion" awards sustained engagement (DeJoy et al., 2010).

QC laboratories contribute success stories through standardized microbiological, physicochemical, and allergen testing, which prevent unsafe batches from reaching the market (International Organization for Standardization (ISO), 2017b; SCCS—Scientific Committee on Consumer Safety, 2021; European Food Safety Authority, 2012; European Parliament and Council, 2009). Similarly, exposure monitoring and health surveillance programs using sensors, diffusion badges, and medical protocols enabled early detection of VOC exceedances, dermatitis, and respiratory sensitization, reducing longterm health risks (Woolfenden, 2010; European Agency for Safety and Health at Work (EU-OSHA), 2020).

Emergency preparedness has also advanced through digital tools, including SDS apps with QR-code scanning for instant hazard information (Bayramova et al., 2023; DeMasi et al., 2022), smart fume hoods, spill detection mats, and Internet of Things (IoT) dashboards that centralize safety data and streamline audits (Pairote et al., 2025).

Cross-functional safety committees reinforced these efforts by conducting structured audits, monitoring safety indicators, reviewing near-misses, and advising on workflow modifications (Gershon et al., 1995; Phimister et al., 2003; Zamani, 2023). Leadership played a decisive role by visibly supporting initiatives, allocating resources, and setting the tone for a shared safety culture (Clarke, 2013; Fruhen et al., 2014).

Results were measurable: nearmiss reporting increased, total incidents dropped by 60%, employee satisfaction rose, and ISO 45001 certification was achieved within 1 year (Edmondson, 1999; Alshreef, 2025; International Organization for Standardization (ISO), 2018a).

These successes demonstrate that leadership, collaboration, training innovation, and digital transformation can elevate safety beyond compliance. Sharing such practices through conferences or training materials helps build industry-wide resilience (Cooper, 2000; Wu et al., 2008; Reason, 2000; Neal and Griffin, 2006).

7.3 Benchmarking industry leaders

Benchmarking industry leaders provides a strategic pathway for cosmetic laboratories to enhance safety, foster innovation, and align with global standards (Patriarca et al., 2018). By observing top performers, smaller enterprises can identify scalable practices that improve their systems (Adekunle, 2025).

Multinationals such as **L'Oréal and Beiersdorf** set benchmarks by integrating safety into corporate culture, R&D pipelines, and sustainability goals. L'Oréal mandates ISO 45001 certification across sites, with executive leadership engaged in Environment, Health, and Safety (EHS) strategy and audits (L'Oréal, 2023a). Their integrated risk management systems consolidate EHS data, inventories, training records, and incidents into centralized platforms, enabling realtime risk visibility, automated compliance alerts, and streamlined audits (L'Oréal, 2021). Complementary digital hazard communication and safety management tools provide multilingual Safety Data Sheets (SDSs), chemical compatibility charts, and emergency response protocols, enabling laboratory personnel to rapidly access critical safety information through mobile devices (L'Oréal, 2021, 2023a; OECD, 2023a).

Beyond technology, leaders invest heavily in **staff development and culture**. Beiersdorf integrates safety into sustainability and innovation training, using internal certification, workshops, leadership briefings, and gamified events to strengthen engagement (Beiersdorf, 2024; Burke et al., 2006). Both companies reinforce accountability by publishing sustainability and safety metrics—incident rates, training participation, and audit results—holding teams responsible for continuous improvement (Beiersdorf, 2024; L'Oréal, 2023a).

Another benchmarking lesson is the structured use of **SMSs** and internal audits. These emphasize proactive hazard identification, CAPA monitoring, and systematic root cause analysis. Audits highlight issues such as expired chemicals, poor labeling, or SOP deviations, with corrective actions tracked centrally for accountability (International Organization for Standardization (ISO), 2018a; OSHA, 2015; International Atomic Energy Agency, 2016).

Production-level safety controls also set benchmarks. Industry leaders apply HACCP principles to monitor critical parameters (temperature, pH, mixing times), ensuring batch integrity (SCCS—Scientific Committee on Consumer Safety, 2021). Before market release, detailed CPSRs consolidate toxicological data, impurities, packaging interactions, and assessor statements, creating a robust foundation for product authorization (European Parliament and Council, 2009; Gądarowska et al., 2022; European Chemicals Agency (ECHA), 2020).

Leaders also integrate predictive toxicology tools, such as QSAR models, the OECD Toolbox, and in silico screening, to anticipate toxicological endpoints when empirical data are lacking, reducing reliance on animal testing while maintaining rigor (Patlewicz et al., 2018; OECD, 2021a).

Smaller laboratories can adapt modular elements of these systems, including:

- Low-cost digital chemical inventories to improve tracking (Adekunle, 2025);
- Internal safety certifications to engage staff (Michael et al., 2005);
- Peer-led safety talks to foster culture at minimal cost (Burke et al., 2006).

Benchmarking does not require replicating large-scale systems. Instead, it offers a vision of excellence that smaller labs can tailor to elevate safety standards, increase regulatory resilience, and build confident working environments (Fernandez-Muniz et al., 2009; Michael et al., 2005).

7.4 Technology-driven best practices

Technological innovations are transforming safety management in cosmetic laboratories, improving hazard communication, emergency preparedness, and responsiveness to complex chemical environments.

One key advancement is the adoption of digital SDS platforms, replacing paper binders with cloud databases accessible from any device. These systems allow rapid retrieval by chemical name or CAS number, flag incompatible substances, and auto-update hazard classifications (Ta et al., 2010; United Nations/European Chemicals Agency (ECHA), 2024a). In emergencies, they provide immediate guidance on first aid, PPE, and evacuation (OSHA, 2012; Ta et al., 2010). Linked innovations include QR-code SDS apps, which reduce response times by giving staff instant hazard access (Bayramova et al., 2023; DeMasi et al., 2022).

Mobile emergency checklist applications complement these systems by guiding staff through step-by-step responses to spills, fires, or inhalation incidents, while documenting events and notifying supervisors (Harvard Office of Environmental Health and Safety (EH&S), 2017; Oklahoma State University Tulsa, Helmerich Research Center, 2013).

Wearable VOC monitors further enhance safety. These badge-sized devices alert users to solvent exposure risks, with advanced models logging personal exposure histories and feeding cloud dashboards for predictive analysis (Deng et al., 2016; Bernasconi et al., 2022; Chen et al., 2012; Reid et al., 2018). A French cosmetics laboratory reduced overexposure incidents by 30% after deploying sensors and relocating fume extraction units (Tsow et al., 2009).

In **QC laboratories**, inline sensors continuously track pH, viscosity, and turbidity, providing early warnings of unsafe deviations (Scott and Wilcock, 2006). Personal monitoring devices, such as diffusion badges, complement this by generating task-specific exposure profiles (American Conference of Governmental Industrial Hygienists, 2021). Combined with structured medical surveillance, these tools support the early detection of dermatitis, respiratory irritation, or sensitization, reinforcing technology as a foundation for occupational health (European Agency for Safety and Health at Work (EU-OSHA), 2020).

Training and reporting have also been digitized. Laboratories now use e-learning modules, quizzes, and simulations to teach hazard communication and emergency response (Hale et al., 2015; Veltri and Pagell, 2007). These are reinforced with drills such as spill or fire exercises (Wu et al., 2008; Wei et al., 2023). Near-miss reporting has shifted to anonymous QR or mobile platforms, improving transparency and engagement (European Agency for Safety and Health at Work (EU-OSHA), 2021). IoT-enabled infrastructure provides further advances: smart fume hoods adjust airflow, spill mats detect leaks, and dashboards centralize realtime data, streamlining audits and trend analysis (Pairote et al., 2025). Predictive analytics and machine learning applied to near-miss and exposure data identify patterns that precede incidents, aligning with EU digital safety initiatives (Pairote et al., 2025). Digital calculators and in silico tools also support formulation safety and substitution decisions, offering hazard classifications, compatibility checks, and systemic exposure estimates (Di Guardo et al., 2025; More et al., 2021). Advanced QSAR models expand predictive toxicology, reducing animal testing while providing early warnings (OECD, 2021a; Kavlock et al., 2009).

Collectively, these innovations create a layered safety ecosystem that ensures up-to-date documentation, transparent exposure monitoring, and standardized emergency responses (Lin et al., 2022). They also empower personnel with real-time decision support, moving beyond static signage to adaptive, interactive tools. As digital transformation accelerates, such practices strengthen safety, accountability, and innovation, pillars of operational excellence in cosmetic laboratories (Bernasconi et al., 2022).

7.5 Realworld case studies in cosmetic safety

One of the most widely documented safety concerns in the cosmetics sector involves talc-based products contaminated with asbestos. Talc and asbestos often occur in close geological proximity, which can lead to cross-contamination if raw material sources are not rigorously controlled. Several case series have demonstrated a clear link between the use of cosmetic talc and the development of mesothelioma in individuals without occupational asbestos exposure (Emory et al., 2020; Moline et al., 2020). In one investigation, asbestos fibers consistent with cosmetic talc exposure were identified in patient tissues, reinforcing the causal association with disease outcomes. These findings illustrate the urgent need for strict supply-chain oversight, advanced analytical screening, and a zero-tolerance approach to contamination in raw materials (Bird and Egilman, 2024).

Another category of cases highlights the unintended risks of preservative reformulation in response to consumer demand for "paraben-free" or "clean" beauty products. Traditional parabens, despite ongoing debate, are well-studied and effective antimicrobial agents. Their removal has sometimes resulted in weaker preservation systems, and in several instances, microbial contamination was detected in products that had passed stability testing prior to release. Recalls have followed the identification of molds such as *Aspergillus sydowii* in liquid foundations marketed as preservative-free, underscoring the consequences of inadequate antimicrobial validation (U.S. Food and Drug Administration, 2024; Katch, 2022). These incidents reveal the dangers of prioritizing market trends over scientific evaluation of product safety.

Microbial contamination also places additional pressure on QC laboratories. Investigations of preservative-free product recalls revealed weaknesses in accelerated stability testing, insufficient challenge testing, and gaps in environmental monitoring during production. Even in cases where health risks to consumers were low, the reputational damage to manufacturers was considerable. These findings emphasize that replacing established preservatives requires not only suitable alternatives but also a comprehensive reevaluation of microbiological testing protocols to ensure safety across the full product lifecycle (Katch, 2022).

Outside of consumer products, lessons in laboratory safety also come from academic research environments. A landmark case involved a fatal laboratory fire caused by the mishandling of a pyrophoric reagent. The researcher involved was not wearing a protective lab coat, and the accident revealed serious lapses in training, supervision, and institutional oversight. The subsequent legal case marked one of the first times that a university faced criminal charges related to laboratory safety practices (Kemsley, 2018). The tragedy catalyzed widespread reforms in laboratory management, highlighting the high stakes of neglecting occupational safety, even in academic contexts.

The longterm implications of this laboratory incident extend to the broader cosmetic science community, where laboratory workers routinely handle reactive solvents, nanomaterials, and VOCs. The accident demonstrated how safety culture, enforcement of PPE, and thorough training are as critical as regulatory frameworks and technical controls. In response, many institutions and companies have strengthened incident reporting mechanisms, implemented systematic safety audits, and invested in continuous training for staff, interns, and students. The recognition that institutional accountability is inseparable from individual responsibility remains one of the most enduring lessons from this case (Kemsley, 2018).

Together, these case studies provide complementary insights into the challenges of cosmetic safety. Talc contamination cases highlight the necessity of advanced raw-material testing and supply-chain vigilance. Preservative-related recalls demonstrate the risks of aligning product design more closely with marketing narratives than with scientific validation. The laboratory fire illustrates the irreplaceable role of culture, training, and accountability in preventing catastrophic outcomes. By integrating these lessons, cosmetic laboratories and manufacturers can move toward more resilient safety frameworks that protect consumers, workers, and industry credibility alike.

7.6 Summary and reflections

In summary, best practices in cosmetic laboratory safety emerge from a dynamic interplay of historical learning, strategic foresight, and innovation adoption. As this chapter has shown, effective safety management is not based on a single element but on a layered, multidisciplinary framework, drawing from incident analysis, technology integration, leadership engagement, and cultural change (Dunn et al., 2023; Ezenwa et al., 2022).

Realworld events—such as fires, spills, expired chemical storage, or PPE misuse—demonstrate the consequences of procedural lapses, inadequate training, or weak inventory systems. Near-miss documentation and corrective actions have proven essential for identifying systemic weaknesses, building institutional memory, and preventing recurrence (International Organization for Standardization (ISO), 2018a; OSHA, 2015; International Atomic Energy Agency, 2016). Transparent reporting systems, especially those enabled by mobile or QR-based tools, strengthen organizational learning and accountability (Geller, 2001; Wei et al., 2023).

At the same time, success stories highlight the benefits of proactive strategies, from PPE programs and blended training approaches to QC safeguards and health surveillance systems that catch noncompliant batches or early signs of occupational illness (International Organization for Standardization (ISO), 2017b; SCCS—Scientific Committee on Consumer Safety, 2021; European Food Safety Authority, 2012; European Agency for Safety and Health at Work (EU-OSHA), 2020). Benchmarks from industry leaders such as L'Oréal and Beiersdorf show the impact of embedding safety into corporate culture, applying HACCP principles in production, and compiling robust CPSRs to support product authorization (L'Oréal, 2023a; European Parliament and Council, 2009; Gądarowska et al., 2022). Their integration of predictive toxicology tools, including QSAR models and in silico platforms, demonstrates how innovation can reduce animal testing while ensuring rigorous risk assessment (Patlewicz et al., 2018; OECD, 2021a).

Technology-driven practices now form a cornerstone of modern safety systems. Digital SDS platforms, QR-coded chemical labeling, wearable VOC sensors, and IoT-enabled dashboards provide realtime hazard visibility and streamlined emergency response (Ta et al., 2010). Predictive analytics and machine learning applied to near-miss data offer preventive insights, while digital training and simulation tools enhance preparedness across all staff levels (Hale et al., 2015; Pairote et al., 2025).

Key enablers of success therefore include:

- **Robust training programs**, combining theoretical, practical, and digital modules that cultivate critical thinking and readiness (Wu et al., 2008; Wei et al., 2023).
- **Deployment of digital tools**, from SDS platforms and wearables to automated exposure monitoring, that close information gaps and enhance decision-making (Ezenwa et al., 2022).
- **A strong safety culture**, driven by leadership and reinforced by recognition systems, where hazard reporting and corrective actions are embraced (Kimble-Hill, 2021).

Organizations that invest holistically—in systems, infrastructure, and people—minimize occupational risks while enhancing product integrity, employee satisfaction, and brand reputation. In a consumer-facing and rapidly evolving industry, safety is inseparable from innovation, ethics, and sustainability. The dual lens of failures and successes creates a powerful learning cycle: incidents provide opportunities to reassess systems and assumptions, while successful interventions offer blueprints for sector-wide improvement and knowledge exchange (Pedrosa et al., 2025; American Chemical Society, 2012; Ezenwa et al., 2022).

Ultimately, by embracing continuous learning, benchmarking excellence, and leveraging technology, laboratories foster environments where safety is not an afterthought but a defining principle of scientific excellence and professional integrity (Ezenwa et al., 2022; A Linden, 2025).

8 Conclusions and recommendations

This chapter has highlighted the multifaceted nature of occupational safety and toxicological risk management in cosmetic industry laboratories. From regulatory compliance and chemical hazard identification to toxicological assessment and emergency preparedness, each element plays a vital role in safeguarding both personnel and end users (Fernandez-Muniz et al., 2009). The integration of green chemistry principles, applied biochemical methods, and sustainability-focused strategies reflects a growing shift toward ethical and responsible innovation (Colberg et al., 2022). Case studies and best practices further illustrate how proactive safety systems can prevent incidents, enhance performance, and align with global regulatory and sustainability standards (Adekunle, 2025).

A recurring theme throughout this chapter is the importance of interdisciplinary integration, linking toxicology, safety culture, and continuous training into a cohesive operational framework (Neal and Griffin, 2006; Reason, 2000). Laboratories that prioritize education, invest in technological tools, and cultivate open communication tend to outperform those that view safety as a static compliance task (Cooper, 2000; Clarke, 2013). Empowering all levels of staff to participate in safety initiatives—from reporting hazards to shaping policy—strengthens both resilience and accountability. These principles must be embedded not only in daily routines but also in longterm strategic planning (Burke et al., 2006; Ezenwa et al., 2022).

Based on the findings and discussion, several key recommendations are proposed for cosmetic laboratories. First, an ongoing toxicological review process should be institutionalized to ensure that all ingredients—new and existing—are regularly evaluated in light of emerging scientific data. This review must incorporate advances in computational toxicology, such as QSAR models, and integrate them with *in vitro* test results and RAX techniques (Ball et al., 2016; Patlewicz et al., 2014). Continuous review supports compliance with evolving regulations and fosters consumer and worker safety.

Second, the substitution of high-risk substances, such as known allergens, endocrine disruptors, or sensitizers, with safer alternatives must be prioritized during formulation and procurement (GreenScreen methodologies; Maertens, 2022). These substitutions not only reduce occupational and consumer risks but also improve regulatory standing and marketability. Embracing the principles of green chemistry—such as using biodegradable solvents, nontoxic surfactants, and plant-derived active ingredients—can lead to more sustainable production practices and reduced environmental impact (Anastas and Zimmerman, 2003).

The digital transformation of SMSs is essential for managing the increasing complexity of cosmetic laboratories. Digital platforms streamline access to SDSs, chemical inventory tracking, incident reporting, and regulatory compliance monitoring. Tools such as ChemInventory, SciShield (formerly BioRAFT), and Quartzy enable realtime data sharing, automated alerts, and centralized documentation, significantly reducing human error and administrative burden (ChemInventory, 2025; SciShield Inc, 2024; Quartzy Inc, 2025).

Mobile-accessible systems improve responsiveness during emergencies and support efficient auditing. Digital trend analysis also helps identify recurring hazards and benchmark safety performance across departments. As laboratories adopt cloud-based and AI-integrated safety tools, SMSs evolve from a reactive framework to a predictive, data-driven system (Park and Kang, 2024).

Beyond digital transformation and AI tools, regulatory and scientific innovations have also reshaped safety practices in the cosmetics sector. Looking to the future, emerging technologies offer powerful tools to enhance laboratory safety. AI-driven safety monitoring systems can identify patterns in incident data, predict risk hotspots, and automate hazard recognition through image and sensor analysis (Park and Kang, 2024; Fan et al., 2024). Realtime exposure analytics, supported by wearable sensors or connected environmental monitoring devices, can alert staff to dangerous conditions before thresholds are breached (Shajari et al., 2023).

In addition to current practices and emerging technologies, ongoing research is necessary to address persistent and emerging toxicological challenges. Scientists in the field of occupational toxicology should strive for ongoing awareness and improvements in the safety of chemical goods. Throughout the upcoming years, more focus will be paid to a few specific concerns that merit it. Certain concerns pertain to toxicology as a whole, whilst others are particularly focused on occupational toxicity. Even though *in vitro* toxicology has already seen some notable advancements (Anadón et al., 2014), it is important to remember that there is still more work to be done and that the safety of people cannot be endangered.

Given that most toxicological data focus on individual chemicals and that individuals are exposed to multiple chemicals at once, the toxicity of mixtures continues to be a concern. This is a serious issue because it would be impossible to test every possible combination and permutation of chemicals that people could be exposed to. Advances in systems toxicology, in silico modeling, and machine learning may help address this challenge, but coordinated efforts in method development and validation are still required (Bloch et al., 2023; Sprinkle and Payne Sturges, 2021).

In addition, the identification of toxicity that may have gone unnoticed in the past as a result of poor assessment methods will receive more attention. It is also possible to predict that the data utilized for occupational chemical hazard assessment will get better with time. Enhancements to hazard assessment models would also have a significant positive impact on toxicology as a whole. Among the tools gaining traction in modern toxicology is physiologically based pharmacokinetic (PBK) modeling, which offers a refined approach to internal exposure estimation. A good example of modern toxicological refinement is the increasing use of PBK modeling. PBK models simulate how a chemical substance is absorbed, distributed, metabolized, and excreted (ADME) in the human body. These models integrate physiological parameters (such as organ volumes and blood flow rates) with chemical-specific properties (such as solubility and metabolic rates) to estimate internal concentrations over time.

To illustrate, one might think of the human body as a network of interconnected reservoirs (organs), with a chemical acting like a dye dropped into the main water supply (the bloodstream). PBK modeling traces how this dye travels to different tanks (liver, kidneys, skin), how much accumulates, how quickly it's processed or excreted, and whether it reaches a toxic threshold in any location. This simulation helps predict internal exposures based on external doses and is especially valuable for nonanimal, in silico safety evaluations (Thiel et al., 2015).

In the cosmetics industry, PBK models are being applied to estimate systemic exposure resulting from dermal absorption of ingredients, particularly in risk assessments for substances with potential endocrine-disrupting or carcinogenic effects (Paini et al., 2019). They also help interpret results from *in vitro* assays by bridging the gap between observed cellular effects and reallife human exposure scenarios. Although data-intensive, PBK models are increasingly supported by publicly available databases and are expected to become a cornerstone of quantitative risk assessment in regulatory toxicology (Caldwell et al., 2012).

Taken together, these developments highlight the need for both institutional commitment and continuous adaptation to ensure the effective protection of laboratory personnel.

The cosmetics industry has seen significant growth in recent years, utilizing a wide range of chemicals to improve the appearance and health of skin, hair, and nails. These substances can be of natural or synthetic origin, and each has specific functions. Safety and efficacy are critical for each ingredient used in the manufacture of cosmetic products, as they must be nonirritating and nontoxic to consumers and workers.

On account of this, the creation of new alternative methods (NAMs) and new genetic regulatory assessment (NGRA) in the cosmetic industry has been a major focus of research and innovation. Consumers' differing opinions about the morality of using animals in products and legislative changes in Europe have been the main forces behind this growth. To guarantee that judgments on consumer safety are made, the primary goal is to undertake risk assessment using uncertainty analysis based on adequate evidence produced by pertinent human NAMs. This strategy seeks to improve consumer safety and transparency while furthering the legal and scientific communities' evolution toward cosmetic regulation.

Despite the promising advances of new approach methodologies (NAMs), their broad implementation in the cosmetics industry faces several challenges. One significant barrier is institutional inertia, as regulatory agencies in many jurisdictions still rely heavily on traditional animal-based toxicity data. The lack of internationally harmonized protocols and validation standards also complicates regulatory acceptance, slowing the integration of NAMs into official safety assessments. In addition, there are logistical and technical hurdles, including the need for high-quality human-relevant data and the limited availability of trained personnel to interpret complex outputs from *in vitro* and in silico systems.

Examples of NAM tools already in use include the OECD QSAR Toolbox, which facilitates RAX and chemical grouping based on molecular structure, and RhE models, such as EpiSkin and SkinEthic, which are widely adopted for skin irritation and corrosion testing. High-throughput screening platforms like ToxCast and microphysiological systems (organ-on-chip) are also being explored for their potential in complex endpoint predictions. Although progress is evident, overcoming these systemic challenges is essential for the widespread, reliable adoption of NAMs in regulatory toxicology and product development within the cosmetics sector (Thomas et al., 2024; Westmoreland et al., 2022; Gilmour et al., 2023).

From the above research, we conclude that it is very important for every company to follow the regulations concerning the safety of employees, as well as to comply with the limits set by the legislation regarding occupational toxicology. Safe working conditions are very important, as well as the training of the staff to avoid any accidents and exposure to risks. The field of occupational toxicology can be constantly enriched with new practices for the protection of workers, as well as with expanded research to identify potential hazards in the cosmetics industry. The evolution of analytical methods is particularly important for research on the toxicology of chemicals with which workers in the cosmetics industry come into contact.

Study Questions

1. How do the EU Cosmetics Regulation (EC No. 1223/2009), MoCRA in the United States, and CSAR in China differ in their approaches to animal testing and product safety requirements?
2. What role do SDSs and the GHS play in ensuring chemical safety in cosmetic laboratories?
3. In what ways do new approach methodologies (NAMs) and next-generation risk assessment (NGRA) transform the traditional toxicological evaluation of cosmetic substances?
4. How can incidents and near-miss reports in cosmetic laboratories contribute to building a proactive safety culture?
5. What are the main challenges associated with regulating "natural" cosmetics, and how do issues such as greenwashing and the lack of validated analytical methods complicate consumer protection?

Glossary

AOP (adverse outcome pathway) Conceptual framework describing the progression from a molecular initiating event to an adverse health effect.
CLP (Classification, Labeling and Packaging Regulation) EU regulation harmonizing classification and labeling of chemicals based on their hazards.
Cosmetovigilance Postmarket monitoring system for identifying, reporting, and evaluating adverse effects from cosmetic products.
CPSR (Cosmetic Product Safety Report) Mandatory EU safety assessment document required before a cosmetic product is marketed.
DNEL (Derived No-Effect Level) Estimated exposure threshold below which no adverse effects are expected.
GHS (Globally Harmonized System of Classification and Labeling of Chemicals) International system for standardized hazard classification and communication.
GLP (Good Laboratory Practice) Quality system ensuring the reliability, integrity, and reproducibility of laboratory studies.
GMP (Good Manufacturing Practice) Standards ensuring that cosmetic products are consistently produced and controlled for quality and safety.
MoCRA (Modernization of Cosmetics Regulation Act) 2022 US law reforming cosmetic regulation, including facility registration, product listing, and safety substantiation.
MoS (margin of safety) Ratio of a toxicological threshold (e.g., NOAEL) to estimated human exposure; used to determine product safety.
NAMs (new approach methodologies) Nonanimal testing strategies including *in vitro* assays, computational models, and integrated approaches.
NGRA (next-generation risk assessment) Risk assessment paradigm combining NAMs, exposure science, and systems toxicology to ensure human safety.
NOAEL (No Observed Adverse Effect Level) Highest tested dose at which no adverse effects are observed in toxicological studies.
PBK (physiologically based kinetic modeling) Computational approach simulating absorption, distribution, metabolism, and excretion of chemicals in humans.
QSAR (quantitative structure–activity relationship) Computational modeling approach predicting chemical activity or toxicity based on molecular structure.
TTC (threshold of toxicological concern) Risk assessment approach setting generic exposure thresholds below which chemicals are considered safe.

Acknowledgments

Not applicable. This work was conducted without external funding or external assistance.

AI Disclosure

During the preparation of this work, the author(s) used ChatGPT to make syntax and grammatical corrections. After using this tool/service, the author(s) reviewed and edited the content as needed and take(s) full responsibility for the content of the publication.

References

EU's digital product passport: advancing transparency and sustainability, 2024. How to Leverage Open Data for Clearer Product Insights and Improved Environmental Practices. https://data.europa.eu/en/news-events/news/eus-digital-product-passport-advancing-transparency-and-sustainability.

Adekunle, K.A., 2025. Operational efficiency meets safety: leveraging industrial management principles to strengthen EHS performance. Multidiscip. J. Healthc. 2 (1), 114–144. https://researchcorridor.org/index.php/mjh/article/view/537.

Adkins, L., Adkins, R.A., 1998. Handbook to life in ancient Greece. Oxford University Press.

Alnuqaydan, A.M., 2024. The dark side of beauty: an in-depth analysis of the health hazards and toxicological impact of synthetic cosmetics and personal care products. Front. Public Health 12, 1439027. doi:10.3389/fpubh.2024.1439027.

Alshreef, B., 2025. The ISO 45001: a systematic review of global adoption trends, outcomes, and barriers (2018–2023). Int. J. Innov. Res. Sci. Stud. 2617-6548. 8 (5), 1127–1136. doi:10.53894/ijirss.v8i5.8970.

Altıokka, İ., 2022. Safety in cosmetics and cosmetovigilance: current regulation in Turkiye. Turk. J. Pharm. Sci. 19 (5), 610–617. doi:10.4274/tjps.galenos.2021.40697.

American Chemical Society, 2012. What Is Safety Culture? Creating Safety Cultures in Academic Institutions, ACS Institute, (Accessed 26 August 2025) Available from: https://institute.acs.org/acs-center/lab-safety/safety-basics-and-ramp/what-is-safety-culture.html.

American Conference of Governmental Industrial Hygienists, 2021. Personal Monitoring and Task-based Exposure Assessment, ACGIH, (Accessed 26 August 2025) Available from: https://www.acgih.org/science/tlv-bei-guidelines/committees/.

American Industrial Hygiene Association, 2020. Laboratory Health and Safety Guidance, AIHA, (Accessed 26 August 2025) Available from: https://www.aiha.org/get-involved/aiha-volunteer-groups/laboratory-safety-committee.

American Red Cross, 2021. First Aid/CPR/AED Participant's Manual. https://www.redcross.org/content/dam/redcross/training-services/first-aid-cpr-aed-participant-manual.pdf.

Anadón, A., Martínez, M.A., Castellano, V., Martínez-Larrañaga, M.R., 2014. The role of in vitro methods as alternatives to animals in toxicity testing. Expert Opin. Drug Metab. Toxicol. 10 (1), 67–79. doi:10.1517/17425255.2014.854329.

Andersen, M.E., 1995. Development of physiologically based pharmacokinetic and physiologically based pharmacodynamic models for applications in toxicology and risk assessment. Toxicol. Lett. 79 (1–3), 35–44. doi:10.1016/0378-4274(95)03355-O.

ANSI/ISEA, 2014. American National Standard for Emergency Eyewash and Shower Equipment (ANSI/ISEA Z358.1–2014). doi:10.1109/IEEESTD.2014.6785142.

AOCS, 2024. Surfactants and Their Applications in Cosmetics. American Oil Chemists' Society. Available from: https://www.aocs.org/resource/an-introduction-to-cosmetic-technology/.

Api, A.M., Basketter, D.A., Cadby, P.A., Cano, M.F., Ellis, G., Gerberick, G.F., Griem, P., McNamee, P.M., Ryan, C.A., Safford, R., 2008. Dermal sensitization quantitative risk assessment (QRA) for fragrance ingredients. Regul. Toxicol. Pharmacol. 10960295. 52 (1), 3–23. doi:10.1016/j.yrtph.2007.10.008.

Atallah, C., Abiad, A.E., Abiad, M.E., Nakad, M., Assaf, J.C., 2025. Bioengineered skin microbiome: the next frontier in personalized cosmetics. Cosmetics. 2079-9284. 12 (5), 205. doi:10.3390/cosmetics12050205.

Axios, 2024. "New Era" of Cosmetics' Regulation: FDA Wields New Powers Over Makeup Companies. Axios. Available from: https://www.axios.com.

Baker, N.A., Chaffin, D.B., 2021. Ergonomics and the prevention of musculoskeletal disorders in laboratories: a review. J. Occup. Rehabil. 31 (1), 1–10. doi:10.1007/s10926-020-09935-9.

Ball, N., Cronin, M.T.D., Shen, J., Blackburn, K., Booth, E.D., Bouhifd, M., Donley, E., Egnash, L., Hastings, C., Juberg, D.R., Kleensang, A., Kleinstreuer, N., Kroese, E.D., Lee, A.C., Luechtefeld, T., Maertens, A., Marty, S., Naciff, J.M., Palmer, J., Pamies, D., Penman, M., Richarz, A.N., Russo, D.P., Stuard, S.B., Patlewicz, G., Van Ravenzwaay, B., Wu, S., Zhu, H., Hartung, T., 2016. Toward good read-across practice (GRAP) guidance. Altex. 18688551. 33 (2), 149–166. Available from: http://www.altex.ch/resources/altex_2016_2_149_166_Ball1.pdf. doi:10.14573/altex.1601251.

Barnes, T.M., Mijaljica, D., Townley, J.P., Spada, F., Harrison, I.P., 2021. Vehicles for drug delivery and cosmetic moisturizers: review and comparison. Pharmaceutics. 19994923. 13 (12). Available from: http://www.mdpi.com/journal/pharmaceutics. doi:10.3390/pharmaceutics13122012.

Barthe, M., Bavoux, C., Finot, F., Mouche, I., Cuceu-Petrenci, C., Forreryd, A., Chérouvrier Hansson, A., Johansson, H., Lemkine, G.F., Thénot, J.-P., Osman-Ponchet, H., 2021. Safety testing of cosmetic products: overview of established methods and new approach methodologies (NAMs). Cosmetics. 2079-9284. 8 (2), 50. doi:10.3390/cosmetics8020050.

Bayramova, A., Edwards, D.J., Roberts, C., Rillie, I., 2023. Constructs of leading indicators: a synthesis of safety literature. J. Saf. Res. 00224375. 85, 469–484. Available from: http://www.sciencedirect.com/science/journal/00224375. doi:10.1016/j.jsr.2023.04.015.

Beauty Labelling Guide, 2022. Key requirements under EU Regulation 1223/2009. Cosmetics Europe. Available from: https://cosmeticseurope.eu/files/8814/6407/5369/Guidelines_on_Cosmetic_Product_Labelling_-_2011.pdf

Beiersdorf, 2024. Sustainability Reporting on Employee Development and Safety Integration. Available from: https://www.beiersdorf.com/sustainability/reporting.

Bergeson, L.L., Hutton, C.N., 2022. NASEM Recommends EPA Conduct Ecological Risk Assessment of UV Filters Found in Sunscreen. Lawrence L. Bergeson & Associates. Available from: https://www.lawbc.com/nasem-recommends-that-epa-conduct-ecological-risk-assessment-of-uv-filters-found-in-sunscreen-including-titanium-oxide-and-zinc-oxide.

Bernasconi, S., Angelucci, A., Aliverti, A., 2022. A scoping review on wearable devices for environmental monitoring and their application for health and wellness. Sensors. 1424-8220. 22 (16), 5994. doi:10.3390/s22165994.

Bird, T., Egilman, D., 2024. Is there asbestos in your makeup? Why women with cancer are suing big beauty brands. The Guardian. June 10. https://www.theguardian.com/lifeandstyle/article/2024/jun/10/is-there-asbestos-in-your-makeup-why-women-with-cancer-are-suing-big-beauty-brands.

Bloch, D., Diel, P., Epe, B., Hellwig, M., Lampen, A., Mally, A., Marko, D., Fernández, M.A.V., Guth, S., Roth, A., Marchan, R., Ghallab, A., Cadenas, C., Nell, P., Vartak, N., van Thriel, C., Luch, A., Schmeisser, S., Herzler, M., Landsiedel, R., Leist, M., Marx-Stoelting, P., Tralau, T., Hengstler, J.G., 2023. Basic concepts of mixture toxicity and relevance for risk evaluation and regulation. Arch. Toxicol. 14320738. 97 (11), 3005–3017. Available from: https://www.springer.com/journal/204. doi:10.1007/s00204-023-03565-6.

Brooks, R., Tassonyi, E., 2023. FDA Regulation of Cosmetics and Personal Care Products: overview of Authority Under the Modernization of Cosmetics Regulation Act of 2022 (MoCRA). Congressional Research Service Report No. R46765. https://crsreports.congress.gov/product/pdf/R/R46765.

Burdock, G.A., 2024. Review of the standards of proof (of safety) for FDA regulated consumer products and how the generally recognized as safe criteria could be applied to cosmetics. Regul. Toxicol. Pharmacol. 02732300. 149, 105603. doi:10.1016/j.yrtph.2024.105603.

Bury, D., Head, J., Keller, D., Klaric, M., Rose, J., 2021. The Threshold of Toxicological Concern (TTC) is a pragmatic tool for the safety assessment: case studies of cosmetic ingredients with low consumer exposure. Regul. Toxicol. Pharmacol. 02732300. 123, 104964. doi:10.1016/j.yrtph.2021.104964.

Caldwell, J.C., Evans, M.V., Krishnan, K., 2012. Cutting edge PBPK models and analyses: providing the basis for future modeling efforts and bridges to emerging toxicology paradigms. J. Toxicol. 16878205. 2012. doi:10.1155/2012/852384.

Carve, M., Nugegoda, D., Allinson, G., Shimeta, J., 2021. A systematic review and ecological risk assessment for organic ultraviolet filters in aquatic environments. Environ. Pollut. 02697491. 268 (Pt B), 115894. doi:10.1016/j.envpol.2020.115894.

Centers for Disease Control and Prevention, 2023. Chemical safety in the workplace. Available from: https://www.cdc.gov/niosh/topics/chemical-safety.

CEPRASRL, 2024. Labelling Information and Instructions According to Article 19 of Regulation (EC) No 1223/2009. Available from: https://www.ceprasrl.it/en/sectors/chemicals-compliance/cosmetic/labelling-info-and-instructions/.

Chatzigianni, M., Pavlou, P., Siamidi, A., Vlachou, M., Varvaresou, A., Papageorgiou, S., 2022. Environmental impacts due to the use of sunscreen products: a mini-review. Ecotoxicology. 0963-9292. 31 (9), 1331–1345. doi:10.1007/s10646-022-02592-w.

ChemInventory, 2025. Laboratory chemical inventory software for real-time tracking and SDS integration. Antipodes Sci. Available from: https://www.cheminventory.net/.

Chemlinked, 2021a. Will China Remove Mandatory Animal Testing for Imported General Cosmetics? Chemlinked by REACH24H. https://cosmetic.chemlinked.com/news/cosmetic-reports/china-lifts-mandatory-animal-testing-general-cosmetics

Chemlinked, 2024. China Announces Full Digitization of Cosmetics Registration and New Ingridient Registration/Notification Materials. Chemlinked. Available from: https://cosmetic.chemlinked.com/news/cosmetic-news/china-announces-full-digitization-of-cosmetics-and-new-ingredient-registrationnotification-materials.

Chemlinked, 2025. China Cosmetic Safety Assessment Regulations. Chemlinked. [Subscription access].

ChemSafetyPro, 2018. What are Margin of Exposure (MOE) and Margin of Safety (MoS) and How to Calculate. Available from: https://www.chemsafetypro.com/Topics/CRA/margin_of_safety_MOS_margin_of_exposure_MOE_difference_chemical_risk_assessment.html.

Chen, C., Campbell, K.D., Negi, I., Iglesias, R.A., Owens, P., Tao, N., Tsow, F., Forzani, E., 2012. A new sensor for the assessment of personal exposure to volatile organic compounds. Atmos. Environ. 54, 679–687. doi:10.1016/j.atmosenv.2012.01.048.

CIR (Cosmetic Ingredient Review), 2023. Safety Assessments. Available from: https://www.cir-safety.org.

CIRS Group, 2024. Understanding Labeling Requirements for Cosmetics in the EU and UK. Available from: https://www.cirs-group.com/en/cosmetics/understanding-labeling-requirements-for-cosmetics-in-the-eu-and-the-uk.

Clarke, S., 2013. Safety leadership: a meta-analytic review of transformational and transactional leadership styles as antecedents of safety behaviours. J. Occup. Organ. Psychol. 0963-1798. 86 (1), 22–49. doi:10.1111/j.2044-8325.2012.02064.x.

CMA ComplianceGate, 2024. Cosmetic Notification Requirements in the European Union: CPNP Explained. ComplianceGate. Available from: https://www.compliancegate.com/cosmetic-notification-requirements-european-union/.

Colberg, J., Hii, K.K., Koenig, S.G., 2022. Importance of green and sustainable chemistry in the chemical industry. Org. Process Res. Dev. 1520586X. 26 (8), 2176–2178. Available from: http://pubs.acs.org/journal/oprdfk. doi:10.1021/acs.oprd.2c00171.

Cooper, M.D., 2000. Towards a model of safety culture. Saf. Sci. 36 (2), 111–136. doi:10.1016/S0925-7535(00)00035-7.

Cornell University EHS, 2020. Administrative Controls—No Cosmetics in Lab. Cornell EHS Safety Manual. Available from: https://ehs.cornell.edu/research-safety/chemical-safety/laboratory-safety-manual/chapter-4-administrative-controls.

CosmeDesk, 2023. Safety Evaluation of Cosmetic Ingredients: Risk Characterization. CosmeDesk Blog. Available from: https://www.cosmedesk.com.

Cosmedesk, 2024a. The Cosmetic Product Safety Report (CPSR). CosmeDesk Blog. Available from: https://www.cosmedesk.com/blog/understanding-cosmetic-legal-safety-requirements-the-cosmetic-product-safety-report-cpsr/

Cosmetic Chemist Safety, 2019. Risks in Cosmetic Formulation Labs. Stop Carcinogens at Work. Available from: https://stopcarcinogensatwork.eu/occupations/cosmetic-chemist/.

Cronin, M.T.D., Cable, S., Desaintes, C., Escher, S.E., Hessel, E., Fritsche, E., Kern, P., Maxwell, G., Ouedraogo, G., Sobanski, T., Wehr, M., White, A., 2026. Report on the European partnership for alternative approaches to animal testing (EPAA) "New Approach Methodology (NAMs) user forum, 30–31 October 2024, Helsinki, Finland. Regul. Toxicol. Pharmacol. 10960295. 164. Available from: https://www.sciencedirect.com/science/journal/02732300. doi:10.1016/j.yrtph.2025.105980.

Crowell, 2023. FDA Launches Cosmetics Direct and Issues Final Guidance on Facility Registration & Product Listings. Crowell & Moring. Available from: https://www.crowell.com/en/insights/client-alerts/fda-launches-cosmetics-direct-and-issues-final-guidance-on-facility-registration-and-product-listings-required-under-mocra.

CTPA (Cosmetic, Toiletry and Perfumery Association), 2023. Natural Ingredients. Available from: https://www.ctpa.org.uk/natural-ingredients.

Darbre, P.D., Harvey, P.W., 2008. Paraben esters: review of recent studies of endocrine toxicity, absorption, esterase and human exposure, and discussion of potential human health risks. J. Appl. Toxicol. 10991263. 28 (5), 561–578. doi:10.1002/jat.1358.

Datta, S., Baudouin, C., Brignole-Baudouin, F., Denoyer, A., Cortopassi, G.A., 2017. The eye drop preservative benzalkonium chloride potently induces mitochondrial dysfunction and preferentially affects LHON mutant cells. Invest. Ophthalmol. Vis. Sci. 58 (4), 2406–2412. doi:10.1167/iovs.16-20903.

DeJoy, D.M., Della, L.J., Vandenberg, R.J., Wilson, M.G., 2010. Making work safer: testing a model of social exchange and safety management. J. Saf. Res. 00224375. 41 (2), 163–171. Available from: http://www.sciencedirect.com/science/journal/00224375. doi:10.1016/j.jsr.2010.02.001.

DeMasi, A., Elston, H., Langerman, N., 2022. Safety data sheets: challenges for authors, expectations for end-users. ACS Chem. Health Saf. 1871-5532. 29 (4), 369–377. doi:10.1021/acs.chas.2c00015.

Deng, Y., Chen, C., Xian, X., Tsow, F., Verma, G., McConnell, R., Fruin, S., Tao, N., Forzani, E., 2016. A novel wireless wearable volatile organic compound (VOC) monitoring device with disposable sensors. Sensors. 1424-8220. 16 (12), 2060. doi:10.3390/s16122060.

Detmer, A., 2010. A Guidance Document on Microbiological Control of Cosmetic Products. Danish Ministry of Environment and Food. Available from: https://www2.mst.dk/udgiv/publications/2010/978-87-92668-66-0/html/helepubl_eng.htm.

Di Guardo, A., Trovato, F., Cantisani, C., Dattola, A., Nisticò, S.P., Pellacani, G., Paganelli, A., 2025. Artificial intelligence in cosmetic formulation: predictive modeling for safety, tolerability, and regulatory perspectives. Cosmetics. 2079-9284. 12 (4), 157. doi:10.3390/cosmetics12040157.

Duffy, M.A., Tronson, N.C., Eisenberg, D., 2021. Supporting mental health and productivity within labs. Neuron. 10974199. 109 (20), 3206–3210. Available from: http://www.cell.com/neuron/home. doi:10.1016/j.neuron.2021.08.021.

Dunn, A.L., Decker, D.M., Cartaya-Marin, C.P., Cooley, J., Finster, D.C., Hunter, K.P., Jacques, D.R.N., Kimble-Hill, A., Maclachlan, J.L., Redden, P., Sigmann, S.B., Situma, C., 2023. Reducing risk: strategies to advance laboratory safety through diversity, equity, inclusion, and respect. J. Am. Chem. Soc. 15205126. 145 (21), 11468–11471. Available from: http://pubs.acs.org/journal/jacsat. doi:10.1021/jacs.3c03627.

Ebmeyer, J., Najjar, A., Lange, D., Boettcher, M., Voß, S., Brandmair, K., Meinhardt, J., Kuehnl, J., Hewitt, N.J., Krueger, C.T., Schepky, A., 2024. Next generation risk assessment: an *ab initio* case study to assess the systemic safety of the cosmetic ingredient, benzyl salicylate, after dermal exposure. Front. Pharmacol. 15, 1345992. doi:10.3389/fphar.2024.1345992.

ECFR (Electronic Code of Federal Regulations), 2022. 21 CFR Part 701: Ingredient Declaration and Net Quantity Requirements. Available from: https://www.ecfr.gov/current/title-21/chapter-I/subchapter-G/part-701.

ECHA (European Chemicals Agency), 2022a. Guidance on the Compilation of Safety Data Sheets (Version 4.0). Available from: https://echa.europa.eu/documents/10162/2324906/sds_en.pdf.

ECHA (European Chemicals Agency), 2023b. Commission Regulation (EU) 2023/2055: Restriction of Microplastics Intentionally Added to Products. Available from: https://echa.europa.eu/hot-topics/microplastics.

ECHA (European Chemicals Agency), 2024a. Guidance on Information Requirements and Chemical Safety Assessment. Available from: https://echa.europa.eu/guidance-documents/guidance-on-information-requirements-and-chemical-safety-assessment.

EcoSistant, 2024. The Role and Obligations of the Responsible Person under Regulation 1223/2009. Available from: https://www.ecosistant.eu.

Ecovia, 2024. Sustainability Schemes and Ethical Labels in Cosmetics Industry. Available from: https://www.ecoviaint.com/sustainability-schemes-cosmetics-industry/.

Edmondson, A., 1999. Psychological safety and learning behavior in work teams. Adm. Sci. Q. 0001-8392. 44 (2), 350–383. doi:10.2307/2666999.

Emory, T.S., Maddox, J.C., Kradin, R.L., 2020. Malignant mesothelioma following repeated exposures to cosmetic talc: a case series of 75 patients. Am. J. Ind. Med. 10970274. 63 (6), 484–489. Available from: http://onlinelibrary.wiley.com/journal/10.1002/(ISSN)1097-0274. doi:10.1002/ajim.23106.

Environmental Working Group (EWG), 2017. "Natural" or Organic Cosmetics? Don't Trust Marketing Claims. Available from: https://www.ewg.org/news-insights/news/natural-or-organic-cosmetics-dont-trust-marketing-claims.

Environmental Working Group (EWG), 2023. The Toxic Twelve Chemicals and Contaminants in Cosmetics. Available from: https://www.ewg.org/the-toxic-twelve-chemicals-and-contaminants-in-cosmetics.

Eskes, C., et al, 2003. The ECVAM international validation study on in vitro tests for skin irritation: validity of the EPISKIN and EpiDerm assays and on the Skin Integrity Function Test. Altern. Lab Anim. 35, 559–601. Available from: https://pubmed.ncbi.nlm.nih.gov/18186667/.

EU SME Centre, 2021. GMP Certificate for Animal Testing Exemption for General Cosmetics. Available from: https://www.eusmecentre.org.cn/publications/gmp-certificate-for-animal-testing-exemption-for-general-cosmetics/.

European Agency for Safety and Health at Work (EU-OSHA), 2020. Health Surveillance at the Workplace: Depending on Risk. Available from: https://osha.europa.eu/en/publications/factsheets/health-surveillance-workplace.

European Agency for Safety and Health at Work (EU-OSHA), 2021. Worker Participation in the Management of Occupational Safety and Health—Qualitative Evidence from ESENER-2. Available from: https://osha.europa.eu/en/publications/worker-participation-management-occupational-safety-and-health

European Agency for Safety and Health at Work (EU-OSHA), 2022. Work-Related Stress: Nature and Management. Available from: https://oshwiki.osha.europa.eu/en/themes/work-related-stress-nature-and-management

European Chemicals Agency (ECHA), 2020. Guidance on Information Requirements and Chemical Safety Assessment. Available from: https://echa.europa.eu/guidance-documents

European Commission. 2020. Commission Regulation (EU) 2020/878 of 18 June 2020 amending Annex II to Regulation (EC) No 1907/2006 of the European Parliament and of the Council concerning the Registration, Evaluation, Authorisation and Restriction of Chemicals (REACH). Official Journal of the European Union, L203, 28–58.

European Commission, 2023. Green Claims—EU Initiative Against Greenwashing. Available from: https://environment.ec.europa.eu/topics/circular-economy/green-claims_en.

European Commission, n.d.a. Cosmetic Product Notification Portal (CPNP). Available from: https://single-market-economy.ec.europa.eu/sectors/cosmetics/cosmetic-product-notification-portal_en

European Committee for Standardization, 2004. EN 14470-1: Safety Storage Cabinets—Part 1: Cabinets for Flammable Liquids.

European Food Safety Authority Scientific Committee, 2025. Guidance on the use of read across for chemical safety assessment. EFSA J. 23 (2), e09586. https://www.efsa.europa.eu/en/efsajournal/pub/9586.

European Food Safety Authority, 2012. Lead dietary exposure in the European population. EFSA J. 10 (7), 2831. https://www.efsa.europa.eu/en/efsajournal/pub/2831.

European Parliament and Council, 2009. Regulation (EC) No 1223/2009 of the European Parliament and of the Council on cosmetic products. Off. J. Eur. Union L342, 59–209. Available from: https://eur-lex.europa.eu/legal-content/EN/TXT/?uri=CELEX%3A32009R1223.

Evans, L., 2024. The green claims directive: the future legal framework for advertising with environmental claims. Eur. Food Feed Law Rev. 19, 174–187.

Ezenwa, S., Talpade, A.D., Ghanekar, P., Joshi, R., Devaraj, J., Ribeiro, F.H., Mentzer, R., 2022. Toward improved safety culture in academic and industrial chemical laboratories: an assessment and recommendation of best practices. ACS Chem. Health Saf. 29 (2), 202–213. doi:10.1021/acs.chas.1c00064.

Fan, Y.L., Hsu, C.H., Wu, J.Y., Tsai, Y.Y., Chen, W.J., Lee, M.S., Hsu, F.R., Liao, L.D., 2024. Enhancing safety with an AI-empowered assessment and monitoring system for BSL-3 facilities. Heliyon 11 (1), e40855. doi:10.1016/j.heliyon.2024.e40855.

Federal Trade Commission (FTC), 2023. Fair Packaging and Labeling Act requirements. Available from: https://www.ftc.gov/legal-library/browse/rules/fair-packaging-labeling-act-regulations-under-section-4-fair-packaging-labeling-act

Federal Trade Commission (FTC), 2025. FTC's Endorsement Guides: What People Are Asking. Available from: https://www.ftc.gov/business-guidance/resources/ftcs-endorsement-guides

Fernandez-Muniz, B., Montes-Peon, J.M., Vazquez-Ordas, C.J., 2009. Relation between occupational safety management and firm performance. Saf. Sci. 47 (7), 980–991. doi:10.1016/j.ssci.2008.10.022.

Ficheux, A.S., Gomez-Berrada, M.P., Roudot, A.C., Ferret, P.J., 2019. Consumption and exposure to finished cosmetic products: a systematic review. Food Chem. Toxicol. 124, 280–299. doi:10.1016/j.fct.2018.11.060.

Filaire, E., Nachat-Kappes, R., Laporte, C., Harmand, M.F., Simon, M., Poinsot, C., 2022. Alternative in vitro models used in the main safety tests of cosmetic products and new challenges. Int. J. Cosmet. Sci. 44 (6), 604–613. doi:10.1111/ics.12803.

Foley, E., 2019. The cosmetic industry: comparing oversight in the European Union and the United States. Creighton Int. Comp. Law J. Available from: https://creighton-intl-comp-law-journal.scholasticahq.com/article/74351.

Ford, R.A., Domeyer, B., Easterday, O., Maier, K., Middleton, J., 2000. Criteria for development of a database for safety evaluation of fragrance ingredients. Regul. Toxicol. Pharmacol. 31 (2 Pt 1), 166–181. doi:10.1006/rtph.1999.1362.

Franco-Gil, M.E., Graça, A., Martins, A., Marto, J., Ribeiro, H.M., 2024. Emollients in dermatological creams: early evaluation for tailoring formulation and therapeutic performance. Int. J. Pharm. 653. Article 123825. doi:10.1016/j.ijpharm.2024.123825.

Fruhen, L.S., Mearns, K.J., Flin, R., Kirwan, B., 2014. Safety intelligence: an exploration of senior managers' characteristics. Saf. Sci. 62, 530–538. doi:10.1016/j.apergo.2013.11.012.

Gądarowska, D., Kalka, J., Daniel-Wójcik, A., Mrzyk, I., 2022. Alternative methods for skin-sensitization assessment. Toxics 10 (12), 740. doi:10.3390/toxics10120740.

Geller, E.S., 2001. The Psychology of Safety Handbook, CRC Press.

Geller, E.S., 2005. Behavior-based safety and occupational risk management. Behav. Modif. 29 (3), 539–561.

Gershon, R.R.M., Vlahov, D., Felknor, S.A., Vesley, D., Johnson, P.C., Delclos, G.L., Murphy, L.R., 1995. Compliance with universal precautions among health care workers at three regional hospitals. Am. J. Infect. Control. 23 (4), 225–236. doi:10.1016/0196-6553(95)90067-5.

Gilmour, N., Kern, P., Casey, W., 2023. Applying a next generation risk assessment framework for skin sensitisation to inconsistent new approach methodology information. ALTEX 40 (3), 439–451. doi:10.14573/altex.2211161.

Goebel, C., Aeby, P., Ade, N., Alépée, N., Aptula, A., Araki, D., et al, 2012. Guiding principles for the implementation of non-animal safety assessment approaches for cosmetics: sskin sensitisation. Regul. Toxicol. Pharmacol. 63 (1), 40–52. doi:10.1016/j.yrtph.2012.02.007.

GOV.UK, 2023. Regulation (EC) No 1223/2009 and Cosmetic Products Enforcement Regulations 2013 (NI/GB). Department for Business, Energy & Industrial Strategy. https://www.gov.uk/government/publications/cosmetic-products-enforcement-regulations-2013/regulation-20091223-and-the-cosmetic-products-enforcement-regulations-2013-great-britain.

Guldenmund, F.W., 2010. (Mis)understanding safety culture and its relationship to safety management. Risk Anal. 30 (10), 1466–1480. doi:10.1111/j.1539-6924.2010.01452.x.

Haber, L.T., Bradley, M.A., Buerger, A.N., Behrsing, H., Burla, S., Clapp, P.W., Dotson, S., Fisher, C., Genco, K.R., Kruszewski, F.H., McCullough, S.D., Page, K.E., Patel, V., Pechacek, N., Roper, C., Sharma, M., Jarabek, A.M., 2024. New approach methodologies (NAMs) for the in vitro assessment of cleaning products for respiratory irritation: workshop report. Front. Toxicol. 6. Article 1431790. doi:10.3389/ftox.2024.1431790.

Hale, A., Borys, D., Else, D., 2015. Management of safety rules and procedures: a review of the literature. Saf. Sci. 80, 151–163. Available from: https://iosh.com/media/rbohgk2k/iosh-research-safety-rules-and-procedures-literature-review-full-report.pdf.

Hansen, S.F., Baun, A., 2012. European regulation affecting nanomaterials—review of limitations and future recommendations. Dose-Response. 10 (3), 364–383. doi:10.2203/dose-response.10-029.Hansen.

Hartlieb, S., Jones, B., 2009. Humanising business through ethical labelling: progress and paradoxes in the UK. J. Bus. Ethics. 88, 583–600. doi:10.1007/s10551-009-0125-x.

Harvard Office of Environmental Health and Safety (EH&S), 2017. Lab Emergency Response Guide. Harvard University EH&S. https://www.ehs.harvard.edu/sites/default/files/lab_emergency_response_guide_0.pdf.

Health Products Regulatory Authority (HPRA), 2024. Obligations of Responsible Persons—CPNP. https://certification-experts.com/gpsr-responsible-person/?gad_source=1&gad_campaignid=21120101984&gclid=CjwKCAiAlfvIBhA6EiwAcErpydUzjya6TZ_jXmffbqQJs-CsnBygzvuqyJGtlIeupFXncqcOx03CcxoCnAIQAvD_BwE

Hughes, J., Ferrett, E., Bale, P., 2020. Introduction to Health and Safety in Construction, sixth ed. Routledge. https://www.taylorfrancis.com/books/mono/10.4324/9780080469720/introduction-health-safety-construction-phil-hughes-ed-ferrett.

International Atomic Energy Agency, 2016. Leadership and Management for Safety: General Safety Requirements No. GSR Part 2. IAEA, Vienna. IAEA Safety Standards Series No. GSR Part 2 https://www-pub.iaea.org/MTCD/Publications/PDF/Pub1750web.pdf.

International Fragrance Association (IFRA), 2023. The IFRA Standards: A Global Risk Management System for Fragrance Safety (49th Amendment). IFRA. https://ifrafragrance.org.

International Labour Office. 2009. Guidelines on occupational safety and health management systems (ILO-OSH 2001), second ed. International Labour Organization. https://www.ilo.org/resource/guidelines-occupational-safety-and-health-management-systems-ilo-osh-2001.

International Organization for Standardization (ISO), 2007. ISO 22716:2007—Cosmetics—Good Manufacturing Practices (Gmp)—guidelines on Good Manufacturing Practices. ISO. https://www.iso.org/standard/36437.html.

International Organization for Standardization (ISO), 2017b. ISO 21149:2017—Cosmetics—Microbiology—Enumeration and Detection of Aerobic Mesophilic Bacteria. ISO. https://www.iso.org/standard/72240.html.

International Organization for Standardization (ISO), 2018a. ISO 45001:2018—Occupational Health and Safety Management systems—Requirements with Guidance for Use. ISO. https://www.iso.org/standard/63787.html.

ISO/IEC, 2017. ISO/IEC 17025:2017—General Requirements for the Competence of Testing and Calibration Laboratories. International Organization for Standardization. https://www.iso.org/standard/66912.html.

ISO, 2021. ISO 10075-1: Ergonomic Principles Related to Mental Workload—Part 1: General Issues and Concepts, Terms and Definitions. International Organization for Standardization. https://www.iso.org/standard/66900.html.

Johnson, P.I., Stapleton, H.M., Mukherjee, B., Hauser, R., Meeker, J.D., 2022. Chemicals of concern in personal care products used by diverse populations. J. Expo. Sci. Environ. Epidemiol. 32 (6), 918–928. doi:10.1038/s41370-022-00485-y.

Jones, G., 2008. Blonde and Blue-Eyed? Globalizing Beauty, c. 1945–c. 1980. Harvard Business School Working Paper No. 09-003. doi:10.1111/j.1468-0289.2007.00388.x.

Jones, S., Kirchsteiger, C., Bjerke, W., 1999. The importance of near miss reporting to further improve safety performance. J. Loss Prev. Process Ind. 12 (1), 59–67. doi:10.1016/S0950-4230(98)00038-2.

Kalofiri, P., Biskanaki, F., Kefala, V., Tertipi, N., Sfyri, E., Rallis, E., 2023. Endocrine disruptors in cosmetic products and the regulatory framework: public health implications. Cosmetics 10, 160. doi:10.3390/cosmetics10060160.

Katch, V., 2022. *The Dirt on "clean Cosmetics"*. Michigan Today. https://michigantoday.umich.edu/2022/03/25/the-dirt-on-clean-cosmetics/

Kaushik, M., Farooq, U., Ali, M.S., Ansari, M.J., Iqbal, Z., Mirza, M.A., 2023. Safety concern and regulatory status of chemicals used in cosmetics and personal care products. Dermato 3 (2), 131–157. doi:10.3390/dermato3020011.

Kavlock, R.J., Austin, C.P., Tice, R.R., 2009. Toxicity testing in the 21st century: implications for human health risk assessment. Risk Anal. 29 (4), 485–487. doi:10.1111/j.1539-6924.2008.01184.x.

Kavlock, R.J., Bahadori, T., Barton-Maclaren, T.S., Gwinn, M.R., Rasenberg, M., Thomas, R.S., 2018. Accelerating the pace of chemical risk assessment. Chem. Res. Toxicol. 31 (5), 287–290. doi:10.1021/acs.chemrestox.7b00339.

Kemsley, J., 2018. 10 years after Sheri Sangji's death, are academic labs any safer? Chem. Eng. News. https://cen.acs.org/safety/lab-safety/10-years-Sheri-Sangjis-death/97/i1.

Khan, M., Bhattacharya, S., Gogoi, S., Ahmad, S., 2024. Concept and requirements of establishing green laboratories: scoping review. Era's J. Med. Res. 11 (2), 260–268. doi:10.24041/ejmr2024.43.

Kimble-Hill, A.C., 2021. Incorporating identity safety into the laboratory safety culture. ACS Chem. Health Saf. 28 (5), 308–315. doi:10.1021/acs.chas.0c00109.

Klaschka, U., 2015. Naturally toxic: natural substances used in personal care products and cosmetics. Environ. Sci. Eur. 27. Article 10. doi:10.1186/s12302-014-0033-2.

Kohli, R., Mittal, A., Mittal, A., 2024. Adverse effects of cosmetics on women's health. BIO Web Conf. 86. Article 01026. doi:10.1051/bioconf/20248601026.

Kroes, R., Renwick, A.G., Feron, V., Galli, C.L., Gibney, M., Greim, H., Guy, R.H., Lhuguenot, J.C., van de Sandt, J.J., 2007. Application of the threshold of toxicological concern (TTC) to the safety evaluation of cosmetic ingredients. Food Chem. Toxicol. 45 (12), 2533–2562. doi:10.1016/j.fct.2007.06.021.

L'Oréal, 2021. Universal Registration Document 2021: Risk Factors and Control Environment. L'Oréal Finance https://loreal-finance.publispeak.com/2021-universal-registration-document/article/151/

L'Oréal, 2023a. Universal Registration Document 2023: Health & Safety Organization; Digital Hazard Communication Systems. L'Oréal Finance. https://www.loreal-finance.comhttps://loreal-finance.publispeak.com/2021-universal-registration-document/article/151/

Lin, X., Wang, Y., Zhang, Q., Li, J., Chen, Y., Wu, T., 2022. Wearable sensor-based monitoring of environmental exposure and health responses, including VOC tracking. Biosensors 12 (12), 1131. doi:10.3390/bios12121131.

Lionetti, N., Rigano, L., 2018. Labeling of cosmetic products: obligations and transparency under EU Regulation 1223/2009. Cosmetics 5 (1), 22. doi:10.3390/cosmetics5010022.

Lv, C., Hou, J., Xie, W., Cheng, H., 2015. Investigation on formaldehyde release from preservatives in cosmetics. Int. J. Cosmet. Sci. 37 (5), 474–478. doi:10.1111/ics.12212.

Lyapina, M., Lyubomirova, K., Kundurzhiev, T., Vizeva, M., 2023. Pilot study of the prevalence of contact sensitization to preservatives as cosmetic ingredients in occupational and educational exposures. Acta Med. Bulg. 50 (3), 29–35. doi:10.2478/AMB-2023-0027.

MacKendrick, N., 2015. Protecting ourselves from chemicals: a study of gender and precautionary consumption. In: Our Chemical Selves: Gender, Toxics, and Environmental Health. UBC Press, p. 58–77.

Maertens, A., 2022. Chapter 1: green chemistry for Green Toxicology. In: Green Toxicology: Making Chemicals Benign by Design. Royal Society of Chemistry, Cambridge, UK, pp. 1–30. doi:10.1039/9781839164392-00001.

Manful, M.E., Ahmed, L., Barry-Ryan, C., 2024. Cosmetic formulations from natural sources: safety considerations and legislative frameworks in the European Union. Cosmetics 11 (3), 72. doi:10.3390/cosmetics11030072.

Martins, A.M., Marto, J.M., 2023. A sustainable life cycle for cosmetics: from design and development to post-use phase. Sustain. Chem. Pharm. 35. Article 101178. doi:10.1016/j.scp.2023.101178.

Mawazi, S.M., Ann, J., Othman, N., Khan, J., Alolayan, S.O., Al Thagfan, S.S., Kaleemullah, M., 2022. A review of moisturizers; history, preparation, characterization and applications. Cosmetics 9 (3), 61. doi:10.3390/cosmetics9030061.

Michael, J.H., Evans, D.D., Jansen, K.J., Haight, J.M., 2005. Management commitment to safety as organizational support: Relationships with non-safety outcomes in wood manufacturing employees. J. Saf. Res. 36 (2), 171–179. doi:10.1016/j.jsr.2005.03.002.

Mishra, S., Petry, T., 2025. New Data Supporting the Use of Read-across in the Safety Assessment of DDDE as a Cosmetic Ingredient. Presentation. CIR Expert Panel for Cosmetic Ingredient Safety. Expert Panel for Cosmetic Ingredient Safety, Washington, DC, United States. 173rd Meeting.

Moline, J., Bevilacqua, K., Alexandri, M., Gordon, R.E., 2020. Mesothelioma associated with the use of cosmetic talc. J. Occup. Environ. Med. 62 (1), 11–17. doi:10.1097/JOM.0000000000001723.

More, S.J., Bampidis, V., Benford, D., Bragard, C., Hernández-Jerez, A.F., Hougaard Bennekou, S., Halldorsson, T.I., Koutsoumanis, K.P., Lambré, C., Machera, K., Naegeli, H., Nielsen, S.S., Schlatter, J.R., Schrenk, D., Silano, V., Turck, D., Younes, M., Benfenati, E., Crépet, A., Te Biesebeek, J.D., Testai, E., Dujardin, B., Dorne, J.L.C.M., Hogstrand, C., EFSA Scientific Committee, 2021. Guidance on the use of the Threshold of Toxicological Concern (TTC) approach. EFSA J. 19 (12), e07033. doi:10.2903/j.efsa.2021.7033.

Najjar, A., Schepky, A., Krueger, C.-T., Dent, M., Cable, S., Li, H., Grégoire, S., Roussel, L., Noël-Voisin, A., Hewitt, N.J., Cardamone, E., 2022. Use of physiologically-based kinetics modelling to reliably predict internal concentrations of the UV filter, homosalate, after repeated oral and topical application. Front. Pharmacol. 12. Article 802514. doi:10.3389/fphar.2021.802514.

National Fire Protection Association (NFPA), 2022. NFPA 45: Standard on Fire Protection for Laboratories Using Chemicals. NFPA. https://www.nfpa.org/codes-and-standards/all-codes-and-standards/list-of-codes-and-standards/detail?code=45.

National Institute for Occupational Safety and Health (NIOSH), 2016. Hierarchy of Controls. Centers for Disease Control and Prevention. https://www.cdc.gov/niosh/topics/hierarchy/default.html

National Institute for Occupational Safety and Health (NIOSH), 2018. About Stress at Work. Centers for Disease Control and Prevention. https://www.cdc.gov/niosh/stress/about/index.html

National Institute for Occupational Safety and Health (NIOSH), 2023. Hierarchy of Controls. CDC. https://www.cdc.gov/niosh/topics/hierarchy/default.html

National Institutes of Health (NIH), 2019. Division of Occupational Health and Safety. https://ors.od.nih.gov/sr/dohs/safety/laboratory/chemicalsafety/Pages/default.aspx.

National Medical Products Administration (NMPA), 2022. The Provisions for Registration and Filing of Cosmetics. NMPA. https://english.nmpa.gov.cn/2022-06/30/c_961747.htm.

NatLaw Review, 2019. FDA & FTC: No Definition for "Natural" Applied to Cosmetics. National Law Review. https://natlawreview.com/article/natural-cosmetics-products-without-clear-definition.

Neal, A., Griffin, M.A., 2006. A study of the lagged relationships among safety climate, safety motivation, safety behavior, and accidents at the individual and group levels. J. Appl. Psychol. 91 (4), 946–953. doi:10.1037/0021-9010.91.4.946.

Nicola, M.R.D., Cattaneo, I., Nathanail, A.V., Carnesecchi, E., Astuto, M.C., Steinbach, M., Williams, A.J., Charles, S., Gestin, O., Lopes, C., Lamonica, D., Tarazona, J.V., Dorne, J.L.C.M., 2023. The use of new approach methodologies for the environmental risk assessment of food and feed chemicals. Curr. Opin. Environ. Sci. Health. 31, 1–8. doi:10.1016/j.coesh.2022.100416.

Nohynek, G.J., Antignac, E., Re, T., Toutain, H., 2010. Safety assessment of personal care products/cosmetics and their ingredients. Toxicol. Appl. Pharmacol. 243 (2), 239–259. doi:10.1016/j.taap.2009.12.001.

NYSCC, 2023. Cosmetic Colorants. NYSCC Blog. Available from: https://nyscc.org/blog/cosmetic-colorants/.

Occupational Safety and Health Administration. 2011. Laboratory safety guidance. (OSHA Publication No. 3404-11R). U.S. Department of Labor. https://www.osha.gov/sites/default/files/publications/OSHA3404LABORATORY-SAFETY-GUIDANCE.pdf.

OECD, 2011. Guidance Notes on Dermal Absorption Studies (OECD Environment, Health and Safety Publications, Series on Testing and Assessment, No. 156). OECD Publishing. https://one.oecd.org/document/ENV/JM/MONO(2011)36/REV1/en/pdf

OECD, 2018. Guidance Document on Good in Vitro Method Practices (GIVIMP). OECD Publishing. doi:10.1787/9789264304796-en.

OECD, 2019a. Guidance Document for Good Laboratory Practice (GLP) Compliance Monitoring. OECD Publishing. (OECD Series on Testing and Assessment, No. 320) https://www.oecd.org/en/topics/sub-issues/testing-of-chemicals/good-laboratory-practice-and-compliance-monitoring.html.

OECD, 2021a. OECD QSAR Toolbox (Version 4.5). Organisation for Economic Co-operation and Development. Computer software https://www.qsartoolbox.org.

OECD, 2023a. Case Study on the Use of Integrated Approaches for Testing and Assessment: Illustrative Example – Cosmetics Industry. OECD Publishing. (OECD Environment, Health and Safety Publications, MONO (2023) 5) https://one.oecd.org/document/ENV/CBC/MONO(2023)5/en/pdf.

Oehlke, K., Behsnilian, D., Mayer-Miebach, E., Weidler, P.G., Greiner, R., Steffen-Heins, A., 2017. Edible solid lipid nanoparticles as carrier system for antioxidants. PLoS ONE. 12 (2), e0171662. doi:10.1371/journal.pone.0171662.

Oklahoma State University Tulsa, Helmerich Research Center, 2013. Laboratory Emergency Response Procedures. Oklahoma State University. https://tulsa.okstate.edu/helmerich-research-center/equipment/docs/hrc-laboratory-emergency-response.pdf.

OSHA, 2012. Hazard Communication Standard: Safety Data Sheets. Occupational Safety and Health Administration. https://www.osha.gov/Publications/OSHA3514.html.

OSHA, 2015. Recommended Practices for Safety and Health Programs. Occupational Safety and Health Administration. https://www.osha.gov/safety-management.

OSHA, 2021. Laboratory Safety Guidance. Occupational Safety and Health Administration. https://www.osha.gov/sites/default/files/publications/OSHA3404laboratory-safety-guidance.pdf.

OSHA, 2023. Laboratory Ergonomics Fact Sheet. Occupational Safety and Health Administration. https://www.osha.gov/sites/default/files/publications/OSHAfactsheet-laboratory-safety-ergonomics.pdf.

Paini, A., Campia, I., Cronin, M.T.D., Asturiol, D., Ceriani, L., Exner, T.E., Gao, W., Gomes, C., Kruisselbrink, J., Martens, M., Meek, M.E.B., Pamies, D., Pletz, J., Scholz, S., Schüttler, A., Spînu, N., Villeneuve, D.L., Wittwehr, C., Worth, A., Luijten, M., 2022. Towards a qAOP framework for predictive toxicology—linking data to decisions. Comput. Toxicol. 21, 100195. doi:10.1016/j.comtox.2021.100195.

Paini, A., Leonard, J.A., Joossens, E., Bessems, J.G.M., Desalegn, A., Dorne, J.L.C.M., Gosling, J.P., Heringa, M.B., Klaric, M., Kliment, T., Kramer, N.I., Loizou, G., Louisse, J., Lumen, A., Madden, J.C., Patterson, E.A., Proença, S., Punt, A., Setzer, R.W., Tan, Y.M., 2019. Next generation physiologically based kinetic (NG-PBK) models in support of regulatory decision making. Comput. Toxicol. 9, 61–72. doi:10.1016/j.comtox.2018.11.002.

Pairote, A., Tipauksorn, P., Suwan, P., Wiwek, A., 2025. Smart Air Control: IoT-Based Ventilation via Smartphone. Paper presented at the Smart Air Control: IoT-Based Ventilation via Smartphone Conference.

Panico, A., Serio, F., Bagordo, F., Grassi, T., Idolo, A., De Giorgi, M., Guido, M., Congedo, M., De Donno, A., 2019. Skin safety and health prevention: an overview of chemicals in cosmetic products. J. Prev. Med. Hyg. 60 (1), E50–E57. doi:10.15167/2421-4248/jpmh2019.60.1.1080.

Pareek, A., Kapoor, D.U., Yadav, S.K., Rashid, S., Fareed, M., Akhter, M.S., Muteeb, G., Gupta, M.M., Prajapati, B.G., 2025. Advancing lipid nanoparticles: a pioneering technology in cosmetic and dermatological treatments. Colloid Interface Sci. Commun. 64, 100814. doi:10.1016/j.colcom.2024.100814.

Park, J., Kang, D., 2024. Artificial intelligence and smart technologies in safety management: a comprehensive analysis across multiple industries. Appl. Sci. 14 (24), 11934. doi:10.3390/app142411934.

Patlewicz, G., Ball, N., Booth, E.D., Hulzebos, E., Zvinavashe, E., Hennes, C., 2014. Use of category approaches, read-across and (Q)SAR: general considerations. Regul. Toxicol. Pharmacol. 68 (3), 353–365. doi:10.1016/j.yrtph.2013.06.002.

Patriarca, R., Di Gravio, G., Costantino, F., Falegnami, A., Bilotta, F., 2018. An analytic framework to assess organizational resilience. Saf. Health Work. 9 (3), 265–276. doi:10.1016/j.shaw.2017.10.005.

Pedrosa, M.H., Salazar, A.K., Cardoso, C., Guedes, J.C., 2025. Study on safety culture following implementation of a near miss management system in traditional manufacturing industry. Safety 11 (1). doi:10.3390/safety11010023.

Phimister, J.R., Oktem, U., Kleindorfer, P.R., Kunreuther, H., 2003. Near-miss incident management in the chemical process industry. Risk Anal. 23 (3), 445–459. doi:10.1111/1539-6924.00326.

Pinto, D., Ciardiello, T., Franzoni, M., Pasini, F., Giuliani, G., Rinaldi, F., 2021. Effect of commonly used cosmetic preservatives on skin resident microflora dynamics. Sci. Rep. 11. Article 8695. doi:10.1038/s41598-021-88039-9.

Princeton University Environmental Health & Safety, 2025. Eye and Face Protection. Princeton University. Available from: https://ehs.princeton.edu/book/export/html/289.

Quartzy Inc., 2025. Quartzy: Lab Inventory and SDS Management Platform. Available from: https://www.quartzy.com

Raies, A.B., Bajic, V.B., 2016. In silico toxicology: computational methods for the prediction of chemical toxicity. Wiley Interdiscip. Rev. Comput. Mol. Sci. 6 (2), 147–172. doi:10.1002/wcms.1240.

Reason, J., 1997. Managing the Risks of Organizational Accidents. first ed. Routledge. doi:10.4324/9781315543543.

Reason, J., 2000. Human error: models and management. BMJ 320 (7237), 768–770. doi:10.1136/bmj.320.7237.768.

Reid, M., Reid, R.D., Oswal, P., Sullivan, K., Bhartia, R., Hug, W.F., 2018. NaDos: a real-time, wearable, personal exposure monitor for hazardous organic vapors. Sens. Actuators B Chem. 255 (Part 3), 2996–3003. doi:10.1016/j.snb.2017.09.122.

Repetto, G., del Peso, A., Zurita, J., 2008. Neutral red uptake assay for the estimation of cell viability/cytotoxicity. Nat. Protoc. 3, 1125–1131. doi:10.1038/nprot.2008.75.

Riesmeier, M., Keute, J., Veall, M.A., et al, 2022. Recipes of Ancient Egyptian kohls more diverse than previously thought. Sci. Rep. 12, 5932. doi:10.1038/s41598-022-08669-0.

Rodrigues, R.M., Stinckens, M., Ates, G., Vanhaecke, T., 2023. Neutral red uptake assay to assess cytotoxicity *in vitro*. Methods Mol. Biol. 2644, 237–245. doi:10.1007/978-1-0716-3052-5_15.

Rovida, C., Alépée, N., Api, A.M., Basketter, D.A., Bois, F.Y., Caloni, F., Corsini, E., Daneshian, M., Eskes, C., Ezendam, J., Fuchs, H., Hayden, P., Hegele-Hartung, C., Hoffmann, S., Hubesch, B., Jacobs, M.N., Jaworska, J., Kleensang, A., Kleinstreuer, N., Lalko, J., et al, 2015. Integrated testing strategies (ITS) for safety assessment. ALTEX 32 (1), 25–40. doi:10.14573/altex.1411011.

Santander Ballestín, S., Luesma Bartolomé, M.J., 2023. Toxicity of different chemical components in sun cream filters and their impact on human health: a review. Appl. Sci. 13 (2). doi:10.3390/app13020712.

Santos, W., Rojas, C., Isidoro, R., Lorente, A., Dias, A., Mariscal, G., Benlloch, M., Lorente, R., 2025. Efficacy of ergonomic interventions on work-related musculoskeletal pain: a systematic review and meta-analysis. J. Clin. Med. 14 (9), 3034. doi:10.3390/jcm14093034.

SCCS – Scientific Committee on Consumer Safety, 2009. Memorandum on Alternative Test Methods in Human Health. European Commission. Available from: https://ec.europa.eu/health/scientific_committees/consumer_safety/docs/sccs_s_001.pdf.

SCCS – Scientific Committee on Consumer Safety, 2019. Guidance on the Safety Assessment of Nanomaterials in Cosmetics. European Commission. Available from: https://health.ec.europa.eu/system/files/2020-10/sccs_o_233_0.pdf.

SCCS – Scientific Committee on Consumer Safety, 2021. Notes of Guidance for the Testing of Cosmetic Ingredients and Their Safety Evaluation (11th Revision). European Commission. Available from: https://health.ec.europa.eu/publications/sccs-notes-guidance-testing-cosmetic-ingredients-and-their-safety-evaluation-11th-revision_en.

SCCS – Scientific Committee on Consumer Safety, 2023. Guidance on the Safety Assessment of Nanomaterials in Cosmetics (2nd Revision). European Commission. Available from: https://health.ec.europa.eu/publications/sccs-guidance-safety-assessment-nanomaterials-cosmetics-2nd-revision_en.

Schaffer, S., 2006. Reading our lips: the history of lipstick regulation in western seats of power. Food Drug Law J. 61 (2), 165–189. https://pubmed.ncbi.nlm.nih.gov/17444030/.

Schug, T.T., Heindel, J.J., Camacho, L., Delclos, K.B., Howard, P., Johnson, A.F., … Walker, N.J., 2013. Designing endocrine disruption out of the next generation of chemicals. Green Chem. 15 (1), 181–198. doi:10.1039/C2GC35055F.

Schulman, P., Roe, E., van Eeten, M., de Bruijne, M., 2004. High reliability and the management of critical infrastructures. J. Conting. Crisis Manag. 12 (1), 14–28. doi:10.1111/j.0966-0879.2004.01201003.x.

SciShield Inc., 2024. Lab Chemical Safety and Compliance Software (formerly BioRAFT). Available from: https://www.scisure.com/

Scott, B., Wilcock, A., 2006. Process analytical technology in the pharmaceutical industry: a toolkit for continuous improvement. PDA J. Pharm. Sci. Technol. 60 (1), 17–53.

Shajari, S., Ahmadi, A., Zhang, Y., Kim, J., 2023. The emergence of AI based wearable sensors for digital health technology: a review. Sensors 23 (23), 9498. doi:10.3390/s23239498.

SpecialChem, 2025. The Ultimate Guide to Cosmetic Preservative Selection. SpecialChem. Available from: https://www.specialchem.com/cosmetics/guide/preservatives-for-cosmetic-formulations

Spielmann, H., Hoffmann, S., Liebsch, M., Botham, P., Fentem, J.H., Eskes, C., Roguet, R., Cotovio, J., Cole, T., Worth, A., Heylings, J., Jones, P., Robles, C., Kandárová, H., Gamer, A., Remmele, M., Curren, R., Raabe, H., Cockshott, A., Gerner, I., Zuang, V., 2007. The ECVAM international validation study on in vitro tests for acute skin irritation: report on the validity of the EPISKIN and EpiDerm assays and on the Skin Integrity Function Test. Altern. Lab Anim. 35 (6), 559–601. doi:10.1177/026119290703500614.

Sprinkle, R.H., Payne Sturges, D.C., 2021. Mixture toxicity, cumulative risk, and environmental justice in United States federal policy, 1980–2016. Environ. Health. 20. Article 104. doi:10.1186/s12940-021-00764-5.

Straut, C.M., Nelson, A., 2020. Improving chemical security with material control and accountability and inventory management. J. Chem. Educ. 97 (7). doi:10.1021/acs.jchemed.9b00844.

Stucki, A.O., Barton-Maclaren, T.S., Bhuller, Y., Henriquez, J., Henry, T., Hirn, Z., et al., 2022. Use of NAMs to meet regulatory requirements: global frameworks, examples, and integration strategies. Front. Toxicol. doi:10.3389/ftox.2022.964553.

Su, Z., Luo, F.-Y., Pei, X.-R., Zhang, F.-L., Xing, S.-X., Wang, G.-L., 2020. Final publication of the "Regulations on the Supervision and Administration of Cosmetics" and new prospectives of cosmetic science in China. Cosmetics 7 (4), 98. doi:10.3390/cosmetics7040098.

Subroto, E., Andoyo, R., Indiarto, R., 2023. Solid lipid nanoparticles: review of the current research on encapsulation and delivery systems for active and antioxidant compounds. Antioxidants 12 (3), 633. doi:10.3390/antiox12030633.

Suter, G.W.I.I., Lizarraga, L.E., 2022. Clearly weighing the evidence in read-across can improve assessments of data-poor chemicals. Regul. Toxicol. Pharmacol. 129, 105111. doi:10.1016/j.yrtph.2021.105111.

Ta, G.C., Mokhtar, M., Mokhtar, A., Ismail, A., Abu Yazid, M.F.B.H., 2010. Analysis of the comprehensibility of chemical hazard communication tools at the industrial workplace. Ind. Health. 48 (6), 835–844. doi:10.2486/indhealth.MS1153.

Tcheremenskaia, O., Battistelli, C.L., Giuliani, A., Benigni, R., Bossa, C., 2019. In silico approaches for prediction of genotoxic and carcinogenic potential of cosmetic ingredients. Comput. Toxicol. 11, 91–100. doi:10.1016/j.comtox.2019.03.005.

Thiel, C., Schneckener, S., Krauss, M., Ghallab, A., Hofmann, U., Kanacher, T., Zellmer, S., Gebhardt, R., Lichtenstein, D., Lippert, J., 2015. A systematic evaluation of the use of physiologically based pharmacokinetic modeling for cross-species extrapolation. J. Pharm. Sci. 104 (1), 191–206. doi:10.1002/jps.24214.

Thomas, R., D'Amico, L., Frederick, A., et al, 2024. EPA Report on statutory and regulatory requirements for vertebrate animal testing and flexibility for implementing new approach methods (NAMs). In: VI, Barriers to Implementation and Use of NAMs. U.S. Environmental Protection Agency, Washington (DC). Available from: https://www.ncbi.nlm.nih.gov/books/NBK614855/.

Tsow, F., Forzani, E., Rai, A., Wang, R., Tsui, R., Mastroianni, S., 2009. A wearable and wireless sensor system for real-time monitoring of toxic environmental volatile organic compounds. IEEE Sens. J. 9 (12), 1734–1740. doi:10.1109/JSEN.2009.2032485.

U.S. Food and Drug Administration, 1938/2011. Federal Food, Drug, and Cosmetic Act, § 201(i), Definition of Cosmetics.

U.S. Food and Drug Administration, 2022c. Small businesses & homemade cosmetics: can I label my cosmetics "natural" or "organic"? Available from: https://www.fda.gov/cosmetics/resources-industry-cosmetics/small-businesses-homemade-cosmetics-fact-sheet.

U.S. Food and Drug Administration, 2024. Suntegrity Skincare Issues Voluntary Recall of Suntegrity Impeccable Skin Sunscreen Foundation Due to Possible Mold Contamination. U.S. Food and Drug Administration. https://www.fda.gov/safety/recalls-market-withdrawals-safety-alerts/suntegrity-skincare-issues-voluntary-recall-suntegrity-impeccable-skin-sunscreen-foundation-multiple.

U.S. Food and Drug Administration, 2025. Modernization of Cosmetics Regulation Act (MoCRA) and Electronic Registration. Available from: https://www.fda.gov/cosmetics/cosmetics-laws-regulations/modernization-cosmetics-regulation-act-2022-mocra

United Nations Environment Programme (UNEP), 2021b. The Precautionary Principle. UNEP. Available from: https://www.unepfi.org/blue-finance/join-us/.

United Nations Environment Programme (UNEP), 2023. Sustainable Consumption and Production Policies: Advancing SDG 12. UNEP. Available from: https://www.unep.org/explore-topics/resource-efficiency/what-we-do/sustainable-consumption-and-production-policies.

United Nations/European Chemicals Agency (ECHA), 2024. REACH Annex II—Safety Data Sheets Requirements. Available from: https://echa.europa.eu/regulations/reach/legislation.

United Nations, 2015. Transforming Our World: The 2030 Agenda for Sustainable Development. Available from: https://sdgs.un.org/2030agenda

University of Minnesota, Environmental Health & Safety, 2025. Chemical Hygiene Plan: PPE Guidelines. University of Minnesota. Available from: https://hsrm.umn.edu/department-environmental-health-safety/lab-research-safety/chemical-hygiene-plan/6-safety-2.

University of North Carolina, Laboratory Safety Manual, 2019. Skin Contact Exposure in Labs. University of North Carolina. Available from: https://ehs.unc.edu/manuals/laboratory/.

Vaillancourt, E., Mohamed, A.A., Ansell, J., Ashikaga, T., Ayad, A., Ayman, H., Valadares Campos, M., Chien, H.-S., Giusti, A., Hatao, M., Hill, F., Khattab, A., Kreiling, R., Lee, A.Y., Li, M., Lin, P., Lin, Y.-C., Mencarelli, V., Milstein, S., Montemayor, B.P., et al., 2025. Highlighting best practices to advance next-generation risk assessment of cosmetic ingredients. NAM J. 1. doi:10.1016/j.namjnl.2025.100020.

van der Zalm, A.J., Barroso, J., Browne, P., et al, 2022. A framework for establishing scientific confidence in new approach methodologies. Arch. Toxicol. 96, 2865–2879. doi:10.1007/s00204-022-03365-4.

Veltri, A., Pagell, M., 2007. A Data-based Evaluation of the Relationship between Occupational Safety and Operating Performance, American Society of Safety Engineers.

Verywell Health, 2025. Giorgi A. Understanding the Role of Surfactants in Cosmetic and Cleaning Products. Verywell Health. Available from: https://www.verywellhealth.com/what-is-a-surfactant-8770258.

Vinardell, M.P., Mitjans, M., 2015. Nanocarriers for delivery of antioxidants on the skin. Cosmetics 2 (4), 342–354. doi:10.3390/cosmetics2040342.

Vinardell, M.P., Mitjans, M., 2017. Alternative methods to animal testing for the safety evaluation of cosmetic ingredients: an overview. Cosmetics 4 (3), 30. doi:10.3390/cosmetics4030030.

Vinken, M., Blanchard, J., Fröhlich, M., Hessel, F., Knapen, D., Rogiers, V., Hengstler, J.G., 2020. The use of adverse outcome pathways in safety assessment. Arch. Toxicol. 94 (6), 1935–1942. doi:10.1007/s00204-020-02670-0.

Vitoux, M.A., Kessal, K., Melik Parsadaniantz, S., Claret, M., Guerin, C., Baudouin, C., Brignole-Baudouin, F., Réaux-Le Goazigo, A., 2020. Benzalkonium chloride-induced direct and indirect toxicity on corneal epithelial and trigeminal neuronal cells: proinflammatory and apoptotic responses in vitro. Toxicol. Lett. 319, 74–84. doi:10.1016/j.toxlet.2019.10.014.

Wang, J., Fu, G., Yan, M., 2020. Investigation and analysis of a hazardous chemical accident in the process industry: triggers, roots, and lessons learned. Processes 8 (4), 477. doi:10.3390/pr8040477.

Wang, Y., Qian, H., 2021. Phthalates and their impacts on human health. Int. J. Environ. Res. Public Health. 18 (14), 7325. doi:10.3390/healthcare9050603.

Westmoreland, C., Bender, H.J., Doe, J.E., Jacobs, M.N., Kass, G.E.N., Madia, F., Mahony, C., Manou, I., Maxwell, G., Prieto, P., Roggeband, R., Sobanski, T., Schütte, K., Worth, A.P., Zvonar, Z., Cronin, M.T.D., 2022. Use of new approach methodologies (NAMs) in regulatory decisions for chemical safety: report from an EPAA Deep Dive Workshop. Regul. Toxicol. Pharmacol. 135, 105261. doi:10.1016/j.yrtph.2022.105261.

Woolfenden, E., 2010. Sorbent-based sampling methods for volatile and semi-volatile organic compounds in air: part 1—sorbent-based air monitoring options. J. Chromatogr. A. 1217 (16), 2674–2684. doi:10.1016/j.chroma.2009.12.042.

World Health Organization, 2023a. International Programme on Chemical Safety (IPCS). World Health Organization. Available from: https://www.who.int/health-topics/chemical-safety#tab=tab_1.

World Health Organization, 2023b. Mental Health at Work: Policy Brief. World Health Organization. https://www.who.int/publications/i/item/9789240057944.

Wu, T.C., Chen, C.H., Li, C.C., 2008. A correlation among safety leadership, safety climate and safety performance. J. Loss Prev. Process Ind. 21 (3), 307–318. doi:10.1016/j.jlp.2007.11.001.

Xu, Y., Ma, D., Li, J., Zhang, J., Wang, Q., Dou, Z., 2026. Quantitative risk assessment method for laboratory safety: based on Mond Index. J. Loss Prev. Process Ind. 99, 105835. doi:10.1016/j.jlp.2025.105835.

Zamani, Z., 2023. Analyzing design and planning trends in medical research laboratories and workplace environments: a benchmarking study. J. Des. Resil. Archit. Plan. 4 (1), 105–121. doi:10.47818/DRArch.2023.v4i1086.

Zhu, H., 2023. Analysis on the Filing of New Cosmetic Ingredients in China: Filing Status of New Cosmetic Ingredients in China from 2021-2023. CIRS Group. Available from: https://www.cirs-group.com/en/cosmetics/analysis-on-the-filing-of-new-cosmetic-ingredients-in-china.

Zohar, D., Polachek, T., 2014. Discourse-based intervention for modifying supervisory communication as leverage for safety climate and performance improvement: a randomized field study. J. Appl. Psychol. 99 (1), 113–124. doi:10.1037/a0034096.

Zohar, D., 2003. Safety climate: conceptual and measurement issues. In: Quick, J.C., Tetrick, L.E., Eds.. Handbook of Occupational Health Psychology. American Psychological Association, pp. 123–142. doi:10.1037/10474-006.

Further reading

Chemlinked, 2021b. China Cosmetic Animal Testing Regulation. Chemlinked. [Subscription access].

Section II

Health benefits of bioactive ingredients from sustainable plant-based sources and their by-products

Chapter 5

Medicinal plants

Eleana Toma[a], **Apostolos Beloukas**[a], **and Sophia Letsiou**[b]
[a]*Department of Biomedical Sciences, School of Health and Care Sciences, University of West Attica, Athens, Greece*
[b]*Department of Food Science and Technology, Faculty of Food Sciences, University of West Attica, Athens, Greece*

1 Introduction

Modern cosmetology and biotechnology are increasingly converging, creating new fields of application and innovation in the cosmetic product sector. At the heart of this evolution are biofunctional cosmetics, which transcend the traditional role of cosmetics as esthetic care products, now offering therapeutic and preventive properties for the skin (Yap and Goh, 2023). The integration of bioactive substances with proven biological activity significantly enhances the value and effectiveness of these products. Medicinal plants play a central role in this new approach, as they constitute a rich source of natural compounds with multiple benefits for skin health and appearance. The use of plants with therapeutic properties has been known since antiquity, both in traditional Greek and Chinese medicine and in Ayurveda (Petrovska, 2012). Today, scientific research has focused on the isolation, analysis, and utilization of these plants' secondary metabolites, with the aim of exploiting them in cosmetology. Such compounds include polyphenols, flavonoids, carotenoids, alkaloids, vitamins (such as C and E), essential oils, and saponins, which confer antioxidant, antiaging, antiinflammatory, and antimicrobial properties to cosmetics. Scientific documentation shows that these compounds can act at the cellular level, interfering with important mechanisms such as the inhibition of oxidation, the enhancement of collagen production, and protection from ultraviolet (UV) radiation. Furthermore, the ability of plant components to penetrate the epidermal layer and reach the dermis makes biofunctional cosmetics active in depth, in contrast to simple cosmetics, which act only superficially. The consumer shift toward natural and plant-based cosmetics is also significant. Modern consumers seek products without parabens, synthetic fragrances, and aggressive chemical substances. Simultaneously, they value transparency in the origin of ingredients and recognize the importance of sustainable production. Medicinal plants provide environmentally friendly and simultaneously effective solutions, enhancing the acceptance of biofunctional cosmetics in the market (Lavuri et al., 2022). Beyond the prevention of premature aging, plant-derived bioactive substances are widely used in cosmetics for specific skin conditions, such as: acne, through antimicrobial and sebum-regulating properties; hydration and regeneration: with the use of polysaccharides and saponins; photoprotection and sunscreens: with carotenoids, flavonoids, and polyphenols; soothing action: with essential oils and terpenes; and whitening and depigmentation: through tyrosinase inhibition and melanin reduction (Qian et al., 2020). The purpose of the present work is to analyze the contribution of bioactive substances from medicinal plants to biofunctional cosmetics through the following key sections: Classification and characterization of plant bioactive compounds; scientific documentation of their mechanisms of action in the skin; examples of plants and cosmetic applications by category of action; and challenges and possibilities for further research in the field of natural cosmetics. Understanding the mode of action of these natural substances and their proper integration into cosmetic products constitutes a dynamic field of scientific and industrial development, which combines the tradition of herbal medicine with the demands of modern cosmetology and dermatology (Goyal and Jerold, 2023).

2 Medicinal plants as a source of bioactives in cosmetics

Medicinal plants are rich in secondary metabolites that interact with the skin's biological processes to deliver functional benefits. These compounds can be extracted from various parts of the plant, including leaves, roots, flowers, and seeds. Key bioactive groups include the following.

Biofunctional Cosmetics for Health. https://doi.org/10.1016/B978-0-443-27500-5.00017-4

2.1 Polyphenols

Polyphenols are among the most complex and, at the same time, most active plant bioactive compounds (Vella et al., 2024). These secondary metabolites are found in small quantities in plants and are classified according to their chemical structure into flavonoids, phenolic acids, and tannins/stilbenes, with flavonoids occupying the first place in popularity (the most well-known group). Flavonoids are a large group of organic compounds mainly found in the plant world and consist of two or more hydroxyl groups attached to an aromatic ring (Michalak, 2022; Zillich et al., 2015). The main property that has made them popular is their antioxidant action on the skin, that is, their ability to carry out reduction reactions. These conclusions are based on *in vitro* studies, which have identified the phenol group as the component of these compounds with the greatest antioxidant activity. The antioxidant activity of polyphenols is attributed to multiple mechanisms, such as the neutralization of free radicals, inhibition of enzymes that degrade the structural proteins of the skin (such as collagenase and elastase), as well as protection against UV radiation, which can cause damage to the skin. As mentioned earlier, these bioactive compounds act against specific skin enzymes, collagenase and elastase, which are responsible for the degradation of structural proteins found distributed in the layers of the skin. According to studies, phloretin, 3-hydroxyphloretin, and quercetin, which are included among polyphenols, are the components that inhibit the action of the destructive skin enzymes. Noteworthy for polyphenolic compounds is also their protective and preventive effect against solar radiation, in addition to antioxidant protection. This type of radiation has been implicated in skin damage, which may even lead to skin cancer. Therefore the use of polyphenols is understandable and clearly justified as ingredients in sunscreens and in any other formulations suggested for application before sun exposure. More specifically, their use in the cosmetic and pharmaceutical industries has increased in modern times as they are able to exert their actions by means of mechanisms that allow them to be released from the formulation in which they are contained, penetrate the epidermal barrier, and act within the dermis layer of the skin. They are also of particular value due to their multiple applications in various conditions such as wounds, inflammatory states, nonpathological conditions such as aging, and skin diseases or conditions of the skin's appendages (Zillich et al., 2015). An important source of these compounds, used as plant extracts and widely known, is tea, especially green tea (*Camellia sinensis* L.). Apart from tea, a fruit known worldwide and massively produced with antioxidant properties is the grape (*Vitis vinifera* L.), which contains anthocyanins, the water-soluble form of flavonoids (Zillich et al., 2015; Liu et al., 2021). As a rule, the higher the percentage of anthocyanins in a plant, the darker its color and the stronger its antioxidant activity (Zillich et al., 2015). In addition, an aromatic plant containing polyphenolic compounds is rosemary (*Rosmarinus officinalis* L.), which is also called *Salvia rosmarinus* based on modern phylogenetic analysis. According to the use of various chromatographic methods, it has been documented that rosemary leaves contain a high concentration of additional secondary metabolites besides polyphenols, such as terpenes, essential oils, and other volatile compounds (de Macedo et al., 2020). In addition, foods with a high polyphenol content include onions, leeks, lettuce, oregano, green tea, apples, cherries, blackcurrants, beans, peaches, apricots, and citrus fruits. The extraction of the plant extract is carried out with the final goal of using it in the cosmetic industry, since it has been proven that the bioactive molecules of polyphenols can penetrate the epidermal barrier and reach the epidermis or even the dermis, thus exerting beneficial and especially antiaging effects on the skin.

2.2 Ascorbic acid (vitamin C)

Vitamin C, also known as ascorbic acid, is an important dietary compound that has a positive impact on the skin by promoting the production of components necessary for maintaining the integrity and normal structure of the skin. In addition, it neutralizes other harmful reactive molecules that slow down the tissue repair process in cases of wounds and burns (Boo, 2022; Zhou et al., 2023). However, before providing a detailed description of the properties of this well-known vitamin, it is useful to present general information that characterizes it. As rightly stated at the beginning of the paragraph, it is one of the dietary substances in human daily life, which cannot be produced endogenously. This specific disadvantage is attributed to the absence of an essential enzyme for the synthesis of vitamin C by the metabolic mechanism and, by extension, the body, oxidase. Therefore the intake of this substance through food is considered necessary, as it is present in sufficient concentrations in numerous foods, especially those of plant origin. The most stable and active form of the vitamin is the reduced form of the molecule, namely, L-ascorbic acid, which does not bind to plasma protein molecules, as is the case with most molecules found in this fluid. The insufficient presence of vitamin C in the body, specifically plasma concentrations below 11 μM, is the cause of the development of scurvy and its associated symptoms. The synthesis of this secondary metabolite has been confirmed to occur in both marine and terrestrial plant organisms. Its antioxidant activity is widely recognized, as it is directly linked to α-tocopherol. Alpha-tocopherol is a compound of great importance as it performs antioxidant functions by protecting low-density lipoprotein and is regenerated by vitamin C. Therefore α-tocopherol cannot act independently without the contribution of vitamin C (Doseděl et al., 2021). It is also worth mentioning that one of the components produced under the regulation of ascorbic acid is collagen. This is an abundant structural protein with antiaging effects in both the human body and other mammals, identified in 28 different types. Due to the aforementioned properties of vitamin C, the cosmeceutical industry has been mobilized to isolate this secondary metabolite from medicinal plants and incorporate it into highly promising dermatological products (Boo, 2022; Zhou et al., 2023). Nevertheless, studies have shown that the administration of ascorbic acid does not always lead to an increase in collagen biosynthesis, which strengthens skin firmness, but mainly in conditions where there is a preexisting deficiency of ascorbic acid or collagen. Furthermore, another issue concerning ascorbic acid involves the difficulty it encounters in penetrating the stratum corneum due to its hydrophilic nature, following topical application. Therefore this condition led the cosmetic industry to develop combined formulations, through clinical trials, composed of ascorbic acid and other bioactive molecules, aiming to increase the effectiveness and potency of ascorbic acid (Boo, 2022). Some of the additional functions of ascorbic acid—apart from its antioxidant action and stimulation of collagen anabolism—include its participation in reactions with carotenoids and antioxidant enzymes, protection of protein thiol groups, reduction of melanin production (protection from discolorations) and the enzyme tyrosinase, and finally protection against oxidative damage caused by UV radiation (Michalak, 2022). In conclusion, it is worth highlighting certain rich sources of vitamin C such as *Kakadu plum* (Michalak, 2022), Acerola (*Malpighia emarginata*) (Olędzki and Harasym, 2024), Camu-Camu (*Myrciaria dubia*) (García-Chacón et al., 2023), and *Carissa carandas* (Dhatwalia et al., 2021). In addition, it is also found in many fruits and vegetables such as sea buckthorn, goji berries, and blackcurrants (Michalak, 2022).

2.3 Carotenoinds

Another category of plant-derived compounds with noteworthy use in the cosmetics industry is carotenoids. Carotenoids are a class of lipophilic pigments responsible for the coloration of many plants, as well as numerous fruits, vegetables, and flowers (Michalak, 2022). They are especially found in plants, though it has recently been discovered that they also occur in microalgae (Aziz et al., 2021). They are divided into two categories: carotenes, which are further subdivided into α-, β-, and γ-carotenes, as well as lycopenes, and, from a chemical point of view, they are composed of carbon atoms (C40) and hydrogen. The second category includes the oxygenated derivatives, xanthophylls, which, in addition to carbon and hydrogen, also contain the element oxygen (Michalak, 2022). These are compounds that the human body is unable to synthesize, and thus they must be obtained through diet in specific quantities. The need for limited consumption arises from the fact that excessive intake may lead to pathological, morphological, or functional conditions. For example, excessive consumption of β-carotene can result in an alteration of the skin's natural color, producing an orange tint. Carotenoids possess and offer a wide range of properties, such as antioxidant and photoprotective effects. The amount of carotenoids contained in plants varies and depends on multiple factors, which must be emphasized and monitored to avoid affecting plant function due to loss of carotenoid content. These factors are related to the plants' exposure to oxidative agents or unsuitable environmental conditions. Plant-based dietary sources rich in carotenoids include mainly carrots, sweet peppers, and pumpkin (Kultys and Kurek, 2022). They are also found in chili peppers, tomatoes, broccoli, spinach, watermelon, and apricots. Fig. 5.1 presents the β-carotene content in foods, with the aim of providing information about the quantity of this component (Michalak, 2022).

Carotenoids are also found in abundant quantities, mainly in sweat and in the sebaceous glands. Their concentration in the human body is influenced by various factors such as season, exposure to UV radiation, smoking, consumption of fruits and vegetables, among others. As previously mentioned, carotenoids possess antioxidant properties, which protect the macromolecules of the cell from the destructive action of free radicals. This property is mainly attributed to the conjugated double bonds of carotenoids and their lipid solubility. They have been identified in all three layers of the skin (epidermis, dermis, subcutaneous tissue), including lycopene, lutein, α-, β-, and γ-carotene, cryptoxanthin, among others. Additional benefits of carotenoids include their ability to reduce the likelihood of developing skin cancer. Following topical application in combination with oral intake (especially of lutein and β-carotene), further advantages arise, such as improvement of skin physiology, hydration, increased elasticity, and photoprotective properties. Finally, oral consumption of lutein, according to studies, ensures protection against erythema resulting from the harmful effects of UV radiation. In conclusion, carotenoids protect both against the action of reactive oxygen species (ROS) and the effects of UV radiation on the skin, as well as against various skin conditions (Michalak, 2022). Therefore the remarkable and beneficial properties of carotenoids have led to increasing demand, resulting in the need for increased production of this bioactive molecule (Ashokkumar et al., 2023).

2.4 Tocopherols and tocotrienols

Another important category of bioactive molecules is vitamin E, which includes eight isoforms: α-, β-, γ-, and δ-tocopherols, as well as the corresponding tocotrienols. These compounds are produced exclusively by photosynthetic organisms, such as

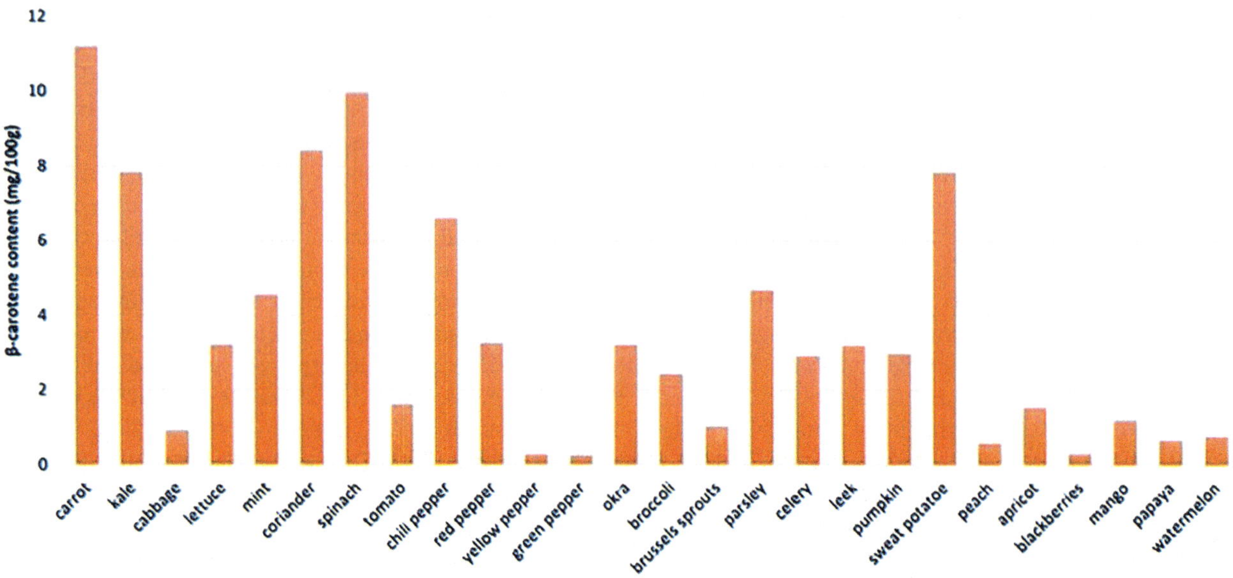

FIG. 5.1 Selected plants that are sources of β-carotene. *(From Michalak, M., 2022. Plant-derived antioxidants: significance in skin health and the ageing process. Int. J. Mol. Sci. 1422-0067. 23 (2), 585. doi:10.3390/ijms23020585.)*

plants and cyanobacteria. They consist of a hydrophobic prenyl group and a polar chromanol ring. The difference between these two types of compounds lies in the prenyl side chains. More specifically, the prenyl side chain of tocopherols is saturated, meaning it contains only single bonds between the atoms, in contrast to the unsaturated chain of tocotrienols, which contains three double bonds. It has been proven that the α-isoform, which is the most active and abundant in the human body, acts by preventing the formation of new free radicals, unlike γ-tocopherol, which exhibits antioxidant activity by neutralizing preexisting free radicals. Tocopherol has also been shown to be absorbed by the skin, which is why its antioxidant properties are utilized in skin care products. However, their role is not only antioxidant but also protective against photoaging, skin cancer (due to antiproliferative properties), and the induction of inflammatory responses. Vitamin E protects against acute and chronic skin damage caused by light exposure. It reduces the production of collagenase, an enzyme that breaks down collagen, limits the synthesis of tyrosinase, and helps prevent rough texture and deep wrinkles. Finally, it is also effectively used on wounds, burns, and surgical injuries. Specifically concerning tocotrienols, their properties in scar healing and in significantly improving damaged skin have been reported (Szewczyk et al., 2021). More specifically, according to literature data, topical or oral administration of tocotrienols accelerated wound healing time. This is due to enhanced protein synthesis, which occurs more rapidly compared to cases without tocotrienol administration, the combating of oxidative factors (ROS), and improved collagen biosynthesis. Nevertheless, the topical action of tocotrienol-containing substances is hindered by the stratum corneum, the outermost layer of the skin. Therefore research and application of alternative delivery methods were conducted, such as encapsulation of tocotrienols in liposomes or nanoemulsions (NEs) (Nair et al., 2022). The cosmetics industry utilizes these innovative strategies for the incorporation of vitamin E isoforms due to their beneficial properties, particularly antioxidant activity (Sharma et al., 2022). Finally, it is worth mentioning certain medicinal plants rich in vitamin E. Some sources include the almond (*Prunus dulcis*) and its oil (Tomishima et al., 2022), aloe vera (*Aloe vera*) (Alven et al., 2021), plant oils, nuts, seeds, greens, and whole grains (Szewczyk et al., 2021).

2.5 Alkaloids

Another important category of plant secondary metabolites, known for their pleiotropic range of biological activities, is the alkaloids. These are chemical compounds primarily based on carbon (C) and contain at least one nitrogen (N) atom, which is the characteristic element of these compounds. Most of these organic compounds are arranged in a heterocyclic form and are derived from amino acids, which serve as the starting materials for their formation (Zhu et al., 2023). However, precursor molecules for the synthesis of these compounds are not always amino acids but can also be other organic compounds. An example of this is the nicotinic alkaloids, which originate from early molecules such as nicotinic acid. Nicotinic alkaloids include both nicotine and anabasine. In addition, another nonamino acid compound that contributes a nitrogen atom (N) for the synthesis of alkaloids in the quinoline and quinazoline groups is anthranilic acid (Bhambhani et al., 2021). The production of these compounds is observed to a greater extent in plants with medicinal properties, but it is not limited to them. In plants, alkaloids exert protective effects and represent nearly 20% of the total secondary metabolite population (Heinrich et al., 2021). The scientific community has also identified alkaloid production in other eukaryotic organisms, such as fungi of the genera *Huperzia* sp., *Phlegmariurus* sp., as well as the endophytic genus *Aspergillus* (Zhu et al., 2023). Furthermore, the production of these low molecular weight compounds has been identified in various kingdoms, including marine organisms. Since the 19th century, alkaloids have been recognized as valuable biological agents in medicine, used to treat various diseases, such as tumor growth inhibition through berberine (BBR) (Bhambhani et al., 2021; Khan et al., 2022). According to existing literature data, numerous plant species recognized as alkaloid sources belong to the families *Berberidaceae, Amaryllidaceae, Liliaceae, Leguminaceae, Papaveraceae, Ranunculaceae,* and *Solanaceae*. It should be clarified that each family and species has the ability to produce different forms of alkaloids, as they arise from different biosynthetic pathways. Typically, most forms derive from a basic alkaloid skeleton, upon which various transformations act, resulting in the creation of different alkaloids. These chemical modifications, utilizing the common alkaloid framework as a substrate, include glycosylation, acylation, reduction, oxidation, and methylation reactions. The differentiation of alkaloids depends on three main factors: the biosynthetic pathway, the chemical organization of functional groups, and their presence in various genera. Regarding alkaloids derived from amino acids as precursor molecules, these include tetrahydroisoquinoline, indole, pyrrolizidine, and piperidine alkaloids. These originate respectively from the amino acids tyrosine, tryptophan, ornithine, and lysine. In addition, other categories of alkaloids include xanthine alkaloids, which include caffeine, as well as steroidal, terpenoid, and chromone derivatives. These alkaloids differ in their biosynthetic origin, as they are not produced from amino acids (Bhambhani et al., 2021). A plant organism that contains alkaloids among other bioactive molecules and is used in cosmetology is myrtle (*Myrtus communis*), belonging to the family *Myrtaceae*. Both topical application and systemic administration have been associated with beneficial dermatological effects on skin areas affected by burns or wounds (Al-Snafi et al., 2024). Furthermore, it has been clarified that both the leaves and coffee beans (*Coffea arabica*), which contain alkaloids such as caffeine, are closely related to the cosmetic field due to their antioxidant, lipolytic, and rejuvenating properties (Ruse et al., 2025). A characteristic example of a plant producing alkaloids with significant medicinal value is the poppy (*Papaver somniferum* L.), which contains alkaloid compounds such as morphine, codeine, noscapine, thebaine, and papaverine. However, to date, its use in cosmetic products has not been recorded despite its medicinal importance (Bhambhani et al., 2021). As shown in Fig. 5.2, the chemical structures of alkaloids and other bioactive molecules exhibit diversity, reflecting their chemical complexity and the wide range of their biological activities.

2.6 Essential oils

Essential oils are a category of compounds containing bioactive ingredients found in various parts of plants. They are popular due to their multiple beneficial properties, and some are well-known for their pleasant fragrance (Michalak, 2022). Specifically, essential oils consist of complex organic compounds soluble in alcohol and ethers but not in water, some of which are present in high quantities while others occur in trace amounts (Sharmeen et al., 2021). Terpenes and other aliphatic compounds play a leading role, while essential oils also contain a significant proportion of hydrocarbons, alcohols, and ketones, among others. These substances, produced as secondary metabolites by specific plant tissues, are used for various medicinal purposes due to their antimicrobial, antiinflammatory, antifungal, and antioxidant effects, and are

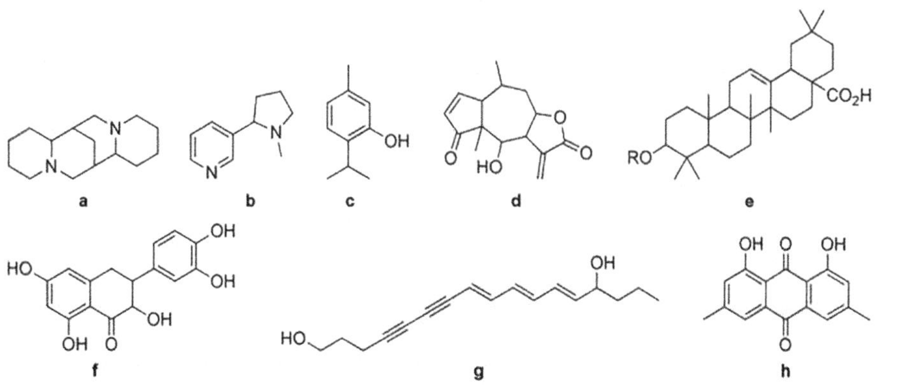

FIG. 5.2 Structures of key plant bioactive compounds: Alkaloids (A, B), monoterpenes (C), sesquiterpenes (D), triterpenes, saponins, steroids (E), flavonoids (F), polyacetylenes (G), and polyketides (H). *(From LiverTox: Clinical and Research Information on Drug-Induced Liver Injury, 2012. Available from: https://www.ncbi.nlm.nih.gov/books/NBK556475/.)*

particularly valued in the field of esthetics (Michalak, 2022; Sharmeen et al., 2021). Apart from the benefits following topical application on the skin, the plants themselves use these secondary metabolites to protect against potential environmental threats such as insects and herbivores (Sharmeen et al., 2021). Regarding their activity and use, mechanisms have been identified that vary and depend on multiple factors. Among these properties, the antioxidant effect stands out, which contributes to the skin's resistance to aging processes. Many skincare products promising fewer imperfections over time include these organic compounds. Such antioxidant components of essential oils, which contribute to the reduction of ROS, include thymol, menthol, linalool, cinnamon, cumin, lemon, clove, mint, basil, oregano, black pepper, patchouli, rosemary, sage, thyme, and ginger. Various extraction methods for essential oils have been applied, with steam distillation being the predominant technique. Focusing on the cosmetics industry, essential oils have significant applications in perfumes and products of renowned companies, and their incorporation is expected to increase in the near future. This is due not only to their multiple beneficial uses but also because they generally do not cause serious side effects, except in some cases (Michalak, 2022). These exceptions include allergic reactions, which may limit the advantages of essential oils in the eyes of consumers (Vostinaru et al., 2020). In addition, although studies on experimental animals have shown low toxicity levels, in some cases, such as essential oils involved in oxidation reactions, skin irritation after topical application has been reported. Toxic effects depend on various factors such as solution concentration, improper storage conditions, and others. Therefore proper storage of vials under suitable conditions is necessary (Vostinaru et al., 2020). A notable disadvantage is that certain essential oils are rare in nature or produced in small quantities. This leads to increased costs both for the industry, which may need to import large amounts from abroad, and for consumers. One of the most widely used and popular essential oils is orange oil, known for its active role in combating skin blemishes. These imperfections include marks, stretch marks, and any other elements that alter the skin's normal appearance and function. The global spread of essential oils' use is also reflected in the revenues of companies operating in this sector (Sharmeen et al., 2021).

2.7 Saponins

Saponins are considered secondary metabolites primarily found in plants. Their production is linked to plant defense, as they contribute to protection against the invasion of pathogenic microorganisms (Kanlayavattanakul et al., 2024). This bioactive compound is responsible for foam formation, as it produces a foamy state when mixed with water. Regarding their chemical composition, it varies depending on the plant species from which they are extracted. However, their amphiphilic nature remains constant. More specifically, the structure of saponins includes a lipophilic part—the aglycone—connected to one or more sugar chains. The hydrophobic backbone is arranged in carbon residue rings, and the number of rings is related to the category of the saponin. The sugar chain linked to the aglycone constitutes the hydrophilic part of the compound and may include glucuronic acid, galacturonic acid, rhamnose, arabinose, xylose, or fructose. Saponins are classified into three types: triterpenoid, steroidal, and alkaloidal. The most commonly found in plants are the triterpenoid saponins, which are formed from six isoprene units (C_5H_8) and often contain up to six rings, comprising 30 carbon atoms in total (C30) (Kanlayavattanakul et al., 2024; Timilsena et al., 2023). In contrast, in steroidal saponins, the hydrophobic part forms 5 or 6 rings based on 27 carbon atoms. Depending on the molecular structure interacting with carbon 22, they are classified as either spirostanes or furostanes (Jiménez et al., 2021). Furthermore, steroidal saponins have been linked to the effective treatment of an inflammatory skin condition: acne (Kanlayavattanakul et al., 2024; Li et al., 2024). These bioactive compounds possess a property that makes them ideal for use in cleaning and cosmetic products: their role as surfactants. Saponins are naturally derived surfactants that reduce surface tension. The strongest surfactant activity has been observed in steroidal structures and in compounds with multiple sugar molecules in the hydrophilic chain. Therefore a directly proportional relationship exists between the number of sugar units and surfactant activity. These amphiphilic substances are highly valuable, as they help form emulsions between liquids with different solubility properties. This feature enables the incorporation of saponins into cosmetic products. The method of extracting saponins from plant materials varies, and the most suitable one must be selected each time to maximize yield. Solvents such as water and alcohols (e.g., methanol, ethanol) are used in simple extraction techniques. However, these methods have shown lower yields. Therefore enhanced extraction techniques—such as ultrasound and microwaves—are often used (Timilsena et al., 2023). A widely used enhanced method is Soxhlet extraction, which is considered effective for isolating bioactive compounds. A notable example of a plant that contains saponins (along with other bioactive compounds) is the genus *Paris polyphylla*, which grows in temperate and tropical zones of Europe and Asia, especially China. It has been used in acne-treatment products due to its antiinflammatory, antimicrobial, and antioxidant effects (Li et al., 2024). Another plant rich in steroidal saponins is the Yucca genus. This genus is primarily found in the United States, Mexico, and Central America and belongs to the *Agavaceae* family. One of its most widely studied and commercially used species is *Yucca schidigera*, which falls into the category of steroidal spirostan saponins. It has demonstrated cytotoxic and antifungal activity. Fig. 5.3 presents the steroidal chemical structure of the secondary metabolite found in *Y. schidigera* to facilitate understanding of its molecular architecture.

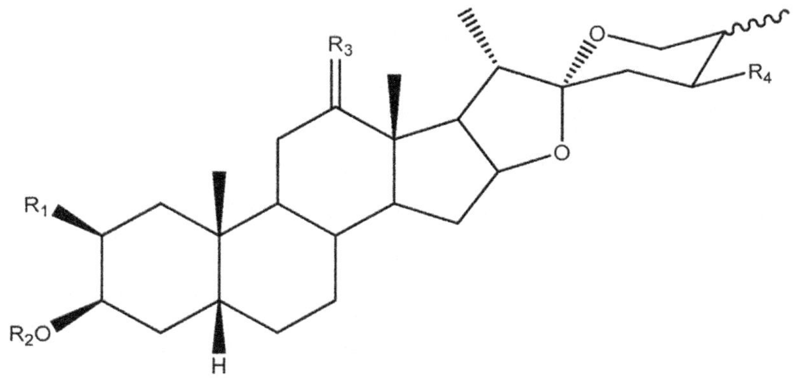

FIG. 5.3 Steroidal spirostane-type chemical structure of the saponin found in the plant *Yucca schidigera*. *(From Jiménez, G.G., Durán, A.G., Macías, F.A., Simonet, A.M., 2021. Structure, bioactivity and analytical methods for the determination of Yucca saponins. Molecules. 14203049. 26 (17). Available from: https://www.mdpi.com/1420-3049/26/17/5251/pdf. doi:10.3390/molecules26175251.)*

In conclusion to this category of bioactive compounds, it is important to mention additional plants from which compounds are isolated with the aim of providing functional properties to cosmetic formulations. These plants include the genera *Acanthopanax senticosus*, *Avena sativa*, *Camellia* spp., *Sanguisorba officinalis*, among others, which are incorporated into specialized skin and hair care products in combination with emollients. The bioactive compounds derived from these plants are classified as functional ingredients, as they significantly contribute to cosmetic formulation technology. Specifically, they perform roles such as forming protective films, gelling, increasing viscosity, stabilizing suspensions, as well as acting as emollient and emulsifying agents (Kanlayavattanakul et al., 2024).

3 Mechanisms of action of medicinal plants

The bioactive compounds from medicinal plants interact with the skin in several ways to deliver therapeutic benefits.

3.1 Antiinflammatory effects

Acute or chronic inflammatory conditions are those that arise following the invasion of foreign agents such as microorganisms, dust particles, viruses, and other elements that can act as antigens, triggering an immune response through the activation of both defensive cells and antimicrobial substances (Arulselvan et al., 2016). The inflammatory state is, therefore, a complex process involving the participation of various cells, the activation of signaling pathways, and the secretion of protective molecules. One of the plants widely known for its multiple beneficial properties is calendula (*Calendula officinalis* L.), also known as marigold, which belongs to the *Asteraceae* family (Vella et al., 2024; García-Chacón et al., 2023) Phenotypically, it is a herbaceous plant with flowers ranging from yellow to orange, capable of thriving in sunny conditions and various soil types. It is a cultivated flower of high significance even in ancient times due to its special properties in addressing multiple ailments. For this reason, it is classified as a medicinal plant. In the modern era, thanks to the secondary metabolites contained in its flowers, this plant is also utilized in the cosmetics industry. Specifically, the bioactive molecules that function as secondary metabolites in calendula are polyphenols (mainly flavonoids), terpenes, and alkaloids. These contribute in many contexts as antioxidants, cardioprotective agents, antimicrobials, cytotoxins, and antiinflammatory agents. The notable antiinflammatory activity is primarily attributed to the properties of terpenes, particularly triterpenes. According to in vivo literature data, this activity is due to the presence of lipophilic triterpene esters. Furthermore, laboratory tests showed that the use of calendula flowers in experimental animals effectively reduced and even treated edema. In addition, plant extracts demonstrated mechanisms that prevent the formation of pro-inflammatory cytokines, known to promote inflammation (Vella et al., 2024). In the cosmetics industry, calendula is mainly used in products designed for sensitive skin types or in cases of skin irritation and itching, offering relief from discomfort. The main component extracted from the plant for its soothing properties is calendula oil. Moreover, the use of this botanical oil has been evaluated as safe, even though its mechanisms of action have not been extensively studied (Silva et al., 2021). Within the context of herbs applied in cosmetology, another notable plant with similar antiinflammatory properties is rosemary (*R. officinalis* L.), belonging to the *Lamiaceae* family. Among its polyphenolic compounds responsible for antiinflammatory action are carnosol, carnosic acid, ursolic acid, oleanolic acid, and micromeric acid. In particular, carnosic acid plays a key role, acting as a switch and inhibitor of the activation of proinflammatory components like NO, which subsequently trigger inflammatory reactions. It is also worth noting that one of the therapeutic properties of rosemary is wound healing. Studies have shown that administration of rosemary extract to laboratory animals (male mice) resulted in decreased healing time for wounds in both diabetic and nondiabetic mice. Moreover, another scientific study conducted on rats with induced wounds and subsequent infection with the fungus *Candida albicans* demonstrated that topical application of a cream containing 4% w/w rosemary significantly accelerated healing compared to a cream with only 2% w/w of the plant's bioactive ingredients. Therefore the effectiveness of the plant in wound healing is undeniably dose-dependent (de Macedo et al., 2020). Another plant with antiinflammatory properties used in cosmetic formulations is turmeric (*Curcuma longa* L.). Turmeric belongs to the *Zingiberaceae* family, like ginger, with which it is often combined to enhance their shared properties. The main bioactive compound responsible for turmeric's antiinflammatory action is curcumin, a polyphenolic compound. This curcuminoid, along with other active compounds, has been utilized for various applications such as treatment on the scalp to prevent inflammation, as well as for skin conditions like infections and itchy irritations. Furthermore, curcumin derivatives—such as tetrahydrocurcuminoid, the reduced form of curcumin—exhibit even stronger antiinflammatory properties, particularly in cosmetics. This derivative also provides significant antioxidant activity and is used as a whitening agent and for combating aging. In conclusion, it is worth highlighting that turmeric, like many other plants with bioactive compounds, offers a wide range of biological actions. Therefore its use is not limited to just antiinflammatory effects but also includes antioxidant, anticancer, and antiaging properties (Messire et al., 2023). In addition, eugenol—being the predominant component of the essential oil of clove (*Syzygium aromaticum* L.)—has demonstrated both antiinflammatory and healing properties in laboratory experiments on mice. These effects were mainly based on mechanisms that influenced the response of proinflammatory cytokines (Haro-González et al., 2021). To summarize, the plants discussed exhibit notable antiinflammatory action through various molecular pathways, making them highly promising candidates for future applications in natural pharmaceutical and cosmetic formulations.

3.2 Antioxidant protection

Antioxidants are molecules or substances that are present in negligible concentrations in the body compared to their substrates and are classified into various categories based on their structure, their solubility in hydrophilic components (e.g., glutathione and ascorbic acid) or in lipophilic elements (e.g., α-tocopherol, β-carotene, lipoic acids, etc.), and their mechanisms of action. They can also be distinguished based on their ability to participate in enzymatic reactions. It is important to note that the mechanism of action of these antioxidant substances varies and follows a sequence involving, first, the prevention of the formation of harmful molecules against the skin, then the inhibition of the action of oxidative substances—that is, those that contribute to the acceleration of premature skin aging—and finally, the repair of skin structure if the previous two stages have been bypassed. The body's primary defense is associated with the prevention of free radical formation. In cases where this preventive step does not occur promptly, the second line of defense involves primarily low molecular weight antioxidants (such as flavonoids, carotenoids, vitamin E, etc.), which play a crucial role in neutralizing the free radicals that have been generated. In the final stage, enzymatic antioxidants catalyze the restoration and repair of tissue damage to the skin. However, it is worth mentioning that harmful molecular agents for the skin are not limited to free radicals; ROS and oxidative stress are equally damaging (Table 5.1). The production and gradual accumulation of these molecules over time result in aging. These reactive species adversely affect the structure and function of cellular components, leading to impaired cellular processes and, ultimately, apoptosis. Among antioxidants, particular emphasis should be placed on

TABLE 5.1 Reactive oxygen species (ROS).

Type of ROS	Chemical formula	Origin	Effect on skin/organism
Superoxide anion	$O_2^{-}\bullet$	Reduction of O_2	Initiates oxidative stress, inflammation
Hydrogen peroxide	H_2O_2	Catalysis of $O_2^{-}\bullet$ by superoxide dismutase (SOD)	Damage to lipids and DNA
Hydroxyl radical	$\bullet OH$	Reduction of H in the presence of a transition metal	Highly cytotoxic, collagen degradation
Singlet oxygen	$^1O_2$	Photochemical reactions, UV radiation	Photoaging, oxidative damage to cells
Hypochlorous acid	HOCl	Neutrophils, myeloperoxidase	Inflammation, tissue damage during immune response

From Md Jaffri, J., 2023. Reactive oxygen species and antioxidant system in selected skin disorders. Malaysian J. Med. Sci. 30 (1), 7–20. doi:10.21315/mjms2023.30.1.2.

those derived from medicinal plants, as they exhibit remarkable protective and functional properties against free radicals (Michalak, 2022).

There is a variety of plants that possess antioxidant activity. One of the widely known oils classified as essential oils is clove oil (*S. aromaticum* L.). It has been distinguished and discussed for its antioxidant benefits, which are attributed to its major component, eugenol (Alfikri et al., 2020). Eugenol, along with other components present in smaller concentrations in clove oil, makes this plant an antioxidant, as they are responsible for the endogenous increase of molecules that combat ROS such as O_2^{-}•, H_2O_2, •OH, $^1O_2$, HOCl, etc. More specifically, from a chemical standpoint, the group responsible for eugenol's antioxidant activity is the hydroxyl group (–OH) embedded in the phenolic compound (Haro-González et al., 2021). Since this oil is a bioactive and biological molecule, it appears to be preferred over other additives that promise similar effects but may have harmful and toxic impacts on health. This essential oil has been assessed and evaluated in terms of various factors related to its efficacy, quality, and antioxidant activity (Alfikri et al., 2020). Another widely known and commonly used plant in everyday routines is green tea (*C. sinensis*). Green tea belongs to the Theaceae family and is popular not only for its antioxidant action but also for its multiple health benefits. Consequently, it has high demand and use despite issues of instability and bioavailability, which have been addressed by the invention and utilization of solvent molecules for extracting its metabolites. The majority of the metabolites responsible for green tea's effects are polyphenolic catechins. Such compounds include epicatechin, epigallocatechin-3, epigallocatechin, and most importantly, epigallocatechin-3-gallate, which is present in the highest concentration. The concentrations of these metabolites vary depending on multiple factors such as the type of tea, growth conditions, extraction process, etc. It is worth mentioning, as noted above, that effective solvents have been developed to extract catechins for use in the cosmetics industry with higher efficiency and fewer side effects. In addition, due to the lipid nature of the skin, it is often difficult or even impossible for any substance to penetrate it unaffected. Therefore catechins are encapsulated in special carrier molecules such as lipid nanoparticles, ethosomes, and niosomes to maximize bioavailability and absorption speed (Alfikri et al., 2020). Moreover, another botanical extract that has attracted attention for over a decade due to its beneficial properties is grape extract (Ferreira et al., 2021). According to statistics and literature, grape extract is noted as the most frequently used active ingredient in cosmetic formulations intended for antiaging (antioxidant) use. The bioactive compound responsible for the strong antioxidant effects in grapes is resveratrol. This is also a polyphenolic compound present in both of its stereoisomeric forms in the aerial parts of the plant. Resveratrol acts through multiple mechanisms, including minimizing the expression of proteins involved in the production of ROS and increasing the synthesis of proteins that counteract these harmful oxygen species. Supporting this, an in vivo study showed that the topical application of a serum containing 1% grape extract twice daily for 4 weeks had a positive effect on skin texture, improving surface uniformity and smoothing imperfections such as wrinkles. Further research summarizes the following data: The extract mainly used in cosmetics is from grape seeds, while the oil has demonstrated emollient properties, providing hydration and elasticity. Finally, grape juice has not been widely used in the cosmetics industry, likely due to the lack of well-documented studies supporting its effects (Ferreira et al., 2021). Concluding with grapes, another plant mentioned above for its antiinflammatory action is rosemary (*R. officinalis* L.). It should be noted that most plants exhibit combined biological activities rather than isolated ones. Rosemary extract shows significant antioxidant capacity mainly linked to its phenolic compounds. The antioxidant action generally focuses on neutralizing free radicals, but secondary metabolites may also biologically regulate apoptosis, cell signaling, and metabolic processing of foreign substances (de Macedo et al., 2020). It is also important to highlight that the photoprotective effect is closely related to antioxidant activity since various forms of radiation promote free radical formation. Specifically, in vivo and *in vitro* experiments demonstrated that rosemary extract combined with citrus extracts increased cell protection by up to 70% after UV exposure, preserving DNA integrity, partially inhibiting free radical formation, and increasing the UV dose required to cause skin damage. Another antioxidant plant is *Andrographis paniculata*, from the *Acanthaceae* family. Its extracts contain flavonoids and phenolic compounds, explaining its antioxidant properties. It has been shown to possess stronger biological activity compared to other antioxidants such as vitamin C. Regarding its mechanism, it primarily involves the inactivation and neutralization of free radicals. Experimentally, *A. paniculata* mimics endogenous enzymes such as superoxide dismutase and catalase in cells susceptible to oxidative stress. These enzymes are crucial for the organism's physiology as natural antioxidant defense mechanisms, making the presence of a plant that mimics such biological activity invaluable for cosmetic use (Messire et al., 2023). Finally, other plant species utilized for maintaining oxidative protection and incorporated into cosmetics include *Butyrospermum parkii*, *Glycine soja*, *Simmondsia chinensis*, and *Helianthus annuus* (Ferreira et al., 2021).

3.3 Antimicrobial properties

Microorganisms, also called microbes, are organisms practically invisible to the naked eye, such as bacteria, fungi, protozoa, and viruses. This category does not include exclusively pathogenic agents but also symbiotic organisms that are present everywhere. They can inhabit multiple environments such as soil, air, surfaces, and even the human body. In humans, the entire collection of microbes colonizing the body is called the microbiome. Although these microorganisms are mostly harmless, they can be opportunistically pathogenic, meaning that when the immune system weakens, they can act harmfully on the host, causing health complications such as infections (Dey and Ray Chaudhuri, 2023). Since microorganisms can grow anywhere, they can also be found in cosmetics due to their favorable composition (water, organic substances). Because of the increasing microbial resistance to antibiotics, scientists have shifted their focus to natural metabolites instead of synthetic chemical compounds. Consequently, plants containing bioactive molecules with antimicrobial properties have increasingly been incorporated into cosmetic formulations. This results in a safe product that creates a feeling of security and trust in consumers. These natural compounds are used as antimicrobials, aiming to inhibit the growth of pathogens in cosmetics. One plant that has demonstrated antimicrobial activity, according to research, is basil (*Ocimum basilicum*) (Rybczyńska-Tkaczyk et al., 2023). Specifically, basil is an herb belonging to the *Lamiaceae* family and possesses a wide range of active and biological properties due to its many bioactive compounds. Various scientific studies report that basil essential oil has contributed to combating many bacterial species, often with stronger effects than common synthetic antibiotics such as ciprofloxacin or gentamicin. The bacteria most sensitive to basil oil and less sensitive to commonly used broad-spectrum antibiotics include *Salmonella, Escherichia coli, Salmonella enterica, Providencia stuartii, coagulase-positive staphylococci,* and *group D streptococci*. To understand the mechanism of action, a comparison is made between the two major bacterial categories, Gram-positive and Gram-negative. Gram-positive bacteria have been shown to be more susceptible to growth inhibition after exposure to the essential oil, unlike Gram-negative bacteria. Basil essential oil has little effect on Gram-negative bacteria, as they possess an outer membrane external to the cell wall, providing protection against hydrophobic external agents. The antimicrobial action of basil essential oil arises from the activity of its main bioactive molecules, such as estragole and linalool. These compounds alter the normal configuration of Gram-positive bacterial membranes, leading to cell death by disrupting the membrane's stability and allowing ATP and potassium ions to leak into the cell (Zhakipbekov et al., 2024). Another well-known plant incorporated in cosmetics for its antimicrobial activity is tea tree (*Melaleuca alternifolia*). Unlike its role as a preservative in cosmetics to prevent microbial growth, its application aims to protect the skin from harmful microbial colonization. Tea tree belongs to the *Myrtaceae* family and is native to Australia. Its essential oil is mainly extracted from the leaves by steam distillation. This oil contains a mixture of over 100 chemical compounds, with terpinen-4-ol being the most biologically active and abundant. Studies have shown that tea tree oil is safe for topical application, which contributes to its acceptance, though safety is limited for certain groups such as children not yet of reproductive age, pregnant or breastfeeding women, and women trying to conceive (Kairey et al., 2023). Therefore tea tree oil is included in many skincare and cosmetic products aimed at relieving dermatological inflammations like acne and other skin conditions. Its mechanism of action is based on the synergistic interaction of its components, including terpenes and alcohols, which modify the membrane components of invading pathogens, weakening them. The lipophilic nature of some compounds, such as cyclic monoterpenes, facilitates their movement into the lipid membrane environment of microorganisms, causing membrane expansion, increased fluidity, and enzyme inhibition. According to literature reviews, antimicrobial activity studies mainly focus on bacteria and fungi rather than viruses, which have been less investigated regarding their susceptibility to tea tree oil. However, studies on enveloped viruses like herpes simplex virus (HSV-1) and influenza have shown positive correlations between tea tree oil application and antiviral efficacy. Enveloped viruses are more sensitive to such agents than nonenveloped ("naked") viruses, which show resistance to many antimicrobials, including tea tree oil. Kairey et al. evaluated the effectiveness of the main chemical compounds of tea tree oil against bacteria, fungi, and nonenveloped viruses, confirming the oil's positive antimicrobial activity. Beyond antimicrobial effects, tea tree oil also contributes to wound healing (Kairey et al., 2023). Another herb widely used for its antimicrobial properties is common thyme. It is a highly valued commercial plant in folk medicine, pharmaceuticals, and cosmetics. Thyme belongs to the Lamiaceae family and is a shrub with aromatic leaves retained year-round. It grows predominantly in Mediterranean regions such as Spain, Greece, parts of Asia, Southern Europe, and North Africa. Thyme's antibacterial actions are primarily attributed to its essential oil. Essential oils consist of complex mixtures of organic compounds such as terpenes, phenols, and alcohols (Gupta et al., 2024). The main active compounds in thyme oil are thymol and carvacrol (Wirtu et al., 2024). Research has confirmed thyme oil's antimicrobial activity, especially against *Streptococcus mutans*. Thymol's mechanism of action against this pathogen involves cell lysis, induction of oxidative stress creating an unfavorable environment for the bacteria, and prevention of resistant bacterial communities known as biofilms (Vassiliou et al., 2023).

Doghish et al. confirmed that thymol, the main component of thyme oil, effectively inhibits the growth of a broad spectrum of bacteria. However, application limitations exist due to thymol's volatility, molecular instability, and lipophilic nature. An effective solution is the use of carriers, such as NEs, to protectively transport the bioactive molecule, ensuring its function without significant hindrance (Doghish et al., 2023). In conclusion, using thyme oil with appropriate delivery systems is justified due to its wide range of activities, including anticancer properties.

3.4 Activation of collagen synthesis and wound healing

Collagen is a crucial protein essential for the elasticity, firmness, and youthfulness of the skin, as well as for its restoration process following tissue damage. It is important to mention that the biosynthesis of collagen, which exists in >27 types, is closely linked to both antiaging effects and the acceleration of wound healing. Therefore plants with antioxidant properties are expected to contribute to the anabolic process of this protein. The highest percentages of collagen formation in the skin concern types I and III collagen, which contribute to the elasticity and cohesion of the skin through their cooperative action, along with type IV collagen, which is present in the skin but in a much smaller amount (5%). It is also worth noting that the biosynthesis of types I and III collagen is inversely proportional to age, resulting in decreased production as age increases (Boo, 2022; Gref et al., 2020). A popular plant used for skin care is aloe vera. This plant belongs to the family *Liliaceae* and is characterized by its green leaves, whose parenchymal tissue inside consists of a clear, gelatinous substance resembling gel. Specifically, the composition of aloe vera consists of three layers. The innermost layer contains a very high water content, approaching 99%, while the remaining percentage consists of solid material containing bioactive compounds. The second layer consists of a latex juice, which is yellow in color and rich in glycosides and anthraquinones. This juice is responsible for the production of a viscous protein. Aloe vera mainly thrives in areas with low humidity, although its cultivation and use have spread to countless regions worldwide. According to bibliographic references, it has been known and referred to as a "gift of nature" due to its applications in various conditions since ancient times, with particular emphasis on its use in medicine (Chelu et al., 2023). The widespread application of raw aloe gel is especially based on wound healing, as the presence and activation of multiple bioactive components in the area of injury contribute positively to other conditions as well. These relate to moisturizing the affected area, reducing stiffness, developing defense against the entry of microorganisms, and relieving pain as much as possible (Panahkhahi, 2010). Aloe is useful for wound care primarily because it activates the mechanism of collagen production. Therefore everything begins with the induction of the proliferation of the cells responsible for producing the structural protein, which are fibroblasts. Fibroblasts are the dominant cells forming part of the connective tissue and are associated with the production of collagen and elastin. Hence, the application of this plant's gel initially increases the number of fibroblasts and, consequently, the production of collagen in larger amounts. According to the research by Hidayat et al., the addition of triatomic oxygen, or ozone, in ointments containing aloe essential oil resulted in increased proliferation of fibroblasts. This increased proliferation leads to enhanced collagen synthesis and further thickening of the dermal tissue compared to the ointment containing only aloe essential oil, without ozone. Therefore ozonated essential oil is considered preferable, as it enhances healing through increased collagen production. In conclusion, many studies confirm that aloe, in any form, contributes to stimulating collagen production and enhancing other biological functions such as healing and protecting the skin tissue (Hidayat et al., 2021). Another medicinal plant containing bioactive molecules necessary for inducing collagen synthesis and wound repair is *Centella asiatica*, which belongs to the family Apiaceae. This plant has been attributed several names from ancient times until today, such as *Hydrocotyle asiatica*, brahmi, mandookaparni, and gotu kola. It is characterized by a soft stem and the ability to grow beyond 2 years (Arribas-López et al., 2022). This plant contains many promising bioactive triterpenoid compounds. These triterpenoids belong to a class of organic compounds possessing amphiphilic properties. More specifically, they consist of a lipophilic aglycone part and a hydrophilic sugar chain. The main bioactive compounds identified are asiatic acid, asiaticoside, madecassoside or brahminoside, and madecassic acid or brahmic acid. The concentration of these compounds depends on multiple factors such as the plant's genetic background, and the extraction process. Experiments on commonly used laboratory animals, such as mice, have confirmed further stimulation of collagen biosynthesis, provided that the maturation of the precursor form procollagen into collagen and finally the assembly of collagen into fibers takes place. The stimulation of collagen synthesis concerned both oral administration and topical application. A correlation has been attributed between the proliferation of fibroblast growth factors, vascular endothelial growth factor, and possibly type I collagen production with tissue repair. The process occurs through the activation of a pathway independent of the kinase TβR2. Arribas-López et al. conducted a review of the existing literature to assess the effectiveness of *C. asiatica* extract in activating factors responsible for skin wound healing. The studies examined involved clinical trials, indicating the involvement of humans rather than laboratory animals. The collected results showed a correlation between the extract and the processes of wound edge contraction through fibroblast action and the formation of granulation tissue containing cells necessary for new epithelium formation. In addition, an acceleration of healing time was observed.

3.5 Skin barrier repair

The skin, as the largest external organ of the human body, constitutes a complex and multidimensional protective system. It is structured into three distinct layers, which, from the outside inward, are: the epidermis, the dermis, and the subcutaneous tissue. However, the concept of protection is especially confined to the epidermal zone, which is further divided into sublayers. These layers follow one another sequentially, beginning with the basal layer, which is in contact with the underlying connective tissue. Next comes the spinous layer, followed by the granular and the clear layers. Finally, the outermost layer is the stratum corneum, which is of paramount importance for the skin's defense and protection (Leo et al., 2022). The stratum corneum contains certain cells that are fully differentiated and have lost their nuclei and organelles, known as corneocytes. These cells contain an abundant protein called keratin, which functions as a protective shield in cooperation with various forms of lipids against numerous factors. Beneath the basal membrane of the epidermis lies the dermis, primarily serving a supportive role for the aforementioned layers. However, it also provides other functions such as thermoregulation, water balance, and vascular supply to the epidermis due to the presence of blood vessels (Bouwstra et al., 2023). The lipids previously mentioned as present in the stratum corneum include ceramides, cholesterol, and fatty acids, which are found in almost equal amounts (Leo et al., 2022). A plant recognized for its strengthening properties on the epidermal barrier is rice (*Oryza sativa*). This grass-like plant belongs to the family Poaceae and is used not only as edible food but also functionally in products aimed at protecting the skin barrier (Zhang et al., 2022). The use of rice is based on the presence of certain components called ceramides, which are also found in the stratum corneum of the skin and significantly contribute to maintaining and protecting the skin barrier. Ceramides are particularly valuable because it has been proven that, with the passage of time and aging, their content in the lipid layer decreases. The consequence of ceramide reduction is water loss from the skin greater than expected, leading to partial disruption of the barrier's balance. A clinical trial conducted by Leo et al. to evaluate the effectiveness of supplements containing rice ceramides confirmed previous experimental data from laboratory animal studies supporting the contribution of rice ceramides to the restoration of the skin barrier. The enhancement of the natural barrier appeared to be based on an increase in the secretion of the sebaceous glands, sebum, which acts preventively against pathogen invasion, similarly to the ceramides of the epidermis.

4 Applications in biofunctional cosmetics

4.1 Acne treatment

Common acne is classified as one of the widely prevalent skin conditions that can affect all age groups indiscriminately, with the highest prevalence among adolescents and young adults (between 18 and 30 years old). The localization of the condition is not limited exclusively to the face, as many may assume, but also occurs on areas of the trunk, such as the neck, upper back, and chest. The clinical manifestations of the condition vary depending on the case and include, besides the common form, acne appearing in newborns and infants, occupational acne, acne with multiple lesions, acute forms, drug-induced acne, and others. However, despite the various heterogeneous manifestations of acne mentioned, common acne accounts for 99% of cases (Kim and Kim, 2024). The condition is evaluated by various factors, including the type of lesion. In cases of blackheads, i.e., open comedones, which are open skin pores exposed to atmospheric air with excessive sebum production, acne falls under the noninflammatory category. Noninflammatory acne also includes whiteheads or closed comedones, where the skin pores are closed and sebum is neither exposed to nor influenced by the external air. On the other hand, inflammatory acne is more critical and severe regarding the damage it causes to the skin, presenting papules, pustules, nodules, and cysts, which later lead to the formation of scar tissue on the epidermal surface (Vasam et al., 2023). Inflammatory acne thus requires special attention, as it demands intensive treatment (Kim and Kim, 2024). The etiological factors causing this skin disease are multiple and not limited to a single factor. These include overproduction of sebum, excessive keratin production exceeding normal levels in the hair follicle area, microbial growth, and the subsequent inflammatory response that follows in each skin type. These factors are interconnected and depend on genetic background, hormone production, and external environmental factors, which determine the pathogenesis and treatment approach. Therapeutic regimens used for acne treatment fall into two categories: one involves topical applications containing active agents such as retinoids and benzoyl peroxide, commonly applied for moderate acne. The second category involves oral medication, including antimicrobial agents and hormones, prescribed by a physician for more severe acne cases. Genetic background significantly influences acne pathogenesis, as increased occurrence has been observed among relatives with the condition. For example, a gene responsible for androgen receptor expression has been directly linked to acne development following mutation. These mutated genes cause hyperactivity of sebaceous glands, which is a causative factor in acne development. Other genetic factors related to immune response also contribute to this skin disorder. Besides genetic factors leading to excessive sebum production, other external influences include diet and weather conditions. Diets rich in high glycemic index foods and dairy products have been shown to correlate with acne development by enhancing the signaling of insulin-like growth factor 1 (IGF-1), which exacerbates sebum formation. In addition, acne is associated with underlying endocrine disorders such as polycystic ovary syndrome and adrenal gland hypertrophy. Regarding the microbiome, several microorganisms affect skin physiology. In particular, overgrowth of bacteria such as *Cutibacterium acnes* and *Staphylococcus epidermidis* releases factors linked to the proinflammatory process, resulting in abnormal synthesis of sebum, keratin, filaggrin, and IGF-1 levels.

As for treatments, the cornerstone agents for improving acne's clinical picture are retinoids of three generations (Tobiasz et al., 2022). Examples include tretinoin (all-trans retinoic acid) and synthetic derivatives like adapalene, tazarotene, trifarotene, alitretinoin, and bexarotene, with tazarotene showing high effectiveness. Benzoyl peroxide is also a key product used alone or in combination with retinoids for maximal lesion repair. Despite classic acne treatments, ongoing research has led to innovative therapies based on phytotherapeutic compounds aimed at acne suppression. Research is driven by challenges such as the side effects of conventional treatments, reduced efficacy, high cost, and antibiotic resistance (Nascimento et al., 2023). For example, tea tree oil (*M. alternifolia*), as discussed earlier, contains bioactive compounds effective in acne management due to its antimicrobial, antiinflammatory, and antioxidant properties, confirmed in vivo (Nascimento et al., 2023). Specifically, studies have shown that topical gels with 5% tea tree oil significantly reduce both the number and severity of acne lesions compared to placebo. However, tea tree oil was less effective than benzoyl peroxide in reducing inflammatory lesions. Combining NEs of tea tree oil with adapalene (a retinoid) in topical gels shows promising therapeutic potential for reducing lesion count and acne severity (Kairey et al., 2023). In addition, a 4-week experimental trial tested a blend of essential oils (3% tea tree, 2% lavender, and jojoba) on acne patients. The intervention group showed significant reductions in *C. acnes*, inflammatory and noninflammatory lesions, and sebum, with minimal side effects limited to transient itching (Nascimento et al., 2023). According to Lee et al., active compounds in tea tree oil such as terpinen-4-ol, α-terpinolene, α-terpinene, and α-terpineol (key terpenes) effectively suppress acne-related bacteria like *C. acnes* and *Staphylococcus aureus*, showing strong antimicrobial properties even at low concentrations without toxic side effects. Another study by Mazzarello et al. concluded that a cream containing 3% tea tree oil, 20% propolis, and 10% aloe vera exhibited stronger effects on acne pathophysiology than established antibiotic products marketed for acne. This enhanced effect was based on greater reductions in acne, scar redness, severity, and overall lesion burden. Thus these studies support tea tree oil's use as a complementary or alternative option in managing various acne types. Another plant whose essential oil is studied for acne treatment is eucalyptus (*Eucalyptus globulus*). Its use stems from multiple properties, including effective scar inhibition associated with acne. Studies confirm the suppressive effect of 1,8-cineole—one of its main components—against pathogenic strains involved in acne, such as *C. acnes*, *S. aureus*, and *S. epidermidis*. Eucalyptus oil not only controls infection but also reduces sebum production. A study showed that a water-based cream with 2% eucalyptus oil was more effective than a commercial acne gel containing 5% benzoyl peroxide (Nurzyńska-Wierdak et al., 2023). Furthermore, cannabis (*Cannabis sativa*) is emerging as a treatment. Cannabidiol (CBD), one of its potent compounds, significantly inhibits lipid overproduction proportional to its concentration. CBD administration reduces mRNA expression for TNF-α and other inflammatory cytokines like IL-1β and IL-6 in sebaceous cells, acting primarily as an antiinflammatory agent in acne prevention (Peyravian et al., 2022). In summary, essential oils successfully used for acne suppression include myrtle (*M. communis Linn.*), lavender (*Lavandula angustifolia Mill.*), oregano (*Origanum vulgare* L.), thyme (*Thymus vulgaris* L.), and lemon (*Citrus limon* L.) oils, usually formulated as creams (Nurzyńska-Wierdak et al., 2023).

4.2 Moisturizers

Skin hydration is a vital process that occurs both endogenously, regulated by the skin's own mechanisms, and exogenously through the topical application of moisturizing products. The endogenous mechanism is based on the presence of the outermost layer of the epidermis, the stratum corneum, which acts beneficially not only as a barrier against foreign invaders but also contributes to the skin's moisture retention mechanism. This layer maintains skin hydration by retaining water molecules originating both from the underlying skin tissues and from the atmosphere. Therefore hydration is an important process that supports the integrity of the epidermal barrier, the activity of enzymes involved in skin function, and the physiological cellular processes related to the removal of dead cells and the differentiation of skin tissue (Liu, 2022). More specifically, a set of chemical factors present in the stratum corneum act homeostatically with regard to the barrier's defensive function and the retention of an appropriate amount of water, contributing to the formation of the natural moisturizing factor (NMF). The function of the stratum corneum largely depends on the acidic environment of the epidermis. A deviation from the skin's normal pH can disrupt the basic functions of the stratum corneum, resulting in a reduced barrier capacity to protect against pathogenic entry, leading to inflammation. Simultaneously, increased water loss occurs, causing dehydration of the skin tissue. Consequently, the mobilization for exogenous skin hydration through topical formulations is necessary both to prevent skin diseases that may arise from barrier dysfunction and to treat them. An example of a skin disorder caused by damage to the integrity of the skin barrier, resulting in reduced hydration, is xerosis (dry skin). This skin condition primarily occurs in older adults due to multifactorial causes that weaken the epidermal barrier. Another condition whose restoration is mainly based on skin hydration is atopic dermatitis. This condition is chronic and recurrent, thus requiring serious and systematic management (Kulthanan et al., 2021). Closing with skin disorders, it is worth mentioning pruritus (itching), psoriasis, and inflammation, which arise due to the absence of NMFs and a thinner stratum corneum layer (Razia et al., 2021).

For the prevention and treatment of skin diseases, plant-based products are therefore developed and offered in the form of skincare formulations. To understand the role of moisturizing creams, it is necessary to explain their function. Moisturizing creams have a dual role: the first is based on creating a protective membrane on the skin's surface that limits water loss through evaporation. The second property relates to humectant elements that help retain water molecules within the stratum corneum. However, the complex structure of the skin barrier limits the ability of moisturizers to penetrate the deeper layers of the epidermis. Therefore colloidal systems such as microemulsions and NEs, as well as particles containing lipids and polymers, have proven effective in delivering moisturizing ingredients into the skin (Razia et al., 2021). For the prevention and treatment of skin diseases, plant-derived products are thus developed and offered as skincare formulations (Liu, 2022). The literature shows that extracts from the leaves, gel, skin, or chemical components of the aloe vera plant have been extensively used in moisturizing skincare products due to their multidimensional mechanisms of action. The experimental study by Razia et al. focused on the moisturizing properties of aloe flowers. It concluded that the use of aloe vera flower extract dissolved in water effectively enhances hydration. This is due to the increased expression of the keratinocyte differentiation marker involucrin (IVL) mediated by the active compound isoorientin (Razia et al., 2021). Finally, according to a study, the extract of wild cherry showed the greatest moisturizing effect among five medicinal plants, with a statistically significant difference compared to the control cream ($P < .05$). Other plant extracts, aside from licorice, also showed higher moisturizing activity. Therefore the findings of this research support the use of plant extracts such as wild cherry in moisturizing cosmetic products (Khazaeli et al., 2011).

4.3 Whitening and brightening products

The skin's color tone varies among individuals and depends on the amount of melanin produced by specialized cells called melanocytes, which deposit melanin into intracellular structures known as melanosomes (Kang et al., 2021). These cells combine two primary functions: the production of pheomelanin, responsible for lighter skin tones, and eumelanin, which gives darker hues to the epidermis. It is clear, therefore, that the distinctive difference in skin tones mainly depends on the amount of eumelanin synthesized. A person genetically predisposed to increased eumelanin biosynthesis will have darker skin, in contrast to a fair-skinned individual who produces limited amounts of this pigment. Both forms of melanin have demonstrated beneficial effects on the skin, with eumelanin playing a distinct protective role (Thawabteh et al., 2023). Specifically, eumelanin has been found to inhibit the penetration of UV rays more effectively than pheomelanin, thus providing an advantage in protecting against skin diseases caused by solar radiation, such as potential skin cancer. However, attention should also be given to pheomelanin, which possesses thermoregulatory properties, helping the body maintain a cooling sensation in high-temperature conditions. This physiological hue and appearance of the skin can be modified under the influence of three main factors: sun exposure, medication intake, and genetic background. It is noteworthy that the pathogenesis of pigmentation disorders does not only involve an increase in skin tone but also a decrease. In the category referring to excessive melanin biosynthesis, known as hyperpigmentation, various hereditary diseases such as Addison's disease are included. Other causative factors of this condition include trauma, psoriatic lesions, atopic eczema, and inflammatory acne. However, all these factors have a low incidence as causes of hyperpigmentation. Sun radiation has been identified as the primary and most significant cause of this skin alteration. Regarding the opposite condition, which leads to decreased melanin production, it occurs after skin injuries caused by heat, trauma, or irritants. This condition, called hypopigmentation, also involves genetically dependent diseases such as albinism. In general, the most conventional treatments for restoring abnormal pigmentation (hyper- or hypopigmentation) rely on pharmaceutical preparations or, occasionally, the topical application of creams to the affected area. However, these recommended treatments have shown drawbacks, including side effects and increased costs. Therefore attention has turned to therapeutic strategies based on medicinal plants. One of the most studied plant extracts widely used for its whitening properties is *Arctostaphylos uva-ursi* (bearberry) (Seo et al., 2012). This plant is rich in bioactive compounds and has been extensively utilized in medicine to treat various pathological conditions. The main biologically active component of *Uva ursi* appears to be hydroquinone (LiverTox: Clinical and Research Information on Drug-Induced Liver Injury, 2012). The addition of a sugar moiety to the hydroquinone molecule results in a compound with modified properties called arbutin. This compound is responsible for the melanin-regulating properties in formulations containing bearberry extract, essential for restoring the skin's normal tone. More specifically, the whitening effect is based on arbutin's ability to effectively inhibit the activity of the enzyme tyrosinase, which plays a crucial role in the metabolic pathway of melanin biosynthesis. This prevents endogenous overproduction of melanin, aligning with the mechanism of action of conventional treatments for pigmentation disorders (similar to the first-mentioned treatment). In addition, licorice is a herb known for its use in treating hyperpigmentation. This plant contains numerous bioactive compounds, including flavonoids and saponins such as liquiritin, liquiritigenin, isoliquiritigenin (ISL), and glycyrrhizin (or glycyrrhizic acid), which confer significant pharmacological and cosmetic benefits. Among these, ISL is specifically associated with suppressing excessive melanin production by inhibiting the gene responsible for encoding tyrosinase (Kang et al., 2021). In summary, the use of bioactive substances from medicinal plants such as liquiritin, hydroquinone, and arbutin proves valuable in the development of cosmetic products with whitening and melanin-regulating properties. Ongoing research into these natural compounds may offer new, safer, and more effective options for managing skin conditions like hyperpigmentation.

4.4 Antiaging products

Skin aging is a process that remains under investigation today due to the complexity of the mechanisms involved in this condition. However, it is widely documented that aging is a nonpathological condition, linearly dependent on age and the passage of time. Besides its negative effects on the skin, aging is associated with an increased frequency of diseases and mortality. It is important to note that the mechanisms involved in skin structural deterioration are triggered by both endogenous and adverse exogenous factors. These gradually lead to the skin developing the following characteristics: initially, there is a reduction in epidermal thickness, which affects the homeostatic function of the epidermal barrier. As previously mentioned regarding the epidermal barrier, thinning of the skin also impacts the immune response. Since the epidermal barrier no longer fully resists pathogen entry, the immune system becomes more susceptible to persistent infections. Moreover, the renewal rate of keratinocytes is disrupted due to limited mitotic divisions of cells located in the basal layer of the epidermis, which further impairs the barrier's maximal function. Reduced synthesis rates of type 1 collagen are also observed, affecting the population of collagen fibers that provide firmness and elasticity to youthful skin. It should not be overlooked that aging is mainly due to the loss of structural and functional properties of the dermis, inevitably resulting in scars, marks, wrinkles, and others. More specifically, from a cellular perspective, senescent cells—those that accumulate over time—exhibit abnormal characteristics not consistent with normal cells. These cells do not proliferate at the usual rate, do not undergo normal cellular and programmed death, and produce substances that create a favorable environment for inflammation and tissue remodeling. A detailed analysis of aging's causes follows by category. Endogenous factors include the inevitable shortening of genetic material, specifically at the chromosome ends called telomeres, during each DNA replication. Also, the continuous accumulation of damage from free radicals, due to normal oxygen production and other molecules, leads to cell and tissue destruction, accelerating aging by inducing oxidative stress. Furthermore, aging depends on hormonal changes that occur with increasing age. Finally, the increased presence of miR-30a, a micro-RNA, leads to keratinocyte alteration, linked to the aging process. Regarding external factors, they are not solely responsible for aging but contribute to its more immediate manifestation, especially in exposed and visible areas such as the face. These factors relate to unprotected sun exposure, daily habits like smoking, alcohol consumption, sleep deprivation, dietary choices, and air pollution. Aging and its signs, such as wrinkles and changes in skin appearance, can cause insecurity and a feeling of lost youth for many women. These changes may affect psychological well-being, lowering self-confidence and causing emotional stress. This problem has been alleviated with the use of various bioactive substances, especially secondary metabolites from medicinal plants like polyphenols, which contribute to slowing aging or improving its symptoms. Polyphenols have long been recognized for their role as antiaging agents. One plant that has attracted interest in cosmetology is the grape (*V. vinifera*), recognized as a valuable tool against aging. Interest in grapes is justified because they contain numerous biologically active compounds belonging to the polyphenol category. Specifically, this plant material is rich in secondary metabolites, including flavonoids such as flavan-3-ols and flavonols, as well as phenolic acids and anthocyanins. In addition, it contains nutrients such as essential fatty acids, amino acids, and vitamins, which enhance its biological activity. Up to nine different plant derivatives can be isolated from grapes and incorporated into cosmetic formulations without causing irritation or harmful effects on the skin, providing consumers with a sense of safety. Among these raw materials, seed extract is the most frequently incorporated into cosmetic products, followed by extracts from other parts of the plant. Market products containing grape extract include wrinkle-reducing face masks, the Red Grape Sheer Glow sunscreen for daily protection, antiaging exfoliants, intensive seed serums, and antiaging body butter, offering comprehensive skin care that combats signs of aging and enhances youthfulness. The use of *V. vinifera* extract in cosmetics with proven antioxidant properties is primarily based on its ability to scavenge free radicals and protect genetic material from their damaging effects. According to literature studies, the isolation of leaf extract from grapes and its topical incorporation has shown effects on genes related to antiaging at the transcriptional level. These data, combined with other related studies, confirm the beneficial and protective action of *V. vinifera* extracts. Nine other top botanical species besides grapes, often used in skincare products aimed at slowing skin aging, include *B. parkii* (shea or *Vitellaria paradoxa*), *G. soja* (soy), *S. chinensis* (jojoba or *Buxus sinensis*), *Theobroma cacao* (cocoa), *C. officinalis* (marigold), *Limnanthes alba* (meadowfoam), *Glycyrrhiza glabra* (licorice), *A. decurrens* (black wattle), and *H. annuus* (sunflower).

4.5 Hair care products

Ensuring both the morphological and functional quality of hair is a critical factor for both an individual's emotional balance and medical disorder management. For this reason, various therapies have been developed and continue to evolve within research frameworks aimed at hair care and maintenance. The hair shaft, from the outside inward, consists of a layer containing macromolecules such as keratin proteins, other related proteins, and structural lipids that act protectively against mechanical and environmental stressors. Internally, the cortex is a very important structure as it determines the hair's flexibility and strength. This middle structure constitutes the majority of the hair mass. The innermost part is the medulla, containing cells that develop in this area and vary depending on hair type. Maintaining healthy hair depends on both daily habits and genetic factors. The balance and combination of these two components reflect the structural integrity of hair. Studies show that diet is a decisive factor for maintaining hair physiology and preventing mass hair loss. More specifically, a diet rich in simple carbohydrates, lipids, and excessive intake of dietary supplements creates favorable conditions for hair loss. High-risk factors for hair health include smoking, exposure to toxic chemicals such as heavy metals, as well as dermatological conditions like atopic dermatitis, dandruff/seborrheic dermatitis, psoriasis, and scalp hair growth disorders. In addition, genetic predisposition, increased endogenous corticosteroid levels, aging, and hormonal changes such as those occurring during menopause have been shown to adversely affect hair density and growth. Also, the loss of a very important factor, 18-methyleicosanoic acid, which is present in hair and gives it hydrophobicity, has been associated with hair health deterioration. This loss usually results from alkaline chemical interventions, including hair dyeing and heat application for hair straightening. Beyond hair loss, other hair dysfunctions can occur, such as dandruff, brittleness, and dryness. These issues affect a significant portion of the population, who continuously seek effective solutions for scalp-related problems. Medicinal plants today offer effective and scientifically documented remedies for these medical issues. One plant with significant benefits for hair care is *Equisetum arvense*, commonly known as horsetail. It contains multiple minerals like silicon, potassium, calcium, manganese, magnesium, and phosphorus, and is also a source of vitamins (A, E, C), dietary fibers, and phytosterols. Furthermore, it contains numerous secondary metabolites such as tannins, alkaloids, saponins, flavonoids, glycosides, and phenolic compounds, including caffeic acid and phenolic esters, which are the bioactive molecules of medicinal plants. All these factors synergistically promote hair growth, combat dandruff and split ends, and effectively hydrate the hair. Another botanical agent that favors hair growth is *Eclipta prostrata*, known as false daisy, belonging to the *Asteraceae* family. It contains a wide range of bioactive metabolites responsible for its extensive therapeutic action. Depending on the plant part used, its application varies for medical or other purposes. The leaves have been shown, after isolation of secondary metabolites with organic petroleum ether, to enhance hair growth when administered to experimental laboratory animals, resulting in faster hair growth and increased hair density. Regarding hair loss treatment, numerous plant extracts have been proposed, such as rosemary (*R. officinalis* L.) and garlic (*Allium sativum*). Their effectiveness is attributed to improved microcirculation and increased diameter of precapillary arterioles. Finally, coconut oil (*Cocos nucifera*) is noteworthy as a protective agent for hair against various damaging factors, stimulating hair and contributing to hair care.

4.6 Sun protection products

The effect of sunlight on the skin, known as photoaging as previously mentioned, is a contributing factor to skin aging. Solar radiation includes three main types of radiation: UV, visible, and infrared (IR), which belong to the category of nonionizing radiation. However, the radiations implicated in skin damage are UV and IR, as they penetrate the skin and cause cellular damage directly related to photoaging. Isolating UV radiation, it can be further classified into UVA (wavelength = 320–400 nm), UVB (280–320 nm), and UVC (100–280 nm). Among these types, UVC is considered the least dangerous and harmful because the ozone layer effectively absorbs most of it. However, UVA and UVB are identified as harmful to skin health due to their short wavelengths and simultaneously very high energy. These features are similar to gamma rays (γ-rays) and X-rays, although those have much smaller wavelengths (10^{-4} nm to 10^{-2} nm for gamma-rays, and 10^{-2} nm to 10^{1} nm for X-rays). Gamma rays and X-rays belong to the category of ionizing radiation, which causes irreversible cellular damage. Regarding IR radiation, it is particularly harmful because it can penetrate deeper skin layers, reaching even the subcutaneous tissue. Prolonged and insufficiently protected sun exposure leads to intracellular modifications such as the accumulation of ROS and pathological alteration of skin proteins like keratin and collagen, among other effects. However, the impacts are closely related to the frequency and wavelength of each form of electromagnetic radiation. More specifically, at the molecular level, increased radiation absorbed as energy by the base pairs of genetic material leads to their mutations and the formation of pyrimidine photoproducts. These photoproducts form complexes that inhibit vital cellular mechanisms required for survival, including DNA replication and transcription. Overall, these radiations cause immune system suppression, prolonged inflammatory responses, and cancer due to photonic damage. To prevent these damages, the use of appropriate cosmetic formulations with sunscreen protection is essential. These are designed to block or reduce the absorption of harmful radiation by the skin. Research focuses on bioactive plant-derived ingredients isolated from medicinal plants, which exhibit strong photoprotective, antioxidant, and antiinflammatory actions. Medicinal plants contain secondary metabolites such as carotenoids, which carry photoactive groups responsible for absorbing radiation in the 330–900 nm and 1000–1100 nm spectra. Another primary factor contributing to absorption and protection in plant tissues is chlorophyll. Carotenoids are particularly effective photoprotective agents because they can absorb and manage light energy in a way that renders it harmless. Specifically, they have a special low-energy state, lower than that of oxygen that can cause damage, thus preventing the formation of dangerous oxygen species that could harm cells. One notable plant with photoprotective properties is *Silybum marianum* (milk thistle). Its main bioactive substance responsible for this activity is silymarin. Its use in creams at a concentration of 10% (w/w) has demonstrated an SPF level close to 9. Regarding silymarin, it was incorporated into sunscreens using solid lipid nanoparticle carriers to achieve maximum stability of the bioactive compound. These sunscreens recorded an SPF index of 14.1 after topical application in vivo conditions. Another plant utilized in sunscreen formulations is *Elaeagnus angustifolia*. The leaf extract was isolated and used at an 8% (w/w) concentration, showing an SPF value of 21.05 with a standard deviation of ±0.85. In addition, extracts of *Moringa oleifera* are rich in polyphenolic compounds, which have potential uses in sunscreen formulations due to their photoprotective properties. Finally, according to research by Abdallah et al., the oil extract from the petals of *Rosa damascena* Mill. (Rosaceae) demonstrated effective shielding from solar radiation. Bioactive compounds from medicinal plants offer natural and effective protection against solar radiation, reducing skin damage. Further research will enhance their use in cosmetics for optimal care, safety, stability, and more.

5 Challenges and considerations

5.1 Extraction and standardization

The adoption of environmentally friendly practices constitutes a major issue for the industry, something that is beginning to be implemented in modern times. A cornerstone of this effort appears to be the utilization of the plant world for the extraction of bioactive compounds, which can be incorporated into many different sectors. More specifically, since plants represent a continuously renewable raw material that does not cause environmental burden, they have attracted scientific interest for ensuring sustainability (Kapadia et al., 2022). There are two categories of high-value chemicals whose isolation can be achieved through various methods. The main difference between these categories lies in the fact that primary metabolites are molecules essential for the survival of plant cells, in contrast to secondary metabolites, which exist to provide additional advantageous characteristics to the cell, such as protective properties. Primary metabolites include fats, proteins, sugars, and nucleic acids, which are stable factors, while secondary ones are more variable. The sequential steps necessary for a bioactive ingredient to exhibit its promised effect in a cosmetic product include: first, the isolation of the substance, which can involve any part of the plant; second, standardization, or the analytical method that ensures the identification of the ingredients and their quantity; and finally, its incorporation into the cosmetic or pharmaceutical product. Isolation of bioactive molecules using solvents is based on solid–liquid extraction. The extract obtained is then processed through various methods such as filtration and evaporation to isolate the bioactive compounds (Cao et al., 2025). Main methods of extracting bioactive substances from plants include hydrodistillation, steam distillation, cold pressing, solvent extraction, Soxhlet extraction, microwave-assisted extraction, ultrasound-assisted extraction (UAE), subcritical water extraction, and supercritical CO_2 extraction. Each method has its own advantages and limitations, depending on the nature of the plant material and the type of bioactive compounds targeted for isolation. The choice of the appropriate technique depends on factors such as efficiency, environmental friendliness, cost, and stability of the extracts. Modern methods such as microwave-assisted and supercritical CO_2 extraction are gaining ground due to their high efficiency and reduced use of toxic solvents. Hydrodistillation is a traditional and less innovative extraction method that primarily uses water and heat. It is also used for extracting low-volatility and water-insoluble molecules but is most commonly employed for extracting hydrophobic compounds with high boiling points. The plant material is submerged in water, and the mixture is heated to boiling. The resulting vapors, containing the plant's volatile components, are condensed in a cooling system and collected as liquid extracts. This method isolates essential oils and other bioactive ingredients. One major advantage of hydrodistillation is the use of water as a solvent, eliminating the risk of toxic residues in the final product. In addition, it has relatively low setup and operational costs, as it does not require an external steam source, unlike other distillation methods. It is especially suitable for heat-sensitive plant materials, which might degrade at high temperatures. Lastly, the use of large-capacity industrial distillers compensates for the method's often limited yield. However, hydrodistillation demands high energy levels, which increases costs and contributes to CO_2 emissions. Its yield is typically low, especially for fresh plant materials, and prolonged exposure to heat may degrade thermo-sensitive compounds and alter their chemical structure. In some cases, a variation called microwave-assisted hydrodistillation is used. This technique has been shown to significantly accelerate extraction and improve the final product yield while also reducing energy consumption. In steam distillation, the plant material is exposed directly to steam, without contacting water. It is mainly used for extracting components from leaves and flowers and is quite similar to hydrodistillation. Advantages include low equipment cost and isolation of pure products free of organic solvent residues. Disadvantages include the lengthy process time, high energy demand, and the effect of temperature on the molecular structure of the compounds to be isolated. In contrast to thermal methods, cold pressing is based on mechanical pressure for the recovery of secondary metabolites, without involving solvents or heat. It is particularly used for extracting bioactive molecules from the peel or seeds of citrus fruits. Since neither heat nor solvent causes degradation, polyphenols and essential oils can be isolated in an unaltered form. The material must pass through screw presses to extract the valuable components with minimal degradation. Other benefits of this method, due to the absence of chemical substances, include a safe and hygienic product, reduced production costs, and less environmental burden. Therefore these advantages make the method highly attractive for industrial use, except when a prior step, known as pretreatment, is required. In solvent extraction, the principle "like dissolves like" applies, meaning the solvent's polarity must match that of the target substance for effective dissolution. Modern solvents follow environmentally friendly practices. "Green solvents" include water, alcohols (e.g., ethanol), diethyl ether, methyltetrahydrofuran, n-butane, and cyclopentyl methyl ether. Harmful organic solvents that require long processing times are avoided. A popular and widely used solvent is ethanol, which has many advantages. This neutral solvent can extract both polar and nonpolar compounds, has antimicrobial properties (preventing contamination), and evaporates easily, simplifying concentration of the extract (Lee et al., 2024). In all cases, the solvent is selected according to the plant and the targeted bioactive compound. An important factor in choosing a suitable solvent is its purity. To avoid impurities that could negatively affect the extraction process, solvents are purified (typically through distillation) to remove unwanted substances. This method is especially recommended for isolating active molecules from heat-sensitive plants. It also helps reduce energy consumption, thus supporting environmental sustainability. The next method is Soxhlet extraction, which is well-known for its ability to process lipophilic molecules as raw materials. Common solvents used include dichloromethane, often combined with acetone or hexane. This method has several advantages and disadvantages. It is established in industry because it yields large quantities of product and is suitable for compounds with a low boiling point and high molecular weight. However, it has disadvantages such as long extraction time, high operational cost due to large energy and solvent use, and reliance on toxic organic solvents, which limits broader application (Cao et al., 2025). Modern (green) extraction methods are at the forefront of research aiming to overcome the limitations of conventional techniques.

5.2 Stability

The stability of bioactive molecules is of critical importance for the efficacy, activity, and safety of final products, as their degradation or alteration can reduce their biological action and potentially cause undesirable reactions. A significant category of secondary metabolites that exhibit high instability is carotenoids. This characteristic is attributed to the presence of multiple bonds in the hydrocarbon chain, which renders the molecules susceptible to various factors such as heat, light, oxygen, and catalysts. These effects consequently lead to oxidation, hydrolysis, and isomerization during the formulation process, both at the extraction stage and during storage. Furthermore, low levels of bioavailability have been reported, indicating limited absorption and utilization of the substance by the organism. For the above reasons, due to the instability and low bioavailability of most secondary metabolites, modern nanotechnology-based strategies have been developed, aiming at eliminating or at least reducing these disadvantages. A significant advantage of nanotechnological systems is that, due to their small size, they can increase the water solubility of compounds that are naturally poorly soluble in water. This is particularly important for many bioactive substances, as increased solubility translates to better absorption by the organism, thereby enhancing their overall bioavailability (Park et al., 2022). The methods include systems such as liposomes, micelles, lipid nanoparticles, polymeric micro- and nanoparticles, as well as nanocapsules, which contribute to improving the stability, protection, and targeted delivery of bioactive molecules. In the case of nanoencapsulation, these systems serve as carriers of the bioactive substances. Despite the effectiveness of this promising approach, the high production cost, the possibility of toxicity occurrence, as well as the risk of nanoparticle incorporation and aggregation, raise certain concerns. Nanoencapsulation systems can be based either on metallic nanoparticles or lipid and polymeric nanoparticles (de Alcantara Lemos et al., 2021). However, toxicity has been detected in both categories. A subcategory of nanoencapsulation, besides those mentioned above, which finds widespread application in cosmetology, is the creation of oil-in-water NEs. Nanoemulsions consist of small lipid spheres within an aqueous solution, carrying the embedded bioactive substance, with diameters ranging from 10 to 200 nm (de Alcantara Lemos et al., 2021). Emulsifiers are commonly added, whose role is significant, as they help reduce surface tension, which is essential when two different phases coexist in one medium. Both high-energy methods, such as high-pressure homogenization, microfluidization, and ultrasonication, and low-energy methods, such as solvent diffusion, are used for NE preparation, chosen according to the system's characteristics and the application requirements (Flieger et al., 2024). In addition, another category of bioactive molecules, consisting of complex mixtures of secondary metabolites and utilizing nanosystems, is essential oils. These are characterized by limited stability, dependence on climatic factors, and increased susceptibility to oxidative reactions. When applying nanotechnological systems, the encapsulation of bioactive substances minimizes their interaction with external environmental factors, which have a higher likelihood of leading bioactive molecules to degradation, alteration of their structure, and bioactivity. Regarding the mechanism of bioactive substance release from the nanocarrier to exert its effect, this can vary depending on the system selected and the applied conditions. More specifically, among the various possible release mechanisms, the one based on carrier erosion stands out, a process in which the carrier itself is degraded, thus allowing the embedded bioactive substance to be released. Nevertheless, release can also occur through other effective ways, such as diffusion of the substance through intervening pores located on the carrier's surface or through pulsatile release, which requires the external application of a magnetic field. In the field of cosmetology, it has been shown that nanoencapsulated essential oils significantly enhance their antioxidant and antimicrobial activity while contributing to the prevention of undesirable effects such as allergic reactions, irritation, and potential toxic effects (Albuquerque et al., 2022). Nanotechnology now plays an important role in maintaining the stability of natural bioactive compounds, especially in fields where quality and efficacy are of great importance, such as pharmaceuticals and cosmetology.

5.3 Safety and adverse reactions

Medicinal plants and the bioactive compounds they contain are used at an exponential rate in modern cosmetology. A significant advantage of these is that they often cause fewer adverse effects, such as toxic reactions and irritations, compared to conventional cosmetics based on synthetic chemical ingredients. It should be clarified that, despite originating from plant products, they may still contain factors, even in small amounts, that pose risks to human health. Cosmetics constitute a favorable environment for the growth of pathogens, as they often contain a high percentage of water, which promotes their proliferation. For this reason, appropriate preservatives are incorporated to prevent contamination and simultaneously extend the shelf life of the formulation. Furthermore, plant-derived products used in cosmetics, such as herbs, may be contaminated with heavy metals through various routes. For example, the extraction process carries contamination risks in industrial production units where it is performed. In addition, herbs grown in terrestrial ecosystems are largely vulnerable to pollution by heavy metals such as nickel, chromium, lead, and others. Specifically, essential oil extracts have been implicated more frequently due to certain levels of essential oils originating from plants like *T. vulgaris* L. and *L. angustifolia* Mill. Heavy metals, which may be "transferred" through bioactive substances, must be taken seriously as they have the capacity to cause serious effects on human health, ranging from allergic contact dermatitis to organ toxicity due to accumulation after entering systemic circulation. Regarding safety issues, the essential oil of *M. alternifolia* (tea tree oil) has attracted scientific attention because of conflicting views concerning its potential risks. More specifically, this oil has been examined and evaluated for its potential to act as an irritant or allergen to the skin. According to conducted studies, tea tree oil ranked 23rd on the list of the most common allergens in Australia based on collected data. Conversely, equally thorough research conducted in North Africa and Europe produced different conclusions regarding the oil's safety, finding a low association with allergic reactions. However, it can be stated with greater certainty, according to the literature, that adulterated forms of the oil, containing some percentage of lower-grade oil, have been linked to adverse reactions. Moreover, oxidized forms of the oil result in reduced efficacy, as the main bioactive compounds responsible for its activity decrease in percentage, while substances associated with skin irritation, such as p-cymene and peroxide, increase. Records have identified zero deaths and increased injuries following the use of the oil by young children, according to data from the United States National Electronic Injury Surveillance System. In conclusion, the use of this oil should be avoided by pregnant women, breastfeeding mothers, and children under 12 years old due to the lack of sufficient conducted studies. Another essential oil for which there are insufficient safety studies is that of the plant hyssop. According to a review of existing literature, this oil, due to its content of active monoterpenic compounds, has been associated with epileptic and neurotoxic effects following high doses in experimental animals. These effects are attributed to the oil's ability to interact with important neurotransmitters and receptors of the central nervous system. In addition, potential allergic reactions and respiratory irritation have been identified due to specific components such as marrubiin. Side effects in humans have not been thoroughly evaluated through clinical trials, and the available knowledge is mainly based on clinical reports and laboratory research. However, the use of the oil at an appropriate dosage not exceeding safe limits is considered safe, with no identified complications or risks. Furthermore, the genus Cymbopogon, which is applied in cosmetology and is generally regarded as safe, shows adverse effects only when dosage limits are exceeded, when soil contamination by heavy metals occurs, or in possible interactions of the plant with certain drugs. Despite the safety profile of this medicinal plant genus, it should be avoided during pregnancy and breastfeeding. In addition, a characteristic example is bergamot essential oil (*Citrus bergamia*), which, despite its stimulatory effect on melanin synthesis through tyrosinase activation, carries a phototoxic risk due to the presence of methoxylated psoralens. Application before exposure to UV radiation can cause photosensitivity and skin reactions, highlighting the importance of safety evaluation even for natural ingredients. In closing, essential oils are generally considered safe with a reduced risk of adverse effects, except in cases of improper storage or use, such as failure to store them in a dark and cool place, which may increase risks. The presence of impurities and oil adulteration, as mentioned above, are also factors contributing to allergenic action, resulting in skin irritations such as contact dermatitis.

5.4 Regulatory compliance

All cosmetic products, prior to reaching consumers, are subject to stringent regulations and quality control procedures. Within these assessments, plant-based cosmetic formulations are thoroughly evaluated regarding their potential risks to consumer health. According to the European Union Cosmetics Regulation (EC) No. 1223/2009, inspections are conducted to detect the possible presence of chemical substances such as heavy metals (mercury, lead, cadmium), plant-protective pharmaceutical compounds, and other substances that may pose toxicological or allergenic hazards. Concurrently, microbiological testing is performed to identify microbial contaminants such as *S. aureus*, *Pseudomonas aeruginosa*, and *E. coli*, given that cosmetics can be contaminated during manufacturing and processing stages. Specifically, this EU regulation mandates microbial stability testing based on ISO 11930:2019 standards. Moreover, within the European Union, cosmetic products placed on the market must undergo a comprehensive safety assessment, with a primary focus on consumer health protection, as stipulated by the legislation of the European Parliament and the Council. Correspondingly, in the United States, cosmetic safety is overseen by the Food and Drug Administration (FDA) under the Federal Food, Drug, and Cosmetic Act and the Fair Packaging and Labeling Act. However, this legislation imposes stricter controls on pharmaceuticals and food products than on botanical ingredients contained in cosmetics. For instance, essential oils—key ingredients in fragrances—are not subject to rigorous FDA regulations; instead, significant responsibility for safety is shifted to the manufacturers. The International Organization for Standardization (ISO), through committee ISO/TC 54, has established international standards for the composition, quality, and labeling of essential oils, thereby substantially contributing to consumer safety and transparency in global trade. Notably, essential oil derived from *R. officinalis* L. (rosemary) is recognized under ISO standard 1342:1988. Beyond regulatory compliance, a crucial factor in the industry's advancement is the protection of innovation, primarily through patenting in the field of plant-based cosmetics. Patents serve as legal mechanisms to safeguard innovative inventions, often focusing on new combinations of botanical extracts or progressive extraction methods, as opposed to traditional isolation of single bioactive molecules. Examples of patented plants used in cosmetology include root extracts of *Pothomorphe*, which act protectively against skin aging and solar damage, as well as extracts from the roots of *G. glabra* and *Sophora flavescens*, utilized for treating hyperpigmentation. It is noteworthy that patents generally do not cover the botanical extracts as natural substances themselves but rather their novel uses, innovative preparation methods, or combinations thereof for specific cosmetic applications.

6 Sustainability

The utilization of medicinal plants, due to their multiple beneficial properties, is fully justified, provided that it does not rely on excessive harvesting or practices approaching exploitation. Otherwise, concerns arise regarding the disruption of biodiversity. To avoid limiting the use of the diverse flora of medicinal plants for commercialization while respecting nature, satisfactory strategies have been proposed and are currently implemented. A widely recognized and predominant approach to prevent the depletion of plant resources involves the collective propagation of plants based on cultivation. This method requires adherence to specific protocols developed by universities or research institutions. However, for such a process to be efficient and effective, it should target plants with high demand and consumption. In other cases, the endeavor would be both unprofitable and unsustainable. Propagation methods may sometimes fail due to reduced seed germination capacity, natural seed dormancy, or difficulties in root development from stem cuttings. Nevertheless, these challenges can be mitigated through cold stratification (exposure to cold and moisture), thermal treatments (heat application), the use of plant hormones to enhance rooting, and smoke-water treatments that promote germination. These methods simulate the natural conditions necessary for plant growth. Regarding propagation techniques, it is also worth mentioning the modern *in vitro* micropropagation method conducted in laboratories, which circumvents the limitations of traditional techniques. Nonetheless, some researchers question the optimality of this method, speculating that medicinal plants are often more effective when cultivated autonomously in their natural environments. An alternative solution is the strengthening of local management, which involves stricter monitoring of altitudinal zones where these plant species grow. This approach protects natural resources while reducing the risk of their overexploitation. Consequently, local populations can rely on nature without depleting it, ensuring a better quality of life for themselves. Another means of protecting flora is by supporting domestic enterprises, mainly through avoiding the commercialization and export of raw plant materials abroad, thus contributing to the enhancement of the local economy and the management of natural resources in an environmentally respectful manner. Furthermore, improved management of plants greatly contributes to sustainability. This strategy aims at the sustainable and equitable harvesting of wild plants and is achieved by providing better conditions for gatherers and protecting nature. To this end, proper methods are implemented, simple regulations established, and information exchanged concerning production and pricing. Finally, strengthening cooperation with neighboring countries facilitates the sale of processed products, opening new markets and boosting the economy, thereby reducing the pressure for uncontrolled harvesting of raw materials.

7 Future perspectives

As mentioned above in the context of the review, the demand for medicinal plants has increased, as their use has been associated with consumers' ecological awareness. The high-value chemical compounds applied in the cosmetics sector are extracted from these plants by various methods, as described in the corresponding chapter. Regarding advanced extraction techniques that fall under the green chemistry strategy, prominent methods include UAE and supercritical CO_2 extraction. However, it is considered important to further develop advanced approaches within the biotechnology field, characterized by reduced energy requirements and environmentally friendly attributes. A potential future perspective involves the application of hybrid extraction techniques that combine advanced methods, such as the integration of ultrasound, microwaves, and supercritical CO_2. Concerning molecular delivery methodologies, these have attracted significant interest in technology research, given that many bioactive molecules possess low water solubility. To achieve effective and targeted action of the desired compound in each formulation, nano- and microsystem-based practices have been developed and are continually evolving to address these challenges as effectively as possible. In the future, particular emphasis is expected to be placed on the use of liposomes and nanocarriers for delivering bioactive molecules in cosmetics. These technologies offer improved control and targeting of active substances, which is especially important for components with low water solubility. Simultaneously, they represent more environmentally friendly options, making them ideal for sustainable applications moving forward. Moreover, the increasing use of natural ingredients in cosmetics raises questions regarding the safety of these products. Despite their appeal, natural origin does not automatically imply the absence of toxicity or allergenic properties. Therefore in the future, stricter measures should be established concerning the analysis, control, and approval of plant-derived cosmetics, including the enactment of specific legislative frameworks tailored to these products. This is an achievable goal that would maximize consumer safety and minimize toxicological risks. Beyond establishing dedicated legislation, the implementation of technical standards and standardization methodologies is required so that the evaluation of natural cosmetics is conducted in a scientifically substantiated manner. Another issue warranting reconsideration within research and development is the use of animals for safety testing of cosmetic products. As ethical awareness and technological capabilities increase, it is expected that alternative methods such as *in vitro* assays and in silico simulations will be further promoted. These methods, used in combination, can provide safe, reliable, and more humane results, contributing to the gradual elimination of animal testing in the cosmetics industry. In conclusion, it is evident that the path toward the development of safe, natural, and sustainable cosmetics lies in technological advancement, regulatory improvement, and maintaining ethical responsibility toward humans and the environment. Hopes rest on new, more environmentally friendly extraction methods, smart technologies for the delivery of active ingredients, and perhaps most importantly, on a regulatory framework that genuinely protects the consumer. Although challenges remain numerous, science appears ready to address them. The future looks promising, provided we continue to proceed with responsibility and vision.

8 Conclusions

The current study conducted a comprehensive review of the modern literature, clearly highlighting the central and continuously increasing role of bioactive substances derived from medicinal plants in the development of cutting-edge biofunctional cosmetics. The initial purpose, which was the in-depth investigation of the beneficial properties of plant extracts through the analysis of in vitro studies that explain their biological mechanisms and their effect on the skin, was fully achieved through a systematic search in scientific databases such as PubMed and ScienceDirect, using targeted keywords. From the thorough review, it was found that medicinal plants indeed constitute an invaluable and multidimensional source of secondary metabolites. Compounds such as polyphenols, flavonoids, carotenoids, alkaloids, vitamins (especially C and E), essential oils, and saponins impart a wide range of therapeutic and protective properties to cosmetic products. Specifically, *in vitro* studies convincingly document their powerful antioxidant activity, protecting cells from oxidative stress; their antiaging capability through the enhancement of collagen and elastin synthesis; their effective antiinflammatory function for soothing irritations; as well as their antimicrobial properties, significant for addressing conditions such as acne. Furthermore, their ability to interfere with critical cellular mechanisms, such as protection from UV radiation and tyrosinase inhibition for reducing hyperpigmentation, was demonstrated. These multiple biological actions make plant bioactives ideal for the development of innovative products addressing a wide range of skin needs, from the prevention of premature aging and deep hydration to the soothing of sensitive skin and the targeted management of acne. The ever-increasing consumer demand for natural, safe, transparent-in-origin, and sustainable cosmetics further enhances the utilization of medicinal plants. This clear market shift toward products free from parabens, synthetic fragrances, and aggressive chemical substances highlights biofunctional cosmetics with plant-derived ingredients as a pioneering, sustainable, and particularly effective solution. This approach not only fully aligns with the most recent scientific developments in dermatology and cosmetology but also responds to contemporary environmental and ethical consumer sensibilities. Despite the impressive progress and immense potential of plant bioactive substances, the field of research in this area remains dynamic and open to further exploration. Future studies are imperative to focus on the standardization of plant extracts, ensuring consistent quality and efficacy; on enhancing the bioavailability of plant ingredients in the skin—perhaps through advanced delivery systems such as nanotechnology—as well as on more extensive and rigorous in vivo clinical trials for the full confirmation of product effectiveness and safety under real-world conditions. The further exploration of unknown plant species, the isolation and characterization of new bioactive molecules, and the understanding of their synergistic actions open new, promising horizons for innovation in cosmetology. In conclusion, the substantial synergy of ancient herbal tradition with modern biotechnological methods offers a dynamic and scientifically substantiated approach to the production of cosmetic products. These products not only improve esthetic appearance but also actively contribute to the health, protection, and functionality of the skin, signaling a bright and promising future for the entire field of dermatology and cosmetology.

References

LiverTox: Clinical and Research Information on Drug-Induced Liver Injury, 2012. Available from: https://www.ncbi.nlm.nih.gov/books/NBK556475/.

Albuquerque, P.M., Azevedo, S.G., de Andrade, C.P., D'Ambros, N.C.D.S., Pérez, M.T.M., Manzato, L., 2022. Biotechnological applications of nanoencapsulated essential oils: a review. Polymers. 20734360. 14 (24). Available from: http://www.mdpi.com/journal/polymers. doi:10.3390/polym14245495.

Alfikri, F.N., Pujiarti, R., Wibisono, M.G., Hardiyanto, E.B., 2020. Yield, quality, and antioxidant activity of clove (*Syzygium aromaticum* L.) bud oil at the different phenological stages in young and mature trees. Scientifica. 2090908X. 2020. Available from: www.hindawi.com/journals/scientifica/. doi:10.1155/2020/9701701.

Al-Snafi, A.E., Teibo, J.O., Shaheen, H.M., Akinfe, O.A., Teibo, T.K.A., Emieseimokumo, N., Elfiky, M.M., Al-kuraishy, H.M., Al-Garbeeb, A.I., Alexiou, A., Papadakis, M., Mahana, H.A.M., Younes, A.M., Elbanna, O.A., Qasem, A.E.A.R., Shahin, I.Y.I., Batiha, G.E.S., 2024. The therapeutic value of *Myrtus communis* L.: an updated review. Naunyn Schmiedebergs Arch. Pharmacol. 14321912. 397 (7), 4579–4600. Available from: https://www.springer.com/journal/210. doi:10.1007/s00210-024-02958-3.

Alven, S., Khwaza, V., Oyedeji, O.O., Aderibigbe, B.A., 2021. Polymer-based scaffolds loaded with aloe vera extract for the treatment of wounds. Pharmaceutics. 1999-4923. 13 (7), 961. doi:10.3390/pharmaceutics13070961.

Arribas-López, E., Zand, N., Ojo, O., Snowden, M.J., Kochhar, T., 2022. A systematic review of the effect of *Centella asiatica* on wound healing. Int. J. Environ. Res. Public Health. 1660-4601. 19 (6), 3266. doi:10.3390/ijerph19063266.

Arulselvan, P., Fard, M.T., Tan, W.S., Gothai, S., Fakurazi, S., Norhaizan, M.E., Kumar, S.S., 2016. Role of antioxidants and natural products in inflammation. Oxid. Med. Cell. Longev. 19420994. 2016. Available from: http://www.hindawi.com/journals/oximed/. doi:10.1155/2016/5276130.

Ashokkumar, V., Flora, G., Sevanan, M., Sripriya, R., Chen, W.H., Park, J.-H., Banu, J.R., Kumar, G., 2023. Technological advances in the production of carotenoids and their applications—a critical review. Bioresour. Technol. 09608524. 367, 128215. doi:10.1016/j.biortech.2022.128215.

Aziz, E., Batool, R., Khan, M.U., Rauf, A., Akhtar, W., Heydari, M., Rehman, S., Shahzad, T., Malik, A., Mosavat, S.H., Plygun, S., Shariati, M.A., 2021. An overview on red algae bioactive compounds and their pharmaceutical applications. J. Complement. Integr. Med. 15533840. 17 (4). Available from: www.degruyter.com/view/j/jcim. doi:10.1515/jcim-2019-0203.

Bhambhani, S., Kondhare, K.R., Giri, A.P., 2021. Diversity in chemical structures and biological properties of plant alkaloids. Molecules. 1420-3049. 26 (11), 3374. doi:10.3390/molecules26113374.

Boo, Y.C., 2022. Ascorbic acid (vitamin C) as a cosmeceutical to increase dermal collagen for skin antiaging purposes: emerging combination therapies. Antioxidants. 2076-3921. 11 (9), 1663. doi:10.3390/antiox11091663.

Bouwstra, J.A., Nădăban, A., Bras, W., McCabe, C., Bunge, A., Gooris, G.S., 2023. The skin barrier: an extraordinary interface with an exceptional lipid organization. Prog. Lipid Res. 01637827. 92, 101252. doi:10.1016/j.plipres.2023.101252.

Cao, S., Liang, J., Chen, M., Chao, X., Wang, X., Qiu, L., Zhao, X., Wenxiao, H., 2025. Comparative analysis of extraction technologies for plant extracts and absolutes. Front. Chem. 2296-2646. 13. doi:10.3389/fchem.2025.1536590.

Chelu, M., Musuc, A.M., Popa, M., Moreno, J.C., 2023. Aloe vera-based hydrogels for wound healing: properties and therapeutic effects. Gels. 2310-2861. 9 (7), 539. doi:10.3390/gels9070539.

de Alcantara Lemos, J., Oliveira, A.E.M.F.M., Araujo, R.S., Townsend, D.M., Ferreira, L.A.M., de Barros, A.L.B., 2021. Recent progress in micro and nano-encapsulation of bioactive derivatives of the Brazilian genus Pterodon. Biomed. Pharmacother. 19506007. 143. Available from: https://www.journals.elsevier.com/biomedicine-and-pharmacotherapy. doi:10.1016/j.biopha.2021.112137.

de Macedo, L.M., Dos Santos, É.M., Militão, L., Tundisi, L.L., Ataide, J.A., Souto, E.B., Mazzola, P.G., 2020. Rosemary (*Rosmarinus officinalis* L., syn *Salvia rosmarinus* spenn.) and its topical applications: a review. Plants. 22237747. 9 (5). Available from: https://www.mdpi.com/2223-7747/9/5/651/pdf. doi:10.3390/plants9050651.

Dey, P., Ray Chaudhuri, S., 2023. The opportunistic nature of gut commensal microbiota. Crit. Rev. Microbiol. 1040-841X. 49 (6), 739–763. doi:10.1080/1040841x.2022.2133987.

Dhatwalia, J., Kumari, A., Verma, R., Upadhyay, N., Guleria, I., Lal, S., Thakur, S., Gudeta, K., Kumar, V., Chao, J.C.-J., Sharma, S., Kumar, A., Manicum, A.-L.E., Lorenzo, J.M., Amarowicz, R., 2021. Phytochemistry, pharmacology, and nutraceutical profile of Carissa species: an updated review. Molecules. 1420-3049. 26 (22), 7010. doi:10.3390/molecules26227010.

Doghish, A., Shehabeldine, A., El-Mahdy, H., Hassanin, M., Al-Askar, A., Marey, S., AbdElgawad, H., Hashem, A., 2023. *Thymus vulgaris* oil nanoemulsion: synthesis, characterization, antimicrobial and anticancer activities. Molecules. 1420-3049. 28 (19), 6910. doi:10.3390/molecules28196910.

Doseděl, M., Jirkovský, E., Macáková, K., Krčmová, L.K., Javorská, L., Pourová, J., Mercolini, L., Remião, F., Nováková, L., Mladěnka, P., 2021. Vitamin c—sources, physiological role, kinetics, deficiency, use, toxicity, and determination. Nutrients. 20726643. 13 (2), 1–36. Available from: https://www.mdpi.com/2072-6643/13/2/615. doi:10.3390/nu13020615.

Ferreira, M.S., Magalhães, M.C., Oliveira, R., Sousa-Lobo, J.M., Almeida, I.F., 2021. Trends in the use of botanicals in anti-aging cosmetics. Molecules. 14203049. 26 (12). Available from: https://www.mdpi.com/1420-3049/26/12/3584/pdf. doi:10.3390/molecules26123584.

Flieger, J., Raszewska-Famielec, M., Radzikowska-Büchner, E., Flieger, W., 2024. Skin protection by carotenoid pigments. Int. J. Mol. Sci. 1422-0067. 25 (3), 1431. doi:10.3390/ijms25031431.

García-Chacón, J.M., Marín-Loaiza, J.C., Osorio, C., 2023. Camu camu (*Myrciaria dubia* (Kunth) McVaugh): an Amazonian fruit with biofunctional properties—a review. ACS Omega. 24701343. 8 (6), 5169–5183. Available from: https://www.pubs.acs.org/journal/acsodf. doi:10.1021/acsomega.2c07245.

Goyal, N., Jerold, F., 2023. Biocosmetics: technological advances and future outlook. Environ. Sci. Pollut. Res. 1614-7499. 30 (10), 25148–25169. doi:10.1007/s11356-021-17567-3.

Gref, R., Deloménie, C., Maksimenko, A., Gouadon, E., Percoco, G., Lati, E., Desmaële, D., Zouhiri, F., Couvreur, P., 2020. Vitamin C–squalene bioconjugate promotes epidermal thickening and collagen production in human skin. Sci. Rep. 2045-2322. 10 (1). doi:10.1038/s41598-020-72704-1.

Gupta, N., Bhattacharya, S., Dutta, A., Tauchen, J., Landa, P., Urbanová, K., Houdková, M., Fernández-Cusimamani, E., Leuner, O., 2024. Synthetic polyploidization induces enhanced phytochemical profile and biological activities in *Thymus vulgaris* L. essential oil. Sci. Rep. 2045-2322. 14 (1). doi:10.1038/s41598-024-56378-7.

Haro-González, J.N., Castillo-Herrera, G.A., Martínez-Velázquez, M., Espinosa-Andrews, H., 2021. Clove essential oil (*Syzygium aromaticum* l. myrtaceae): extraction, chemical composition, food applications, and essential bioactivity for human health. Molecules. 14203049. 26 (21). Available from: https://www.mdpi.com/1420-3049/26/21/6387/pdf. doi:10.3390/molecules26216387.

Heinrich, M., Mah, J., Amirkia, V., 2021. Alkaloids used as medicines: structural phytochemistry meets biodiversity—an update and forward look. Molecules. 1420-3049. 26 (7), 1836. doi:10.3390/molecules26071836.

Hidayat, A.T., Arifin, M.T., Nur, M., Muniroh, M., Susilaningsih, N., Subramanian, S., 2021. Ozonated aloe vera oil effective increased the number of fibroblasts and collagen thickening in the healing response of full-thickness skin defects. Int. J. Inflamm. 2042-0099. 2021, 1–8. doi:10.1155/2021/6654343.

Jiménez, G.G., Durán, A.G., Macías, F.A., Simonet, A.M., 2021. Structure, bioactivity and analytical methods for the determination of *Yucca saponins*. Molecules. 14203049. 26 (17). Available from: https://www.mdpi.com/1420-3049/26/17/5251/pdf. doi:10.3390/molecules26175251.

Kairey, L., Agnew, T., Bowles, E.J., Barkla, B.J., Wardle, J., Lauche, R., 2023. Efficacy and safety of *Melaleuca alternifolia* (tea tree) oil for human health—a systematic review of randomized controlled trials. Front. Pharmacol. 16639812. 14. Available from: http://www.frontiersin.org/Pharmacology. doi:10.3389/fphar.2023.1116077.

Kang, M.H., Jang, G.Y., Ji, Y.J., Lee, J.H., Choi, S.J., Hyun, T.K., Kim, H.D., 2021. Antioxidant and anti-melanogenic activities of heat-treated licorice (Wongam, *Glycyrrhiza glabra* × *guralensis*) extract. Curr. Issues Mol. Biol. 14673045. 43 (2), 1171–1187. Available from: https://www.mdpi.com/1467-3045/43/2/83/pdf. doi:10.3390/cimb43020083.

Kanlayavattanakul, M., Mersni, D., Lourith, N., 2024. Plant-derived saponins and their prospective for cosmetic and personal care products. Bot. Stud. 1999-3110. 65 (1). doi:10.1186/s40529-024-00438-8.

Kapadia, P., Newell, A.S., Cunningham, J., Roberts, M.R., Hardy, J.G., 2022. Extraction of high-value chemicals from plants for technical and medical applications. Int. J. Mol. Sci. 14220067. 23 (18). Available from: http://www.mdpi.com/journal/ijms. doi:10.3390/ijms231810334.

Khan, H., Alam, W., Alsharif, K.F., Aschner, M., Pervez, S., Saso, L., 2022. Alkaloids and colon cancer: molecular mechanisms and therapeutic implications for cell cycle arrest. Molecules. 1420-3049. 27 (3), 920. doi:10.3390/molecules27030920.

Khazaeli, P., Sharififar, F., Amiri, F., Heravi, G., 2011. Evaluation of moisturizing effect of methanolic extract of five medicinal plants incorporated into cream bases using impedance and extensiometry methods. J. Drugs Dermatol. 15459616. 10 (10), 1116–1121. Available from: http://jddonline.com/articles/download_article/1616.

Kim, H.J., Kim, Y.H., 2024. Exploring acne treatments: from pathophysiological mechanisms to emerging therapies. Int. J. Mol. Sci. 1422-0067. 25 (10), 5302. doi:10.3390/ijms25105302.

Kulthanan, K., Tuchinda, P., Nitiyarom, R., Chunharas, A., Chantaphakul, H., Aunhachoke, K., Chularojanamontri, L., Rajatanavin, N., Jirapongsananuruk, O., Vichyanond, P., Chatchatee, P., Sangsupawanich, P., Wananukul, S., Singalavanija, S., Trakanwittayarak, S., Rerkpattanapipat, T., Thongngarm, T., Wisuthsarewong, W., Limpongsanurak, W., Kamchaisatian, W., Noppakun, N., 2021. Clinical practice guidelines for the diagnosis and management of atopic dermatitis. Asian Pac. J. Allergy Immunol. 22288694. 39 (3), 145–155. Available from: https://apjai-journal.org/wp-content/uploads/2021/09/4_AP-010221-1050-No-Supplement.pdf. doi:10.12932/AP-010221-1050.

Kultys, E., Kurek, M.A., 2022. Green extraction of carotenoids from fruit and vegetable byproducts: a review. Molecules. 14203049. 27 (2). Available from: https://www.mdpi.com/1420-3049/27/2/518/pdf. doi:10.3390/molecules27020518.

Lavuri, R., Jabbour, C.J.C., Grebinevych, O., Roubaud, D., 2022. Green factors stimulating the purchase intention of innovative luxury organic beauty products: implications for sustainable development. J. Environ. Manage. 03014797. 301, 113899. doi:10.1016/j.jenvman.2021.113899.

Lee, J.E., Jayakody, J.T.M., Kim, J.I., Jeong, J.W., Choi, K.M., Kim, T.S., Seo, C., Azimi, I., Hyun, J.M., Ryu, B.M., 2024. The influence of solvent choice on the extraction of bioactive compounds from Asteraceae: a comparative review. Foods. 23048158. 13 (19). Available from: www.mdpi.com/journal/foods. doi:10.3390/foods13193151.

Leo, T.K., Tan, E.S.S., Amini, F., Rehman, N., Ng, E.S.C., Tan, C.K., 2022. Effect of rice (*Oryza sativa* L.) ceramides supplementation on improving skin barrier functions and depigmentation: an open-label prospective study. Nutrients. 2072-6643. 14 (13), 2737. doi:10.3390/nu14132737.

Li, L., Zhang, J., Cheng, W., Feiqian, D., Wang, C., Quan, A., 2024. Saponins of *Paris polyphylla* for the improvement of acne: anti-inflammatory, antibacterial, antioxidant and immunomodulatory effects. Molecules. 1420-3049. 29 (8), 1793. doi:10.3390/molecules29081793.

Liu, J., Zhou, H., Song, L., Yang, Z., Qiu, M., Wang, J., Shi, S., 2021. Anthocyanins: promising natural products with diverse pharmacological activities. Molecules. 1420-3049. 26 (13), 3807. doi:10.3390/molecules26133807.

Liu, J.K., 2022. Natural products in cosmetics. Nat. Prod. Bioprospect. 21922209. 12 (1). Available from: https://www.springer.com/journal/13659. doi:10.1007/s13659-022-00363-y.

Messire, G., Serreau, R., Berteina-Raboin, S., 2023. Antioxidant effects of catechins (EGCG), andrographolide, and curcuminoids compounds for skin protection, cosmetics, and dermatological uses: an update. Antioxidants. 2076-3921. 12 (7), 1317. doi:10.3390/antiox12071317.

Michalak, M., 2022. Plant-derived antioxidants: significance in skin health and the ageing process. Int. J. Mol. Sci. 1422-0067. 23 (2), 585. doi:10.3390/ijms23020585.

Nair, A.B., Gorain, B., Pandey, M., Jacob, S., Shinu, P., Aldhubiab, B., Almuqbil, R.M., Elsewedy, H.S., Morsy, M.A., 2022. Tocotrienol in the treatment of topical wounds: recent updates. Pharmaceutics. 19994923. 14 (11). Available from: http://www.mdpi.com/journal/pharmaceutics. doi:10.3390/pharmaceutics14112479.

Nascimento, T., Gomes, D., Simões, R., Miguel, M.D.G., 2023. Tea tree oil: properties and the therapeutic approach to acne—a review. Antioxidants. 2076-3921. 12 (6), 1264. doi:10.3390/antiox12061264.

Nurzyńska-Wierdak, R., Pietrasik, D., Walasek-Janusz, M., 2023. Essential oils in the treatment of various types of acne—a review. Plants. 2223-7747. 12 (1), 90. doi:10.3390/plants12010090.

Olędzki, R., Harasym, J., 2024. Acerola (*Malpighia emarginata*) anti-inflammatory activity—a review. Int. J. Mol. Sci. 1422-0067. 25 (4), 2089. doi:10.3390/ijms25042089.

Panahkhahi, M., 2010. Station-based deconstructed training model for teaching procedural skills to medical students: a quasi-experimental study. Adv. Med. Educ. Pract. 1179-7258. 1, 17–23. doi:10.2147/AMEP.S13750.

Park, H., Otte, A., Park, K., 2022. Evolution of drug delivery systems: from 1950 to 2020 and beyond. J. Control. Release. 18734995. 342, 53–65. Available from: www.elsevier.com/locate/jconrel. doi:10.1016/j.jconrel.2021.12.030.

Petrovska, B.B., 2012. Historical review of medicinal plants' usage. Pharmacogn. Rev. 09762787. 6 (11), 1–5. doi:10.4103/0973-7847.95849.

Peyravian, N., Deo, S., Daunert, S., Jimenez, J.J., 2022. The anti-inflammatory effects of cannabidiol (CBD) on acne. J. Inflamm. Res. 1178-7031. 15, 2795–2801. doi:10.2147/jir.s355489.

Qian, W., Liu, W., Zhu, D., Cao, Y., Tang, A., Gong, G., Hua, S., 2020. Natural skin-whitening compounds for the treatment of melanogenesis (Review). Exp. Ther. Med. 1792-0981. 20 (1), 173–185. doi:10.3892/etm.2020.8687.

Razia, S., Park, H., Shin, E., Shim, K.-S., Cho, E., Kim, S.-Y., 2021. Effects of aloe vera flower extract and its active constituent isoorientin on skin moisturization via regulating involucrin expression. Vitro Mol. Dock. Stud. Molecules. 1420-3049. 26 (9), 2626. doi:10.3390/molecules26092626.

Ruse, G., Jîjie, A.R., Moacă, E.A., Pătrașcu, D., Ardelean, F., Jojic, A.A., Ardelean, S., Tchiakpe-Antal, D.S., 2025. *Coffea arabica*: an emerging active ingredient in dermato-cosmetic applications. Pharmaceuticals. 14248247. 18 (2). Available from: https://www.mdpi.com/journal/pharmaceuticals. doi:10.3390/ph18020171.

Rybczyńska-Tkaczyk, K., Grenda, A., Jakubczyk, A., Kiersnowska, K., Bik-Małodzińska, M., 2023. Natural compounds with antimicrobial properties in cosmetics. Pathogens. 2076-0817. 12 (2), 320. doi:10.3390/pathogens12020320.

Seo, D.H., Jung, J.H., Lee, J.E., Jeon, E.J., Kim, W., Park, C.S., 2012. Biotechnological production of arbutins (α- and β-arbutins), skin-lightening agents, and their derivatives. Appl. Microbiol. Biotechnol. 14320614. 95 (6), 1417–1425. doi:10.1007/s00253-012-4297-4.

Sharma, A., Kuhad, A., Bhandari, R., 2022. Novel nanotechnological approaches for treatment of skin-aging. J. Tissue Viability. 0965206X. 31 (3), 374–386. doi:10.1016/j.jtv.2022.04.010.

Sharmeen, J.B., Mahomoodally, F.M., Zengin, G., Maggi, F., 2021. Essential oils as natural sources of fragrance compounds for cosmetics and cosmeceuticals. Molecules. 14203049. 26 (3). Available from: http://www.mdpi.com/journal/molecules. doi:10.3390/molecules26030666.

Silva, D., Ferreira, M.S., Sousa-Lobo, J.M., Cruz, M.T., Almeida, I.F., 2021. Anti-inflammatory activity of *Calendula officinalis* l. flower extract. Cosmetics. 20799284. 8 (2). Available from: https://www.mdpi.com/2079-9284/8/2/31/pdf. doi:10.3390/cosmetics8020031.

Szewczyk, K., Chojnacka, A., Górnicka, M., 2021. Tocopherols and tocotrienols—bioactive dietary compounds; what is certain, what is doubt? Int. J. Mol. Sci. 1422-0067. 22 (12), 6222. doi:10.3390/ijms22126222.

Thawabteh, A.M., Jibreen, A., Karaman, D., Thawabteh, A., Karaman, R., 2023. Skin pigmentation types, causes and treatment—a review. Molecules. 14203049. 28 (12). Available from: http://www.mdpi.com/journal/molecules. doi:10.3390/molecules28124839.

Timilsena, Y.P., Phosanam, A., Stockmann, R., 2023. Perspectives on saponins: food functionality and applications. Int. J. Mol. Sci. 1422-0067. 24 (17), 13538. doi:10.3390/ijms241713538.

Tobiasz, A., Nowicka, D., Szepietowski, J.C., 2022. *Acne vulgaris*—novel treatment options and factors affecting therapy adherence: a narrative review. J. Clin. Med. 2077-0383. 11 (24), 7535. doi:10.3390/jcm11247535.

Tomishima, H., Luo, K., Mitchell, A.E., 2022. The almond (*Prunus dulcis*): chemical properties, utilization, and valorization of coproducts. Annu. Rev. Food Sci. Technol. 19411421. 13, 145–166. Available from: http://www.annualreviews.org/journal/food. doi:10.1146/annurev-food-052720-111942.

Vasam, M., Korutla, S., Bohara, R.A., 2023. *Acne vulgaris*: a review of the pathophysiology, treatment, and recent nanotechnology based advances. Biochem. Biophys. Rep. 24055808. 36, 101578. doi:10.1016/j.bbrep.2023.101578.

Vassiliou, E., Awoleye, O., Davis, A., Mishra, S., 2023. Anti-inflammatory and antimicrobial properties of thyme oil and its main constituents. Int. J. Mol. Sci. 1422-0067. 24 (8), 6936. doi:10.3390/ijms24086936.

Vella, F.M., Pignone, D., Laratta, B., 2024. The Mediterranean species *Calendula officinalis* and *Foeniculum vulgare* as valuable source of bioactive compounds. Molecules. 1420-3049. 29 (15), 3594. doi:10.3390/molecules29153594.

Vostinaru, O., Heghes, S.C., Filip, L., 2020. Safety profile of essential oils. IntechOpen. doi:10.5772/intechopen.91363.

Wirtu, S.F., Ramaswamy, K., Maitra, R., Chopra, S., Mishra, A.K., Jule, L.T., 2024. Isolation, characterization and antimicrobial activity study of *Thymus vulgaris*. Sci. Rep. 20452322. 14 (1). Available from: https://www.nature.com/srep/. doi:10.1038/s41598-024-71012-2.

Yap, W.H., Goh, B.H., 2023. Editorial: biofunctional molecule exploratory research on application in food and health. Molecules. 14203049. 28 (13). Available from: http://www.mdpi.com/journal/molecules. doi:10.3390/molecules28135089.

Zhakipbekov, K., Turgumbayeva, A., Akhelova, S., Bekmuratova, K., Blinova, O., Utegenova, G., Shertaeva, K., Sadykov, N., Tastambek, K., Saginbazarova, A., Urazgaliyev, K., Tulegenova, G., Zhalimova, Z., Karasova, Z., 2024. Antimicrobial and other pharmacological properties of *Ocimum basilicum*, Lamiaceae. Molecules. 1420-3049. 29 (2), 388. doi:10.3390/molecules29020388.

Zhang, Y., Cai, C., Yunfu, G., Shi, Y., Gao, X., 2022. Microplastics in plant-soil ecosystems: a meta-analysis. Environ. Pollut. 02697491. 308, 119718. doi:10.1016/j.envpol.2022.119718.

Zhou, Y., Phan, A.D.T., Akter, S., Bobasa, E.M., Seididamyeh, M., Sivakumar, D., Sultanbawa, Y., 2023. Bioactive properties of Kakadu plum-blended products. Molecules. 14203049. 28 (6). Available from: http://www.mdpi.com/journal/molecules. doi:10.3390/molecules28062828.

Zhu, J., Song, L., Shen, S., Wanxin, F., Zhu, Y., Liu, L., 2023. Bioactive alkaloids as secondary metabolites from plant endophytic Aspergillus genus. Molecules. 1420-3049. 28 (23), 7789. doi:10.3390/molecules28237789.

Zillich, O.V., Schweiggert-Weisz, U., Eisner, P., Kerscher, M., 2015. Polyphenols as active ingredients for cosmetic products. Int. J. Cosmet. Sci. 0142-5463. 37 (5), 455–464. doi:10.1111/ics.12218.

Chapter 6

Aromatic plants and herbs

Konstantina Tsikrika[a], Eleftherios Kotos[a], Elpida Mantzakopoulou[a], Pol Gimenez-Gil[a], Ronald Halim[b], Charalambos Proestos[a], and Dimitrios Argyropoulos[c]

[a]*Laboratory of Food Chemistry, Department of Chemistry, National and Kapodistrian University of Athens, Athens, Greece*

[b]*UCD Algae Group, School of Biosystems and Food Engineering, University College Dublin, Dublin, Ireland*

[c]*d-Lab: Digital Agriculture and Bioresources, School of Biosystems and Food Engineering, University College Dublin, Dublin, Ireland*

1 Introduction

Medicinal and aromatic plants (MAPs) are vital sources of bioactive compounds for pharmaceuticals, cosmetics, natural health products, and the food industry (Brendler and Brinckmann, 2023). The World Health Organization recognizes their importance in achieving global health objectives, particularly in promoting accessible and natural healthcare solutions (World Health Organisation, 2023).

In Europe alone, >1300 medicinal plant species are utilized, with approximately 90% harvested from wild populations (Chen et al., 2016; Socaci et al., 2020), while the global market for herbal products is projected to reach almost USD 105 billion by 2026, with a compound annual growth rate of 6.5% (Bareetseng, 2022). This trend is largely driven by consumer preference for natural, sustainable alternatives to synthetic additives, particularly in food preservation, where plant-derived antioxidants and antimicrobials are increasingly favored. In addition, the food industry is adopting these natural compounds to replace synthetic preservatives, aligning with market preferences and boosting competitiveness (Socaci et al., 2020).

However, the expanding MAP industry generates substantial waste (Marcelino et al., 2023b), estimated at 30 million tons annually (Wei et al., 2022). Despite containing valuable nutrients and bioactive compounds, residues from herbs are frequently disposed of through stacking, landfilling, or incineration, resulting not only in resource wastage but also in significant environmental pollution (de Elguea-culebras et al., 2022). Particularly in essential oil (EO) production, where yields are often low (typically < 5% of processed biomass), large volumes of residual plant material remain underutilized (Kong et al., 2019).

The circular economy model offers a promising solution by transforming waste into valuable resources (Choudhury et al., 2018). Defined as a regenerative system that minimizes waste through reuse, recycling, and sustainable design, this approach aligns with global sustainability goals (Geissdoerfer et al., 2017). Following these principles, MAP by-products can be repurposed into antimicrobial agents, biofertilizers, animal feed additives, or even nutraceuticals, reducing environmental impact while creating economic value. Nonetheless, the valorization of by-products from distillation and drying processes presents a significant challenge (Taghouti et al., 2022).

Extraction efficiency of bioactive compounds from MAPs highly depends on method selection and the operational parameters, such as extraction duration, temperature, solid-to-liquid ratio (S/L), and pH (Lampakis et al., 2021). Although traditional solid–liquid extraction (SLE) techniques remain widely used, emerging green technologies, viz. ultrasound-assisted extraction (UAE), microwave-assisted extraction (MAE), supercritical fluid extraction (SFE), and pulsed electric field (PEF), improve yield and sustainability (Ameer et al., 2017; Kant and Kumar, 2022).

This chapter evaluates the state-of-the-art in novel extraction methods for MAPs and MAP-derived by-products, demonstrating superior efficiency compared to conventional methods, industrial scalability, and environmental sustainability of cutting-edge extraction techniques. The analysis was conducted through a systematic review of peer-reviewed publications (primarily from the last decade) selected from Elsevier's Scopus database. The study focused on the most widely used MAPs, identified through targeted keyword searches ("extraction," "medicinal plants," "aromatic plants," "herbs," etc.) combined with Boolean operators. Following rigorous screening to ensure relevance, the selected publications were categorized by four key parameters: (1) extraction method, (2) target bioactive compounds, (3) plant species, and (4) operational conditions, enabling direct comparison between conventional and innovative extraction technologies. The chapter

Biofunctional Cosmetics for Health. https://doi.org/10.1016/B978-0-443-27500-5.00010-1

identifies optimal extraction parameters for maximizing bioactive recovery and discusses future research directions to further advance waste valorization in the MAP industry, with particular emphasis on scaling green technologies and utilizing underutilized by-product streams.

2 Novel extraction methods for MAPs

2.1 Ultrasound-assisted extraction

UAE employs sonic waves in the frequency range of 20–2000 kHz. The primary mechanism behind this process is acoustic cavitation, where ultrasonic (US) waves generate regions of alternating compression and expansion in a liquid medium, leading to the formation and collapse of microscopic bubbles (Paniwnyk, 2017; Tsikrika et al., 2022). During the expansion phase, these bubbles grow as they absorb dissolved gases, followed by a violent collapse that produces localized high temperatures, extreme pressures, and shock waves. This phenomenon disrupts plant cell walls, enhancing their permeability and facilitating the release of intracellular components into the extraction solvent (Dhanani et al., 2017; Khan et al., 2022).

UAE can be performed using two main approaches: direct and indirect UAE. In direct UAE, a US probe is immersed into the sample–solvent mixture, whereas indirect UAE employs a US bath US radiation, which can handle multiple samples simultaneously though at a lower intensity compared to direct sonication. The efficiency of UAE depends on several parameters, including temperature, solvent type, sonication cycle, homogenization granularity, and extraction duration (Weggler et al., 2020).

UAE offers significant advantages over conventional methods by enabling lower temperatures and solvent consumption, while enhancing both the extraction efficiency and selectivity, resulting in improved purity of the extracted compounds (da Silva et al., 2022). Its ability to operate under mild thermal conditions makes it particularly suitable for thermolabile phytochemicals. In addition, this method minimizes solvent usage, reduces extraction time, as well as carbon and water footprints (Chemat et al., 2017; Tsikrika et al., 2022).

Findings of recent studies on the application of UAE in MAPs are summarized. The antioxidant and antimicrobial activity of two *Crocus sativus* L. tepal extracts—one with flavonoid aglycons and the other with glycosides—compared to *Melissa officinalis* (a strong antioxidant) and propolis (a potent antimicrobial) was investigated (Kakouri et al., 2017). Total phenolic content ranged from 5.5 to 39.0 mg CAE/g, while antioxidant activity (2,2-diphenyl-1-picrylhydrazyl, DPPH and 2,2′-azino-bis(3-ethylbenzothiazoline-6-sulfonic acid), ABTS assays) showed IC_{50} values of 14.17–203.88 μg/mL and 10.15–81.58 μg/mL, respectively. Liquid chromatography with diode array detection coupled to mass spectrometry (LC-DAD/MS) identified major compounds, and antimicrobial tests against six bacterial species revealed the aglycon-rich tepal extract was most effective, even against resistant strains like *Listeria monocytogenes* and *Salmonella enterica*, with activity at just 1.5 mg (Table 6.1).

Sarfarazi et al. (2022) describe UAE as a viable alternative to traditional methods for extracting saffron bioactives, namely, picrocrocin, safranal, and crocin, as it offers a faster and more straightforward approach compared to conventional techniques, enhancing the extraction efficiency. The authors employed a four-factor, five-level full factorial central composite design (CCD) for the optimization of the extraction method. Response surface methodology (RSM) and artificial bee colony analysis showed that optimal conditions were an ethanol concentration of 58.58% or 53.07%, an extraction time of 6.85 min or 7.32 min, a duty cycle of 0.82 or 0.93, and an amplitude of 91.11% or 100%, respectively.

Regarding rosemary, utilizing US for the extraction of antioxidants enhances the yields in comparison to extraction by stirring. These findings also suggest that the choice of solvent plays a significant role when customizing an US extraction method for a particular material. Specifically, ethanol proves to be more effective for dried plant material as opposed to fresh ones. Furthermore, US extraction has demonstrated effectiveness even when scaling up to a solvent volume of 125 liters, signifying the potential for commercial-scale applications of ultrasound in this context (Paniwnyk et al., 2009). An effective technique to extract carnosic acid and rosmarinic acid from *Rosmarinus officinalis* was proposed by Zu et al. (2012). Under the idealized conditions, this method achieved a commendable extraction efficiency for the two phenolcarboxylic acids. In comparison with alternative methods, their suggested approach offers superior extraction efficiency and notably shorter extraction durations.

Caser et al. (2023) found that extracts acquired through UAE from fresh lavender (*Lavandula angustifolia*) flowers exhibited superior performance compared to the US extracts from dried flowers across various investigated parameters, except for total antioxidant capacity. The application of UAE in water proved to be highly effective in extracting bioactive compounds with potential health benefits. Therefore they concluded that UAE holds much promise for plant-derived products with advantageous health effects. Girbu et al. (2023) performed UAE on the same plant. Their thin-layer

TABLE 6.1 Summary of recent research on ultrasound-assisted extraction of medicinal and aromatic plants.

Plant (matrix)	Extraction conditions	Extractor	Optimum conditions	Key results	Author(s)
Aloe vera (leaf skin)	Time: 0.1–36.9 min Frequency: 20 kHz Solvent: EtOH	US horn-type cavitation extractor	UAE for 30 min; 65% sonication power; EtOH 80%	Max extraction of aloin A was 4.33 mg/g and aloin B 4.46 mg/g, and the extraction yield was 9.43%	(Behaiyn et al., 2023)
Aristotelia serrata (leaves)	Time: 10 min Frequency: 24 kHz Temperature: 50°C Solvent: EtOH/H_2O 1:1	UP200S US processor unit	UAE for 17.12 min; US intensity of 0.52 W/mL; EtOH 74%	The yield increased by 13% after UAE under the optimized conditions IC_{50} for butyrylcholinesterase enzyme and radical scavenging activity was found to be 26.2 μg/mL, respectively	(Majid and Silva, 2020)
Crocus sativus (stigmas)	Time: 2–10 min Frequency: 20 kHz Temperature: < 30°C Solvent: EtOH	SONOPULS HD 3200 US homogenizer	RSM analysis: UAE for 6.85 min; 91.11% US amplitude; EtOH 58.58% ABC analysis: UAE for 7.32 min; 100% US power; EtOH 53.07%	Max extraction of crocetin esters	(Sarfarazi et al., 2022)
Crocus sativus (tepals)	Time: 20 min Frequency: 35 kHz Temperature: 25 ± 1°C Solvent: petroleum ether, MeOH	US bath	Not specified	The yield was 18 ± 6 mg/g for hydrolyzed and 51 ± 4 mg/g for nonhydrolyzed extract The TPC was 31 ± 3 mg caffeic acid equivalents/g for nonhydrolyzed tepal extract and 5.5 ± 0.9 mg CAE/g for hydrolyzed tepal extract	(Ganorkar et al., 2022)
Eichhornia crassipes (leaves, stems, and roots)	Time: 10–50 min Frequency: 24 kHz Temperature: 20°C Solvent: H_2O	UP200Ht sonicator unit	UAE for 30 min; 50% US amplitude; 30% US pulse ratio; 20 mL H_2O	Stem yield 3.1% Highest TPC in leaves (8.89 mg GAE/g)	(Ganorkar et al., 2022)
Gymnema sylvestre (leaves)	Time: 10 min Frequency: 26 kHz Temperature: 40°C Solvent: EtOH with enzyme cocktail	Hielscher US unit	5.5 pH; 5.5 mL enzyme, 65°C, 150 min incubation	Max yield 36.51% TFC 56.6 mg RE/g TPC 111.3 mg GAE/g DPPH 71.22%	Saeed et al., 2022
Larrea cuneifolia (leaves)	Time: 15, 38, 60 min Frequency: 20 kHz Temperature: 40°C Solvent: NADES	Cleanson US bath	UAE for 42 min; plant–solvent ratio of 75 mg/mL	UAE using NADES resulted in high extractability for both polar and weakly polar phenolic compounds	(Espino et al., 2018)
Lavandula angustifolia (flowers)	Time: 15 min Frequency: 23 kHz Temperature: – Solvent: water	Sarl Reus US extractor	Not specified	TPC 662.29–781.01 mg GAE/100 g DB DPPH: 26.82–34.95 μmol TE/g DB; ABTS: 29.08–33.00 μmol TE/g DB	(Caser et al., 2023)
Lavandula angustifolia Mill. (stalks and flowers)	Time: 0–120 min Frequency: 35 kHz Temperature: 60°C Solvent: EtOH 96%, EtOH 70%, ethylacetate	A Raypa UC-150	UAE for 45 min; 96% EtOH	96% ethanol extraction yielded 3.3% triterpenic acids (1% pomolic acid, DW) Ethyl acetate selectively extracted flower compounds, enriching triterpenic acids to 67.8% (16.2% pomolic acid) 70% EtOH led to higher extraction yields (14.2–17.0% DB), but the content of UA (0.6% DB) and OA (0.3% DB) was lower	(Girbu et al., 2023)

Continued

TABLE 6.1 Summary of recent research on ultrasound-assisted extraction of medicinal and aromatic plants—cont'd

Plant (matrix)	Extraction conditions	Extractor	Optimum conditions	Key results	Author(s)
Pimpinella anisum L. (seeds)	Time: 0–60 min Frequency: 35 kHz Temperature: < 30°C Solvent: 0.5% w/v brine	Bandelin US bath	US pretreatment for 44.28 min	US pretreatment to ohmic-assisted hydrodistillation (US-OH) method resulted in a shorter total extraction time compared to plain hydrodistillation and was 28% more efficient US-OH method had lower energy consumption (0.180 kW h/g EO) and higher TPC (11.65 GAE/g EO). Results showed that the quality of EO	(Jafari et al., 2022)
Rhodiola rosea L., *Rhodiola crenulata*, and *Rhodiola quadrifida* (root and rhizome)	Time: 15, 45, and 60 minutes Frequency: – Temperature: 40°C and 60°C Solvent: MeOH/water (3:1 and 1:3)	Laboratory sonicator	UAE for 60 min; 40°C	*R. rosea* salidroside: 0.6% (0.3–1.5%), and the sum of rosin, rosarin, and rosavin, expressed as rosin, was 1.4% (0.6–2.6%) *R. crenulata* salidroside: 0.8% (0.01–1.6%) *R. quadrifida* salidroside 1.1% (0.6–2.4%)	(Ajdert et al., 2022)
Rosmarinus officinalis	Time: 30 min Frequency: 50 kHz Power: 100, 150, 200, and 250 W Temperature: 20°C Solvent: Ionic liquid in H_2O, H_2O, 1 M NaBr, 80% EtOH, 1 M [C8mim]Br	KQ-250DB US Wash unit	UAE for 30 min; 221 W; 1:20 solid-to-liquid ratio	The verification tests under those conditions resulted in an actual extraction efficiency of 98.91% ± 1.3% Higher efficiency and shorter extraction time for the extraction of carnosic acid and rosmarinic acid from *R. officinalis* compared to conventional methods	(Zu et al., 2012)
Rosmarinus officinalis	Time: 10 min Frequency: – Temperature: 40°C Solvent: H_2O or EtOH/H_2O 1:1	UP400S US unit	EtOH as solvent	UAE reduced the extraction of flavonoids in comparison with maceration Flavonoids: 16.29–24.99 mg CE/g DB. Antioxidant activity: 5.55–10.60 mmol TE Flavonoids: 17.45–25.06 mg CE/g DB (EtOH) vs. 15.90–21.23 mg CE/g DB (H_2O)	(Munekata et al., 2020)
Rosmarinus officinalis (leaves)	Time: 15–120 min Frequency: 20 kHz Temperature: 25°C, 35°C, 50°C Solvent: EtOH or MeOH	Sonics & Materials Inc. sonicator	MeOH for rosmarinic acid extraction; EtOH for carnosic acid extraction	Rosmarinic acid: 1.2 mg/g DB (MeOH) vs. 0.2 mg/g DB (EtOH) Carnosic acid: 6.41 mg/g (EtOH) vs. 4.27 mg/g (MeOH) Yield extraction: 100% (30 min) vs. 80% (45 min)	(Paniwnyk et al., 2009)
Syzygium aromaticum (buds)	Time: Varied Frequency: 53 kHz Temperature: Varied Solvent: ethanol	KUDOS US bath	UAE for 31 min; 30°C; 7% plant concentration	Predicted yield: 22.86% Experimental yield: 22.43%	(Tekin et al., 2015)
Thymus serpyllum L.	Time: 40, 55, and 70 min Frequency: 40 kHz Temperature: 50°C, 65°C, and 80°C Solvent: EtOH 45%, 60%, and 75% + water	Bath sonicator (EUP540A, Euinstruments, France)	UAE for 70 min; 70.28°C; 45% EtOH	Total extraction yield: 30.37% TPC: 4.3619 g GAE/100 g	(Mrkonjić et al., 2021)
Thymus vulgaris	Time: 10 min Frequency: – Temperature: 40°C Solvent: H_2O or EtOH/H_2O 1:1	UP400S US unit	H_2O as solvent	Flavonoids: 10.42–15.22 mg CE/g DB Antioxidant activity: 5.15–8.35 mmol TE (water)	(Munekata et al., 2020)
Vaccinium sect. Cyanococcus (leaves)	Time: 45 min Frequency: 20 kHz Temperature: 65°C Solvent: NADES	Waterbath sonicator	UAE for 45 min; 65°C; solvent-to-sample ratio of 15% v/w	Total phenol content: 135 ± 1 mg GAE/g DB Antioxidant activity: 153 ± 0 mg TEAC/g DB	(Santos-Martín et al., 2023)

chromatography analysis of the extracted compounds revealed significant levels of ursolic acid and oleanolic acid. When compared with Soxhlet extraction, the UAE method yielded lower extraction quantities. However, it offered the advantages of gentler extraction conditions, a shorter extraction duration, and higher selectivity for triterpenic acids.

The recovery of valuable constituents, particularly polyphenols, was significantly influenced by the extraction conditions, when ultrasound was applied to thyme (*Thymus vulgaris*) (Munekata et al., 2020). Considering the extraction method (conventional extraction vs. UAE) and solvent (water vs. 50:50 hydroethanolic solution) used, the most noteworthy extract was derived utilizing UAE with water as the solvent. This extract demonstrated improved extraction of carotenoids, high antioxidant activity, inhibitory effects on *S. enterica*, stimulatory impacts on *Lactobacillus casei*, and substantial in vitro antiinflammatory activity compared to that obtained with conventional methods.

Mrkonjić et al. (2021) investigated the extraction of polyphenols from wild thyme (*Thymus serpyllum* L.) filter-tea by-product via UAE. To optimize the extraction process, a three-level, three-variable face-centered central composite experimental design, utilizing RSM, was implemented. The independent variables selected comprised temperature (50°C, 65°C, and 80°C), extraction duration (40, 55, and 70 min), and ethanol concentration (45%, 60%, and 75%). The chosen responses were total extraction yield (Y) and total phenolic content (TPC), alongside antioxidant activity. The experimental results were fitted to a second-order polynomial model, with the goodness of fit evaluated through regression analysis and analysis of variance. A strong correlation between the experimental and predicted values was observed, indicating that the developed models could facilitate multiresponse optimization aimed at maximizing the yields of targeted responses while enhancing the antioxidant potential of *T. serpyllum* liquid extracts. Moreover, the application of UAE demonstrated advantages in comparison to conventional SLE with respect to antioxidant activity, total extraction yield, and TPC. The authors concluded that *T. serpyllum* by-product possesses the potential to serve as a raw material to produce extracts rich in antioxidants.

Behaiyn et al. (2023) found that in the UAE of *Aloe vera* leaf skins, elevating the ethanol concentration and extending the sonication duration changed the extraction yield. This research proposes that UAE is an efficient, secure, and economically viable approach to maximize aloin extraction from *A. vera* leaf skins.

A UAE extraction technique was reported as fine-tuned for the leaves of *Vaccinium sect. Cyanococcus* (Santos-Martín et al., 2023). These extraction parameters facilitated the successful retrieval of phenolic compounds from blueberry leaves, as confirmed by spectrophotometric assessments and chromatographic identification of a wide range of individual phenolic compounds.

Another study illustrated that UAE proved to be an efficient and dependable approach for inhibiting the butyrylcholinesterase enzyme (anti-BChE activity), an enzyme involved in memory impairment, while enhancing the levels of antioxidant compounds from *Aristotelia serrata* (wineberry or makomako, a small deciduous shrub of New Zealand) leaves (Majid and Silva, 2020). Ganorkar et al. (2022) studied UAE as a waste valorization method for leaves, stems, and roots of water hyacinth (*Eichhornia crassipes*), comparing organic solvent to water extraction mainly for acquiring shikimic acid. UAE was more efficient compared to conventional extraction, resulting in a higher yield, TPC, and antioxidant activity.

A combined method of UAE and natural deep eutectic solvents (NADES) was employed to extract phenolic compounds from *Larrea cuneifolia,* an Argentinian autochthonous plant (Espino et al., 2018). This approach was assessed based on its alignment with sustainability principles, achieving low values of environmental pollution potential, as evidenced by a Green Certificate. Additionally, the extraction efficiency was compared with conventional solvents, revealing that NADES demonstrated exceptional extractability for both polar and weakly polar phenolic compounds.

Gavrila et al. (2023) employed a US pretreatment on thyme leaves to augment the thymol concentration and the extraction efficiency of the EO acquired via microwave-assisted hydro-distillation (MWHD). In contrast to conventional hydrodistillation (HD), the sequential application of US pretreatment and microwave (MW) extraction led to a reduction in extraction duration by 72%. Upon the application of US pretreatment (US amplitude at 70%), the EO yield was observed to be 23% greater in comparison to the extraction conducted without pretreatment (2.67 ± 0.06 g EO/100 g DM for the MWHD with ultrasound pretreatment vs. 2.18 ± 0.07 g EO/100 g DM for the MWHD devoid of pretreatment).

A novel technique using UAE in conjunction with enzyme-mediation and optimized by RSM was performed for extracting bioactive compounds from *Gymnema sylvestre*, a herb of the family Apocynaceae found in many regions of Asia and Africa (Saeed et al., 2022). The authors highlight that the method was not only effective but also eco-friendly and cost-effective.

2.2 Microwave-assisted extraction

The utilization of MW in food processing has attracted considerable attention in recent decades. Various advantages over traditional thermal treatment methods exist, such as energy savings from volumetric heating, reduced processing time and cost, sustainability, and the potential for automation or online connectivity to analytical instrumentation. MW applications include pasteurization, sterilization, drying, or thawing of food products, often used alongside thermal methods (Ekezie et al., 2017; Guzik et al., 2022).

MW technology operates on the principle of electromagnetic field transmission and vertical oscillation within a wavelength range of 1 mm to 1 m, corresponding to frequencies from 0.3 to 300 GHz. Unlike traditional thermal methods relying on convection, conduction, and radiative heat transfer, MWs induce volumetric heating based on the dielectric properties of the target material (Bingham et al., 2001; Venkatesh and Raghavan, 2004; Vollmer, 2004). Microwave heating occurs through two primary mechanisms: (1) dipole rotation, where polar molecules (like water) rapidly align with the oscillating electromagnetic field, generating molecular friction and heat, and (2) ionic conduction, where charged particles (e.g., salts) collide under field-induced motion. While nonpolar compounds respond weakly to MWs, the prevalence of polar molecules—especially water—in biological materials enables efficient energy absorption and volumetric heating (Sun et al., 2016; Yoshikawa, 2020).

MAE is a blend of MWs and traditional SLE; the mechanism of extraction at the cellular level in MAE is characterized by a unique interplay of heat and mass transfer phenomena, where the interaction induces the release of thermal energy into the liquid medium, aiding in the extraction of the desired compounds through molecular ionic conduction and dipole rotation (Alslaibi et al., 2013). In contrast to traditional conductive heating methods, MWs possess the capability to rapidly heat the entire sample uniformly, thereby augmenting extraction efficiency (Alara et al., 2021). Furthermore, the utilization of binary mixtures comprising organic solvents and water enhances the efficiency of extraction via MAE when compared with individual organic solvents. Agitation during the extraction process is identified as an additional beneficial factor during MAE, as it accelerates the rate of solvent transfer, especially in instances where concentrated polyphenols are entrapped within plant material (Lee et al., 2016).

Table 6.2 outlines the main findings of recent research on the application of MAE on MAPs. Sarfarazi et al. (2020) extracted key saffron compounds, namely, picrocrocin, safranal, and crocin, by MAE, utilizing RSM. A CCD was employed to optimize extraction variables, including temperature (45°C–125°C), duration (10–30 min), and ethanol concentration (0–100 v/v%). Through the RSM optimization algorithm, the ideal conditions were found to be a temperature of 95.91°C, a duration of 30 min, and an ethanol concentration of 59.59%, while high-performance liquid chromatography (HPLC) analysis identified four crocetin esters in the optimized saffron extract. The use of MAE for the extraction of valuable compounds from saffron tepals, which could find applications in the food, pharmaceutical, or cosmetic sectors, employing RSM, was also assessed by Cerdá-Bernad et al. (2022). A CCD was utilized to optimize extraction parameters, including temperature, duration, and ethanol concentration. The extracts were evaluated for TPC and flavonoid content, as well as antioxidant capacity (oxygen radical absorbance capacity, ORAC and hydroxyl radical scavenging capacity, HOSC assays), yielding maximum values of 126.20 ± 2.99 mg gallic acid equivalents (GAE)/g dry matter; 8.05 ± 0.11 mg catechin equivalents (CE)/g dry matter; 6219 ± 246 μmol Trolox equivalent antioxidant capacity (TEAC)/dry matter; and 3131 ± 205 μmol TEAC/dry matter, respectively. The results suggested that the optimal extraction conditions involved a combination of low temperature (25°C) and extended extraction time (5 min) using ethanol as the solvent (100%). The authors concluded that MAE was proven to be an effective method for isolating bioactive compounds from saffron floral by-products with minimal energy consumption. Najafi et al. (2022) examined the impact of various extraction methods on the antioxidant properties of saffron (*C. sativus* L.). Saffron stigmas underwent extraction using water, ethanol, methanol, and their combinations via maceration extraction, ultrasonic-assisted extraction (UAE), MAE, and the combination of UAE with MAE. The findings revealed that the sample extracted using methanol/water (50:50) with the combination of UAE and MAE methods exhibited the highest TPC (31.56 mg/g GAE) and antioxidant activity (83.24% inhibition).

"Green" extraction methodologies, specifically bead milling extraction, UAE, and MAE, were evaluated for their efficacy in recovering a high-value extract from thyme (*T. vulgaris* L.) (Adhar et al., 2022). Among all the eco-friendly extraction techniques examined, MAE emerged as the most effective method in terms of extraction yield (20.84% ± 0.51), thymol concentration (731.71 mg/g), TPC (23.53 ± 1.83 mg (GAE)/g of extract), and flavonoid (6.22 ± 0.35 mg of quercetin equivalent (QE/g of extract) contents. Furthermore, the thyme extract obtained through MAE exhibited the most pronounced antioxidant activity when compared with the other extracts tested.

Gonzalez-Rivera et al. (2023) combined US and MW irradiation extraction (US-IMWAE) for the valorization of lavender and rosemary. Their findings indicate that the environmentally friendly US-IMWAE extraction method yields higher quantities of EOs with desirable composition profiles suitable for industries such as cosmetics, fragrances, perfumes, as well as pharmaceutical and medical applications. The presence of a high concentration of rosmarinic acid and TPC in the hydrosols obtained using the US-IMWAE method underscores its significant potential. Furthermore, US-IMWAE offers environmental benefits, flexibility, controllability, and the capacity to overcome scale-up challenges in ultrasound and MW-assisted industrial processes.

As reported by Choudhary et al. (2021), MAE was found to have higher yields compared to Soxhlet extraction for *Chenopodium album*, a globally spread MAP, yielding 6.83%–14.56% as opposed to 3.38%–9.53%, respectively. The investigation revealed that MAE significantly increased the concentration of secondary metabolites in all extracts compared to Soxhlet. MAE proved to be a superior extraction technique for *C. album* in contrast to Soxhlet extraction.

TABLE 6.2 Summary of recent research on microwave-assisted extraction of medicinal and aromatic plants.

Author(s)	Plant matrix	Extraction conditions	Extractor	Optimum conditions	Key results
(Choudhary et al., 2021)	*Chenopodium album*	200 W; 50°C; 18 min; petroleum ether; ethyl acetate; MeOH; EtOH; H_2O; H_2O	Magnetic shaker	Aqueous extraction	• Yield (%): petroleum ether (6.83), ethyl acetate (8.58), methanol (12.15), hydroalcoholic (10.12), aqueous (14.56) • MAE significantly increased secondary metabolite levels
(Mustapa et al., 2015)	*Clinacanthus nutans* Lindau (leaves and stems)	300 W max power; 2.45 GHz; EtOH/H_2O	CEMDiscover microwave oven	EtOH/H_2O mixture	• High yield obtained • TPC: 11.30 ± 0.39 mg GAE/g DM • Flavonoid content: 4.66 ± 0.20 mg GAE/g
(Sarfarazi et al., 2020)	*Crocus sativus* L. (stigmas)	2.45 GHz; 1000 W max output power; 45°C–125°C; 10–30 min; 0%–100% EtOH	MicroSYNTH microwave apparatus	MAE for 30 min, 95.91°C, 59.59% EtOH	• Optimal extraction conditions determined by response surface methodology
(Cerdá-Bernad et al., 2022)	*Crocus sativus* L. (tepals)	500 psi with 300 W max output power; 0.5–5 min; 25°C–100°C; 0%–100% EtOH.	Discover SP-CEMMWsystem	MAE for 5 min, 25°C, 100% EtOH	• TPC: 126.20 ± 2.99 mg GAE/g dw • TFC: 8.05 ± 0.11 mg CE/g dw • ORAC: 6219 ± 246 μmol TEAC/dw • HOSC: 3131 ± 205 μmol TEAC/dw
(Najafi et al., 2022)	*Crocus sativus* L. (stigmas)	Power level of 30%; 2 min; H_2O; EtOH; MeOH; 50:50 H_2O/EtOH; 50:50 H_2O/MeOH	Conventional microwave oven	UAE combined with MAE; 50:50 H_2O/MeOH	• Maximum TPC and antioxidant activity achieved with a methanol/water mixture • Combined UAE–MAE showed highest performance
(Gonzalez-Rivera et al., 2023)	*Lavandula angustifolia* Mill. (leaves and stems) *Salvia rosmarinus* Schleid. (leaves and stems)	S/L ratio 1:10, 60 min, 300 W	MW antenna	MAE for 60 min; S/L ratio 1:10; 300 W	• Increased EO yield, linalool, and linalyl acetate content (lavender) • Increased eucalyptol and α-/β-pinene content (rosemary) • Highest cellulose, lowest lignin in solid residues (lavender)
(Binello et al., 2017)	*Melissa officinalis* L.	20 bar; 100°C; 500 W max power; 10 min; EtOH, EtOH/H_2O; H_2O	Closed multimode reactor	EtOH as solvent	• Best extraction yield of polyphenols and rosmarinic acid with ethanol
(Bellumori et al., 2016)	*Rosmarinus officinalis*	S/L ratio 1:10, 10 min, 100% EtOH	Closed multimode reactor under N_2 (20 bar) at 100°C	MAE for 10 min; 100% EtOH; S/L ratio 1:10	• Maximum extraction yield: 20% • Total phenols yield: 184.2 mg/g dried extract, 36.6 mg/g dried leaves
(Adhar et al., 2022)	*Thymus vulgaris* L. (leaves)	Constant power of 250 W; 78°C; vapor pressure of 15 bars; 2 h	Microwave reactor	MAE for 2 h; 250 W, 78°C, 15 bars	• Extraction yield: 20.84% ± 0.51 • Thymol concentration: 731.71 mg/g • TPC: 23.53 ± 1.83 mg GAE/g extract • Flavonoid: 6.22 ± 0.35 mg QE/g extract • Highest antioxidant effect compared to other extracts

Mustapa et al. (2015) investigated different extraction methods to determine the most effective approach for extracting phytochemical compounds from *Clinacanthus nutans* Lindau, a popular medicinal plant in Southeast Asia. While Soxhlet extraction exhibited the highest overall yield, it employed high temperatures and a longer duration, leading to some limitations in terms of selectivity for specific bioactive compounds. In contrast, MAE and pressurized MAE (P-MAE) demonstrated shorter extraction times and enhanced selectivity, with MAE achieving high yields of polyphenols and flavonoids. On the contrary, supercritical carbon dioxide extraction was the most efficient method for phytosterol extraction, particularly β-sitosterol. These findings emphasize that the Soxhlet method, while yielding high quantities, may not be the most efficient and selective technique for extracting specific bioactive compounds from *C. nutans*.

Single-step MAE for 10 min in ethanol and a mixture of ethanol/water (7:3 v/v) yielded approximately 16% w/w when used for extracting phenolic compounds from lemon balm (*M. officinalis* L.) leaves, while MAE in pure water gave the highest extraction yield (~31% w/w) (Binello et al., 2017). Similarly, MAE single extraction step for polyphenols from rosemary leaves exhibited yields of 18%–21% w/w in water and ethanol (Bellumori et al., 2016).

MAE technology showcases high efficiency in terms of time compared to conventional extraction methods, coupled with a reasonable cost and the generation of substantial quantities of bioactive compounds, even under standard pressure conditions. The efficacy of the extraction process is contingent upon various factors, including temperature, duration of radiation exposure, intensity of energy input, choice of solvent, and their interplay (Nour et al., 2021). Nonetheless, there are specific limitations associated with its applicability for extracting certain bioactive compounds, such as polyphenols, particularly concerning the potential impact of certain variables on its effectiveness, including the duration and power of MW exposure, the purity and surface area of the sample, and the composition of the sample matrix (Alara et al., 2021).

2.3 Supercritical fluid extraction

A supercritical fluid (SF), often referred to as a dense gas, exhibits physical properties that combine characteristics of both gases and liquids when it reaches its critical point. The critical region is defined by specific temperature and pressure conditions. SFs typically behave like gases but also possess the solvent properties associated with liquids. One of the most familiar examples of an SF is carbon dioxide (CO_2), which transitions into a supercritical state at pressures exceeding 7380 kPa and temperatures above 31.1°C (Khan et al., 2022).

Over the last two decades, there has been a significant focus on employing near-critical and supercritical carbon dioxide as a solvent, especially in industries such as food, pharmaceuticals, and perfumes. CO_2 stands out as an excellent solvent choice due to its nontoxic, nonexplosive nature, widespread availability, and ease of removal from extracted products (Simándi et al., 1998).

The process of SFE relies on three key stages: (1) the dissolution or resolution of analytes by supercritical CO_2, (2) the sweeping of these analytes, and (3) the subsequent trapping of analytes. As high-pressure liquid CO_2 is introduced into the extraction chamber, it permeates and dissolves within the sample matrix, resolving the primarily nonpolar analytes. The supercritical CO_2, carrying the extracted analytes, is then captured, after which the CO_2 is evaporated, leading to the separation of the extract (Ray et al., 2023). Organic cosolvents can be incorporated into SFE to recover polar compounds. This, however, can add complexity to the purification and recycling of carbon dioxide, resulting in elevated costs. Consequently, this approach is rarely employed in commercial uses of SFE (Manjare and Dhingra, 2019).

A summary of studies on SFE of MAPs is presented in Table 6.3. According to an early study by Carvalho et al. (2005), extracts derived from rosemary (*R. officinalis*) leaves through SFE, at 300 bar and 40°C, displayed greater antioxidant activity in comparison with extracts obtained via low-pressure distillation. Although the low-pressure extraction yielded a larger quantity of extract, its antioxidant activity was found to be inferior to that of the SFE extract. In another study investigating aromatic extracts from fresh rosemary samples, SFE was found to be the most favorable method due to its significantly lower energy consumption and carbon emissions (Moura et al., 2022). Specifically, SFE required 290 MJ per g of extract, whereas the hydrodistillation method consumed 363 MJ/g. Conversely, when aiming to obtain 1 g of α-pinene, SFE exhibited lower selectivity and resulted in higher energy consumption and carbon emissions.

Although SFE proved superior to other methods (MAE, P-MAE, and Soxhlet) for phytosterol and β-sitosterol extraction from snake grass (*C. nutans* Lindau), a tropical MAP predominantly grown in Southeast Asia, Mustapa et al. (2015) reported that it yielded significantly lower amounts. These findings were attributed to the nonpolar nature of carbon dioxide as a solvent, which is less suitable for extracting the numerous polar compounds found in *C. nutans* oil, including chlorophyll and polyphenols. This observation led them to conclude that supercritical extraction for *C. nutans* may not be economically viable.

Variations in pressure and temperature during CO_2-SFE of clove EO allowed selective extraction of nonpolar compounds, predominantly oxygenated monoterpenes, as reported by de Oliveira et al. (2016). The authors found that, depending on the operating conditions of temperature and pressure, the characteristics of the extracted oil can change. The highest yield was achieved at 50°C and 300 bar. This is the first report of the phytotoxic effect of clove EOs obtained with CO_2 SFE against invasive plant species *Mimosa pudica* and *Senna obtusifolia*.

Mrkonjić et al. (2024) elucidated the chemical profile and assessed the antioxidant and antimicrobial activities of the EO and lipid extracts derived from *T. serpyllum* L. herbal dust, utilizing HD, Soxhlet, and SFE. Furthermore, a comparative analysis of the chemical profiles of the resulting EO and extracts was conducted, alongside the evaluation of antioxidant,

TABLE 6.3 Summary of recent research on supercritical fluid extraction and subcritical fluid extraction of medicinal and aromatic plants.

Author(s)	Plant matrix	Extraction conditions	Extractor	Optimum conditions	Key results
(Phan et al., 2020)	*Callisia fragrans* (leaves)	Time: 3 h Pressure: 100, 150, 200, and 250 bar Temperature: 40, 45, 50, and 60°C Flow: 12, 14, 16, 18, and 20 g/min	Custom-made CO_2 SFE setup	20 g/min flow rate	• TPC: 87.42 mg/g • IC_{50}: 243.83 μM/g • Max antioxidant activity at 20 g/min: 192.58 μM TE/g
(Morsy, 2020)	*Carum copticum* L.	Time: 1.5 h Pressure: 104 and 167 bar Temperature: 40°C Flow: 0.882 g/h	Lab-scale SFE ISCO SFX 220 unit	167 bar	• Yield increased from 1.38% to 2.78%. • Thymol yield: 1.77 g/100 g db
(Mustapa et al., 2015)	*Clinacanthus nutans Lindau*	Time: 2 h Pressure: 350 bar Temperature: 60°C Flow: 9 kg/h	Custom-made CO_2 SFE setup	350 bar; 60°C	• Low yield (3.19%); high flavonoid (5.88 mg/g) and β-sitosterol (0.83 mg/g) content
(Goleroudbary and Ghoreishi, 2016)	*Corrected Text: Crocus sativus* L.	Time: varied Pressure: varied Temperature: varied Flow: varied	Custom-made CO_2 SFE setup	Crocin: SFE for 110 min; 44°C; 193 bar Safranal: SFE for 122 min; 92°C; 213 bar	• Crocin recovery: 32.67%, 1.836 mg/min • Safranal: 91.76%, 1.652 mg/min
(Nerome et al., 2016)	*Crocus sativus* L.(spice)	Time: varied Pressure: 200–400 bar Temperature: 40–80°C Flow: 2.04 g/min	Custom-made CO_2 SFE setup	Crocins: 80°C; 300 bar Safranal: 80°C; 400 bar	• Extracted picrocrocin, safranal, and α-crocin; methanol → picrocrocin and safranal; water → α-crocin
(Nejad-Sadeghi et al., 2015)	*Dracocephalum kotschyi*	Time: varied Pressure: varied Temperature: varied Flow: varied	Custom-made CO_2 SFE setup	SFE for 100 min; 240 bar; 60°C; 6.8 g/s	• Yield: 2.81% (predicted), 2.72% (actual) • CO_2 flow and time most significant
(Rahimi et al., 2011)	*Matricaria recutita* L.	Time: 7 h Pressure: 250 bar Temperature: 40°C Flow: 0.4158 kg/h	Model 7071 Applied Separations, SFE unit	SFE form 200 min; 40°C; 200 bar; 0.24012 kg/h	• Best yield at 40°C/200 bar
(Carvalho et al., 2005)	*Rosmarinus officinalis* (leaves)	Time: 3 h Pressure: 100, 150, 200, 250, 300 bar Temperature: 30°C and 40°C Flow: 0.32 kg/h	Model 7071 Applied Separations, SFE unit	40°C; 250–300 bar	• High antioxidant activity at 250–300 bar/40°C • Lowest antioxidant activity at 30°C/150 bar
(Glisic et al., 2011)	*Salvia officinalis L*	Time: – Pressure: 150 and 300 bar Temperature: 50°C Flow: 0.4 kg/h	Semibatch Autoclave Engineers Screening System	300 bar; 50°C	• Maximum extract and unique compounds at 300 bar

Continued

TABLE 6.3 Summary of recent research on supercritical fluid extraction and subcritical fluid extraction of medicinal and aromatic plants—cont'd

Author(s)	Plant matrix	Extraction conditions	Extractor	Optimum conditions	Key results
(de Oliveira et al., 2016)	*Syzygium aromaticum*	Time: 0.5 h + 2 h Pressure: 100, 200, 300 bar Temperature: 40°C and 50°C Flow: 0.32 kg/h	Model 7071 Applied Separations, SFE unit	40°C; 100 bar	• Oil yield: 13.14% at 40°C/100 bar
(Milovanovic et al., 2022)	*Taraxacum officinale* (seeds)	Time: – Pressure: 100, 200, 300, and 450 bar Temperature: 40°C and 60°C Flow: 9.0 kg/h	SITEC SFE unit	100 bar; 40°C	• TPC: 5.5–12.1 mg GAE/g • Best antioxidant activity (64.4%) at 100 bar/40°C • CC_{50} = 385.8 μg/mL
(Mrkonjić et al., 2024)	*Thymus serpyllum* L.	Time: 3 h Pressure: 100, 225, and 350 bar Temperature: 40°C, 50°C, and 60°C Flow: 0.2, 0.3, and 0.4 kg/h	HPEP	350 bar; 50°C; 0.3 kg/h	• Yield: 2.93% • High DPPH/ABTS activity at high/low P–T • MIC = 0.31–0.83 mg/mL
(Morsy, 2020)	*Thymus vulgaris* L.	Time: 1.5 h Pressure: 104, 167 bar Temperature: 40°C Flow: 0.882 g/h	Lab-scale SFE ISCO SFX 220 unit	167 bar	• Yield: 1.28% • Thymol: 1.06 g/100 g db • High selectivity at 167 bar
(Fu et al., 2023)	*Uncaria rhynchophylla*	Time: 0.5, 1, and 1.5 h Pressure: 200, 250, and 300 bar Temperature: 35°C, 40°C, and 45°C Flow: 1 mL/min	Waters SFE system	SFE for 60–90 min; 250 bar; 40°C.	• Alkaloids appear after 60–90 min • Pressure and temperature increase improve yield

antibacterial, and antifungal activities of the lipid extracts. Based on the antioxidant and antimicrobial activities, as well as the yield and selectivity of monoterpenes, SFE demonstrated significant advantages over traditional extraction methods. In addition, the SFE extracts could be regarded as having considerable potential for applications within the pharmaceutical and cosmetic sectors, as well as serving as viable alternatives to synthetic additives in the food industry.

A mathematical model for SFE recovery of chamomile (*Matricaria recutita*) was presented by Rahimi et al. (2011). They subsequently compared the model's outcomes with experimental data and found that there was a strong agreement between the model's predictions and the actual experimental results. In addition, they explored the impact of particle diameter on the extraction yield and observed that the extraction yield displayed a weak dependence on particle diameter.

A study by Glisic et al. (2011) assessed the use of SFE after the application of UAE on sage (*S. officinalis* L.) to obtain concentrated diterpenes, as these compounds exhibit high antioxidant activity. The authors concluded that UAE as a pretreatment followed by CO_2 SFE resulted in two valuable products: the US extract, which is rich in sugars and has immunomodulatory properties, and the SF extract, which had high levels of diterpenes and sesquiterpenes.

Milovanovic et al. (2022) optimized the SFE of dandelion (*Taraxacum officinale*) seeds by varying operating pressures within the range of 100 to 450 bar and temperatures ranging from 40°C to 60°C. Their findings demonstrated that higher pressure resulted in an increased extraction rate. Conversely, elevating the temperature led to a reduction in the extraction rate; when the temperature was raised from 40°C to 60°C, there was a significant decline in extraction yields at 100 and 200 bar, while at 300 and 450 bar, the increase in temperature had a minimal impact on the final yield. Nejad-Sadeghi et al. (2015) carried out the optimization of five crucial process parameters: pressure, temperature, average particle size, CO_2 flow rate, and dynamic extraction time for SFE of EOs from *Dracocephalum kotschyi* Boiss, an Iranian medicinal plant, member of the Lamiaceae family. Their optimization led to the attainment of a practical extraction yield of 2.72% by weight, which represents a significant achievement in the extraction of EO from that valuable medicinal plant.

Morsy (2020) concluded that SFE at 40°C and 167 bar proved to be the optimal method for obtaining thymol-rich extracts with highly favorable sensory attributes from *Carum copticum* L. (ajwain) and *T. vulgaris* L. (thyme). In the case of ajwain, the SFE extract obtained at this pressure was particularly well-received, characterized by its spicy, pungent, and aromatic odor, notable for the absence of any burnt notes. Similarly, the sensory characteristics (spicy, pungent, herbaceous, and phenol-like) scores for the thyme SFE extract, obtained under the same conditions, were also significantly higher. In contrast, aroma analysis revealed noteworthy adverse changes in the aroma of thyme EO.

Higher yields of all the constituents from saffron (*C. sativus*) were obtained using SFE with an entrainer compared to a conventional liquid solvent method (Nerome et al., 2016). These yields increased with rising temperature for all components. In addition, higher pressure resulted in larger quantities of 4-hydroxy-2,6,6-trimethyl-1-cyclohexene-1-carboxaldehyde and safranal in the extract, in line with their expectations. However, the maximum amounts of picrocrocin, α-crocin, and deglycosylated crocin were obtained at 300 bar, with the quantity extracted at 400 bar being approximately half. In another study, also on *C. sativus*, safranal and crocin were experimentally extracted from saffron using SFE and modified SFE using methanol as an entrainer (Goleroudbary and Ghoreishi, 2016). By employing the optimal conditions, the authors achieved a mean experimental recovery of 90.03% by weight for safranal and 33.05% by weight for crocin, which closely matched the values predicted by their model.

The optimum SFE conditions of *Callisia fragrans*, a Vietnamese MAP used in traditional medicine, were determined as a CO_2 flow rate of 20 g/min, an extraction temperature of 45°C, and a pressure of 200 bar, with ethanol as a cosolvent at a 14% concentration (Phan et al., 2020).

2.4 Subcritical water extraction

Subcritical water extraction (SWE), also referred to as pressurized hot water extraction, superheated water extraction, pressurized liquid extraction, or even accelerated solvent extraction when water is used as the solvent, is an extraction method employing pressurized water as the extractant within a temperature range spanning from 100°C to 374°C (Plaza and Turner, 2015). The application of high pressure in the extraction process is essential for retaining water in its liquid state. Subcritical conditions have an impact on the thermodynamic properties of water, including the strength and arrangement of hydrogen bonds. Under these subcritical conditions, elevated temperatures reduce the strength of hydrogen bonds in water, subsequently leading to a decrease in the polarity and dielectric constant of water (Carr et al., 2011). Consequently, the polarity of water becomes akin to that of organic solvents like ethanol and methanol at room temperature, leading to an augmented solubility of nonpolar substances in water. Furthermore, the elevated temperature associated with subcritical conditions results in reduced water viscosity and surface tension, which, in turn, promotes greater diffusivity and enhanced mass transport (Hassas-Roudsari et al., 2009).

The process of SWE involves three key steps: initially, the target analyte is separated from the plant material; next, subcritical water infiltrates the plant material, facilitating the dissolution of solutes in the water; and finally, the solute is extracted from the plant matrix (Teo et al., 2010). The extraction process encompasses both thermodynamic and kinetic elements, meaning that the efficiency of extraction is impacted by three interconnected factors: solubility, mass transfer, and the matrix effect. Each of these distinct stages in SWE is governed by various parameters, including temperature, pressure, time, flow rate, and other factors chosen for the extraction (Gilbert-López et al., 2017).

Table 6.4 summarizes the findings of recent studies on SWE of MAPs. Halim et al. (2021) explored the yields of EOs from SWE of kaffir lime (*Citrus hystrix*) using both univariate and multivariate methodologies. They developed and validated a regression model based on the experimental design. The study revealed that SWE of *C. hystrix* leaves at elevated temperatures (160°C and 180°C) generated a greater quantity of EO compounds compared to SWE at 140°C and hydrodistillation.

TABLE 6.4 Recent research on subcritical water extraction of medicinal and aromatic plants.

Author(s)	Medicinal plant	Extraction conditions	Extractor	Optimum conditions	Key results
(Halim et al., 2021)	*Citrus hystrix* (leaves)	Time: 20–40 min Temperature: 140°C–180°C Sample/solvent ratio: 0.025–0.175 g/mL	Static-mode batch fluid extraction unit	SWE for 29 min; 0.75 mm particle size; 0.025 g/mL ratio; 174°C	• Yield: 2.14 ± 0.03% (w/w)
(Song and Ko, 2022)	*Coriandrum sativum* L.(seeds)	Time: 5–20 min Temperature: 110°C–200°C Sample/solvent ratio: –	Dionex Model 350 Accelerated Solvent Extractor	Not specified	• Geraniol: 1.22 ± 0.22 mg/g • Linalool oxide: 0.30 ± 0.09 mg/g • Better extraction than conventional methods
(Esmaeelian et al., 2020)	*Crocus sativus* L. (corms)	Time: 10–30 min Temperature: 100°C–180°C Sample/solvent ratio: –	In-house-built SW extractor	SWE for 21.99 min; 180°C	• DPPH IC_{50}: 61.67 mg/kg • TPC: 816.34 mg GAE/100 g DB
(Ahmadian-Kouchaksaraie and Niazmand, 2017)	*Crocus sativus* L. (petals)	Time: 20–60 min Temperature: 120°C–160°C Sample/solvent ratio: 0.025–0.05 g/mL	In-house-built SW extractor	SWE for 54 min; 159°C; 0.028 g/mL	• TPC: 1616 mg/100 g • TFC: 239 mg/100 g • DPPH: 86.05% • FRAP: 5.1 mM
(Sarfarazi et al., 2019)	*Crocus sativus* L. (stigmas)	Time: 5–15 min Temperature: 105°C–125°C Sample/solvent ratio: –	In-house-built SW extractor	SWE for 7.32 min; 105°C	• Not numerically detailed
(Nastić et al., 2018)	*Geranium macrorrhizum* (leaves)	Time: 30 min Temperature: 60°C–200°C Sample/solvent ratio: 0.025	In-house-built SW extractor	Not specified	• DPPH: 197.0 ± 4.3 mg TE/g DB
(Šeremet et al., 2021)	*Glechoma hederacea* L.	Time: 5 min Temperature: 200°C Sample/solvent ratio: 0.01 g/mL	In-house-built SW extractor	SWE for 5 min; 200°C, 5 min, 0.01 g/mL	• TPC: 60.1 mg GAE/g dmb • AA: 0.280–0.349 mmol Trolox/g dmb
(Machmudah et al., 2022)	*Moringa oleifera*	Time: 30 min Temperature: 140°C Sample/solvent ratio: –	In-house-built SW extractor	140°C, 5 MPa	• TPC: 82.26 mg GAE/g DB
(Nastić et al., 2018)	*Morus nigra* (leaves)	Time: 30 min Temperature: 60°C–200°C Sample/solvent ratio: 0.025	In-house-built SW extractor	160°C	• TPC: 61.89 ± 5.67 mg • GAE/g DB • DPPH: 68.88 ± 5.73 mg TE/g DB
(Aćimović et al., 2021)	*Satureja kitaibelii*	Time: 30 min Temperature: 130°C Sample/solvent ratio: 0.033 g/mL	In-house-built SW extractor	130°C, 0.033 g/mL	• Syringic acid: 37.88 mg/g • Caffeic acid: 18.06 mg/g • Epicatechin: 10.04 mg/g • AhgA: 30.72%
(Nastić et al., 2018)	*Teucrium chamaedrys* (flower)	Time: 30 min Temperature: 60°C–200°C Sample/solvent ratio: 0.025	In-house-built SW extractor	160°C	• TPC: 176.74 ± 3.41 mg GAE/g DB • DPPH: 196.12 ± 2.12 mg TE/g DB

An increase in extraction temperature enhanced the efficiency of phenolic compound extraction from *Moringa oleifera*, *Sauropus androgynus*, and *Sesbania grandiflora,* MAPs broadly distributed in Asian countries, by SWE, while elevated extraction pressure facilitated a faster extraction process (Machmudah et al., 2022). Higher temperatures promote the breaking of phenolic compound bonds within the plant biomass, and increased pressure enhances the interaction between the plant biomass and the subcritical water. Notably, the levels of extracted polyphenols could reach 82.26 (140°C, 50 bar), 75.32 (160°C, 50 bar), and 78.91 (160°C, 100 bar) mg of GAE/g of dry weight for *M. oleifera, S. androgynus*, and *S. grandiflora*, respectively. Based on these findings, they deemed this type of extraction technique both practical and effective for extracting phenolic compounds from the above MAPs.

Findings of the study by Nastić et al. (2018) establish that SWE at different temperatures applied to medicinal plants, namely, black mulberry (*Morus nigra* L.), wall germander (*Teucrium chamaedrys* L.), wild geranium (*Geranium macrorrhizum* L.), and comfrey (*Symphytum officinale* L.), holds significant potential as an extraction method for compounds with antioxidant, antimicrobial, and cytotoxic characteristics. SWE at 160°C and 10 bar exhibited the highest levels of phenols and antioxidant activity, while chlorogenic acid, gallic acid, and protocatechuic acid were the main phenolic acids in the extracts of the studied MAPs, especially in the case of *G. macrorrhizum*. The extracts also showed activity against eight tested microbial strains, with *Staphylococcus aureus* and *Aspergillus niger* being the most sensitive to SWE, while cytotoxic activity against cancerous cells derived from human cervix carcinoma, human rhabdomyosarcoma, and murine fibroblast was also observed. All the MAP extracts obtained by SWE had better bioactivity as compared to extracts obtained by other extraction techniques.

In a study conducted by Aćimović et al. (2021), phenolic compounds were effectively extracted from *Satureja kitaibelii,* or Rtanj tea, a native species of the Carpathian mountain chain on the Balkan Peninsula, using SWE. The resulting crude extract contained a substantial quantity of phenolic antioxidants. Moreover, the *S. kitaibelii* extract demonstrated commendable antioxidant properties and exhibited various biological attributes, including antiinflammatory and antihyperglycemic activities. Additionally, the tested extract displayed a potent antimicrobial effect against Gram-positive bacteria, yeasts, and fungi.

Šeremet et al. (2021) effectively employed RSM to optimize the production of phenolic extracts abundant in antioxidants via SWE of *Glechoma hederacea* L., also infamous as ground ivy, a native Croatian species. The actual results for TPC and antioxidant capacity closely aligned with the anticipated values. It was observed that the sample-to-solvent ratio exerted the most significant impact on all the assessed responses.

A two-factor, three-level full-factorial CCD was formulated to establish the correlation between the independent process variables during SWE, namely, extraction time and temperature, and the dependent variables, viz. picrocrocin, safranal, and crocin contents in saffron (*C. sativus*) extracts (Sarfarazi et al., 2019). Through this design, the optimal conditions were identified as an extraction temperature of 105°C and an extraction time of 7.32 min. The models exhibited close agreement between predicted and experimental results, highlighting the robust predictive capability of their model. Esmaeelian et al. (2020) also utilized CCD for *C. sativus* to attain the optimal subcritical water extraction process conditions, which were found to be 180°C and 21.99 min. A strong alignment between the experimental results and the predictions was observed, indicating the effectiveness of the suggested conditions and the dependability of the CCD analysis. Furthermore, microdilution and disc diffusion tests substantiate that the SC-SWE extract possesses antibacterial properties.

Ahmadian-Kouchaksaraie and Niazmand (2017) investigated supercritical carbon dioxide (SC-CO_2) extraction as a green method to obtain antioxidants from *C. sativus* petals. Using a Box–Behnken design (BBD) and RSM, the optimal conditions were determined as 62°C, 47 min, and 164 bar, maximizing phenolic content (1423 mg/100 g), flavonoids (180 mg/100 g), anthocyanins (103.4 mg/100 g), and antioxidant activity (74.5% DPPH scavenging, 3.9 mM ferric reducing antioxidant power (FRAP)). Experimental results matched predictions, confirming the model's accuracy. Principal component analysis further clarified interactions between antioxidant properties, demonstrating BBD's effectiveness in optimizing extraction. Song and Ko (2022) observed that the primary terpene in *Coriandrum sativum* seeds is oxygenated monoterpene, and SWE allowed for a rapid extraction process at a relatively low temperature. The study noted the transformation of linalool into linalool oxide as the extraction temperature increased during the SWE process. Furthermore, it was found that monoterpene yields are significantly affected by variations in their chemical structures and SWE conditions. The results also demonstrated the superior effectiveness of SWE compared to conventional extraction methods. SWE, in particular, reduced the extraction time when compared with methods involving methanol, hexane, hot water, and hydrodistillation.

2.5 Pulsed electric fields

PEF has been utilized as an extraction technology to obtain beneficial and bioactive substances from medicinal plants and their by-products, such as phenolic compounds, dietary fibers, and pigments. PEF is an eco-friendly method that operates at low temperatures, requires minimal energy, and is compatible with environmentally friendly solvents (Athanasiadis et al.,

2021). PEF, whether applied independently or in conjunction with processes like sonication or SFs, minimizes the negative effects of traditional heating processes, serving as a viable alternative to traditional extraction methods. It has been effectively employed to separate, stabilize, and dehydrate important compounds from plants without altering their inherent properties, as it has minimal impact on the nutritional elements, bioactive compounds, and the visual characteristics of the product. In addition, PEF has been proposed as a method to induce stress in plant cells, thereby promoting the production of active components (Ranjha et al., 2021).

PEF is an extraction process that relies on short-lived electrical pulses lasting a few seconds and ranging from 20 kV/cm to 80 kV/cm. At these electrical power levels, the electric fields create pores in the plant tissue membranes. Consequently, this causes a temporary or permanent change in the membrane's semipermeability at the plant's interface, known as "electroporation," facilitating the release of bound bioactive compounds at room temperature (Garavand et al., 2019).

This nonthermal extraction process prevents the degradation, hydrolysis, and polymerization of the target compounds. Because of its capacity to electroporate cell membranes, PEF is often utilized as a preliminary treatment to improve the recovery of bioactive materials before applying a subsequent conventional or innovative extraction process (Ranjha et al., 2021). Consequently, PEF extraction of plant-derived materials shows great promise for the recovery of phenolic compounds, vitamins, and other valuable components (Barba et al., 2015).

In contrast to conventional extraction methods, PEF facilitates the efficient and straightforward identification, classification, and analysis of bioactive elements. PEF-assisted extraction results in higher yields while using fewer solvents and less energy, ultimately saving a significant amount of time compared to conventional extraction approaches (Ghoshal, 2023).

PEF technology finds widespread use in various applications. These include the inactivation of microorganisms at high specific energy input levels, the preprocessing of plant materials for subsequent downstream procedures at lower to moderate specific energy input levels, and even the direct extraction of plant materials. To improve the extent of extraction in a particular solid-liquid system, a range of PEF parameters must be carefully adjusted. These parameters encompass the intensity of the electric field, the characteristics of the pulse (such as its shape, width, and frequency), and the duration of the application (Genovese et al., 2024).

Table 6.5 summarizes recent studies on PEF extraction applied to MAPs, highlighting its classification as a green extraction technique for phytochemicals. Athanasiadis et al. (2021) demonstrated that PEF significantly enhances the extraction of total polyphenols from sage (*Salvia officinalis* L.) leaves, achieving a 73.23% increase in yield compared to conventional methods. Under optimized conditions—using a 25% aqueous ethanol solvent and a 100 μs pulse duration—PEF not only improved polyphenol recovery but also boosted the extraction efficiency of rosmarinic acid by up to 403.12%. In addition, the study revealed that PEF-treated extracts exhibited greater resistance to oxidation, further underscoring the method's potential for preserving bioactive compounds. These findings position PEF as a sustainable and efficient extraction technique, with promising applications in the production of high-quality functional foods and cosmetics.

The effect of PEF application as a pretreatment strategy for EO extraction was assessed on eucalyptus, rosemary, and thyme leaves (Barros et al., 2022). The initial PEF pretreatment was systematically applied to eucalyptus and rosemary leaves 2 weeks postharvest, utilizing a 2 kV/cm electric field with a specific energy of approximately 10 kJ/kg, and subsequently followed by EO extraction via HD with distillation durations of 30 and 60 min. The most favorable outcomes were observed in PEF pretreated samples subjected to 30 min of HD, demonstrating an upward trend in the average extraction yield of approximately 17% and 11% for eucalyptus and rosemary, respectively, when contrasted with samples where no PEF was administered. The optimization of the PEF pretreatment process was also investigated, with the aim of maximizing the yield of EO extracted from dry thyme leaves while minimizing energy consumption across various distillation durations. It was observed that for the specified plant material, an electric field of 1 kV/cm with an energy input of 0.4 kJ/kg and an HD duration of 30 min, following PEF application, could achieve an extraction yield that was up to 40% greater than that obtained through conventional methods.

An earlier study investigated the impact of high-voltage PEF on the extraction of key components in saffron, with a focus on color (crocin), flavor (safranal), and taste (picrocrocin) (Pourzaki et al., 2013). Under standardized conditions of 25°C, the results revealed significant improvements in these components. Notably, when using a 5 kV voltage, 100 pulses, and a 35-ms pulse width in accordance with ISO 3632-2 guidelines, there was a 14.1% increase in color, a 15.5% enhancement in bitterness, and a 10.2% rise in taste.

PEF followed by UAE was applied to Greek MAPs, namely, *Olea europaea* L. leaves and unripe fruit, *M. officinalis* L. leaves, *Cistus incanus* L. spp. *creticus* leaves, *Vitis vinifera* L. cv. "Xinomavro" leaves, marc, and fruits, *Aronia melanocarpa* L. fruits, *Punica granatum* L. peel, and *C. sativus* L. petals (Ziagova et al., 2022). A solvent ratio of 1:20 g plant material/mL water, 5 min of PEF, followed by 30 min of US, resulted in the maximum extraction efficiency. The authors also reported high TPC levels for *M. officinalis* L. and *P. granatum* L. (155 mg GAE/g dry weight and 208 mg GAE/g dry weight, respectively), while, apart from *C. sativus* L. petals and *V. vinifera* L. marc, all the other extracts exhibited high antioxidant capacity.

TABLE 6.5 Summary of recent research on the extraction of medicinal and aromatic plants using pulsed electric fields.

Author(s)	Plant matrix	Extraction conditions	Extractor	Optimum conditions	Results
(Pourzaki et al., 2013)	Dried saffron stigma	Temperature: 25°C; pulse frequency: 0.1–10 Hz; pulse width: 10–100 ms; max voltage output: 5 kV; current voltage: 33 A	High-voltage pulse generator	Pulse number: 35; pulse width: 100 ms; electric field strength:5 kV.	• 5.76% increase in color, 7.5% increase in bitterness, and 5.9% increase in taste. • Greater pulse width achieves greater extraction.
(Athanasiadis et al., 2021)	Sage leaves	Temperature: 7°C and 15°C, average relative humidity: 75%	High voltage power generator	Pulses of 100 μs; PEF: 0.7–3.0 kV/cm; energy input: 1.0–20.0 kJ/kg.	• Increased mass transfer; identified volatiles: eucalyptol, β-thujone, camphor, borneol; best phenolics at 100 μs.
(Carpentieri et al., 2021)	*Origanum vulgare* L. *Thymus serpyllum* L.	Electric field strength (E_{opt}): 5 kV/cm Total specific energy input (Wt): 40 kJ/kg	High-voltage pulsed power (25 kV–500A) generator	5 kV/cm	• 33% increase in limonene in EtOH extracts; limited impact overall.
(Barros et al., 2022)	Eucalyptus, rosemary, and thyme leaves	Voltage of 10 kV, frequency of 5 Hz, pulse width of 10 μs, and field strength of 2 kV/cm	Batch treatment chamber	Thyme: PEF for 30 min; 1 kV/cm; 0.4 kJ/kg.	• 30 min PEF: 17% (eucalyptus) and 11% (rosemary) higher yield; 30% higher TPC in eucalyptus; thyme yield ↑40%.
(Ziagova et al., 2022)	*Olea europaea* L. *leaves and unripe fruit, Melissa officinalis* L. *leaves, Cistus incanus* L. *ssp. creticus leaves, Vitis vinifera* L. *cv "Xinomavro" leaves, marc, and fruits, Aronia melanocarpa* L. *fruits, Punica granatum* L. *peel, and Crocus sativus* L. *petals*	Time: 3–6 min; 0.5–2 kW; alternating current	Custom made PEF apparatus	PEF for 5 min, 1:20 plant-to-solvent ratio.	• High TPC in *Melissa officinalis, Punica granatum*; antioxidant activity ~ 90% in aqueous extracts
(Mpakos et al., 2024)	*Cannabis sativa leaves*	0.8 kV/cm electric fieldstrength; 20 min; pulse duration of 55 μs; pulse period of 550 μs	Two custom stainless-steel chambers, a mode/arbitrary waveform generator, a digital oscilloscope, and a high-voltage power generator.	0.9 kV/cm, 10 μs pulse duration, 1000 μs period, 25 min; 50% EtOH/H_2O (20:1L:S).	• A pulse duration of 10 μs, a pulse period of 1000 μs, and an electric field strength of 0.9 kV/cm for 25 min were the optimal conditions • A 50% (v/v) mixture of EtOH/H_2O in a 20:1 liquid-to-solid ratio the most efficient solvent. • The optimal conditions resulted in ~ 75% higher TPC levels • Some individual polyphenols showed an increase of up to ~ 300%
(Bozinou et al., 2019)	*Moringa oleifera* leaves	Max voltage of 25 kV; electric field strength (*E*) of 7 kV/cm; 40 min	Static bench scale system	PD = 20 ms PI = 100 μs 40 min PEF	• PEF for 40 min resulted in the highest extraction of total phenols at a PD of 20 msec and a PI of 100 μs

Carpentieri et al. (2021) reported the comparative effects of PEF and UAE on the degree of cellular disintegration of oregano (*Origanum vulgare* L.) and wild thyme (*T. serpyllum* L.), as well as the extractability of phenolic compounds during the subsequent hydroalcoholic extraction (0%–50% ethanol in water, v/v) conducted for up to 4 h. The rate of phenolic compound extraction exhibited a decline over time and was accurately predicted ($R^2 = 0.898–0.989$) by Peleg's model. The application of either PEF or US treatment prior to SLE allowed for the reduction of both the duration and concentration of ethanol required to attain equivalent recovery yields of phenolic compounds. Under optimized conditions for PEF (3 kV/cm, 10 kJ/kg) and US (400 W, 20 min) treatments, the extracts derived from either PEF or US pretreated herb samples demonstrated enhanced TPC (36% on average) and antioxidant activity (FRAP) (36% on average) compared to SLE, particularly when employing 25% ethanol as the solvent.

Recently, Mpakos et al. (2024) reported that the optimized conditions for PEF extraction of polyphenols from *Cannabis sativa* L. leaves were as follows: a pulse duration of 10 μs, a pulse period of 1000 μs, and an electric field strength of 0.9 kV/cm after 25 min of treatment, while the most efficient solvent was a 50% (*v/v*) mixture of ethanol and water in a 20:1 liquid-to-solid ratio. Under these conditions, TPC increased by 75%, and FRAP and DPPH antioxidant activity values increased by 74% and 71%, respectively, compared to untreated samples and individual polyphenols exhibited an increment of 300% compared to the untreated samples.

PEF was found to be the best extraction method when applied to *M. oleifera* leaves, as compared to MAE, UAE, boiling water extraction, and plain water maceration (control) (Bozinou et al., 2019). The levels of total phenols were the highest upon PEF treatment for 40 min at 20 ms PD and 100 μs PI.

3 Conclusion

Extraction is a critical step in isolating bioactive compounds from natural sources. The efficiency, selectivity, and methodology of extraction significantly influence phytoconstituent purity, yield, residual matrix content, cost-effectiveness, and scalability. Conventional extraction methods often suffer from low specificity, poor reproducibility, and suboptimal yields, driving the need for advanced techniques. Modern extraction techniques—such as US-, MW-, PEF-, and SF-assisted extraction—demonstrate clear advantages over conventional methods across several critical parameters; they consistently show enhanced extraction efficiency through improved cell disruption mechanisms and better compound solubility. They also offer superior selectivity by enabling targeted recovery of specific bioactive classes through tunable operational parameters, reduce processing times compared to conventional methods while maintaining or improving extract quality. Environmentally, they represent a substantial advancement through substantially reduced solvent requirements, lower energy consumption, and minimal generation of hazardous waste. Their scalability has been demonstrated across various plant matrices, with particular success in aromatic herbs and medicinal species.

Recent research has extensively examined MAP species across diverse plant organs, with leaves being the most studied (e.g., *A. vera*, *T. vulgaris*), followed by flowers (e.g., *C. sativus*) and roots (e.g., *Rhodiola rosea*). Notably, the Lamiaceae family, including thyme and rosemary, has been a focal point due to its rich bioactive profile. However, the valorization of by-products remains underexplored, presenting a significant opportunity for future research. Further validation is still needed to optimize the extraction techniques; critical parameters like temperature, pressure, extraction time, enzyme selection, and pH must be carefully controlled to ensure consistent results.

Growing environmental awareness has also spurred interest in green chemistry within natural product research, emphasizing eco-friendly processes (e.g., SFE's recyclable CO_2 and UAE's low-water workflows). Future studies should prioritize by-product utilization and systematic comparisons across plant families and parts to unlock the full potential of MAP-derived bioactives.

Acknowledgments

This research was partially funded by the SARG of the National and Kapodistrian University of Athens (research grant: 14053) and by the Horizon Europe Framework Programme (HORIZON) for research and innovation under the Marie Sklodowska-Curie MSCA Staff Exchanges Grant Agreement 101086323 (Project acronym: NanoCosmos) (Fig. 6.1). Views and opinions expressed, however, are those of the author(s) only and do not necessarily reflect those of the European Union or the Research Executive Agency. Neither the European Union nor the granting authority can be held responsible for them.

Funded by the
European Union

FIG. 6.1 Partially funded by SARG of the National and Kapodistrian University of Athens (research grants: 14053 and European Union). Research was partially funded by SARG of the National and Kapodistrian University of Athens (research grants: 14053) and by the Horizon Europe Framework Programme (HORIZON) for research and innovation under the Marie Sklodowska-Curie MSCA Staff Exchanges Grant agreement 101086323 (Project acronym: NanoCosmos). Views and opinions expressed are however those of the author(s) only and do not necessarily reflect those of the European Union or the Research Executive Agency. Neither the European Union nor the granting authority can be held responsible for them."

References

Aćimović, M., Šeregelj, V., Šovljanski, O., Šaponjac, V.T., Švarc Gajić, J., Brezo-Borjan, T., Pezo, L., 2021. In vitro antioxidant, antihyperglycemic, anti-inflammatory, and antimicrobial activity of *Satureja kitaibelii* Wierzb. ex Heuff. subcritical water extract. Ind. Crops Prod. 09266690. 169, 113672. doi:10.1016/j.indcrop.2021.113672.

Adhar, M., HadjKacem, B., Périno-Issartier, S., Amor, I.B., Feki, A., Gargouri, J., Gargouri, A., Tounsi, S., Chemat, F., Allouche, N., 2022. Thymol-enriched extract from *Thymus vulgaris* L. leaves: green extraction processes and antiaggregant effects on human platelets. Bioorg. Chem. 00452068. 125, 105858. doi:10.1016/j.bioorg.2022.105858.

Ahmadian-Kouchaksaraie, Z., Niazmand, R., 2017. Supercritical carbon dioxide extraction of antioxidants from *Crocus sativus* petals of saffron industry residues: optimization using response surface methodology. J. Supercrit. Fluids. 08968446. 121, 19–31. doi:10.1016/j.supflu.2016.11.008.

Ajdert, P., Jan, L., Burman, R., 2022. Liquid chromatographic method for the quantification of salidroside and cinnamyl alcohol glycosides for quality control of golden root (*Rhodiola rosea* L.). J. Appl. Res. Med. Aromat. Plants 26, 100364. doi:10.1016/j.jarmap.2021.100364.

Alara, O.R., Abdurahman, N.H., Ukaegbu, C.I., 2021. Extraction of phenolic compounds: a review. Curr. Res. Food Sci. 26659271. 4, 200–214. Available from: https://www.journals.elsevier.com/current-research-in-food-science. doi:10.1016/j.crfs.2021.03.011.

Alslaibi, T.M., Abustan, I., Ahmad, M.A., Foul, A.A., 2013. A review: production of activated carbon from agricultural byproducts via conventional and microwave heating. J. Chem. Technol. Biotechnol. 10974660. 88 (7), 1183–1190. doi:10.1002/jctb.4028.

Ameer, K., Shahbaz, H.M., Kwon, J.H., 2017. Green extraction methods for polyphenols from plant matrices and their byproducts: a review. Compr. Rev. Food Sci. Food Saf. 15414337. 16 (2), 295–315. Available from: http://www.interscience.wiley.com/jpages/1541-4337. doi:10.1111/1541-4337.12253.

Athanasiadis, V., Lakka, A., Palaiogiannis, D., Pappas, V.M., Bozinou, E., Ntourtoglou, G., Makris, D.P., Dourtoglou, V.G., Lalas, S.I., 2021. Pulsed electric field and *Salvia officinalis* L. Leaves: a successful combination for the extraction of high value added compounds. Foods 23048158. 10 (9). Available from: https://www.mdpi.com/2304-8158/10/9/2014/pdf. doi:10.3390/foods10092014.

Barba, F.J., Parniakov, O., Pereira, S.A., Wiktor, A., Grimi, N., Boussetta, N., Saraiva, J.A., Raso, J., Martin-Belloso, O., Witrowa-Rajchert, D., Lebovka, N., Vorobiev, E., 2015. Current applications and new opportunities for the use of pulsed electric fields in food science and industry. Food Res. Int. 09639969. 77, 773–798. Available from: https://www.elsevier.com/inca/publications/store/4/2/2/9/7/0. doi:10.1016/j.foodres.2015.09.015.

Bareetseng, S., 2022. The worldwide herbal market: trends and opportunities. J. Biomed. Res. Environ. Sci. 27662276. 3 (5), 575–584. doi:10.37871/jbres1482.

Barros, M., Redondo, L., Rego, D., Serra, C., Miloudi, K., 2022. Extraction of essential oils from plants by hydrodistillation with pulsed electric fields (PEF) pre-treatment. Appl. Sci. 2076-3417. 12 (16), 8107. doi:10.3390/app12168107.

Behaiyn, S., Ebrahimi, S.N., Rahimi, M., Behboudi, H., 2023. Response surface methodology optimization extraction of aloins from *Aloe vera* leaf skin by ultrasonic horn sonicator and cytotoxicity evaluation. Ind. Crops Prod. 09266690. 202, 117043. doi:10.1016/j.indcrop.2023.117043.

Bellumori, M., Innocenti, M., Binello, A., Boffa, L., Mulinacci, N., Cravotto, G., 2016. Selective recovery of rosmarinic and carnosic acids from rosemary leaves under ultrasound- and microwave-assisted extraction procedures. C. R. Chim.. 1878-1543. 19 (6), 699–706. doi:10.1016/j.crci.2015.12.013.

Binello, A., Cravotto, G., Boffa, L., Stevanato, L., Bellumori, M., Innocenti, M., Mulinacci, N., 2017. Efficient and selective green extraction of polyphenols from lemon balm. C. R. Chim. 1878-1543. 20 (9-10), 921–926. doi:10.1016/j.crci.2017.06.003.

Bingham, E., Cohrssen, B., Powell, C.H., 2001. Radio-Frequency and Microwave Radiation Patty's Toxicology. Wiley. doi:10.1002/0471435139.tox101.

Bozinou, E., Karageorgou, I., Batra, G., Dourtoglou, V.G., Lalas, S.I., 2019. Pulsed electric field extraction and antioxidant activity determination of *Moringa oleifera* dry leaves: a comparative study with other extraction techniques. Beverages. 2306-5710. 5 (1), 8. doi:10.3390/beverages5010008.

Brendler, T., Brinckmann, J.A., 2023. Export Guide to Medicinal and Aromatic Plant Ingredients and Products. American Herbal Products Association (AHPA) / United Plant Savers.

Carpentieri, S., Mazza, L., Nutrizio, M., Jambrak, A.R., Ferrari, G., Pataro, G., 2021. Pulsed electric fields- and ultrasound-assisted green extraction of valuable compounds from *Origanum vulgare* L. and *Thymus serpyllum* L.. Int. J. Food Sci. Technol. 13652621. 56 (10), 4834–4842. Available from: http://onlinelibrary.wiley.com/journal/10.1111/(ISSN)1365-2621. doi:10.1111/ijfs.15159.

Carr, A.G., Mammucari, R., Foster, N.R., 2011b. A review of subcritical water as a solvent and its utilisation for the processing of hydrophobic organic compounds. Chem. Eng. J. 13858947. 172 (1), 1–17. doi:10.1016/j.cej.2011.06.007.

Carvalho, R.N., Moura, L.S., Rosa, P.T.V., Meireles, M.A.A., 2005. Supercritical fluid extraction from rosemary (*Rosmarinus officinalis*): kinetic data, extract's global yield, composition, and antioxidant activity. J. Supercrit. Fluids 35 (3), 197–204. doi:10.1016/j.supflu.2005.01.009.

Caser, M., Mélanie Falla, N., Demasi, S., Scariot, V., 2023. From fresh to dried lavender flower: changes in phytochemical profile according to drying method. Horticulturae. 2311-7524. 9 (6), 700. doi:10.3390/horticulturae9060700.

Cerdá-Bernad, D., Baixinho, J.P., Fernández, N., Frutos, M.J., 2022. Evaluation of microwave-assisted extraction as a potential green technology for the isolation of bioactive compounds from saffron (*Crocus sativus* L.) floral by-products. Foods 23048158. 11 (15). Available from: https://www.mdpi.com/journal/foods. doi:10.3390/foods11152335.

Chemat, F., Rombaut, N., Meullemiestre, A., Turk, M., Perino, S., Fabiano-Tixier, A.S., Abert-Vian, M., 2017. Review of green food processing techniques. Preservation, transformation, and extraction. Innov. Food Sci. Emerg. Technol. 14668564. 41, 357–377. Available from: http://www.elsevier.com/locate/ifset. doi:10.1016/j.ifset.2017.04.016.

Chen, S.L., Yu, H., Luo, H.M., Wu, Q., Li, C.F., Steinmetz, A., 2016. Conservation and sustainable use of medicinal plants: problems, progress, and prospects. Chin. Med. (United Kingdom) 17498546. 11 (1). Available from: http://www.cmjournal.org/. doi:10.1186/s13020-016-0108-7.

Choudhary, N., Chatterjee, M., Kumar, S., Singh, G., Suttee, A., 2021. Effect of conventional method and microwave assisted extraction on phytoconstituents of *Chenopodium album*. Mater. Today Proc. 22147853. 45, 5362–5367. doi:10.1016/j.matpr.2021.01.947.

Choudhury, S., Hongliang, H., Larkin, P., Meinke, H., Shabala, S., Ahmed, I., Zhou, M., 2018. Agronomical, biochemical and histological response of resistant and susceptible wheat and barley under BYDV stress. PeerJ. 2167-8359. 6 (5), e4833. doi:10.7717/peerj.4833.

da Silva, R.F., Carneiro, C.N., Cheila, C.B., Gomez, F.J.V., Espino, M., Boiteux, J., Fernández, M.D.L.Á., Silva, M.F., de S. Dias, F., 2022. Sustainable extraction bioactive compounds procedures in medicinal plants based on the principles of green analytical chemistry: a review. Microchem. J. 0026265X. 175. Available from: https://www.elsevier.com/inca/publications/store/6/2/0/3/9/1. doi:10.1016/j.microc.2022.107184.

de Elguea-culebras, G.O., Bravo, E.M., Sánchez-Vioque, R., 2022. Potential sources and methodologies for the recovery of phenolic compounds from distillation residues of Mediterranean aromatic plants. An approach to the valuation of by-products of the essential oil market – a review. Ind. Crops Prod. 09266690. 175. Available from: https://www.elsevier.com/inca/publications/store/5/2/2/8/2/5. doi:10.1016/j.indcrop.2021.114261.

de Oliveira, M.S., da Costa, W.A., Pereira, D.S., Botelho, J.R.S., de Alencar Menezes, T.O., de Aguiar Andrade, E.H., da Silvada Silva, S.H.M., da Silva Sousa Filho, A.P., de Carvalho, R.N., 2016. Chemical composition and phytotoxic activity of clove (*Syzygium aromaticum*) essential oil obtained with supercritical CO_2. J. Supercrit. Fluids. 08968446. 118, 185–193. doi:10.1016/j.supflu.2016.08.010.

Dhanani, T., Sonal Shah, N.A.G., Kumar, S., 2017. Effect of extraction methods on yield, phytochemical constituents and antioxidant activity of *Withania somnifera*. Arab. J. Chem. 18785352. 10, S1193. doi:10.1016/j.arabjc.2013.02.015.

Ekezie, F.G.C., Sun, D.W., Han, Z., Cheng, J.H., 2017. Microwave-assisted food processing technologies for enhancing product quality and process efficiency: a review of recent developments. Trends Food Sci. Technol. 09242244. 67, 58–69. Available from: http://www.elsevier.com/wps/find/journaldescription.cws_home/601278/description#description. doi:10.1016/j.tifs.2017.05.014.

Esmaeelian, M., Jahani, M., Einafshar, S., Feizy, J., 2020. Optimization of experimental parameters in subcritical water extraction of bioactive constituents from the saffron (*Crocus sativus* L.) corm based on response surface methodology. J. Food Meas. Charact. 2193-4126. 14 (4), 1822–1832. doi:10.1007/s11694-020-00429-w.

Espino, M., Fernández, M.D.L.Á., Gomez, F.J.V., Boiteux, J., Silva, M.F., 2018. Green analytical chemistry metrics: towards a sustainable phenolics extraction from medicinal plants. Microchem. J. 0026265X. 141, 438–443. Available from: https://www.elsevier.com/inca/publications/store/6/2/0/3/9/1. doi:10.1016/j.microc.2018.06.007.

Fu, Q., Dong, W., Ge, D., Ke, Y., Jin, Y., 2023. Supercritical fluid-based method for selective extraction and analysis of indole alkaloids from *Uncaria rhynchophylla*. J. Chromatogr. A 1710, 464410. doi:10.1016/j.chroma.2023.464410.

Ganorkar, P.V., Jadeja, G.C., Desai, M.A., 2022. Extraction of shikimic acid from water hyacinth (*Eichhornia crassipes*) using sonication: an approach towards waste valorization. J. Environ. Manag. 10958630. 305. Available from: https://www.sciencedirect.com/journal/journal-of-environmental-management. doi:10.1016/j.jenvman.2021.114419.

Garavand, F., Rahaee, S., Vahedikia, N., Jafari, S.M., 2019. Different techniques for extraction and micro/nanoencapsulation of saffron bioactive ingredients. Trends Food Sci. Technol. 09242244. 89, 26–44. Available from: http://www.elsevier.com/wps/find/journaldescription.cws_home/601278/description#description. doi:10.1016/j.tifs.2019.05.005.

Gavrila, A.I., Chisega-Negrila, C.G., Maholea, L., Gavrila, M.L., Parvulescu, O.C., Popa, I., 2023. Enhancing the extraction process efficiency of thyme essential oil by combined ultrasound and microwave techniques. Agronomy 20734395. 13 (9). Available from: https://www.mdpi.com/journal/agronomy/. doi:10.3390/agronomy13092331.

Geissdoerfer, M., Savaget, P., Bocken, N.M.P., Hultink, E.J., 2017. The circular economy – a new sustainability paradigm? J. Clean. Prod. 09596526. 143, 757–768. doi:10.1016/j.jclepro.2016.12.048.

Genovese, J., Rocculi, P., Miklavčič, D., Mahnič-Kalamiza, S., 2024. The forgotten method? Pulsed electric field thresholds from the perspective of texture analysis. Food Res. Int. 09639969. 176, 113869. doi:10.1016/j.foodres.2023.113869.

Ghoshal, G., 2023. Comprehensive review on pulsed electric field in food preservation: gaps in current studies for potential future research. Heliyon. 24058440. 9 (6), e17532. doi:10.1016/j.heliyon.2023.e17532.

Gilbert-López, B., Plaza, M., Mendiola, J.A., Ibáñez, E., Herrero, M., 2017. Subcritical Water Extraction and Neoformation of Antioxidants Water Extraction of Bioactive Compounds: From Plants to Drug Development. Elsevier, Spain, pp. 109–130. Available from: https://www.sciencedirect.com/book/9780128093801. doi:10.1016/B978-0-12-809380-1.00004-8.

Girbu, V., Organ, A., Grinco, M., Cotelea, T., Ungur, N., Barba, A., Kulcitki, V., 2023. Identification, quantitative determination and isolation of pomolic acid from lavender (*Lavandula angustifolia* Mill.) wastes. Sustain. Chem. Pharm. 23525541. 33, 101140. doi:10.1016/j.scp.2023.101140.

Glisic, S.B., Ristic, M., Skala, D.U., 2011. The combined extraction of sage (*Salvia officinalis* L.): ultrasound followed by supercritical CO_2 extraction. Ultrason. Sonochem. 13504177. 18 (1), 318–326. Available from: https://www.elsevier.com/inca/publications/store/5/2/5/4/5/1. doi:10.1016/j.ultsonch.2010.06.011.

Goleroudbary, M.G., Ghoreishi, S.M., 2016. Response surface optimization of Safranal and Crocin extraction from *Crocus sativus* L. via supercritical fluid technology. J. Supercrit. Fluids. 08968446. 108, 136–144. doi:10.1016/j.supflu.2015.10.024.

Gonzalez-Rivera, J., Campanella, B., Pulidori, E., Bramanti, E., Tiné, M.R., Bernazzani, L., Onor, M., Bàrberi, P., Duce, C., Ferrari, C., 2023. From volatiles to solid wastes: towards the full valorization of lavender and rosemary by simultaneous in situ microwaves and ultrasounds irradiation extraction. Ind. Crops Prod. 09266690. 194, 116362. doi:10.1016/j.indcrop.2023.116362.

Guzik, P., Kulawik, P., Zając, M., Migdał, W., 2022. Microwave applications in the food industry: an overview of recent developments. Crit. Rev. Food Sci. Nutr. 15497852. 62 (29), 7989–8008. Available from: https://www.tandfonline.com/loi/bfsn20. doi:10.1080/10408398.2021.1922871.

Halim, N.A.A., Abidin, Z.Z., Siajam, S.I., Hean, C.G., Harun, M.R., 2021. Optimization studies and compositional analysis of subcritical water extraction of essential oil from *Citrus hystrix* DC. leaves. J. Supercrit. Fluids 08968446. 178. Available from: https://www.journals.elsevier.com/the-journal-of-supercritical-fluids. doi:10.1016/j.supflu.2021.105384.

Hassas-Roudsari, M., Chang, P.R., Pegg, R.B., Tyler, R.T., 2009. Antioxidant capacity of bioactives extracted from canola meal by subcritical water, ethanolic and hot water extraction. Food Chem. 03088146. 114 (2), 717–726. doi:10.1016/j.foodchem.2008.09.097.

Jafari, R., Zandi, M., Ganjloo, A., 2022. Effect of ultrasound and microwave pretreatments on extraction of anise (*Pimpinella anisum* L.) seed essential oil by ohmic-assisted hydrodistillation. J. Appl. Res. Med. Aromat. Plants 31, 100418. doi:10.1016/j.jarmap.2022.100418.

Kakouri, E., Daferera, D., Paramithiotis, S., Astraka, K., Drosinos, E.H., Polissiou, M.G., 2017. Crocus sativus L. tepals: the natural source of antioxidant and antimicrobial factors. J. Appl. Res. Med. Aromat. Plants 22147861. 4, 66–74. Available from: http://www.journals.elsevier.com/journal-of-applied-research-on-medicinal-and-aromatic-plants/. doi:10.1016/j.jarmap.2016.09.002.

Kant, R., Kumar, A., 2022. Review on essential oil extraction from aromatic and medicinal plants: techniques, performance and economic analysis. Sustain. Chem. Pharm. 23525541. 30, 100829. doi:10.1016/j.scp.2022.100829.

Khan, M.K., Hassan, S., Imran, M., Ahmad, M.H., 2022. Extraction of Bioactive Compounds from Clove (*Syzygium aromaticum*) Clove (*Syzygium aromaticum*): Chemistry, Functionality and Applications. Elsevier, Pakistan, pp. 405–417. Available from: https://www.sciencedirect.com/book/9780323851770. doi:10.1016/B978-0-323-85177-0.00010-0.

Kong, W., Huang, C., Shi, J., Li, Y., Jiang, X., Duan, Q., Huang, Y., Duan, Y., Zhu, X., 2019. Recycling of Chinese herb residues by endophytic and probiotic fungus *Aspergillus cristatus* CB10002 for the production of medicinal valuable anthraquinones. Microb. Cell Fact. 1475-2859. 18 (1). doi:10.1186/s12934-019-1150-9.

Lampakis, D., Skenderidis, P., Leontopoulos, S., 2021. Technologies and extraction methods of polyphenolic compounds derived from pomegranate (*Punica granatum*) peels. a mini review. Processes. 2227-9717. 9 (2), 236. doi:10.3390/pr9020236.

Lee, C.S., Binner, E., Winkworth-Smith, C., John, R., Gomes, R., Robinson, J., 2016. Enhancing natural product extraction and mass transfer using selective microwave heating. Chem. Eng. Sci. 00092509. 149, 97–103. Available from: http://www.journals.elsevier.com/chemical-engineering-science/. doi:10.1016/j.ces.2016.04.031.

Machmudah, S., Fitriana, M.W., Fatbamayani, N., Wahyudiono, H.K., Winardi, S., Goto, M., 2022. Phytochemical compounds extraction from medicinal plants by subcritical water and its encapsulation via electrospraying. Alex. Eng. J. 11100168. 61 (3), 2116–2128. doi:10.1016/j.aej.2021.07.033.

Majid, H., Silva, F.V.M., 2020. Improvement of butyrylcholinesterase enzyme inhibition and medicinal properties of extracts of *Aristotelia serrata* leaves by ultrasound extraction. Food Bioprod. Process. 09603085. 124, 445–454. Available from: http://www.elsevier.com/wps/find/journaldescription.cws_home/713883/description#description. doi:10.1016/j.fbp.2020.10.004.

Manjare, S.D., Dhingra, K., 2019. Supercritical fluids in separation and purification: a review. Mater. Sci. Energy Technol. 25892991. 2 (3), 463–484. Available from: https://www.keaipublishing.com/en/journals/materials-science-for-energy-technologies/. doi:10.1016/j.mset.2019.04.005.

Marcelino, S., Gaspar, P.D., Paço, A., 2023. Sustainable waste management in the production of medicinal and aromatic plants—a systematic review. Sustainability (Switzerland) 20711050. 15 (18). Available from: http://www.mdpi.com/journal/sustainability/. doi:10.3390/su151813333.

Milovanovic, S., Grzegorczyk, A., Świątek, Ł., Dębczak, A., Tyskiewicz, K., Konkol, M., 2022. Dandelion seeds as a new and valuable source of bioactive extracts obtained using the supercritical fluid extraction technique. Sustain. Chem. Pharm. 23525541. 29, 100796. doi:10.1016/j.scp.2022.100796.

Morsy, N.F.S., 2020. Production of thymol rich extracts from ajwain (*Carum copticum* L.) and thyme (*Thymus vulgaris* L.) using supercritical CO2. Ind. Crops Prod. 09266690. 145. Available from: https://www.elsevier.com/inca/publications/store/5/2/2/8/2/5. doi:10.1016/j.indcrop.2019.112072.

Moura, B., Monteiro, H., Mata, T.M., Martins, A.A., 2022. Life cycle energy and carbon emissions of essential oil extraction from Rosemary. Energy Rep. 23524847. 8, 291–297. Available from: http://www.journals.elsevier.com/energy-reports/. doi:10.1016/j.egyr.2022.01.063.

Mpakos, D., Chatzimitakos, T., Athanasiadis, V., Mantiniotou, M., Bozinou, E., Lalas, S.I., 2024. Optimization of pulsed electric field-based extraction of bioactive compounds from *Cannabis sativa* leaves. Analytica 26734532. 5 (1), 90–106. Available from: https://www.mdpi.com/journal/analytica. doi:10.3390/analytica5010006.

Mrkonjić, Ž., Kaplan, M., Milošević, S., Božović, D., Sknepnek, A., Miletić, D., Lazarević Mrkonjić, I., Rakić, D., Zeković, Z., Pavlić, B., 2024. Green extraction approach for isolation of bioactive compounds in wild thyme (*Thymus serpyllum* L.) herbal dust—chemical profile, antioxidant and antimicrobial activity and comparison with conventional techniques. Plants. 2223-7747. 13 (6), 897. doi:10.3390/plants13060897.

Mrkonjić, Ž., Rakić, D., Olgun, E.O., Canli, O., Kaplan, M., Teslić, N., Zeković, Z., Pavlić, B., 2021. Optimization of antioxidants recovery from wild thyme (*Thymus serpyllum* L.) by ultrasound-assisted extraction: multi-response approach. J. Appl. Res. Med. Aromat. Plants. 22147861. 24, 100333. doi:10.1016/j.jarmap.2021.100333.

Munekata, P.E.S., Alcántara, C., Žugčić, T., Abdelkebir, R., Collado, M.C., García-Pérez, J.V., Jambrak, A.R., Gavahian, M., Barba, F.J., Lorenzo, J.M., 2020. Impact of ultrasound-assisted extraction and solvent composition on bioactive compounds and in vitro biological activities of thyme and rosemary. Food Res. Int. 18737145. 134. Available from: https://www.elsevier.com/inca/publications/store/4/2/2/9/7/0. doi:10.1016/j.foodres.2020.109242.

Mustapa, A.N., Martin, Á., Mato, R.B., Cocero, M.J., 2015. Extraction of phytocompounds from the medicinal plant *Clinacanthus nutans* Lindau by microwave-assisted extraction and supercritical carbon dioxide extraction. Ind. Crops Prod. 09266690. 74, 83–94. Available from: https://www.elsevier.com/inca/publications/store/5/2/2/8/2/5. doi:10.1016/j.indcrop.2015.04.035.

Najafi, Z., Zahran, H.A., Yeşilçubuk, N.Ş., Gürbüz, H., 2022. Effect of different extraction methods on saffron antioxidant activity, total phenolic and crocin contents and the protective effect of saffron extract on the oxidative stability of common vegetable oils. Grasas Y Aceites 19884214. 73 (4). Available from: https://grasasyaceites.revistas.csic.es/index.php/grasasyaceites/article/view/1960. doi:10.3989/GYA.0783211.

Nastić, N., Švarc-Gajić, J., Delerue-Matos, C., Barroso, M.F., Soares, C., Moreira, M.M., Morais, S., Mašković, P., Srček, V.G., Slivac, I., Radošević, K., Radojković, M., 2018. Subcritical water extraction as an environmentally-friendly technique to recover bioactive compounds from traditional Serbian medicinal plants. Ind. Crops Prod. 09266690. 111, 579–589. Available from: https://www.elsevier.com/inca/publications/store/5/2/2/8/2/5. doi:10.1016/j.indcrop.2017.11.015.

Nejad-Sadeghi, M., Taji, S., Goodarznia, I., 2015. Optimization of supercritical carbon dioxide extraction of essential oil from *Dracocephalum kotschyi* Boiss: an endangered medicinal plant in Iran. J. Chromatogr. A. 00219673. 1422, 73–81. doi:10.1016/j.chroma.2015.10.040.

Nerome, H., Ito, M., Machmudah, S., Wahyudiono, H.K., Goto, M., 2016. Extraction of phytochemicals from saffron by supercritical carbon dioxide with water and methanol as entrainer. J. Supercrit. Fluids. 08968446. 107, 377–383. doi:10.1016/j.supflu.2015.10.007.

Nour, A.H., Oluwaseun, A.R., Nour, A.H., Omer, M.S., Ahmed, N., 2021. Microwave-Assisted Extraction of Bioactive Compounds (Review). IntechOpen. doi:10.5772/intechopen.96092.

Paniwnyk, L., 2017. Applications of ultrasound in processing of liquid foods: a review. Ultrason. Sonochem. 13504177. 38, 794–806. doi:10.1016/j.ultsonch.2016.12.025.

Paniwnyk, L., Cai, H., Albu, S., Mason, T.J., Cole, R., 2009. The enhancement and scale up of the extraction of anti-oxidants from *Rosmarinus officinalis* using ultrasound. Ultrason. Sonochem. 13504177. 16 (2), 287–292. doi:10.1016/j.ultsonch.2008.06.007.

Phan, L.T.M., Nguyen, K.T.P., Vuong, H.T., Tran, D.D., Nguyen, T.X.P., Hoang, M.N., Mai, T.P., Nguyen, H.H., 2020. Supercritical fluid extraction of polyphenols from Vietnamese *Callisia fragrans* leaves and antioxidant activity of the extract. J. Chem. 20909071. 2020. Available from: http://www.hindawi.com/journals/chem/contents/. doi:10.1155/2020/9548401.

Plaza, M., Turner, C., 2015. Pressurized hot water extraction of bioactives. TrAC Trends Anal. Chem. 01659936. 71, 39–54. doi:10.1016/j.trac.2015.02.022.

Pourzaki, A., Mirzaee, H., Hemmati Kakhki, A., 2013. Using pulsed electric field for improvement of components extraction of saffron (*Crocus sativus*) stigma and its pomace. J. Food Process. Preserv. 01458892. 37 (5), 1008–1013. doi:10.1111/j.1745-4549.2012.00749.x.

Rahimi, E., Prado, J.M., Zahedi, G., Meireles, M.A.A., 2011. Chamomile extraction with supercritical carbon dioxide: mathematical modeling and optimization. J. Supercrit. Fluids. 08968446. 56 (1), 80–88. doi:10.1016/j.supflu.2010.11.008.

Ranjha, M.M.A.N., Kanwal, R., Shafique, B., Arshad, R.N., Irfan, S., Kieliszek, M., Kowalczewski, P.Ł., Irfan, M., Khalid, M.Z., Roobab, U., Aadil, R.M., 2021. A critical review on pulsed electric field: a novel technology for the extraction of phytoconstituents. Molecules 14203049. 26 (16). Available from: https://www.mdpi.com/1420-3049/26/16/4893/pdf. doi:10.3390/molecules26164893.

Ray, A., Dubey, K.K., Marathe, S.J., Singhal, R., 2023. Supercritical fluid extraction of bioactives from fruit waste and its therapeutic potential. Food Biosci. 22124306. 52. Available from: http://www.journals.elsevier.com/food-bioscience/. doi:10.1016/j.fbio.2023.102418.

Saeed, R., Ahmed, D., Mushtaq, M., 2022. Ultrasound-aided enzyme-assisted efficient extraction of bioactive compounds from *Gymnema sylvestre* and optimization as per response surface methodology. Sustain. Chem. Pharm. 23525541. 29, 100818. doi:10.1016/j.scp.2022.100818.

Santos-Martín, M., Cubero-Cardoso, J., González-Domínguez, R., Cortés-Triviño, E., Sayago, A., Urbano, J., Fernández-Recamales, Á., 2023. Ultrasound-assisted extraction of phenolic compounds from blueberry leaves using natural deep eutectic solvents (NADES) for the valorization of agrifood wastes. Biomass Bioenergy. 09619534. 175, 106882. doi:10.1016/j.biombioe.2023.106882.

Sarfarazi, M., Jafari, S.M., Rajabzadeh, G., Feizi, J., 2019. Development of an environmentally-friendly solvent-free extraction of saffron bioactives using subcritical water. LWT. 00236438. 114, 108428. doi:10.1016/j.lwt.2019.108428.

Sarfarazi, M., Jafari, S.M., Rajabzadeh, G., Galanakis, C.M., 2020. Evaluation of microwave-assisted extraction technology for separation of bioactive components of saffron (*Crocus sativus* L.). Ind. Crops Prod. 09266690. 145. Available from: https://www.elsevier.com/inca/publications/store/5/2/2/8/2/5. doi:10.1016/j.indcrop.2019.111978.

Sarfarazi, M., Rajabzadeh, Q., Tavakoli, R., Ibrahim, S.A., Jafari, S.M., 2022. Ultrasound-assisted extraction of saffron bioactive compounds; separation of crocins, picrocrocin, and safranal optimized by artificial bee colony. Ultrason. Sonochem. 18732828. 86. Available from: https://www.elsevier.com/inca/publications/store/5/2/5/4/5/1. doi:10.1016/j.ultsonch.2022.105971.

Šeremet, D., Jokić, S., Aladić, K., Vojvodić Cebin, A., Božac, N., Mandura, A., Komes, D., 2021. Optimization of heat-, microwave-assisted and subcritical water extraction of phenolic compounds from ground ivy (*Glechoma hederacea* L.) using response surface methodology. J. Appl. Res. Med. Aromat. Plants. 22147861. 25, 100346. doi:10.1016/j.jarmap.2021.100346.

Simándi, B., Oszagyán, M., Lemberkovics, É., Kéry, Á., Kaszács, J., Thyrion, F., Mátyás, T., 1998. Supercritical carbon dioxide extraction and fractionation of oregano oleoresin. Food Res. Int. 09639969. 31 (10), 723–728. doi:10.1016/s0963-9969(99)00051-4.

Socaci, S.A., Fărcaş, A.C., Tofană, M., 2020. Functional ingredients derived from aromatic plants. In: Florou-Paneri, P., Christaki, E., Giannenas, I. (Eds.), Feed Additives. Elsevier, pp. 133–146. doi:10.1016/B978-0-12-814700-9.00008-X.

Song, E.J., Ko, M.J., 2022. Extraction of monoterpenes from coriander (*Coriandrum sativum* L.) seeds using subcritical water extraction (SWE) technique. J. Supercrit. Fluids 08968446. 188. Available from: https://www.journals.elsevier.com/the-journal-of-supercritical-fluids. doi:10.1016/j.supflu.2022.105668.

Sun, J., Wang, W., Yue, Q., 2016. Review on microwave-matter interaction fundamentals and efficient microwave-associated heating strategies. Materials 1996-1944. 9 (4), 231. doi:10.3390/ma9040231.

Taghouti, I., Cristobal, R., Brenko, A., Stara, K., Markos, N., Chapelet, B., Hamrouni, L., Buršić, D., Bonet, J.-A., 2022. The market evolution of medicinal and aromatic plants: a global supply chain analysis and an application of the Delphi method in the Mediterranean area. Forests. 1999-4907. 13 (5), 808. doi:10.3390/f13050808.

Tekin, K., Akalın, M.K., Şeker, M.G., 2015. Ultrasound bath-assisted extraction of essential oils from clove using central composite design. Ind. Crops Prod. 77, 954–960. doi:10.1016/j.indcrop.2015.09.071.

Teo, C.C., Tan, S.N., Yong, J.W.H., Hew, C.S., Ong, E.S., 2010. Pressurized hot water extraction (PHWE). J. Chromatogr. A. 00219673. 1217 (16), 2484–2494. doi:10.1016/j.chroma.2009.12.050.

Tsikrika, K., Chu, B.S., Bremner, D.H., Lemos, A., 2022. Effect of ultrasonic treatment on enzyme activity and bioactives of strawberry puree. Int. J. Food Sci. Technol. 13652621. 57 (3), 1739–1747. Available from: http://onlinelibrary.wiley.com/journal/10.1111/(ISSN)1365-2621. doi:10.1111/ijfs.15550.

Venkatesh, M.S., Raghavan, G.S.V., 2004. An overview of microwave processing and dielectric properties of agri-food materials. Biosyst. Eng. 15375110. 88 (1), 1–18. doi:10.1016/j.biosystemseng.2004.01.007.

Vollmer, M., 2004. Physics of the microwave oven. Phys. Educ. 0031-9120. 39 (1), 74–81. doi:10.1088/0031-9120/39/1/006.

Weggler, B.A., Gruber, B., Teehan, P., Jaramillo, R., Dorman, F.L., 2020. Inlets and sampling. Sep. Sci. Technol. 12, 141–203. Available from: http://www.elsevier.com/wps/find/bookdescription.cws_home/BS_S760/description#description. doi:10.1016/B978-0-12-813745-1.00005-2.

Wei, L.S., Goh, K.W., Hamid, N.K.A., Kari, Z.A., Wee, W., Van Doan, H., 2022. A mini-review on co-supplementation of probiotics and medicinal herbs: application in aquaculture. Front. Vet. Sci. 22971769. 9. Available from: https://journal.frontiersin.org/journal/veterinary-science. doi:10.3389/fvets.2022.869564.

World Health Organisation, 2023. 75 Years of Improving Public Health. World Health Organisation.

Yoshikawa, N., 2020. Mechanism of Microwave Heating of Matter RF Power Semiconductor Generator Application in Heating and Energy Utilization. Springer Singapore, Japan, pp. 71–89. Available from: http://dx.doi.org/10.1007/978-981-15-3548-2. doi:10.1007/978-981-15-3548-2_3.

Ziagova, M.G., Mavromatidou, C., Samiotis, G., Amanatidou, E., 2022. Total phenolic content and antioxidant capacity of Greek medicinal and aromatic plant extracts using pulsed electric field followed by ultrasounds extraction process. J. Food Process. Preserv. 17454549. 46 (7). Available from: http://onlinelibrary.wiley.com/journal/10.1111/(ISSN)1745-4549. doi:10.1111/jfpp.16639.

Zu, G., Zhang, R., Yang, L., Chunhui, M., Yuangang, Z., Wang, W., Zhao, C., 2012. Ultrasound-assisted extraction of carnosic acid and rosmarinic acid using ionic liquid solution from *Rosmarinus officinalis*. Int. J. Mol. Sci. 1422-0067. 13 (9), 11027–11043. doi:10.3390/ijms130911027.

Chapter 7

Herbal tea, cocoa, and coffee

Theodora Adamantidi, Athena Venieri, Maria Kioiloglou, Antigoni Bourgani, Konstantina Kyprou, Anastasia Pilakouri, and Alexandros Tsoupras
Hephaestus Laboratory, School of Chemistry, Faculty of Sciences, Democritus University of Thrace, Kavala University Campus, Kavala, Greece

1 Introduction

Natural products have long been recognized as important aspects of human health and wellness, where plant-derived extracts have played pivotal roles in both traditional medicine and modern therapeutic applications (Wang et al., 2024; Liu et al., 2023; Anoraga et al., 2024; Freitas et al., 2024). Over the past decades, a marked shift toward the utilization of many natural bioactive agents in the cosmetic and cosmeceutical industries has been observed. This shift is driven by current consumer demand for safer, sustainable, and multifunctional ingredients with less side effects and more effective outcomes. Among these, plant-based beverages like herbal teas, cocoa, and coffee have attracted considerable scientific and industrial interest due to their remarkable phytochemical composition and well-documented biological activity (Wang et al., 2024; Liu et al., 2023; Anoraga et al., 2024; Freitas et al., 2024).

Historically, the utilization of plant extracts and infusions for cosmetic applications dates back thousands of years, mainly in ancient civilizations across Asia, South America, and the Mediterranean region. Infusions from leaves, flowers, or other aerial plant parts were traditionally consumed not only for their sensory properties, but also for their antioxidant, antiinflammatory, and antimicrobial therapeutic effects (Wang et al., 2024; Liu et al., 2023; Anoraga et al., 2024; Freitas et al., 2024). Tea plants have been classified, based on their chlorophyll and anthocyanin content, into albino, yellow, and "Zijuan," whereas, through different processing techniques, six types of tea were identified and examined, namely, black, green, oolong, white, dark, and yellow tea, all of which presented diverse flavor and aroma profiles (Wang et al., 2022; Zhao et al., 2022).

Commercial teas prepared from *Camellia sinensis*, such as common green and black tea, have been extensively consumed in East Asia for centuries and are among the most widely studied plant beverages worldwide (Wang et al., 2022). Their bioactivity is primarily attributed to their polyphenolic compounds, such as catechins [e.g., epigallocatechin gallate (EGCG)], flavonoids, or—in the case of black tea—oxidation-derived compounds, including theaflavins and thearubigins, which reportedly contribute to strong antioxidant and photoprotective effects relevant to skin health (Wang et al., 2022; Zhao et al., 2022). In parallel, herbal infusions obtained from non-*C. sinensis* plants, including *Sideritis scardica* (Greek mountain tea), have been long utilized in Mediterranean regions for their medicinal effects. Their bioactive profile is well characterized by their phenolic acids (e.g., caffeic and ferulic acid derivatives), flavonoids (e.g., apigenin and luteolin), phenylethanoid glycosides, and terpenoids, which contribute to antioxidant, antiinflammatory, and neuroprotective benefits (Żyżelewicz et al., 2020). Similarly, chamomile (*Matricaria chamomilla*) has been widely exploited in traditional medicinal and cosmetic approaches for its soothing and dermatological benefits. Its bioactive composition, predominantly comprising apigenin, α-bisabolol, and chamazulene compounds, is widely known for its antiirritant, antiinflammatory, and wound healing effects and is utilized for sensitive and damaged skin applications (El Mihyaoui et al., 2022).

Beyond herbal teas, cocoa and coffee represent two globally consumed plant-derived products with notable bioactivity and, therefore, promising cosmetic benefits. Cocoa, isolated from the seeds of *Theobroma cacao*, has a long history of use dating back to Mesoamerican civilizations, with its major producers being Brazil, Cameroon, Ivory Coast, Ecuador, Ghana, Indonesia, and Nigeria. It exhibits a rich phytochemical profile dominated by flavanols such as epicatechin and catechin, along with procyanidins (PCs) and methylxanthines (e.g., theobromine), which are associated with potent antioxidant

Biofunctional Cosmetics for Health. https://doi.org/10.1016/B978-0-443-27500-5.00009-5

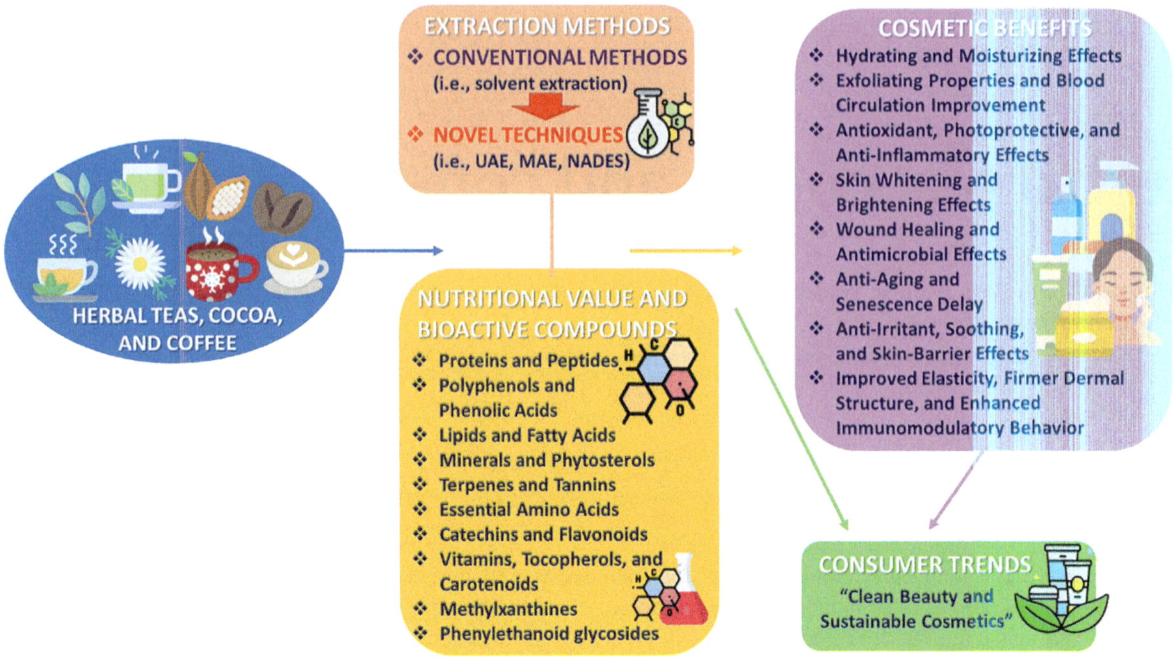

FIG. 7.1 Herbal tea, cocoa, and coffee bioactives: extraction methods, pharmacological properties, and cosmetic applications following clean beauty consumer trends. *(Parts of this figure were obtained from the open access free platform of https://www.flaticon.com/ (accessed on February 13, 2026).)*

capacity, improved immunomodulatory activity, and microcirculation, as well as remarkable skin-protective effects (Wang et al., 2024; Anoraga et al., 2024; Tušek et al., 2024). On the contrary, coffee, obtained from roasted seeds of the *Rubiaceae* family *Coffea* genus species and cultivated especially in Brazil, is one of the most consumed beverages globally and contains a complex mixture of bioactives like chlorogenic acids (CGAs), caffeine, trigonelline, diterpenes (e.g., cafestol, kahweol), and melanoidins formed during roasting. These constituents exert vast antioxidant, antiinflammatory, and photoprotective effects, supporting their incorporation into cosmetics and cosmeceuticals targeting skin aging (Wang et al., 2024; Freitas et al., 2024; Amiri et al., 2024; Makiso et al., 2024).

Recently, the incorporation of extracts derived from herbal teas, cocoa, and coffee into cosmetic formulations has gained increasing attention. Their free radical scavenging activity, modulation of inflammation-related pathways, hydrating action, and sustained protection against ultraviolet (UV) radiation-induced damage, alongside scientific advances in their extraction technologies, controlled release methods (e.g., nanoformulations), and bioactive stability preservation, further enhance their applicability in topical formulations targeting skin health (Wang et al., 2024; Amiri et al., 2024; Gălbău et al., 2024; Oussou et al., 2023).

The aim of this study is to present a comprehensive discussion on the most consumed herbal teas, cocoa, and coffee. Particular emphasis is given to their nutritional composition and bioactive profiles, followed by an examination of the most utilized extraction technologies. The mechanisms through which these constituents contribute to skin health and biofunctional cosmetic performance are further examined, alongside current commercial cosmetic and cosmeceutical applications based on nut-derived agents. Finally, safety concerns, limitations, challenges, and future perspectives are also outlined within the framework of sustainability and the circular economy. The key highlights of this comprehensive review are visually summarized in the graphical abstract (Fig. 7.1).

2 Nutritional composition and bioactive profile of herbal tea, cocoa, and coffee

Plant-derived infusions, including herbal teas, cocoa, and coffee, are well-recognized for their complex biochemical composition and significant biological activity. These plant matrices contain a diverse array of macronutrients, micronutrients, and bioactive phytochemicals that contribute to their nutritional value and functional properties. Although their exact composition varies depending on botanical origin, geographical conditions, processing methods, and extraction techniques, they share a common biological profile (e.g., phenolic acids, alkaloids, and other secondary metabolites) with strong antioxidant, antiinflammatory, moisturizing, and skin-protective effects (El-Saadony et al., 2025; Michalak, 2022; Chandrasekara and Shahidi, 2018).

From a botanical perspective, herbal teas can be classified into two main categories: those derived from *C. sinensis*, including green and black tea, and those obtained from other plant species (herbal infusions), such as chamomile (*M. chamomilla*) and Greek mountain tea derived from *S. scardica*. Cocoa is isolated from the seeds of *T. cacao*, while coffee originates from roasted seeds of *Coffea* species. Despite differences in origin and processing, all these plant materials enclose a wide array of bioactives relevant to cosmetic applications (Wang et al., 2024; Liu et al., 2023; Oussou et al., 2023; El-Saadony et al., 2025; Michalak, 2022; Chandrasekara and Shahidi, 2018).

In general, herbal teas are typically low in macronutrients due to their aqueous preparation but are rich in soluble phytochemicals, whereas cocoa exhibits a high lipid content relevant to its cocoa butter content, and coffee contains minimal macronutrients but is a significant source of bioactives (Wang et al., 2024; Liu et al., 2023; Oussou et al., 2023; El-Saadony et al., 2025; Michalak, 2022; Chandrasekara and Shahidi, 2018). Table 7.1 provides a thorough overview of the various extraction techniques utilized for chamomile, highlighting the key bioactive compounds targeted in each method.

Beyond their basic nutritional composition, herbal tea, cocoa, and coffee plant matrix-derived products are particularly valued for their rich phytochemical profiles. Tea infusions isolated from *C. sinensis* are characterized by high levels of catechins (e.g., EGCG), flavonoids, terpenes, terpenoids, and, in the case of black tea, oxidation products, including theaflavins and thearubigins (Wang et al., 2022; Zhao et al., 2022; Uba et al., 2022; Wang et al., 2011; da Silva Aragão et al., 2025). Greek mountain tea (*S. scardica*) also exhibits an abundant phytochemical profile, mainly comprising phenylethanoid glycosides, flavonoids (e.g., apigenin, luteolin), and several phenolic acids (Żyżelewicz et al., 2020; Pavlova et al., 2021; Tsibranska et al., 2011), while chamomile (*M. chamomilla*) contains a plethora of flavonoids like apigenin as well, alongside terpenoids (e.g., α-bisabolol, chamazulene) (El Mihyaoui et al., 2022; Sarma et al., 2023).

TABLE 7.1 Proximate nutritional composition of herbal teas, cocoa, and coffee.

Nutrient	Herbal tea[a]			Cocoa[a] (*Theobroma cacao*)	Coffee[a] (*Coffea* species)
	Camellia sinensis (green and black tea leaves)	Greek mountain tea (*Sideritis scardica*)	Chamomile (*Matricaria chamomilla*)		
Moisture	11.302 ± 0.467	–	14.89	~3.0–15.0	~1–10
Protein	11.725 ± 0.247	5–12.0 ± 0.5	19.06	3.26–28.0	~8–11
Total lipid/fat	4.946 ± 0.177	1.9 ± 0.2 (<3)	10.89	11.0–23.0	~0.5–3.0
Monounsaturated fatty acids (MUFAs)	~53.6–58.4	13.86 ± 21.17 (max value: 38.31% oleic acid)	~12.9 (oleic acid)	~ > 32 (mainly oleic acid)	~8–12 (mainly oleic acid, 8.22%)
Polyunsaturated fatty acids (PUFAs)	~22.3–24.2	7.49 ± 11.14 (min: 20.36% linoleic acid and 1.18% γ-linolenic acid)	~65.5 (linoleic and α-linoleic acid)	~ < 3 (mainly linoleic acid)	~35–45 (mainly linoleic acid, 43.39%)
Saturated fatty acids (SFAs)	~18.6–21.5	5.97 ± 7.07 (min: 1.25% capric acid and max: 19.71% palmitic acid)	~11.3–30.2 (palmitic and stearic acid)	~60 (mainly palmitic and stearic acids)	~40–50 (mainly palmitic acid, 36.57%, and stearic acid, 7.37%)
Carbohydrates	64.893 ± 0.516	50.6–65	33.16	9.0–28.0	~58.0–85.0
Fiber	1.729 ± 0.141	–	13.89	16.89–60.60	High content (mainly cellulose 24.5% and hemicellulose 29.7%)
Ash	5.406 ± 0.035	5.5 ± 0.1–9	8.26	3.70–11.42	~3.0–5.0
References	(Uba et al., 2022; Wang et al., 2011)	(Pavlova et al., 2021; Ognyanov et al., 2021; Shabani et al., 2022)	(Joseph et al., 2024; Bora et al., 2025)	(Razola-Díaz et al., 2023; Soares and Oliveira, 2022; Torres-Moreno et al., 2015)	(Bobková et al., 2022; Liu et al., 2022)

**Percentage out of the total fatty acids (FAs).
[a]*Proximate percentage concentration (%).*

Cocoa from *T. cacao* is especially rich in flavanols (e.g., epicatechin, catechin), PCs, methylxanthines (e.g., theobromine), and several lipid constituents, which contribute to its emollient properties (Anoraga et al., 2024; Razola-Díaz et al., 2023; Soares and Oliveira, 2022; Torres-Moreno et al., 2015). In contrast, coffee (*Coffea* species) contains CGA, caffeine, diterpenes (e.g., cafestol and kahweol), and melanoidins, which are strongly associated with antiinflammatory, antioxidant, antimicrobial, and photoprotective activities (Freitas et al., 2024; Amiri et al., 2024; Bobková et al., 2022; Liu et al., 2022; Ali and Bhowmik, 2025).

In addition to their polyphenol and alkaloid content, these plant matrices also contain vitamins (e.g., vitamin E, B-complex vitamins), minerals (e.g., potassium, magnesium, iron), and other health-promoting bioactive metabolites and volatile compounds, such as amino and organic acids. However, many of these are either retained or concentrated in the by-products generated during processing, highlighting their potential for green valorization in cosmetics and cosmeceuticals (Wang et al., 2024; Gălbău et al., 2024; Oussou et al., 2023; El-Saadony et al., 2025; Michalak, 2022). The structures of the major bioactives present in herbal teas (e.g., *C. sinensis* (green and black), chamomile, and Greek mountain tea), cocoa, and coffee are shown in Fig. 7.2, while their potential cosmetic and cosmeceutical properties are summarized in Table 7.2.

2.1 Herbal tea (C. sinensis—green and black tea, Greek mountain tea, and chamomile) brief bioactive profile and green extraction methods

Herbal teas represent a diverse group of plant-derived infusions characterized by a wide array of phytochemicals with strong health-promoting activity. Tea infusions from *C. sinensis* green are rich in catechins, whereas black tea presents a higher concentration of oxidation products such as theaflavins and thearubigins. In contrast, *S. scardica* tea comprises flavonoids, phenylethanoid glycosides, and phenolic acids, while chamomile contains primarily flavonoids and terpenoids (Liu et al., 2023; Wang et al., 2022; El Mihyaoui et al., 2022; Chandrasekara and Shahidi, 2018; Pavlova et al., 2021). Microwave-assisted extraction (MAE), for example, under the optimal parameters of 87.9% (v/v) ethanol, 2 min, and

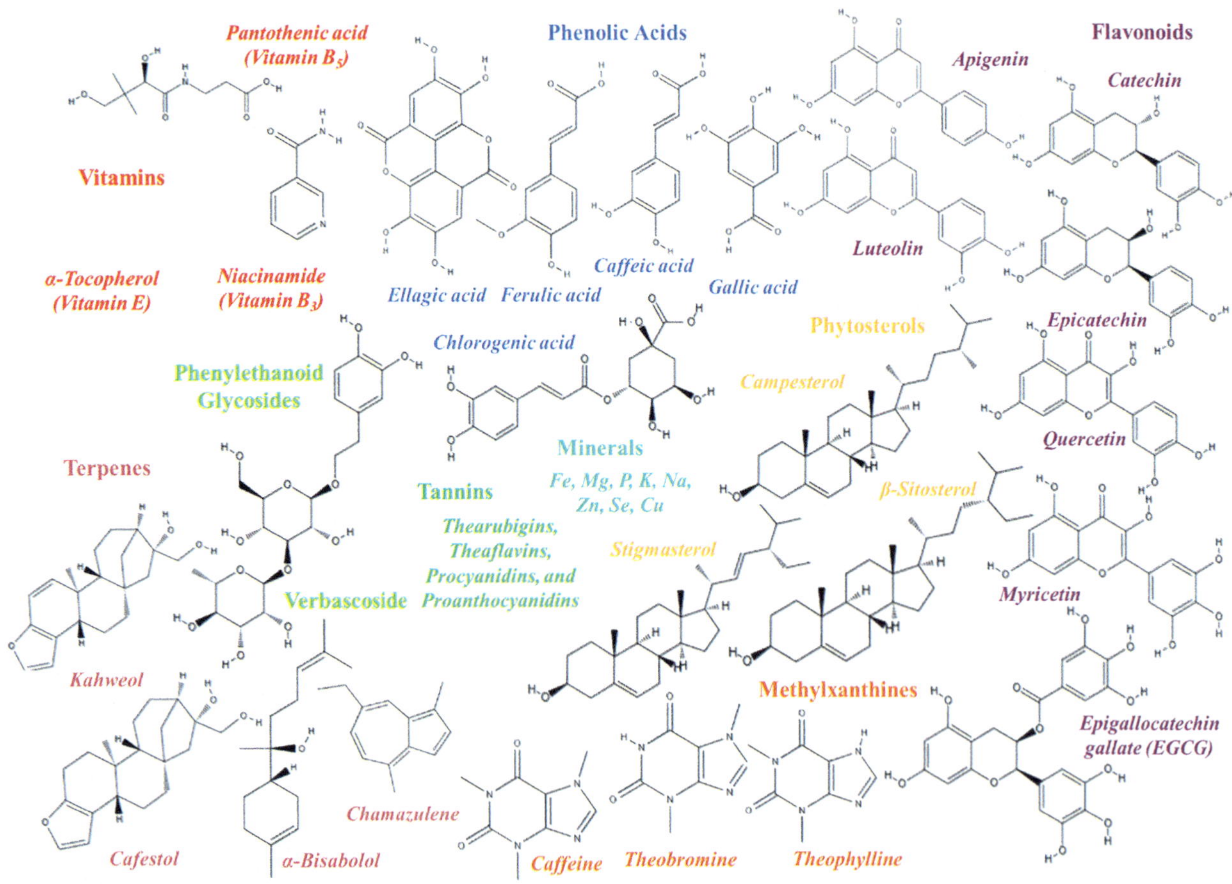

FIG. 7.2 Main representatives of each bioactive class present in herbal teas, cocoa, and coffee extracts. *(Parts of this figure (structure of bioactive molecules) were obtained from the open access free platform of https://www.molview.org/ (accessed on February 27, 2026).)*

TABLE 7.2 Bioactive compounds in herbal teas, cocoa, and coffee with potential cosmetic and cosmeceutical applications.

Bioactive compounds	Indicative source	Cosmetic and cosmeceutical function	References
Phenolic acids (e.g., ellagic, caffeic, (di) caffeoylquinic, feruloylquinic, gallic, syringic, sinapic, protocatechuic, ferulic, and chlorogenic acids)	Herbal teas, including Greek mountain tea, chamomile, *Camellia sinensis* (green and black tea), cocoa, and coffee	Antioxidant, antiaging, barrier repair, moisturizing, and antiinflammatory properties	(Liu et al., 2023; El Mihyaoui et al., 2022; Makiso et al., 2024; Uba et al., 2022; Soares and Oliveira, 2022; Ali and Bhowmik, 2025; Bouloumpasi et al., 2024)
Flavonoids (e.g., apigenin, luteolin, quercetin, naringenin, myricetin, rutin, kaempferol, and their derivatives)	Herbal teas, including Greek mountain tea, chamomile, *Camellia sinensis* (green and black tea), cocoa, and coffee	Antioxidant, antiglycation, antiaging, barrier repair, moisturizing, and antiinflammatory properties	(Liu et al., 2023; El Mihyaoui et al., 2022; Makiso et al., 2024; Uba et al., 2022; Soares and Oliveira, 2022; Ali and Bhowmik, 2025; Bouloumpasi et al., 2024)
Flavonoid catechins [e.g., EGCG, epigallocatechin (EGC), and epicatechin-3-gallate (ECG)]	Herbal teas (mainly green tea *Camellia sinensis*), cocoa, and coffee	Photoprotective, antiaging, antiinflammatory, and radical scavenging properties	(Liu et al., 2023; El Mihyaoui et al., 2022; Makiso et al., 2024; Uba et al., 2022; Soares and Oliveira, 2022; Ali and Bhowmik, 2025; Bouloumpasi et al., 2024)
Phenylethanoid glycosides (e.g., verbascoside, isoverbascoside, acetophenone, 1-phenylethanol, L-phenylalanine)	Herbal teas (*Camellia sinensis,* green tea, and *Sideritis scardica*)	Antioxidant, neuro-stimulant, and antiinflammatory action	(Bouloumpasi et al., 2024; Dong et al., 2012)
Tannins (complex tannin molecules like thearubigins and theaflavins), procyanidins, and proanthocyanidins	Theaflavins and thearubigins in *Camellia sinensis* black tea, while procyanidins (condensed tannins) are present in cocoa Little (in the form of flavonoids or catechins) to negligible content in *S. scardica* and *M. chamomilla,* and as ellagitannins or gallotannins in coffee	Moisturizing, barrier repair, antioxidant action, and antiinflammatory effects	(Liu et al., 2023; Soares and Oliveira, 2022; Ali and Bhowmik, 2025)
Terpenes (e.g., chrysophanol, cafestol, kahweol) and terpenoids (e.g., α-bisabolol, chamazulene)	Chamomile is rich in sesquiterpenoids like α-bisabolol and chamazulene Triterpenoids are present in *C. sinensis* and diterpenoids in *S. scardica*Chrysophanol is mainly present in cocoaDiterpenes (e.g., cafestol, kahweol) are present in coffee	Wound healing, antiinflammatory, structural support, biomimetic emollient, sebum regulation, and moisturizing properties	(Liu et al., 2023; El Mihyaoui et al., 2022; Uba et al., 2022; Soares and Oliveira, 2022; Ali and Bhowmik, 2025; Bouloumpasi et al., 2024)
Methylxanthines (e.g., caffeine, theobromine, theophylline)	*Camellia sinensis* (green and black tea), cocoa (mainly theobromine), and coffee	Photoprotective, antiaging, antiinflammatory, and radical scavenging properties	(Soares and Oliveira, 2022; Ali and Bhowmik, 2025; Bag et al., 2022)
Minerals (e.g., iron, sodium, magnesium, potassium, zinc, calcium, selenium)	Herbal teas, including Greek mountain tea, chamomile, and *Camellia sinensis* (green and black tea), cocoa, and coffee	Skin metabolism support, barrier repair, and enzyme support	(El-Saadony et al., 2025; Soares and Oliveira, 2022; Klepacka et al., 2021; Janda et al., 2020)
Vitamins (e.g., B_1, B_2, B_3, B_5, B_6, B_9, B_{12}, D_2, and E)	Herbal teas, including Greek mountain tea, chamomile, and *Camellia sinensis* (green and black tea), cocoa, and coffee	Natural UV filters, antiskin photoaging, and antioxidant effects	(El-Saadony et al., 2025; Chandrasekara and Shahidi, 2018; Soares and Oliveira, 2022; Ali and Bhowmik, 2025)
Carotenoids and pigments (e.g., β-carotene, lutein, zeaxanthin, chlorophylls, melanoidins)	Theaflavins in nonfermented herbal teasMelanoidin pigments in coffeeAnthocyanins in cocoa	Antioxidant, UV protection, colorant, and antipigmentation benefits	(Liu et al., 2023; Soares and Oliveira, 2022; Ali and Bhowmik, 2025; Bag et al., 2022)
Fatty acids (e.g., palmitic, stearic, oleic, linoleic, linolenic)	Herbal teas, including Greek mountain tea, chamomile, and *Camellia sinensis* (green and black tea), cocoa, and coffee	Moisturizing, antioxidant, antiaging, and antiinflammatory agents	(Wang et al., 2011; Shabani et al., 2022; Bora et al., 2025; Soares and Oliveira, 2022; Torres-Moreno et al., 2015; Liu et al., 2022)
Essential amino acids (e.g., isoleucine, leucine, valine, threonine, lysine, methionine)	Herbal teas, including Greek mountain tea, chamomile, and *Camellia sinensis* (green and black tea), cocoa, and coffee	Antiaging, antioxidant, and skin hydration properties	(Liu et al., 2023; El Mihyaoui et al., 2022; Uba et al., 2022; Shabani et al., 2022; Soares and Oliveira, 2022; Bag et al., 2022; Mazzafera et al., 2019)
Phytosterols (e.g., β-sitosterol, brassicasterol, stigmasterol, campesterol)	Herbal teas, including Greek mountain tea, chamomile, and *Camellia sinensis* (green and black tea), cocoa, and coffee	Skin barrier repair, antiinflammatory, antioxidant, immunomodulatory, and antiaging effects	(El Mihyaoui et al., 2022; Oracz et al., 2014; Kamgang Nzekoue et al., 2020; Patel et al., 2023; Aboutabl et al., 2002)

100°C, led to a 12.29% extraction yield, total phenolic content (TPC) of 121.76 mg gallic acid equivalents (GAE)/g dry weight (d.w.), 81.87 mg/g d.w. isoscutellarein, and 113.50 mg/g d.w. hypolaetin derivatives (ISC DER and HYP DER, respectively) (Bouloumpasi et al., 2024).

The extraction yield of green tea antioxidant polyphenols was notably improved under the combination of ultrasound-assisted extraction (UAE) and deep eutectic solvents, especially choline chloride (ChCl)–glycerol. Under the optimal extraction conditions of a 36:1 mL/g liquid-to-solid ratio, 461.5 W ultrasonic power, and 21 min ultrasonic time, the highest TPC value of 243 ± 7 mg GAE/g d.w. was achieved. Moreover, the four major catechins of green tea, including epicatechin (EC), epigallocatechin (EGC), epicatechin gallate (ECG), and EGCG, were identified as expected in the extracts and exhibited high antioxidant activity (Luo et al., 2020).

Regarding chamomile extraction, bioactives were extracted from its ligulate flowers using several green methods, including UAE, MAE, and subcritical water extraction (SWE), as well as conventional techniques like Soxhlet extraction. Especially in SWE extracts, a total extraction yield of 49.70% and a TPC of 151.45 mg epicatechin equivalents/mL under moderate subcritical conditions, alongside a high flavonoid (e.g., apigenin, catechins, luteolin) and phenolic acid content (e.g., gallic acid and CGA), was achieved, which was associated with the high antioxidant, antimicrobial, and antitumor activity of chamomile (Cvetanović et al., 2015). Interestingly, traditional extraction methods like maceration or Soxhlet extraction are currently being replaced by greener, more effective, and sustainable techniques like MAE, UAE, SWE, enzyme-assisted extraction (EAE), supercritical fluid extraction (SFE, mainly with CO_2), and natural deep eutectic solvent (NADES) use, which reportedly contribute to a remarkable ~ 40% reduction in energy consumption (Plyduang et al., 2026).

2.2 Cocoa brief bioactive profile and green extraction methods

Cocoa, derived from *T. cacao*, is a rich source of bioactives with significant relevance to both nutritional and cosmetic applications. Its phytochemical composition is dominated by several flavonoids (e.g., catechins), PCs, methylxanthines (e.g., caffeine, theobromine), and lipids with high emollient and skin conditioning properties. The concentration and content of cocoa agents are notably influenced by postharvest processing steps, including drying, fermentation, roasting, and alkalization, which may lead to partial degradation of flavonols and the formation of degradation by-products, such as melanoidins, which also exhibit antioxidant activity (Anoraga et al., 2024; Tušek et al., 2024; Oussou et al., 2023; Soares and Oliveira, 2022; Oracz et al., 2014).

MAE extraction under the optimal conditions of 855 W, 3.06 min, and 50 mL/g yielded a TPC of 2.724 mg GAE/g, total saponin content of 0.241 mg escin equivalents/g, alongside the ferric reducing antioxidant power (FRAP), 2,2-diphenyl-1-picrylhydrazyl (DPPH), and 2,2'-azino-bis-(3-ethylbenzothiazoline-6-sulfonic acid) of 81.966, 99.680, and 90.890 μmol Trolox equivalents (TE)/g, respectively (Jurado-Beizaga et al., 2026). Similarly, a combined UAE–EAE method at an enzyme concentration of 1.0% (v/v) combined with an ultrasonication amplitude of 80% produced the highest yields of bioactive compounds, including a TPC of 286.97 ± 1.01 mg GAE/g, total flavonoid content of 42.20 ± 0.28 mg caffeic acid equivalents/g, PC of 7.76 ± 0.30 mg PC/g, DPPH value of 132.31 ± 0.72, and FRAP value of 125.88 ± 0.24 μM TE/g. Furthermore, the extract also demonstrated significant tyrosinase and collagenase inhibitory action, with half-maximal inhibitory concentration (IC50) values of 1.32 ± 0.07 and 1.26 ± 0.02 mg/mL, respectively (Sunanta et al., 2026).

Cocoa bean shell (CBS) bioactives have been successfully isolated using MAE, UAE, EAE, SFE CO_2, SWE, NADES, pressurized liquid extraction, and pulsed electric field (PEF) extraction, with UAE and MAE being the most effective techniques for theobromine extraction. In addition, the encapsulation of its bioactives for achieving controlled release in cosmetic or nutraceutical applications has been evaluated mainly using maltodextrin mixed with gum Arabic, chitosan, and whey protein through spray drying or freeze-drying procedures (Alvarez-Yanamango et al., 2025).

2.3 Coffee brief bioactive profile and green extraction methods

Coffee, obtained from the roasted seeds of *Coffea* species, is a complex matrix rich in bioactives with diverse biological activities. The predominant phytochemicals included in coffee extracts are phenolic acids, mainly CGAs, as well as caffeine, diterpenes like cafestol and kahweol, trigonelline, and melanoidins formed during roasting—compounds that demonstrate several antioxidant, scavenging, antiinflammatory, and photoprotective effects (Amiri et al., 2024; Makiso et al., 2024; Oussou et al., 2023; Mazzafera et al., 2019; Kamgang Nzekoue et al., 2020). The extraction of coffee bioactives is commonly achieved through aqueous methods (e.g., brewing or infusion), which are effective for extracting polar constituents such as caffeine and CGAs (Zhang et al., 2022; Vera et al., 2026). Moreover, organic solvent extraction using methanol, ethanol, or acetone is also widely applied for enhancing the recovery of thermolabile phenolic acids and diterpenes (Sabino et al., 2025).

Supercritical CO_2 extraction is a promising technology for caffeine extraction, but it is a procedure requiring a large amount of CO_2 to achieve a high decaffeination degree. As a result, a pressure swing extraction method, where the pressure varied up and down, was employed to achieve a high degree of decaffeination with less CO_2 supply. Applying 353 K, 30 MPa, and 80% of the CO_2 supply resulted in nearly 100% decaffeination when compared with the pressure constant operation (at 30 MPa), while using the pressure swing technique led to comparable caffeine extraction without the water-soaking pretreatment (Hiraga et al., 2025). MAE extraction was utilized for the selective decaffeination of Gayo Aceh Arabica coffee, mainly focusing on the simultaneous caffeine reduction and CGA preservation. Alongside response surface methodology and under the optimal conditions of 450 W microwave power, 10 min of extraction time, and a feed-to-solvent ratio of 0.125 g/mL, MAE led to a 68.97% decrease in caffeine and an 88.25% CGA retention (high selectivity ratio of 1.74), revealing superior efficacy compared to solvent-based or SFE with CO_2 (Yuniati et al., 2025).

In general, UAE results in a polyphenol and antioxidant compound increase using low energy consumption, whereas MAE is highly efficient for accelerating mass transfer and bioactive agent release. Furthermore, high-pressure extraction is suitable for achieving higher phenolic yields and accelerating cold brewing processes, while cold atmospheric plasma extraction notably increases both the phenolic content and the antioxidant activity of coffee extracts (Vera et al., 2026).

3 Health-promoting properties of herbal tea, cocoa, and coffee extracts

Extracts derived from herbal teas, cocoa, and coffee exhibit a wide range of biological activities, which are highly relevant to skin health, cosmetics, and cosmeceutical applications. These effects are primarily attributed to their rich composition of phenolic acids, flavonoids, methylxanthines, catechins, and other secondary metabolites, which effectively modulate key molecular pathways widely involved in oxidative stress, inflammation, cellular aging, and skin barrier function (Wang et al., 2024; Gălbău et al., 2024; Oussou et al., 2023; El-Saadony et al., 2025; Michalak, 2022). The numerous health-promoting activities of herbal tea (*C. sinensis* green and black tea, *S. scardica*, and chamomile), cocoa, and coffee extracts are discussed in the following subsections. An overview of how these herbal teas of *Camellia sinensis* tea, *S. scardica* tea, and chamomile, cocoa, and coffee bioactives, can contribute to several health-promoting defenses is depicted in Fig. 7.3.

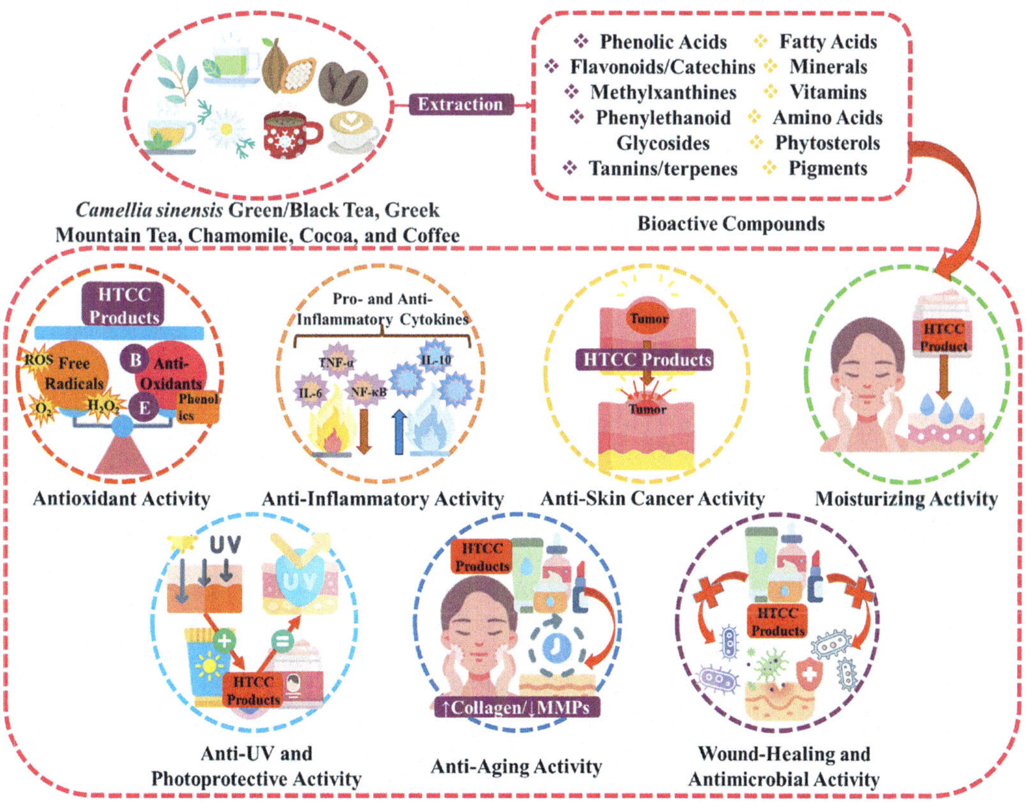

FIG. 7.3 Health-promoting effects of herbal teas, cocoa, and coffee bioactives. *(Parts of this figure were obtained from the open access free platform of https://www.freepik.com/ (Accessed 3 March 2026).)*

3.1 Antioxidant activity

C. sinensis leaf extracts have garnered mass attention due to their antioxidant, radical scavenging, and general health-promoting profile. Organic solvent extraction using methanol, DPPH assay analysis (ascorbic acid as the positive control), and gas chromatography–mass spectrometry profiling demonstrated that the *C. sinensis* methanolic extracts had IC_{50} values of 69.51 μg/mL, with caffeine being the main compound identified (74.47%) (Hasan et al., 2024). Interestingly, *C. sinensis,* due to its higher phenolic content, revealed higher photostability, antioxidant activity, and antiinflammatory value than both chamomile and Açaí (*Euterpe oleracea*) tea infusions (Garbossa and Campos, 2016). For *S. scardica*, recently, five NADESs composed of betaine, glycerol, glucose, urea, citric acid, and sucrose were evaluated for their extraction efficacy, where a mixture of betaine–glycerol–glucose (BGG4) revealed comparable or even superior extraction efficacy and antioxidant activity compared to 70% ethanol. In addition, CGA, verbascoside, and non-, mono-, and diacetylated allosyl hypolaetin glycosides were identified as the main constituents, with promising antioxidant activity for use in future cosmetics (Zissi et al., 2025). Similarly, chamomile also demonstrates strong antioxidant activity with a half-maximal effective concentration (EC_{50}) of 2.07 mg/mL in the DPPH assay (Reddy et al., 2025).

Depositing catechin and epicatechin bioactives in the stratum corneum, following a 6% topical application of aqueous cocoa powder 1 and 2 h after the application, led to an increase in both agents at 2 h, while higher epicatechin than catechin levels were detected from the cocoa powder at both time points, revealing cocoa's strong antioxidant activity and benefits toward systemic circulation and endothelium well-functioning (Draelos et al., 2024). Coffee silverskin, a coffee roasting by-product, contains high amounts of dietary fiber (49% insoluble/7% soluble), 19% proteins, ~ 5 g/100 g potassium, ~ 2 g/100 g magnesium, ~ 0.6 g/100 g calcium, several vitamins, low fat (2.4%), 1.25 g/100 g caffeine, 246 mg/100 g CGA, and 5.68 mg/100 g 5-hydroxymethylfurfural. Due to its phytochemical-rich profile, silverskin extracts protected erythrocytes from oxidative stress-induced hemolysis and, at higher extract concentrations, offered a prooxidant effect (Costa et al., 2018).

3.2 Antiinflammatory activity

Camelia sinensis green tea is mainly characterized by its catechin content and, especially, the presence of EGCG. Several studies notably report that its extract offers synergistic antioxidant and antiinflammatory activities, as, at concentrations between 12.5 and 25 μM, it inhibited the effect of reactive oxygen species (ROS) by up to 50%–60% when exposed to skin-damaging constituents such as nitroprusside, dihydrorhodamine, and inflammatory mediators like tumor necrosis factor α (TNF-α) (Febrinasari et al., 2025). *C. sinensis* polyphenols significantly improve microcirculation, inhibiting nitric oxide (NO), prostaglandin, thromboxane, and leukotriene inflammatory activity, soothing inflammation, reducing the swelling around the eyes, and accelerating wound and skin eruption healing (Koch et al., 2019). Furthermore, *S. scardica* reveals vast antiinflammatory and anticancer effects targeting the nuclear factor κB (NF-κB)-NOD-like receptor protein 3 inflammasome cascade (Yücer et al., 2025), while reportedly, it also targets other redox-sensitive molecular pathways such as the nuclear factor erythroid 2-related factor 2 (Nrf2), mitogen-activated protein kinase (MAPK), and phosphoinositide 3-kinase/protein kinase B (PI3K/Akt) cascades, making it a promising ingredient for future cosmetic applications (Papanikolaou et al., 2024).

Integrating *M. chamomilla* extracts into facial soaps, skin repair lotions, shampoos, sunscreens, skincare products, conditioners, and scalp serums has led to several antiinflammatory effects, such as a reduction in scalp irritation (Dai et al., 2023). Chamomile-based formulations also help manage dermatological conditions such as dandruff or psoriasis due to their soothing and antimicrobial effects (Tiwari et al., 2023; Chen et al., 2024). Emerging evidence suggests that chamomile oil polyphenols can support skin microbiome balance when incorporated into probiotic-infused cosmetics, strengthening skin barrier function and lowering inflammation, which may be associated with acne and rosacea (Cvetanović Kljakić et al., 2023; Choi et al., 2024). *M. chamomilla* also significantly reduced interleukin 22 (IL-22), TNF-α, and lipopolysaccharide-stimulated elevation of HaCaT cell inflammation, an activity highly correlated with PI3K/Akt/mTOR and *p38* MAPK inflammatory pathways, suggesting its potential as a therapeutic strategy against psoriasis (Tiwari et al., 2023; Chen et al., 2024).

Cocoa has been considered a great pain relief agent, widely linked to the downregulation of inflammatory responses induced by mediators like cyclooxygenase-2, NF-κB, IL-1β, IL-6, IL-2, TNF-α, and MAPK. Cocoa extracts, especially those abundant in flavonoids and catechins, are able to reduce the activity of several proinflammatory cytokines, including IL-1β, IL-6, and TNF-α, as well as other chemokines, ROS, and NO, decreasing macrophage TNF-α secretion, monocyte chemoattractant protein 1, and IL-6 and IL-8 production (De Feo et al., 2020). In addition, topical antiinflammatory studies on *Coffee* species extracts revealed that coffee could significantly decrease myeloperoxidase and *N*-acetyl-β-d-glycosaminidase-induced inflammation. Other studies showed that unabsorbed spent coffee grounds applied to RAW 264.7 macrophages could suppress NO production by 55%, modulating IL-10, C–C and C–X–C motif chemokine ligands 17 and 9 (CCL-17 and CXCL9, respectively), as well as IL-1β and IL-5 cytokines, providing a soothing effect (Santos et al., 2021).

3.3 Antiskin cancer activity

C. sinensis green tea, abundant in polyphenols, is correlated with a wide array of target organs for human cancer prevention. Green tea EGCG or the Polyphenon E mixture led to a 60% increase in free EGCG's systemic availability, suppressed the UV_B-mediated increase in epidermal thickness and transepidermal water loss (TEWL), and restored the UV_B-mediated decrease in the total antioxidant capacity in both skin and blood, minimizing the risk of photocarcinogenesis (Afaq and Katiyar, 2011). Reportedly, green tea polyphenols' oral administration or topical EGCG application could suppress skin tumor development in mice via the induction of the IL-2 immunomodulatory cytokine, the IL-2-dependent DNA repair following a repair mechanism based on nucleotide excision, the inhibition of the resulting UV-induced immunosuppression, the inhibition of angiogenic factors, and the stimulation of cytotoxic T cells in a tumor microenvironment, as potential photocarcinogenesis inhibitors (Katiyar et al., 2007). Similarly, *S. scardica* extracts exhibit strong cytotoxicity against various cancer cell lines, such as B16 melanoma cells, where its diterpenoid, siderol, may inhibit cell proliferation synergistically with standard treatments, acting as a potent inhibitor of aggressive, metastatic cancers like melanoma (Tasheva et al., 2023; İşitez, 2026). Moreover, German chamomile (*Matricaria recutita* L.) flowers exerted significant cytotoxic activity on melanoma cells, revealing an IC_{50} value of 40.7 μg/mL, which was almost twofold higher than on epidermoid carcinoma cells with an IC_{50} value of 71.4 μg/mL (Sak et al., 2017).

Cocoa has also demonstrated significant anticarcinogenic activity in melanoma cell lines (A-375 and B16–F10), reducing the viability and proliferation of all cells without damaging fibroblast cells. Furthermore, it increased paclitaxel activity on A-375 by suppressing cell proliferation and increasing oxidative stress (Mello et al., 2022). In addition, topical cocoa extract application or oral consumption may help protect the skin from UV-induced oxidative damage by downregulating proinflammatory cytokines like IL-2 and inhibiting NF-κB signaling (Draelos et al., 2024). On the contrary, regarding coffee's cosmetic value, topical caffeine application may notably increase the sun protection factor (SPF) of sunscreens by 25%, offering significant protection against photocarcinogenesis (Elias et al., 2023). In animal models, topical caffeine or EGCG application may also reduce the number of malignant squamous cell carcinomas by 72% and 66%, respectively, thereby inhibiting sunlight-induced skin cancer in humans (Lu et al., 2002).

3.4 Moisturizing properties

C. sinensis green tea EGCG (12.5 and 25 μM), owing to its vast antioxidant activity, could effectively improve skin moisture via the natural moisturizing factors. Filaggrin was notably elevated by EGCG compared to 10 μg/mL retinol, while transglutaminase-1 and hyaluronic acid synthases 1 and 2 were also augmented (Kim et al., 2018). Moreover, 6.0% w/w of *C. sinensis* green tea glycolic leaf extract, used in a study involving 24 volunteers (25–40 years old) with Fitzpatrick types II and III on their forearm skin, led to upregulated skin moisture and a significant reduction in skin roughness (Gianeti et al., 2013). *S. scardica* Greek mountain tea also contributed a notable increase in skin hydration, preventing TEWL and inhibiting collagenase and elastase (Żyżelewicz et al., 2020). Interestingly, nanoformulations of tea tree oil, lavender oil, rosemary oil, and chamomile oil have resulted in enhanced skin hydration, reduced oxidative damage, and boosted collagen synthesis, contributing to skin regeneration and overall skin health promotion (Reddy et al., 2025). *M. chamomilla*, due to its emollient action, may offer reduced TEWL, enhanced skin elasticity, and calmer broken microblood vessels (Dai et al., 2023).

Cocoa butter could be an effective moisturizer for topical cream formulations, as it enhances hydration and nourishment, providing effortless spreadability, high occlusivity, and exceptional anti-UV benefits (Purushothaman et al., 2025). Furthermore, upcycled cocoa pod husks contain polysaccharides, which can be formulated into products capable of upregulating skin hydration by over 50% (52.48%) while concurrently maintaining stable moisture levels for up to 4 weeks (Tantapakul et al., 2024; Anatachodwanit et al., 2025). Following, spent coffee ground oil extracted via SFE CO_2 and incorporated into a nonionic oil/water cream formulation (10%) led to a hydration boost, increasing skin barrier function, elevating sebum levels, and lowering TEWL (Ribeiro et al., 2013). Moreover, caffeine improves microcirculation and hydration by stimulating blood flow to the skin's surface, allowing better oxygen and nutrient delivery to the tissues (Ruse et al., 2025), as well as by increasing the electrical potential across the skin, enhancing electroosmosis (Emmetsberger et al., 2018).

3.5 Anti-UV and photoprotective properties

In vitro testing of *C. sinensis* green tea extract, especially owing to its catechin and polyphenol content, resulted in an SPF value of 27.4 at a 15% concentration (very high protection) (Putri et al., 2025). Other clinical trials reveal that the topical application of 2.5%–5% green tea polyphenols can decrease UV-induced redness (erythema) by up to 66% (Palatty et al., 2013). SSE's photoprotective, hyaluronidase- and elastase-inhibiting potential, as well as its antioxidant, antimelanogenic, and anti-UV_B properties, make it a significant candidate for use in cosmetic products against skin aging (Sklirou et al., 2021). The topical application of *M. chamomilla* extracts, which are rich in coumarins and flavonoids, enhances skin hydration, restores skin barrier function, improves photostability, and offers protection against UV-induced damage and premature aging, leading to clinical improvement in several skin-related conditions (Garbossa and Campos, 2016; Nóbrega et al., 2013). In addition, chamomile's natural brightening and conditioning properties make it an excellent agent for UV-protective lighters and sprays (Padule et al., 2022; Gautam et al., 2024).

Cocoa may exhibit reparative activity against UV_B-initiated damage in human fibroblasts by notably enhancing antioxidant enzymes like superoxide dismutase and glutathione peroxidase (GP_X) (Lee et al., 2024). It also exhibits significant biological action, leading to a decrease in basal ROS levels and NO and modulating cell cycle function in the absence of UV_B exposure by increasing the G2/M phase (da Silva Prade et al., 2024). Coffee extracts reveal anti-UV and photoprotective properties as well. *Coffea arabica* flavonoid and terpene agents may accelerate UV_B absorption by protecting fibroblast cells (da Silva Prade et al., 2024), whereas CGAs present in coffee prevent UVA-induced skin photoaging by primarily regulating collagen metabolism and apoptosis in human dermal fibroblasts (Rodrigues et al., 2023). Caffeine also acts as a sunscreen adjuvant, absorbing UV radiation (primarily in the 260–300 nm range) and increasing SPF values by ~ 25% when added to standard formulations (Rodrigues et al., 2023).

3.6 Antiaging activity

C. sinensis polyphenols and flavonoids are indicators of green tea's great antioxidant and antiaging activity, as they protect against ROS and delay the progression of skin aging (Febrinasari et al., 2025). Clinical trials showed that a 6% green tea extract applied topically for 4 weeks significantly improved skin roughness and reduced fine line depth (Febrinasari et al., 2025). Moreover, 24 Korean females between the ages of 30 and 59 years with fine wrinkles at the lateral canthal lines received 2.5 mg of *C. sinensis*, leading to a 36.3% wrinkle improvement (Hong et al., 2013). Skin-aging-related studies have revealed that *S. scardica* extracts contain collagenase, inhibit advanced glycation end product formation, and lower UVB-induced matrix metalloproteinase-1 (MMP-1) expression because of three flavonoid compounds with an uncommon 8-hydroxyl moiety, namely, isoscutellarein, 4′-O-methylhypolaetin, and 4′-O-methylisoscutellarein (Sato et al., 2022). Furthermore, Roman chamomile extracts, after being treated with ethyl acetate as a solvent, led to a remarkable inhibition of hyaluronidase, elastase, tyrosinase, and melanin, demonstrating excellent antioxidant, whitening, and antiaging properties (Sui et al., 2025).

Cocoa powder could enhance skin moisture and, therefore, reduce facial wrinkles, as reported in a 12-week clinical trial and in vitro studies. Cocoa powder successfully promoted water retention, enhanced antioxidant enzyme activities, promoted hyaluronic acid production in H_2O_2-treated keratinocytes (KCs), and inhibited the expression of MMP-1. Supporting the in vitro findings, aged skin displayed marked improvement in skin hydration and wrinkle formation reduction after 12 weeks of cocoa powder consumption (Lee et al., 2024). Furthermore, in moderately photoaged Korean women with visible facial wrinkles (43–86 years old) undergoing a 24-week trial, regular cocoa flavanol consumption led to the reduction of facial wrinkles and restoration of skin elasticity, preventing the progression of photoaging (Yoon et al., 2016). In addition, CGA, pyrocatechol, and 3,4,5-tricaffeoyl quinic acid isolated from *C. arabica* at concentrations up to 50 μg/mL maintained ~ 90% viability. Chlorogenic acid and 3,4,5-tricaffeoyl quinic acid notably increased type-I procollagen levels, while treated cells also revealed an MMP basal expression level similar to the control cells (downregulation of MMP-1, MMP-3, and MMP-9 and upregulation of procollagen synthesis), highlighting coffee's potential as a therapeutic agent against induced photoaging (Santos et al., 2021).

3.7 Wound healing and antimicrobial activity

C. sinensis EGCG content is widely associated with cutaneous wound healing, antiangiogenic, and antiinflammatory effects. In a double-blind, randomized, controlled clinical trial with 62 human volunteers, EGCG reduced mast cells (1–3 weeks), increased M2 macrophages, and downregulated both the vascular endothelial growth factor A and cluster of differentiation 31 (week 1 and weeks 1–2 after direct application). Direct application decreased scar thickness (1–3 weeks) and also increased scar elasticity (4 weeks), revealing its vast potential as a wound healing agent (Ud-Din et al., 2019; Xu et al., 2021). Caffeic acid and EGCG present in herbal *C. sinensis* tea exhibit several antimicrobial properties against a plethora of microbial strains, both Gram-positive and Gram-negative (Boudou et al., 2025).

S. scardica exhibited vast antimicrobial activity against Gram-negative bacteria *Haemophilus* sp. and *Pasteurella multocida*, as well as the Gram-positive *Corynebacterium pseudotuberculosis* (MIC: 40–640 μg/mL). *Candida albicans* and *Pseudomonas aeruginosa* growth was inhibited by all extracts, while *Klebsiella pneumoniae* and *Escherichia coli* strains were the most resistant microorganisms (Tadić et al., 2012). Chamazulene, apigenin, and α-bisabolol are present at high concentrations in chamomile and are capable of enhancing burn wound healing by promoting tissue regeneration, reducing wound size, and increasing collagen deposition. Moreover, chamomile extracts exhibit potent antimicrobial activity, specifically against a spoilage agent called *Alicyclobacillus* spp., including its species such as *A. acidoterrestris*, *A. herbarium*, *A. acidophilus*, *A. hesperidium*, and *A. sendaiensis*, as well as microbial strains such as *S. aureus*, *P. aeruginosa*, and *E. coli* (de Oliveira et al., 2024; Herman et al., 2013). In addition, chamomile extracts have been shown to accelerate KC migration and fibroblast proliferation, two key processes in tissue repair and wound closure (Sah et al., 2022; Niknam et al., 2021).

Cocoa bean and cocoa pod husk extracts are able to increase the number of fibroblasts, mainly stimulating the production of the transforming growth factor-β, a critical factor for collagen synthesis and tissue remodeling, as well as enhancing closure rates, increasing epithelial thickness, and elevating vessel proliferation (Edo et al., 2023; Rahayu et al., 2024). Moreover, cocoa by-products such as "wood vinegar" from cocoa pod shells exhibit inhibitory activity against fungi like *C. albicans* and *Aspergillus niger*, whereas cocoa extracts demonstrate inhibitory activity against common skin pathogens like *Staphylococcus aureus* and *Staphylococcus epidermidis* (Desvita et al., 2022). Interestingly, in *S. aureus* and *S. epidermidis*-infected wound rabbit skin models, a cocoa ethanolic extract cream of 8% improved wound recovery to 72.7% and 86.1% from the original rates of the base cream (23.5% and 34.7%) (Tunjung-Sari et al., 2016). Regarding coffee, topical CGA benefited the wound healing procedure in carbopol hydrogels with 10% extract from green and roasted press cake. Both extracts notably reduced the wound area size, but green coffee offered the greatest wound reduction, outlining its important role in wound healing regulation through inflammatory response downregulation (Rodrigues et al., 2023). Coffee has also demonstrated ideal antimicrobial effects against both Gram-positive and Gram-negative bacteria. Its extract did not reveal any activity against *C. albicans* and *P. aeruginosa*, but presented positive results ranging from 31.5 (*K. pneumoniae*) to 250 μg/mL (*S. aureus*) against all other tested microorganisms, including *S. aureus*, *S.* epidermidis, *K. pneumoniae*, and *E. coli* (Santos et al., 2021).

4 Applications of herbal tea, cocoa, and coffee extracts in the cosmetic and cosmeceutical industry

4.1 Skincare, haircare, and body care applications

Herbal tea (*C. sinensis*, *S. scardica*, and *M. chamomilla*), cocoa, and coffee extracts have been widely integrated into cosmetic and cosmeceutical formulations across both the skincare and haircare sectors, contributing not only to product performance but also to product stability (Dai et al., 2023; Tasheva et al., 2023; Martínez-Inda et al., 2025; Koch et al., 2019).

In skincare applications, these extracts are extensively utilized in emulsions, serums, creams, gels, and masks targeting oxidative stress, inflammation, and premature skin aging. Polyphenol-rich extracts from green tea (especially abundant in EGCG) and coffee may effectively neutralize ROS, preventing lipid peroxidation and oxidative stress-induced damage (Gianeti et al., 2013; Martínez-Inda et al., 2025). Moreover, catechins and CGAs inhibit MMPs, making them potent candidates for antiwrinkle formulations (Kim et al., 2018; Rodrigues et al., 2023). Antiinflammatory and soothing applications are predominantly correlated with chamomile and Greek mountain tea, as their rich flavonoid (e.g., apigenin, luteolin) and terpenoid content (e.g., α-bisabolol) modulate inflammatory pathways (e.g., NF-κB), reducing erythema or irritation (El Mihyaoui et al., 2022; Yücer et al., 2025). Furthermore, cocoa, and particularly cocoa butter, are central ingredients in moisturizing and barrier-repair formulations, which reduce TEWL and enhance skin hydration (Purushothaman et al., 2025; Lee et al., 2024). In parallel, coffee-derived lipids and diterpenes may also contribute to emollient properties, improving skin texture and softness (Liu et al., 2022). Finally, green tea and coffee are frequently incorporated as complementary agents to conventional UV filters commonly used in sunscreens or after-sun products (Amiri et al., 2024; Anatachodwanit et al., 2025; Putri et al., 2025).

Considering haircare applications, these plant-derived extracts notably contribute to scalp health and hair fiber, protein, or lipid protection. Tea constituents have successfully been integrated into many haircare applications as surfactants, foaming agents, emulsifiers, antioxidants, antimicrobial agents, and preservatives, primarily cleaning and removing excessive sebum from hair and scalp (Sang et al., 2023). In addition, caffeine present in coffee extracts has been associated with hair follicle activity stimulation, actively promoting hair growth by improving microcirculation and counteracting dihydrotestosterone at the follicular level. As a result, caffeine is frequently included in antihair loss shampoos, lotions, serums, and foams (Szendzielorz and Spiewak, 2025). Regarding cocoa's haircare significance, a hair growth cream formula based on cocoa pod peel water fraction effectively stimulated (12.5%) hair growth activity, depending on the hair length data, without any signs of irritation (Mustarichie et al., 2022).

As for body care applications, these extracts are increasingly utilized in targeted formulations, including anticellulite and body-contouring products, due to their ability to temporarily enhance skin firmness and reduce the appearance of cellulite. Interestingly, methylxanthines, mainly caffeine, theobromine, and theophylline, exhibit notable lipolytic action by triggering triglyceride breakdown in adipocytes and enhancing microcirculation (Santos et al., 2021; Garcia et al., 2021).

4.2 Examples from commercial products using herbal tea, cocoa, and coffee extracts

Herbal tea, cocoa, and coffee-derived ingredients are widely utilized in commercial cosmetics and cosmeceuticals due to their multifaceted properties. These agents can be found in a wide range of formulations, including moisturizers, facial oils, antiaging creams, hair conditioners, body care products, and sunscreens or other UV-protective formulations (Dai et al., 2023; Tasheva et al., 2023; Martínez-Inda et al., 2025; Koch et al., 2019). Table 7.3 includes commercial nut and nut by-product-based cosmetic and cosmeceutical products.

TABLE 7.3 Commercial herbal tea, cocoa, or coffee-derived cosmetic and cosmeceutical products.

Cosmetic product	Cosmetic use	Key ingredient	Beneficial impact	References
NEOGEN—Green Tea Real Fresh Foam Cleanser	Foam cleanser	*Camellia sinensis* leaf water and *C. sinensis* leaf	Gentle impurity removal, antiacne, antioxidant, exfoliant, skin-brightening, and soothing properties	(Neogen Green Tea Real Fresh Foam Cleanser, n.d.)
NUXE—Body Rêve de thé Exalting Fragrant Water	Fragrant water	*Camellia sinensis* flower extract	Antimicrobial, antioxidant, nourishing, freshness, and rejuvenating effects	(Nuxe body Rêve de thé Exalting Fragrant Water, n.d.)
STARSKIN—Silkmud™ Green Tea Clay Anti-Aging Liftaway Mud Face Sheet Mask	Face sheet mask	*Camellia sinensis* leaf powder	Gentle impurity removal, antioxidant, exfoliant, skin-brightening, and soothing effects	(STARSKIN SilkmudTM Green Tea Clay Anti-Aging Liftaway Mud Face Sheet Mask, n.d.)
KORRES—Olympus Tea Cleansing Foaming Cream	Foaming cream	*Sideritis scardica* flower, leaf, and stem extract	Makeup removal, gentle cleansing, exfoliant, skin brightening, soothing, and antioxidant properties	(Korres Olympus Tea Cleansing Foaming Cream, n.d.)
APIVITA—Tonic Mountain Tea Tonifying Shower Gel	Shower gel	*Sideritis scardica* flower, leaf, and stem extract	Antiseptic, antioxidant, soothing, and antiinflammatory effects	(Apvita Tonic Mountain Tea Tonifying Shower Gel, n.d.)
APIVITA—Suncare Anti-Wrinkle Face Cream Olive & 3D Pro-Algae SPF50	Suncare face cream	*Sideritis scardica* flower, leaf, and stem extract	Antiaging, antiwrinkle, moisturizing, UV-protective, antioxidant, skin brightening, and soothing properties	(Apivita Suncare Anti-Wrinkle Face Cream Olive & 3D Pro-Algae Spf50, n.d.)
BIOLAND—Argan Conditioner	Hair conditioner	*Matricaria chamomilla* flower oil	Moisturizing, rejuvenating, resistance boosting, hair brightening, antioxidant, and exfoliant	(BioLand Argan Conditioner, n.d.)
EARTHWISE BEAUTY—Nap in the Meadow Face Serum	Face serum	*Matricaria chamomilla* flower oil	Moisturizing, refreshing, antioxidant, skin brightening, soothing, and cleansing effects	(Earthwise Beauty Nap In The Meadow Face Serum, n.d.)
FREZYDERM—Chamomile Bath	Liquid solution	*Matricaria chamomilla* extract	Soothing, antiirritation, suitable for atopic dermatitis or dry skin individuals, and soothing effects	(Frezyderm Chamomile Bath, n.d.)
APIVITA—Cocoa Butter Lip Balm	Lip balm	*Theobroma cacao* seed butter	Antioxidant, antiinflammatory, emollient, perfuming, soothing, and sunscreen effects	(Apivita Cocoa Butter, n.d.)
NIVEA—Cocoa Nourish	Moisture serum	*Theobroma cacao* seed butter	Antioxidant, moisturizing, and deep cleansing effects	(Nivea Cocoa Nourish, n.d.)
NUXE—Contour Des Yeux Prodigieux Anti-Fatigue Moisturizing Eye Cream	Eye cream	*Theobroma cacao* callus powder	Dark circle minimization, puffiness reduction, antioxidant, and skin brightening properties	(Nuxe Contour Des Yeux Prodigieux Anti-Fatigue Moisturizing Eye Cream, n.d.)

Cosmetic product	Cosmetic use	Key ingredient	Beneficial impact	References
ESSENCE—Coffee to Glow Coffee Body Scrub	Body scrub	*Coffea arabica* seed powder	Dead skin cell removal, exfoliant, nourishing, moisturizing, antioxidant, and soothing effects	(Essence Coffee To Glow Coffee Body Scrub, n.d.)
AVON—Ageless Restoring Overnight Gel	Overnight gel mask	*Coffea arabica* leaf/ seed extract and *Camellia sinensis* leaf extract	Antiaging, antiwrinkle, antioxidant, skin brightening, and soothing properties	(Avon Ageless Restoring Overnight Gel, n.d.)
COSMEDIX—Protect UV Broad Spectrum SPF30 Moisturizing Spray	Moisturizing spray	*Coffea arabica* leaf/ seed extract and *Camellia sinensis* leaf extract	UV-protective, moisturizing, antiacne, antioxidant, skin brightening, and soothing effects	(Cosmedix Protect Uv Broad Spectrum Spf 30 Moisturizing Spray, n.d.)
LA VIE EN ROSE—Bikini Cream	Body cream	Caffeine, *Theobroma cacao* seed butter, and *Camellia sinensis* leaf extract	Skin firmness, anticellulite, antioxidant, and soothing properties	(La vie en rose Bikini Cream ingredients (Explained), n.d.)
COCOSOLIS—Skin Anti-Cellulite Dry Oil	Dry body oil	*Coffea arabica* seed oil	Skin firmness, anticellulite, antioxidant, and soothing properties	(Cocosolis Skin Anti-cellulite Dry Oil, n.d.)

5 Limitations, challenges, and future perspectives

Despite the significant potential of herbal tea (*C. sinensis*, *S. scardica*, and *M. chamomilla*), cocoa, and coffee extracts in cosmetic and cosmeceutical applications, several persistent limitations and challenges must be addressed to ensure their effective and safe application. One of the primary challenges lies in the variability of their chemical composition, which is, in general, influenced by factors such as plant species, geographical origin, cultivation practices, harvesting conditions, and postharvesting processing. This variability may pose challenges in the full identification of bioactive content, as well as in achieving standardization and reproducibility at an industrial level (Vikhe et al., 2025; Batovska et al., 2025; Crozier et al., 2011).

Another critical limitation is the stability of bioactives, as many key constituents in these plant matrices, such as catechins, flavonoids, and CGAs, are highly sensitive to environmental factors, including extreme light, temperature, oxygen, and pH conditions. The degradation of these thermolabile compounds may ultimately lead to final product formulations with less or no expected bioactivity, compromised bioavailability, and reduced effectiveness (Chandrasekara and Shahidi, 2018; Kosińska et al., 2012).

Selecting the appropriate extraction method also presents challenges, as while conventional techniques are widely employed, the frequent use of organic solvents or other inefficiencies may pose several environmental challenges. Therefore even though green extraction methods like MAE, UAE, EAE, PEF, SFE, and SWE offer improved efficacy and selectivity, their broad utilization is often limited by cost, scalability, and industrial applicability aspects (Vera et al., 2026; Cao et al., 2025). Furthermore, safety and regulatory considerations also remain a nonnegligible challenge. The use of certain organic solvents, potential allergenicity concerns, and raw material variability, as well as the lack of well-designed clinical studies to confirm their efficacy and safety toward humans, are of significant importance and must be considered prior to their broader application (Vikhe et al., 2025; Batovska et al., 2025; Crozier et al., 2011).

Future perspectives in this field are focused on the development of standardized extracts with fully identified bioactive profiles, as well as the application of green and sustainable technologies (e.g., MAE, UAE) and green solvents (e.g., NADES) (El-Saadony et al., 2025; Alvarez-Yanamango et al., 2025; Vera et al., 2026; Martínez-Inda et al., 2025; Cao et al., 2025). Moreover, advances in formulation science, including the incorporation of nanotechnology-based delivery systems (e.g., nanoemulsions, liposomes, and encapsulation technologies), are expected to enhance the stability, bioavailability, and sustained and targeted delivery of bioactives (Niu et al., 2022; Sitarek et al., 2024; Kavin et al., 2025). In addition, valorizing agroindustrial by-products such as spent coffee grounds, cocoa shells, and tea residues is a promising approach for the sustainable and cost-effective production and isolation of bioactives (Oussou et al., 2023; Kamgang Nzekoue et al., 2020; Sabino et al., 2025; Rahayu et al., 2024; Desvita et al., 2022; Mustarichie et al., 2022).

Of interest are also studies indicating that there are some natural bioactives in herbal teas that strongly and with high specificity affect the thromboinflammatory pathway of platelet-activating factor (PAF), including catechin, quercetin, and other bioflavonoids, as well as several polar lipids (glycolipids and phospholipids bearing unsaturated fatty acids in their structure, especially monounsaturated or omega-3 ones) (Tsoupras et al., 2020). Especially for the bioflavonoids from these sources, like catechin and quercetin, when assessed in mixtures against the PAF pathway, they showed much higher antiinflammatory activities in human platelets (a classic human cell model for assessing the anti-PAF effect of a natural compound) (Tsoupras et al., 2019), compared to the activities that they showed on their own, suggesting potent synergy by the copresence of these flavonoids in mixtures like the extracts from these natural herb sources (Chrysikopoulou et al., 2025). Moreover, molecular docking assessment has shown high affinity for the binding of these flavonoids on specific sites of the specific PAF membrane receptor (PAF receptor) and thus by blocking the binding of PAF on its receptor, provides a structure–activity relationship explanation for the specificity against this inflammatory pathway associated with the antiinflammatory activities of the bioflavonoids present in these natural herb sources (Tsiapali et al., 2025). Taking into account that PAF and its inflammatory signaling are highly implicated in chronic inflammatory complications, including those of the skin like melanoma and skin cancer (Tsoupras et al., 2024), the strong antiinflammatory potential of the extracts from these herbal teas, and their appropriate utilization in biofunctional cosmetic applications, further suggest preventive and protective properties for such formulation products based on these bioactive ingredients against skin inflammation, erythema, melanoma, and skin cancer. Nevertheless, more well-designed clinical trials, alongside interdisciplinary research and innovation, will be essential for unlocking the full potential of herbal teas, cocoa, and coffee and their potent anti-PAF properties.

6 Conclusions

Herbal teas, cocoa, and coffee constitute rich sources of bioactives, including polyphenols, flavonoids, and methylxanthines, which demonstrate significant antioxidant, antiinflammatory, antiaging, and photoprotective properties. Their diverse phytochemical profiles, alongside advanced extraction, identification, quantification, and formulation technologies, support their growing use in cosmetics and cosmeceuticals targeting skin protection, hydration, and barrier function. However, limitations and challenges related to bioavailability, stability, and composition variability still persist. Future research must therefore focus on developing standardized extracts, sustainable extraction methodologies, and advanced delivery systems to enhance their efficacy and industrial applicability. Overall, herbal tea, cocoa, and coffee ingredients represent a natural, sustainable approach for the development of next-generation cosmetics and cosmeceuticals.

Acknowledgments

The authors would like to thank the School of Chemistry of the Faculty of Sciences at the Democritus University of Thrace for their continuous support.

Conflicts of interest

The authors declare no conflicts of interest.

Funding

This research received no external funding.

Author contributions

A.T. was involved in conceptualization, methodology, validation, visualization, supervision, and project administration. A.T. and T.A. were involved in writing—review and editing. All authors contributed to software, investigation, and writing—original draft preparation and have read and agreed to the published version of the manuscript.

References

Aboutabl, E.A., Nassar, M.I., Elsakhawy, F.M., Maklad, Y.A., Osman, A.F., El-Khrisy, E.A.M., 2002. Phytochemical and pharmacological studies on *Sideritis taurica* Stephan ex Willd. J. Ethnopharmacol. 03788741. 82 (2-3), 177–184. doi:10.1016/s0378-8741(02)00172-1.

Afaq, F., Katiyar, S.K., 2011. Polyphenols: skin photoprotection and inhibition of photocarcinogenesis. Mini-Rev. Med. Chem. 18755607. 11 (14), 1200–1215. Available from: http://www.eurekaselect.com/633/journal/mini-reviews-medicinal-chemistry. doi:10.2174/138955751111091200.

Ali, M.A., Bhowmik, S., 2025. Bioactive compounds in coffee husk: extraction, functional properties, applications, and sustainable approach in circular economy. RSC Sustain. 27538125. 3 (10), 4410–4425. Available from: https://www.rsc.org/journals-books-databases/about-journals/rsc-sustainability/#scope. doi:10.1039/d5su00531k.

Alvarez-Yanamango, E., Obregon, D., Ibañez, A., 2025. A comprehensive review of the development of green extraction methods and encapsulation of theobromine from cocoa bean shells for nutraceutical applications. Food Eng. Rev. 1866-7910. 17 (4), 1083–1104. doi:10.1007/s12393-025-09425-6.

Amiri, R., Akbari, M., Moradikor, N., 2024. Bioactive potential and chemical compounds of coffee. Prog. Brain Res. 288, 23–33. Available from: https://www.sciencedirect.com/science/bookseries/00796123. doi:10.1016/bs.pbr.2024.06.011.

Anatachodwanit, A., Chanpirom, S., Tree-Udom, T., Kitthaweesinpoon, S., Jiamphun, S., Aryuwat, O., Tantapakul, C., Vinardell, M.P., Sripisut, T., 2025. Upcycled cocoa pod husk: a sustainable source of phenol and polyphenol ingredients for skin hydration, whitening, and anti-aging. Life. 2075-1729. 15 (7), 1126. doi:10.3390/life15071126.

Anoraga, S.B., Shamsudin, R., Hamzah, M.H., Sharif, S., Saputro, A.D., 2024. Cocoa by-products: a comprehensive review on potential uses, waste management, and emerging green technologies for cocoa pod husk utilization. Heliyon. 24058440. 10 (16), e35537. doi:10.1016/j.heliyon.2024.e35537.

Apivita Cocoa Butter, n.d. https://incidecoder.com/products/apivita-cocoa-butter. Accessed 13 Apr 2026.

Apivita Suncare Anti-Wrinkle Face Cream Olive & 3D Pro-Algae Spf50, n.d. https://incidecoder.com/products/apivita-suncare-anti-wrinkle-face-cream-olive-3d-pro-algae-spf50. Accessed 13 Apr 2026.

Apvita Tonic Mountain Tea Tonifying Shower Gel, n.d. https://incidecoder.com/products/apvita-tonic-mountain-tea-tonifying-shower-gel. Accessed 13 Apr 2026.

Avon Ageless Restoring Overnight Gel, n.d. https://incidecoder.com/products/avon-ageless-restoring-overnight-gel-2. Accessed 13 Apr 2026.

Bag, S., Mondal, A., Majumder, A., Banik, A., 2022. Tea and its phytochemicals: hidden health benefits & modulation of signaling cascade by phytochemicals. Food Chem. 03088146. 371, 131098. doi:10.1016/j.foodchem.2021.131098.

Batovska, D., Panova, N., Gerasimova, A., Tumbarski, Y., Ivanov, I., Dincheva, I., Yotkovska, I., Gentscheva, G., Nikolova, K., 2025. Chamomile matters: species- and producer-dependent variation in Bulgarian *Matricaria recutita* L. and *Chamaemelum nobile* L. essential oils and their cosmetic potential. Cosmetics. 2079-9284. 12 (3), 123. doi:10.3390/cosmetics12030123.

BioLand Argan Conditioner, n.d. https://incidecoder.com/products/bioland-argan-conditioner. Accessed 13 Apr 2026.

Bobková, A., Poláková, K., Demianová, A., Belej, Ľ., Bobko, M., Jurčaga, L., Gálik, B., Novotná, I., Iriondo-DeHond, A., 2022. Comparative analysis of selected chemical parameters of *Coffea arabica*, from cascara to silverskin. Foods. 2304-8158. 11 (8), 1082. doi:10.3390/foods11081082.

Bora, B., Yin, T., Zhang, B., Altan, C.O., Benjakul, S., 2025. Comparison between Indian and commercial chamomile essential oils: chemical compositions, antioxidant activities and preventive effect on oxidation of Asian seabass visceral depot fat oil. Food Chem. X. 25901575. 26, 102292. doi:10.1016/j.fochx.2025.102292.

Boudou, F., Belakredar, A., Keziz, A., Alsaeedi, H., Cornu, D., Bechelany, M., Barhoum, A., 2025. Camellia sinensis phytochemical profiling, druglikeness, and antibacterial activity against gram-positive and gram-negative bacteria: in vitro and in silico insights. Front. Chem. 2296-2646. 13. doi:10.3389/fchem.2025.1555574.

Bouloumpasi, E., Koskeridou, A., Irakli, M., Karioti, A., Tsivelika, N., Chatzopoulou, P., 2024. Bioactive compounds of green phenolic extracts obtained via microwave-assisted extraction of *Sideritis* species grown in Greece. Molecules. 1420-3049. 29 (23), 5612. doi:10.3390/molecules29235612.

Cao, S., Liang, J., Chen, M., Chao, X., Wang, X., Qiu, L., Zhao, X., Wenxiao, H., 2025. Comparative analysis of extraction technologies for plant extracts and absolutes. Front. Chem. 2296-2646. 13. doi:10.3389/fchem.2025.1536590.

Chandrasekara, A., Shahidi, F., 2018. Herbal beverages: bioactive compounds and their role in disease risk reduction - A review. J. Tradit. Complement. Med. 22254110. 8 (4), 451–458. doi:10.1016/j.jtcme.2017.08.006.

Chen, G., Lv, C., Nie, Q., Li, X., Lv, Y., Liao, G., Liu, S., Ge, W., Chen, J., Du, Y., 2024. Essential oil of *Matricaria chamomilla* alleviates psoriatic-like skin inflammation by inhibiting PI3K/Akt/mTOR and p38 MAPK signaling pathway. Clin. Cosmet. Investig. Dermatol. 11787015. 17, 59–77. Available from: https://www.dovepress.com/getfile.php?fileID=95834. doi:10.2147/CCID.S445008.

Choi, H.Y., Lee, Y.J., Kim, C.M., Lee, Y.M., 2024. Revolutionizing cosmetic ingredients: harnessing the power of antioxidants, probiotics, plant extracts, and peptides in personal and skin care products. Cosmetics 20799284. 11 (5). Available from: https://www.mdpi.com/journal/cosmetics. doi:10.3390/cosmetics11050157.

Chrysikopoulou, V., Rampaouni, A., Koutsia, E., Ofrydopoulou, A., Mittas, N., Tsoupras, A., 2025. Anti-inflammatory, antithrombotic and antioxidant efficacy and synergy of a high-dose vitamin C supplement enriched with a low dose of bioflavonoids; in vitro assessment and in vivo evaluation through a clinical study in healthy subjects. Nutrients. 2072-6643. 17 (16), 2643. doi:10.3390/nu17162643.

Cocosolis Skin Anti-cellulite Dry Oil, n.d. https://incidecoder.com/products/cocosolis-skin-anti-cellulite-dry-oil. Accessed 13 Apr 2026.

Cosmedix Protect Uv Broad Spectrum Spf 30 Moisturizing Spray, n.d. https://incidecoder.com/products/cosmedix-protect-uv-broad-spectrum-spf-30-moisturizing-spray. Accessed 13 Apr 2026.

Costa, A.S.G., Alves, R.C., Vinha, A.F., Costa, E., Costa, C.S.G., Nunes, M.A., Almeida, A.A., Santos-Silva, A., Oliveira, M.B.P.P., 2018. Nutritional, chemical and antioxidant/pro-oxidant profiles of silverskin, a coffee roasting by-product. Food Chem. 18737072. 267, 28–35. Available from: https://www.elsevier.com/locate/foodchem. doi:10.1016/j.foodchem.2017.03.106.

Crozier, A., Ashihara, H., Tomás-Barbéran, F., 2011. Teas, Cocoa and Coffee: Plant Secondary Metabolites and Health Teas, Cocoa and Coffee: Plant Secondary Metabolites and Health. Wiley-Blackwell, United Kingdom, pp. 1–252. Available from: http://onlinelibrary.wiley.com/book/10.1002/9781444347098. doi:10.1002/9781444347098.

Cvetanović Kljakić, A., Radosavljević, M., Zengin, G., Yan, L., Gašić, U., Kojić, P., Torbica, A., Belović, M., Zeković, Z., 2023. New biological and chemical insights into optimization of chamomile extracts by using artificial neural network (ANN) model. Plants. 2223-7747. 12 (6), 1211. doi:10.3390/plants12061211.

Cvetanović, A., Švarc-Gajić, J., Mašković, P., Savić, S., Nikolić, L., 2015. Antioxidant and biological activity of chamomile extracts obtained by different techniques: perspective of using superheated water for isolation of biologically active compounds. Ind. Crops Prod. 09266690. 65, 582–591. doi:10.1016/j.indcrop.2014.09.044.

da Silva Aragão, N., Marques, M.N., de Lima, B.R., de Aguiar Queiros, A., de Souza, E.B., Júnior, R.C.P., Paxiúba Duncan, W., Aguiar, J.P.L., de Souza Marinho, V., do Amaral Souza, F.D.C., 2025. Integrated chemical profiling of Camellia sinensis teas marketed in Brazil: physicochemical, mineral, and volatile compound characterization. Food Chem. Adv. 2772753X. 9, 101154. doi:10.1016/j.focha.2025.101154.

da Silva Prade, J., da Silva D'ávila, C.M., da Silva, T.C., et al., 2024. Cocoa (*Theobroma cacao* L.) photobiological effect on human fibroblast cells (HFF-1) exposed to ultraviolet B (UVB) radiation. J. Toxicol. Environ. Health A. doi:10.1080/15287394.2024.2439535.

Dai, Y.-L., Ying, L., Wang, Q., Niu, F.-J., Kun-Wei, L., Wang, Y.-Y., Wang, J., Zhou, C.-Z., Gao, L.-N., 2023. Chamomile: a review of its traditional uses, chemical constituents, pharmacological activities and quality control studies. Molecules. 1420-3049. 28 (1), 133. doi:10.3390/molecules28010133.

De Feo, M., Paladini, A., Ferri, C., Carducci, A., Pinto, R.D., Varrassi, G., Grassi, D., 2020. Anti-Inflammatory and anti-nociceptive effects of cocoa: a review on future perspectives in treatment of pain. Pain Ther. 2193-8237. 9 (1), 231–240. doi:10.1007/s40122-020-00165-5.

de Oliveira, P.R.S., Pretes, N.S., Ribeiro, A.C., Castro, J.C., Garcia, F.P., Nakamura, C.V., Bona, E., Mikcha, J.M.G., Junior, M.M., de Abreu Filho, B.A., 2024. Comparative assessment of antibacterial activity of *Matricaria chamomilla* L. extract, nisin and of its combination against Alicyclobacillus spp. Food Microbiol. 10959998. 124. Available from: https://www.sciencedirect.com/science/journal/07400020. doi:10.1016/j.fm.2024.104597.

Desvita, H., Faisal, M., Mahidin, S., 2022. Antimicrobial potential of wood vinegar from cocoa pod shells (*Theobroma cacao* L.) against *Candida albicans* and *Aspergillus Niger*. Mater. Today Proc. 22147853. 63, S210. doi:10.1016/j.matpr.2022.02.410.

Dong, F., Yang, Z., Baldermann, S., Kajitani, Y., Ota, S., Kasuga, H., Imazeki, Y., Ohnishi, T., Watanabe, N., 2012. Characterization of l-phenylalanine metabolism to acetophenone and 1-phenylethanol in the flowers of *Camellia sinensis* using stable isotope labeling. J. Plant Physiol. 01761617. 169 (3), 217–225. doi:10.1016/j.jplph.2011.12.003.

Draelos, Z.D., Draelos, M.M., Feng, S., Madera, Z., Chen, M., 2024. Topical antioxidant cocoa polyphenol skin penetration. J. Cosmet. Dermatol. 14732165. 23 (12), 4072–4076. Available from: http://onlinelibrary.wiley.com/journal/10.1111/(ISSN)1473-2165. doi:10.1111/jocd.16637.

Earthwise Beauty Nap In The Meadow Face Serum, n.d. https://incidecoder.com/products/earthwise-beauty-nap-in-the-meadow-face-serum. Accessed 13 Apr 2026.

Edo, G.I., Samuel, P.O., Oloni, G.O., Ezekiel, G.O., Onoharigho, F.O., Oghenegueke, O., Nwachukwu, S.C., Rapheal, O.A., Ajokpaoghene, M.O., Okolie, M.C., Ajakaye, R.S., Ndudi, W., Igbodo, P.C., 2023. Review on the biological and bioactive components of cocoa (*Theobroma cacao*). insight on food, health and nutrition. Nat. Resour. Hum. Health 25831194. 3 (4), 426–448. Available from: https://www.nrfhh.com/pdf-174302-96666?filename=Review%20on%20the%20Biological.pdf. doi:10.53365/nrfhh/174302.

El Mihyaoui, A., da Silva, J.C.G.E., Charfi, S., Emilia Candela Castillo, M., Lamarti, A., Arnao, M.B., 2022. Chamomile (*Matricaria chamomilla* L.): a review of ethnomedicinal use, phytochemistry and pharmacological uses. Life. 2075-1729. 12 (4), 479. doi:10.3390/life12040479.

El-Saadony, M.T., Saad, A.M., Mohammed, D.M., Alkafaas, S.S., El-Mageed, T.A.A., Fahmy, M.A., Ahmed, A.E., Algopishi, U.B., Abu-Elsaoud, A.M., Mosa, W.F.A., AbuQamar, S.F., El-Tarabily, K.A., 2025. Plant bioactive compounds: extraction, biological activities, immunological, nutritional aspects, food application, and human health benefits—A comprehensive review. Front. Nutr. 2296861X. 12. Available from: https://journal.frontiersin.org/journal/nutrition. doi:10.3389/fnut.2025.1659743.

Elias, M.L., Israeli, A.F., Madan, R., 2023. Caffeine in skincare: its role in skin cancer, sun protection, and cosmetics. Indian J. Dermatol. 19983611. 68 (5), 546–550. Available from: http://www.e-ijd.org. doi:10.4103/ijd.ijd_166_22.

Emmetsberger, J., Ionita-Manzatu, V., Mammone, T., 2018. Caffeine enhances epidermal hydration by increasing the transepithelial electric potential and electroosmosis. J. Am. Acad. Dermatol. 01909622. 79 (3), AB60. doi:10.1016/j.jaad.2018.05.278.

Essence Coffee To Glow Coffee Body Scrub, n.d. https://incidecoder.com/products/essence-coffee-to-glow-coffee-body-scrub. Accessed 13 Apr 2026.

Febrinasari, R.P., Benedictus, B., Tan, K., Mardhiati, Y., Putri, S.K., Choiri, S., Wahyuni, D.S.C., 2025. Green tea as a cosmetic agent for skin aging: a scoping review. Avicenna J. Phytomed. 22287949. 14 (5), 1393–1407. Available from: http://ajp.mums.ac.ir/. doi:10.22038/ajp.2025.25449.

Freitas, V.V., Borges, L.L.R., Vidigal, M.C.T.R., Dos Santos, M.H., Stringheta, P.C., 2024. Coffee: a comprehensive overview of origin, market, and the quality process. Trends Food Sci. Technol. 09242244. 146. Available from: https://www.sciencedirect.com/science/journal/09242244. doi:10.1016/j.tifs.2024.104411.

Frezyderm Chamomile Bath, n.d. https://incidecoder.com/products/frezyderm-chamomile-bath. Accessed 13 Apr 2026.

Gălbău, C.Ş., Irimie, M., Neculau, A.E., Dima, L., da Silva, L.P., Vârciu, M., Badea, M., 2024. The potential of plant extracts used in cosmetic product applications—antioxidants delivery and mechanism of actions. Antioxidants 20763921. 13 (11). Available from: https://www.mdpi.com/journal/antioxidants. doi:10.3390/antiox13111425.

Garbossa, W.A.C., Campos, P.M.B.G.M., 2016. Euterpe oleracea, *Matricaria chamomilla*, and *Camellia sinensis* as promising ingredients for development of skin care formulations. Ind. Crops Prod. 09266690. 83, 1–10. Available from: https://www.elsevier.com/inca/publications/store/5/2/2/8/2/5. doi:10.1016/j.indcrop.2015.11.026.

Garcia, L.B., Pires, G.A., Oliveira, D.A.J., Silva, L.A.O., Gomes, A.F., Amaral, J.G., Pereira, G.R., Ruela, A.L.M., 2021. Incorporation of glycolic extract of cocoa beans (*Theobroma cacao* L.) into microemulsions and emulgels for skincare. Ind. Crops Prod. 09266690. 161. Available from: https://www.elsevier.com/inca/publications/store/5/2/2/8/2/5. doi:10.1016/j.indcrop.2020.113181.

Gautam, D.G., Shelke, P.G., Hatwar, P.R., Bakal, R.L., Shinde, N.M., 2024. Phytochemicals in hair care: a review of natural ingredients and their applications. GSC Biol. Pharm. Sci. 25813250. 29 (2), 331–340. doi:10.30574/gscbps.2024.29.2.0449.

Gianeti, M.D., Mercurio, D.G., Campos, P.M.B.G.M., 2013. The use of green tea extract in cosmetic formulations: not only an antioxidant active ingredient. Dermatol. Ther. 15298019. 26 (3), 267–271. doi:10.1111/j.1529-8019.2013.01552.x.

Hasan, M.R., Haque, M.M., Hoque, M.A., Sultana, S., Rahman, M.M., Shaikh, M.A.A., Sarker, M.K.U., 2024. Antioxidant activity study and GC-MS profiling of *Camellia sinensis* Linn. Heliyon. 24058440. 10 (1), e23514. doi:10.1016/j.heliyon.2023.e23514.

Herman, A., Herman, A.P., Domagalska, B.W., Młynarczyk, A., 2013. Essential oils and herbal extracts as antimicrobial agents in cosmetic emulsion. Indian J. Microbiol. 00468991. 53 (2), 232–237. Available from: http://www.springerlink.com/content/0046-8991/. doi:10.1007/s12088-012-0329-0.

Hiraga, Y., Yoshida, C., Aoki, K., Watanabe, M., 2025. Efficient decaffeination of green coffee beans using pressure swing supercritical CO_2 extraction. Innov. Food Sci. Emerg. Technol. 14668564. 104, 104154. doi:10.1016/j.ifset.2025.104154.

Hong, Y.H., Jung, E.Y., Shin, K.S., Yu, K.W., Chang, U.J., Suh, H.J., 2013. Tannase-converted green tea catechins and their anti-wrinkle activity in humans. J. Cosmet. Dermatol. 14732165. 12 (2), 137–143. doi:10.1111/jocd.12038.

İşitez, N., 2026. The anticancer potential of *Sideritis akmanii* extract in melanoma cells via oxidative stress and cytokine regulation. Health Sci. Q. 2791-6022. 6 (1), 175–184. doi:10.26900/hsq.3006.

Janda, K., Jakubczyk, K., Baranowska-Bosiacka, I., Kapczuk, P., Kochman, J., Rębacz-Maron, E., Gutowska, I., 2020. Mineral composition and antioxidant potential of coffee beverages depending on the brewing method. Foods. 2304-8158. 9 (2), 121. doi:10.3390/foods9020121.

Joseph, A., Olakunle, F., Gimba, U., et al., 2024. Studies on nutritional and medicinal properties of chamomile flower, pumpkin fruit and maca root. Afr. J. Biol. Chem. Phys. Sci. 3, 88–97.

Jurado-Beizaga, E., Alvarez-Yanamango, E., Herrera-Calderon, O., Ibañez, A., 2026. Optimisation of the microwave-assisted extraction process of bioactive compounds with antioxidant activity from cocoa pod husk (Theobroma cacao L.). Sustain. Food Technol. 2753-8095. 4 (2), 1869–1882. doi:10.1039/d5fb00924c.

Kamgang Nzekoue, F., Khamitova, G., Angeloni, S., Nácher Sempere, A., Tao, J., Maggi, F., Xiao, J., Sagratini, G., Vittori, S., Caprioli, G., 2020. Spent coffee grounds: a potential commercial source of phytosterols. Food Chem. 03088146. 325, 126836. doi:10.1016/j.foodchem.2020.126836.

Katiyar, S., Elmets, C.A., Katiyar, S.K., 2007. Green tea and skin cancer: photoimmunology, angiogenesis and DNA repair. J. Nutr. Biochem. 09552863. 18 (5), 287–296. doi:10.1016/j.jnutbio.2006.08.004.

Kavin, T., Murugaiyah, V., Tan, J.K., Kassim, M.N.I., Ramakrishna, S., Vigneswari, S., 2025. Eco-friendly synthesis of silver nanoparticles using *Coffea arabica* husk for enhanced antibacterial and anti-cancer applications. Biomass Bioenergy. 09619534. 194, 107625. doi:10.1016/j.biombioe.2025.107625.

Kim, E., Hwang, K., Lee, J., Han, S.Y., Kim, E.-M., Park, J., Cho, J.Y., 2018. Skin protective effect of epigallocatechin gallate. Int. J. Mol. Sci. 1422-0067. 19 (1), 173. doi:10.3390/ijms19010173.

Klepacka, J., Tońska, E., Rafałowski, R., Czarnowska-Kujawska, M., Opara, B., 2021. Tea as a source of biologically active compounds in the human diet. Molecules. 1420-3049. 26 (5), 1487. doi:10.3390/molecules26051487.

Koch, W., Zagórska, J., Marzec, Z., Kukula-Koch, W., 2019. Applications of tea (*Camellia sinensis*) and its active constituents in cosmetics. Molecules. 1420-3049. 24 (23), 4277. doi:10.3390/molecules24234277.

Korres Olympus Tea Cleansing Foaming Cream, n.d. https://incidecoder.com/products/korres-olympus-tea-cleansing-foaming-cream. Accessed 13 Apr 2026.

Kosińska, A., Xie, Y., Diering, S., Héritier, J., Andlauer, W., 2012. Stability of phenolic compounds isolated from cocoa, green tea and strawberries in Hank's Balanced Salt Solution under cell culture conditions. Pol. J. Food Nutr. Sci. 1230-0322. 62 (2), 91–96. doi:10.2478/v10222-011-0048-y.

La vie en rose Bikini Cream ingredients (Explained), n.d. https://incidecoder.com/products/la-vie-en-rose-bikini-cream. Accessed 13 Apr 2026.

Lee, S.G., Nguyen, N.H., Lee, Y.I., Jung, I., Kim, I.A., Jang, H., Shin, H., Lee, J.H., 2024. The role of cacao powder in enhancing skin moisture and reducing wrinkles: a 12-week clinical trial and in vitro study. Curr. Issues Mol. Biol. 14673045. 46 (11), 12574–12587. Available from: https://www.mdpi.com/journal/cimb. doi:10.3390/cimb46110746.

Liu, Y., Chen, M., Yimin, L., Feng, X., Chen, Y., Lin, L., 2022. Analysis of lipids in green coffee by ultra-performance liquid chromatography–time-of-flight tandem mass spectrometry. Molecules. 1420-3049. 27 (16), 5271. doi:10.3390/molecules27165271.

Liu, Y., Guo, C., Zang, E., Shi, R., Liu, Q., Zhang, M., Zhang, K., Minhui, L., 2023. Review on herbal tea as a functional food: classification, active compounds, biological activity, and industrial status. J. Future Foods. 27725669. 3 (3), 206–219. doi:10.1016/j.jfutfo.2023.02.002.

Lu, Y.P., Lou, Y.R., Xie, J.G., Peng, Q.Y., Liao, J., Yang, C.S., Huang, M.T., Conney, A.H., 2002. Topical applications of caffeine or (-)-epigallocatechin gallate (EGCG) inhibit carcinogenesis and selectively increase apoptosis in UVB-induced skin tumors in mice. Proc. Natl. Acad. Sci. U. S. A. 99 (19), 12455–12460. doi:10.1073/pnas.182429899.

Luo, Q., Zhang, J.R., Li, H.B., Wu, D.T., Geng, F., Corke, H., Wei, X.L., Gan, R.Y., 2020. Green extraction of antioxidant polyphenols from green tea (*Camellia sinensis*). Antioxidants 20763921. 9 (9), 1–15. Available from: https://www.mdpi.com/2076-3921/9/9/785/pdf. doi:10.3390/antiox9090785.

Makiso, M.U., Tola, Y.B., Ogah, O., Endale, F.L., 2024. Bioactive compounds in coffee and their role in lowering the risk of major public health consequences: a review. Food Sci. Nutr. 20487177. 12 (2), 734–764. Available from: https://onlinelibrary.wiley.com/journal/10.1002/%28ISSN%292048-7177. doi:10.1002/fsn3.3848.

Martínez-Inda, B., Jiménez-Moreno, N., Esparza, I., Ancín-Azpilicueta, C., 2025. Coffee and cocoa by-products as valuable sources of bioactive compounds: the influence of ethanol on extraction. Antioxidants. 2076-3921. 14 (1), 42. doi:10.3390/antiox14010042.

Mazzafera, P., Schimpl, F., Kiyota, E., 2019. Proteins of coffee beans: recent advances. In: Farah, A., Farah, A. (Eds.), Coffee: Production, Quality and Chemistry. The Royal Society of Chemistry, pp. 429–444. doi:10.1039/9781782622437-00429.

Mello, G.H.D., D'Ávila, C.M.D.S., Viana, A.R., Krause, L.M.F., Cadoná, F.C., 2022. Cocoa presents cytotoxicity against melanoma cancer cell lines (A-375 e B16-F10) and improves chemotherapy activity by increasing oxidative stress. J. Food Biochem. 17454514. 46 (12). Available from: http://onlinelibrary.wiley.com/journal/10.1111/(ISSN)1745-4514. doi:10.1111/jfbc.14512.

Michalak, M., 2022. Plant-derived antioxidants: significance in skin health and the ageing process. Int. J. Mol. Sci. 1422-0067. 23 (2), 585. doi:10.3390/ijms23020585.

Mustarichie, R., Hasanah, A.N., Wilar, G., Gozali, D., Saptarini, N.M., Constantino, V.R.-L., 2022. New hair growth cream formulation with cocoa pod peel (*Theobroma cacao* L.). Sci. World J. 1537-744X. 2022, 1–7. doi:10.1155/2022/2299725.

Neogen Green Tea Real Fresh Foam Cleanser, n.d. https://incidecoder.com/products/neogen-green-tea-real-fresh-foam-cleanser. Accessed 13 Apr 2026.

Niknam, S., Tofighi, Z., Faramarzi, M.A., Abdollahifar, M.A., Sajadi, E., Dinarvand, R., Toliyat, T., 2021. Polyherbal combination for wound healing: *Matricaria chamomilla* L. and *Punica granatum* L. Daru J. Pharm. Sci. 20082231. 29 (1), 133–145. Available from: https://rd.springer.com/journal/40199. doi:10.1007/s40199-021-00392-x.

Niu, L., Ziqiang, L., Fan, W., Zhong, X., Peng, M., Liu, Z., 2022. Nano-strategies for enhancing the bioavailability of tea polyphenols: preparation, applications, and challenges. Foods. 2304-8158. 11 (3), 387. doi:10.3390/foods11030387.

Nivea Cocoa Nourish, n.d. https://incidecoder.com/products/nivea-cocoa-nourish. Accessed 13 Apr 2026.

Nóbrega, A.T., Wagemaker, T.A., Maia Campos, P.M., 2013. Antioxidant activity of *Matricaria chamomilla* L. extract and clinical efficacy of cosmetic formulations containing this extract and its isolated compounds: actividade antioxidante do extracto de *Matricaria chamomilla* L. e eficácia clínica de formulações cosméticas contendo este extracto e seus compostos isolados. J. Biomed. Biopharm. Res. 10, 249–261. doi:10.19277/BBR.10.2.69.

Nuxe body Rêve de thé Exalting Fragrant Water, n.d. https://incidecoder.com/products/nuxe-body-reve-de-the-exalting-fragrant-water. Accessed 13 Apr 2026.

Nuxe Contour Des Yeux Prodigieux Anti-Fatigue Moisturizing Eye Cream, n.d. https://incidecoder.com/products/nuxe-contour-des-yeux-prodigieux-anti-fatigue-moisturizing-eye-cream. Accessed 13 Apr 2026.

Ognyanov, M., Remoroza, C.A., Schols, H.A., Petkova, N.T., Georgiev, Y.N., 2021. Structural study of a pectic polysaccharide fraction isolated from "mountain tea" (*Sideritis scardica* Griseb.). Carbohydr. Polym. 01448617. 260, 117798. doi:10.1016/j.carbpol.2021.117798.

Oracz, J., Nebesny, E., Żyżelewicz, D., 2014. Effect of roasting conditions on the fat, tocopherol, and phytosterol content and antioxidant capacity of the lipid fraction from cocoa beans of different *Theobroma cacao* L. cultivars. Eur. J. Lipid Sci. Technol. 1438-7697. 116 (8), 1002–1014. doi:10.1002/ejlt.201300474.

Oussou, K.F., Guclu, G., Kelebek, H., Selli, S., 2023. Valorization of cocoa, tea and coffee processing by-products-wastes. Adv. Food Nutr. Res. 107, 91–130. Available from: http://www.elsevier.com/wps/find/bookdescription.cws_home/704624/description#description. doi:10.1016/bs.afnr.2023.03.003.

Padule, K., Shinde, S., Chitlange, S., Giram, P., Nagore, D., 2022. The advancement of herbal-based nanomedicine for hair. Cosmetics. 2079-9284. 9 (6), 118. doi:10.3390/cosmetics9060118.

Palatty, P.L., Baliga, M.S., Rajeev, A.G., Haniadka, R., Bhat, H.P., Pai, K.S.R., Rai, M.P., Geevarughese, N.M., Arora, R., 2013. *Camellia sinensis* (Tea) in the Prevention of UV-induced Carcinogenesis: A Mechanistic Overview Bioactive Dietary Factors and Plant Extracts in Dermatology. Humana Press Inc, India, pp. 367–384. Available from: http://www.springer.com/in/book/9781627031677. doi:10.1007/978-1-62703-167-7_34.

Papanikolaou, K., Kouloridas, K., Rosvoglou, A., Gatsas, A., Georgakouli, K., Deli, C.K., Draganidis, D., Argyropoulou, A., Michailidis, D., Fatouros, I.G., Jamurtas, A.Z., 2024. Characterization of the *Sideritis scardica* extract SidTea+™ and its effect on physiological profile, metabolic health and redox biomarkers in healthy adults: a randomized, double-blind, placebo-controlled study. Molecules. 1420-3049. 29 (5), 1113. doi:10.3390/molecules29051113.

Patel, P.K., Sarma, R., Gogoi, B., Singh, S.K., Handique, N., Babu, A., 2023. Phytosterol composition in the oil of bi-clonal seed stocks of tea (*Camellia sinensis* L.) in north east India. J. Plant. Crops. 2454-8480. 51 (3), 128–132. doi:10.25081/jpc.2023.v51.i3.8339.

Pavlova, M., Dyankova, S., Solak, A., et al., 2021. Antioxidant activity of Mursalski tea (*Sideritis scardica* Griseb.) extracts. J Mt Agric Balk 24, 484–500. https://www.researchgate.net/publication/357569069.

Plyduang, T., Monton, C., Suksaeree, J., 2026. Sustainable green extraction approaches for herbal phytochemicals supporting environmentally friendly and climate responsive product development. Sustain. Chem. Clim. Action. 27728269. 8, 100184. doi:10.1016/j.scca.2026.100184.

Purushothaman, V.K., Wen, T.J., Anne, M., Kayarohanam, S., Saleem, T.S.M., Chellammal, H.S.J., Janakiraman, A.K., 2025. Cocoa butter as an effective moisturizer for topical cream. J. Nat. Remedies 23203358. 25 (2), 391–401. Available from: https://informaticsjournals.co.in/index.php/jnr/article/download/45897/32288. doi:10.18311/jnr/2025/45897.

Putri, M., Hariati, A., Basir, A.A., 2025. Sunscreen cream formulation from green tea extract (*Camellia sinensis*) and SPF value test. Int. J. Health Sci. 2987-0836. 3 (3), 522–530. doi:10.59585/ijhs.v3i3.794.

Rahayu, Y.C., Setiawatie, E.M., Rahayu, R.P., Cholid, Z., Rachmawati, D., Sulistyani, E., Hamidah, S., 2024. Wound healing potential of cocoa pod husk (*Theobroma cacao* L.) extract gel on tooth extraction socket in rats. Malays. J. Med. Health Sci. 26369346. 20, 11–16. Available from: DPR240723-004431.

Razola-Díaz, M.D.C., Aznar-Ramos, M.J., Verardo, V., Melgar-Locatelli, S., Castilla-Ortega, E., Rodríguez-Pérez, C., 2023. Exploring the nutritional composition and bioactive compounds in different cocoa powders. Antioxidants. 2076-3921. 12 (3), 716. doi:10.3390/antiox12030716.

Reddy, B.H.V., Hussain, S.M.S., Hussain, M.S., Kumar, R.N., Gupta, J., 2025. Essential oils in cosmetics: antioxidant properties and advancements through nanoformulations. Pharmacol. Res. Nat. Prod. 29501997. 6. Available from: https://www.sciencedirect.com/journal/pharmacological-research-natural-products. doi:10.1016/j.prenap.2025.100192.

Ribeiro, H., Marto, J., Raposo, S., Agapito, M., Isaac, V., Chiari, B.G., Lisboa, P.F., Paiva, A., Barreiros, S., Simões, P., 2013. From coffee industry waste materials to skin-friendly products with improved skin fat levels. Eur. J. Lipid Sci. Technol. 1438-7697. 115 (3), 330–336. doi:10.1002/ejlt.201200239.

Rodrigues, R., Oliveira, M.B.P.P., Alves, R.C., 2023. Chlorogenic acids and caffeine from coffee by-products: a review on skincare applications. Cosmetics 20799284. 10 (1). Available from: https://www.mdpi.com/journal/cosmetics. doi:10.3390/cosmetics10010012.

Ruse, G., Jîjie, A.R., Moacă, E.A., Pătraşcu, D., Ardelean, F., Jojic, A.A., Ardelean, S., Tchiakpe-Antal, D.S., 2025. *Coffea arabica*: an emerging active ingredient in dermato-cosmetic applications. Romania Pharm. 14248247. 18 (2). Available from: https://www.mdpi.com/journal/pharmaceuticals. doi:10.3390/ph18020171.

Sabino, N.L., Fogarin, H.M., Murillo-Franco, S.L., Bérgamo, M.O., Moreno, L.V., da Silva, D.D.V., Funari, C.S., Dussán, K.J., 2025. Investigating the influence of solvents and extraction methods on the efficacy of phenolic compound recovery from spent coffee grounds. Sep. Purif. Technol. 13835866. 362, 131793. doi:10.1016/j.seppur.2025.131793.

Sah, A., Naseef, P.P., Kuruniyan, M.S., Jain, G.K., Zakir, F., Aggarwal, G., 2022. A comprehensive study of therapeutic applications of chamomile. Pharmaceuticals. 1424-8247. 15 (10), 1284. doi:10.3390/ph15101284.

Sak, K., Nguyen, T.H., Viet Duc, H., Thi Thao, D., Raal, A., Schumacher, U., 2017. Cytotoxic effect of chamomile (*Matricaria recutita*) and marigold (*Calendula officinalis*) extracts on human melanoma SK-MEL-2 and epidermoid carcinoma KB cells. Cogent Med. 2331-205X. 4 (1), 1333218. doi:10.1080/2331205x.2017.1333218.

Sang, S.H., Akowuah, G.A., Liew, K.B., Lee, S.K., Keng, J.W., Lee, S.K., Yon, J.A.L., Tan, C.S., Chew, Y.L., 2023. Natural alternatives from your garden for hair care: revisiting the benefits of tropical herbs. Heliyon 24058440. 9 (11). Available from: http://www.journals.elsevier.com/heliyon/. doi:10.1016/j.heliyon.2023.e21876.

Santos, É.M.D., Macedo, L.M.D., Tundisi, L.L., Ataide, J.A., Camargo, G.A., Alves, R.C., Oliveira, M.B.P.P., Mazzola, P.G., 2021. Coffee by-products in topical formulations: a review. Trends Food Sci. Technol. 09242244. 111, 280–291. Available from: http://www.elsevier.com/wps/find/journaldescription.cws_home/601278/description#description. doi:10.1016/j.tifs.2021.02.064.

Sarma, N., Gogoi, R., Begum, T., Lal, M., Perveen, K., Alsahikh, N.A., Alsulami, J.A., 2023. A study on the chemical profile of cultivated chamomile (*Matricaria chamomilla* L.) flower essential oil from North East India with special emphasis on its pharmacological importance. J. Essent. Oil-Bear. Plants 0972060X. 26 (3), 745–760. Available from: http://www.tandfonline.com/loi/teop20?open=16&repitition=0#vol_16. doi:10.1080/0972060X.2023.2239289.

Sato, F., Wong, C.P., Furuya, K., Kuzu, C., Kimura, R., Udo, T., Honda, H., Yang, J., 2022. Anti-skin aging activities of *Sideritis scardica* and 3 flavonoids with an uncommon 8-hydroxyl moiety. Nat. Prod. Commun. 1934-578X. 17 (5). doi:10.1177/1934578x221094910.

Shabani, L., Beadini, S., Beadini, N., Hajrullai-Musliu, Z., 2022. Analysis of the fatty acid content of *Sideritis scardica* Gris. using GC-FID. Thalassia Salent. 44, 147–154. doi:10.1285/i15910725v44p147.

Sitarek, P., Merecz-Sadowska, A., Sikora, J., Osicka, W., Śpiewak, I., Picot, L., Kowalczyk, T., 2024. Exploring the therapeutic potential of *Theobroma cacao* L.: insights from in vitro, in vivo, and nanoparticle studies on anti-inflammatory and anticancer effects. Antioxidants. 2076-3921. 13 (11), 1376. doi:10.3390/antiox13111376.

Sklirou, A.D., Angelopoulou, M.T., Argyropoulou, A., Chaita, E., Boka, V.I., Cheimonidi, C., Niforou, K., Mavrogonatou, E., Pratsinis, H., Kalpoutzakis, E., Aligiannis, N., Kletsas, D., Trougakos, I.P., Skaltsounis, A.L., 2021. Phytochemical study and in vitro screening focusing on the anti-aging features of various plants of the Greek flora. Antioxidants. 2076-3921. 10 (8), 1206. doi:10.3390/antiox10081206.

Soares, T.F., Oliveira, M.B.P.P., 2022. Cocoa by-products: characterization of bioactive compounds and beneficial health effects. Molecules 14203049. 27 (5). Available from: https://www.mdpi.com/1420-3049/27/5/1625/pdf. doi:10.3390/molecules27051625.

STARSKIN SilkmudTM Green Tea Clay Anti-Aging Liftaway Mud Face Sheet Mask, n.d. https://incidecoder.com/products/starskin-silkmud-tm-green-tea-clay-anti-aging-liftaway-mud-face-sheet-mask. Accessed 13 Apr 2026.

Sui, L., Wang, Y., Zhang, X., Yuan, M., Hong, J., Jinlian, L., 2025. Phytochemicals of Roman chamomile: antioxidant, anti-aging, and whitening activities of distillation residues. Open Life Sci. 2391-5412. 20 (1). doi:10.1515/biol-2025-1177.

Sunanta, P., Leksawasdi, N., Sommano, S.R., Taesuwan, S., Rachtanapun, P., Techapun, C., Sumonsiri, N., Khemacheewakul, J., 2026. Valorization of cocoa bean shell into high-value bioactive extracts as functional food ingredients using green extraction techniques: enzyme-assisted and ultrasound-assisted methods. Appl. Food Res. 27725022. 6 (1), 101813. doi:10.1016/j.afres.2026.101813.

Szendzielorz, E., Spiewak, R., 2025. Caffeine as an active molecule in cosmetic products for hair loss: its mechanisms of action in the context of hair physiology and pathology. Molecules. 1420-3049. 30 (1), 167. doi:10.3390/molecules30010167.

Tadić, V., Bojović, D., Arsić, I., Đorđević, S., Aksentijevic, K., Stamenić, M., Janković, S., 2012. Chemical and antimicrobial evaluation of supercritical and conventional *Sideritis scardica* Griseb., Lamiaceae extracts. Molecules. 1420-3049. 17 (3), 2683–2703. doi:10.3390/molecules17032683.

Tantapakul, C., Khat-udomkiri, N., Sitthichai, P., Chomsak, A., Thananusak, N., Phukhatmuen, P., Vinardell, M.P., Sripisut, T., 2024. Exploring the physicochemical properties of polysaccharides extracted from cocoa pod husk waste and their efficacy in skin hydration. Ind. Crops Prod. 09266690. 222, 119940. doi:10.1016/j.indcrop.2024.119940.

Tasheva, K., Georgieva, A., Denev, P., Dimitrova, L., Dimitrova, M., Misheva, S., Petkova-Kirova, P., Lazarova, M., Petrova, M., 2023. Antioxidant and antitumor potential of micropropagated balkan endemic *Sideritis scardica* griseb. Plants. 2223-7747. 12 (23), 3924. doi:10.3390/plants12233924.

Tiwari, V., More, S., Gulia, S., Sunder Selwyn, T., Ramachandran, M., 2023. Assessing medicinal plant extracts in strengthening anti-dandruff shampoo: an analysis using multi-criteria decision-making techniques. Int. J. Pharm. Qual. Assur. 0975-9506. 14 (04), 1136–1143. doi:10.25258/ijpqa.14.4.48.

Torres-Moreno, M., Torrescasana, E., Salas-Salvadó, J., Blanch, C., 2015. Nutritional composition and fatty acids profile in cocoa beans and chocolates with different geographical origin and processing conditions. Food Chem. 03088146. 166, 125–132. doi:10.1016/j.foodchem.2014.05.141.

Tsiapali, O.I., Kontaxi, N.I., Pavlidis, K., Ofrydopoulou, A., Prokopiou, V., Letsiou, S., Kosheleva, R.I., Mitropoulos, A., Tsoupras, A., 2025. Anti-inflammatory and antioxidant properties of anti-UV creams enriched with natural extracts from avocado, apple, and kiwi by-products, with and without nanobubbles. Cosmetics 20799284. 12 (5). Available from: https://www.mdpi.com/journal/cosmetics. doi:10.3390/cosmetics12050231.

Tsibranska, I., Tylkowski, B., Kochanov, R., Alipieva, K., 2011. Extraction of biologically active compounds from *Sideritis* ssp. L. Food Bioprod. Process. 09603085. 89 (4), 273–280. doi:10.1016/j.fbp.2010.10.004.

Tsoupras, A., Adamantidi, T., Finos, M.A., Philippopoulos, A., Detopoulou, P., Tsopoki, I., Kynatidou, M., Demopoulos, C.A., 2024. Re-assessing the role of platelet activating factor and its inflammatory signaling and inhibitors in cancer and anti-cancer strategies. Front. Biosci. Landmark 27686698. 29 (10). Available from: https://www.imrpress.com/journal/FBL/29/10. doi:10.31083/j.fbl2910345.

Tsoupras, A., Lordan, R., Harrington, J., Pienaar, R., Devaney, K., Heaney, S., Koidis, A., Zabetakis, I., 2020. The effects of oxidation on the antithrombotic properties of tea lipids against PAF, thrombin, collagen, and ADP. Foods. 2304-8158. 9 (4), 385. doi:10.3390/foods9040385.

Tsoupras, A., Zabetakis, I., Lordan, R., 2019. Platelet aggregometry assay for evaluating the effects of platelet agonists and antiplatelet compounds on platelet function in vitro. MethodsX. 22150161. 6, 63–70. doi:10.1016/j.mex.2018.12.012.

Tunjung-Sari, A.B., Wahyudi, T., Mufida, D.C., et al., 2016. Use of cocoa ethanolic extract for treatment of Staphylococcal infection in rabbit-skin model. Pelita Perkeb. Coffee Cocoa Res. J. 32, 34–42. doi:10.22302/iccri.jur.pelitaperkebunan.v32i1.214.

Tušek, K., Valinger, D., Jurina, T., Sokač Cvetnić, T., Gajdoš Kljusurić, J., Benković, M., 2024. Bioactives in cocoa: novel findings, health benefits, and extraction techniques. Separations. 2297-8739. 11 (4), 128. doi:10.3390/separations11040128.

Uba, J.O., Onyeike, E.N., Ogunka-Nnoka, C.U., Ikewuchi, C.C., 2022. Bioactive and nutrient composition of *Camellia sinensis* (Tea plant) leaves. J. Med. Plants Stud. 23940530. 10 (6), 06–14. doi:10.22271/plants.2022.v10.i6a.1481.

Ud-Din, S., Foden, P., Mazhari, M., Al-Habba, S., Baguneid, M., Bulfone-Paus, S., McGeorge, D., Ardeshir Bayat, A.D.-B., 2019. Randomized trial shows the role of zonal priming and direct topical application of epigallocatechin-3-gallate in the modulation of cutaneous scarring in human skin. J. Invest. Dermatol. 0022202X. 139 (8), 1680. doi:10.1016/j.jid.2019.01.030.

Vera, W., Quevedo-Olaya, J.L., Samaniego-Rafaele, C., Culqui-Arce, C., Jesús Sánchez-Chero, M., Quispe-Santivañez, G.W., Salvador-Reyes, R., 2026. Emerging technologies for sustainable extraction and valorization of bioactive compounds from coffee beans and by-products: principles, bioactivity enhancement, and industrial perspectives. Biomass. 2673-8783. 6 (2), 18. doi:10.3390/biomass6020018.

Vikhe, D.S., Kape, S., Gaikwad, R., Jamdhade, M., 2025. Standardizing herbal cosmetics: analytical approaches, regulatory complexities, and emerging trends. Int. J. Pharm. Sci. 03. doi:10.5281/zenodo.15152062.

Wang, C., Han, J., Yuting, P., Wang, X., 2022. Tea (*Camellia sinensis*): a review of nutritional composition, potential applications, and omics research. Appl. Sci. 2076-3417. 12 (12), 5874. doi:10.3390/app12125874.

Wang, Q., Gui-Lin, H., Qiu, M.-H., Cao, J., Xiong, W.-Y., 2024. Coffee, tea, and cocoa in obesity prevention: mechanisms of action and future prospects. Curr. Res. Food Sci. 26659271. 8, 100741. doi:10.1016/j.crfs.2024.100741.

Wang, Y., Sun, D., Chen, H., Qian, L., Ping, X., 2011. Fatty acid composition and antioxidant activity of tea (*Camellia sinensis* L.) seed oil extracted by optimized supercritical carbon dioxide. Int. J. Mol. Sci. 1422-0067. 12 (11), 7708–7719. doi:10.3390/ijms12117708.

Xu, F.W., Lv, Y.L., Zhong, Y.F., Xue, Y.N., Wang, Y., Zhang, L.Y., Hu, X., Tan, W.Q., 2021. Beneficial effects of green tea EGCG on skin wound healing: a comprehensive review. Molecules 14203049. 26 (20). Available from: https://www.mdpi.com/1420-3049/26/20/6123/pdf. doi:10.3390/molecules26206123.

Yoon, H.S., Kim, J.R., Park, G.Y., Kim, J.E., Lee, D.H., Lee, K.W., Chung, J.H., 2016. Cocoa flavanol supplementation influences skin conditions of photo-aged women: a 24-week double-blind, randomized, controlled trial. J. Nutr. 15416100. 146 (1), 46–50. Available from: http://jn.nutrition.org/content/146/1/46.full.pdf. doi:10.3945/jn.115.217711.

Yücer, R., Schröder, A., Topçu, G., Efferth, T., 2025. Identification of anti-inflammatory and anti-cancer compounds targeting the NF-κB-NLRP3 inflammasome pathway from a phytochemical library of the Sideritis genus. J. Ethnopharmacol. 03788741. 338 (Pt 2), 119074. doi:10.1016/j.jep.2024.119074.

Yuniati, Y., Ningtyas, R.W., Saraswati, E., Agustini, M., Mahfud, M., 2025. Simultaneous extraction of caffeine and chlorogenic acid from Arabica coffee using microwave-assisted extraction. Food Chem. Adv. 2772753X. 9, 101158. doi:10.1016/j.focha.2025.101158.

Zhang, L., Wang, X., Manickavasagan, A., Lim, L.-T., 2022. Extraction and physicochemical characteristics of high pressure-assisted cold brew coffee. Future Foods. 26668335. 5, 100113. doi:10.1016/j.fufo.2022.100113.

Zhao, T., Chao, L., Wang, S., Song, X., 2022. Green tea (*Camellia sinensis*): a review of its phytochemistry, pharmacology, and toxicology. Molecules. 1420-3049. 27 (12), 3909. doi:10.3390/molecules27123909.

Zissi, L., Dimaki, V.D., Birba, V.S., Galani, V.C., Magafa, V., Hatziantoniou, S., Lamari, F.N., 2025. Natural deep eutectic solvents as green alternatives for extracting bioactive compounds from sideritis taxa with potential cosmetic applications. Antioxidants 20763921. 14 (1). Available from: https://www.mdpi.com/journal/antioxidants. doi:10.3390/antiox14010068.

Żyżelewicz, D., Kulbat-Warycha, K., Oracz, J., Żyżelewicz, K., 2020. Polyphenols and other bioactive compounds of sideritis plants and their potential biological activity. Molecules. 1420-3049. 25 (16), 3763. doi:10.3390/molecules25163763.

Chapter 8

Spices

Rony Aad and Simone Vesentini
Politecnico di Milano, Department of Electronics, Information, and Bioengineering, Milan, Italy

1 Introduction

In recent years, the cosmetics industry has witnessed a notable shift toward biofunctional cosmetics, a category of products that extend beyond traditional esthetics to deliver tangible physiological and health benefits to the skin. These products typically incorporate bioactive compounds known for their antioxidant, antiaging, UV-protective, antiinflammatory, antimicrobial, wound healing, and antiwrinkle properties (Guldiken et al., 2018; Yang and Ling, 2025). Unlike pharmaceuticals, biofunctional cosmetics remain within the cosmetic classification while offering therapeutic-like benefits, placing them within the emerging "cosmeceutical" domain, a fast-growing segment of the global personal care market (Dureja et al., 2005). Biofunctional cosmetics respond to increasing consumer demands for solutions addressing premature aging, oxidative stress, sensitive skin, pigmentation disorders, and environmentally induced skin damage (Naser, 2021). The active ingredients used in these formulations are generally perceived as safe, multifunctional, and supported by growing scientific evidence of efficacy (Lau et al., 2024). Among these, bioactives derived from natural sources, including spices, are gaining particular attention for their dual role in health promotion and cosmetic performance.

The cosmetics industry is recognized as one of the fastest-growing global sectors (Liu, 2022). In recent years, this industry has undergone a significant transformation, marked by a clear shift toward natural-based products (Alves et al., 2020). This transition reflects a broader paradigm shift driven by rising consumer awareness of chemical safety concerns, environmental sustainability, and regulatory pressures that increasingly discourage or restrict the use of harmful synthetic chemicals.

Consumers now actively seek products marketed as natural, clean, or green, which are commonly associated with lower toxicity, improved skin compatibility, and ecological responsibility (Dini and Laneri, 2021). In response, numerous brands have reformulated their products to eliminate synthetic preservatives, parabens, sulfates, and artificial fragrances, replacing them with plant-derived alternatives (Martins et al., 2025). Alongside consumer and regulatory drivers, the natural/organic cosmetics market has expanded substantially over the last five years, with recent estimates placing its value around USD 32–42 billion in 2023–2024 and projecting steady growth through 2030. Asia–Pacific remains the fastest-growing region, with strong momentum in Korea and India (Grand View Research, n.d.). Multiple overviews and application-focused reviews document the growing incorporation of spice-derived actives across topical and oral formats, ranging from essential oils and polyphenol-rich extracts to terpenoids and alkaloids, addressing their mechanisms of action, safety considerations, and formulation strategies (Fuloria et al., 2022; Ulanowska and Olas, 2021; Nabavi et al., 2015; Javed et al., 2024; Mandal et al., 2023). Within this evolving landscape, spices, long valued in culinary and medicinal traditions, are emerging as a particularly promising class of cosmetic ingredients. Their multifunctional bioactivity and compatibility with sustainability-oriented formulation make them strong candidates for integration into next-generation biofunctional cosmetics (Mandal et al., 2023).

2 Spices: Definition and cosmetic relevance

The definition of "spices" remains relatively imprecise across both scholarly and dictionary sources. Some definitions conflate spices with herbs, while others emphasize aromatic seeds or classify dried fruits as spices. According to Sinha, both spices and herbs are angiosperms, meaning plants whose reproductive organs are borne in flowers and whose seeds are enclosed within fruits (Sinha, 2007). The Codex Classification, Section 028, provides a more detailed description, defining spices as "aromatic seeds, buds, roots, bark, pods, berries, or other fruits … used in small quantities to season, flavor, or add aroma to food," typically in dried form (Codex, 19933). Similarly, other authors describe spices and herbs broadly as plant-derived substances that impart flavor and aroma, while acknowledging that the boundary between them is often ambiguous. In general, spices may originate from roots, rhizomes, stems, bark, flowers, fruits, or seeds, whereas herbs usually refer to the soft, nonwoody leafy

Biofunctional Cosmetics for Health. https://doi.org/10.1016/B978-0-443-27500-5.00016-2

parts of plants (FS, n.d.). The classification "Spices and Dried Aromatic Herbs" further includes dried components or mixtures of plants used for flavoring, coloring, or imparting aroma, whether whole, broken, ground, or blended (Douglas et al., 2005).

For this chapter, a working definition, inspired by the literature discussed above, is adopted: **spices are plant-derived substances obtained from nonleafy plant parts, such as seeds, roots, bark, buds, fruits, and rhizomes, used primarily in dried form**. In contrast, herbs are excluded from this definition, as they refer to leafy tissues. Only bioactive compounds derived from spices and their potential applications in cosmetics will be considered.

To ground this definition in an authoritative classification, Table 1 presents the list of spices recognized in the Codex Alimentarius Classification (CXA 004-1993, Group 028), along with their botanical names and source parts. These will serve as the basis for subsequent discussions of their bioactive compounds, traditional, and modern cosmetic and health applications.

It is worth noting, as shown in Table 8.1, however, that certain entries in the Codex list, most notably saffron (derived from the stigmas of *Crocus sativus* L.), do not strictly conform to the above working definition, as they originate from floral

TABLE 8.1 Spices with botanical names and source type (Codex, 1993).

Spice	Botanical name	Source type
Allspice (Pimento)	*Pimenta dioica*	Dried fruit (berry)
Angelica seed	*Angelica archangelica, Angelica sylvestris*	Dried seed
Anise seed	*Pimpinella anisum*	Dried seed
Annatto	*Bixa orellana*	Seed coat
Black cumin	*Nigella sativa*	Seeds
Calamus	*Acorus calamus*	Rhizome
Caper	*Capparis spinosa*	Flower bud
Caraway	*Carum carvi*	Dried seed
Cardamom	*Elettaria cardamomum*	Seed capsule
Cassia bark	*Cinnamomum cassia*	Bark
Cassia buds	*Cinnamomum cassia*	Flower buds
Celery seed	*Apium graveolens*	Seed
Chilli-type pepper	*Capsicum (annuum, frutescens, Chinese)*	Dried fruit/pod
Cinnamon	*Cinnamomum zeylanicum, C. cassia*	Bark
Clove	*Syzygium aromaticum*	Flower bud
Coriander seeds	*Coriandrum sativum*	Dried seed
Cumin	*Cuminum cyminum*	Dried seed
Dill seeds	*Anethum graveolens*	Dried seed
Fennel seeds	*Foeniculum vulgare*	Dried seed
Fenugreek	*Trigonella foenum-graecum*	Dried seed
Galangal	*Alpinia galanga, Alpinia officinarum*	Rhizome
Ginger	*Zingiber officinale*	Rhizome
Grains of paradise	*Aframomum melegueta*	Dried seed
Juniper	*Juniperus communis*	Dried berry
Liquorice	*Glycyrrhiza glabra*	Root
Lovage	*Levisticum officinale*	Seed
Mace	*Myristica fragrans*	Aril (seed covering)
Nutmeg	*Myristica fragrans*	Seed
Pepper (pepper/white)	*Piper nigrum*	Dried fruit/seed
Poppy seeds	*Papaver somniferum*	Seed
Long pepper	*Piper longum*	Dried fruit
Saffron	*Crocus sativus*	Stigmas
Sumac	*Rhus coriaria* L.	Dried fruit (berry)
Turmeric	*Curcuma longa*	Rhizome
Vanilla	*Vanilla planifolia*	Dried fermented pod

structures rather than the typical nonleafy parts such as seeds, roots, bark, or rhizomes. Similar exceptions include floral- or fruit-derived materials such as cloves, capers, and vanilla, which undergo specific postharvest processing (e.g., curing or fermentation) to develop their characteristic aromas. Nevertheless, these substances are explicitly classified as spices under the Codex standard (CXS 326-2017) owing to their long-established culinary, aromatic, and functional roles, and are therefore retained within this classification.

Spices have long been prized not only for their culinary value but also for their therapeutic applications, and modern research confirms that varieties such as turmeric, cinnamon, clove, ginger, saffron, and black pepper contain a rich array of bioactive phytochemicals, including curcuminoids, piperine, gingerols, eugenol, cinnamaldehyde, terpenes, and flavonoids (Kalasariya et al., 2024; Papadopoulou et al., 2025). These compounds are directly relevant to skin health, where they contribute to antioxidant protection against reactive oxygen species (ROS), antiinflammatory activity that reduces irritation and inflammation, antimicrobial effects against acne-causing and pathogenic bacteria, photoprotective actions through UV absorption or ROS neutralization, and wound healing properties mediated by the stimulation of collagen synthesis and skin regeneration pathways (Pereira, 2018; Papadopoulou et al., 2024). For instance, curcumin demonstrates potent antiinflammatory, wound healing, and antioxidant functions, while crocin, derived from saffron, has been investigated for its antipigmentation and skin-brightening potential (Kalasariya et al., 2024; Papadopoulou et al., 2024; Morganti et al., 2019). Today, advances in analytical and biomedical methodologies enable the scientific validation and optimization of these spice-derived compounds, ensuring their safe, effective, and sustainable integration into modern cosmetic formulations (Papadopoulou et al., 2025). The next section explores the specific phytochemicals derived from these spices, their mechanisms of action, and their relevance to cosmetic skin care.

While the next section delves into the phytochemical composition and biological activity of spice-derived compounds, it is important to recognize that their use in skin care is not new. Across ancient cultures, spices have served as key ingredients in cosmetic rituals and dermatological preparations. These traditional practices, outlined in Box 1, form the cultural and empirical foundation for modern scientific interest in their bioactivity.

BOX 1 Historical use of spices in traditional cosmetic and dermatological practices

Ancient Egypt

One of the earliest records of the cosmetic use of spices originates from ancient Egypt. Plant-based resins and essential oils, especially myrrh and frankincense, were formulated into unguents and ointments for skin protection, ritual purification, and embalming purposes (Parish and Crissey, 1988; Jain and Chaudhri, 2009). Botanical residue analyses of burial artifacts confirm the widespread use of aromatic compounds, pigments, and essential oils (McMullen and Dell'Acqua, 2023). Saffron and turmeric were also noted for their skin-enhancing and antiinflammatory properties, while cloves were primarily valued for their fragrance (Fig. 8.1) (McMullen and Dell'Acqua, 2023).

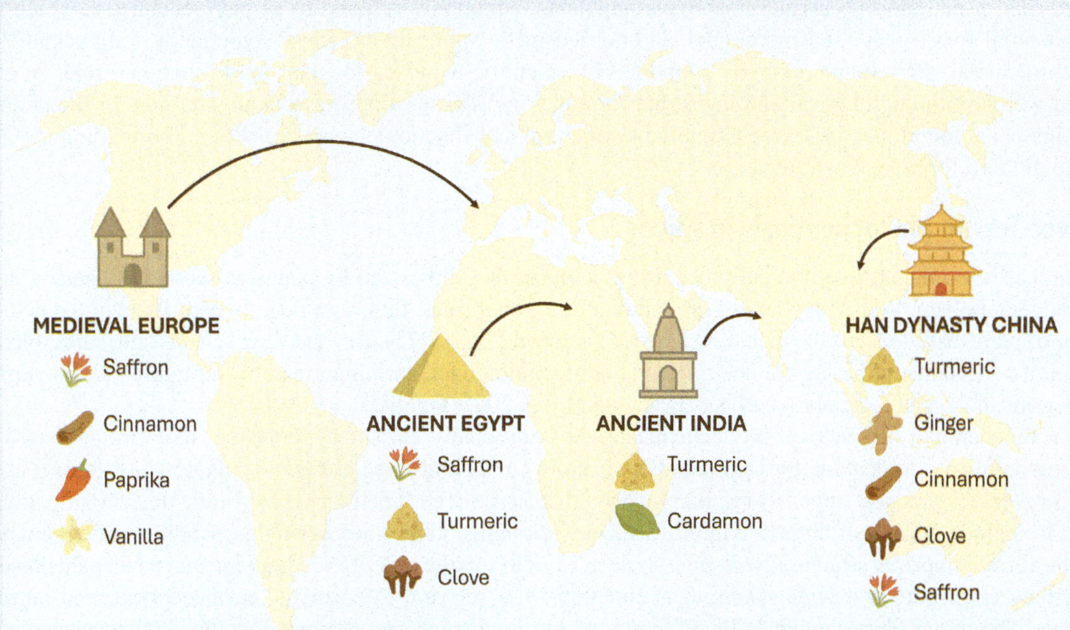

FIG. 8.1 Historical origins and cultural dissemination of key spices used for cosmetic and health purposes. This image illustrates a map of the world along with icons referring to the different cultures that used spices in cosmetics in the past. Also, it shows a selection of the spices that they incorporated into their products.

Continued

BOX 1 Historical use of spices in traditional cosmetic and dermatological practices—cont'd

India (Ayurveda)
In Indian Ayurvedic medicine, spices have long been integral to beauty rituals. Turmeric (*Curcuma longa*), in particular, was revered for its antiseptic, antiinflammatory, and complexion-brightening properties (Turmeric: The Genus Curcuma, n.d.). Classical texts describe its use in facial masks and pastes, alongside sandalwood and cardamom, for soothing and aromatic functions (Singh et al., 2025). Modern dermatologic reviews confirm turmeric's continued relevance in skin care, linking traditional knowledge with current scientific validation (Fuloria et al., 2022).

China (traditional Chinese medicine)
In traditional Chinese medicine, aromatic botanicals were incorporated into topical and ingestible cosmetic remedies as early as the Han dynasty (Han et al., 2021). The *Bencao Gangmu* by Li Shizhen outlines dermatologic uses for turmeric (antiinflammatory, brightening) (Li et al., 2010), ginger (circulatory stimulant) (Shahrajabian et al., 2019), cinnamon (warming, circulation) (Tan et al., 2021), cloves (antiseptic, analgesic) (Batiha et al., 2020), and saffron (skin tone enhancement) (Yang et al., 2023). These ingredients were used in ointments and decoctions, often for both cosmetic and therapeutic outcomes (McMullen and Dell'Acqua, 2023).

Greece, Rome, and Medieval Europe
The Greco-Roman world utilized a wide array of spice-derived botanicals in grooming and perfumery. Saffron, myrtle, and cinnamon appear in elite fragrance and ointment formulations, as supported by archaeometric analyses of Roman *unguentaria* (Cosano et al., 2023). Medieval European traditions preserved and adapted these practices as the spice trade expanded, introducing Eastern spices into Western pharmacopoeia and cosmetic formulas (McMullen and Dell'Acqua, 2023).

Colonial and Early Modern Europe
The colonial period introduced New World spices such as vanilla, allspice, and paprika into European perfumery and skincare. These were incorporated into increasingly refined creams and lotions, particularly in perfumery hubs like Grasse, France. Spice extracts were often blended with florals and citrus oils, reflecting both therapeutic intent and olfactory sophistication (McMullen and Dell'Acqua, 2023).

Across regions and centuries, from ancient Egypt to classical Greece and colonial France, spices provided a shared cultural and therapeutic foundation for cosmetic practices. These historical traditions offer valuable insights into the enduring appeal and dermatologic relevance of plant-based actives, laying the groundwork for their modern application in biofunctional cosmetics.

3 Spice-derived bioactive compounds and their relevance to skin health

Spices are rich in naturally occurring bioactive compounds, commonly referred to as phytochemicals, which hold significant potential for cosmetic, cosmeceutical, and nutricosmetic applications. These compounds, long acknowledged in traditional medicine, are now increasingly supported by scientific evidence for their multifunctional roles in enhancing health and wellness through topical and ingestible formulations. This section presents an overview of the major classes of phytochemicals found in spices, discussing their structural and functional characteristics and providing key examples relevant to modern formulation strategies.

3.1 Overview of phytochemicals in spices

Phytochemicals are nonnutritive, naturally occurring compounds synthesized by plants as secondary metabolites during growth and metabolism. While they do not serve direct nutritional roles, they significantly contribute to the color, aroma, and flavor of plant-based materials, including spices (Yang and Ling, 2025). Beyond their sensory attributes, phytochemicals exhibit a wide range of biological activities, including antioxidant, antiinflammatory, antimicrobial, photoprotective, antiaging, anticancer, and regenerative effects (Yang and Ling, 2025; Guldiken et al., 2018).

From a biochemical perspective, phytochemicals are traditionally classified into three main groups based on their biosynthetic pathways: terpenoids (or isoprenoids), phenolic compounds, and nitrogen-containing alkaloids (Gupta et al., 2020). However, for practical applications, particularly in spice-derived functional ingredients, this classification is often expanded to include additional bioactive families such as saponins, glycosides, phenylpropanoids, and coumarins. Each of these families comprises structurally distinct molecules with unique and often complementary mechanisms of action. Together, they contribute to a wide spectrum of functionalities relevant to cosmetic, cosmeceutical, and nutricosmetic applications. The major phytochemicals found in commonly used spices are presented alongside their respective chemical families in Table 8.2. The major families are discussed in detail, with selected examples of individual phytochemicals highlighted and examined for their relevance to cosmetic applications and multifunctional properties.

TABLE 8.2 Major spice-derived phytochemicals and their families.

Phytochemical	Spice source(s)	Phytochemical family	References
Curcumin	Turmeric	Phenolics	(Hewlings and Kalman, 2017)
Gingerol	Ginger	Phenolics	(Srinivasan, 2017)
Eugenol	Clove, allspice	Phenolics	(Ulanowska and Olas, 2021)
Cinnamaldehyde	Cinnamon, cassia bark	Phenylpropanoids	(Sharma et al., 2016)
Piperine	Black pepper, long pepper	Alkaloids	(Srinivasan, 2007)
Capsaicin	Chili pepper	Alkaloids	(Reddy et al., 2024)
Thymoquinone	Black cumin	Terpenoid	(Karaman, 2020)
Cuminaldehyde	Cumin	Phenylpropanoids	(Bai et al., 2025)
Anethole	Anise seed, fennel	Phenolics	(Andarwulan and Shetty, 1999)
Linalool	Coriander	Terpenoid	(Shahidi and Hossain, 2018)
Myristicin	Nutmeg, mace	Phenylpropanoids	(Okiki et al., 2023)
Diosgenin	Fenugreek	Saponin	(Shahidi and Hossain, 2018)
Glabridin	Liquorice	Phenolics	(Pastorino et al., 2018)
Crocin	Saffron	Carotenoid	(Hosseinzadeh and Nassiri-Asl, 2013)
Vanillin	Vanilla	Phenolics	(Shahidi and Hossain, 2018)

3.2 Phenolics

Spices are rich sources of structurally diverse phenolic compounds, which include both polyphenols and simple phenols. Over 500 polyphenols have been identified across plant-based foods, including fruits, vegetables, coffee, cocoa, wine, and notably, herbs and spices (Lazaridis et al., 2024a; Singh and Yadav, 2022). In spices, representative phenolics include curcumin (turmeric), gingerol (ginger), eugenol (clove and allspice), anethole (anise seed and fennel), glabridin (licorice), and vanillin (vanilla), as reported in Table 8.2.

Phenolics are plant-derived secondary metabolites characterized by one or more hydroxyl groups attached to an aromatic ring. They are typically divided into subclasses such as phenolic acids, flavonoids, stilbenes, lignans, phenolic alcohols, and polyphenols (Abbas et al., 2017). Among these, phenolic acids, including hydroxycinnamic acids (e.g., caffeic, ferulic, sinapic acids) and hydroxybenzoic acids (e.g., vanillic, syringic acids), are commonly found in high concentrations in spices like clove, cinnamon, turmeric, and saffron (Kumar and Goel, 2019; Saraswathi et al., 2020).

Phenolics occur in both free and bound forms. Free phenolics are readily extractable and soluble in organic or aqueous solvents, while bound phenolics are covalently linked to cell wall macromolecules and may exhibit even greater antioxidant and antiinflammatory activities (Singh et al., 2025; Kumar and Goel, 2019; Wang et al., 2020). Spices, as complex plant matrices, have phenolic content influenced by factors such as drying, processing, and extraction methods (Lazaridis et al., 2024b).

Beyond their traditional culinary functions, enhancing flavor, aroma, and color, phenolic compounds are increasingly recognized for their health-promoting properties, particularly in cosmetic and dermatological applications (de Lima Cherubim et al., 2020). These bioactive molecules exhibit a broad spectrum of biological activities, including antioxidant, antiinflammatory, antimicrobial, photoprotective, and antiaging effects, which collectively contribute to cellular defense, repair, and homeostasis in skin health. Notably, spice-derived phenolics, such as curcumin, gingerol, eugenol, and anethole, have been shown to exert significant pharmacological effects, including antioxidant, antiinflammatory, and anticancer activities (Singh and Yadav, 2022).

Recent reviews highlight the growing potential of these compounds not only in traditional medicine but also as natural and safer alternatives to synthetic ingredients in modern cosmeceutical formulations (Singh and Yadav, 2022). Their mechanisms of action include scavenging ROS, chelating transition metals, modulating inflammatory and oxidative pathways, and inhibiting skin-aging enzymes such as matrix metalloproteinases (MMPs), collagenase, elastase, and tyrosinase (de Lima Cherubim et al., 2020). In addition, phenolics can enhance skin barrier integrity, reduce UV-induced damage, and improve dermal elasticity, making them ideal for use in antiaging creams, sunscreens, serums, and skin-brightening products. Their compatibility with various delivery systems, such as emulsions, hydrogels, and nanocarriers, further supports their effective incorporation into natural, plant-based skincare formulations that align with the growing consumer demand for clean-label cosmetics.

Curcumin (diferuloylmethane), the principal bioactive phenolic compound in turmeric (*C. longa*), has garnered significant attention in dermatology and cosmetic science due to its multifunctional bioactivities, including antioxidant, anti-inflammatory, antimicrobial, antineoplastic, and skin-brightening effects (Vaughn et al., 2016; Grynkiewicz and Ślifirski, 2012). Chemically, curcumin ((1E,6E)-1,7-bis(4-hydroxy-3-methoxyphenyl)-1,6-heptadiene-3,5-dione) (Fig. 8.2) is a diarylheptanoid with two methoxy-phenolic aromatic rings connected by a seven-carbon linker and a β-diketone moiety, structural features responsible for its ability to scavenge free radicals, chelate metal ions, and modulate redox-sensitive signaling pathways, which are crucial for preventing oxidative skin damage (Priyadarsini, 2013).

Curcumin's antioxidant role in skin health has been supported by clinical and mechanistic studies. In a human trial conducted in 2020, curcumin supplements were administered to 308 participants, resulting in an approximate 50% reduction in malondialdehyde levels, a biomarker of lipid peroxidation, demonstrating its systemic oxidative stress-lowering potential (Jakubczyk et al., 2020). This antioxidant efficacy is largely attributed to the methoxy ($-OCH_3$) groups on its aromatic rings, as curcumin has shown higher radical scavenging activity than its analogues (Jayaprakasha et al., 2006). In addition, it downregulates inflammatory mediators such as NF-κB and cyclooxygenase-2 (COX-2), helping to reduce redness, irritation, and swelling associated with chronic skin conditions (Vaughn et al., 2016; Kant et al., 2014).

Topically, curcumin exhibits photoprotective effects by reducing Ultraviolet induced oxidative damage and enhancing DNA repair mechanisms (Sharma et al., 2022; Kasprzak-Drozd et al., 2024). It also supports wound healing and skin regeneration by promoting fibroblast proliferation, collagen synthesis, and transforming growth factor β1 (TGF-β1) modulation (Kasprzak-Drozd et al., 2024; Yen et al., 2018; Chen et al., 2021). Furthermore, curcumin's ability to inhibit tyrosinase, the key enzyme in melanin biosynthesis, underlies its skin-brightening and antipigmentation potential (Jiang et al., 2013). Through the suppression of MMP-1 and MMP-9 (MMPs), curcumin helps maintain the structural integrity of collagen and elastin, reinforcing its antiaging role in cosmeceutical formulations (Kasprzak-Drozd et al., 2024).

Given these properties, curcumin is increasingly incorporated into modern skincare products (Box 2), including creams (Zaman and Akhtar, 2013), masks (Azizah, n.d.), serums (Pratiwi et al., 2021), and cleansers (Lim et al., 2023), with demonstrated efficacy in improving hyperpigmentation, skin tone, and overall dermal health (Kryst, 2023). Nanoformulations have further improved its topical stability and bioavailability, enhancing its practical use in cosmetic science (Yallapu et al., 2015). For formulation and quality control, curcumin is typically extracted using organic solvents (e.g., ethanol, methanol, acetone) and identified via UV–Vis spectroscopy (λmax ~ 420–425 nm), Furier Transform Infrared and High Performance Liquid Chromatography, allowing reliable analysis of its purity and concentration in skincare applications (Priyadarsini, 2014; Ciuca and Racovita, 2023).

Gingerol, chemically known as [6]-gingerol (5-hydroxy-1-(4-hydroxy-3-methoxyphenyl)decan-3-one) (Fig. 8.3), is a phenolic ketone and the principal pungent bioactive compound found in the rhizome of *Zingiber officinale* (ginger). It

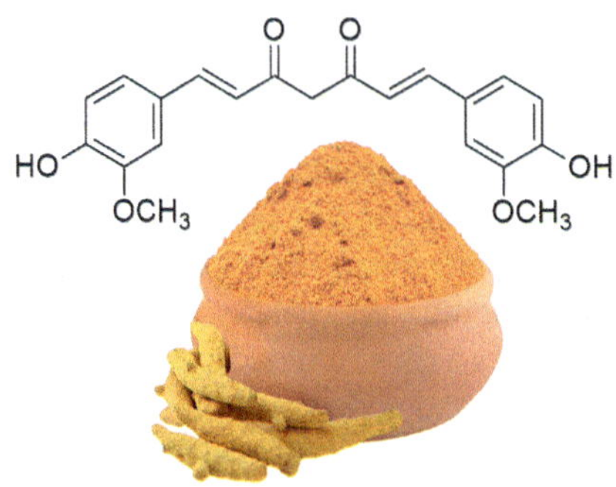

FIG. 8.2 Turmeric and its bioactive compound: curcumin. The rhizomes of curcuma are shown in this image along with its powder, and the chemical formula of curcumin ((1E,6E)-1,7-bis(4-hydroxy-3-methoxyphenyl)-1,6-heptadiene-3,5-dione) is illustrated, highlighting its functional groups responsible for its properties.

BOX 2 Traditional use of turmeric in modern soap making

Did you know that turmeric is still incorporated into artisanal cosmetic products today? One example is **Khan el Saboun**, one of Lebanon's oldest traditional soap manufacturers, which continues to craft natural soaps infused with turmeric (Khan Al-Saboun., 2024.). This illustrates how the long-recognized skin-beneficial properties of turmeric remain valued in contemporary skincare formulations.

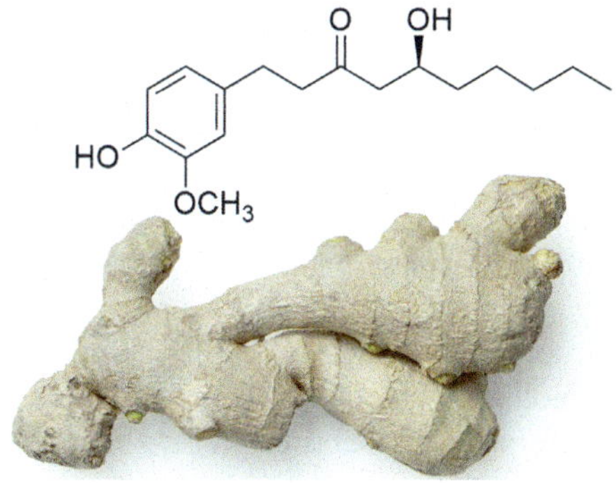

FIG. 8.3 Ginger and its bioactive compound: gingerol. The ginger rhizome is shown in this image along with the chemical structure of [6]-gingerol (5-hydroxy-1-(4-hydroxy-3-methoxyphenyl)decan-3-one), highlighting its functional groups responsible for its properties.

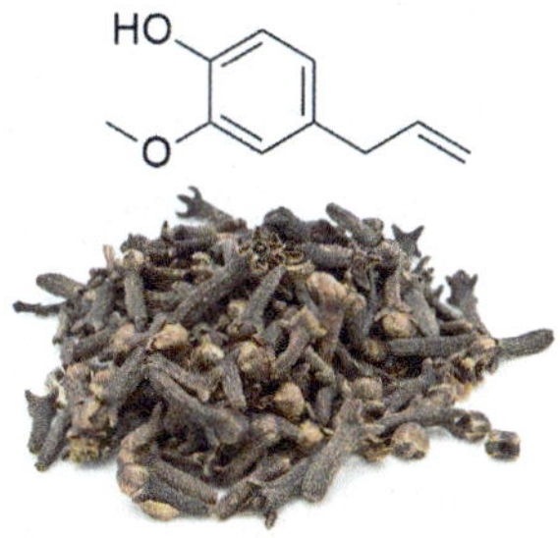

FIG. 8.4 Clove and its bioactive compound: eugenol. Cloves are shown in this image along with the chemical structure of eugenol (4-allyl-2-methoxyphenol), highlighting its functional groups responsible for its properties.

exhibits potent antioxidant, antiinflammatory, and antimicrobial properties (Alhanshali and Khachemoune, 2024; Samota et al., 2024). These activities support skin health by combating oxidative stress, protecting against photoaging, and alleviating conditions such as acne, inflammatory dermatitis, and pigmentation disorders.

Gingerol protects skin cells by scavenging ROS, modulating inflammatory pathways, and reducing redness (Alhanshali and Khachemoune, 2024; Samota et al., 2024). Beyond skincare, gingerol has been linked to improved blood circulation and stimulation of hair growth, making it particularly valuable in haircare formulations (M. Penkar et al., 2023). In addition, its incorporation into both traditional and modern products, ranging from face serums (Patidar et al., n.d.) and herbal soaps (Kinanti et al., 2024) to functional beverages and supplements (Zagórska et al., 2023; Shaukat et al., 2023), demonstrates its versatility across cosmetic and health-related formulations. Recent studies and product developments continue to explore gingerol's incorporation into innovative cosmetic, cosmeceutical, and nutraceutical formulations, highlighting its growing relevance as a bioactive ingredient for cosmetics and health.

Eugenol, chemically known as 4-allyl-2-methoxyphenol (Fig. 8.4), is an amphipathic phenolic compound predominantly derived from the dried flower buds of *Syzygium aromaticum* (clove). It is also present in smaller amounts in allspice, cinnamon, and nutmeg (Lazaridis et al., 2024a). Eugenol exhibits strong antioxidant, antiinflammatory, and antimicrobial activities (Ulanowska and Olas, 2021). By scavenging free radicals, limiting ROS, and inhibiting proinflammatory mediators, it protects cellular components such as lipids, proteins, and DNA from oxidative damage. These effects translate into valuable dermatological benefits, enhancing skin protection, resilience, and resistance to skin problems (Ulanowska and Olas, 2021).

In addition to its antioxidant and antiinflammatory roles, eugenol also demonstrates antimicrobial activity against various bacteria and fungi through mechanisms that disrupt microbial cell integrity. This property enhances its usefulness in cosmetic formulations, both by contributing to product preservation and by supporting skin protection (Marchese et al., 2017).

In summary, spice-derived phenolics such as curcumin, gingerol, and eugenol illustrate the diverse bioactivities that make this class of compounds highly valuable in cosmetics, cosmeceuticals, and nutricosmetics. While these examples emphasize antioxidant, antiinflammatory, antimicrobial, and skin-brightening effects, other phenolics from spices, including anethole, glabridin, and vanillin, are also important contributors to skin protection, pigmentation control, and antiaging. Collectively, these bioactives safeguard the skin from oxidative and inflammatory stress while enhancing its resilience and overall appearance, making them versatile functional ingredients across topical skincare, advanced cosmeceutical products, and ingestible formulations designed to promote beauty from within.

3.3 Terpenoids

Terpenoids, also known as isoprenoids, are a structurally diverse class of natural products derived from five-carbon isoprene units. They represent one of the largest families of phytochemicals, with over 80,000 identified compounds across the plant kingdom (Christianson, 2017). In plants, terpenoids serve multiple ecological functions, including pigmentation, aroma, growth regulation, and defense against pathogens. In spices, representative terpenoids include thymoquinone (black cumin), linalool (coriander), and various monoterpenes and sesquiterpenes found in cinnamon and nutmeg (Shahidi and Hossain, 2018). Terpenoids are commonly classified according to the number of isoprene units into monoterpenes (C10), sesquiterpenes (C15), diterpenes (C20), triterpenes (C30), and higher homologues (Nagegowda and Gupta, 2020). This structural variability underlies their broad biological activities. Many terpenoids are volatile, contributing to the characteristic aroma and flavor of spices, while others act as pigments or precursors to hormones such as gibberellins and abscisic acid (Nagegowda and Gupta, 2020).

Beyond their sensory roles, terpenoids are increasingly recognized as multifunctional bioactives with therapeutic and cosmetic potential. Compounds such as thymoquinone from *Nigella sativa* exhibit antioxidant, antiinflammatory, antimicrobial, and wound healing properties (Nasiri et al., 2022; Hannan et al., 2021). Linalool, a monoterpene alcohol found in many essential oils, shows antimicrobial, antioxidant, and antiinflammatory activities (Box 3). In cosmetics, it enhances product preservation and skin protection while reducing the need for high essential oil concentrations that may cause irritation (Herman et al., 2016). These activities collectively contribute to skin protection and regeneration.

BOX 3 Case study: Linalool—a spice-derived terpenoid with photoprotective activity

Linalool, a naturally occurring monoterpenoid alcohol abundant in coriander (*Coriandrum sativum*), cinnamon leaf (*Cinnamomum zeylanicum*), and other aromatic spices, has been shown to possess significant photoprotective and antioxidant properties in human skin cells. In a study by Gunaseelan et al. (2017), human dermal fibroblasts were pretreated with linalool prior to UVB irradiation to evaluate its potential to mitigate oxidative and inflammatory damage (Fig. 8.5) (Gunaseelan et al., 2017).

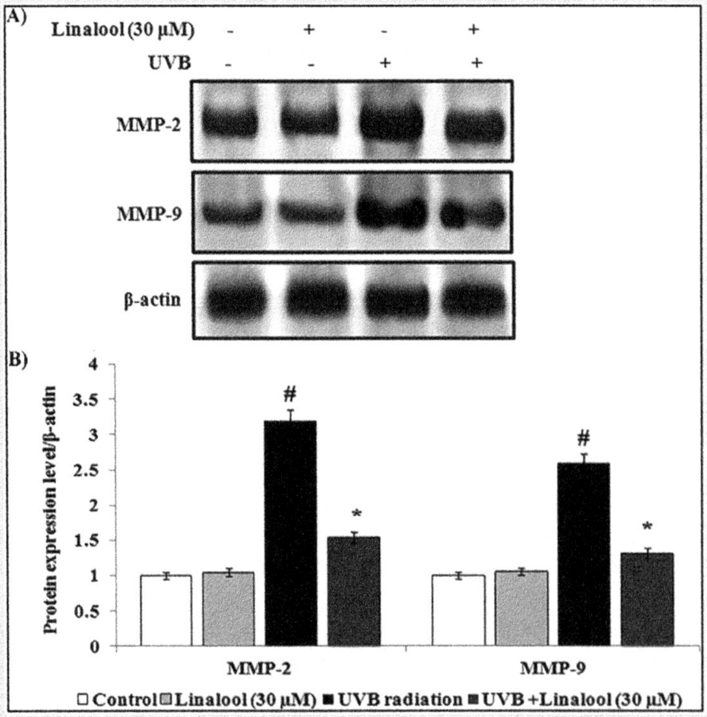

FIG. 8.5 Photoprotective activity of linalool in human dermal fibroblasts (HDFs) (Gunaseelan et al., 2017). (A) Effect of linalool on UVB-induced expression of matrix metalloproteinases (MMP-2 and MMP-9) in HDFs. (B) Densitometric analysis represents means ± SD from three immunoblots, expressed as relative band density normalized to β-actin levels. Values not sharing a common marking (# and *) differ significantly at $P < 0.05$ (DMRT). Linalool pretreatment attenuated UVB-induced oxidative and inflammatory responses, preserving collagen integrity and cell viability. (*From Gunaseelan, S., Balupillai, A., Govindasamy, K., Ramasamy, K., Muthusamy, G., Shanmugam, M., Thangaiyan, R., Robert, B.M., Nagarajan, R.P., Ponniresan, V.K., Rathinaraj, P., Slominski, A.T., 2017. Linalool prevents oxidative stress activated protein kinases in single UVB-exposed human skin cells. PLOS ONE. 1932-6203. 12 (5), e0176699. https://doi.org/10.1371/journal.pone.0176699. Licensed under CC BY 4.0. No modifications were made.*)

Exposure to UVB (20 mJ cm^{-2}) markedly increased intracellular ROS production, lipid peroxidation, and depletion of endogenous antioxidant defenses [superoxide dismutase (SOD), catalase (CAT), glutathione peroxidase (GPx), glutathione (GSH)]. Pretreatment with linalool effectively restored antioxidant enzyme activities and reduced oxidative stress biomarkers, demonstrating its strong redox-modulatory capacity. Moreover, linalool inhibited the phosphorylation of MAPKs (ERK, JNK, p38) and prevented NF-κB activation by stabilizing IκBα, leading to a significant reduction in proinflammatory mediators [TNF-α, interleukin-6 (IL-6), COX-2] and MMPs (MMP-2 and MMP-9).

These effects collectively attenuated UVB-induced collagen degradation, mitochondrial dysfunction, and DNA oxidative lesions (8-oxoG formation), preserving cell viability and dermal structural integrity. The authors concluded that linalool exerts its photoprotective effect through the coordinated suppression of oxidative and inflammatory signaling, reinforcing skin resilience to UV stress and supporting its inclusion in natural photoprotective and antiaging formulations.

Mechanistically, terpenoids act by scavenging ROS, modulating inflammatory mediators, stabilizing cell membranes, and promoting collagen synthesis and tissue repair (Javed et al., 2024). Certain terpenoids also exhibit inhibitory effects on skin-aging enzymes such as elastase, collagenase, and tyrosinase, reinforcing their utility in antiaging and skin-brightening applications (Binic et al., 2013). The versatility of terpenoids has enabled their integration into diverse cosmetic and dermatological formulations, including moisturizers, antiaging creams, sunscreens, haircare products, and makeup. Their lipophilic nature enhances skin penetration, while advanced delivery systems such as nanoemulsions, liposomes, and hydrogels further improve their stability, bioavailability, and controlled release of actives (Deveci, 2025). As natural, plant-derived ingredients, terpenoids align with the growing demand for clean-label, multifunctional actives in cosmetics, cosmeceuticals, and nutricosmetics.

Thymoquinone (2-isopropyl-5-methyl-1,4-benzoquinone) (Fig. 8.6), the principal bioactive constituent of *N. sativa* (black cumin), exhibits a wide spectrum of activities, including antioxidant, antiinflammatory, antimicrobial, and wound healing properties (Christianson, 2017). It has demonstrated therapeutic potential in skin disorders such as eczema, psoriasis, acne, vitiligo, and impaired wound healing, as well as in protecting against skin pigmentation (Nasiri et al., 2022; Aljabre et al., 2015). Mechanistically, thymoquinone scavenges ROS and activates cellular antioxidant defenses, leading to increased activity of enzymes such as SOD, CAT, and GPx. These effects help reduce lipid peroxidation and protect cellular components from oxidative damage (Hannan et al., 2021; Fatima Shad et al., 2021). It also downregulates NF-κB, COX-2, and proinflammatory cytokines such as TNF-α and IL-6, thereby reducing inflammatory responses and contributing to protection against chronic skin disorders (Hannan et al., 2021).

Thymoquinone has demonstrated broad-spectrum antimicrobial activity, showing significant effects against Gram-positive bacteria such as *Staphylococcus aureus*, Gram-negative bacteria, including *Escherichia coli* and *Pseudomonas aeruginosa*, as well as the pathogenic yeast *Candida albicans* (Forouzanfar et al., 2014). These activities highlight its potential role as a bioactive compound for skin protection and as a supportive ingredient in cosmetic formulations. In addition, thymoquinone accelerates wound healing by promoting keratinocyte proliferation, angiogenesis, and collagen deposition, ultimately enhancing tissue repair and skin elasticity (Kmail et al., 2023; Sallehuddin et al., 2020). Modern product development has explored the incorporation of thymoquinone into topical creams, oils, and nanoformulations, which enhance its stability, penetration, and bioavailability. These advances support its potential role in preventing photoaging, preserving collagen, improving skin hydration, and promoting wound repair (Evanti et al., 2025).

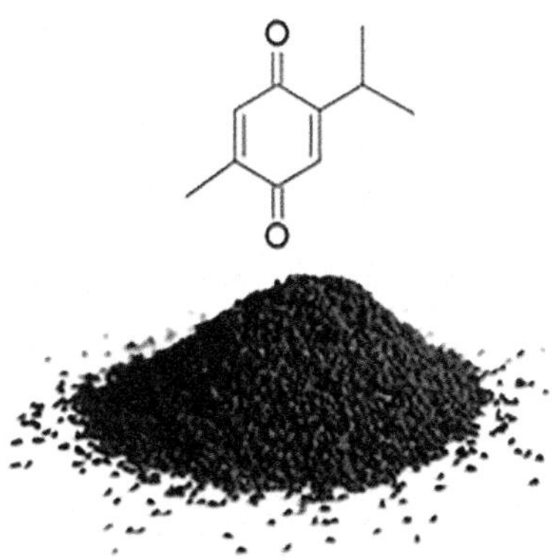

FIG. 8.6 Black cumin and its bioactive compound: thymoquinone. Black cumin seeds are shown in this image along with the chemical structure of thymoquinone (2-isopropyl-5-methyl-1,4-benzoquinone), highlighting its functional groups responsible for its properties.

3.4 Alkaloids

Alkaloids are nitrogen-containing cyclic organic compounds derived from amino acids and widely distributed across spices, herbs, and medicinal plants (Letchuman et al., 2025). In cosmetics, they are valued for their antioxidant, antiinflammatory, antimicrobial, analgesic, and regenerative properties, which complement the activities of other phytochemical groups such as phenolics and terpenoids (Letchuman et al., 2025; Nagappan et al., 2012). These bioactivities contribute to skin protection, improved microcirculation, and tissue renewal, supporting overall skin health and appearance (Stępniowska et al., n.d.).

Alkaloids are incorporated into various cosmetic and dermatological formulations, including creams, lotions, tonics, masks, and antiaging or anticellulite products, due to their ability to stimulate circulation, reduce inflammation, and enhance skin tone (Stępniowska et al., n.d.). Among spice-derived alkaloids, piperine and capsaicin are particularly significant for modern cosmetic and cosmeceutical applications because of their multifunctional actions and favorable safety profiles.

Piperine (1-[5-(1,3-benzodioxol-5-yl)-1-oxo-2,4-pentadienyl] piperidine) (Fig. 8.7) is the principal piperidine alkaloid in *Piper nigrum* L. (black pepper) and represents a key cosmetic bioactive (Srinivasan, 2007). It exhibits antiinflammatory, antioxidant, and anticellulite properties and is used in face creams, lotions, tonics, and soaps (Stępniowska et al., n.d.). Mechanistically, piperine influences adipogenic transcription factors such as peroxisome proliferator-activated receptor gamma (PPARγ), SREBP-1c, and CCAAT/enhancer-binding protein beta, leading to the downregulation of genes responsible for adipocyte differentiation and lipid accumulation (Park et al., 2012). This mechanism underlies its role in slowing fat deposition and improving skin firmness and texture.

In addition, piperine enhances dermal penetration and absorption of active ingredients, a property leveraged in various topical and transdermal formulations (Platel and Srinivasan, 2000). It is also incorporated into detergents and soaps, as well as in antinail-biting preparations, where it provides a mild sensory deterrent without causing irritation (Wadhwa et al., 2014). Its multifunctionality and low toxicity make it an attractive natural additive for anticellulite and rejuvenating cosmetics, aligning with the trend toward plant-based actives in sustainable formulations.

Capsaicin ((6E)-N-[(4-hydroxy-3-methoxyphenyl)methyl]-8-methyl-6-nonenamide) (Fig. 8.8) is a proto-alkaloid derived from chili peppers (*Capsicum* spp.) (Reddy et al., 2024; Stępniowska et al., n.d.). It possesses analgesic, antioxidant, thermogenic, antibacterial, and circulation-stimulating properties that are exploited in cosmetics and dermatological care (Saraswathi et al., 2020). At low concentrations ($\leq$0.025%), capsaicin is incorporated into lip products (glosses and lipsticks) to promote a fuller appearance through transient vasodilation (Boudreau et al., 2009), as well as into hair masks, shampoos, and scalp treatments to enhance microcirculation and support hair growth (Lee et al., 2003).

It is also used in anticellulite and slimming balms, where it enhances blood flow and stimulates lipolysis, a process that breaks down fat cells (Stępniowska et al., n.d.). In animal and cell models, capsaicin has been shown to reduce adipocyte lipid content and suppress the expression of PPARγ and CCAAT/enhancer-binding protein alpha, supporting its potential as a fat-reducing agent (Joo et al., 2010; Lee et al., 2011). Furthermore, its antioxidant activity delays lipid peroxidation and the oxidation of fatty components in emulsions, improving cosmetic shelf stability (Ahuja et al., 2006). These combined effects make capsaicin a multifunctional ingredient in topical products aimed at skin firming, circulation enhancement, and scalp revitalization.

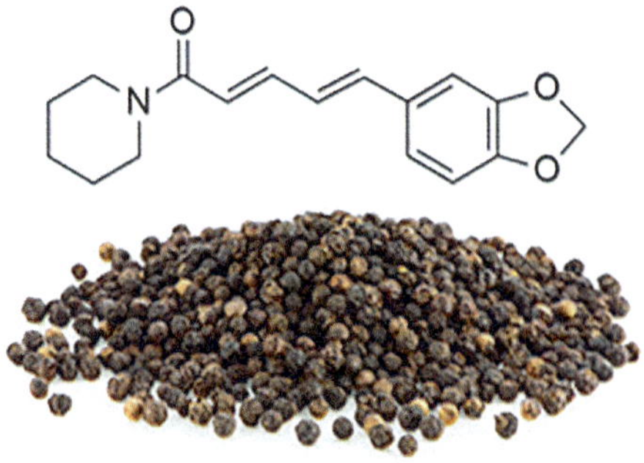

FIG. 8.7 Black pepper and its bioactive compound: piperine. Black pepper is shown in this image along with the chemical structure of piperine (1-[5-(1,3-benzodioxol-5-yl)-1-oxo-2,4-pentadienyl] piperidine), highlighting its functional groups responsible for its properties.

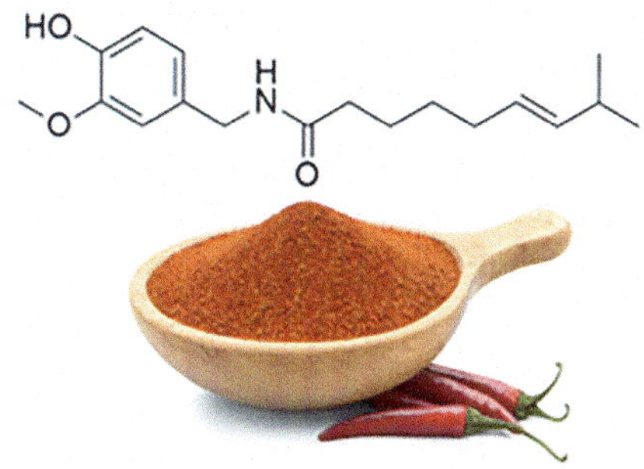

FIG. 8.8 Chili pepper and its bioactive compound: capsaicin. Chili pepper is shown in this image along with the chemical structure of capsaicin ((6E)-N-[(4-hydroxy-3-methoxyphenyl)methyl]-8-methyl-6-nonenamide), highlighting its functional groups responsible for its properties.

3.5 Other bioactives

In addition to the major phytochemical classes, spices contain several minor yet functionally significant compounds, including essential oils, saponins, glycosides, phenylpropanoids, coumarins, and carotenoids. These bioactives collectively enhance both the therapeutic efficacy and sensory qualities of cosmetic formulations. Essential oils, volatile aromatic compounds typically obtained through distillation, are abundant in spices such as cinnamon (cinnamaldehyde), ginger (zingiberene), cumin (cuminaldehyde), nutmeg (myristicin), and black pepper (β-caryophyllene). They exhibit antimicrobial, antioxidant, antiinflammatory, and aromatherapeutic properties that improve both product performance and user experience (Shahidi and Hossain, 2018). Saponins, naturally occurring glycosides with surface-active and foaming properties, are found in fenugreek and similar spice plants. They demonstrate mild cleansing, antiinflammatory, and skin-soothing effects, making them valuable in cleansers, shampoos, and gentle emulsions (Timilsena et al., 2023). Glycosides, such as glabridin and glycyrrhizin from licorice, act as depigmenting and antiinflammatory agents while enhancing the solubility, stability, and delivery of other active ingredients in formulations (Tian et al., 2008; Bartnik and Facey, 2023). Phenylpropanoids, including cinnamic acid derivatives, cinnamaldehyde, cuminaldehyde, and myristicin, display UV-absorbing, antioxidant, antimicrobial, and circulation-stimulating effects, supporting skin protection, photostability, and antiaging functionality (Neelam and Sharma, 2020). Coumarins are naturally occurring aromatic lactones widely distributed in plants such as cassia cinnamon (*Cinnamomum cassia*) and licorice (*Glycyrrhiza glabra*), where they contribute to the characteristic sweet fragrance. In addition to their aromatic qualities, coumarins possess notable antioxidant and antimicrobial properties, enhancing their value in pharmaceutical, cosmetic, and food applications (Sharifi-Rad et al., 2021). Finally, carotenoids, such as crocin from saffron (*C. sativus*), are natural pigments known for their potent antioxidant and photoprotective properties. Crocin effectively shields skin lipids from UVA- and pollution-induced oxidation, helping to maintain skin radiance and resilience against environmental stress (Maoka, 2020; Fagot et al., 2018). Collectively, these bioactives enhance the functionality, stability, and sensory appeal of spice-derived cosmetic products, forming a foundation for multifunctional formulations that combine efficacy with sensorial benefits. Among them, cinnamaldehyde and cuminaldehyde stand out as key phenylpropanoid representatives and are examined in detail hereafter for their individual characteristics and cosmetic relevance.

Cinnamaldehyde, chemically known as (2E)-3-phenylprop-2-enal (Fig. 8.9), is the principal phenylpropanoid compound found in *Cinnamomum verum* (cinnamon) and is largely responsible for its characteristic aroma and biological activity (Sharma et al., 2016). It exhibits potent antimicrobial, antioxidant, and antiinflammatory properties, making it highly valuable in cosmetic and dermatological formulations (Doyle and Stephens, 2019). As the dominant constituent of cinnamon essential oil, cinnamaldehyde contributes to the strong antioxidant potential of cinnamon extracts, which have been shown to neutralize free radicals, chelate metal ions, and enhance endogenous antioxidant enzyme activity.

These mechanisms help protect skin cells from oxidative stress, inflammation, and premature aging (Singh and Yadav, 2022). In addition, cinnamaldehyde demonstrates notable antibacterial and antifungal efficacy even at low concentrations, supporting its use as a natural preservative and bioactive enhancer in topical products (Doyle and Stephens, 2019; Sharma et al., 2016). It also promotes local microcirculation, aiding in skin revitalization and improved nutrient delivery. Recent advances in nanoencapsulation and emulsion-based systems have enhanced its stability, bioavailability, and controlled release, facilitating incorporation into diverse cosmetic formulations without compromising sensory attributes (Nabavi et al., 2015; Hill et al., 2013). Altogether, the multifunctional bioactivity and formulation adaptability of cinnamaldehyde position it as a promising natural ingredient for next-generation cosmetic and cosmeceutical applications.

Cuminaldehyde, chemically identified as 4-isopropylbenzaldehyde (Fig. 8.10), is the major bioactive constituent of *Cuminum cyminum* (green cumin) and exhibits strong antioxidant, antimicrobial, and antiinflammatory properties (Bai et al., 2025; Hajlaoui et al., 2010). These bioactivities make it an important multifunctional compound in the context of cosmetic and dermatological formulations. By inhibiting tyrosinase activity and stabilizing its structure through strong ligand binding, cuminaldehyde helps regulate melanin synthesis and counteracts oxidative stress, thereby promoting even skin tone, protecting cellular components, and supporting overall skin integrity and resilience (Baruah et al., 2025). In vitro studies demonstrate that cumin essential oil, which contains a high proportion of cuminaldehyde (~48.8%), exerts strong antiinflammatory activity by suppressing multiple inflammatory mediators. It downregulates the expression of pro-inflammatory cytokines such as IL-1 and IL-6, as well as inducible nitric oxide synthase (iNOS) and COX-2, while inhibiting the phosphorylation of JNK, ERK, and NF-κB signaling pathways in lipopolysaccharide (LPS)-stimulated macrophages (Wei et al., 2015).

Moreover, cuminaldehyde itself acts as a competitive inhibitor of 15-lipoxygenase (LOX), an enzyme responsible for leukotriene biosynthesis, thereby mitigating lipid peroxidation and inflammatory responses (Tomy et al., 2014). In addition to its antiinflammatory role, cumin essential oil exhibits potent antimicrobial and antifungal activity, effectively inhibiting *C. albicans* and other skin-associated pathogens (Hajlaoui et al., 2010; Minooeianhaghighi et al., 2017). These combined antioxidant, antimicrobial, and antiinflammatory effects highlight cuminaldehyde as a multifunctional bioactive compound suitable for incorporation into cosmetic and cosmeceutical formulations aimed at skin protection, rejuvenation, and balance (Baruah et al., 2025; Ebada, 2017).

Overall, the diverse range of bioactive compounds present in spices highlights their remarkable relevance in modern cosmetic, cosmeceutical, and nutricosmetic formulations. Acting synergistically, these natural molecules provide potent antioxidant, antiinflammatory, antimicrobial, photoprotective, and regenerative effects that support skin protection, renewal, and overall health. Their multifunctionality extends beyond therapeutic benefits, enhancing product stability, safety, and sensory appeal while aligning with the global shift toward natural, sustainable, and scientifically validated ingredients. Together, these properties illustrate how spice-derived phytochemicals bridge traditional botanical knowledge with innovative formulation science, offering safe and effective solutions for skin care and wellness. The following section explores the mechanisms of action through which these compounds exert their protective and restorative effects on the skin.

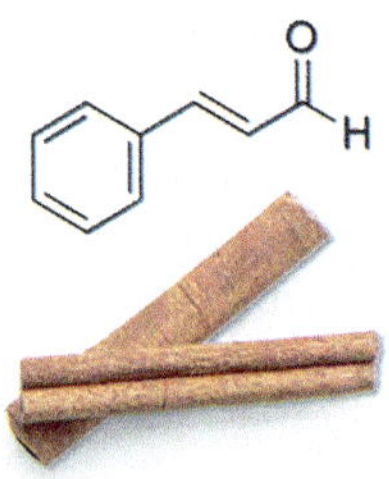

FIG. 8.9 Cinnamon and its bioactive compound: cinnamaldehyde. Cinnamon is shown in this image along with the chemical structure of cinnamaldehyde ((2E)-3-phenylprop-2-enal), highlighting its functional groups responsible for its properties.

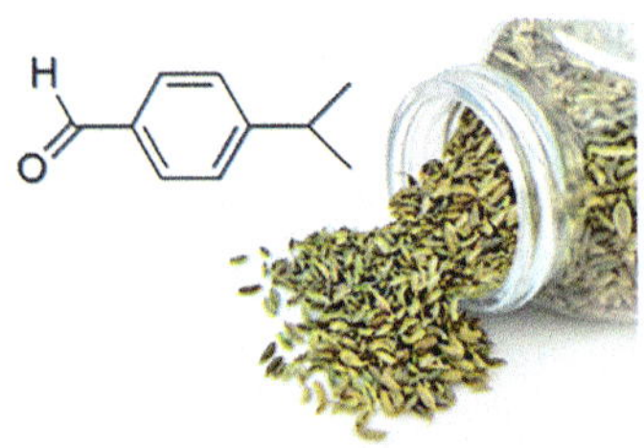

FIG. 8.10 Cumin and its bioactive compound: cuminaldehyde. Cumin seeds are shown in this image along with the chemical structure of cuminaldehyde (4-isopropylbenzaldehyde), highlighting its functional groups responsible for its properties.

3.6 Mechanisms of action and skin benefits

Phytochemicals derived from spices exhibit a broad range of biofunctional properties that support skin health and cosmetic efficacy. These naturally occurring compounds, including polyphenols, terpenoids, alkaloids, and others, modulate several cellular and molecular pathways relevant to dermatological protection, repair, and rejuvenation. Despite their structural diversity, their effects frequently converge on common biological targets, offering multifunctional benefits through antioxidant, antiinflammatory, antimicrobial, photoprotective, and regenerative mechanisms. Below is an overview of the key mechanisms through which spice-derived phytochemicals exert their activity.

3.6.1 *Antioxidant activity*

The antioxidant activity of spice-derived phytochemicals underpins many of their cosmetic and systemic health benefits. As detailed earlier, oxidative stress represents a key contributor to skin aging, pigmentation irregularities, and inflammation. Spice-derived phytochemicals counteract these effects primarily through ROS neutralization, metal chelation, and enzyme regulation.

Polyphenols act through hydrogen atom transfer and single-electron transfer mechanisms, directly scavenging reactive oxygen and nitrogen species. Their structural motifs, particularly hydroxyl and methoxy groups on aromatic rings, enhance radical-stabilizing capacity and explain their high antioxidant potential (Makris and Boskou, 2014). They also chelate transition metals such as Fe^{2+} and Cu^{2+}, thereby preventing Fenton-type reactions responsible for free-radical generation and lipid peroxidation (Quideau et al., 2011).

In oxidative environments, excessive ROS disrupt mitochondrial function and damage nucleic acids, proteins, and membrane lipids, ultimately impairing cellular homeostasis. Antioxidant phytochemicals mitigate these effects by stabilizing redox signaling pathways and maintaining equilibrium between pro-oxidant and antioxidant forces (Gulcin, 2020).

Terpenoids complement these effects by upregulating endogenous antioxidant enzymes such as SOD, CAT, and GPx, helping restore the skin's redox balance and resilience to environmental stressors (Lazaridis et al., 2024a; de Cássia da Silveira E Sá et al., 2013). Alkaloids contribute to skin protection by mitigating oxidative stress through modulation of redox signaling pathways, enhancing endogenous antioxidant defenses, and reducing oxidative damage to lipids and proteins (Macáková et al., 2019).

Through these combined actions, spice-derived phytochemicals provide multifaceted protection against oxidative damage, forming the biochemical basis for their use in cosmetic formulations aimed at skin rejuvenation and in functional foods or nutraceuticals promoting systemic antioxidant defense.

3.6.2 *Antiinflammatory activity*

As noted in the discussion of phytochemicals earlier, chronic inflammation underlies multiple dermatological conditions, including acne, eczema, and premature aging. Spice bioactives alleviate inflammatory stress primarily by suppressing key proinflammatory pathways and modulating cytokine activity.

Polyphenols exert antiinflammatory effects by suppressing the activation of the transcription factor NF-κB and downregulating proinflammatory enzymes such as COX-2 and LOX, thereby reducing the production of inflammatory mediators, including prostaglandins and cytokines (Guldiken et al., 2018). They also modulate MAPK and JAK/STAT signaling, leading to decreased proinflammatory cytokine production and attenuated immune-cell activation (Yahfoufi et al., 2018).

Terpenoids exert similar effects through the MAPK and JNK signaling cascades, decreasing cytokine expression (TNF-α, IL-1β, IL-6) and attenuating skin redness and irritation (Trepa et al., 2024). In addition, several monoterpenes and sesquiterpenes suppress iNOS and modulate antioxidant–inflammatory cross-talk, thereby enhancing tissue recovery and limiting oxidative–inflammatory cycles (de Cássia da Silveira E Sá et al., 2013).

Alkaloids modulate NF-κB signaling and suppress iNOS expression, thereby attenuating inflammatory responses and supporting skin barrier function (Duan et al., 2022; Kim et al., 2003; Prosser et al., 2013; Li et al., 2023). Through these complementary mechanisms, spice-derived phytochemicals help restore cutaneous immune homeostasis and provide a molecular rationale for their incorporation into cosmeceutical formulations.

3.6.3 *Antimicrobial activity*

As discussed previously, many spice-derived phytochemicals possess potent antimicrobial and antiseptic activities essential for maintaining a balanced skin microbiota. Their efficacy is attributed to the multitarget disruption of microbial physiology.

Phenolic compounds act by damaging microbial membranes, increasing permeability, and inhibiting enzymatic and metabolic functions, ultimately leading to cell lysis (Burt, 2004). They additionally interfere with quorum sensing and microbial communication systems, thereby reducing virulence factor production and biofilm stability. This interference is particularly relevant in controlling opportunistic skin pathogens such as *S. aureus* and *Cutibacterium acnes*, both implicated in acne and atopic conditions (Khan et al., 2014).

Terpenoids exert their antimicrobial action mainly through the disruption of microbial cell membranes, increasing permeability and causing leakage of cellular contents, ultimately leading to the loss of viability and cell lysis (Guimarães et al., 2019).

Alkaloids demonstrate antibacterial effects by targeting multiple cellular processes, including the inhibition of nucleic acid and protein synthesis, disruption of membrane potential, and suppression of virulence factors and biofilm formation (Cushnie et al., 2014). Together, these mechanisms support the use of spice-derived phytochemicals as multifunctional agents that not only suppress pathogenic microorganisms but also help preserve the skin's commensal microbiota, an increasingly recognized determinant of skin health and cosmetic integrity (Belkaid and Segre, 2014).

3.6.4 Photoprotective activity

Consistent with observations in the sections on phenolics and terpenoids, several spice bioactives confer photoprotective benefits by attenuating the oxidative and inflammatory consequences of UV exposure. Their effects arise from a coordinated modulation of antioxidant, antiinflammatory, and melanogenic pathways that preserve epidermal and dermal integrity under photostress conditions.

Phenolic compounds play a dual role in photoprotection by absorbing UV radiation and inhibiting tyrosinase activity, which reduces melanin overproduction and prevents hyperpigmentation (de Lima Cherubim et al., 2020; Han et al., 2007). In addition, they activate the Nrf2/Keap1 antioxidant pathway, which upregulates genes encoding heme oxygenase-1, glutathione S-transferase, and NAD(P)H:quinone oxidoreductase 1, key enzymes that strengthen the skin's redox defense and promote repair of UV-induced oxidative lesions (Chaiprasongsuk and Panich, 2022).

Terpenoids exert complementary photoprotective effects by modulating NF-κB and MAPK signaling, reducing the release of inflammatory mediators, and maintaining redox balance in keratinocytes and fibroblasts (Herman et al., 2016; Kumar et al., 2022).

Alkaloids demonstrate photoprotective activity by reducing UV-induced oxidative stress, preventing DNA strand breaks, and modulating NF-κB and apoptotic signaling pathways to preserve cellular integrity and viability (Verma et al., 2017).

3.6.5 Regenerative and wound healing effects

The regenerative capacity of spice-derived compounds, detailed earlier for thymoquinone, curcumin, and piperine, is linked to their ability to stimulate cell proliferation, angiogenesis, and extracellular matrix remodeling.

Polyphenols enhance keratinocyte migration and collagen synthesis, promoting wound closure and dermal remodeling via the regulation of TGF-β-mediated pathways (Javed et al., 2024). In in vivo studies, curcumin-loaded hydrogels have been shown to accelerate re-epithelialization, promote organized collagen deposition, and reduce scar formation through the activation of TGF-β1 signaling (Chen et al., 2025).

Terpenoids stimulate fibroblast proliferation, collagen synthesis, and angiogenic responses through the modulation of TGF-β, fibroblast growth factor 2, and vascular endothelial growth factor signaling, supporting dermal repair and regeneration (Javed et al., 2024; Trepa et al., 2024). In vivo, thymoquinone-loaded nanoemulgels significantly accelerated wound closure, increased epithelial thickness, and enhanced collagen deposition and maturation compared with untreated controls (Algahtani et al., 2021).

Alkaloids facilitate tissue repair by promoting angiogenesis, enhancing collagen deposition, and modulating inflammatory cytokines, thereby supporting effective wound healing and tissue regeneration (Fetse et al., 2014; Alsareii et al., 2023).

Taken together, the molecular mechanisms underlying the activity of spice-derived phytochemicals explain their multifunctional behavior in cosmetic and dermatological formulations. By simultaneously modulating oxidative balance, inflammatory signaling, microbial integrity, UV response, and tissue regeneration, these compounds provide comprehensive skin protection and renewal. Understanding these interconnected pathways not only validates the long-standing use of spices in traditional beauty systems but also guides the scientific development of biofunctional cosmetics that integrate natural efficacy with advanced formulation design. An overview of representative spice-derived compounds, their key skin-related mechanisms, and cosmetic applications is summarized in Table 8.3.

TABLE 8.3 Cosmeceutical attributes of spices: Key phytochemicals, skin actions, indications, and formulations.

Spice	Key phytochemical (class)	Principal biophysical/skin-related properties	Conditions treated/ benefits	Forms used in cosmetics
Turmeric (*Curcuma longa*)	Curcumin (phenolic polyphenol)	Potent antioxidant; antiinflammatory; tyrosinase inhibition; promotes collagen synthesis and wound repair	Hyperpigmentation, photoaging, wound healing, loss of firmness	Extract, nanoemulsion, hydrogel, essential oil, powder
Ginger (*Zingiber officinale*)	Gingerol (phenolic ketone)	Antioxidant; antiinflammatory; antimicrobial; improves microcirculation	Photoaging, acne, puffiness, dullness	Extract, essential oil, serum, powder
Clove (*Syzygium aromaticum*)	Eugenol (phenolic)	Antioxidant; antiinflammatory; antimicrobial; mild analgesic	Acne, irritation, microbial control, product preservation	Essential oil, extract
Cinnamon (*Cinnamomum verum*)	Cinnamaldehyde (phenylpropanoid)	Antioxidant; antimicrobial; circulation-stimulating; antiinflammatory	Acne-prone skin, revitalization, product preservation	Essential oil, extract, nanoemulsion
Black Pepper (*Piper nigrum*)	Piperine (alkaloid)	Antioxidant; antiinflammatory; enhances skin penetration of actives	Improved delivery, firming, anticellulite, rejuvenation	Essential oil, extract, cream
Chili Pepper (*Capsicum* spp.)	Capsaicin (alkaloid)	Antioxidant; thermogenic; circulation-stimulating; analgesic	Lip plumping, anticellulite, scalp stimulation	Extract, balm, lotion
Black Cumin (*Nigella sativa*)	Thymoquinone (terpenoid quinone)	Antioxidant; antiinflammatory; antimicrobial; wound healing	Acne, eczema, dermatitis, photoaging	Black seed oil, extract, nanoemulgel
Cumin (*Cuminum cyminum*)	Cuminaldehyde (phenylpropanoid)	Antioxidant; antiinflammatory; antimicrobial; tyrosinase inhibition	Uneven tone, irritation, microbial imbalance	Essential oil, extract
Fennel/Anise (*Foeniculum vulgare, Pimpinella anisum*)	Anethole (phenolic ether)	Antioxidant; mild antiinflammatory; antimicrobial	Puffiness, mild irritation, tone balance	Essential oil, extract
Coriander (*Coriandrum sativum*)	Linalool (terpenoid alcohol)	Antioxidant; antiinflammatory; photoprotective	UV-induced stress, irritation, redness	Essential oil, extract, nanoemulsion
Nutmeg (*Myristica fragrans*)	Myristicin (phenylpropanoid)	Antioxidant; antibacterial; circulation-enhancing	Blemish-prone skin, dullness, uneven texture	Powder, essential oil, extract
Fenugreek (*Trigonella foenum-graecum*)	Saponins (diosgenin)	Moisturizing; barrier-restoring; antiinflammatory	Dryness, irritation, barrier recovery	Seed powder, extract
Liquorice (*Glycyrrhiza glabra*)	Glabridin (phenolic isoflavan)	Depigmenting (tyrosinase inhibition); antioxidant; antiinflammatory	Hyperpigmentation, redness, uneven tone	Extract, glycoside-rich fraction
Saffron (*Crocus sativus*)	Crocin (carotenoid glycoside)	Potent antioxidant; photoprotective; brightening; antiaging	Dullness, pigmentation, photoaging	Extract, infused oil, powder
Vanilla (*Vanilla planifolia*)	Vanillin (phenolic aldehyde)	Antioxidant; soothing; aromatic; mild antimicrobial	Sensory enhancement, soothing care, antioxidant protection	Extract, aromatic base, essential oil

4 Phytochemicals extraction and formulations

Spice-derived bioactives have gained attention in modern cosmeceutical science due to their multifunctional properties, making them valuable natural agents for skin protection and rejuvenation (Ali et al., 2021). Recent years have witnessed a strong shift toward eco-friendly, plant-based cosmetics, driven by consumer preference for ingredients perceived as natural, sustainable, and safe (Dini and Laneri, 2021). This has catalyzed the growth of the "green beauty" movement, promoting formulations with minimal synthetic additives and responsible sourcing. Botanical extracts, essential oils, and spice-derived actives are now central to mainstream and niche cosmetic lines, valued for both functionality and sensory appeal (Sharmeen et al., 2021; Michalak, 2023). Plant-based ingredients dominate the cosmeceutical market because of their multitarget biological actions, biocompatibility, and low toxicity. Phenolic- and terpenoid-rich extracts counter oxidative and inflammatory processes that underlie photoaging, acne, and dermatitis, improving overall skin health (Singh and Yadav, 2022). Essential oils from spices such as black pepper, cardamom, and star anise are incorporated into serums, cleansers, and gels not only for fragrance but also for exfoliating, toning, and detoxifying effects (Mandal et al., 2023; Durczyńska and Żukowska, 2024). From a market standpoint, botanical ingredients have come to represent purity, transparency, and efficacy within the cosmetic industry. Advances in formulation and delivery technologies now enable natural bioactives to perform on par with, or even surpass, synthetic ingredients, reinforcing their position as key drivers of modern cosmetic innovation. Consequently, spice-derived actives are increasingly featured in diverse skincare products such as creams, serums, facial oils, gels, and exfoliating masks designed to target different cosmetic and health needs.

4.1 Extraction and preparation of spice phytochemicals

A wide spectrum of extraction strategies has been explored for isolating bioactive compounds from spices, ranging from traditional solvent-based techniques to advanced green and biotechnological processes. The choice of method determines not only the extraction yield but also the purity, stability, and cosmetic compatibility of the recovered phytochemicals. Conventional methods such as maceration, percolation, decoction, and distillation remain widely used for their simplicity and established efficacy in producing essential oils and oleoresins. However, emerging approaches, including ultrasound- and microwave-assisted extraction, enzyme-assisted extraction (EAE), and supercritical or pressurized fluid systems, offer substantial improvements in efficiency, selectivity, and sustainability. These modern methods minimize solvent use, reduce processing time and energy demands, and better preserve thermolabile or oxidation-sensitive actives. The principal extraction techniques, their operational principles, major spice applications, and cosmetic relevance are summarized in Table 8.4.

4.1.1 Additional green and emerging extraction approaches

Beyond the key solvent-based and distillation techniques, recent advances in extraction technology have introduced more sustainable and efficient approaches for isolating spice-derived phytochemicals. Accelerated solvent extraction (ASE) utilizes elevated temperature and pressure to enhance solvent diffusion, providing rapid and reproducible yields with reduced solvent consumption. EAE applies hydrolytic enzymes, such as cellulase and pectinase, to degrade plant cell walls, facilitating the release of bound flavonoids and phenolic acids, an approach that aligns well with the "green chemistry" principles favored in natural cosmetic production. Similarly, pressurized hot water extraction (PHWE) employs subcritical water as a clean solvent capable of dissolving both polar and moderately nonpolar phytochemicals without leaving chemical residues. Traditional variants, such as infusion or mild digestion, remain used in artisanal or small-scale contexts but generally offer lower yields and limited selectivity compared with modern alternatives. The range of available extraction techniques, their principles, and relevance to cosmetic applications are summarized in Table 8.4 (López-Salazar et al., 2023; Bitwell et al., 2023; Akhtar et al., 2019; Chemat et al., 2019).

4.2 Incorporation into cosmetic product types

Spice-derived phytochemicals have gained increasing prominence across the cosmetic, cosmeceutical, and nutricosmetic sectors due to their multifunctional biological activities and natural consumer appeal (Table 8.5). Their incorporation into formulations depends largely on physicochemical characteristics, such as solubility, polarity, volatility, and stability, as well as on their intended mechanism of action, whether to restore skin homeostasis, prevent photoaging, or promote overall dermal vitality.

TABLE 8.4 Summary of key extraction methods used to obtain bioactive compounds from spices, highlighting their operational type, main features, and relevance to formulation development in cosmetics, cosmeceuticals, and nutricosmetics (López-Salazar et al., 2023; Bitwell et al., 2023; Akhtar et al., 2019; Chemat et al., 2019).

Extraction method	Type	Key features	Advantages/cosmetic relevance	Limitations
Maceration/ percolation	Conventional (solvent-based)	Soak or slowly percolate powdered plant material in a suitable solvent at ambient or mild temperature.	Simple, low-cost; compatible with hydroalcoholic tinctures; minimal equipment.	Long time, higher solvent consumption; possible degradation/oxidation without an inert atmosphere.

Extraction method	Type	Key features	Advantages/cosmetic relevance	Limitations
Decoction/ digestion/ infusion	Conventional (aqueous)	Boiling or mild heating in water (decoction/digestion) or brief hot-solvent contact (infusion).	Food-grade, safe for simple aqueous cosmetics; extracts water-soluble phenolics and tannins.	Low selectivity and yields; unsuitable for heat-labile volatiles.
Soxhlet extraction	Conventional (hot solvent, continuous)	Cyclic reflux for exhaustive extraction.	Good recovery of nonpolar oleoresins/terpenoids; reproducible loads.	High temperature/long exposure; larger solvent use; not "green."
Steam/hydro-distillation	Conventional (volatile oils)	Steam volatilizes essential oils; condensate separates oil and water.	Produces perfume-grade essential oils for antimicrobial/aroma uses.	Energy-intensive; not suitable for nonvolatile or thermolabile, nonoily actives.
Pressurized liquid extraction (PLE/ASE)	Modern/ "green(er)"	Elevated temperature (typically 50°C–200°C) and pressure keep the solvent liquid and enhance mass transfer.	Rapid, efficient, lower solvent volumes; good reproducibility.	Specialized equipment; high T/P can degrade sensitive actives if not optimized.
Ultrasound-assisted extraction (UAE)	Modern/green	Acoustic cavitation disrupts cell walls, improves solvent penetration, and mass transfer.	Faster extraction, lower energy; gentle for thermo-labile phenolics; scalable.	Requires optimization (solvent, power, duty cycle, time) to avoid oxidation or overextraction.
Microwave-assisted extraction (MAE)	Modern/green	Rapid volumetric heating of the solvent/plant matrix releases intracellular compounds.	Very fast; reduced solvent and energy use; often higher yields; preserves bioactivity when parameters controlled.	Risk of hot-spots/overheating; careful control of solvent type, power, time, and particle size required.
Supercritical CO_2 extraction (SFE)	Modern/green (solvent-residue-free)	Supercritical CO_2 (often with an ethanol modifier) extracts nonpolars; tunable by P/T.	High-purity essential oils/ oleoresins; no solvent residues, ideal for premium cosmetics.	High CAPEX; limited efficiency for polar phenolics without a cosolvent.
Enzyme-assisted extraction (EAE)	Modern/ biocatalytic	Cell wall enzymes (cellulase/ pectinase/hemicellulase) liberate bound phenolics/glycosides.	Mild, eco-friendly; can boost phenolic yield and antioxidant activity; fits "clean beauty."	Enzyme cost/specificity; longer steps and optimization needed.
Pressurized hot water extraction (PHWE/ subcritical water)	Modern/ solvent-free	Water at 100°C–200°C under ~ 10–15 MPa behaves like a mid-polarity solvent.	Green, residue-free; selective extraction of antioxidants/phenolics; good for cosmetic actives.	Thermal degradation risk at high T; requires a pressure-rated system.

TABLE 8.5 Illustrative examples of spice-derived cosmetic, cosmeceutical, and nutricosmetic products.

Product name	Active phytochemical(s)	Primary function	Formulation type	References
Kiehl's Turmeric & Cranberry Seed Masque	Turmeric	Antioxidant, glow-enhancing	Cream mask	(Kiehls, n.d.)
Himalaya Dental Cream	Cinnamon	Antimicrobial, gum protection	Herbal toothpaste	(Himalaya Wellness, n.d.)
Vicco Turmeric Cream	Turmeric	Antiacne, healing	Oil-in-water emulsion	(Vicco Turmeric, n.d.)
Biotique Bio Clove Purifying Face Pack	Clove	Blemish control, antibacterial	Herbal clay mask	(Biotique, n.d.)
Kama Ayurveda Kumkumadi Brightening Serum	Saffron	Brightening, antiaging	Oil-based serum	(Kama Ayurveda, n.d.)
Dabur Red Toothpaste	Clove	Antibacterial oral care	Herbal toothpaste	(Dabur Red Toothpaste, n.d.)
Meriva® Curcumin Capsules	Curcumin	Systemic antioxidant, skin radiance	Oral nutricosmetic supplement	(Star Labs France, n.d.)

In topical cosmetics and cosmeceuticals, spice-derived actives are formulated into creams, gels, serums, emulsions, masks, and oils, each designed to optimize targeted delivery and sensory attributes. Emulsions and lotions provide controlled hydration and efficient dispersion of both hydrophilic and lipophilic actives, while hydrogels and gels enable nongreasy, fast-absorbing applications suitable for oily or sensitive skin. Clay and peel-off masks act as concentrated systems for exfoliation and detoxification, whereas oil-based serums enhance penetration of lipid-soluble actives and offer emollient, barrier-restoring benefits (Parhi, 2019).

In nutricosmetics, spice phytochemicals are incorporated into capsules, functional beverages, or fortified foods, acting systemically to enhance skin tone, elasticity, and antioxidant defense. Ingredients such as curcumin, piperine, and polyphenolic extracts demonstrate synergistic bioactivity when coformulated with vitamins, collagen peptides, or carotenoids, thereby supporting dermal health and the skin–gut axis (Hegde et al., 2023; Agrawal et al., 2024).

Recent advances in delivery technologies have expanded the potential of spice bioactives across all product categories. Nanocarrier-based systems, including nanoemulsions, liposomes, phytosomes, and solid lipid nanoparticles (SLNs), improve solubility, protect sensitive compounds from photochemical and oxidative degradation, and enhance dermal or intestinal absorption. These platforms also allow controlled or sustained release, increasing bioavailability and therapeutic efficacy (Manickam et al., 2020; Shukla et al., 2024). Such nanotechnological strategies bridge traditional botanical knowledge with modern evidence-based formulation science, enabling the design of multifunctional cosmetics and cosmeceuticals that deliver both esthetic and therapeutic benefits (Parhi, 2019; Agrawal et al., 2024).

5 Conclusion and future perspectives

Spices have long been valued across civilizations not only for their culinary importance but also for their medicinal and cosmetic applications. Modern scientific research has confirmed that widely used spices such as turmeric, cinnamon, clove, ginger, saffron, and black pepper are rich sources of bioactive phytochemicals, including curcuminoids, gingerols, piperine, eugenol, cinnamaldehyde, terpenes, flavonoids, and related secondary metabolites. These compounds contribute to the characteristic color, aroma, and flavor of spices while also exhibiting diverse biological activities that are increasingly relevant to cosmetic science. As consumer demand shifts toward natural and multifunctional ingredients, spices have emerged as valuable reservoirs of bioactive molecules for the development of cosmetics, cosmeceuticals, and nutricosmetics. Spice-derived phytochemicals represent a promising class of bioactives that bridge traditional ethnobotanical knowledge with modern cosmetic innovation. Their multifunctional activities, including antioxidant, antiinflammatory, antimicrobial, photoprotective, and regenerative effects, make them highly valuable ingredients for skincare and beauty formulations. The overall pathway from raw spice materials to the development of biofunctional beauty products is summarized in Fig. 8.11, which illustrates the transformation of spice-derived raw materials through sequential stages of extraction, purification, standardization, and formulation, ultimately leading to commercial products in cosmetics, cosmeceuticals, and nutricosmetics.

In this context, spices can be broadly defined as plant-derived substances obtained from nonleafy plant parts, including seeds, roots, bark, buds, fruits, and rhizomes, generally used in dried form. Their functional value is largely attributed to phytochemicals, which are secondary metabolites synthesized by plants during growth and metabolism. Although not directly involved in primary nutrition, these compounds play important ecological roles in plants and contribute significantly to the biological and functional properties of spice-derived materials. These phytochemicals exert multiple mechanisms of action that are highly relevant to dermatological and cosmetic applications. Their antioxidant capacity enables the neutralization of ROS and the mitigation of oxidative stress associated with skin aging and environmental exposure. In addition, many spice-derived compounds exhibit antiinflammatory, antimicrobial, photoprotective, and regenerative properties, contributing to improved skin protection, wound healing, barrier function, and antiaging performance. Consequently, these natural molecules are increasingly incorporated into cosmetic formulations as multifunctional active ingredients. The extraction and utilization of these bioactives rely on a range of technologies. While conventional techniques such as solvent extraction and steam distillation remain widely employed, increasing attention is being directed toward greener and more sustainable approaches. Emerging extraction technologies, including supercritical fluid extraction, ultrasound-assisted extraction, microwave-assisted extraction, and EAE, allow improved efficiency, reduced solvent use, and better preservation of sensitive phytochemicals. Such advances support the broader transition toward sustainable and biobased cosmetic innovation. At the formulation level, recent developments in delivery technologies are further expanding the applicability of spice-derived bioactives. Nanocarrier systems such as nanoemulsions, liposomes, phytosomes, and SLNs can enhance the solubility, stability, and bioavailability of hydrophobic phytochemicals while protecting them from degradation. These delivery platforms also enable controlled or sustained

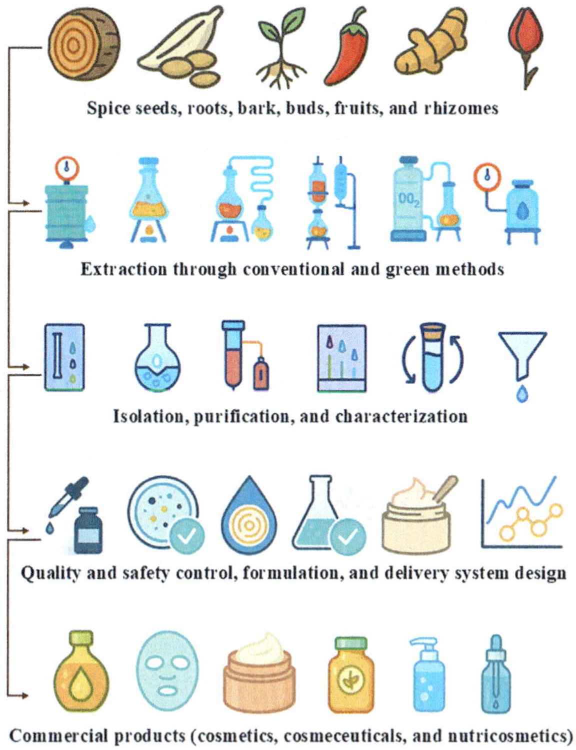

Spice seeds, roots, bark, buds, fruits, and rhizomes
Extraction through conventional and green methods
Isolation, purification, and characterization
Quality and safety control, formulation, and delivery system design
Commercial products (cosmetics, cosmeceuticals, and nutricosmetics)

FIG. 8.11 From raw spices to biofunctional commercial products. Illustrated workflow showing the transformation of spice-derived raw materials (seeds, roots, bark, buds, fruits, and rhizomes) through sequential stages of extraction, purification, standardization, and formulation, leading to the development of commercial products encompassing cosmetics, cosmeceuticals, and nutricosmetics. Each stage represents a critical step in isolating, characterizing, and optimizing bioactive compounds for safe and effective skin health and beauty applications.

release, improving dermal absorption and overall efficacy. By integrating nanotechnology with botanical ingredients, modern formulation science is effectively bridging traditional plant knowledge with advanced cosmetic design. Despite their considerable potential, several challenges remain for the effective integration of spice-derived compounds into cosmetic products. These include:

Color and sensory esthetics: Many spice-derived compounds present formulation challenges due to their intense natural pigmentation and characteristic aromas. Pigmented molecules, such as curcumin and capsanthin, can alter the visual appearance of cosmetic products or cause temporary skin staining, while strong-smelling constituents, like eugenol and cinnamaldehyde, may reduce sensory acceptance. Achieving the desired color balance and fragrance profile without compromising efficacy remains a critical aspect of product design.

Chemical and physical stability: Numerous spice bioactives are sensitive to light, heat, and oxygen, leading to degradation and loss of potency over time. Their thermolabile nature limits conventional processing and storage conditions. Ensuring chemical stability through protective formulation approaches is essential to maintaining efficacy and shelf life in finished cosmetic products.

Bioavailability and skin penetration: The low water solubility and poor membrane permeability of many hydrophobic compounds, including curcumin, piperine, and thymoquinone, restrict their biological effectiveness. This limited bioavailability poses a major obstacle to achieving sufficient concentrations at target skin layers or systemic sites when used in topical or oral formats.

Safety and regulatory compliance: While spice phytochemicals are generally regarded as safe, some constituents can cause irritation or sensitization, particularly at higher concentrations. Maintaining safe exposure levels, ensuring proper labeling, and adhering to international cosmetic and nutraceutical regulations are essential to guarantee product safety and consumer trust.

Standardization and extract variability: The chemical composition of spice extracts can vary substantially depending on the botanical source, growing conditions, and extraction technique. Such variability can influence both biological activity and product consistency. Establishing standardized extraction procedures and robust quality control systems is therefore necessary for reproducibility and large-scale commercialization.

Nevertheless, growing scientific evidence supporting the biological efficacy of spice-derived phytochemicals continues to accelerate their adoption in cosmetic and health-related formulations. At the same time, the cosmetics industry is undergoing a major shift toward sustainability, transparency, and plant-based innovation, with leading companies increasingly prioritizing renewable raw materials, biodegradable ingredients, and green chemistry principles in product development. For example, according to L'Oréal Groupe's 2024 Universal Registration Document, 66% of the ingredients used in its formulas were bio-based, derived from abundant minerals, or obtained through circular processes, while 92% of its bio-based ingredients were traceable and sustainably sourced, reflecting the industry's broader commitment to environmentally responsible cosmetic formulations (L'Oréal Groupe, 2025). In this context, spice-derived phytochemicals represent a particularly promising category of naturally sourced bioactives that align with the cosmetics industry's transition toward sustainable and biobased ingredients, offering multifunctional biological activity while supporting the development of innovative and environmentally responsible cosmetic formulations. Within this evolving landscape, biofunctional cosmetics, formulations that combine esthetic benefits with biologically active ingredients, are gaining increasing importance. Spice-derived phytochemicals are particularly well positioned to contribute to this sector due to their multifunctional activities, natural origin, and compatibility with emerging green technologies. Future progress will likely involve further optimization of green extraction methods, improved standardization of botanical extracts, and the continued development of advanced delivery systems capable of maximizing the stability and bioavailability of these compounds. Overall, spice-derived bioactives represent a compelling intersection between traditional botanical knowledge and contemporary cosmetic science. Their chemical diversity and multifunctional biological properties offer significant opportunities for the development of safe, effective, and sustainable cosmetic formulations. Continued interdisciplinary research integrating phytochemistry, dermatology, biotechnology, and formulation science will be essential to fully harness the potential of these natural resources. As innovation progresses, spices are likely to play an increasingly important role in shaping the next generation of green, biobased cosmetic technologies.

AI disclosure

During the preparation of this work, the author(s) used ChatGPT (OpenAI) to enhance the readability and language of the text. After utilizing this tool, the author(s) reviewed and edited the content as needed and take(s) full responsibility for the content of the publication.

References

Abbas, M., Saeed, F., Anjum, F.M., Afzaal, M., Tufail, T., Bashir, M.S., Ishtiaq, A., Hussain, S., Suleria, H.A.R., 2017. Natural polyphenols: an overview. Int. J. Food Prop. 15322386. 20 (8), 1689–1699. Available from: https://www.tandf.co.uk/journals/titles/10942912.asp. doi:10.1080/10942912.2016.1220393.

Agrawal, R., Jurel, P., Deshmukh, R., Harwansh, R.K., Garg, A., Kumar, A., Singh, S., Guru, A., Kumar, A., Kumarasamy, V., 2024. Emerging trends in the treatment of skin disorders by herbal drugs: traditional and nanotechnological approach. Pharmaceutics 19994923. 16 (7). Available from: http://www.mdpi.com/journal/pharmaceutics. doi:10.3390/pharmaceutics16070869.

Ahuja, K.D.K., Kunde, D.A., Ball, M.J., Geraghty, D.P., 2006. Effects of capsaicin, dihydrocapsaicin, and curcumin on copper-induced oxidation of human serum lipids. J. Agric. Food Chem. 00218561. 54 (17), 6436–6439. doi:10.1021/jf061331j.

Akhtar, I., Javad, S., Yousaf, Z., Iqbal, S., Jabeen, K., 2019. Microwave assisted extraction of phytochemicals an efficient and modern approach for botanicals and pharmaceuticals. J. Pharm. Sci. 1011601X. 32 (1), 223–230. Available from: http://www.pjps.pk/wp-content/uploads/pdfs/32/1/Paper-32.pdf.

Algahtani, M.S., Ahmad, M.Z., Shaikh, I.A., Abdel-Wahab, B.A., Nourein, I.H., Ahmad, J., 2021. Thymoquinone loaded topical nanoemulgel for wound healing: formulation design and in-vivo evaluation. Molecules 14203049. 26 (13). Available from: https://www.mdpi.com/1420-3049/26/13/3863/pdf. doi:10.3390/molecules26133863.

Alhanshali, L., Khachemoune, A., 2024. Clinical dermatologic applications of ginger: a focused review. Int. J. Dermatol. 0011-9059. 63 (4), 438–442. doi:10.1111/ijd.16963.

Ali, A., Wu, H., Ponnampalam, E.N., Cottrell, J.J., Dunshea, F.R., Suleria, H.A.R., 2021. Comprehensive profiling of most widely used spices for their phenolic compounds through lc-esi-qtof-ms2 and their antioxidant potential. Antioxidants 20763921. 10 (5). Available from: https://www.mdpi.com/2076-3921/10/5/721/pdf. doi:10.3390/antiox10050721.

Aljabre, S.H.M., Alakloby, O.M., Randhawa, M.A., 2015. Dermatological effects of *Nigella sativa*. J. Dermatol. Dermatol. Surg. 23522410. 19 (2), 92–98. doi:10.1016/j.jdds.2015.04.002.

Alsareii, S.A., Ahmad, J., Umar, A., Ahmad, M.Z., Shaikh, I.A., 2023. Enhanced in vivo wound healing efficacy of a novel piperine-containing bioactive hydrogel in excision wound rat model. Molecules 14203049. 28 (2). Available from: http://www.mdpi.com/journal/molecules. doi:10.3390/molecules28020545.

Alves, A., Sousa, E., Kijjoa, A., Pinto, M., 2020. Marine-derived compounds with potential use as cosmeceuticals and nutricosmetics. Molecules. 1420-3049. 25 (11), 2536. doi:10.3390/molecules25112536.

Andarwulan, N., Shetty, K., 1999. Phenolic content in differentiated tissue cultures of untransformed and *Agrobacterium*-transformed roots of anise (*Pimpinella anisum* L.). J. Agric. Food Chem. 0021-8561. 47 (4), 1776–1780. doi:10.1021/jf981214r.

Azizah, L., n.d. Effectiveness of an organic mask of moringa leaves (*Moringa oleifera*) and Turmeric (*Curcuma longa*) for facial care.

Bai, Y., Qier, M., Junni, Q., Chula, S., 2025. The chemical composition of cumin (*Cuminum cyminum* L.) analyzed by UPLC-Q-Orbitrap MS and GC-MS. Nat. Prod. Commun. 1934-578X. 20 (4). doi:10.1177/1934578x251328280.

Bartnik, M., Facey, P., 2023. Glycosides Pharmacognosy: Fundamentals, Applications, and Strategies, second ed., Elsevier, Poland, pp. 103–165. Available from: https://www.sciencedirect.com/book/9780443186578. doi:10.1016/B978-0-443-18657-8.00001-3.

Baruah, T.J., Dutta, S.P., Das, P.P., Darjee, M.S., Deka, D., Bora, J., Malik, S., Das, A., 2025. Computational and biochemical evidence reveal cuminaldehyde as a potent tyrosinase inhibitor. Discover Chem. 3005-1193. 2 (1). doi:10.1007/s44371-025-00311-y.

Batiha, G.E.S., Alkazmi, L.M., Wasef, L.G., Beshbishy, A.M., Nadwa, E.H., Rashwan, E.K., 2020. Syzygium aromaticum l. (myrtaceae): traditional uses, bioactive chemical constituents, pharmacological and toxicological activities. Biomolecules 2218273X. 10 (2). Available from: https://www.mdpi.com/2218-273X/10/2/202/pdf. doi:10.3390/biom10020202.

Belkaid, Y., Segre, J.A., 2014. Dialogue between skin microbiota and immunity. Science 10959203. 346 (6212), 954–959. Available from: http://www.sciencemag.org/content/346/6212/954.full.pdf. doi:10.1126/science.1260144.

Binic, I., Lazarevic, V., Ljubenovic, M., Mojsa, J., Sokolovic, D., 2013. Skin ageing: natural weapons and strategies. Evid. Based Complement. Alternat. Med. 1741-427X. 2013, 1–10. doi:10.1155/2013/827248.

Biotique, n.d. CLOVE Oil Control Anti-Blemish Face Pack 75g. Available from: https://global.biotique.com/products/clove-oil-control-anti-blemish-face-pack-75g-jar.

Bitwell, C., Indra, S.S., Luke, C., Kakoma, M.K., 2023. A review of modern and conventional extraction techniques and their applications for extracting phytochemicals from plants. Sci. Afr. 24682276. 19. Available from: https://www.journals.elsevier.com/scientific-african. doi:10.1016/j.sciaf.2023.e01585.

Boudreau, S.A., Wang, K., Svensson, P., Sessle, B.J., Arendt-Nielsen, L., 2009. Vascular and psychophysical effects of topical capsaicin application to orofacial tissues. J. Oral Facial Pain Headache 23330376. 23 (3), 253–264. Available from: https://jop.quintessenz.de/63bc/jop_2009_03_s0253.pdf.

Burt, S., 2004. Essential oils: their antibacterial properties and potential applications in foods—a review. Int. J. Food Microbiol. 01681605. 94 (3), 223–253. doi:10.1016/j.ijfoodmicro.2004.03.022.

Chaiprasongsuk, A., Panich, U., 2022. Role of phytochemicals in skin photoprotection via regulation of Nrf2. Front. Pharmacol. 1663-9812. 13. doi:10.3389/fphar.2022.823881.

Chemat, F., Abert-Vian, M., Fabiano-Tixier, A.S., Strube, J., Uhlenbrock, L., Gunjevic, V., Cravotto, G., 2019. Green extraction of natural products. Origins, current status, and future challenges. TrAC Trends Anal. Chem. 18793142. 118, 248–263. Available from: https://www.elsevier.com/locate/trac. doi:10.1016/j.trac.2019.05.037.

Chen, J., Liu, S., Tang, Y., Guan, X., Wang, Y., Qike, L., Shaozhi, F., 2025. Curcumin-loaded hydrogels promote skin wound healing. Soft Matter. 1744-683X. 21 (37), 7184–7203. doi:10.1039/d5sm00621j.

Chen, K., Pan, H., Dongxu, J., Yunjian, L., Duan, H., Pan, W., 2021. Curcumin-loaded sandwich-like nanofibrous membrane prepared by electrospinning technology as wound dressing for accelerate wound healing. Mater. Sci. Eng. C. 09284931. 127, 112245. doi:10.1016/j.msec.2021.112245.

Christianson, D.W., 2017. Structural and chemical biology of terpenoid cyclases. Chem. Rev. 15206890. 117 (17), 11570–11648. Available from: http://pubs.acs.org/journal/chreay. doi:10.1021/acs.chemrev.7b00287.

Ciuca, M.D., Racovita, R.C., 2023. Curcumin: overview of extraction methods, health benefits, and encapsulation and delivery using microemulsions and nanoemulsions. Romania Int. J. Mol. Sci. 14220067. 24 (10). Available from: http://www.mdpi.com/journal/ijms. doi:10.3390/ijms24108874.

Codex Alimentarius Commission (CAC). 1993. Classification of Foods and Animal Feeds (CXA 004-1993), Group 028: Spices. Food and Agriculture Organization of the United Nations (FAO) and World Health Organization (WHO).

Cosano, D., Román, J.M., Lafont, F., Arrebola, J.R.R., 2023. Archaeometric identification of a perfume from roman times. Heritage 25719408. 6 (6), 4472–4491. Available from: https://www.mdpi.com/journal/heritage. doi:10.3390/heritage6060236.

Cushnie, T.P.T., Cushnie, B., Lamb, A.J., 2014. Alkaloids: an overview of their antibacterial, antibiotic-enhancing and antivirulence activities. Int. J. Antimicrob. Agents 18727913. 44 (5), 377–386. Available from: https://www.elsevier.com/locate/ijantimicag. doi:10.1016/j.ijantimicag.2014.06.001.

Dabur Red Toothpaste, n.d. DABUR RED TOOTHPASTE - 200g - Annachi Supermarket.

de Cássia da Silveira E Sá, R., Andrade, L.N., de Sousa, D.P., 2013. A review on anti-inflammatory activity of monoterpenes. Molecules. 1420-3049. 18 (1), 1227–1254. doi:10.3390/molecules18011227.

de Lima Cherubim, D.J., Martins, C.V.B., Fariña, L.O., da Silva de Lucca, R.A., 2020. Polyphenols as natural antioxidants in cosmetics applications. J. Cosmet. Dermatol. 14732165. 19 (1), 33–37. Available from: http://onlinelibrary.wiley.com/journal/10.1111/(ISSN)1473-2165. doi:10.1111/jocd.13093.

Deveci, E., 2025. Nanoemulsions in cosmetics: enhancing efficacy and stability. J. Dermatol. Sci. Cosmet. Technol. 2950306X. 2 (3), 100107. doi:10.1016/j.jdsct.2025.100107.

Dini, I., Laneri, S., 2021. The new challenge of green cosmetics: natural food ingredients for cosmetic formulations. Molecules. 1420-3049. 26 (13), 3921. doi:10.3390/molecules26133921.

Douglas, M., Heyes, J., Smallfield, B., Herbs, spices and essential oils: post-harvest operations in developing countries. (2005),

Doyle, A.A., Stephens, J.C., 2019. A review of cinnamaldehyde and its derivatives as antibacterial agents. Fitoterapia 18736971. 139. Available from: https://www.elsevier.com/locate/fitote. doi:10.1016/j.fitote.2019.104405.

Duan, Z., Xie, H., Shasha, Y., Wang, S., Yang, H., 2022. Piperine derived from *Piper nigrum* L. inhibits LPS-induced inflammation through the MAPK and NF-κB signalling pathways in RAW264.7 cells. Foods. 2304-8158. 11 (19), 2990. doi:10.3390/foods11192990.

Durczyńska, Z., Żukowska, G., 2024. Properties and applications of essential oils: a review. J. Ecol. Eng. 2299-8993. 25 (2), 333–340. doi:10.12911/22998993/177404.

Dureja, H., Kaushik, D., Gupta, M., Kumar, V., Lather, V., 2005. Cosmeceuticals: an emerging concept. Indian J. Pharmacol. 02537613. 37 (3), 155–159. Available from: http://www.ijp-online.com/. doi:10.4103/0253-7613.16211.

Ebada, M.E., 2017. Cuminaldehyde: a potential drug candidate. J. Pharmacol. Clin. Res. 24735574. 2 (2). doi:10.19080/JPCR.2017.02.555585.

Evanti, A., Wargasetia, T., Gunadi, J., 2025. Role of *Nigella sativa* L. seed (black cumin) in preventing photoaging (review). Biomed. Rep. 2049-9434. 23 (2), 1–13. doi:10.3892/br.2025.2009.

Fagot, D., Pham, D.M., Laboureau, J., Planel, E., Guerin, L., Nègre, C., Donovan, M., Bernard, B.A., 2018. Crocin, a natural molecule with potentially beneficial effects against skin ageing. Int. J. Cosmet. Sci. 0142-5463. 40 (4), 388–400. doi:10.1111/ics.12472.

Fatima Shad, K.F., Soubra, W., Cordato, D.J., 2021. The role of thymoquinone, a major constituent of *Nigella sativa*, in the treatment of inflammatory and infectious diseases. Clin. Exp. Pharmacol. Physiol. 14401681. 48 (11), 1445–1453. Available from: http://onlinelibrary.wiley.com/journal/10.1111/(ISSN)1440-1681. doi:10.1111/1440-1681.13553.

Fetse, J., Kyekyeku, J., Dueve, E., Mensah, K., 2014. Wound healing activity of total alkaloidal extract of the root bark of *Alstonia boonei* (Apocynaceae). Br. J. Pharm. Res. 22312919. 4 (23), 2642–2652. doi:10.9734/bjpr/2014/13952.

Forouzanfar, F., Bazzaz, B.S.F., Hosseinzadeh, H., 2014. Black cumin (*Nigella sativa*) and its constituent (thymoquinone): a review on antimicrobial effects. Iran. J. Basic Med. Sci. 20083874. 17 (12), 929–938. Available from: http://ijbms.mums.ac.ir/pdf_3862_470d114ad2a349430c8c8be2190bc312.html.

FS, n.d. Spices and Herbs. Available from: https://www.fs.usda.gov/wildflowers/ethnobotany/food/spices.shtml.

Fuloria, S., Mehta, J., Chandel, A., Sekar, M., Rani, N.N.I.M., Begum, M.Y., Subramaniyan, V., Chidambaram, K., Thangavelu, L., Nordin, R., Wu, Y.S., Sathasivam, K.V., Lum, P.T., Meenakshi, D.U., Kumarasamy, V., Azad, A.K., Fuloria, N.K., 2022. A comprehensive review on the therapeutic potential of *Curcuma longa* Linn. in relation to its major active constituent curcumin. Front. Pharmacol. 16639812. 13. Available from: http://www.frontiersin.org/Pharmacology. doi:10.3389/fphar.2022.820806.

Grand View Research, n.d. Natural Cosmetics Market Size, Share & Growth Report 2030. Available from: https://www.grandviewresearch.com/industry-analysis/natural-cosmetics-market.

Grynkiewicz, G., Ślifirski, P., 2012. Curcumin and curcuminoids in quest for medicinal status. Acta Biochim. Pol. 1734-154X. 59 (2). doi:10.18388/abp.2012_2139.

Guimarães, A.C., Meireles, L.M., Lemos, M.F., Guimarães, M.C.C., Endringer, D.C., Fronza, M., Scherer, R., 2019. Antibacterial activity of terpenes and terpenoids present in essential oils. Molecules 14203049. 24 (13). Available from: https://www.mdpi.com/1420-3049/24/13/2471/pdf. doi:10.3390/molecules24132471.

Gulcin, İ., 2020. Antioxidants and antioxidant methods: an updated overview. Arch. Toxicol. 14320738. 94 (3), 651–715. Available from: https://link.springer.de/link/service/journals/00204/index.htm. doi:10.1007/s00204-020-02689-3.

Guldiken, B., Ozkan, G., Catalkaya, G., Ceylan, F.D., Yalcinkaya, I.E., Capanoglu, E., 2018. Phytochemicals of herbs and spices: health versus toxicological effects. Food Chem. Toxicol. 18736351. 119, 37–49. Available from: https://www.elsevier.com/locate/foodchemtox. doi:10.1016/j.fct.2018.05.050.

Gunaseelan, S., Balupillai, A., Govindasamy, K., Ramasamy, K., Muthusamy, G., Shanmugam, M., Thangaiyan, R., Robert, B.M., Nagarajan, R.P., Ponniresan, V.K., Rathinaraj, P., Slominski, A.T., 2017. Linalool prevents oxidative stress activated protein kinases in single UVB-exposed human skin cells. PLOS ONE. 1932-6203. 12 (5), e0176699. doi:10.1371/journal.pone.0176699.

Gupta, J., Sharma, S., Sharma, N.R., Kabra, D., 2020. Phytochemicals enriched in spices: a source of natural epigenetic therapy. Arch. Pharm. Res. 19763786. 43 (2), 171–186. Available from: http://www.springerlink.com/content/0253-6269. doi:10.1007/s12272-019-01203-3.

Hajlaoui, H., Mighri, H., Noumi, E., Snoussi, M., Trabelsi, N., Ksouri, R., Bakhrouf, A., 2010. Chemical composition and biological activities of Tunisian *Cuminum cyminum* L. essential oil: a high effectiveness against Vibrio spp. strains. Food Chem. Toxicol. 02786915. 48 (8-9), 2186–2192. doi:10.1016/j.fct.2010.05.044.

Han, B., Chong, J., Sun, Z., Jiang, X., Xiao, Q., Zech, J., Roberts, P., Rao, H., Yang, Y., 2021. The rise of the cosmetic industry in ancient China: insights from a 2700-year-old face cream. Archaeometry. 0003-813X. 63 (5), 1042–1058. doi:10.1111/arcm.12659.

Han, X., Shen, T., Lou, H., 2007. Dietary polyphenols and their biological significance. Int. J. Mol. Sci. 1422-0067. 8 (9), 950–988. doi:10.3390/i8090950.

Hannan, M.A., Rahman, M.A., Sohag, A.A.M., Uddin, M.J., Dash, R., Sikder, M.H., Rahman, M.S., Timalsina, B., Munni, Y.A., Sarker, P.P., Alam, M., Mohibbullah, M., Haque, M.N., Jahan, I., Hossain, M.T., Afrin, T., Rahman, M.M., Tahjib-Ul-arif, M., Mitra, S., Oktaviani, D.F., Khan, M.K., Choi, H.J., Moon, I.S., Kim, B., 2021. Black cumin (*Nigella sativa* L.): a comprehensive review on phytochemistry, health benefits, molecular pharmacology, and safety. Nutrients 20726643. 13 (6). Available from: https://www.mdpi.com/2072-6643/13/6/1784/pdf. doi:10.3390/nu13061784.

Hegde, M., Girisa, S., BharathwajChetty, B., Vishwa, R., Kunnumakkara, A.B., 2023. Curcumin formulations for better bioavailability: what we learned from clinical trials thus far? ACS Omega 24701343. 8 (12), 10713–10746. Available from: https://pubs.acs.org/journal/acsodf. doi:10.1021/acsomega.2c07326.

Herman, A., Tambor, K., Herman, A., 2016. Linalool affects the antimicrobial efficacy of essential oils. Curr. Microbiol. 0343-8651. 72 (2), 165–172. doi:10.1007/s00284-015-0933-4.

Hewlings, S., Kalman, D., 2017. Curcumin: a review of its effects on human health. Foods. 2304-8158. 6 (10), 92. doi:10.3390/foods6100092.

Hill, L.E., Taylor, T.M., Gomes, C., 2013. Antimicrobial efficacy of poly(DL-lactide-co-glycolide) (PLGA) nanoparticles with entrapped cinnamon bark extract against *Listeria monocytogenes* and *Salmonella typhimurium*. J. Food Sci. 17503841. 78 (4), N626. doi:10.1111/1750-3841.12069.

Himalaya Wellness, n.d. Himalaya BOTANIQUE Complete Care Toothpaste - Simply Cinnamon - 150 g. Available from: https://himalayawellness.eu/products/himalaya-botanique-complete-care-toothpaste-simply-cinnamon-150g.

Hosseinzadeh, H., Nassiri-Asl, M., 2013. Avicenna's (Ibn Sina) *The Canon of Medicine* and saffron (*Crocus sativus*): a review. Phytother. Res. 0951418X. 27 (4), 475–483. doi:10.1002/ptr.4784.

Jain, N.K., Chaudhri, S.K., 2009. History of cosmetics. Asian J. Pharm. 0973-8398. 3 (3), 164. doi:10.4103/0973-8398.56292.

Jakubczyk, K., Drużga, A., Katarzyna, J., Skonieczna-Żydecka, K., 2020. Antioxidant potential of curcumin—a meta-analysis of randomized clinical trials. Antioxidants. 2076-3921. 9 (11), 1092. doi:10.3390/antiox9111092.

Javed, S., Mangla, B., Salawi, A., Sultan, M.H., Almoshari, Y., Ahsan, W., 2024. Essential oils as dermocosmetic agents, their mechanism of action and nanolipidic formulations for maximized skincare. Cosmetics 20799284. 11 (6). Available from: https://www.mdpi.com/journal/cosmetics. doi:10.3390/cosmetics11060210.

Jayaprakasha, G.K., Rao, L.J., Sakariah, K.K., 2006. Antioxidant activities of curcumin, demethoxycurcumin and bisdemethoxycurcumin. Food Chem. 03088146. 98 (4), 720–724. doi:10.1016/j.foodchem.2005.06.037.

Jiang, Y., Zhiyun, D., Xue, G., Chen, Q., Yujing, L., Zheng, X., Conney, A., Zhang, K., 2013. Synthesis and biological evaluation of unsymmetrical curcumin analogues as tyrosinase inhibitors. Molecules. 1420-3049. 18 (4), 3948–3961. doi:10.3390/molecules18043948.

Joo, J.I., Kim, D.H., Choi, J.W., Yun, J.W., 2010. Proteomic analysis for antiobesity potential of capsaicin on white adipose tissue in rats fed with a high fat diet. J. Proteome Res. 15353907. 9 (6), 2977–2987. doi:10.1021/pr901175w.

Kalasariya, H.S., Maya-Ramírez, C.E., Cotas, J., Pereira, L., 2024. Cosmeceutical significance of seaweed: a focus on carbohydrates and peptides in skin applications. Phycology 26739410. 4 (2), 276–313. Available from: https://www.mdpi.com/journal/phycology. doi:10.3390/phycology4020015.

Kama Ayurveda, n.d. Kumkumadi Silky Serum 50 Ml | Kama Ayurveda. Available from: https://www.kamaayurveda.com/ww/en/p/kumkumadi-silky-serum-50-ml–000000000065221702.

Kant, V., Gopal, A., Pathak, N.N., Kumar, P., Tandan, S.K., Kumar, D., 2014. Antioxidant and anti-inflammatory potential of curcumin accelerated the cutaneous wound healing in streptozotocin-induced diabetic rats. Int. Immunopharmacol. 18781705. 20 (2), 322–330. Available from: https://www.elsevier.com/locate/intimp. doi:10.1016/j.intimp.2014.03.009.

Karaman, K., 2020. Characterization of *Saccharomyces cerevisiae*-based microcarriers for encapsulation of black cumin seed oil: stability of thymoquinone and bioactive properties. Food Chem. 03088146. 313, 126129. doi:10.1016/j.foodchem.2019.126129.

Kasprzak-Drozd, K., Niziński, P., Hawrył, A., Gancarz, M., Hawrył, D., Oliwa, W., Pałka, M., Markowska, J., Oniszczuk, A., 2024. Potential of curcumin in the management of skin diseases. Int. J. Mol. Sci. 1422-0067. 25 (7), 3617. doi:10.3390/ijms25073617.

Khan Al-Saboun. 2024. Turmeric Honey Soap - 100g. Available from: https://khanalsaboun.net/product/turmeric-honey-soap-100g/?v=82a9e4d26595.

Khan, M.S.A., Ahmad, I., Cameotra, S.S., Botha, F., 2014. Sub-MICs of *Carum copticum* and *Thymus vulgaris* influence virulence factors and biofilm formation in *Candida* spp. BMC Complement. Altern. Med. 14726882. 14 (1). Available from: http://www.biomedcentral.com/1472-6882/14/337. doi:10.1186/1472-6882-14-337.

Kiehls, n.d. Finest Apothecary Skincare, Hair Care, & Body Care - Kiehl's. Available from: https://www.kiehls.com/.

Kim, C.S., Kawada, T., Kim, B.S., Han, I.S., Choe, S.Y., Kurata, T., Yu, R., 2003. Capsaicin exhibits anti-inflammatory property by inhibiting IkB-a degradation in LPS-stimulated peritoneal macrophages. Cell. Signal. 15 (3), 299–306. doi:10.1016/S0898-6568(02)00086-4.

Kinanti, A.P., Darmawan, M.A., Muryanto, M., Gozan, M., 2024. Formulation of herbal solid soap with illipe oil as raw material with ginger extract as antibacterial. AIP Conf. Proc. 15517616. 3080 (1). http://scitation.aip.org/content/aip/proceeding/aipcp. doi:10.1063/5.0198974.

Kmail, A., Said, O., Saad, B., 2023. How thymoquinone from *Nigella sativa* accelerates wound healing through multiple mechanisms and targets. Curr. Issues Mol. Biol. 1467-3045. 45 (11), 9039–9059. doi:10.3390/cimb45110567.

Kryst, J., 2023. Cosmetics containing turmeric in the light of the results of scientific research. Aesthetic Cosmetol. Med. 27193241. 12 (5), 169–174. doi:10.52336/acm.2023.016.

Kumar, K.J.S., Vani, M.G., Wang, S.Y., 2022. Limonene protects human skin keratinocytes against UVB-induced photodamage and photoaging by activating the Nrf2-dependent antioxidant defense system. Environ. Toxicol. 15227278. 37 (12), 2897–2909. Available from: http://onlinelibrary.wiley.com/journal/10.1002/(ISSN)1522-7278. doi:10.1002/tox.23646.

Kumar, N., Goel, N., 2019. Phenolic acids: natural versatile molecules with promising therapeutic applications. Biotechnol. Rep. 2215017X. 24, e00370. doi:10.1016/j.btre.2019.e00370.

L'Oréal Groupe, 2025. Universal Registration Document. L'Oréal Groupe. Available from: https://www.loreal-finance.com/system/files/2025-03/2024_Universal_Registration_Document_LOREAL.pdf.

Lau, M., Gollogly, J.M., Wang, J.Y., Jagdeo, J., 2024. Cosmeceuticals for antiaging: a systematic review of safety and efficacy. Arch. Dermatol. Res. 1432069X. 316 (5). Available from: https://www.springer.com/journal/403. doi:10.1007/s00403-024-02908-2.

Lazaridis, D.G., Karabagias, V.K., Karabagias, I.K., Andritsos, N.D., Giannakas, A.E., 2024b. Physicochemical and phytochemical characterization of green coffee, cinnamon clove, and nutmeg EEGO, and aroma evaluation of the raw powders. Eur. Food Res. Technol. 14382385. 250 (1), 83–96. Available from: https://www.springer.com/journal/217. doi:10.1007/s00217-023-04367-x.

Lazaridis, D.G., Kitsios, A.P., Koutoulis, A.S., Malisova, O., Karabagias, I.K., 2024a. Fruits, spices and honey phenolic compounds: a comprehensive review on their origin, methods of extraction and beneficial health properties. Antioxidants 20763921. 13 (11). Available from: https://www.mdpi.com/journal/antioxidants. doi:10.3390/antiox13111335.

Lee, M., Kim, C., Kim, I., Kim, Y., 2011. Effects of capsaicin on lipid catabolism in 3T3-L1 adipocytes. Phytother. Res. 0951-418X. 25 (6), 935–939. doi:10.1002/ptr.3339.

Lee, W.S., Ahn, H.J., Kim, Y.H., 2003. The effect of coapplication of capsaicin and minoxidil on the murine hair growth. Korean J. Dermatol. 41 (4), 451–460.

Letchuman, S., Madhuranga, H.D.T., Madhurangi, B.L.N.K., Premarathna, A.D., Saravanan, M., 2025. Alkaloids unveiled: a comprehensive analysis of novel therapeutic properties, mechanisms, and plant-based innovations. Intell. Pharm. 2949866X. 3 (4), 268–276. Available from: https://www.keaipublishing.com/en/journals/intelligent-pharmacy/. doi:10.1016/j.ipha.2024.09.007.

Li, J., Wang, H., Zhang, L., An, N., Wan, N., Gao, Q., Yang, Y., 2023. Capsaicin affects macrophage anti-inflammatory activity via the MAPK and NF-κB signaling pathways. Int. J. Vitam. Nutr. Res. 0300-9831. 93 (4), 289–297. doi:10.1024/0300-9831/a000721.

Li, R., Xiang, C., Zhang, X., Guo, D.A., Min, Y., 2010. Chemical analysis of the chinese herbal medicine turmeric (*Curcuma longa* L.). Curr. Pharm. Anal. 15734129. 6 (4), 256–268. doi:10.2174/157341210793292356.

Lim, C.T., Hasham@Hisam, R., Sabtu, R., 2023. Formulation and characterization of herbal cleansing gel from turmeric extract-loaded nanostructured lipid carriers. J. Bioprocess. Biomass Technol. 2976-3177. 2 (1), 25–30. doi:10.11113/bioprocessing.v2n1.25.

Liu, J.K., 2022. Natural products in cosmetics. Nat. Prod. Bioprospect. 21922209. 12 (1). Available from: https://www.springer.com/journal/13659. doi:10.1007/s13659-022-00363-y.

López-Salazar, H., Camacho-Díaz, B.H., Ocampo, M.L.A., Jiménez-Aparicio, A.R., 2023. Microwave-assisted extraction of functional compounds from plants: a review. BioResources 19302126. 18 (3), 6614–6638. Available from: https://bioresources.cnr.ncsu.edu/wp-content/uploads/2023/07/BioRes_18_3_6583_Bahrin_KMSAL_Review_Mechan_Bamboo_Pole_Building_Eng_22575.pdf. doi:10.15376/biores.18.3.Lopez-Salazar.

Macáková, K., Afonso, R., Saso, L., Mladěnka, P., 2019. The influence of alkaloids on oxidative stress and related signaling pathways. Free Radic. Biol. Med. 08915849. 134, 429–444. doi:10.1016/j.freeradbiomed.2019.01.026.

Makris, D.P., Boskou, D., 2014. Plant-derived Antioxidants as Food Additives. CABI Publishing, pp. 169–190. doi:10.1079/9781780642666.0169.

Mandal, D., Sarkar, T., Chakraborty, R., 2023. Critical review on nutritional, bioactive, and medicinal potential of spices and herbs and their application in food fortification and nanotechnology. Appl. Biochem. Biotechnol. 0273-2289. 195 (2), 1319–1513. doi:10.1007/s12010-022-04132-y.

Manickam, V., Sundar, V., Panchangam, R.L., Amiti, K.A.S., Tamizhselvi, R., 2020. Nanotechnology in Delivery and Targeting of Phytochemicals. Springer Science and Business Media LLC, pp. 211–264. doi:10.1007/978-3-030-44921-6_6.

Maoka, T., 2020. Carotenoids as natural functional pigments. J. Nat. Med. 1340-3443. 74 (1), 1–16. doi:10.1007/s11418-019-01364-x.

Marchese, A., Barbieri, R., Coppo, E., Orhan, I.E., Daglia, M., Nabavi, S.F., Izadi, M., Abdollahi, M., Nabavi, S.M., Ajami, M., 2017. Antimicrobial activity of eugenol and essential oils containing eugenol: a mechanistic viewpoint. Crit. Rev. Microbiol. 15497828. 43 (6), 668–689. doi:10.1080/1040841X.2017.1295225.

Martins, A.M., Silva, A.T., Marto, J.M., 2025. Advancing cosmetic sustainability: upcycling for a circular product life cycle. Sustainability. 2071-1050. 17 (13), 5738. doi:10.3390/su17135738.

McMullen, R.L., Dell'Acqua, G., 2023. History of natural ingredients in cosmetics. Cosmetics 20799284. 10 (3). Available from: https://www.mdpi.com/journal/cosmetics. doi:10.3390/cosmetics10030071.

Michalak, M., 2023. Plant extracts as skin care and therapeutic agents. Int. J. Mol. Sci. 1422-0067. 24 (20), 15444. doi:10.3390/ijms242015444.

Minooeianhaghighi, M.H., Sepehrian, L., Shokri, H., 2017. Antifungal effects of *Lavandula binaludensis* and *Cuminum cyminum* essential oils against *Candida albicans* strains isolated from patients with recurrent vulvovaginal candidiasis. J. Mycol. Med. 11565233. 27 (1), 65–71. doi:10.1016/j.mycmed.2016.09.002.

Morganti, P., Morganti, G., Colao, C., 2019. Biofunctional textiles for aging skin. Biomedicines. 2227-9059. 7 (3), 51. doi:10.3390/biomedicines7030051.

Nabavi, S., Di Lorenzo, A., Izadi, M., Sobarzo-Sánchez, E., Daglia, M., Nabavi, S., 2015. Antibacterial effects of cinnamon: from farm to food, cosmetic and pharmaceutical industries. Nutrients. 2072-6643. 7 (9), 7729–7748. doi:10.3390/nu7095359.

Nagappan, T., Segaran, T., Wahid, M., Ramasamy, P., Vairappan, C., 2012. Efficacy of carbazole alkaloids, essential oil and extract of *Murraya koenigii* in enhancing subcutaneous wound healing in rats. Molecules 1420-3049. 17 (12), 14449–14463. doi:10.3390/molecules171214449.

Nagegowda, D.A., Gupta, P., 2020. Advances in biosynthesis, regulation, and metabolic engineering of plant specialized terpenoids. Plant Sci. 01689452. 294, 110457. doi:10.1016/j.plantsci.2020.110457.

Naser, W., 2021. The cosmetic effects of various natural biofunctional ingredients against skin aging: a review. Int. J. Appl. Pharm. 0975-7058. 13 (1), 10–18. doi:10.22159/ijap.2021v13i1.39806.

Nasiri, N., Nezhad, M.I., Sharififar, F., Khazaneha, M., Najafzadeh, M.J., Mohamadi, N., 2022. The therapeutic effects of nigella sativa on skin disease: a systematic review and meta-analysis of randomized controlled trials. Evid. Based Complement. Alternat. Med. 17414288. 2022. Available from: http://www.hindawi.com/journals/ecam/contents.html. doi:10.1155/2022/7993579.

Neelam, A.K., Sharma, K.K., 2020. Phenylpropanoids and its derivatives: biological activities and its role in food, pharmaceutical and cosmetic industries. Crit. Rev. Food Sci. Nutr. 15497852. 60 (16), 2655–2675. Available from: https://www.tandfonline.com/loi/bfsn20. doi:10.1080/10408398.2019.1653822.

Okiki, P.A., Nwobi, C.P., Akpor, O.B., Adewole, E., Agbana, R.D., 2023. Assessment of nutritional and medicinal properties of nutmeg. Sci. Afr. 24682276. 19. Available from: https://www.journals.elsevier.com/scientific-african. doi:10.1016/j.sciaf.2023.e01548.

Papadopoulou, D., Chrysikopoulou, V., Rampaouni, A., Tsoupras, A., 2024. Antioxidant and anti-inflammatory properties of water kefir microbiota and its bioactive metabolites for health promoting bio-functional products and applications. AIMS Microbiol. 2471-1888. 10 (4), 756–811. doi:10.3934/microbiol.2024034.

Papadopoulou, S.N.A., Anastasiou, E.A., Adamantidi, T., Ofrydopoulou, A., Letsiou, S., Tsoupras, A., 2025. A comprehensive review on the beneficial roles of vitamin D in skin health as a bio-functional ingredient in nutricosmetic, cosmeceutical, and cosmetic applications. Appl. Sci. 2076-3417. 15 (2), 796. doi:10.3390/app15020796.

Parhi, R., 2019. The Role of Phytocompounds in Cosmeceutical Applications. Informa UK Limited, pp. 139–160. doi:10.1201/9780429259968-11.

Parish, L.C., Crissey, J.T., 1988. Cosmetics: a historical review. Clin. Dermatol. 0738081X. 6 (3), 1–4. doi:10.1016/0738-081X(88)90024-7.

Park, U.H., Jeong, H.S., Jo, E.Y., Park, T., Yoon, S.K., Kim, E.J., Jeong, J.C., Um, S.J., 2012. Piperine, a component of black pepper, inhibits adipogenesis by antagonizing PPARγ activity in 3T3-L1 cells. J. Agric. Food Chem. 15205118. 60 (15), 3853–3860. doi:10.1021/jf204514a.

Pastorino, G., Cornara, L., Soares, S., Rodrigues, F., Oliveira, M.B.P.P., 2018. Liquorice (*Glycyrrhiza glabra*): a phytochemical and pharmacological review. Phytother. Res. 10991573. 32 (12), 2323–2339. Available from: http://onlinelibrary.wiley.com/journal/10.1002/(ISSN)1099-1573. doi:10.1002/ptr.6178.

Patidar, M., Deshmukh, N., Mandloi, N., Patidar, B., Pillai, D.S., n.d. Formulation and evaluation of face serum containing phytosome of gingerol oil, *Carica papaya* pulp extract and *Aloe vera* gel.

Penkar, G.M., Salkar, M.R., Chavan, P.S., Ambade, M.S., Parab, S.A., Sawant, M.M., Japgap, V.A., 2023. Formulation and evaluation of herbal hair serum in treatment of various hair- related problems. Res. J. Pharmacogn. Phytochem. 0975-4385. 105–110. doi:10.52711/0975-4385.2023.00016.

Pereira, L., 2018. Seaweeds as a source of bioactive substances and skin care therapy—cosmeceuticals, algotherapy, and thalassotherapy. Cosmetics. 2079-9284. 5 (4), 68. doi:10.3390/cosmetics5040068.

Platel, K., Srinivasan, K., 2000. Influence of dietary spices and their active principles on pancreatic digestive enzymes in albino rats. Nahrung/Food. 0027-769X. 44 (1), 42–46. doi:10.1002/(sici)1521-3803(20000101)44:1<42::aid-food42>3.0.co;2-d.

Pratiwi, D., Sidoretno, W.M., Aisah, N., 2021. The combination of turmeric (*Curcuma domestica*) rhizome extract and collagen in a serum formulation as an antioxidant. Borneo J. Pharm. 26214814. 4 (1), 36–42. doi:10.33084/bjop.v4i1.1578.

Priyadarsini, K., 2014. The chemistry of curcumin: from extraction to therapeutic agent. Molecules. 1420-3049. 19 (12), 20091–20112. doi:10.3390/molecules191220091.

Priyadarsini, K.I., 2013. Chemical and structural features influencing the biological activity of curcumin. Curr. Pharm. Des. 13816128. 19 (11), 2093–2100. doi:10.2174/138161213805289228.

Prosser, G.A., Copp, J.N., Mowday, A.M., Guise, C.P., Syddall, S.P., Williams, E.M., Horvat, C.N., Swe, P.M., Ashoorzadeh, A., Denny, W.A., Smaill, J.B., Patterson, A.V., Ackerley, D.F., 2013. Creation and screening of a multi-family bacterial oxidoreductase library to discover novel nitroreductases that efficiently activate the bioreductive prodrugs CB1954 and PR-104A. Biochem. Pharmacol. 18732968. 85 (8), 1091–1103. doi:10.1016/j.bcp.2013.01.029.

Quideau, S., Deffieux, D., Douat-Casassus, C., Pouységu, L., 2011. Plant polyphenols: chemical properties, biological activities, and synthesis. Angew. Chem. Int. Ed. 1433-7851. 50 (3), 586–621. doi:10.1002/anie.201000044.

Reddy, D.N., Mylabathula, M.M., Al-Rajab, A.J., 2024. Industrial Demand and Applications of Capsaicin Capsaicinoids: From Natural Sources to Biosynthesis and Their Clinical Applications. Springer Nature, India, pp. 249–291. Available from: https://link.springer.com/book/10.1007/978-981-99-7779-6. doi:10.1007/978-981-99-7779-6_12.

Sallehuddin, N., Nordin, A., Bt Hj Idrus, R., Fauzi, M.B., 2020. Nigella sativa and its active compound, thymoquinone, accelerate wound healing in an in vivo animal model: a comprehensive review. Int. J. Environ. Res. Public Health. 1660-4601. 17 (11), 4160. doi:10.3390/ijerph17114160.

Samota, M.K., Rawat, M., Kaur, M., Garg, D., 2024. Gingerol: extraction methods, health implications, bioavailability and signaling pathways. Sustain. Food Technol. 2753-8095. 2 (6), 1652–1669. doi:10.1039/d4fb00135d.

Saraswathi, K., Arumugam, P., Sivaraj, C., 2020. Pharmacological activities of differential parts of selected Essential Indian Spices. J. Pharmacogn. Phytochem. 22784136. 9 (2), 2024–2033. doi:10.22271/phyto.2020.v9.i2ag.11151.

Shahidi, F., Hossain, A., 2018. Bioactives in spices, and spice oleoresins: phytochemicals and their beneficial effects in food preservation and health promotion. J. Food Bioact. 2637-8779. 3, 8–75. doi:10.31665/jfb.2018.3149.

Shahrajabian, M.H., Sun, W., Cheng, Q., Shahrajabian, M.H., Sun, W., Cheng, Q., 2019. Pharmacological uses and health benefits of ginger (*Zingiber officinale*) in traditional Asian and ancient Chinese medicine and modern practice. Notulae Sci. Biol. 20673264. 11 (3), 309–319. Available from: https://www.notulaebiologicae.ro/index.php/nsb. doi:10.15835/NSB11310419.

Sharifi-Rad, J., Cruz-Martins, N., López-Jornet, P., Lopez, E.P.F., Harun, N., Yeskaliyeva, B., Beyatli, A., Sytar, O., Shaheen, S., Sharopov, F., Taheri, Y., Docea, A.O., Calina, D., Cho, W.C., 2021. Natural coumarins: exploring the pharmacological complexity and underlying molecular mechanisms. Oxid. Med. Cell. Longev. 19420994. 2021. Available from: http://www.hindawi.com/journals/oximed/. doi:10.1155/2021/6492346.

Sharma, A., Kuhad, A., Bhandari, R., 2022. Novel nanotechnological approaches for treatment of skin-aging. J. Tissue Viability. 0965206X. 31 (3), 374–386. doi:10.1016/j.jtv.2022.04.010.

Sharma, U.K., Sharma, A.K., Pandey, A.K., 2016. Medicinal attributes of major phenylpropanoids present in cinnamon. BMC Complement. Altern. Med. 14726882. 16 (1). Available from: http://www.biomedcentral.com/bmccomplementalternmed/. doi:10.1186/s12906-016-1147-4.

Sharmeen, J., Mahomoodally, F., Zengin, G., Maggi, F., 2021. Essential oils as natural sources of fragrance compounds for cosmetics and cosmeceuticals. Molecules. 1420-3049. 26 (3), 666. doi:10.3390/molecules26030666.

Shaukat, M.N., Nazir, A., Fallico, B., 2023. Ginger bioactives: a comprehensive review of health benefits and potential food applications. Antioxidants. 2076-3921. 12 (11), 2015. doi:10.3390/antiox12112015.

Shukla, S., Mhaske, A., Shukla, R., 2024. Nanocarriers for the Delivery of Cosmeceuticals Nanotechnology Based Delivery of Phytoconstituents and Cosmeceuticals. Springer Singapore, India, pp. 305–328. Available from: https://link.springer.com/book/9789819953141. doi:10.1007/978-981-99-5314-1_10.

Singh, N., Brown, A.N., Gold, M.H., 2025. Ayurvedic ingredients in dermatology: a call for research. J. Cosmet. Dermatol. 14732165. 24 (2). Available from: http://onlinelibrary.wiley.com/journal/10.1111/(ISSN)1473-2165. doi:10.1111/jocd.16673.

Singh, N., Yadav, S.S., 2022. A review on health benefits of phenolics derived from dietary spices. Curr. Res. Food Sci. 26659271. 5, 1508–1523. Available from: https://www.journals.elsevier.com/current-research-in-food-science. doi:10.1016/j.crfs.2022.09.009.

Sinha, N.K. (Ed.), 2007. Handbook of Food Products Manufacturing. Wiley-Interscience, Hoboken, NJ.

Srinivasan, K., 2007. Black pepper and its pungent principle piperine: a review of diverse physiological effects. Crit. Rev. Food Sci. Nutr. 1040-8398. 47 (8), 735–748. doi:10.1080/10408390601062054.

Srinivasan, K., 2017. Ginger rhizomes (*Zingiber officinale*): a spice with multiple health beneficial potentials. PharmaNutrition. 22134344. 5 (1), 18–28. doi:10.1016/j.phanu.2017.01.001.

Star Labs France, n.d. CURCUMIN TURMENIC MERIVA®. Available from: https://starlabsfrance.fr/products/curcumin-turmenic-meriva%c2%ae.

Stępniowska, A., Cieplińska, P., Fac, W., Górska, J., n.d. Selected alkaloids used in the cosmetics industry.

Tan, H.Y., Nabil, W.N.N., Xu, H.X., 2021. Clinical research on cinnamomi cortex: a scoping review. Chin. Med. Cult. 25899473. 4 (4), 243–250. Available from: https://journals.lww.com/CMC/pages/aboutthejournal.aspx. doi:10.4103/CMAC.CMAC_42_21.

Tian, M., Yan, H., Row, K.H., 2008. Extraction of glycyrrhizic acid and glabridin from licorice. Int. J. Mol. Sci. 14220067. 9 (4), 571–577. Available from: http://www.mdpi.net/ijms/papers/i9040571.pdf. doi:10.3390/ijms9040571.

Timilsena, Y.P., Phosanam, A., Stockmann, R., 2023. Perspectives on saponins: food functionality and applications. Int. J. Mol. Sci. 1422-0067. 24 (17), 13538. doi:10.3390/ijms241713538.

Tomy, M.J., Dileep, K.V., Prasanth, S., Preethidan, D.S., Sabu, A., Sadasivan, C., Haridas, M., 2014. Cuminaldehyde as a lipoxygenase inhibitor: in vitro and in silico validation. Appl. Biochem. Biotechnol. 0273-2289. 174 (1), 388–397. doi:10.1007/s12010-014-1066-0.

Trepa, M., Sułkowska-Ziaja, K., Kała, K., Muszyńska, B., 2024. Therapeutic potential of fungal terpenes and terpenoids: application in skin diseases. Molecules. 1420-3049. 29 (5), 1183. doi:10.3390/molecules29051183.

Turmeric, n.d. Turmeric The Genus Curcuma. 28.

Ulanowska, M., Olas, B., 2021. Biological properties and prospects for the application of eugenol—a review. Int. J. Mol. Sci. 1422-0067. 22 (7), 3671. doi:10.3390/ijms22073671.

Vaughn, A.R., Branum, A., Sivamani, R.K., 2016. Effects of turmeric (*Curcuma longa*) on skin health: a systematic review of the clinical evidence. Phytother. Res. 10991573. 1243–1264. Available from: http://onlinelibrary.wiley.com/journal/10.1002/(ISSN)1099-1573. doi:10.1002/ptr.5640.

Verma, A., Kushwaha, H.N., Srivastava, A.K., Srivastava, S., Jamal, N., Srivastava, K., Ray, R.S., 2017. Piperine attenuates UV-R induced cell damage in human keratinocytes via NF-kB, Bax/Bcl-2 pathway: an application for photoprotection. J. Photochem. Photobiol. B Biol. 18732682. 172, 139–148. Available from: https://www.elsevier.com/locate/jphotobiol. doi:10.1016/j.jphotobiol.2017.05.018.

Vicco Turmeric, n.d. VICCO TURMERIC (crème 70g) Vicco.

Wadhwa, S., Singhal, S., Rawat, S., 2014. Bioavailability enhancement by piperine: a review. Asian J. Biomed. Pharm. Sci. 4 (36), 1–8.

Wang, Z., Shiyang, L., Shenghan, G., Lin, S., 2020. Review of distribution, extraction methods, and health benefits of bound phenolics in food plants. J. Agric. Food Chem. 0021-8561. 68 (11), 3330–3343. doi:10.1021/acs.jafc.9b06574.

Wei, J., Zhang, X., Yang, B., Miao, R., Zhang, Z., Hailan, S., 2015. Anti-inflammatory effects of cumin essential oil by blocking JNK, ERK, and NF-κB signaling pathways in LPS-stimulated RAW 264.7 cells. Evid. Based Complement. Alternat. Med. 1741-427X. 2015, 1–8. doi:10.1155/2015/474509.

Yahfoufi, N., Alsadi, N., Jambi, M., Matar, C., 2018. The immunomodulatory and anti-inflammatory role of polyphenols. Nutrients. 2072-6643. 10 (11), 1618. doi:10.3390/nu10111618.

Yallapu, M.M., Nagesh, P.K.B., Jaggi, M., Chauhan, S.C., 2015. Therapeutic applications of curcumin nanoformulations. AAPS J. 15507416. 17 (6), 1341–1356. Available from: http://www.springerlink.com/content/1550-7416/. doi:10.1208/s12248-015-9811-z.

Yang, W., Qiu, X., Qinghua, W., Chang, F., Zhou, T., Zhou, M., Pei, J., 2023. Active constituents of saffron (*Crocus sativus* L.) and their prospects in treating neurodegenerative diseases (review). Exp. Ther. Med. 1792-0981. 25 (5). doi:10.3892/etm.2023.11934.

Yang, Y., Ling, W., 2025. Health benefits and future research of phytochemicals: a literature review. J. Nutr. 00223166. 155 (1), 87–101. doi:10.1016/jtjnut.2024.11.007.

Yen, Y., Chi-Ming, P., Liu, C., Chen, Y., Chen, Y., Liang, C., Hsieh, J., Huang, H., Chen, Y., 2018. Curcumin accelerates cutaneous wound healing via multiple biological actions: the involvement of TNF-α, MMP-9, α-SMA, and collagen. Int. Wound J. 1742-4801. 15 (4), 605–617. doi:10.1111/iwj.12904.

Zagórska, J., Pietrzak, K., Kukula-Koch, W., Czop, M., Laszuk, J., Koch, W., 2023. Influence of diet on the bioavailability of active components from *Zingiber officinale* using an in vitro digestion model. Foods. 2304-8158. 12 (21), 3897. doi:10.3390/foods12213897.

Zaman, S.U., Akhtar, N., 2013. Effect of turmeric (*Curcuma longa* Zingiberaceae) extract cream on human skin sebum secretion. Trop. J. Pharm. Res. 1596-9827. 12 (5). doi:10.4314/tjpr.v12i5.1.

Chapter 9

Marine and freshwater plants

Marina Seferli, Theodora Adamantidi, Athena Venieri, and Alexandros Tsoupras
Hephaestus Laboratory, School of Chemistry, Faculty of Sciences, Democritus University of Thrace, Kavala University Campus, Kavala, Greece

1 Introduction

Aquatic plant microorganisms and macroorganisms, including marine macroalgae, microalgae, cyanobacteria, and freshwater macrophytes, represent a promising yet underutilized source of bioactive compounds for biofunctional and cosmeceutical applications (Puchkova et al., 2021). Such organisms have evolved in highly dynamic environments characterized by fluctuating nutrient availability, salinity, tidal exposure, and intense solar radiation. Their long-term adaptation to these stressors has resulted in distinctive metabolic pathways that generate structurally diverse secondary metabolites with potent biological activities relevant to skin health (Jimoh and Kambizi, 2022; Pooja et al., 2020).

Compared with terrestrial plants, aquatic species exhibit a high content of antioxidants, pigments, complex polysaccharides, phenolics, carotenoids, polar lipids (PLs), mono- and poly-unsaturated fatty acids (MUFAs and PUFAs), amino acids, and other stress-responsive molecules. Their inherent defenses against oxidative stress, microbial invasion, ultraviolet (UV) exposure, and environmental fluctuations translate into skin-relevant benefits, such as antiinflammatory activity, photoprotection, tissue regeneration, enhanced hydration, and delayed skin aging. These properties align with current cosmetic trends favoring natural ingredients with minimal chemical additives and marked therapeutic value (Jimoh and Kambizi, 2022; Pooja et al., 2020; Conde et al., 2021; Seferli et al., 2025).

Microalgae have recently emerged as valuable sources of compounds with antioxidant, antiinflammatory, and regenerative effects. They synthesize carotenoids and pigments such as astaxanthin, phycobiliproteins like C-phycocyanin, essential fatty acids, bioactive PLs, polysaccharides, vitamins, phenolics, and other metabolites as adaptive responses to environmental stress (Conde et al., 2021; Borowitzka, 2013; Ambati et al., 2014; Puchkova et al., 2021). Such metabolites have mitigated oxidative damage, modulate inflammatory signaling, protect against UV-induced injury, support collagen synthesis (Jayawardhana et al., 2023), enhance hydration, and prevent skin cancer-related malfunctions (Puchkova et al., 2021; Chinjoo and Golzary, 2025). However, challenges such as chemical instability, poor solubility, and limited skin permeability necessitate the development of advanced delivery systems, including encapsulation and carriers like liposomes, nanoparticles, and biopolymer-based systems, to enhance their topical bioavailability (Ulber, 2021; Conde et al., 2021; Menaa et al., 2021; Koukouraki et al., 2020; Shiels et al., 2021).

Marine macroalgae (seaweed), belonging to the *Chlorophyta* (green algae), *Phaeophyceae* (brown algae), and *Rhodophyta* (red algae) phyla, also constitute a major reservoir of bioactive ingredients with a long history of use in food, medicine, and cosmetics (Borowitzka, 2013; Ambati et al., 2014; Puchkova et al., 2021). Their metabolites include polysaccharides (e.g., alginates, carrageenans, agar, and ulvans), polyphenols such as phlorotannins, carotenoids, proteins, lipids, and minerals. Modern research has elucidated the molecular mechanisms supporting their traditional applications, revealing their moisturizing, antioxidant, antiinflammatory, antimicrobial, and photoprotective properties (Dong et al., 2020; Pimentel et al., 2018; Lourenço-Lopes et al., 2020). For instance, phlorotannins offer potent antioxidant and antienzymatic activities that protect dermal collagen and elastin from degradation (Chen et al., 2011; Hempel et al., 2023). Furthermore, pigments like fucoxanthin, chlorophylls, and phycoerythrin provide both coloration and antiaging effects, while macroalgal polysaccharides function as natural moisturizers, film formers, stabilizers, and delivery-enhancing excipients in cosmetic formulations (Pimentel et al., 2018).

Biofunctional Cosmetics for Health. https://doi.org/10.1016/B978-0-443-27500-5.00026-5

Freshwater aquatic plants, though less explored than marine species, also possess crucial cosmeceutical potential. Species such as *Nelumbo nucifera* (lotus), *Nymphaea lotus* (Egyptian water lily), *Nasturtium officinale* (watercress), and *Hydrocotyle vulgaris* (marsh pennywort) produce unique phytochemicals, including flavonoids and other phenolic bioactives, polysaccharides, carotenoids, PLs, fatty acids, and alkaloids, that support antioxidant, antiinflammatory, antimicrobial, soothing, moisturizing, whitening, and antiaging properties (Seferli et al., 2024; Dash et al., 2013; Dhanasinghe et al., 2025). Their traditional use in Ayurveda, traditional Chinese medicine, and African ethnobotany for skin purification, wound healing, and the treatment of inflammatory dermatoses (Zheng et al., 2004) is increasingly supported by modern analytical, phytochemical, and mechanistic dermal protection-related studies (Seferli et al., 2024, 2025; Gupta et al., 2009).

Beyond their rich biochemical profiles, aquatic plants offer notable advantages in sustainability and production efficiency. Microalgae and macroalgae can be cultivated in controlled systems requiring minimal freshwater, arable land, or fertilizers (Couteau, 2016; Morais et al., 2021). Their ability to thrive in saline or nutrient-poor environments, coupled with rapid growth rates and sensitivity to environmental modulation, enables scalable, high-yield production of specific bioactive molecules (Seferli et al., 2024; Klimek-Szczykutowicz et al., 2018; Tungmunnithum et al., 2021). This supports the broader framework of blue biotechnology (Costa et al., 2023), which integrates marine and aquatic bioresources into the development of innovative, sustainable, and eco-responsible cosmetics of high value (Sabeena Farvin and Jacobsen, 2013; Bocanegra et al., 2009).

Some aquatic species also produce molecules that are rare or absent in terrestrial plants. Fucoidans, sulfated polysaccharides from brown algae, exhibit strong antiaging and skin-repairing effects. For example, astaxanthin, a marine-derived carotenoid, offers exceptional antioxidant and UV-protective activity, whereas mycosporine-like amino acids (MAAs) act as natural UV filters with high photostability. Phycobiliproteins, found in cyanobacteria and red algae, provide antioxidant capacity and serve as natural colorants, while additional metabolites contribute to cellular detoxification via metal chelation and reactive species neutralization, effects that may translate into skin detoxification and enhanced cellular defense (Jimoh and Kambizi, 2022; Pooja et al., 2020; Dagnino-Leone et al., 2022; Sotelo et al., 2021).

From a formulation standpoint, extracts from aquatic plants provide multifunctional benefits as both active ingredients and structural components that improve stability, texture, and delivery efficiency. Their versatility enables the development of formulations that combine esthetic enhancement with dermatological function, aligning with consumer preferences for natural, effective, and environmentally responsible skin health-based products (Dhanasinghe et al., 2025; Castangia et al., 2016).

Collectively, the biochemical richness, environmental adaptability, and sustainability advantages of several microalgae, macroalgae, and freshwater aquatic plants underscore their transformative potential in modern cosmetic science. This chapter provides a comprehensive overview of their broader classification, bioactive profiles, mechanisms of action, health-promoting benefits, and potential applications in the cosmetics industry, combining scientific insights with industrial perspectives. Commercial formulations, formulation challenges, limitations, and future perspectives are discussed as well. Through this synthesis, the chapter emphasizes the transformative role of aquatic bioresources in developing the next generation of natural, functional, and environmentally responsible cosmetics.

2 Classification and bioactive potential of microalgae, macroalgae, and freshwater aquatic plants

Microalgae, macroalgae, cyanobacteria, and freshwater aquatic plant-based organisms represent diverse groups of photosynthetic or partially photosynthetic organisms with notable biotechnological relevance. Their taxonomic classification strongly influences their biochemical profiles, ecological roles, and broader applicability in cosmetic formulations (Puchkova et al., 2021; Pooja et al., 2020; Dagnino-Leone et al., 2022; Sotelo et al., 2021). The following subsections provide a structured classification-based overview of these groups and highlight the bioactive molecules that define their cosmetic potential.

2.1 Microalgae and cyanobacteria

Microalgae and cyanobacteria are unicellular or simple multicellular microorganisms capable of efficient photosynthesis. Their rapid growth, metabolic flexibility, simple cellular structure, adaptability to various environmental and cultivation conditions, and high content of bioactive metabolites make them key candidates for sustainable ingredient production in cosmetic product manufacture. Such agents biosynthesize pigments, MUFAs and PUFAs, PLs (phospholipids and glycolipids), polysaccharides, peptides, and antioxidant molecules (i.e., phenolics and carotenoids) that contribute to photoprotection, inflammation control, antioxidant defense, and extracellular matrix (ECM) support (Conde et al., 2021; Koukouraki et al., 2020; Shiels et al., 2021; Mourelle et al., 2017; Nowruzi et al., 2020).

These organisms successfully regulate oxidative stress through the modulation of reactive oxygen species (ROS), modulate pro- and antiinflammatory cytokines, and support cellular repair pathways that promote skin homeostasis and antiaging effects. At the tissue level, microalgal metabolites stimulate collagen and elastin synthesis, enhance hydration, and improve barrier integrity, resulting in skin regeneration and dermal balance protection (Favas et al., 2021). Their cultivation in photobioreactors requires minimal land and freshwater, enabling controlled, eco-friendly production and targeted optimization of desired metabolites (Mourelle et al., 2017; Nowruzi et al., 2020; Favas et al., 2021).

Microalgae are primarily classified as *Cyanophyceae* (blue–green algae), *Chlorophyceae* (green algae), *Porphyridiophyceae* (red algae), and *Bacillariophyceae* (including the diatoms). Blue–green algae include *Arthrospira platensis* and *Arthrospira maxima* species, with *A. platensis,* otherwise known as *Spirulina platensis*, being the maincomponent. *S. platensis* is a filamentous cyanobacterium rich in phycocyanin, γ-linolenic acid (GLA), polysaccharides, vitamins, carotenoids, PLs, and trace minerals (e.g., zinc, selenium, and iron) (Conde et al., 2021; Shiels et al., 2021; Ragusa et al., 2021). Its main metabolite, C-phycocyanin, provides potent antiinflammatory and antioxidant effects by reducing free radicals and inflammatory cytokines such as tumor necrosis factor α (TNF-α) and interleukin-1β (IL-1β), as well as antiplateletactivating factor (anti-PAF) activities (Conde et al., 2021; Koukouraki et al., 2020; Shiels et al., 2021). Moreover, its high GLA content supports the skin barrier, elasticity, and moisture retention, decreasing transepidermal water loss (TEWL). Spirulina polysaccharides can also enhance hydration while stimulating fibroblasts, contributing to ECM regeneration. Finally, it contains a variety of antioxidant nutrients like β-carotene, tocopherols, and B-complex vitamins, which protect the skin from oxidative damage, support cell repair, and contribute to efficient energy metabolism in skin tissues (Ragusa et al., 2021; Ramos et al., 2025; Gunes et al., 2017).

Green microalgae predominantly include *Chlorella* species, *Haematococcus pluvialis,* and *Dunaliella salina. Chlorella vulgaris* contains high levels of chlorophyll, essential amino acids, peptides, polysaccharides, vitamins, and minerals. Chlorophyll derivatives counteract UV-induced oxidative stress and environmental pollution, supporting skin clarity maintenance. In addition, peptides and amino acids are capable of stimulating collagen production and strengthening the dermal matrix, preserving skin firmness and structural integrity. Cell wall polysaccharides, such as β-1,3-glucan, improve barrier repair, reduce TEWL, and promote elastin and fibronectin expression, improving overall skin texture. Its wide range of micronutrients, including B-complex vitamins, trace minerals, and PUFAs, also contributes to skin vitality by supporting microcirculation, improving tissue oxygenation, and offering a brighter, more even complexion. Due to its detoxifying properties, *C. vulgaris* is frequently included in cosmetics designed for skin exposed to pollution, oxidative stress, or signs of fatigue (Agustina et al., 2021; Putri et al., 2021; Hidhayati et al., 2025).

Following green microalgae *H. pluvialis*, it is the most concentrated natural source of astaxanthin, a red ketocarotenoid with exceptional antioxidant capacity. Astaxanthin is capable of protecting mitochondrial integrity, preventing lipid peroxidation, and inhibiting inflammatory cytokines and matrix metalloproteinases (MMPs), while enhancing firmness, reducing wrinkles, and improving skin tone and smoothness. Due to its lipophilic nature, astaxanthin is well-suited for advanced topical delivery systems such as emulsions, lipid nanoparticles, and concentrated serums (Cheng and Shah, 2023; Tominaga et al., 2012; Marino et al., 2020). Moreover, green microalgae *D. salina* is well-known for the production of high amounts of β-carotene, providing antioxidant, eye protection, and anticancer benefits (Vieira et al., 2020). When incorporated in cosmetics and cosmeceuticals, its extract counteracts skin aging under intense solar irradiation, particularly attributed to its antiglycation and antiinflammatory properties (Vieira et al., 2020; Havas et al., 2022).

Red algae are mainly represented by *Porphyridium* species, which in turn produce phycoerythrin and PUFAs with notable antiviral (antiherpes), antibacterial, antiinflammatory, antioxidant, and immunomodulatory properties. These species exhibit remarkable antioxidant capacity against oxidative stress, protecting against premature aging and offering prolonged elasticity when integrated into cosmetics and cosmeceuticals. Furthermore, they are also used as coloring agents, retaining their color stability even within a pH range of 4–5 (Chinjoo and Golzary, 2025; Agustina et al., 2020). Finally, *Bacillariophyceae* diatoms, including *Phaeodactylum tricornutum*, are primarily responsible for the production of eicosapentaenoic acid (EPA) and fucoxanthin metabolites involved in improving insulin resistance, as well as providing anticancer, antimicrobial, antioxidant, antiinflammatory, and cardioprotective benefits (Chinjoo and Golzary, 2025; Nieri et al., 2023). Fig. 9.1 illustrates the main classification, representative species, and metabolites of microalgae and cyanobacteria.

At this point, it must be mentioned that microalgae constitute a rich source of bioactive PLs that exhibit potent antiinflammatory and antithrombotic properties, largely attributed to their ability to inhibit PAF and modulate PAF/PAF-receptor (PAFR)-related pathways. The most active microalgal lipids include phospholipids enriched with ω-3 PUFAs, such as α-linolenic acid (ALA), EPA, and docosahexaenoic acid (DHA), esterified at the *sn-2* position of the glycerol backbone, as well as sulfo-glycolipids, including 3-sulfoquinovosyl diacylglycerols (SQDGs) (see Fig. 9.2), for which a patent has been reported demonstrating activity against skin inflammation via anti-PAF mechanisms (Conde et al., 2021; Koukouraki et al., 2020; Shiels et al., 2021).

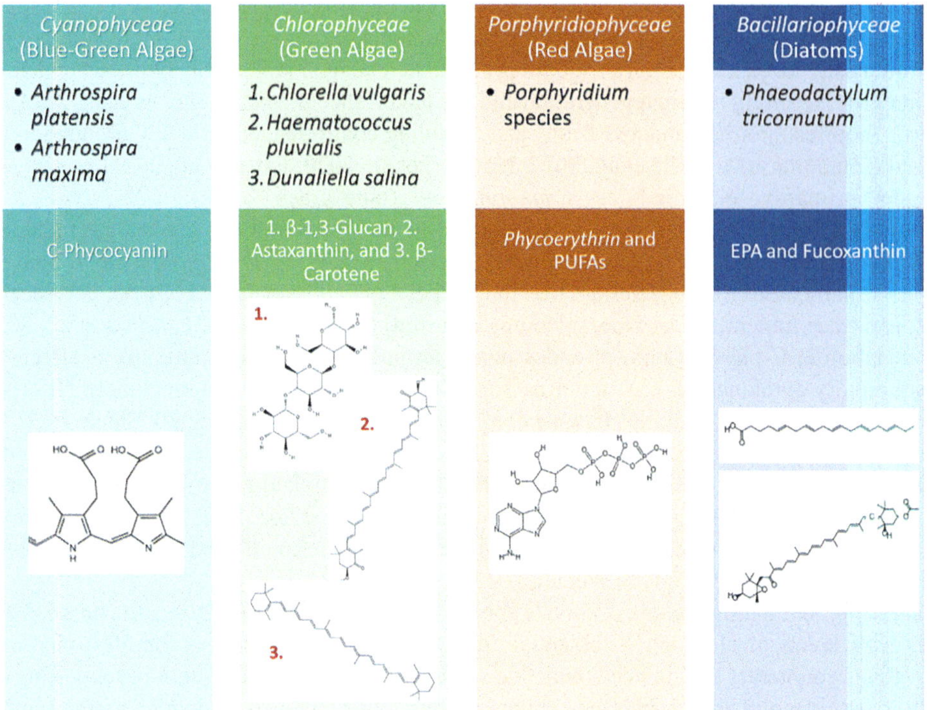

FIG. 9.1 Classification, representative species, and associated metabolites of the main microalgae and cyanobacteria species. *(Source: Authors' creation, while all structures used in this figure were obtained from the free open-access platforms: https://molview.org/ and https://www.sigmaaldrich.com/ (Assessed 24 October 2025).)*

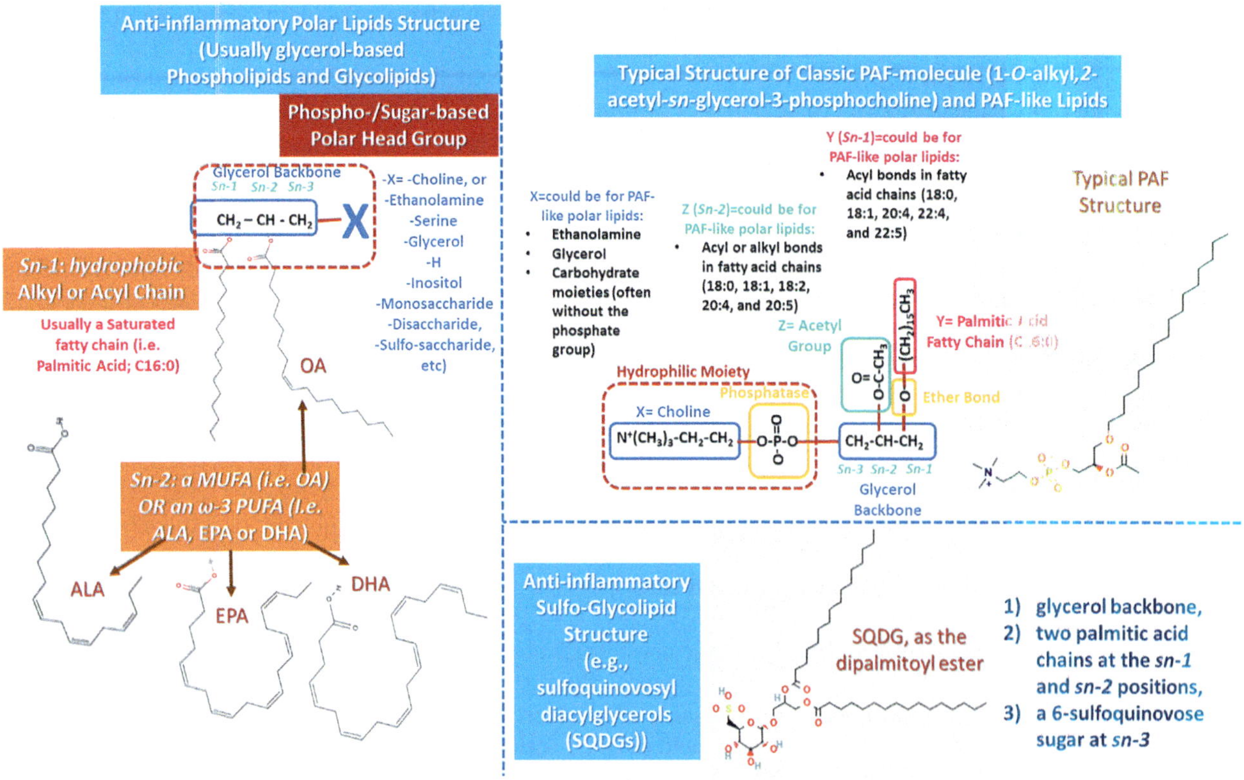

FIG. 9.2 Representative structures of microalgae bioactive polar lipids with MUFA (OA) or a ω-3 PUFA (EPA, DHA, or ALA) at the *sn-2* position of their glycerol backbones, as well as PAF-like lipids and sulfo-glycolipids like sulfoquinovosyl-diacylglycerols (SQDGs). *(Source: Authors' creation, while all structures used were obtained from the free open-access platforms: https://molview.org/ and https://pubchem.ncbi.nlm.nih.gov/ (Assessed 24 October 2025).)*

Extracts of PLs from species such as *Chlorococcum* and *Spirulina* have demonstrated strong in vitro, ex vivo, and preclinical anti-PAF, antiinflammatory, and antithrombotic activities, including inhibition of PAF-induced platelet aggregation and attenuation of inflammatory cytokine production. Such PLs appear to exert their anti-PAF effects through several complementary mechanisms, including the direct antagonism or interference with PAF/PAFR binding due to structural homology with PAF's molecular structure, suppression of enzymatic PAF biosynthesis, reduction of oxidative stress, and modulation of gut microbiota. These findings highlight microalgae as a promising dietary and nutraceutical source of natural PAF inhibitors for cosmetic and cosmeceutical applications (Conde et al., 2021; Koukouraki et al., 2020; Shiels et al., 2021) (Fig. 9.1).

2.2 Macroalgae (seaweeds)

Marine macroalgae (seaweeds) are multicellular, photosynthetic organisms classified into green (Chlorophyta), brown (Phaeophyta), and red (Rhodophyta). Adapted to dynamic marine environments with high UV exposure, fluctuating salinity, microbial pressure, and oxidative stress, they have developed sophisticated biochemical defense systems and produce a wide array of secondary metabolites. Although not essential for primary metabolism, these molecules support ecological resilience and have attracted increasing interest in functional dermatology, cosmetics, and cosmeceuticals (Havas et al., 2022; Zouboulis and Hoenig, 2019; Russell-Goldman and Murphy, 2020).

Macroalgae are particularly rich in bioactives relevant to skin care. Brown algae synthesize sulfated polysaccharides, such as fucoidans, which exhibit hydrating, antiinflammatory, and wound healing effects. Red algae are a major source of carrageenans, which enhance moisture retention and form protective films on the skin, while green algae produce ulvans that reinforce the barrier function and exert immunomodulatory activity (Corinaldesi et al., 2017).

Beyond polysaccharides, macroalgae generate polyphenolic compounds, most notably phlorotannins in brown algae, which demonstrate strong antioxidant capacity, inhibit collagen-degrading enzymes, and show antimicrobial properties. Marine algae also contain carotenoids such as fucoxanthin that protect skin cells from oxidative stress and regulate lipid metabolism. In addition, red algae produce MAAs, natural UV-absorbing agents that provide endogenous photoprotection. Terpenoids and halogenated compounds further contribute antimicrobial, antiaging, and antifungal properties (Corinaldesi et al., 2017; Siahaan et al., 2022). The biosynthesis of these metabolites is strongly influenced by environmental cues. UV exposure stimulates the production of photoprotective and antioxidant agents, while pathogen contact induces defensive terpenoids and halogenated molecules. This chemically responsive behavior underscores their ecological adaptation and their relevance as models for skin protection under environmental stress (Corinaldesi et al., 2017; Siahaan et al., 2022).

Structurally, several macroalgal agents contain sulfate, bromide, or iodide substitutions, contributing to high solubility, stability, and enhanced bioactivity. Their polysaccharides, often of high molecular weight and polyanionic nature, provide excellent film-forming and moisture retention effects, making them well-suited for protective and hydrating formulations (Nimisha and Singh, 2024). In cosmetology, these marine-derived compounds support multiple skin functions: they reduce oxidative stress and photoaging, improve hydration and elasticity, accelerate tissue repair, and modulate inflammatory signaling. Their integration into cosmetic products is further facilitated by sustainable extraction technologies, like enzyme-assisted and supercritical fluid extraction, which preserve bioactivity while minimizing environmental impact (Corinaldesi et al., 2017; Siahaan et al., 2022; Nimisha and Singh, 2024).

Macroalgae (seaweeds) are classified as *Chlorophyceae* (green algae), *Phaeophyceae* (brown algae), and *Rhodophyceae* (red algae). *Chlorophyceae* (green algae) are predominantly represented by *Ulva* and *Cladophora* species. *Ulva* species (sea lettuce) are easily recognized by their thin, leaf-like structures known as thalli and their remarkable tolerance to changing environmental conditions, such as fluctuations in salinity and nutrient availability. *Ulva* species contain ulvans, unique sulfated heteropolysaccharides with antioxidant, immunomodulatory, and antiinflammatory properties. Ulvans enhance hydration, promote epithelial regeneration, stimulate fibroblasts and keratinocytes, and strengthen the skin barrier (Ruslan et al., 2021; Saleem et al., 2024). *Ulva* species also contain chlorophylls, carotenoids such as lutein, polyphenols, and amino acids that protect against oxidative damage and inhibit matrix-degrading enzymes. Its rapid compatibility and growth with sustainable aquaculture make *Ulva* a promising eco-friendly cosmetic resource (Dini, 2023). Moreover, *Ulva* extracts influence the activity of proinflammatory cytokines like IL-6 and TNF-α, suggesting their potential application in soothing irritated or sensitive skin (Łęska et al., 2018). Similarly, *Cladophora* species reportedly possess a high supply of antioxidants, chlorophylls, fatty acids, and peptides capable of retaining skin hydration and improving skin elasticity, beneficial as cosmetic moisturizing and firming agents (Fabrowska et al., 2015, 2017).

Phaeophyceae (brown algae), represented by *Laminaria*, *Fucus,* and *Pylaiella* species, are typically found in temperate to cold coastal waters and thrive in environments characterized by strong tidal movement, cool temperatures, and high nutrient availability (López-Hortas et al., 2021). *Laminaria* species, including *Laminaria digitata* and *Laminaria japonica*, are distinguished by their rich polysaccharide content of alginates, laminarin, and fucoidans. Alginates provide hydration and soothing effects through gel-forming properties, while laminarin, a β-glucan-type, offers antiinflammatory, antioxidant, and immunomodulatory benefits. Fucoidans regulate inflammation, stimulate collagen synthesis, inhibit MMPs, and support tissue regeneration (Resende et al., 2021). *Fucus,* mainly *Fucus vesiculosus* (bladderwrack), contains phlorotannins, unique polyphenols with marked antioxidant and antienzymatic activity, as well as vitamins, essential nutrients (e.g., iodine, trace minerals), and fucoxanthin, which offers photoprotection and lipid stabilization. These species are widely used in antiaging, firming, and detoxifying formulations (Muñoz-Quintana et al., 2024; Kalasariya et al., 2025; Pereira, 2018). In addition, *Pylaiella* species extracts have been used in cosmetic formulations due to their rich composition of bioactive compounds such as polysaccharides, alginic acid, and mannitol (Bogdan et al., 2025).

Rhodophyceae (red algae) are predominantly recognized by *Palmaria*, *Ceramium*, and *Polysiphonia* species. *Palmaria palmata* (dulse) is native to the cold coastal waters of the North Atlantic and North Pacific and is rich in carrageenans, free amino acids, small peptides (e.g., taurine, glycine, and asparagine), phycoerythrin, and MAAs, components that collectively support cellular hydration and osmotic balance, while also stimulating protein synthesis within the dermis (Sawant Desai and Kelkar Mane, 2023; Kasanah et al., 2022). Carrageenans provide hydration, film formation, and barrier reinforcement, while MAAs absorb UV radiation and protect from photooxidative stress, promoting collagen and elastin synthesis and improving elasticity and regeneration (Kalasariya et al., 2022). In addition, phycoerythrin, a red-colored phycobiliprotein, has also demonstrated antioxidant and antiinflammatory potential in preliminary studies in topical formulations (Sawant Desai and Kelkar Mane, 2023; Kasanah et al., 2022; Kalasariya et al., 2022). Similarly, *Ceramium* spp. include lipids, proteins, and various secondary metabolites with vast antioxidant and antimicrobial potential as active cosmetic and cosmeceutical ingredients (Bazes et al., 2006), whereas *Polysiphonia* spp. possess a rich content of antioxidants and phycobiliproteins valued for future cosmetic products (Al-Amro et al., 2019). Fig. 9.3 illustrates the main classification and representative species of macroalgae (seaweeds).

2.3 Freshwater aquatic plants

Freshwater aquatic plants provide a distinct phytochemical profile, specifically shaped by their adaptation to dynamic freshwater environments. They often accumulate trace elements and produce phenolics, flavonoids, peptides, and pigments that support skin protection, repair, structure, appearance, and overall wellness (Seferli et al., 2024; Pooja et al., 2020). Representative aquatic and wetland plants explored for their cosmetic and cosmeceutical potential include *N. nucifera*, *Lemna* sp., *Ipomoea aquatica* Forsk., *N. officinale*, *Eleocharis dulcis*, *Bacopa monnieri*, *Enhydra fluctuans* Lour., *Rotula aquatica* Lour., *Pistia stratiotes*, *Nymphaea nouchali*, *Hedychium coronarium*, *Hydrilla verticillata*, and *Eichhornia crassipes* (Fig. 9.4) (Seferli et al., 2024; Pooja et al., 2020).

Lemna minor, commonly known as duckweed, accumulates micronutrients and heavy metals, activating antioxidant enzymes such as peroxidases and catalases. Although Lemna has a relatively simple structure, it demonstrates complex biochemical behavior in response to environmental conditions, making it a promising source of bioactive compounds with potential skin benefits (Seferli et al., 2024; Pooja et al., 2020). It produces a wide array of phenolic acids, flavonoids, peptides, proteins, amino acids, and chlorophyll derivatives, supporting antioxidant activities, the neutralization of oxidative stress, skin protection from environmental damage, skin microbiota management, collagen formation, and barrier repair. *Lemna* is promising for the development of detoxifying, soothing, and microbiome-balancing topical cosmetic products (Seferli et al., 2024; Pooja et al., 2020). Similarly, *N. nucifera* (sacred lotus) has also revealed great antioxidant, antifungal, antimicrobial, and antiinflammatory properties, incorporated in natural cosmetic cream formulations, particularly due to its high flavonoid, phenolic, alkaloid, and polysaccharide content (Siddhi and Khamkar, 2025; Seferli et al., 2024).

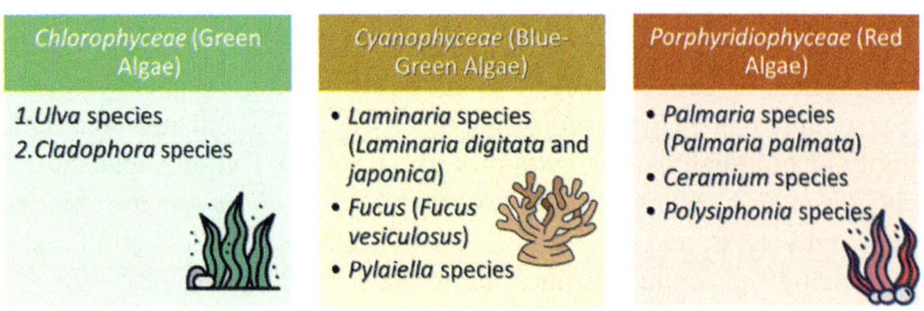

FIG. 9.3 Overview of the main macroalgal groups and representative species. *(Source: Authors' creation, while all icons used in this figure were obtained from the free open-access platform: https://www.flaticon.com/ (Assessed 24 October 2025).)*

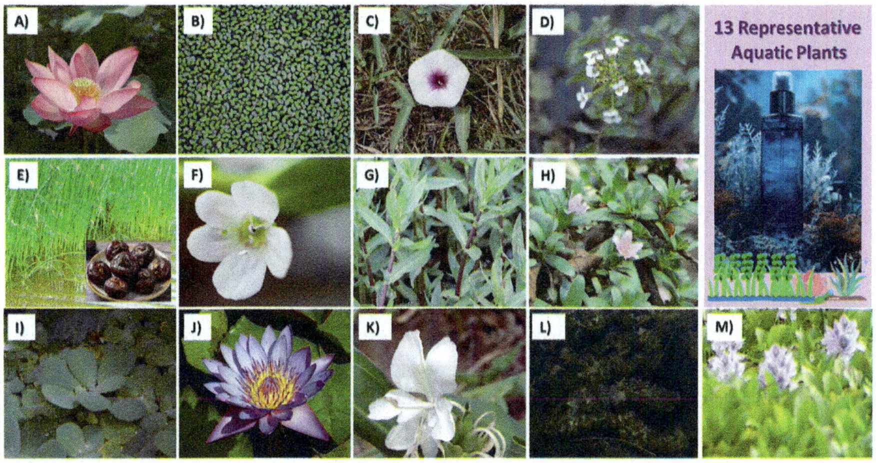

FIG. 9.4 Representative images of the afore-selected aquatic and wetland plants explored for their cosmetic and cosmeceutical potential: (A) *Nelumbo nucifera*, (B) *Lemna* sp., (C) *Ipomoea aquatica* Forsk., (D) *Nasturtium officinale*, (E) *Eleocharis dulcis*, (F) *Bacopa monnieri*, (G) *Enhydra fluctuans* Lour., (H) *Rotula aquatica* Lour., (I) *Pistia stratiotes*, (J) *Nymphaea nouchali*, (K) *Hedychium coronarium*, (L) *Hydrilla verticillata*, and (M) *Eichhornia crassipes*. *(Source: All figures of the aquatic plants were obtained from the free open-access platforms: https://www.freepik.com/, https://pixabay.com/ and https://www.shutterstock.com/. As for Rotula aquatica Lour., credits for this figure belong to https://commons.wikimedia.org/wiki/user:Vinayaraj (Accessed 24 October 2025).)*

Recent research by Seferli et al. (2025) has highlighted that the freshwater aquatic plants *Lemna* sp., especially *L. minor* and *N. nucifera,* are valuable sources of amphiphilic bioactives with notable antioxidant, antiinflammatory, and antithrombotic properties. These activities are attributed to their rich content of carotenoids and phenolic constituents, as well as PL fractions, particularly phospholipids and glycolipids. The PLs exhibit characteristic fatty acid profiles, including monoenes and ω-3 PUFAs, especially ALA esterified predominantly at the *sn-2* position of the glycerol backbone, enhancing their biological potency. Such amphiphilic bioactive molecules demonstrate significant anti-PAF activities, which contribute to the mitigation of PAF-mediated inflammatory cascades, while their carotenoids and phenolics provide strong protection against oxidative stress and skin inflammation (Seferli et al., 2024, 2025).

I. aquatica has reportedly been used for ages in Polynesian cosmetopoeia as an effective hair and scalp cosmetic treatment, revealing a regulatory effect on dermal papilla cells (Ajao and Sadgrove, 2024). Moreover, cosmetic formulations integrating *N. officinale* extracts exhibited pH values suitable for the skin, playing a critical role in maintaining skin health and integrity, providing a hydrating effect, and safeguarding skin health mainly against environmental stressors (Klimek-Szczykutowicz et al., 2025). Although less studied for its cosmetic value, *E. dulcis* has demonstrated notable emulsifying and stabilizing properties for water-in-oil emulsions, showcasing its great potential as a future cosmetic agent (Gu et al., 2024). As a skin-conditioning agent, *B. monnieri* has presented vast antioxidant, antiinflammatory, and antimicrobial properties, further promoting its use as a natural preservative and active ingredient in cosmetic applications (Yadav et al., 2022).

E. fluctuans is currently being researched for its potential use in cosmetics, mainly due to its strong antioxidant and antiinflammatory properties, which are relevant for addressing skin concerns like aging, hyperpigmentation, and inflammation (Barua et al., 2021). Furthermore, *R. aquatica* and *P. stratiotes* have demonstrated analgesic, antiinflammatory, and antioxidant activity with great medicinal properties, supporting their future use as cosmetic ingredients (Seferli et al., 2024; Pooja et al., 2020). Blue lotus, *N. nouchali*, comprises volatile compounds and a characteristic aroma perception, holding promising potential in the cosmetic and perfumery industries (Wu et al., 2025). Similarly, *H. coronarium* essential oil, beyond its antiaging, antimicrobial, antiinflammatory, and antioxidant effects, is valued in the perfume industry for its floral scent. It is an attractive anticollagenase agent as well, indicating its future use in antiwrinkle formulations (Tammasorn et al., 2023a).

H. verticillata, a submerged freshwater plant known for its fine, branched structure, bioaccumulates trace elements and metals and detoxifies water via chelation and intracellular sequestration. It contains polyphenols, flavonoids, carotenoids, and chlorophylls that reduce oxidative damage and inflammation, while contributing to both cellular protection and tissue regeneration when applied topically (Prabha et al., 2019). *H. verticillata* also exhibits antimicrobial action and supports hydration, cell turnover, and antiaging signaling, making it relevant for antipollution, antiaging, antiinflammatory, and protective skincare products (Prabha et al., 2019; Shrivastava and Srivastava, 2021). Finally, *E. crassipes* (water hyacinth) contains polyphenols, flavonoids, sterols, glycosides, amino acids, and minerals, displaying antibacterial, antiinflammatory, and antioxidant activities. It exhibits great inhibitory effects against *S. aureus* and *P. acnes*, supporting acne-prone and sensitive skin applications, while it also promotes collagen metabolism, enhances skin hydration, and inhibits MMPs, thereby enhancing skin firmness and elasticity (Lalitha and Jayanthi, 2014; Bakrim et al., 2022). Despite being invasive, its biochemical richness and sustainability potential position it as a valuable dermocosmetic agent (Lalitha and Jayanthi, 2014; Ben Bakrim et al., 2022).

3 Bioactives and health-promoting constituents in microalgae, macroalgae, and freshwater aquatic plants for skincare applications

Microalgae, macroalgae, and freshwater aquatic plants comprise a plethora of bioactive constituents, which exert remarkable health-promoting properties useful for the formation of cosmetic and cosmeceutical formulations. Due to their antiinflammatory, antioxidant, antiaging, antibacterial, and immunomodulatory profiles, they may serve as important cosmetic agents in future innovative cosmetics and cosmeceuticals (Conde et al., 2021; Koukouraki et al., 2020; Shiels et al., 2021). Fig. 9.5 and the following subsections list the main classes of bioactive compounds found in both algae and aquatic plants.

3.1 Bioactives and health-promoting constituents in microalgae

3.1.1 Carotenoids, natural pigments, and colorants

Carotenoids are yellow–orange, fat-soluble antioxidants and provitamin A sources. Key commercial molecules include β-carotene, astaxanthin, lutein, zeaxanthin, lycopene, and bixin (Mourelle et al., 2017; Terao, 1989). *D. salina* accumulates ~14% β-carotene (dry weight), while *H. pluvialis* is the richest natural source of astaxanthin (Cordero et al., 1996; Guerin et al., 2003). Their ROS-reducing and skin-regenerating effects support their use in antiaging formulations (Mourelle et al., 2017; Guerin et al., 2003; OUCI, 2025). Encapsulation of astaxanthin in liposomes, nanoemulsions, or poly(lactic-co-glycolic acid) nanoparticles enhances stability, skin permeation, and UV-protective antioxidant activity. These delivery systems also improve astaxanthin's photostability, a major limitation in its free form (Hama et al., 2012; Sun et al., 2020; Hu et al., 2019).

Microalgal pigments offer great biodegradable alternatives to synthetic dyes. Phycocyanin (blue) from *Spirulina* and carotenoids such as lutein and zeaxanthin from *Chlorella* (yellow-to-orange tones) provide coloration along with antioxidant and photoprotective benefits (Pulz and Gross, 2004). They are used in lipsticks, eyeshadows, and tinted moisturizers

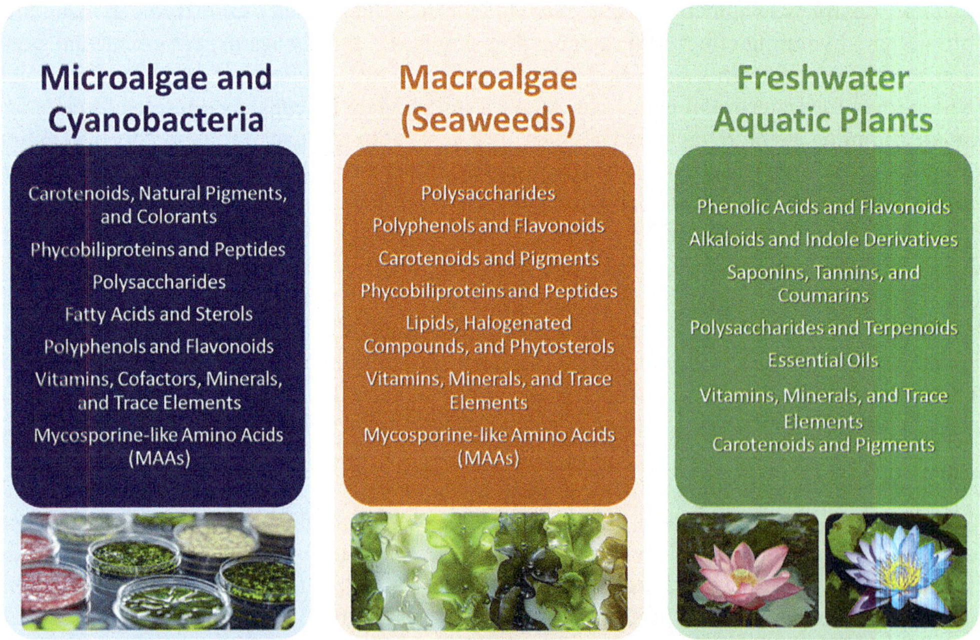

FIG. 9.5 Bioactive compounds found in microalgae, macroalgae, and aquatic plants. *(Source: Authors' creation, while all figures were obtained from the free open-access platforms https://www.freepik.com/ and https://pixabay.com/ (Accessed 24 October 2025).)*

(Khan et al., 2018). Regulatory acceptance of microalgal pigments is expanding due to their safety profile, while their biodegradability further enhances their market appeal as clean-label ingredients (Conde et al., 2021; Koukouraki et al., 2020; Shiels et al., 2021; Safafar et al., 2015).

3.1.2 Phycobiliproteins and peptides

Phycobiliproteins, including phycocyanin and phycoerythrin, mainly from *Arthrospira* and *Porphyridium*, are used in food coloring, cosmetics, and diagnostics (Quiñones et al., 2020; Spolaore et al., 2006). Hyalurosome encapsulation enhances their stability, dermal penetration, antioxidant activity, and keratinocyte proliferation, while improving phycocyanin bioavailability (Castangia et al., 2016; Byeon et al., 2017).

Protein hydrolysates from *Chlorella* and *Arthrospira* exhibit antiinflammatory, hydration-promoting, and antioxidant effects (Goossens, 2011; Chinjoo and Golzary, 2025). *Chlorella* peptides reduce UVB-induced MMP-1 expression and restore collagen synthesis (Chen et al., 2011). Interestingly, *Arthrospira* extracts regulate aquaporin-3, hyaluronic acid synthase 3, filaggrin, and *Smit* genes, improving hydration and osmotic stress tolerance (TKS, 2025). Limitations include peptide heterogeneity, allergenicity, and the high costs of isolating individual bioactive peptides. However, standardization remains a major industrial challenge (Tang et al., 2025; Günal-Köroğlu et al., 2025).

3.1.3 Polysaccharides

Microalgal polysaccharides, like alguronic acid from *Solazyme/Porphyridium,* improve skin hydration, elasticity, and cell renewal, supporting their use in antiaging products. Their high molecular weight often limits their capability of deeply penetrating the skin barrier, so formulation optimization is required (Tsaloglou et al., 2016; Juncan et al., 2021; Schramm and Weiß, 2024). Microalgae species also secrete bioactive exopolysaccharides (EPS), which provide hydration, film formation, antiinflammatory effects, and prebiotic-like support for the skin microbiome (Chinjoo and Golzary, 2025; Joelyna et al., 2024; Morais et al., 2022).

3.1.4 Fatty acids and sterols

Microalgae provide PUFAs, including DHA, EPA, and GLA, that moisturize and restore the skin barrier (Ohse et al., 2015; Ma et al., 2016; Santin et al., 2021). *Nannochloropsis* and *Monodus subterraneus* are notable sources of linolenic acids relevant for skincare (Ma et al., 2016). In addition, microalgae sterols include ergosterol, brassicasterol, and stigmasterol, which exhibit notable antiinflammatory and barrier repair effects (Volkman, 2016; Fagundes et al., 2020).

3.1.5 Polar lipids

Microalgae are abundant sources of PLs, including phospholipids, glycolipids, and betainolipids, that contain high levels of ω-3 PUFAs such as ALA, EPA, and DHA, typically esterified at the *sn-2* position, a configuration correlated with enhanced bioactivity. Glycolipids like SQDGs, monogalactosyl diacylglycerols, and digalactosyl diacylglycerols are rich in chloroplast-rich microalgae (mainly green microalgae like *Chlorococcum* sp. and *Spirulina*), contributing to membrane structure and biological function. Numerous studies demonstrate that microalgal PLs exert potent antiinflammatory and antithrombotic effects, largely by modulating or inhibiting the PAF cascade, with specific PL species acting as natural PAF antagonists, suppressing PAF- and thrombin-induced platelet aggregation (Conde et al., 2021; Koukouraki et al., 2020; Shiels et al., 2021; Safafar et al., 2015).

3.1.6 Polyphenols (microalgal phenolics) and flavonoids

Although less abundant than in microalgae, some microalgae produce gallic, caffeic, ferulic, and *p*-coumaric acid, which provide antioxidant, antimicrobial, and antiinflammatory activity and can synergize with carotenoids for UV protection. Cinnamaldehydes, resveratrol, and various flavonoids and flavonoid derivatives, such as naringenin, apigenin, luteolin, rutin, kaempferol, quercetin, catechin, and epicatechin, also comprise microalgae species (Del Mondo et al., 2022).

3.1.7 Vitamins, cofactors, minerals, and trace elements

Microalgae are rich sources of vitamins B complex (B_1, B_2, B_3, B_6, and B_{12}), C, K_1, and E (tocopherols), which reportedly provide antioxidant defense, collagen stabilization, and skin-brightening effects (especially vitamin B_3). Its mineral and trace element content, particularly selenium, zinc, and magnesium, also supports antioxidant enzyme activity, improves barrier function, and regulates inflammation by suppressing proinflammatory mediators (Koyande et al., 2019; Guil-Guerrero and Prates, 2025).

3.1.8 Mycosporine-like amino acids

Although macroalgae are the major source of MAAs, microalgae also partially produce these major skincare-relevant molecules. Predominantly found in cyanobacteria, common MAAs in microalgae include shinorine, porphyra-334, and mycosporine-glycine, which are natural UV-absorbing compounds with sun protection factor-like effects and remarkable antiphotoaging, anti-UV, and, concurrently, antiaging activity (Peng et al., 2023).

3.2 Bioactives and health-promoting constituents in macroalgae

Macroalgae contain diverse polysaccharides, polyphenols, pigments, proteins, peptides, lipids, vitamins, and minerals. Composition varies by phylum, namely, *Chlorophyta* (green algae), *Phaeophyceae* (brown algae), and *Rhodophyta* (red algae), as well as among species, geographic origin, and environmental conditions (El-Beltagi et al., 2022; Hermund et al., 2022).

3.2.1 Polysaccharides

Macroalgae polysaccharides serve as moisturizers, emulsifiers, stabilizers, and film-formers in cosmetic formulations. Brown algae contain alginate, fucoidan, and laminarin, while red algae contain carrageenans and agar. Green algae, on the contrary, mainly synthesize ulvans and sulfated polysaccharides. These compounds are capable of forming hydrogels that create a film over the skin, retaining moisture and enhancing barrier function (Senevirathne et al., 2010; Athukorala et al., 2006). Fucoidans extracted from *F. vesiculosus* and *Saccharina japonica* have demonstrated remarkable hyaluronidase inhibitory activity, helping preserve the integrity of the ECM and counteract skin aging (Zhang et al., 2010). Ulvans (*Ulva lactuca*) provide hydration, elasticity, and notable antioxidant properties (2018).

3.2.2 Polyphenols

Phlorotannins, abundant in brown algae, exhibit strong antioxidant, antiinflammatory, UV-protective, and antienzymatic activities. These phloroglucinol oligomers can inhibit tyrosinase, collagenase, and elastase, supporting antiaging, skin-brightening, antiwrinkle, antihyperpigmentation, and antiphotoaging effects (Yoon et al., 2008; Cotas et al., 2020). For example, phlorotannin-rich extracts from *Ecklonia cava* and *F. vesiculosus* effectively scavenge ROS and nitric oxide radicals (NO•) in vitro, highlighting their potential as multifunctional cosmetic ingredients (Couteau, 2016; Wang et al., 2015). Red and green algae also contain phenolic compounds, albeit in lower concentrations, which contribute to their antioxidant and antimicrobial effects. Interestingly, polyphenol content increases under environmental stress, influencing extract variability (Morais et al., 2021).

3.2.3 Pigments

Macroalgal pigments, mainly including chlorophylls, carotenoids (e.g., fucoxanthin and astaxanthin), and phycobiliproteins (e.g., phycoerythrin and phycocyanin), offer antioxidant and photoprotective benefits. Fucoxanthin, beyond modulating melanogenesis pathways, absorbs UV radiation and protects fibroblasts from ROS formation and photo-induced damage (Morais et al., 2021; Ko et al., 2011). Chlorophyll derivatives (e.g., pheophytin-a) reveal antioxidant and antiinflammatory properties, whereas red algae phycobiliproteins serve as natural colorants and antioxidants (Dong et al., 2020). These are used in sunscreens, antiaging creams, and skin-brightening formulations (Dong et al., 2020).

3.2.4 Proteins and peptides

Macroalgal proteins and derived peptides offer biofunctional properties, including elasticity, hydration, and ECM regeneration, which are highly important for moisturizers and bioactive carriers in topical cosmetic formulations. Green algae, such as *U. lactuca*, contain aosaine, an elastin-mimetic protein that enhances skin elasticity (2018). Enzymatic hydrolysates stimulate collagen, elastin, and glycosaminoglycan synthesis in fibroblasts, thereby supporting antiwrinkle and skin-firming effects (Couteau, 2016; Wang et al., 2015).

Lectins, found specifically in red algae, have also been revealed to possess immunomodulatory, antiinflammatory, antitumor, and skin-repairing signaling properties. Furthermore, macroalgal antimicrobial peptides include ulvan-binding and defensin-like peptides, which provide skin microbiome balance and support antiacne formulations (Habibie et al., 2023; de Arruda et al., 2023).

3.2.5 Lipids, halogenated compounds, phytosterols, vitamins, and minerals

Especially in red and brown algae, halogenated bromophenols, iodinated and chlorinated terpenes have revealed vast antimicrobial, antiinflammatory, and antioxidant properties. Moreover, macroalgae lipid sterols (e.g., fucosterol, clionasterol, campesterol) and fatty acids contribute to photoprotective and antiinflammatory activities (Gressler et al., 2010). Sterols can reduce MMP expression and enhance procollagen type I production in UVB-exposed fibroblasts (Wang et al., 2015).

Vitamins (A, C, E, and B-complex) and minerals (such as magnesium, zinc, and iron) act as antioxidants and enzymatic cofactors essential for skin homeostasis (Alparslan et al., 2018). Species such as *U. lactuca*, *Caulerpa lentillifera*, and *F. vesiculosus* are rich in these micronutrients, enhancing their cosmetic appeal (Kim, 2011; Pereira et al., 2013).

3.2.6 Mycosporine-like amino acids

Macroalgae are a major source of MAAs with significant skincare-relevant benefits. Common in red algae are shinorine, porphyra-334, and palythine, which are natural UV filters with strong photoprotective, anti-ROS, antiphotoaging, and anti-UV properties (Peng et al., 2023; Vaz et al., 2025).

3.3 Bioactives and health-promoting constituents in aquatic plants

3.3.1 Phenolic acids and flavonoids

N. nucifera and *Nymphaea* spp. contain phenolic acids (e.g., gallic, chlorogenic, and ferulic acids) and flavonoids (e.g., quercetin, kaempferol, and myricetin) (Tungmunnithum et al., 2021; CIR-Safety, 2025). These molecules function as antioxidants by donating hydrogen atoms or electrons to neutralize free radicals and inhibit enzymes such as tyrosinase, elastase, and collagenase through metal-ion chelation (Dhanasinghe et al., 2025). For example, *N. nucifera* leaf extract inhibits 59% of tyrosinase activity at 100 μg/mL, outperforming arbutin, a conventional whitening agent (Seferli et al., 2024, 2025).

3.3.2 Alkaloids, indole derivatives, saponins, tannins, and coumarins

Watercress (*N. officinale*) contains indole alkaloids, such as indole-3-acetonitrile-4-methoxy-2-S-D-glucopyranoside (IAMG), which enhance fibroblast migration and collagen synthesis, while reducing MMP-1 expression under UVB stress (Al-Snafi, 2020; Panahi Kokhdan et al., 2021). This suggests a dual antiphotoaging and wound healing role mediated through mitogen-activated protein kinase (MAPK) and tumor growth factor β (TGF-β) signaling modulation (Klimek-Szczykutowicz et al., 2018).

Common in *N. nucifera* and *N. nouchali* are saponins and tannins (e.g., ellagitannins and gallotannins), providing notable surfactant, astringent, skin-cleansing, antiinflammatory, antiacne, and antioxidant effects as important enhancers of skin penetration (Seferli et al., 2024; Jiang et al., 2018). Aquatic plant coumarins, such as scopoletin and umbelliferone in *E. crassipes,* have demonstrated antioxidant, depigmenting, and mild photoprotective potential as future effective cosmetic agents (Seferli et al., 2024).

3.3.3 Polysaccharides, terpenoids, and essential oils

Polysaccharides, especially from lotus root and water lily petals, offer great hydration, film formation, and soothing action (Abelti et al., 2023; Afrin et al., 2024). *H. coronarium* produces monoterpenes (e.g., 1,8-cineole, linalool, and β-pinene) and sesquiterpenes with pronounced antielastase and anticollagenase activity (Tammasorn et al., 2023). Rhizome absolutes inhibit collagenase by up to 95.7%, surpassing EGCG, supporting their potential as an antiwrinkle cosmetic ingredient (Russell-Goldman and Murphy, 2020).

3.3.4 Carotenoids and vitamins

Aquatic plants synthesize β-carotene, lutein, astaxanthin, and vitamin E derivatives that protect against UV-induced oxidative stress and lipid peroxidation (Anonymous, 2005). These compounds complement sunscreen products by absorbing UV radiation, mitigating antioxidant defense, and contributing to antiinflammatory responses in UV-exposed skin (Seferli et al., 2024, 2025; CIR-Safety, 2025).

3.3.5 Polar lipids

Freshwater aquatic plants such as *N. nucifera* and *Lemna* sp. are emerging sources of bioactive PLs. Their amphiphilic lipid fractions contain phospholipids and glycolipids enriched with monoenes and ω-3 PUFAs, particularly ALA in the *sn-2* position of the glycerol backbone, a structural feature associated with enhanced antiinflammatory activity. Such PLs, alongside their co-extracted phenolics and carotenoids, contribute to the strong antioxidant, antithrombotic, and antiinflammatory properties observed in vitro. Several glycolipid and phospholipid species demonstrated the ability to inhibit PAF-induced platelet activation, indicating potential protective effects against oxidative stress and skin inflammation via their anti-PAF mechanisms. As observed by Seferli et al. (2025), extracts, particularly from *Lemna* sp., showed potent antiplatelet activity against PAF and adenosine diphosphate (ADP) (Seferli et al., 2024, 2025).

4 Health-promoting properties, cosmetic applications, and formulation roles of microalgae, macroalgae, and aquatic plant bioactives

Microalgae, macroalgae, and aquatic plants have emerged as high-value cosmetic resources due to their rich repertoire of bioactive compounds and well-documented skin-beneficial effects. Their vast antioxidant, antiinflammatory, photoprotective, moisturizing, and antiaging properties translate directly into multiple cosmetic functions, ranging from environmental defense and deep moisturization to pigmentation control, barrier restoration, and wrinkle reduction (Kalasariya et al., 2022; Pooja et al., 2020; Guil-Guerrero and Prates, 2025). Such agents, often comprising pigments, polysaccharides, peptides, lipids, sterols, and other secondary metabolites, enable diverse formulation roles, including hydration enhancement, film formation, viscosity modulation, firmness enhancement, stabilization, and sensory optimization. Their compatibility with green extraction, renewable cultivation, and clean-beauty standards further amplifies their relevance in contemporary cosmetic science (Kalasariya et al., 2022; Pooja et al., 2020; Guil-Guerrero and Prates, 2025).

Driven by consumer demand for natural and sustainable actives, the cosmetics industry has increasingly integrated algae- and aquatic plant-derived ingredients into commercial products and patented formulations (Pooja et al., 2020; Mago et al., 2025). Many brands currently rely on microalgal, macroalgal, and aquatic plant bioactives to support claims related to wrinkle reduction, UV protection, soothing effects, acne control, and skin-tone improvement. At the same time, ongoing research and development (R&D) continues to validate these ingredients through in vitro, in vivo, and ex vivo models, contributing to a growing array of research-backed cosmetic agents. Table 9.1 summarizes representative commercial products, highlighting their cosmetic uses, their algal or aquatic plant constituents involved, and their skin health-promoting benefits (Kalasariya et al., 2022; Pooja et al., 2020; Guil-Guerrero and Prates, 2025; Mago et al., 2025).

4.1 Health-promoting properties and cosmetic applications of microalgae bioactive constituents

Microalgae have emerged as an important source of bioactive compounds for cosmetic and cosmeceutical products. Their bioactive agents, including pigments, lipids, polysaccharides, proteins, vitamins, and MAAs, are used for various skin-related purposes, such as providing antioxidant protection, hydration, photoprotection, and antiaging effects (Conde et al., 2021; Koukouraki et al., 2020; Shiels et al., 2021; Mourelle et al., 2017; Prates, 2025; Martínez-Ruiz et al., 2022). These organisms can be cultivated in controlled environments with low land and freshwater requirements, aligning with the sustainability goals of the modern cosmetic industry (Table 9.2) (Jaber, 2025).

4.2 Antiaging and antioxidant effects

Oxidative stress is a major driver of skin aging, contributing to collagen degradation, elastin fragmentation, and wrinkle formation. Microalgal carotenoids like astaxanthin (*H. pluvialis*) and β-carotene (*D. salina*) exhibit strong free radical scavenging activity and inhibit lipid peroxidation in dermal cells. Microalgal antioxidants have also demonstrated antiglycation activity, helping prevent collagen stiffening and loss of elasticity (Guerin et al., 2003; Higuera-Ciapara et al., 2006). Interestingly, topical formulations containing astaxanthin improved skin elasticity and reduced wrinkle depth by modulating oxidative pathways and inhibiting MMPs (Tominaga et al., 2012b). In addition, phycobiliproteins from *S. platensis* and polyphenolic compounds from *C. vulgaris* provide antioxidant protection, supporting their inclusion in antiaging serums and creams (Conde et al., 2021; Chinjoo and Golzary, 2025; Koukouraki et al., 2020; Shiels et al., 2021; Miranda et al., 1998).

TABLE 9.1 Commercial products and research-backed cosmetic agents derived from microalgae, macroalgae, and/or freshwater aquatic plants.

Cosmetic product	Cosmetic use	Microalgae, macroalgae, or aquatic plant source/ ingredient	Beneficial impact	References
Algenist—Green Microalgae Retinol[+] Regenerating Serum	Retinol serum	*Chlorella vulgaris* extract and *Parachlorella beijerinckii* EPSs	Antiaging, antiacne, antioxidant, exfoliant, soothing, and hydrating properties	(Algenist, 2025)
REN—Atlantic Kelp and Microalgae Anti-Fatigue Toning Body Oil	Body oil	*Gelidium cartilagineum* and *Laminaria digitata*	Improves skin elasticity, toning, and firmness, also offering muscle fatigue relief	(Good Vibes Pharmacy, 2025)
THE DEWY SKIN—Microalgae Potion Face and Lip Serum	Face and lip serum	Microalgae and plankton extract	Brightening, antiacne, exfoliating, soothing, melanin-modulating, toning, and strengthening effects	(Amazon, 2025b)
Ahava—Dunaliella Algae Peel-Off Mask	Peel-off mask	*Dunaliella salina* algae extract	Nourishing, moisturizing, antiwrinkle, antifine line, and antioxidant effects	(*Dunaliella*, 2025)
Very MWL Annabella—*Haematococcus Pluvialis* Facial Repair Mask	Facial repair mask	*Haematococcus pluvialis*, *Chondrus crispus*, and *Undaria pinnatifida*	Moisturizing, nourishing, antioxidant, and skin-soothing properties	(VERYMWL, 2025)
La Prairie—Cellular Swiss Ice Crystal Oil	Dry oil	*Chlamydomonas nivalis*	Antiaging, glowing, and skin-moisturizing effects	(Bletapharm, 2025)
Sea Laria—A-GEL	Skin gel	*Gracilaria* sp.	Skin-hydrating, soothing, wound healing, and scar/rash-alleviating properties	(Sealaria, 2025)
Gelyma—Helionori	Water and concentrated active algae ingredients	*Porphyra umbilicalis* (MAAs) extract	UVA filtering, antiphotoaging, and sunburn-protective active ingredient	(HELIONORI, 2025)
L'Oréal—Pure Clay Glow Scrub (Foam Wash, Red)	Exfoliating scrub	*Palmaria palmata* extract	Sebum-reducing, deep-cleansing, detoxifying, and skin-brightening effects	(L'Oréal Paris, 2025)
Patyka—Sacred Lotus Face Cream	Face cream	*Nelumbo nucifera* (Sacred lotus)	Skin-brightening, revitalizing, relieving, and soothing effects	(Real Beauty Outlet, 2025)
Daughter Earth—Sacred Lotus and Vanilla Body Butter	Body butter	*Nelumbo nucifera* (sacred lotus)	Skin-nourishing, hydrating, radical scavenging, and emollient properties	(Amazon, 2025a)
Revolution Skincare—Aloe Vera and Water Lily Soothing Face Mask	Face mask	*Nymphaea alba* extract	Irritation-calming, revitalizing, skin-soothing, and moisturizing effects	(Notino, 2025)
FarmHouse Fresh—Watercress Hydration Cascade Gelée Moisturizer	Gelée moisturizer	*Nasturtium officinale* extract	Moisturizing, antioxidant, and skin-brightening effects	(FarmHouse Fresh, 2025)
Fable & Mane—MahaMane Smooth and Shine Hair Oil	Hair oil	*Bacopa monnieri* leaf extract	Hair-smoothening, brightening, antifrizzing, and glowing properties	(MahaMane, 2025)
Laneige—Retinol Firming Cream Treatment	Firming cream	*Hedychium coronarium* root extract	Skin-nourishing, hydrating, antiaging, smoothing, and antiwrinkle properties	(LANEIGE, 2025)

TABLE 9.2 Bioactives in microalgae with potential cosmetic and cosmeceutical applications.

Bioactive compounds	Indicative microalgae source	Cosmetic and cosmeceutical function	References
Chlorophylls	*Chlorella vulgaris* and *Arthrospira* sp.	Colorant or antioxidant ingredients	(Pagels et al., 2020, 2021)
MAAs	*Porphyra* and *Chondrus* sp.	Natural UV filters, antiphotoaging, and antioxidant agents	(Peng et al., 2023)
β-Carotene	*Dunaliella salina*	Antiaging, antioxidant, and provitamin A agents	(Mourelle et al., 2017; Terao, 1989)
Astaxanthin	*Haematococcus pluvialis*	Antiaging, UV protection, and antioxidant properties	(Guerin et al., 2003; Hama et al., 2012; Sun et al., 2020; Hu et al., 2019)
Lutein	*Chlorella* and *Arthrospira* sp.	Antioxidant and skin protection	(Guerin et al., 2003)
Zeaxanthin	*Nannochloropsis, Chlorella*	Antipigmentation and antioxidant benefits	(Ma et al., 2016; Navalho et al., 2025)
Phenolic compounds and polyphenols	*Chlamydomonas, Chlorella,* and *Arthrospira* sp.	Antioxidant, antiglycation, and antiinflammatory properties	(Del Mondo et al., 2022)
Vitamins and minerals	Most microalgae species	Skin-renewal, antifatigue, cellular metabolism support, soothing, and antiinflammatory effects	(Koyande et al., 2019; Guil-Guerrero and Prates, 2025)
PUFAs (DHA, EPA, γ-linolenic acid)	*Nannochloropsis, Monodus subterraneus,* and *Ulkenia* sp.	Moisturizing, skin barrier restoration, and antiinflammatory agents	(Ohse et al., 2015; Ma et al., 2016; Santin et al., 2021)
Phycobiliproteins (phycocyanin and phycoerythrin)	*Arthrospira, Porphyridium*	Colorant, antioxidant, and fluorescent labeling effects	(Quiñones et al., 2020; Spolaore et al., 2006; Byeon et al., 2017)
Phytosterols (ergosterol, brassicasterol, and stigmasterol)	*Nannochloropsis* and *Monodus subterraneus*	Barrier repair, antiinflammatory, and antiaging ingredients	(Volkman, 2016; Fagundes et al., 2020)
Stable isotopically labeled compounds (13C, 15N, 2H)	General microalgae	Research, structural determination, and metabolic studies	(Tang et al., 2025)
Peptides/protein hydrolysates	*Chlorella* and *Arthrospira* sp.	Antiaging, antioxidant, and skin hydration properties	(Goossens, 2011; TKS, 2025; Chinjoo and Golzary, 2025; Chen et al., 2011; Tang et al., 2025; Günal-Köroğlu et al., 2025)
Polysaccharides (alguronic acid, porphyridium, and EPSs)	*Solazyme* and *Porphyridium* sp.	Moisturizing, elasticity, cell renewal, film-forming, hydration, and thickening agents	(Tsaloglou et al., 2016; Juncan et al., 2021; Schramm and Weiß, 2024)
Polar lipids (phospholipids and glycolipids)	*Chlorococcum* and *Spirulina* sp.	Anti-PAF, antiinflammatory, and antithrombotic	(Conde et al., 2021; Koukouraki et al., 2020; Shiels et al., 2021)

4.3 Photoprotection and environmental stress defense

Exposure to UV radiation leads to DNA damage, photoaging, and hyperpigmentation. Microalgal MAAs, such as shinorine and porphyra-334, absorb UV radiation between 310 and 360 nm and dissipate it safely as heat, functioning as natural sunscreens (Rastogi and Sinha, 2009). They also suppress inflammatory mediators and protect against UV-induced apoptosis in keratinocytes (Conde et al., 2000). Carotenoids and chlorophyll derivatives provide additional photoprotection by quenching singlet oxygen and ROS generated by UV exposure. Some microalgal extracts also exhibit antipollution chelating activity, reducing heavy-metal-induced oxidative stress (Novoveská et al., 2019). Several microalgal extracts are now incorporated into "urban defense" skincare formulations to protect against particulate matter and blue light emitted by electronic devices (Natura-Tec, 2025).

4.4 Skin hydration and barrier reinforcement

Microalgal polysaccharides significantly improve skin hydration and barrier function. Sulfated polysaccharides from *Porphyridium cruentum* and EPSs from *C. vulgaris* have high water-binding capacities and form protective films on the skin's surface (Plaza et al., 2009; De Jesus Raposo et al., 2013). These compounds reduce TEWL and enhance stratum corneum flexibility, functioning similarly to hyaluronic acid (Cristofoli et al., 2023). Microalgal polysaccharides specifically enhance skin smoothness and notably improve tactile sensory properties in cosmetics. Furthermore, microalgal lipids rich in PUFAs also support the structural integrity of the epidermal barrier and modulate inflammation, making them valuable in barrier repair and moisturizing (Pereira et al., 2012).

4.5 Soothing, antiinflammatory, and microbiome-balancing properties

Species such as *Nannochloropsis oculata* and *S. platensis* produce bioactive peptides and polysaccharides with antiinflammatory activity through the downregulation of proinflammatory cytokines, including IL-1β and TNF-α in dermal fibroblasts (Pham et al., 2016). These extracts are suitable for formulations targeting sensitive or reactive skin. Moreover, microalgal metabolites support the skin microbiome by inhibiting opportunistic pathogens while also promoting beneficial commensals, aligning with current trends in probiotic and microbiome-friendly cosmetics (Mourelle et al., 2017). Microalgal antiinflammatory components may also reduce erythema, accelerate diabetic wound healing, and support postprocedure skin recovery (Conde et al., 2021; Chinjoo and Golzary, 2025; Koukouraki et al., 2020; Shiels et al., 2021; Pei et al., 2025).

Especially from Koukouraki et al. (2020), a patent against skin inflammation for the sulfo-glycolipids (SQDG) of Spirulina, as well as for other phosphor- and glycol lipids with liquid chromatography - mass spectometry (LC–MS) results for their structures, was demonstrated. All extracts revealed strong anti-PAF and antithrombin activities in washed rabbit platelets activated by PAF and thrombin. Phycocyanobilin exhibited the strongest inhibitory effects on PAF/thrombin-induced platelet aggregation, with a more pronounced antithrombin effect, followed by notable anti-PAF inhibitory indices of the total lipid extracts. Through high-performance liquid chromatography separation of the *Spirulina* lipid extracts into lipid subclasses' fractions, specific PL fractions of glycolipids and PAF-like phosphatidylcholine moieties exhibited the strongest anti-PAF effects, while at higher concentrations, they also showed high anti-PAF agonistic and platelet-aggregatory effects (Koukouraki et al., 2020).

4.6 Formulation and technological aspects

Integrating microalgal extracts into cosmetic formulations presents challenges related to stability, solubility, and odor masking. Modern encapsulation methods, such as liposomes, nanoemulsions, and biopolymer microcapsules, enhance the stability and delivery of sensitive compounds such as carotenoids and MAAs (Vieira et al., 2020; Prieto and Lagaron, 2024). These systems protect active ingredients from oxidation and facilitate controlled release upon topical application. In addition, microalgal fractions can also function as natural colorants and mild thickeners. Recent advances in bioreactor cultivation and strain selection have enabled the production of extracts tailored for optimal cosmetic performance and formulation compatibility (Martínez-Ruiz et al., 2022).

4.7 Emerging and synergistic applications

Innovative formulations increasingly combine microalgal actives with other natural agents to achieve synergistic effects. For instance, *Chlorella* extracts combined with hyaluronic acid improve hydration and firmness more than either ingredient alone (Chinjoo and Golzary, 2025). Similarly, astaxanthin-enriched emulsions fortified with green tea polyphenols provide enhanced antioxidant synergy (OyetakinWhite et al., 2012). Microalgal actives are also being explored for blue-light protection and skin tone evening in hybrid skincare-makeup products (Georgieva et al., 2024). As consumer interest in natural, multifunctional cosmetics grows, microalgae are becoming cornerstone ingredients in next-generation formulations emphasizing efficacy, sustainability, and biocompatibility (Becker, 2013).

5 Health-promoting properties and cosmetic applications of macroalgae bioactive constituents

The extensive application of macroalgal compounds in the cosmetic and cosmeceutical industries is driven by their diverse biological activities, including antiaging, antioxidant, UV-protecting, moisturizing, whitening, and antiinflammatory effects. Their multifunctionality stems from the synergistic interactions among macroalgal polysaccharides, polyphenols, lipids, pigments, proteins, vitamins, and minerals. Together, these compounds make macroalgae a versatile, green source for developing advanced skin and hair care products (Table 9.3) (Kalasariya et al., 2022).

5.1 Antioxidant activity

Oxidative stress, primarily induced by ROS, accelerates skin aging, inflammation, and pigmentation. Macroalgal secondary metabolites, such as polyphenols, carotenoids, vitamins, and peptides, exhibit robust antioxidant properties through ROS scavenging, metal chelation, and lipid peroxidation inhibition (Admassu et al., 2018; Plaza et al., 2008). Phlorotannins extracted from *E. cava* and fucoidans from *F. vesiculosus* reduce ROS-induced fibroblast damage, thereby preventing collagen degradation and dermal elasticity loss (Kim, 2016). Carotenoids, such as fucoxanthin and astaxanthin, effectively quench singlet oxygen and inhibit UV-induced lipid peroxidation, contributing to the maintenance of skin integrity (Sabeena Farvin and Jacobsen, 2013; Ko et al., 2011). Ulvans from *U. lactuca* and phenolic compounds from *Porphyra/Pyropia* species further enhance radical scavenging capacity and antioxidant enzyme activity, confirming the antioxidant potential of macroalgae in topical products (Wang et al., 2009; Jing et al., 2021; Wijesinghe and Jeon, 2012; Pereira et al., 2009).

TABLE 9.3 Bioactives in macroalgae with potential cosmetic and cosmeceutical applications.

Bioactive compounds	Indicative macroalgae source	Cosmetic and cosmeceutical function	References
Phlorotannins, fucoidans, carotenoids (e.g., fucoxanthin, chlorophylls), and sterols (e.g., fucosterol)	*Fucus vesiculosus* and *Ascophyllum nodosum* (Brown)	Antioxidant, antiaging, UV protection, tyrosinase inhibition, moisturizing, and anticellulite properties	(Sabeena Farvin and Jacobsen, 2013; Cotas et al., 2020; Wijesinghe and Jeon, 2012; Qiu et al., 2022)
Phlorotannins, polysaccharides, pigments, and carotenoids	*Ecklonia cava*, *E. stolonifera*, and *Saccharina japonica* (brown)	Antiphotoaging, collagen-boosting, hyaluronidase-inhibiting, antiinflammatory, and antioxidant ingredients	(Wijesinghe and Jeon, 2012; Taboada et al., 2010; FAO, 2025)
MAAs and essential amino acids	*Porphyra*, *Gracilaria*, and *Palmaria* sp. (red)	UV protection, antiphotoaging, antiinflammatory, and antioxidant effects	(Peng et al., 2023; Vaz et al., 2025)
Proteins, peptides, and lectins	*Gracilaria* sp.	Cell signaling and wound healing agents	(Habibie et al., 2023; de Arruda et al., 2023)
Fucoxanthin, phlorotannins, and alginates	*Sargassum* and *Turbinaria* sp. (brown)	Photoprotection, antiaging, and moisturizing benefits	(Sabeena Farvin and Jacobsen, 2013; Taboada et al., 2010; Kang et al., 2013)
Vitamins, cofactors, and trace minerals	*Ulva lactuca*, *Caulerpa lentillifera* (green), and *Fucus vesiculosus* (brown)	Antioxidants and enzymatic cofactors that are essential for skin homeostasis	(Kim, 2011; Pereira et al., 2013)
Carrageenans and polysaccharides	*Kappaphycus alvarezii* (red)	Wound healing, hair care, and skin barrier improvement	(Torres et al., 2019)
Sulfated polysaccharides, amino acids, and phenolics	*Porphyra/Pyropia* spp. (red)	Antioxidant, antiinflammatory, UV protection, and moisturizing effects	(Jing et al., 2021; Fernando and Kim, 2018)
Ulvans, aosaine (protein), vitamins (A, B, C, E), and trace minerals	*Ulva lactuca* and *Caulerpa lentillifera* (green)	Hydration, antiwrinkle, elasticity, and antioxidant properties	(Pereira et al., 2013; Courtois, 2009)
Polysaccharides, brominated metabolites, fatty acids, and flavonoids	*Asparagopsis armata* (red)	Antiacne, antibacterial, antiinflammatory, and antioxidant effects	(Siao et al., 2015)
Polyphenols, flavonoids, and meroditerpenes	*Ericaria amentacea* (brown)	Photoprotection, antiaging, antioxidant, and antiinflammatory benefits	(Bocanegra et al., 2009)

5.2 Antiaging activity

Macroalgal compounds counteract both intrinsic and extrinsic skin aging by stimulating collagen and elastin synthesis, inhibiting MMPs, and strengthening the skin's moisture-retention capacity. Fucoidans and phlorotannins from brown algae, like *F. vesiculosus* and *E. cava,* suppress MMP-1 and elastase activity, preserving the structural integrity of the dermal ECM (Qiu et al., 2022; Draelos, 2018). Bioactive peptides from green algae, including aosaine from *U. lactuca*, act as signaling molecules that promote collagen type I synthesis and improve skin firmness (Courtois, 2009). Sterols, such as fucosterol, commonly found in brown macroalgae, modulate fibroblast proliferation and ECM deposition, contributing to skin regeneration and rejuvenation (Taboada et al., 2010). Some macroalgal extracts also reduce glycation-induced stiffness of collagen fibers, providing antisugar and antiyellowing benefits (Pei et al., 2025; Dhahri et al., 2022; Barbosa et al., 2021). Furthermore, polysaccharides from *Sargassum muticum* enhance hyaluronic acid preservation and moisture retention, reinforcing their relevance in antiaging skincare formulations (Thiyagarasaiyar et al., 2020).

5.3 Moisturizing and skin barrier function

Macroalgal polysaccharides, like alginate, carrageenan, and ulvan, possess exceptional water retention capacity. These polymers form protective films on the skin's surface, reduce TEWL, and maintain hydration levels (Wang et al., 2009; Chrapusta et al., 2017). Moreover, they promote ceramide synthesis, strengthening the skin's lipid barrier. Fucoidan from *F. vesiculosus* and laminarin from *S. japonica* improve skin elasticity, texture, and hydration in clinical settings, validating their effectiveness as natural moisturizing agents in dermocosmetics (Pimentel et al., 2018; Qiu et al., 2022).

5.4 Whitening and tyrosinase inhibition

Hyperpigmentation results from excessive melanin production mediated by tyrosinase. Macroalgal extracts, especially polyphenol-rich fractions such as phlorotannins, exhibit potent tyrosinase inhibitory and antimelanogenic activity. For example, phlorotannins from *E. cava* reduce melanin synthesis in B16F10 melanoma cells, producing a visible skin-brightening effect (Wijesinghe and Jeon, 2012). Similarly, extracts of *F. vesiculosus* suppress tyrosinase activity and modulate melanocyte signaling (Cotas et al., 2020). Sulfated polysaccharides from red algae (e.g., *Porphyra/Pyropia* species) also inhibit melanin formation in vitro, representing a natural and safe alternative to synthetic skin-lightening agents (Torres et al., 2019; Jing et al., 2021).

5.5 Antiinflammatory activity

Chronic inflammation contributes to various dermatological disorders such as erythema, photoaging, and acne. Macroalgal metabolites, including fucoidans, phlorotannins, carotenoids, and peptides, exert significant antiinflammatory effects by modulating key cytokines and signaling pathways. These compounds inhibit TNF-α, IL-6, and nitrogen oxide (NO) production in keratinocytes and macrophages (Senevirathne et al., 2010; Khansari et al., 2009). Microalgae, additionally, soothe irritation, reduce redness, and support skin recovery after cosmetic procedures or sun exposure. *F. vesiculosus* fucoidans downregulate UVB-induced cyclooxygenase-2 (COX-2) expression, alleviating erythema and photoinduced inflammation (Pimentel et al., 2018). Phlorotannins modulate nuclear factor kappa B and MAPK signaling cascades, providing robust antiinflammatory efficacy (Cotas et al., 2020).

5.6 UV-protective activity

Macroalgal pigments and polyphenols play a crucial role in protecting the skin from harmful UV radiation. Carotenoids (e.g., fucoxanthin and astaxanthin), chlorophylls, and phycobiliproteins can absorb UV radiation and dissipate the energy as heat, thereby preventing the generation of ROS (Pimentel et al., 2018; Ko et al., 2011). Phlorotannin-rich extracts from *E. cava* provide dual protection by absorbing UVB radiation and neutralizing ROS, thereby shielding dermal fibroblasts from photooxidative damage (Wijesinghe and Jeon, 2012). Similarly, fucoidans and carotenoids from *F. vesiculosus* exhibit UV absorbance and DNA-protective properties. In addition, fucoxanthin from *S. muticum* demonstrates photoprotective and antioxidant activities, highlighting the potential of macroalgal compounds as natural sunscreen agents (Pimentel et al., 2018; Lourenço-Lopes et al., 2020).

5.7 Slimming and anticellulite activity

Macroalgal compounds are increasingly incorporated into body-contouring cosmetics targeting adipose tissue metabolism and cellulite. Fucoidans and polyphenols from brown algae influence genes associated with adipogenesis and lipolysis. Fucoidans inhibit preadipocyte differentiation and stimulate lipolytic enzyme activity, reducing subcutaneous fat accumulation, as well as enhancing overall skin smoothness and offering improved microcirculation in cellulite-prone areas (Bedoux et al., 2014; Couteau, 2016). Consequently, brown algae extracts are used in topical slimming creams and body-firming products, contributing to improved skin firmness and reduced cellulite appearance. These results demonstrate the versatility of macroalgal bioactives in addressing esthetic and physiological aspects of skin health (Bedoux et al., 2014; Couteau, 2016).

6 Health-promoting properties and cosmetic applications of freshwater aquatic plant bioactive constituents

Aquatic plants, including freshwater macrophytes and hydrophytes, represent an emerging source of bioactive compounds for cosmetic and cosmeceutical applications. Their unique adaptation to submerged or semi-submerged environments promotes the production of protective metabolites such as phenolic acids, flavonoids, polysaccharides, carotenoids, vitamins, minerals, and essential oils. These molecules exhibit antioxidant, antiinflammatory, whitening, moisturizing, and photoprotective properties, positioning aquatic plants as sustainable and eco-friendly alternatives to terrestrial botanicals (Chaudhary et al., 2020; Academy, 2023; Seferli et al., 2024, 2025; Tungmunnithum et al., 2021; Tammasorn et al., 2023; Kim et al., 2011).

Common genera used in cosmetic formulations include *N. officinale* (watercress), *H. coronarium*, *N. nucifera*, *Nymphaea* (water lily), *E. crassipes* (water hyacinth), and *L. minor* (duckweed). Extracts of these species possess a rich repertoire of phytochemicals. These bioactive extracts are currently increasingly incorporated into cosmetic preparations, due to their antioxidant, antiaging, photoprotective, antiwrinkle, antimicrobial, skin-whitening, and wound healing properties (Table 9.4) (Chaudhary et al., 2020; Academy, 2023; Seferli et al., 2024, 2025; Tungmunnithum et al., 2021; Tammasorn et al., 2023; Kim et al., 2011).

TABLE 9.4 Bioactives in aquatic plants with potential cosmetic and cosmeceutical applications.

Bioactive compounds	Indicative aquatic plant source	Cosmetic and cosmeceutical function	References
IAMG, flavonoids, and other phenolic bioactives, carotenoids, essential oils, and MAAs	*Nasturtium officinale*, *Lemna minor*, and *Nelumbo nucifera*	Antiinflammatory, antioxidant, antiaging, UV protection, wound healing, fibroblast migration	(Paudel and Panth, 2015; Chaudhary et al., 2020; Seferli et al., 2024, 2025)
Terpenoids, alkaloids, and indole derivatives	*Nelumbo nucifera* and *Eichhornia crassipes*	Fibroblast migration, collagen synthesis, and MMP-1 expression reduction	(Al-Snafi, 2020; Bakrim et al., 2022; Panahi Kokhdan et al., 2021)
Saponins, tannins, and coumarins	*Hydrilla verticillata* and *Nasturtium officinale*	Surfactant, astringent, skin-cleansing, antiinflammatory, antiacne, antiwrinkle, and antioxidant effects	(Seferli et al., 2024; Prabha et al., 2019; Jiang et al., 2018)
Carotenoids, vitamins, trace minerals, and pigments	*Nelumbo nucifera*, *Eichhornia crassipes*, *Hydrilla verticillata*, and *Lemna minor*	UV-protective, antiaging, antiwrinkle, skin-brightening, antioxidant, and anti-photoaging activity	(Paudel and Panth, 2015; Seferli et al., 2024, 2025; Shrivastava and Srivastava, 2021; Lalitha and Jayanthi, 2014; Bakrim et al., 2022; Anonymous, 2005)
Ellagic acid, flavonoids, and rhizome/leaf absolutes	*Hedychium coronarium*	Antiwrinkle, antielastase, antihyaluronidase, antimicrobial (antiacne)	(Tammasorn et al., 2023)
Nuciferine, O-nornuciferine, roemerine, flavonoids, and other phenolic bioactives	*Nelumbo nucifera*	Antiinflammatory, antioxidant, whitening (tyrosinase/DOPA oxidase inhibition), antiaging (elastase inhibition)	(Seferli et al., 2024, 2025; Nguyen et al., 2012; Ha et al., 2010)
Flavonoids, phenolic bioactives, glycosides	*Nymphaea lotus*/*N. nouchali*	Antiaging, antiinflammatory, antioxidant, antiwrinkle	(Tungmunnithum et al., 2021)
Polysaccharides, glycosides, flavonoids, phenolic bioactives	Various aquatic plants	Moisturization, antioxidative, antiaging, skin barrier enhancement	(Lall, 2020; Lall, 2022)
Polar lipid bioactives (phospholipids and glycolipids with MUFAs/PUFAs in their structures)	*Lemna minor* and *Nelumbo nucifera*	Antiinflammatory and skin-health-promoting effects	(Seferli et al., 2024, 2025)

6.1 Antiaging and antiwrinkle applications

A primary cosmetic application of aquatic plant bioactives is the mitigation of skin aging and wrinkle formation. Compounds such as flavonoids, polyphenols, and glycosides modulate the activity of MMPs, including MMP-1, MMP-2, and MMP-9, which degrade collagen, elastin, and hyaluronic acid in the ECM (Academy, 2023; Tammasorn et al., 2023). Water lily (*Nymphaea* spp.) extracts inhibit elastase activity and upregulate sirtuin 2 (*SIR2*) gene expression, enhancing fibroblast longevity and reducing oxidative stress (Tungmunnithum et al., 2021). Similarly, *H. coronarium* rhizome absolutes show significant anticollagenase activity, preserving dermal structure and elasticity (Tammasorn et al., 2023). *N. nucifera* leaf, flower, and seed extracts inhibit elastase activity more effectively than the reference compound adenosine, demonstrating strong antiwrinkle potential, while they enhance superoxide dismutase and catalase activity in skin cells, providing additional antioxidant defense (Seferli et al., 2024, 2025; Kim et al., 2011).

6.2 Photoprotection and skin health

Photoprotective properties of aquatic plant bioactives, especially pigments and phenolics, are relevant in formulations aimed at preventing photoaging. IAMG from *N. officinale* mitigates UVB-induced photodamage by promoting fibroblast migration, reducing MMP-1 expression, and restoring type I procollagen levels. Such compounds can be formulated using encapsulation or stabilizing delivery systems to improve their dermal bioavailability and prevent the degradation of photosensitive phytochemicals (Chaudhary et al., 2020). Flavonoids from lotus and water lily absorb UV radiation, reduce ROS formation, and prevent DNA damage in keratinocytes, whereas carotenoids from duckweed provide additional photoprotective effects by quenching singlet oxygen (Seferli et al., 2024; Afrin et al., 2024; Lee et al., 2015). Extracts from *E. crassipes* have shown UVB-protective potential linked to their antioxidant capacity (Lalitha and Jayanthi, 2014; Bakrim et al., 2022).

6.3 Antioxidant, antiinflammatory, antimicrobial, and antiacne applications

Aquatic plants contain bioactive flavonoids, triterpenoids, and polysaccharides that modulate proinflammatory pathways. Lotus extracts inhibit the production of TNF-α, IL-1β, and NO in macrophages and keratinocytes. Water lily extracts alleviate erythema and irritation by suppressing COX-2 expression and reactive nitrogen species (Seferli et al., 2024; Osama et al., 2023).

Aquatic plant bioactives also exhibit significant antimicrobial activity, particularly against acne-related bacteria. *H. coronarium* leaf extracts inhibit *Cutibacterium acnes*, surpassing even clindamycin in some assays (Tammasorn et al., 2023). Their flavonoid (e.g., quercetin, kaempferol), phenolic acid (e.g., caffeic, ferulic, ellagic, and gallic acid), and carotenoid content offers a dual redox behavior, generating ROS that exert both antimicrobial and antioxidant effects (Tammasorn et al., 2023). *N. nucifera* extracts also reveal significant activity against Gram-positive acne pathogens, supporting their incorporation into gels, creams, or emulsions for acne treatment (Academy, 2023; Kim et al., 2011). In addition, lotus leaf alkaloids have demonstrated remarkable antimicrobial, antiacne, and sebum-regulating effects (Paudel and Panth, 2015).

As highlighted by Seferli et al. (2025), extracts, especially those derived from *Lemna* sp., demonstrated high antiplatelet activity against PAF and ADP. LC–MS analyses confirmed the presence of PLs rich in MUFAs and ω-3 PUFAs, with a favorable ω-6/ω-3 ratio, highly associated with potent antiinflammatory activity. Furthermore, high levels of total phenolics and carotenoids were also observed, aligning with the strong antioxidant capacity of both species (Seferli et al., 2024, 2025).

6.4 Whitening and brightening formulations

Aquatic plant bioactives modulate melanogenesis, supporting skin-whitening applications. *N. nucifera* seed, leaf, and flower extracts inhibit L-3,4-dihydroxyphenylalanine (DOPA) oxidase activity, reducing melanin synthesis effectively, even when tyrosinase inhibition is modest. Combining DOPA oxidase inhibition and antioxidant activity creates a synergistic mechanism for skin brightening, pigmentation control, and antimelanogenesis effects, suitable for incorporation into serums, creams, or encapsulated formulations (Kim et al., 2011).

6.5 Moisturization and skin barrier enhancement

Polysaccharides and glycosides from aquatic plants serve as natural humectants and film-forming agents, promoting hydration and enhancing skin barrier function (Chaudhary et al., 2020; Tungmunnithum et al., 2021). Their high water-binding capacity and antioxidant activity protect the skin from oxidative stress while maintaining moisture levels. Polysaccharides from seagrasses (*Cymodocea nodosa*) and water lilies have been incorporated into hydrogels and nanoemulsions, demonstrating multifunctional efficacy in several cosmetic and cosmeceutical applications (Chaudhary et al., 2020; Tungmunnithum et al., 2021).

7 Limitations, challenges, and future perspectives

The commercial and scientific potential of microalgae (and cyanobacteria), macroalgae (seaweeds), and freshwater aquatic or wetland plants is substantial, yet multiple limitations, as well as unresolved challenges, still restrict their wide-scale integration into cosmetic and cosmeceutical formulations. A major constraint lies in biomass productivity, cultivation efficacy, and species-specific growth/harvesting requirements, which differ widely among taxa, for instance, between *H. pluvialis, D. salina,* and *N. nucifera*. The production of high-value metabolites often depends on stress-induced pathways that reduce biomass yield and increase production costs associated with pollution. Controlled cultivation systems, including photobioreactors or biorefinery systems, may mitigate environmental fluctuations but remain energy-intensive and high-cost-requiring solutions, demanding technological optimization for industrial scalability (Motta et al., 2025; Kumar et al., 2024; Omweno et al., 2024; Samoraj et al., 2024).

Another significant challenge is the heterogeneity and instability of bioactive compounds, which complicates standardization. Carotenoids, phlorotannins, polysaccharides, and alkaloids can degrade under light, heat, or oxygen, leading to variable cosmetic efficacy. Matrix complexity in species like *Porphyridium, Fucus, Ecklonia, Ulva,* and *N. officinale* further complicates purification and batch-to-batch reproducibility (Motta et al., 2025; Jimoh and Kambizi, 2022; Bogdan et al., 2025; Khan et al., 2018; Thiyagarasaiyar et al., 2020; Kumar et al., 2024). Encapsulation methods, such as liposomes or nanoemulsions, improve stability and skin penetration but, unfortunately, concurrently increase formulation costs while requiring regulatory evaluation (Riseh et al., 2021; Vieira et al., 2020; Feng et al., 2023). In addition, extraction and purification limitations also restrict commercial adoption. Conventional organic-solvent extractions may not align with clean beauty standards (e.g., use of nongreen solvents), whereas green extraction methods (e.g., supercritical fluid CO_2, ultrasound-assisted extraction) require high costs and specialized equipment without always achieving optimal sufficient bioactive (e.g., polysaccharides, sterols, phenolics) yields (Motta et al., 2025; Jimoh and Kambizi, 2022; Karabulut et al., 2024).

Regulatory and safety challenges remain central concerns. Although both microalgae and macroalgae are generally considered safe, species-specific contaminants, such as heavy metals or toxins, pose a risk, particularly in open cultivation systems. Macroalgae such as *Fucus* (Klick, 1993) or *Asparagopsis* (Hutchings et al., 2024) may accumulate brominated metabolites or iodine at levels requiring strict purification and quality control. Moreover, aquatic plants like *E. crassipes* and *H. verticillata* are historically classified as invasive species in certain regions, complicating regulatory approval and sustainable-sourcing frameworks (Harun et al., 2021; Silveira et al., 2025).

From an industrial cosmetic standpoint, consumer perception and market positioning influence commercial success. While marine-based and algae-derived ingredients are strongly associated with premium (mostly Korean) skincare, aquatic plant extracts lack equivalent market recognition. Bridging this gap requires fully evaluating the antiinflammatory mechanistic profile, signaling modulation, enzyme inhibition, and dermal penetration properties, while providing more robust clinical demonstrations to substantiate claims related to their high cosmetic value (Motta et al., 2025; Jimoh and Kambizi, 2022; Bogdan et al., 2025). Looking forward, biotechnological advances will play a decisive role. Genetic engineering, strain selection, and even CRISPR-driven innovations may significantly upregulate bioactive yields and promote the importance of controlled biosynthesis aligned with circular economy principles (Dhokane et al., 2023; De Saeger et al., 2024; Bayır et al., 2025).

Future perspectives in cosmetic science point toward multifunctional, environmentally resilient, and clinically validated bioactives. A shift toward precision cosmetology, mainly targeting skin microbiome modulation, oxidative stress networks, proinflammatory mediator signaling, and ECM remodeling, aligns with microalgae, macroalgae, and aquatic plant molecular diversity. Continued interdisciplinary research and collaborations across marine biology, biotechnology, dermatological research, and formulation chemistry will be essential to fully unlock the cosmetic, cosmeceutical, and therapeutic potential of these organisms (Motta et al., 2025; Jimoh and Kambizi, 2022; Bogdan et al., 2025; Khan et al., 2018; Thiyagarasaiyar et al., 2020; Kumar et al., 2024).

8 Conclusions

Microalgae, macroalgae, and aquatic plants represent a rapidly expanding frontier in cosmetic R&D due to their exceptional biochemical diversity and demonstrable skin benefits. Their pigments, polysaccharides, peptides, phenolics, MUFAs and PUFAs, carotenoids, PLs, vitamins, and other secondary metabolites provide several activities, ranging from antioxidant and photoprotective effects to moisturizing, antiinflammatory, and antiaging properties, supporting their integration into next-generation skincare formulations. Growing consumer preference for natural, green, and scientifically validated ingredients further accelerates industry investment in algal and aquatic-plant technologies.

Despite clear advantages, challenges related to biomass production, compound stability, regulatory acceptance, and economic feasibility must be addressed to ensure broader, more consumer preference-based commercialization. Advances in cultivation engineering, metabolic optimization, green extraction, and clinical validation will be critical to overcoming such challenges and limitations. With continued innovation, these biological resources are poised to become foundational ingredients in high-performance, eco-responsible cosmetic products.

Acknowledgments

The authors would like to thank the School of Chemistry of the Faculty of Sciences at the Kavala University Campus of the Democritus University of Thrace and the Fisheries Research Institute of the Hellenic Agricultural Organization-DIMITRA (ELGO-DIMITRA) at Nea Peramos, Kavala, Greece, for their continuous support.

Author contributions

A.T. was involved in conceptualization, methodology, validation, visualization, supervision, and project administration. A.T., M.S., T.A., and V.A. were involved in investigation. A.T., M.S., and T.A. were involved in writing—review and editing. All authors contributed to software and writing—original draft preparation and have read and agreed to the published version of the manuscript.

Conflicts of interest

The authors declare no conflicts of interest.

Funding

This research received no external funding.

References

Abelti, A.L., Teka, T.A., Bultosa, G., 2023. Review on edible water lilies and lotus: future food, nutrition and their health benefits. Appl. Food Res. 27725022. 3 (1), 100264. doi:10.1016/j.afres.2023.100264.

Academy, M., 2023. Evaluation of in vitro anti-acne activity of methanolic extracts of *Cyperus rotundus* and *Nymphaea nouchali*. Int. J. Community Med. Public Health. doi:10.18203/2394-6040.IJCMPH20230201.

Admassu, H., Gasmalla, M.A.A., Yang, R., Zhao, W., 2018. Bioactive peptides derived from seaweed protein and their health benefits: antihypertensive, antioxidant, and antidiabetic properties. J. Food Sci. 0022-1147. 83 (1), 6–16. doi:10.1111/1750-3841.14011.

Afrin, A., Abedin, M.Z., Esrafil, M., Reza, M.S.A., Zubair, M.A., 2024. Composition and antioxidant properties of water lily (*Nymphaea nouchali*) tuber and development of composite biscuits. Food Human. 29498244. 2, 100227. doi:10.1016/j.foohum.2024.100227.

Agustina, S., Aidha, N.N., Oktarina, E., 2021. The extraction of antioxidants from *Chlorella vulgaris* for cosmetics. IOP Conf. Ser. Mater. Sci. Eng. 1757-8981. 1011 (1), 012057. doi:10.1088/1757-899x/1011/1/012057.

Agustina, S., Aidha, N.N., Oktarina, E., Setiawati, I., 2020. Antioxidant activity of *Porphyridium cruentum* water extracts for cosmetic cream. IOP Conf. Ser. Mater. Sci. Eng. 1757899X. 980 (1). https://iopscience.iop.org/journal/1757-899X. doi:10.1088/1757-899X/980/1/012042.

Ajao, A.A.-N., Sadgrove, N.J., 2024. Cosmetopoeia of African plants in hair treatment and care: topical nutrition and the antidiabetic connection? Diversity. 1424-2818. 16 (2), 96. doi:10.3390/d16020096.

Al-Amro, A.A., Al-Mutlaq, M.A., Al-Moauthe, S., Al-Tukhaif, N., Othaimeen, R.B., Al-Mutairi, N., Al-Rashed, S., Al-Malki, F., Haq, S.H., 2019. Antioxidant activity of Rhodophyta algae Polysiphonia and Laurencia collected from the Arabian Gulf. Asian J. Appl. Sci. 19963343. 12 (2), 71–75. doi:10.3923/ajaps.2019.71.75.

Al-Snafi, A.E., 2020. A review on *Nasturtium officinale*: a potential medicinal plant. IOSR J. Pharm. 10, 33–43.

Algenist, 2025. Green Microalgae Retinol + Serum—Reduce Wrinkles & Rejuvenate Skin—Algenist https://www.algenist.com/products/green-microalgae-retinol-regenerating-serum?srsltid=AfmBOopsCZEcICawkefU6lPveFFFAEgUHNTjsdGDzndhXte1eBLruY9h

Alparslan, L., Şekeroğlu, N., Kijjoa, A., 2018. The potential of marine resources in cosmetics. Curr. Perspect. Med. Aromat. Plants. 2619-9645. 1 (2), 53–66. doi:10.38093/cupmap.488904.

Amazon, 2025a. Daughter Earth: sacred Lotus & Vanilla Body Butter | hydrating Blend of Vitamin E Moringa & Cotton Seed Oil | locks Moisture & Soothes Troubled Skin | post Shower Apply | lipid Barrier For Skin | 100ml. Amazon.in: Beauty. https://www.amazon.in/DAUGHTER-EARTH-Sacred-Vanilla-Butter/dp/B0895G3TWP

Amazon, 2025b. The Dewy Skin, Face & Lip Pigmentation Serum for Oily Acne Prone Skin | reduces Dark Spots, Blemishes, Acne Marks, Tanning, Open Pores, Blackheads, Whiteheads | 10 ML | serum for Men and Women: Amazon.in: Beauty https://www.amazon.in/Dewy-Skin-Microalgae-Potion-Anti-Blemish/dp/B0C3ZXTYYV

Ambati, R.R., Moi, P.S., Ravi, S., Aswathanarayana, R.G., 2014. Astaxanthin: sources, extraction, stability, biological activities and its commercial applications—a review. Mar. Drugs. 16603397. 12 (1), 128–152. Available from: http://www.mdpi.com/1660-3397/12/1/128/pdf. doi:10.3390/md12010128.

Anonymous, 2005. Trends in Food Science and Technology. Trends Food Sci. Technol. 09242244. 16 (10), 479–480. doi:10.1016/j.tifs.2005.09.002.

Athukorala, Y., Kim, K.N., Jeon, Y.J., 2006. Antiproliferative and antioxidant properties of an enzymatic hydrolysate from brown alga, *Ecklonia cava*. Food Chem. Toxicol. 02786915. 44 (7), 1065–1074. doi:10.1016/j.fct.2006.01.011.

Bakrim, W.B., Ezzariai, A., Karouach, F., Sobeh, M., Kibret, M., Hafidi, M., Kouisni, L., Yasri, A., 2022. *Eichhornia crassipes* (Mart.) Solms: a comprehensive review of its chemical composition, traditional use, and value-added products. Front. Pharmacol. 1663-9812. 13. doi:10.3389/fphar.2022.842511.

Barbosa, M., Fernandes, F., João Carlos, M., Valentão, P., Andrade, P.B., 2021. Adding value to marine invaders by exploring the potential of *Sargassum muticum* (Yendo) Fensholt phlorotannin extract on targets underlying metabolic changes in diabetes. Algal Res. 22119264. 59, 102455. doi:10.1016/j.algal.2021.102455.

Barua, A., Alam, M.S., Junaid, M., Akter, Y., Afrose, S.S., Sharmin, T., Akter, R., Hosen, S.M.Z., 2021. Phytochemistry, traditional uses and pharmacological properties of enhydra fluctuans lour: a comprehensive review. Curr. Pharm. Biotechnol. 18734316. 22 (8), 1061–1068. Available from: https://www.eurekaselect.com/CDN/download.php?param=Sk9VjUk5gBTFyMvQ6kVO7L0NjQQin8yMpi84bLzAxwMD2ZHLgnBkjZnx68YX1BwbfGlj1YXR2pb2d4vcgGRmhfHx6mNjqMwZtGFiANTYd5ZDxNkNyjM0aYmI40OGtU4MkzNk0OGUbzMmuQ4OfQTcVYTcVYl&key=VWlxn-RWluuZE8UtQAVNEgc2REZZkzVJQrTMyeRDMj1Rjbc1N6DV2nLTQh3MzrItMdjM1dNjQAzMjsNERh2VEseATcVYbTcVY. doi:10.2174/1389201021666200922161529.

Bayır, A., Saoula, S., Almansour, A., Wang, D., Bayır, M., Uzun, B.N., Turhan, S., Arslan, H., Arslan, G., 2025. CRISPR-based genetic improvement of aquaculture species. Fishes. 2410-3888. 10 (2), 84. doi:10.3390/fishes10020084.

Bazes, A., Silkina, A., Defer, D., Bernède-Bauduin, C., Quéméner, E., Braud, J.P., Bourgougnon, N., 2006. Active substances from *Ceramium botryocarpum* used as antifouling products in aquaculture. Aquaculture. 00448486. 258 (1-4), 664–674. Available from: http://www.journals.elsevier.com/aquaculture/. doi:10.1016/j.aquaculture.2006.04.017.

Becker, E.W., 2013. Handbook of microalgal culture biotechnology and applied phycology. In: Richmond, A. (Ed.), Microalgae in Human and Animal Nutrition. Oxford Scientific Research Publishing, Oxford, pp. 312–351.

Bedoux, G., Hardouin, K., Burlot, A.S., Bourgougnon, N., 2014. Bioactive components from seaweeds: cosmetic applications and future development. Adv. Bot. Res. 71, 345–378. doi:10.1016/B978-0-12-408062-1.00012-3.

Bletapharm, 2025. Bletapharm | la Prairie Cellular Swiss Ice Crystal Dry Oil 30ML.https://www.bletapharm.gr/product/14822/la-prairie-cellular-swiss-ice-crystal-dry-oil-30ml.

Bocanegra, A., Bastida, S., Benedí, J., Ródenas, S., Sánchez-Muniz, F.J., 2009. Characteristics and nutritional and cardiovascular-health properties of seaweeds. J. Med. Food. 1096620X. 12 (2), 236–258. doi:10.1089/jmf.2008.0151.

Bogdan, C., Molnar, M., Dima, E.I., Olteanu, A.A., Safta, D.A., Moldovan, M.L., 2025. Marine macroalgae in topical formulations: bioactive compounds, variability, analytical challenges and skin benefits. Pharmaceutics. 19994923. 17 (9). Available from: http://www.mdpi.com/journal/pharmaceutics. doi:10.3390/pharmaceutics17091143.

Borowitzka, M.A., 2013. High-value products from microalgae-their development and commercialisation. J. Appl. Phycol. 09218971. 25 (3), 743–756. doi:10.1007/s10811-013-9983-9.

Byeon, S.Y., Cho, M.K., Shim, K.H., Kim, H.J., Song, H.G., Shin, H.S., 2017. Development of a spirulina extract/alginate-imbedded pcl nanofibrous cosmetic patch. J. Microbiol. Biotechnol. 17388872. 27 (9), 1657–1663. Available from: http://www.jmb.or.kr/journal/download.php?Filedir=./submission/Journal/027/&num=8665. doi:10.4014/jmb.1701.01025.

Castangia, I., Manca, M.L., Catalán-Latorre, A., Maccioni, A.M., Fadda, A.M., Manconi, M., 2016. Phycocyanin-encapsulating hyalurosomes as carrier for skin delivery and protection from oxidative stress damage. J. Mater. Sci. Mater. Med. 15734838. 27 (4), 1–10. Available from: www.wkap.nl/journalhome.htm/0957-4530. doi:10.1007/s10856-016-5687-4.

Chaudhary, R., Kumar, S., Malik, J., Singh, G., Siroliya, V.K., 2020. A review of the phytochemical and pharmacological potential of the watercress plant (*Nasturtium officinale*): a medicinal plant. Int. J. Pharm. Biol. Sci. Arch. 10 (9), 33–43.

Chen, C.L., Liou, S.F., Chen, S.J., Shih, M.F., 2011. Protective effects of Chlorella-derived peptide on UVB-induced production of MMP-1 and degradation of procollagen genes in human skin fibroblasts. Regul. Toxicol. Pharmacol. 10960295. 60 (1), 112–119. doi:10.1016/j.yrtph.2011.03.001.

Cheng, X., Shah, M., 2023. Astaxanthin from Haematococcus: production, applications, and advances. In: Jacob-Lopes, E., Queiroz, M.I., Maroneze, M.M., Zepka, L.Q. (Eds.), Handbook of Food and Feed from Microalgae. Academic Press, pp. 221–236. doi:10.1016/B978-0-323-99196-4.00033-4.

Chinjoo, N., Golzary, A., 2025. Microalgae: revolutionizing skin repair and enhancement. Biotechnol. Rep. 2215017X. 47, e00911. doi:10.1016/j.btre.2025.e00911.

Chrapusta, E., Kaminski, A., Duchnik, K., Bober, B., Adamski, M., Bialczyk, J., 2017. Mycosporine-like amino acids: potential health and beauty ingredients. Mar. Drugs. 1660-3397. 15 (10), 326. doi:10.3390/md15100326.

CIR-Safety, 2025. Safety Assessment of *Nelumbo nucifera*-Derived Ingredients as Used in Cosmetics | cosmetic Ingredient Review. https://www.cir-safety.org/panelbook/safety-assessment-nelumbo-nucifera-derived-ingredients-used-cosmetics-1

Conde, F.R., Churio, M.S., Previtali, C.M., 2000. The photoprotector mechanism of mycosporine-like amino acids. Excited-state properties and photostability of porphyra-334 in aqueous solution. J. Photochem. Photobiol. B Biol. 10111344. 56 (2-3), 139–144. doi:10.1016/s1011-1344(00)00066-x.

Conde, T.A., Zabetakis, I., Tsoupras, A., Medina, I., Costa, M., Silva, J., Neves, B., Domingues, P., Domingues, M.R., 2021. Microalgal Lipid extracts have potential to modulate the inflammatory response: a critical review. Int. J. Mol. Sci. 1422-0067. 22 (18), 9825. doi:10.3390/ijms22189825.

Cordero, B., Otero, A., Patiño, M., Arredondo, B.O., Fabregas, J., 1996. Astaxanthin production from the green alga *Haematococcus pluvialis* with different stress conditions. Biotechnol. Lett. 01415492. 18 (2), 213–218. doi:10.1007/BF00128682.

Corinaldesi, C., Barone, G., Marcellini, F., Dell'Anno, A., Danovaro, R., 2017. Marine microbial-derived molecules and their potential use in cosmeceutical and cosmetic products. Mar. Drugs. 1660-3397. 15 (4), 118. doi:10.3390/md15040118.

Costa, J.P., Custódio, L., Reis, C.P., 2023. Exploring the potential of using marine-derived ingredients: from the extraction to cutting-edge cosmetics. Mar. Drugs. 1660-3397. 21 (12), 620. doi:10.3390/md21120620.

Cotas, J., Leandro, A., Monteiro, P., Pacheco, D., Figueirinha, A., Gonçalves, A.M.M., da Silva, G.J., Pereira, L., 2020. Seaweed phenolics: from extraction to applications. Mar. Drugs. 1660-3397. 18 (8), 384. doi:10.3390/md18080384.

Courtois, J., 2009. Oligosaccharides from land plants and algae: production and applications in therapeutics and biotechnology. Curr. Opin. Microbiol. 13695274. 12 (3), 261–273. doi:10.1016/j.mib.2009.04.007.

Couteau, C., Coiffard, L., 2016. Chapter 14—seaweed application in cosmetics. In: Eds., Fleurence, J., Levine, I. Seaweed in Health and Disease Prevention, Academic Press, San Diego, pp. 423–441. doi:10.1016/B978-0-12-802772-1.00014-2.

Cristofoli, N.L., Lima, A.R., da Costa, A.M.R., Evtyugin, D., Silva, C., Varela, J., Vieira, M.C., 2023. Structural characterization of exopolysaccharides obtained from *Porphyridium cruentum* exhausted culture medium. Food Bioprod. Process. 09603085. 138, 162–171. Available from: http://www.elsevier.com/wps/find/journaldescription.cws_home/713883/description#description. doi:10.1016/j.fbp.2023.02.001.

Dagnino-Leone, J., Figueroa, C.P., Castañeda, M.L., Youlton, A.D., Vallejos-Almirall, A., Agurto-Muñoz, A., Pavón Pérez, J., Agurto-Muñoz, C., 2022. Phycobiliproteins: structural aspects, functional characteristics, and biotechnological perspectives. Comput. Struct. Biotechnol. J. 20010370. 20, 1506–1527. Available from: www.csbj.org. doi:10.1016/j.csbj.2022.02.016.

Dash, B.K., Sen, M.K., Alam, K., Hossain, K., Islam, R., Banu, N.A., Rahman, S., Jamal, A.H.M., 2013. Antibacterial activity of *Nymphaea nouchali* (Burm. f) flower. Ann. Clin. Microbiol. Antimicrob. 14760711. 12 (1). Available from: http://www.ann-clinmicrob.com/content/12/1/27. doi:10.1186/1476-0711-12-27Bangladesh.

de Arruda, M.C.S., da Silva, M.R.O.B., Cavalcanti, V.L.R., Brandao, R.M.P.C., Marques, D.D.A.V., de Lima, L.R.A., Porto, A.L.F., Bezerra, R.P., 2023. Antitumor lectins from algae: a systematic review. Algal Res. 22119264. 70. Available from: http://www.sciencedirect.com/science/journal/aip/22119264. doi:10.1016/j.algal.2022.102962.

De Jesus Raposo, M.F., De Morais, R.M.S.C., De Morais, A.M.M.B., 2013. Health applications of bioactive compounds from marine microalgae. Life Sci. 18790631. 93 (15), 479–486. doi:10.1016/j.lfs.2013.08.002.

De Saeger, J., Vandelannoote, E.C., Lee, H., Park, J., Blomme, J., 2024. Genome editing in macroalgae: advances and challenges. Front. Genome Ed. 2673-3439. 6. doi:10.3389/fgeed.2024.1380682.

Del Mondo, A., Sansone, C., Brunet, C., 2022. Insights into the biosynthesis pathway of phenolic compounds in microalgae. Comput. Struct. Biotechnol. J. 20010370. 20, 1901–1913. doi:10.1016/j.csbj.2022.04.019.

Dhahri, M., Alghrably, M., Mohammed, H.A., Badshah, S.L., Noreen, N., Mouffouk, F., Rayyan, S., Qureshi, K.A., Mahmood, D., Lachowicz, J.I., Jaremko, M., Emwas, A.H., 2022. Natural polysaccharides as preventive and therapeutic horizon for neurodegenerative diseases. Pharmaceutics. 19994923. 14 (1). Available from: https://www.mdpi.com/1999-4923/14/1/1/pdf. doi:10.3390/pharmaceutics14010001.

Dhanasinghe, J.C., Ubeysinghe, N.S., De Silva, I.C., 2025. Antioxidant activity and anti-tyrosinase activity of *Nelumbo nucifera* Gaertn. flower extract encapsulated in layered double hydroxide. Curr. Appl. Sci. Technol. 25869396. 25 (4). Available from: https://li01.tci-thaijo.org/index.php/cast/article/download/262003/179662. doi:10.55003/cast.2025.262003.

Dhokane, D., Shaikh, A., Yadav, A., Giri, N., Bandyopadhyay, A., Dasgupta, S., Bhadra, B., 2023. CRISPR-based bioengineering in microalgae for production of industrially important biomolecules. Front. Bioeng. Biotechnol. 2296-4185. 11. doi:10.3389/fbioe.2023.1267826.

Dini, I., 2023. The potential of algae in the nutricosmetic sector. Molecules. 1420-3049. 28 (10), 4032. doi:10.3390/molecules28104032.

Dong, M., Jiang, Y., Wang, C., Yang, Q., Jiang, X., Zhu, C., 2020. Determination of the extraction, physicochemical characterization, and digestibility of sulfated polysaccharides in seaweed—*Porphyra haitanensis*. Mar. Drugs. 1660-3397. 18 (11), 539. doi:10.3390/md18110539.

Draelos, Z.D., 2018. The science behind skin care: moisturizers. J. Cosmet. Dermatol. 14732165. 17 (2), 138–144. Available from: http://onlinelibrary.wiley.com/journal/10.1111/(ISSN)1473-2165. doi:10.1111/jocd.12490.

Dunaliella, 2025. Dunaliella algae peel-off mask. AHAVA Global https://global.ahava.com/products/dunaliella-algae-peel-off-mask

El-Beltagi, H.S., Mohamed, A.A., Mohamed, H.I., Ramadan, K.M.A., Barqawi, A.A., Mansour, A.T., 2022. Phytochemical and potential properties of seaweeds and their recent applications: a review. Mar. Drugs. 16603397. 20 (6). Available from: https://www.mdpi.com/1660-3397/20/6/342/pdf?version=1653475780. doi:10.3390/md20060342.

Fabrowska, J., Kapuścińska, A., Łęska, B., Feliksik-Skrobich, K., Nowak, I., 2017. In vivo studies and stability study of *Cladophora glomerata* extract as a cosmetic active ingredient. Acta Pol. Pharm. Drug Res. 00016837. 74 (2), 633–641. Available from http://www.ptfarm.pl/pub/File/Acta_Poloniae/2017/Nr%202/633.pdf.

Fabrowska, J., Łęska, B., Schroeder, G., 2015. Freshwater *Cladophora glomerata* as a new potential cosmetic raw material. Chemik 00092886. 69 (8), 491–497. Available from http://www.chemikinternational.com/wp-content/uploads/2015/09/8_15_Fabrowska_GB.pdf.

Fagundes, M.B., Vendruscolo, R.G., Wagner, R., 2020. Chapter 21 - Sterols from microalgae. In: Jacob-Lopes, E., Maroneze, M.M., Queiroz, M.I., Zepka, L.Q. (Eds.), Handbook of Microalgae-Based Processes and Products. Academic Press, pp. 573–596. ISBN: 9780128185360. doi:10.1016/B978-0-12-818536-0.00021-X.

FAO, 2025. A guide to the seaweed industry. https://www.fao.org/4/y4765e/y4765e00.htm

FarmHouse Fresh, 2025. Watercress Hydration Cascade® Gelée Moisturizer. https://farmhousefreshgoods.com/products/watercress-hydration-cascade-moisturizer

Favas, R., Morone, J., Martins, R., Vasconcelos, V., Lopes, G., 2021. Cyanobacteria and microalgae bioactive compounds in skin-ageing: potential to restore extracellular matrix filling and overcome hyperpigmentation. J. Enzyme Inhib. Med. Chem. 1475-6366. 36 (1), 1829–1838. doi:10.1080/14756366.2021.1960830.

Feng, Y., Zarei, V., Mousavipour, N., 2023. Provision and assessment properties of nanoliposomes containing macroalgae extracts of *Sargassum boveanume* and *Padina pavonica*. LWT. 00236438. 175, 114194. doi:10.1016/j.lwt.2022.114194.

Fernando, P.S., Kim, J., 2018. Algal polysaccharides: potential bioactive substances for cosmeceutical applications. Crit. Rev. Biot. 1–15. doi:10.1080/07388551.2018.1503995.

Georgieva, Z., Karcheva, Z., Toshkova-Yotova, T., Georgieva, A., Toshkova, R., Petrova, D., Zhiponova, M., Chaneva, G., 2024. Blue light enhances the antioxidant, antimicrobial, and antitumor potential of the green microalgae *Coelastrella* sp. BGV. Plants. 2223-7747. 13 (23), 3295. doi:10.3390/plants13233295.

Good Vibes Pharmacy, 2025. Ren Atlantic Kelp and Microalgae Anti-Fatigue Toning Body Oil 100ML 1+1. Good Vibes Pharmacy. https://www.goodvibespharmacy.com/el/products/ren-atlantic-kelp-and-microalgae-anti-fatigue-toning-body-oil-100ml-11

Goossens, A., 2011. Contact-allergic reactions to cosmetics. J Allergy (Cairo). doi:10.1155/2011/467071.

Gressler, V., Yokoya, N.S., Fujii, M.T., Colepicolo, P., Filho, J.M., Torres, R.P., Pinto, E., 2010. Lipid, fatty acid, protein, amino acid and ash contents in four Brazilian red algae species. Food Chem. 03088146. 120 (2), 585–590. doi:10.1016/j.foodchem.2009.10.028.

Gu, Y., Shuai, L., Yang, J., Jiang, W., Yang, X., 2024. Investigation of self-assembly of daucosterol from eleocharis dulcis peel with γ-oryzanol for stabilized water-in-oil emulsion gels. LWT. 00236438. 213, 117070. doi:10.1016/j.lwt.2024.117070.

Guerin, M., Huntley, M.E., Olaizola, M., 2003. Haematococcus astaxanthin: applications for human health and nutrition. Trends Biotechnol. 01677799. 21 (5), 210–216. doi:10.1016/s0167-7799(03)00078-7.

Guil-Guerrero, J.L., Prates, J.A.M., 2025. Microalgae bioactives for functional food innovation and health promotion. Foods. 23048158. 14 (12). Available from: www.mdpi.com/journal/foods. doi:10.3390/foods14122122.

Günal-Köroğlu, D., Karabulut, G., Ozkan, G., Yılmaz, H., Gültekin-Subaşı, B., Capanoglu, E., 2025. Allergenicity of alternative proteins: reduction mechanisms and processing strategies. J. Agric. Food Chem. 0021-8561. 73 (13), 7522–7546. doi:10.1021/acs.jafc.5c00948.

Gunes, S., Tamburaci, S., Dalay, M.C., Gurhan, I.D., 2017. In vitro evaluation of *Spirulina platensis* extract incorporated skin cream with its wound healing and antioxidant activities. Pharm. Biol. 1388-0209. 55 (1), 1824–1832. doi:10.1080/13880209.2017.1331249.

Gupta, A., Kumar, R., Upadhyay, N.K., Surekha, P., Roy, P.K., 2009. Synthesis, characterization and efficacy of chemically crosslinked PVA hydrogels for dermal wound healing in experimental animals. J. Appl. Polym. Sci. 0021-8995. 111 (3), 1400–1408. doi:10.1002/app.28990.

Ha, J.Y., Lee, K., Park, J., Dong, A., Shin, H.S., 2010. Cytoprotective activity of lotus (*Nelumbo nucifera* Gaertner) leaf extracts on the mouse embryonic fibroblast cell. Food Sci. Biotechnol. 12267708. 19 (5), 1171–1176. doi:10.1007/s10068-010-0167-y.

Habibie, A., Raharjo, T.J., Swasono, R.T., Retnaningrum, E., 2023. Antibacterial activity of active peptide from marine macroalgae *Chondrus crispus* protein hydrolysate against *Staphylococcus aureus*. Pharmacia. 04280296. 70 (4), 983–992. Available from: https://pharmacia.pensoft.net/. doi:10.3897/pharmacia.70.e112215.

Hama, S., Takahashi, K., Inai, Y., Shiota, K., Sakamoto, R., Yamada, A., Tsuchiya, H., Kanamura, K., Yamashita, E., Kogure, K., 2012. Protective effects of topical application of a poorly soluble antioxidant astaxanthin liposomal formulation on ultraviolet-induced skin damage. J. Pharm. Sci. 00223549. 101 (8), 2909–2916. doi:10.1002/jps.23216.

Harun, I., Pushiri, H., Amirul-Aiman, A.J., Zulkeflee, Z., 2021. Invasive water hyacinth: ecology, impacts and prospects for the rural economy. Plants. 2223-7747. 10 (8), 1613. doi:10.3390/plants10081613.

Havas, F., Krispin, S., Cohen, M., Loing, E., Farge, M., Suere, T., Attia-Vigneau, J., 2022. A *Dunaliella salina* extract counteracts skin aging under intense solar irradiation thanks to its antiglycation and anti-inflammatory properties. Mar. Drugs. 1660-3397. 20 (2), 104. doi:10.3390/md20020104.

HELIONORI, 2025. HELIONORI®—GELYMA http://www.gelyma.com/helionori.html

Hempel, M.D.S.S., Colepicolo, P., Zambotti-Villela, L., 2023. Macroalgae biorefinery for the cosmetic industry: basic concept, green technology, and safety guidelines. Phycology. 2673-9410. 3 (1), 211–241. doi:10.3390/phycology3010014.

Hermund, D.B., Torsteinsen, H., Vega, J., Figueroa, F.L., Jacobsen, C., 2022. Screening for new cosmeceuticals from brown algae *Fucus vesiculosus* with antioxidant and photo-protecting properties. Mar. Drugs. 1660-3397. 20 (11), 687. doi:10.3390/md20110687.

Hidhayati, N., Purba, L.D.A., Firman, N.F.A., Admirasari, R., Rahman, D.Y., Agustini, N.W.S., Maryati, M., Anam, K., Prayitno, J., 2025. Current status and future prospects of Chlorella as raw materials in cosmeceuticals: cultivation, extraction, and commercial applications. J. Appl. Phycol. 0921-8971. 37 (1), 343–354. doi:10.1007/s10811-024-03372-1.

Higuera-Ciapara, I., Félix-Valenzuela, L., Goycoolea, F.M., 2006. Astaxanthin: a review of its chemistry and applications. Crit. Rev. Food Sci. Nutr. 1040-8398. 46 (2), 185–196. doi:10.1080/10408690590957188.

Hu, F., Liu, W., Yan, L., Kong, F., Wei, K., 2019. Optimization and characterization of poly(lactic-co-glycolic acid) nanoparticles loaded with astaxanthin and evaluation of anti-photodamage effect in vitro. R. Soc. Open Sci. 2054-5703. 6 (10), 191184. doi:10.1098/rsos.191184.

Hutchings, J.L., Grebneva, Y., Dilmetz, S.J., Pincher, D.W.M., Hoffmann, P., 2024. Analytical methods for the analysis of bromoform in red seaweed *Asparagopsis armata* and *Asparagopsis taxiformis*—a review. Algal Res. 22119264. 79. Available from: https://www.sciencedirect.com/science/journal/22119264. doi:10.1016/j.algal.2024.103478.

Jaber, I.G., 2025 Microalgae: natural Ingredients For Beauty Products. TecScience. https://tecscience.tec.mx/en/biotechnology/microalgae-in-the-cosmetic-industry/

Jayawardhana, H.H.A.C.K., Jayawardena, T.U., Sanjeewa, K.K.A., Liyanage, N.M., Nagahawatta, D.P., Lee, H.G., Kim, J.I., Jeon, Y.J., 2023. Marine algal polyphenols as skin protective agents: current status and future prospectives. Mar. Drugs. 16603397. 21 (5). Available from: http://www.mdpi.com/journal/marinedrugs. doi:10.3390/md21050285.

Jiang, X., Hansen, H.C.B., Strobel, B.W., Cedergreen, N., 2018. What is the aquatic toxicity of saponin-rich plant extracts used as biopesticides? Environ. Pollut. 18736424. 236, 416–424. Available from: www.elsevier.com/inca/publications/store/4/0/5/8/5/6. doi:10.1016/j.envpol.2018.01.058.

Jimoh, M.O., Kambizi, L., 2022. Aquatic phytotherapy: prospects, challenges and bibliometric analysis of global research output on medicinal aquatic plants from 2011-2020. In: Lall, N. (Ed.), Medicinal Plants for Cosmetics, Health and Diseases. CRC Press, South Africa, pp. 507–522. Available from: https://www.routledge.com/Medicinal-Plants-for-Cosmetics-Health-and-Diseases/Lall/p/book/9781003108375. doi:10.1201/9781003108375-26.

Jing, R., Guo, K., Zhong, Y., Wang, L., Zhao, J., Gao, B., Ziyi, Y., Chen, Y., Xuenan, L., Nuo, X., Xuan, X., 2021. Protective effects of fucoidan purified from *Undaria pinnatifida* against UV-irradiated skin photoaging. Ann. Transl. Med. 23055839. 9 (14), 1185. doi:10.21037/atm-21-3668.

Joelyna, F.A., Hadiyanto, Khoironi, A., Pratama, W.D., 2024. The utilization of exopolysaccharide (EPS) from microalgae *Chlorella vulgaris* in microplastic removal. IOP Conf. Ser. Earth Environ. Sci. 1755-1307. 1414 (1), 012017. doi:10.1088/1755-1315/1414/1/012017.

Juncan, A.M., Moisă, D.G., Santini, A., Morgovan, C., Rus, L.L., Vonica-țincu, A.L., Loghin, F., 2021. Advantages of hyaluronic acid and its combination with other bioactive ingredients in cosmeceuticals. Molecules. 14203049. 26 (15). Available from: https://www.mdpi.com/1420-3049/26/15/4429/pdf. doi:10.3390/molecules26154429.

Kalasariya, H.S., Pereira, L., Cotas, J., 2025. Carbohydrates and proteins from seaweed: a promising frontier in skin cosmeceuticals. In: Thalassotherapy Cosmeceuticals, Vol. 2, pp. 222–244. CRC Press. Available from: https://www.taylorfrancis.com/books/edit/10.1201/9781003399285. doi:10.1201/9781003399285-14.

Kalasariya, H.S., Pereira, L., Patel, N.B., 2022. Pioneering role of marine macroalgae in cosmeceuticals. Phycology. 2673-9410. 2 (1), 172–203. doi:10.3390/phycology2010010.

Kang, M.C., Kim, K.N., Kang, S.M., Yang, X., Kim, E.A., Song, C.B., Nah, J.W., Jang, M.K., Lee, J.S., Jung, W.K., Jeon, Y.J., 2013. Protective effect of dieckol isolated from *Ecklonia cava* against ethanol caused damage in vitro and in zebrafish model. Environ. Toxicol. Pharmacol. 18727077. 36 (3), 1217–1226. doi:10.1016/j.etap.2013.09.018.

Karabulut, G., Purkiewicz, A., Goksen, G., 2024. Recent developments and challenges in algal protein and peptide extraction strategies, functional and technological properties, bioaccessibility, and commercial applications. Compr. Rev. Food Sci. Food Saf. 1541-4337. 23 (3). doi:10.1111/1541-4337.13372.

Kasanah, N., Ulfah, M., Imania, O., Hanifah, A.N., Marjan, M.I.D., 2022. Rhodophyta as potential sources of photoprotectants, antiphotoaging compounds, and hydrogels for cosmeceutical application. Molecules. 14203049. 27 (22). Available from: http://www.mdpi.com/journal/molecules. doi:10.3390/molecules27227788.

Khan, M.I., Shin, J.H., Kim, J.D., 2018. The promising future of microalgae: current status, challenges, and optimization of a sustainable and renewable industry for biofuels, feed, and other products. Microb. Cell Fact. 14752859. 17 (1). Available from: http://www.microbialcellfactories.com/home/. doi:10.1186/s12934-018-0879-x.

Khansari, N., Shakiba, Y., Mahmoudi, M., 2009. Chronic inflammation and oxidative stress as a major cause of age- related diseases and cancer. Recent Pat. Inflamm. Allergy Drug Discov. 1872213X. 3 (1), 73–80. doi:10.2174/187221309787158371.

Kim, S.-K., 2011. Marine Cosmeceuticals: Trends and Prospects. CRC Press.

Kim, S.-K., 2016. Marine Cosmeceuticals: Trends and Prospects, CRC Press.

Kim, T., Kim, H.J., Cho, S.K., Kang, W.Y., Baek, H., Jeon, H.Y., Kim, B., Kim, D., 2011. Nelumbo nucifera extracts as whitening and anti-wrinkle cosmetic agent. Korean J. Chem. Eng. 02561115. 28 (2), 424–427. doi:10.1007/s11814-010-0357-6.

Klick, S., 1993. The release of volatile halocarbons to seawater by untreated and heavy metal exposed samples of the brown seaweed *Fucus vesiculosus*. Mar. Chem. 03044203. 42 (3-4), 211–221. doi:10.1016/0304-4203(93)90013-e.

Klimek-Szczykutowicz, M., Malinowska, M.A., Gałka, A., Blažević, I., Đulović, A., Paprocka, P., Wrzosek, M., Szopa, A., 2025. *Nasturtium officinale* microshoot culture multiplied in plantform bioreactor—phytochemical profiling and biological activity. Molecules. 1420-3049. 30 (4), 936. doi:10.3390/molecules30040936.

Klimek-Szczykutowicz, M., Szopa, A., Ekiert, H., 2018. Chemical composition, traditional and professional use in medicine, application in environmental protection, position in food and cosmetics industries, and biotechnological studies of *Nasturtium officinale* (watercress)—a review. Fitoterapia. 0367326X. 129, 283–292. doi:10.1016/j.fitote.2018.05.031.

Ko, S.-C., Cha, S.-H., Heo, S.-J., Lee, S.-H., Kang, S.-M., Jeon, Y.-J., 2011. Protective effect of *Ecklonia cava* on UVB-induced oxidative stress: in vitro and in vivo zebrafish model. J. Appl. Phycol. 0921-8971. 23 (4), 697–708. doi:10.1007/s10811-010-9565-z.

Koukouraki, P., Tsoupras, A., Sotiroudis, G., Demopoulos, C.A., Sotiroudis, T.G., 2020. Antithrombotic properties of Spirulina extracts against platelet-activating factor and thrombin. Food Biosci. 22124292. 37, 100686. doi:10.1016/j.fbio.2020.100686.

Koyande, A.K., Chew, K.W., Rambabu, K., Tao, Y., Chu, D.T., Show, P.L., 2019. Microalgae: a potential alternative to health supplementation for humans. Food Sci. Hum. Wellness. 22134530. 8 (1), 16–24. Available from: www.keaipublishing.com/en/journals/food-science-and-human-wellness/. doi:10.1016/j.fshw.2019.03.001.

Kumar, C., Sharma, M., Kaur, M., Arya, S.K., Khatri, M., 2024. Cultivation of Algae: Techniques and Challenges. Springer Science and Business Media LLC, pp. 43–65. doi:10.1007/978-981-97-1662-3_3.

L'Oréal Paris, 2025 Pure Clay Foam Wash Red. https://www.loreal-paris.co.uk/pure-clay/foam-wash-red

Lalitha, P., Jayanthi, P., 2014. Antiaging activity of the skin cream containing ethyl acetate extract of *Eichhornia crassipes* (Mart.) Solms. Int. J. PharmTech Res. 09744304. 6 (1), 29–34. Available from http://sphinxsai.com/2014/PharmTech/PDF/PT=05(29-34)JM14.pdf.

Lall, N., 2020. Aquatic Plants: Pharmaceutical and Cosmetic Applications. CRC Press. doi:10.1201/9780429429095.

Lall, N., 2022. Medicinal Plants for Cosmetics, Health and Diseases. CRC Press. doi:10.1201/9781003108375.

LANEIGE, 2025. LANEIGE | retinol Firming Cream Treatment. SEPHORA https://www.sephora.gr/p/retinol-firming-cream-treatment-664534.html

Lee, D.B., Kim, D.H., Je, J.Y., 2015. Antioxidant and cytoprotective effects of lotus (*Nelumbo nucifera*) leaves phenolic fraction. Prev. Nutr. Food Sci. 22878602. 20 (1), 22–28. Available from: http://pdf.medrang.co.kr/paper/pdf/PNF/2015/020/PNF020-01-04.pdf. doi:10.3746/pnf.2015.20.1.22.

Łęska, B., Messyasz, B., Schroeder G., 2018. Application of algae biomass and algae extracts in cosmetic formulations. In: Chojnacka, K., PP., W., Schroeder, G., Michalak, I. (Eds.), Algae Biomass: Characteristics and Applications: Towards Algae-based Products. Springer International Publishing, Cham, pp. 89–101. doi:10.1007/978-3-319-74703-3_8.

López-Hortas, L., Flórez-Fernández, N., Torres, M.D., Ferreira-Anta, T., Casas, M.P., Balboa, E.M., Falqué, E., Domínguez, H., 2021. Applying seaweed compounds in cosmetics, cosmeceuticals and nutricosmetics. Mar. Drugs. 1660-3397. 19 (10), 552. doi:10.3390/md19100552.

Lourenço-Lopes, C., Fraga-Corral, M., Jimenez-Lopez, C., Pereira, A.G., Garcia-Oliveira, P., Carpena, M., Prieto, M.A., Simal-Gandara, J., 2020. Metabolites from macroalgae and its applications in the cosmetic industry: a circular economy approach. Resources. 2079-9276. 9 (9), 101. doi:10.3390/resources9090101.

Ma, X.N., Chen, T.P., Yang, B., Liu, J., Chen, F., 2016. Lipid production from Nannochloropsis. Mar. Drugs. 16603397. 14 (4). Available from: http://www.mdpi.com/1660-3397/14/4/61/pdf. doi:10.3390/md14040061.

Mago, Y., Sharma, Y., Thakran, Y., Mishra, A., Tewari, S., Kataria, N., 2025. Next-generation organic beauty products obtained from algal secondary metabolites: a sustainable development in cosmeceutical industries. Mol. Biotechnol. 1073-6085. 67 (8), 2881–2901. doi:10.1007/s12033-023-00841-9.

MahaMane, 2025. MahaMane Smooth & Shine Hair Oil | Fable & Mane ≡ SEPHORA https://www.sephora.gr/p/mahamane-smooth-shine-hair-oil-P10048344.html

Marino, T., Iovine, A., Casella, P., Martino, M., Chianese, S., Larocca, V., Musmarra, D., Molino, A., 2020. From *Haematococcus pluvialis* microalgae a powerful antioxidant for cosmetic applications. Chem. Eng. Trans. 22839216. 79, 271–276. Available from: https://www.aidic.it/cet/20/79/046.pdf. doi:10.3303/CET2079046.

Martínez-Ruiz, M., Martínez-González, C.A., Kim, D.-H., Santiesteban-Romero, B., Reyes-Pardo, H., Villaseñor-Zepeda, K.R., Meléndez-Sánchez, E.R., Ramírez-Gamboa, D., Díaz-Zamorano, A.L., Sosa-Hernández, J.E., Coronado-Apodaca, K.G., María Gámez-Méndez, A., Iqbal, H.M.N., Parra-Saldivar, R., 2022. Microalgae bioactive compounds to topical applications products—a review. Molecules. 1420-3049. 27 (11), 3512. doi:10.3390/molecules27113512.

Menaa, F., Wijesinghe, U., Thiripuranathar, G., Althobaiti, N.A., Albalawi, A.E., Khan, B.A., Menaa, B., 2021. Marine algae-derived bioactive compounds: a new wave of nanodrugs? Mar. Drugs. 16603397. 19 (9). Available from: https://www.mdpi.com/1660-3397/19/9/484/pdf. doi:10.3390/md19090484.

Miranda, M.S., Cintra, R.G., Barros, S.B.M., Mancini-Filho, J., 1998. Antioxidant activity of the microalga *Spirulina maxima*. Braz. J. Med. Biol. Res. 0100-879X. 31 (8), 1075–1079. doi:10.1590/s0100-879x1998000800007.

Morais, M.G., Santos, T.D., Moraes, L., Vaz, B.S., Morais, E.G., Costa, J.A.V., 2022. Exopolysaccharides from microalgae: production in a biorefinery framework and potential applications. Bioresour. Technol. Rep. 2589014X. 18, 101006. doi:10.1016/j.biteb.2022.101006.

Morais, T., Cotas, J., Pacheco, D., Pereira, L., 2021. Seaweeds compounds: an ecosustainable source of cosmetic ingredients? Cosmetics. 2079-9284. 8 (1), 8. doi:10.3390/cosmetics8010008.

Motta, D.N., Torres, V.G.S., de Queiroz Hermino, V.L., Neves, S.M.B., de Oliveira, L.V.V., Carvalho, R.P., da Silva, E.P., 2025. Challenges of microalgae production: from the laboratory to large scale. In: Severo, I.A., Ordóñez, J.C., Mariano, A.B., Vargas, J.V.C. (Eds.), Microalgae Horizons. Grand Challenges in Biology and Biotechnology. Springer, Cham, pp. 11–21. Part F426. doi:10.1007/978-3-031-84282-5_2.

Mourelle, M.L., Gómez, C.P., Legido, J.L., 2017. The potential use of marine microalgae and cyanobacteria in cosmetics and thalassotherapy. Cosmetics. 20799284. 4 (4). Available from: https://www.mdpi.com/2079-9284/4/4/46/pdf. doi:10.3390/cosmetics4040046.

Muñoz-Quintana, M., Padrón-Sanz, C., Dolbeth, M., Arenas, F., Vasconcelos, V., Lopes, G., 2024. Revealing the potential of *Fucus vesiculosus* Linnaeus for cosmetic purposes: chemical profile and biological activities of commercial and wild samples. Mar. Drugs. 1660-3397. 22 (12), 548. doi:10.3390/md22120548.

Natura-Tec, 2025. A Look at Microalgae-Based Actives for Modern Cosmetics | natura-Tec. https://www.deverauxspecialties.com/blog/a-look-at-microalgae-based-actives-for-modern-cosmetics/

Navalho, S., Ferrer-Ledo, N., Barbosa, M.J., Varela, J., 2025. Nannochloropsis lipids and polyunsaturated fatty acids: potential applications and strain improvement. Mar. Drugs. 1660-3397. 23 (3), 128. doi:10.3390/md23030128.

Nguyen, K.H., Ta, T.N., Pham, T.H.M., Nguyen, Q.T., Pham, H.D., Mishra, S., Nyomba, B.L.G., 2012. Nuciferine stimulates insulin secretion from beta cells—an in vitro comparison with glibenclamide. J. Ethnopharmacol. 18727573. 142 (2), 488–495. doi:10.1016/j.jep.2012.05.024.

Nieri, P., Carpi, S., Esposito, R., Costantini, M., Zupo, V., 2023. Bioactive molecules from marine diatoms and their value for the nutraceutical industry. Nutrients. 2072-6643. 15 (2), 464. doi:10.3390/nu15020464.

Nimisha, Singh, A., 2024. Exploring marine-derived bioactives for innovative cosmeceutical applications: a review. J. Appl. Nat. Sci. 2231-5209. 16 (2), 478–494. doi:10.31018/jans.v16i2.5433.

Notino, 2025. Revolution Skincare London. Revolution Skincare Aloe Vera & Water Lily Soothing Face Mask | Notino.co.uk. WwwNotinoCoUk. https://www.notino.co.uk/revolution-skincare/revolution-skincare-aloe-vera-water-lily-soothing-face-mask/.

Novoveská, L., Ross, M.E., Stanley, M.S., Pradelles, R., Wasiolek, V., Sassi, J.F., 2019. Microalgal carotenoids: a review of production, current markets, regulations, and future direction. Mar. Drugs. 16603397. 17 (11). Available from: https://www.mdpi.com/1660-3397/17/11/640/pdf. doi:10.3390/md17110640.

Nowruzi, B., Sarvari, G., Blanco, S., 2020. The cosmetic application of cyanobacterial secondary metabolites. Algal Res. 22119264. 49, 101959. doi:10.1016/j.algal.2020.101959.

Ohse, S., Derner, R.B., Ávila Ozório, R., Corrêa, R.G., Furlong, E.B., Cesar, P., Cunha, R., 2015. Lipid content and fatty acid profiles in ten species of microalgae. Idesia (Arica) 33 (1), 93–101. doi:10.4067/S0718-34292015000100010.

Omweno, J.O., Argwings, O., Sieberi, B.M., Angima, M., Ondieki, P.M., 2024. Utilization of aquatic plants and microalgae for sustainable aquaculture production and potential biotechnological applications. TEBT. 3009-0806. 2 (2), 57–71. doi:10.53623/tebt.v2i2.451.

Osama, M., Wei, C.R., Saleem, R., Unar, A.A., Unar, K., Siyal, F.J., Shaikh, B., Baig, S.G., Siddiq, A., 2023. Aquatic plants with anti-inflammatory and anti-oxidant activities. J. Surv. Fish. Sci. 3802–3806. doi:10.53555/sfs.v10i1.1738.

OUCI, 2025. Polysaccharide Applications in Cosmetic http://ouci.dntb.gov.ua/en/works/7XkgZ3M9/

OyetakinWhite, P., Tribout, H., Baron, E., 2012. Protective mechanisms of green tea polyphenols in skin. Oxid. Med. Cell. Longev. 1942-0900. 2012, 1–8. doi:10.1155/2012/560682.

Pagels, F., Pereira, R.N., Vicente, A.A., Guedes, A.C., 2021. Extraction of pigments from microalgae and cyanobacteria—a review on current methodologies. Appl. Sci. 2076-3417. 11 (11), 5187. doi:10.3390/app11115187.

Pagels, F., Salvaterra, D., Amaro, H.M., Guedes, A.C., 2020. Pigments from microalgae. In: Jacob-Lopes, E., Maroneze, M.M., Queiroz, M.I., Zepka, L.Q. (Eds.), Handbook of Microalgae-Based Processes and Products: Fundamentals and Advances in Energy, Food, Feed, Fertilizer, and Bioactive Compounds. Elsevier, Portugal, pp. 465–492. Available from: https://www.elsevier.com/books/handbook-of-microalgae-based-processes-and-products/jacob-lopes/978-0-12-818536-0. doi:10.1016/B978-0-12-818536-0.00018-X.

Panahi Kokhdan, E., Khodabandehloo, H., Ghahremani, H., Doustimotlagh, A.H., 2021. A narrative review on therapeutic potentials of watercress in human disorders. Evid. Based Complement. Altern. Med. 17414288. 2021. Available from: http://www.hindawi.com/journals/ecam/contents.html. doi:10.1155/2021/5516450.

Paudel, K.R., Panth, N., 2015. Phytochemical profile and biological activity of *Nelumbo nucifera*. Evid. Based Complement. Altern. Med. 2015. doi:10.1155/2015/789124.

Pei, J., Kanwal, S., Sivaramakrishnan, R., Katelakha, K., 2025. Therapeutic potential of microalgae-derived natural compounds in diabetic wound healing: a comprehensive review. Heliyon. 24058440. 11 (4), e42723. doi:10.1016/j.heliyon.2025.e42723.

Peng, J., Guo, F., Liu, S., Fang, H., Zhenshang, X., Wang, T., 2023. Recent advances and future prospects of mycosporine-like amino acids. Molecules. 1420-3049. 28 (14), 5588. doi:10.3390/molecules28145588.

Pereira, H., Barreira, L., Figueiredo, F., Custódio, L., Vizetto-Duarte, C., Polo, C., Rešek, E., Engelen, A., Varela, J., 2012. Polyunsaturated fatty acids of marine macroalgae: potential for nutritional and pharmaceutical applications. Mar. Drugs. 1660-3397. 10 (9), 1920–1935. doi:10.3390/md10091920.

Pereira, L., 2018. Seaweeds as source of bioactive substances and skin care therapy—cosmeceuticals, algotheraphy, and thalassotherapy. Cosmetics. 2079-9284. 5 (4), 68. doi:10.3390/cosmetics5040068.

Pereira, L., Amado, A.M., Critchley, A.T., van de Velde, F., Ribeiro-Claro, P.J.A., 2009. Identification of selected seaweed polysaccharides (phycocolloids) by vibrational spectroscopy (FTIR-ATR and FT-Raman). Food Hydrocoll. 0268005X. 23 (7), 1903–1909. Available from: https://www.journals.elsevier.com/food-hydrocolloids. doi:10.1016/j.foodhyd.2008.11.014.

Pereira, L., Gheda, S.F., Ribeiro-Claro, P.J.A., 2013. Analysis by vibrational spectroscopy of seaweed polysaccharides with potential use in food, pharmaceutical, and cosmetic industries. Int. J. Carbohydr. Chem. 1687-9341. 2013, 1–7. doi:10.1155/2013/537202.

Pham, T.X., Park, Y.K., Lee, J.Y., 2016. Anti-inflammatory effects of spirulina platensis extract via the modulation of histone deacetylases. Nutrients. 20726643. 8 (6). Available from: http://www.mdpi.com/2072-6643/8/6/381/pdf. doi:10.3390/nu8060381.

Pimentel, F., Alves, R., Rodrigues, F., Oliveira, M.P.P., 2018. Macroalgae-derived ingredients for cosmetic industry—an update. Cosmetics. 2079-9284. 5 (1), 2. doi:10.3390/cosmetics5010002.

Plaza, M., Cifuentes, A., Ibanez, E., 2008. In the search of new functional food ingredients from algae. Trends Food Sci. Technol. 09242244. 19 (1), 31–39. doi:10.1016/j.tifs.2007.07.012.

Plaza, M., Herrero, M., Cifuentes, A., Ibáñez, E., 2009. Innovative natural functional ingredients from microalgae. J. Agric. Food Chem. 0021-8561. 57 (16), 7159–7170. doi:10.1021/jf901070g.

Pooja, K., Rani, S., Rana, V., Pal, G.K., 2020. Aquatic plants as a natural source of antimicrobial and functional ingredients. In: Prakash, B. (Ed.), Functional and Preservative Properties of Phytochemicals. Elsevier, India, pp. 93–118. Available from: https://www.sciencedirect.com/book/9780128185933. doi:10.1016/B978-0-12-818593-3.00003-8.

Prabha, S.P., Karthik, C., Chandrika, S.H., 2019. Phytol—a biosurfactant from the aquatic weed *Hydrilla verticillata*. Biocatal. Agric. Biotechnol. 18788181. 17, 736–742. Available from: http://www.journals.elsevier.com/biocatalysis-and-agricultural-biotechnology/. doi:10.1016/j.bcab.2019.01.026.

Prates, J.A.M., 2025. Applications of bioactive compounds from marine microalgae in health, cosmetics, and functional foods. Appl. Sci. 2076-3417. 15 (11), 6144. doi:10.3390/app15116144.

Prieto, C., Lagaron, J.M., 2024. Nanoencapsulation and nanocoating of bioactives of application interest in food, nutraceuticals and pharma. Nanomaterials. 2079-4991. 14 (3), 313. doi:10.3390/nano14030313.

Puchkova, T.V., Khapchaeva, S.A., Zotov, V.S., Lukyanov, A.A., Solovchenko, A.E., 2021. Marine and freshwater microalgae as a sustainable source of cosmeceuticals. Mar. Biol. J. 24999776. 6 (1), 67–81. doi:10.21072/mbj.2021.06.1.06.

Pulz, O., Gross, W., 2004. Valuable products from biotechnology of microalgae. Appl. Microbiol. Biotechnol. 0175-7598. 65 (6), 635–648. doi:10.1007/s00253-004-1647-x.

Putri, T.W., Nursida, N.F., Raya, I., 2021. Antioxidant activity of *Chlorella vulgaris* used as an antioxidant cream. J. Phys. Conf. Ser. 1742-6588. 1899 (1), 012030. doi:10.1088/1742-6596/1899/1/012030.

Qiu, S.-M., Aweya, J.J., Liu, X., Liu, Y., Tang, S., Zhang, W., Cheong, K.-L., 2022. Bioactive polysaccharides from red seaweed as potent food supplements: a systematic review of their extraction, purification, and biological activities. Carbohydr. Polym. 01448617. 275, 118696. doi:10.1016/j.carbpol.2021.118696.

Quiñones, C.F., Reinado, R.C., Niño, A.E., Fernández-Acero, F.J., 2020. Microalgae: molecular biology, proteomics and applications. In: Prime Archives in Molecular Biology. Vide Leaf, pp. 1–65. doi:10.37247/PAMB.1.2020.45.

Ragusa, I., Nardone, G.N., Zanatta, S., Bertin, W., Amadio, E., 2021. Spirulina for skin care: a bright blue future. Cosmetics. 2079-9284. 8 (1), 7. doi:10.3390/cosmetics8010007.

Ramos, S.D.P., Bürck, M., Costa, S.F.F.D., Assis, M., Braga, A.R.C., 2025. Spirulina as a key ingredient in the evolution of eco-friendly cosmetics. BioTech. 26736284. 14 (2). Available from: https://www.mdpi.com/journal/biotech. doi:10.3390/biotech14020041.

Rastogi, R.P., Sinha, R.P., 2009. Biotechnological and industrial significance of cyanobacterial secondary metabolites. Biotechnol. Adv. 07349750. 27 (4), 521–539. doi:10.1016/j.biotechadv.2009.04.009.

Real Beauty Outlet, 2025. Sacred Lotus Face Cream. https://real-beauty-outlet.myshopify.com/products/sacred-lotus-face-cream

Resende, D.I.S.P., Ferreira, M., Magalhães, C., Lobo, J.M.S., Sousa, E., Almeida, I.F., 2021. Trends in the use of marine ingredients in anti-aging cosmetics. Algal Res. 22119264. 55, 102273. doi:10.1016/j.algal.2021.102273.

Riseh, R.S., Skorik, Y.A., Thakur, V.K., Pour, M.M., Tamanadar, E., Noghabi, S.S., 2021. Encapsulation of plant biocontrol bacteria with alginate as a main polymer material. Int. J. Mol. Sci. 1422-0067. 22 (20), 11165. doi:10.3390/ijms222011165.

Ruslan, F.S., Susanti, D., Noor, N.M., Aminudin, N.I., Taher, M., 2021. Bioactive compounds, cosmeceutical and nutraceutical applications of green seaweed species (Chlorophyta). Squalen Bull. Mar. Fish. Postharvest Biotechnol. 24069272. 16 (1), 41–55. Available from: https://www.bbp4b.litbang.kkp.go.id/squalen-bulletin/index.php/squalen/article/view/514/pdf. doi:10.15578/squalen.514.

Russell-Goldman, E., Murphy, G.F., 2020. The pathobiology of skin aging: new insights into an old dilemma. Am. J. Pathol. 15252191. 190 (7), 1356–1369. Available from: http://ajp.amjpathol.org/. doi:10.1016/j.ajpath.2020.03.007.

Sabeena Farvin, K.H.S., Jacobsen, C., 2013. Phenolic compounds and antioxidant activities of selected species of seaweeds from Danish coast. Food Chem. 03088146. 138 (2-3), 1670–1681. doi:10.1016/j.foodchem.2012.10.078.

Safafar, H., Van Wagenen, J., Møller, P., Jacobsen, C., 2015. Carotenoids, phenolic compounds and tocopherols contribute to the antioxidative properties of some microalgae species grown on industrial wastewater. Mar. Drugs. 1660-3397. 13 (12), 7339–7356. doi:10.3390/md13127069.

Saleem, R., Osama, M., Khadim, S., Farooqi, U., Advani, R.S., Unar, K., Unar, A.A., Baloch, N., Siyal, F.J., Shaikh, B., Zafar, J., Fatima, F., 2024. A systematic review to unveil therapeutic potential of some common green seaweeds. J. Surv. Fish. Sci. 92–97. doi:10.53555/sfs.v11i3.2341.

Samoraj, M., Çalış, D., Trzaska, K., Mironiuk, M., Chojnacka, K., 2024. Advancements in algal biorefineries for sustainable agriculture: biofuels, high-value products, and environmental solutions. Biocatal. Agric. Biotechnol. 18788181. 58, 103224. doi:10.1016/j.bcab.2024.103224.

Santin, A., Russo, M.T., Ferrante, M.I., Balzano, S., Orefice, I., Sardo, A., 2021. Highly valuable polyunsaturated fatty acids from microalgae: strategies to improve their yields and their potential exploitation in aquaculture. Molecules. 1420-3049. 26 (24), 7697. doi:10.3390/molecules26247697.

Sawant Desai, S., Kelkar Mane, V., 2023. Biotechnological Advances in Cosmetic Industry. Scrivener Publishing LLC (Wiley and Sons), pp.103–136. doi:10.1002/9781119792888.ch3.

Schramm, S., Weiß, D., 2024. Bioluminescence—The Vibrant Glow of Nature and its Chemical Mechanisms. ChemBioChem. 1439-4227. 25 (9). doi:10.1002/cbic.202400106.

Sealaria, 2025 A-gel. https://sealaria.com/product/a-gel-2/

Seferli, M., Kotanidou, C., Lefkaki, M., Adamantidi, T., Panoutsopoulou, E., Finos, M.A., Krey, G., Kamidis, N., Stamatis, N., Anastasiadou, C., Tsoupras, A., 2024. Bioactives of the freshwater aquatic plants, *Nelumbo nucifera* and lemna minor, for functional foods, cosmetics and pharmaceutical applications, with antioxidant, anti-inflammatory and antithrombotic health promoting properties. Appl. Sci. 2076-3417. 14 (15), 6634. doi:10.3390/app14156634.

Seferli, M., Lefkaki, M., Manousakis, V., Ofrydopoulou, A., Shiels, K., Saha, S.K., Krey, G., Kamidis, N., Stamatis, N., Anastasiadou, C., Tsoupras, A., 2025. Amphiphilic bioactives of freshwater aquatic plants *Nelumbo nucifera* (Indian Lotus) and Lemna sp. with antioxidant, anti-inflammatory and antithrombotic activities: in vitro study. Pharmaceuticals. 1424-8247. 18 (6), 835. doi:10.3390/ph18060835.

Senevirathne, M., Ahn, C.B., Je, J.Y., 2010. Enzymatic extracts from edible red algae, *Porphyra tenera*, and their antioxidant, anti-acetylcholinesterase, and anti-inflammatory activities. Food Sci. Biotechnol. 12267708. 19 (6), 1551–1557. doi:10.1007/s10068-010-0220-x.

Shiels, K., Tsoupras, A., Lordan, R., Nasopoulou, C., Zabetakis, I., Murray, P., Saha, S.K., 2021. Bioactive lipids of marine microalga *Chlorococcum* sp. SABC 012504 with anti-inflammatory and anti-thrombotic activities. Mar. Drugs. 1660-3397. 19 (1), 28. doi:10.3390/md19010028.

Shrivastava, M., Srivastava, S., 2021. Application and research progress of *Hydrilla verticillata* in ecological restoration of water contaminated with metals and metalloids. Environ. Chall. 26670100. 4, 100177. doi:10.1016/j.envc.2021.100177.

Siahaan, E.A., Agusman, Pangestuti, R., Shin, K.H., Kim, S.K., 2022. Potential cosmetic active ingredients derived from marine by-products. Mar. Drugs. 16603397. 20 (12). Available from: http://www.mdpi.com/journal/marinedrugs. doi:10.3390/md20120734.

Siao, A.C., Hou, C.W., Kao, Y.H., Jeng, K.C., 2015. Effect of sesamin on apoptosis and cell cycle arrest in human breast cancer MCF-7 cells. Asian Pac. J. Cancer Prev. 15137368. 16 (9), 3779–3783. Available from: http://www.apocpcontrol.org/paper_file/issue_abs/Volume16_No9/3779-3783%201.19%20An-Ci%20Siao.pdf. doi:10.7314/APJCP.2015.16.9.3779.

Siddhi, G., Khamkar, S.P., 2025. Formulation and evaluation of anti-fungal cream using *Nelumbo nucifera* and *Azadirachta indica* leaves extracts. Int. J. Sci. Res. Technol. doi:10.5281/zenodo.15401169.

Silveira, M.J., Michelan, T.S., de Carvalho Harthman, V., 2025. Invasive *Hydrilla verticillata* impacts native aquatic plants at family and species levels. Aquat. Ecol. 15735125. 59 (2), 657–669. Available from: https://www.springer.com/journal/10452. doi:10.1007/s10452-025-10186-x.

Sotelo, C.G., Blanco, M., Ramos, P., Vázquez, J.A., Perez-Martin, R.I., 2021. Sustainable sources from aquatic organisms for cosmeceuticals ingredients. Cosmetics. 20799284. 8 (2). Available from: https://www.mdpi.com/2079-9284/8/2/48/pdf. doi:10.3390/cosmetics8020048.

Spolaore, P., Joannis-Cassan, C., Duran, E., Isambert, A., 2006. Commercial applications of microalgae. J. Biosci. Bioeng. 13891723. 101 (2), 87–96. doi:10.1263/jbb.101.87.

Sun, R., Xia, N., Xia, Q., 2020. Non-aqueous nanoemulsions as a new strategy for topical application of astaxanthin. J. Dispersion Sci. Technol. 41 (12), 1777–1788. doi:10.1080/01932691.2019.1635027.

Taboada, C., Millán, R., Míguez, I., 2010. Composition, nutritional aspects and effect on serum parameters of marine algae *Ulva rigida*. J. Sci. Food Agric. 0022-5142. 90 (3), 445–449. doi:10.1002/jsfa.3836.

Tammasorn, P., Charoensup, W., Bunrod, A., Kanjanakawinkul, W., Chaiyana, W., 2023. Promising anti-wrinkle applications of aromatic extracts of *Hedychium coronarium* J. Koenig via antioxidation and collagenase inhibition. Pharmaceuticals. 1424-8247. 16 (12), 1738. doi:10.3390/ph16121738.

Tang, Y., Nie, T., Zhang, L., Liu, X., Deng, H., 2025. Peptides in cosmetics: from pharmaceutical breakthroughs to skincare innovations. Cosmetics. 2079-9284. 12 (3), 107. doi:10.3390/cosmetics12030107.

Terao, J., 1989. Antioxidant activity of β-carotene-related carotenoids in solution. Lipids. 0024-4201. 24 (7), 659–661. doi:10.1007/bf02535085.

Thiyagarasaiyar, K., Goh, B.H., Jeon, Y.J., Yow, Y.Y., 2020. Algae metabolites in cosmeceutical: an overview of current applications and challenges. Mar. Drugs. 16603397. 18 (6). Available from: https://www.mdpi.com/1660-3397/18/6/323/pdf. doi:10.3390/md18060323.

TKS, 2025. A Novel Biotechnological Active Ingredient, Derived from the Microalga Spirulina, Increases Hydration and Reduces Osmotic Stress in Skin Cells—TKS | Publisher, Event Organiser, Media Agency. TKS Publisher. https://www.teknoscienze.com/tks_article/a-novel-biotechnological-active-ingredient-derived-from-the-microalga-spirulina-increases-hydration-and-reduces-osmotic-stress-in-skin-cells/.

Tominaga, K., Hongo, N., Karato, M., Yamashita, E., 2012. Cosmetic benefits of astaxanthin on humans subjects. Acta Biochim. Pol. 1734154X. 59 (1), 43–47. Available from: http://www.actabp.pl/pdf/1_2012/43.pdf. doi:10.18388/abp.2012_2168.

Torres, M.D., Flórez-Fernández, N., Domínguez, H., 2019. Integral utilization of red seaweed for bioactive production. Mar. Drugs. 1660-3397. 17 (6), 314. doi:10.3390/md17060314.

Tsaloglou, M.N., et al., 2016. Microalgae: Current Research and Applications. Caister Academic Press, Harvard University, Cambridge, MA. doi:10.21775/9781910190272.

Tungmunnithum, D., Kongsawadworakul, P., Hano, C., 2021. A cosmetic perspective on the antioxidant flavonoids from *Nymphaea lotus* L. Cosmetics. 2079-9284. 8 (1), 12. doi:10.3390/cosmetics8010012.

Ulber, R., editor, 2021. Bioactive Compounds from Brown Algae. Multidisciplinary Digital Publishing Institute. doi:10.3390/books978-3-0365-2469-6.

Vaz, B.M.C., Contieri, M.S., Leite, C.T.S., de Souza Mesquita, L.S., Conde, A., Oliveira, J.P., Pinto, D.C.G.A., Ventura, S.P.M., 2025. Efficient extraction and purification of mycosporines-like amino acids (MAAs) following a multiproduct biorefinery approach. Sep. Purif. Technol. 13835866. 363, 132200. doi:10.1016/j.seppur.2025.132200.

VERYMWL, 2025 Annabella Haematococcus Pluvialis Facial Repair Mask - VERYMWL https://www.verymwl.com/en/very-mwl-annabella-haematococcus-pluvialis-facial-repair-mask/

Vieira, M.V., Pastrana, L.M., Fuciños, P., 2020. Microalgae encapsulation systems for food, pharmaceutical and cosmetics applications. Mar. Drugs. 16603397. 18 (12). Available from: https://www.mdpi.com/1660-3397/18/12/644. doi:10.3390/md18120644.

Volkman, J.K., 2016. Sterols in microalgae. In: Borowitzka, M.A., Beardall, J., Raven, J.A. (Eds.), The Physiology of Microalgae. Springer International Publishing, Cham, pp. 485–505. doi:10.1007/978-3-319-24945-2_19.

Wang, H.M.D., Chen, C.C., Huynh, P., Chang, J.S., 2015. Exploring the potential of using algae in cosmetics. Bioresour. Technol. 18732976. 184, 355–362. Available from: www.elsevier.com/locate/biortech. doi:10.1016/j.biortech.2014.12.001.

Wang, T., Jónsdóttir, R., Ólafsdóttir, G., 2009. Total phenolic compounds, radical scavenging and metal chelation of extracts from Icelandic seaweeds. Food Chem. 03088146. 116 (1), 240–248. doi:10.1016/j.foodchem.2009.02.041.

Wijesinghe, W.A.J.P., Jeon, Y.J., 2012. Biological activities and potential industrial applications of fucose rich sulfated polysaccharides and fucoidans isolated from brown seaweeds: a review. Carbohydr. Polym. 01448617. 88 (1), 13–20. doi:10.1016/j.carbpol.2011.12.029.

Wu, P., Zong, D., Yang, L., Jia, X., Lili, Q., Yihong, W., Chunping, X., 2025. Volatile compounds and characteristic aroma perception in blue lotus (*Nymphaea nouchali* var. caerulea) three processed products: insights from flavoromics and molecular docking. LWT. 00236438. 229, 118193. doi:10.1016/j.lwt.2025.118193.

Yadav, U., Thakur, K., Vishwakarma, B., Jha, A., 2022. To study the effects of *Bacopa monnieri* and *Momordica charantia* as natural preservatives on herbal cream. Genius J. X, 95–102.

Yoon, N.Y., Kim, H.R., Chung, H.Y., Choi, J.S., 2008. Anti-hyperlipidemic effect of an edible brown algae, *Ecklonia stolonifera*, and its constituents on poloxamer 407-induced hyperlipidemic and cholesterol-fed rats. Arch. Pharm. Res. 19763786. 31 (12), 1564–1571. doi:10.1007/s12272-001-2152-8.

Zhang, Z., Wang, F., Wang, X., Liu, X., Hou, Y., Zhang, Q., 2010. Extraction of the polysaccharides from five algae and their potential antioxidant activity in vitro. Carbohydr. Polym. 01448617. 82 (1), 118–121. doi:10.1016/j.carbpol.2010.04.031.

Zheng, B., Zheng, J., Zeng, S., 2004. Study on three functional components of Chinese main lotus seed varieties. Inst. Food Sci. Technol. 26, 158–160.

Zouboulis, C.C., Hoenig, L.J., 2019. Skin aging revisited. Clin. Dermatol. 18791131. 37 (4), 293–295. Available from: www.elsevier.com/locate/clindermatol. doi:10.1016/j.clindermatol.2019.04.012.

Further reading

Kim, S.-K., 2015. Handbook of Marine Microalgae: Biotechnology Advances. Academic Press, pp. 1–585. doi:10.1016/C2013-0-19117-9.

Chapter 10

Vegetables and vegetable biowaste

Despoina Pantazi, Maria Nektaria Magkoulia, and Kassiani Lalexou
Laboratory of Biochemistry, Department of Chemistry, University of Ioannina, Ioannina, Greece

1 Introduction

Plants have evolved to resist sunlight by producing secondary metabolites that either neutralize its negative effects or use it to perform photochemical processes. Similarly, human skin has an innate photoprotective and antioxidant defense mechanism. A current scientific strategy is to develop sunscreen formulations that incorporate safe photostable secondary metabolites, provide broad ultraviolet A (UVA) and ultraviolet B (UVB) protection, reduce oxidative stress, and improve natural skin protection mechanisms, thereby preserving and rejuvenating the intrinsic photochemical barrier (Korkina et al., 2018).

Vegetables play a key role in human diets and are composed of primary metabolites (such as carbohydrates, lipids, and amino acids) and secondary metabolites with important biological functions. They help plants defend themselves against biotic and abiotic factors and are essential for their interaction with other organisms and the environment. Their use in humans has been associated with positive health outcomes, as epidemiological studies have shown a reduced risk of cardiovascular disease, stroke, and some cancers. This benefit is attributed mainly to fiber but also to compounds with high antioxidant activity, such as carotenoids and various flavonoid classes. These molecules support cell antioxidant protection, promote cardiovascular health, and assist in neuroprotective mechanisms (Barbulova et al., 2015).

The use of bioactive phytochemicals derived from waste produced by fresh produce is generating growing interest in the agrifood and cosmetics sectors, with a focus on green extraction techniques that are sustainable. Methods such as ultrasonic extraction, microwave-assisted extraction (MAE), supercritical liquid extraction, and pulsed electric field extraction minimize dependence on harmful solvents and reduce energy consumption, while ensuring high efficiency plant regeneration. Plant compounds such as carotenoids, polyphenols, glucosinolates, and betalains have antioxidant and antiinflammatory properties, protecting the skin from UV light and oxidative stress. Their inclusion in skincare formulations offers a natural and safe alternative to synthetic antioxidants, while promoting a circular economy and minimizing environmental waste (Fig. 10.1). This approach increases the efficacy of skin care products and promotes sustainable industrial practices (Valisakkagari et al., 2024).

2 Categories of natural bioactive compounds

2.1 Polyphenols

Polyphenols have become important food additives. In the last decade, numerous studies have confirmed their role in the prevention of degenerative diseases, including cardiovascular diseases and cancer (Scalbert et al., 2005). These metabolites of secondary plant metabolism have strong antioxidant, antiinflammatory, antimicrobial, and antiviral properties, which make them attractive phytochemicals for medicinal products and cosmetics (Ignat et al., 2010).

Polyphenols are secondary metabolites of plants found widely in vegetables and medicinal herbs (medicinal and aromatic plants) and serve as a vital source of bioactive substances with health benefits (Gurib-Fakim, 2005; Kaur and Das, 2011). These compounds are produced by two primary metabolic pathways: shikimate and acetic acid, which include a wide range of classes of compounds, such as phenolic acids, coumarins, lignins, flavonoids, proanthocyanidins, and stilbenes (Sánchez-Moreno, 2002; Bravo, 2009). There is extensive epidemiological evidence that polyphenol intake helps to prevent chronic oxidative stress-related diseases, including cardiovascular disease, cancer, neurodegenerative diseases (e.g., Alzheimer's and Parkinson's), type 2 diabetes, and infectious diseases (Teixeira et al., 2013; Lutz et al., 2019). Their biological effects include antioxidant, antiinflammatory, antimicrobial, and anticancer protection, although their effectiveness varies according to the

Biofunctional Cosmetics for Health. https://doi.org/10.1016/B978-0-443-27500-5.00014-9

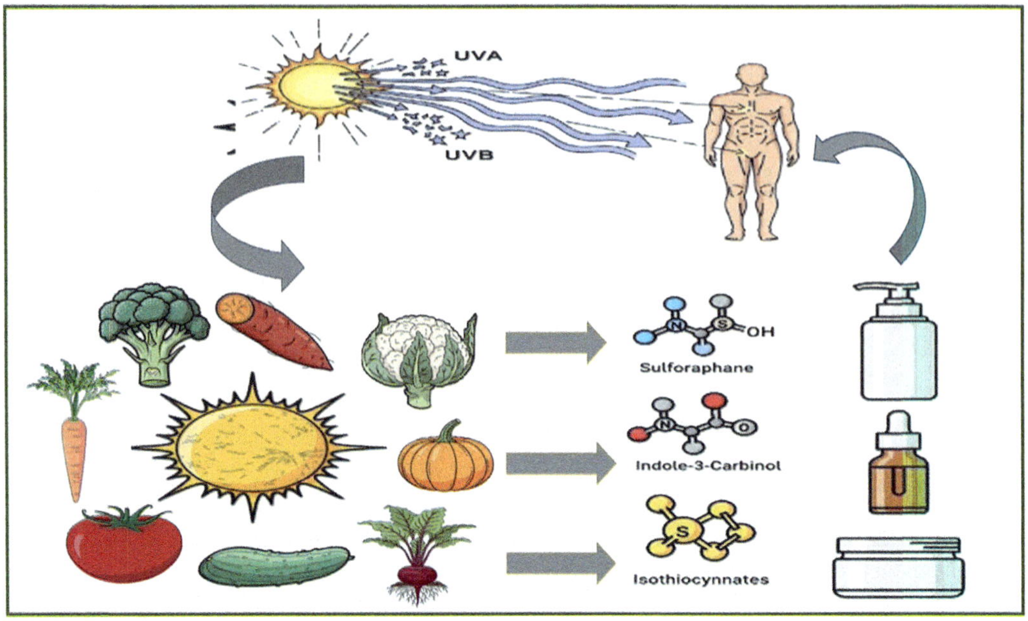

FIG. 10.1 Bioactive vegetable compounds in cosmetics. *(Prepared using mindthegraph.com, Accessed 24 September 2025.)*

type of compound, its concentration, and bioavailability (Bravo, 2009). In addition, the polyphenol content of vegetables varies considerably, with a higher concentration in darker varieties such as red and black beans, Brussels sprouts, and onions (Bravo, 2009). Notably, phenolic acids, including galactocyanins, salicylic acid, caffeic acid, and chlorogenic acids, have potent antioxidant and antiinflammatory properties, while derivatives such as resveratrol, anthocyanins, and proanthocyanidins have cardioprotective and antiinflammatory properties (Pinto et al., 2021). In addition, the intake of polyphenol-rich vegetables and extracts may inhibit inflammatory processes, reduce pathogen growth, and improve innate antioxidant defenses, making them particularly useful for cosmetic and biofunctional products (Pinto et al., 2021).

2.2 Carotenoids

Carotenoids are natural, brightly colored pigments of plants found in >600 plant species, and they are responsible for the coloration of fruits, vegetables, and leaves (Krinsky and Johnson, 2005). In addition to their esthetic function, they have important biological properties, as their intake is linked to protection against chronic diseases and the promotion of good skin health (Krinsky and Johnson, 2005; Stahl and Sies, 2012). These fat soluble substances include beta-carotene, lycopene, and lutein, which have potent photoprotective and antiinflammatory effects that help reduce the UV sensitivity of the skin. The main dietary sources of these compounds are carrots and tomatoes (Stahl and Sies, 2012). Environmental and technological factors, such as heat, light, and processing methods, influence the isomerization of carotenoids, which results in structural changes and even degradation. Geometric *cis–trans* isomers differ in their absorption spectra and their coloring intensity, and the number of conjugated double bonds is directly correlated with their antioxidant activity. Isomer analysis and separation are mainly carried out by high-performance liquid chromatography, which facilitates the precise identification of fruits and vegetables (Khoo et al., 2011).

Dietary intake of carotenoids has become an important factor in the protection of the skin against UV radiation, and the potential for the topical application of plant compounds has also been examined. The unique ability of carotenoids to extinguish excited molecules has aroused interest in their biological, nutritional, and medical functions (Stahl and Sies, 2012). When exposed to UV light, photosensitive compounds are activated and, in the presence of molecular oxygen, can form singlet oxygen, a highly reactive species that damages biomolecules such as DNA, proteins, and lipids, and contributes to oxidative stress. Although there is no specific enzyme for the deactivation of singlet oxygen, its neutralization occurs through small molecules with a quenching effect, with carotenoids being the most important natural quenchers. Their mechanism is based on the transfer of excitatory energy from the oxygen molecule to the carotenoid, which then releases this energy as heat and returns to its original state, completing the catalytic cycle. This process is considered quasienzymatic since the carotenoid does not change and may be repeated. Their rapid response rate, close to the diffusion limit, makes them highly effective against singlet oxygen, with the most potent of these being lycopene (Di Mascio et al., 1989).

2.3 Glucosinolates and isothiocyanates

Vegetables of the families *Brassicaceae*, *Capparaceae*, and *Caricaceae*, including broccoli, Brussels sprouts, arugula, kale, bok choy, and radishes, are rich in glucosinolates (Miao et al., 2021). These compounds are synthesized from glucose and amino acids and are composed of the thioglycoside group of the beta-dibasic acid and the ester N-hydroxysulfate with different side chains (Aghajanzadeh et al., 2019). Glucosinolates can be classified according to their amino acid precursor group into aliphatic, indole, and aromatic groups, with progoitrin, sinigrin, and glucoraphanin being the most prominent examples (Halkier and Gershenzon, 2006). These compounds have been shown to have important antioxidant activity (Cabello-Hurtado et al., 2011), antiinflammatory activity (Ruiz-Alcaraz et al., 2022), and anticarcinogenic activity (Cuellar-Núñez et al., 2020). They also have a positive impact on heart disease (Esteve, 2020) and musculoskeletal disorders (Connolly et al., 2021). Their levels may be affected by genetic and environmental factors, and cooking and processing practices may also affect the final yield and product characteristics (Redha et al., 2023). Glucosinolates are noted for their relative stability; however, enzymatic hydrolysis by myrosinase under mechanical or thermal conditions, which results in the formation of isothiocyanate compounds, may be observed (Barba et al., 2016). A similar process occurs in the human gastrointestinal tract, where gut microbial and myrosinase enzymes contribute to glucosinolate breakdown into bioactive isothiocyanates (Narbad and Rossiter, 2018). These compounds, such as sulforaphane (SF) and indole-3-carbinol (I3C), have been the subject of scientific interest because of their recognized antioxidant and anticancer properties (Akbari and Namazian, 2020). Their role in antiinflammatory, antiallergic, and antineoplastic activities also highlights their potential to prevent chronic diseases. In particular, I3C has been associated not only with anticancer effects but also with antihypertensive and antiarrhythmic properties (Redha et al., 2023).

2.4 Vitamins and minerals

Vitamins and minerals in vegetables are key regulators of skin health (Pullar et al., 2017). Vitamin C, present in high concentrations in normal skin, contributes to collagen synthesis and provides antioxidant protection against photoaging (Pullar et al., 2017). Vitamin E, folic acid, and other trace elements similarly increase cell renewal and enhance the elasticity of the skin (Pullar et al., 2017). Their combined intake via diet or topical application is a strategy of major cosmetic and therapeutic interest (Pullar et al., 2017). Vitamin C is soluble in water and is essential for humans because it cannot be synthesized endogenously, due to the lack of the enzyme gulonolactone oxidase, in many other animals (Nishikimi et al., 1994). It is present in fruits and vegetables, but its content is reduced by cooking, processing, and storage (Jeffery et al., 2003). Vitamin C is crucial to collagen synthesis and tissue strength and contributes to the repair and regeneration of the skin (Jeffery et al., 2003). It also acts as a potent antioxidant, protecting cells against oxidative stress and promoting dermal fibroblasts to proliferate, which is important for wound healing (Jeffery et al., 2003). Vitamin C intake increases during inflammation and injury, suggesting that supplementation may improve tissue regeneration (Pullar et al., 2017). Vitamin C deficiency leads to scurvy, which is characterized by symptoms such as tiredness, bleeding, inability to heal wounds, and severe complications (Nishikimi et al., 1994). Studies show that despite the availability of fruits and vegetables, vitamin deficiency is common in different populations, underlining the importance of vitamins for health and tissue regeneration (Pullar et al., 2017).

3 Characteristics of vegetables and their effects

3.1 Broccoli

Broccoli *(Brassica oleracea* var. *italica*) of the Brassicaceae family is a major source of bioactive ingredients such as glucosinolates (glucoraphanin), flavonoids (quercetin, kaempferol), vitamins (C, A, and B complexes), carotenoids (lutein), and minerals (potassium, selenium) (Bechara et al., 2022; Finley et al., 2001). Its use is associated with several skin-related benefits, both through diet and topical application (Moskwa et al., 2023). Of particular interest is SF, a glucoraphanin degradation product, which has been shown to reduce the harmful effects of ultraviolet radiation and susceptibility to erythema (Kerns et al., 2021; Talalay et al., 2007). Its antioxidant and possibly anticancer properties in the skin are well-studied (Moskwa et al., 2023).

Lutein also protects against photoaging and reduces the wrinkling caused by UVB radiation (Lim et al., 2013). Quercetin helps to maintain skin structure by inhibiting collagen degradation (Shin et al., 2019) and kaempferol combines antioxidant, antiinflammatory, and antitumor properties to increase protection against sun damage (Moreno et al., 2006; Özyürek et al., 2009).

3.2 Tomatoes

Tomato (*Solanum lycopersicum* L., syn. *Lycopersicon esculentum* Mill.), a member of the Solanaceae family, is one of the most widely consumed and highly nutritious vegetables in the world (Ali et al., 2020; Kurina et al., 2021). Tomatoes are rich in vitamins (C, E), minerals (K), carotenoids (lycopene, beta-carotene), phytosterols (beta-sitosterol, campesterol, stigmasterol), and phenolic compounds (kaempferol, quercetin, lutein, ferulic acid, chlorogenic acid, and caffeic acid). Among these, lycopene has been shown to be a powerful antioxidant with proven skin-protective effects: it reduces harmful UV radiation and inflammation, prevents DNA damage, and helps reduce tumor growth (Fazekas et al., 2003; Heo et al., 2021). Clinical trials have shown that tomato paste intake (40 g per day, corresponding to 16 mg lycopene) increases carotenoid levels in the skin and plasma, while reducing UVB-induced inflammation (Moskwa et al., 2023). Regular consumption or topical application of tomato extracts before exposure to UV light appears to be protective and reduces the risk of developing cancerous skin tumors (Fazekas et al., 2003; Heo et al., 2021).

3.3 Carrots

Carrots (*Daucus carota* L.), a member of the Apiaceae family, are among the most widely cultivated root vegetables in the world, originating in Asia (Lm et al., 2020). They have a rich nutritional profile, containing vitamins (A, C, E, K, H, and B), minerals (calcium, potassium, iron, copper, phosphorus, magnesium, zinc, and cobalt), and bioactive substances such as folic acid, malic acid, inositol, and pectin (Moskwa et al., 2023). Carotenoids are of major importance: beta-carotene (0.53–4.96 mg per 100 g), lutein, zeaxanthin, and lycopene (0.15–9.02 mg per 100 g). Luteolin, also present in carrots, has been reported to be a photoprotective agent (Stahl et al., 2005). Carrot oil has antiaging properties, with high antioxidant activity and a 6.92 SPF, making it a promising cosmetic ingredient (Singh et al., 2018). In addition, methanol extract from red carrots (*D. carota* L., R4G series) has been shown to be rich in anthocyanins with potent antioxidant and antiinflammatory properties and has major potential to prevent aging of the skin (Bianconi et al., 2020).

3.4 Cucumber

Cucumber (*Cucumis sativus* L.), a member of the family Cucurbitaceae, is a widely consumed vegetable worldwide (Naureen et al., 2022). In Ayurvedic medicine, its fruits, seeds, and leaves are used to prevent aging of the skin (Mukherjee et al., 2011, 2012). Due to its high water content (over 96%), it has a cooling and soothing effect, which makes it useful for the relief of skin problems such as sunburn (Naureen et al., 2022). Its chemical composition includes carbohydrates, proteins, minerals (Ca, P, Fe), enzymes (protease, ascorbate oxidase, succinic dehydrogenase, and malate dehydrogenase), and ascorbic acid (Naureen et al., 2022). The pulp and peel extracts were found to be rich in lactic acid (7–8% w/w) and possess strong antioxidant properties (Sotiroudis et al., 2010).

In addition, the methanolic extract of cucumber seeds has been shown to have significant antioxidant and photoprotective potential (Gill et al., 2009). In cucumber leaves, lutein appears to be involved in the inhibition of melanogenesis and tyrosinase activity. Studies have shown that the methanolic extract of cucumber has photoprotective effects against UVA and UVB radiation through mechanisms related to its antioxidant activity (Kai et al., 2008).

3.5 Cauliflower

Cauliflower, a member of the Brassicaceae family, is a major source of secondary metabolites, predominantly glucosinolates and polyphenols, which have potent antioxidant, anticancer, and cardiovascular activities (Ahmed and Ali, 2013). The enzymatic degradation of glucosinolates leads to the formation of bioactive compounds, of which SF is the most prominent and has been identified as a key substance in the promotion of health (Abbaoui et al., 2018). Studies in animal models and cell lines have shown that SF exerts chemoprotective activity against UV irradiation through mechanisms, including modulation of signaling pathways, independent of NF-κB, and inhibition of the activation of NF-κB (Valisakkagari et al., 2024). Cauliflower modulates the transcription factor AP-1 (Valisakkagari et al., 2024). Sulforaphane rich extracts, such as broccoli root extracts, are proposed as a promising strategy to reduce skin cancer growth following exposure to UV light (Valisakkagari et al., 2024). Furthermore, the polyphenols in cruciferous vegetables, such as caffeic acid and luteolin, have a protective effect on the skin by reducing DNA damage, apoptotic death, oxidative stress, and photoaging via the SIRT3, reactive oxygen species (ROS), and mitogen-activated protein kinase (MAPK) pathways (Mu et al., 2021).

3.6 Beetroot

Beetroot contains bioactive ingredients such as betacyanins, carotenoids, phenolic acids, and flavonoids, which have antiinflammatory, antihypertensive, antibacterial, and anticancer properties (Zin et al., 2020). Betalains, organic pigments classified as betacyanins and betaxanthins, have strong antioxidant activity and help to neutralize free radicals, while also having anticancer properties (Azeredo, 2008). Studies have shown that betalains reduce skin cancer development in animal models and inhibit tumor and papilloma growth (Valisakkagari et al., 2024). In addition, compounds such as caffeic acid and rutin found in beetroot enhance skin protection by regulating key molecular pathways, reducing cyclooxygenase-2 (COX-2) expression, NF-κB, and matrix metalloproteinase (MMP), and increasing the synthesis of p53 and collagen (Balupillai et al., 2018). Overall, beetroot phytochemicals are emerging as promising chemotherapeutic agents against skin cancer (Valisakkagari et al., 2024).

3.7 Sweet potato

Sweet potatoes are an important source of bioactive substances such as anthocyanins, flavonoids, and phenolic acids, which have antioxidant and antiinflammatory properties and are protective against cardiovascular diseases, neurodegenerative disorders, and cancer (Liu et al., 2019). The main active substances are cyanidin, myricetin, and caffeic acid, which bind to peroxide radicals and help protect skin cells (Valisakkagari et al., 2024). Anthocyanin extract from purple-fleshed sweet potatoes has been shown in mouse models to reduce oxidative stress and skin inflammation by inhibiting NF-κB activation and MAPK phosphorylation, as well as enhancing antioxidant enzyme activity (Zhi et al., 2019). Cyanidin helps protect HaCaT keratinocytes by reducing the production of ROS, caspase-3, Bcl-2, and p53, while myricetin protects keratinocytes from UVB damage by reducing the development of dermal edema and skin cancer (Jung et al., 2010). In addition, beta-carotene inhibits apoptosis and reduces the MMP associated with aging, whereas coumaric acid enhances antioxidant protection by activating Nrf2 and reducing the expression of inflammatory cytokines (Wertz et al., 2004). Overall, the phytochemicals in sweet potatoes have multidimensional protective effects on skin health and aging (Valisakkagari et al., 2024).

3.8 Pumpkin

Pumpkin is cultivated worldwide, and its skin, pulp, and seeds are rich in phytochemical constituents such as flavonoids, carotenoids, phytosterols, and phenolic compounds. These compounds are associated with antiinflammatory, anticancer, antibacterial, and antidiabetic effects (Kaur et al., 2019). According to Valisakkagari et al. (2024), pumpkin-derived syringic acid exerts protective activity against damage to the skin caused by UVB by inhibiting key biomarkers such as prostaglandin E2, MMP-1, and COX-2. Based on these findings, syringic acid may be a promising candidate for treating UVB-induced skin lesions through modulation of molecular pathways involved in cellular damage (Valisakkagari et al., 2024).

In addition, against UVA-induced skin damage, the combination of phenolic acids-with syringic acid reduces cell cycle arrest, oxidative damage, accumulation of ROS, protein Keap1, and malondialdehyde (Sun et al., 2022). Pumpkin acid mixture controls cell cycle proteins (p53, p21, and p16), increases collagen secretion, and enhances cell survival by increasing the activity of intracellular antioxidants such as glutathione, glutathione peroxidase, superoxide dismutase, and catalase (Sun et al., 2022).

Pumpkin seed extract prevents cytotoxicity and slows cellular aging in normal NIH-3T3 fibroblasts induced by doxorubicin (Muntafiah et al., 2017). Because tocopherol is bound to the cytochrome CYP3A4, it protects the cells and has antiaging properties (Muntafiah et al., 2017). Plant-derived compounds, especially tocopherol from pumpkin seeds, have been shown to possess strong antiaging properties and require further research (Muntafiah et al., 2017).

4 Isolation of natural bioactive compounds

In the food, biochemistry, and pharmaceuticals industries, the process of extracting bioactive compounds from plant materials is of key importance (Valisakkagari et al., 2024). Traditional methods such as Soxhlet extraction, maceration, and steam distillation use organic solvents such as methanol, ethanol, and water, which are often associated with high energy consumption, long processing times, and negative impacts on the environment (Valisakkagari et al., 2024).

To overcome the limitations of these traditional methods, advanced green extraction methods have been developed to achieve sustainability using mild conditions, substitute solvents, and lower energy consumption (Valisakkagari et al., 2024). Such techniques include high hydrostatic pressure extraction, MAE, ultrasound-assisted extraction (UAE), supercritical fluid extraction (SFE), and subcritical water extraction, all of which allow for high yields of extracts with low impact on the environment (Valisakkagari et al., 2024).

4.1 Microwave-assisted extraction

MAE uses nonionizing electromagnetic radiation from 300 MHz to 300 GHz to heat plant samples (Bagade and Patil, 2019). Heating activates polar solvents through ionic conduction and dipole rotation, increasing the solvents' diffusion in the cells (Vinatoru et al., 2017). Heat causes the evaporation of moisture and pressure build-up in the cell walls, leading to cell rupture and facilitating the release of bioactive compounds (Marić et al., 2018).

MAE systems are divided into open, operating under atmospheric conditions, and closed, applying high pressure and temperature to extract the material more quickly (Llompart et al., 2019). The efficiency of MAE is determined by factors such as microwave strength, temperature, duration, and solvent content (Panja, 2017). This technique offers cost-efficiency, reduced solvent consumption, and shorter extraction times (Panja, 2017; Rifna et al., 2021). The main drawback is the low yield when using nonpolar solvents (Panja, 2017). MAE is an efficient method for the recovery of plant compounds with a limited impact on the environment (Bagade and Patil, 2019). Its use in cosmetic and pharmaceutical products improves the quality and sustainability of extracts (Llompart et al., 2019).

4.2 Ultrasound-assisted extraction

UAE is a sustainable and green extraction method that reduces processing time and retains bioactive compounds at room temperature (Chemat et al., 2016). The technique uses ultrasonic frequencies of approximately 20 kHz and a power density of 10–1000 W per cm^2 to generate compression and rarefaction waves in a liquid medium (Chemat et al., 2016). The formation of microscopic bubbles releases energy and increases the pressure and temperature, facilitating the extraction (Valisakkagari et al., 2024). The process involves diffusion, disrupting cell walls and increasing the penetration of the solvent, ultimately improving extraction efficiency (Valisakkagari et al., 2024). This method is mainly used in liquid–solid or liquid–liquid systems for the extraction of bioactive compounds (Rifna et al., 2021). One limitation of the method is the potential formation of hydrogen (H) and hydroxyl (OH) radicals by water vapor decomposition at high temperatures and pressures (Rifna et al., 2021). Low frequency (20–40 kHz) and low temperature enhance performance and minimize solvent resistance (Valisakkagari et al., 2024).

Overall, this technique offers energy efficiency, short extraction times, and minimal phytochemical degradation (Chemat et al., 2016), making it an effective and sustainable method for extracting bioactive compounds from plant samples (Chemat et al., 2016).

4.3 Supercritical fluid extraction

SFE is a technique that utilizes temperature and pressure close to the critical point of solvents to reach their supercritical state (Luca et al., 2022). Supercritical CO_2 is considered safe, chemically inert, inexpensive, and nonflammable, and it offers excellent solvating power under pressure (Valisakkagari et al., 2024). In a supercritical state, CO_2 combines gas and liquid characteristics and facilitates rapid and efficient extraction (Valisakkagari et al., 2024).

Cosolvents, such as ethanol, may be added to increase the polarity of the solvent, enabling the extraction of polar phytochemicals (Rovetto and Aieta, 2017). This process allows CO_2 to reach critical levels at 31.1°C and 7.38 MPa and then return to its gaseous state at mild temperatures, allowing the solvent to be easily recovered (Arumugham et al., 2021). Accelerated extraction and reduced solvent consumption are characteristics of the process (Arumugham et al., 2021).

This method is limited primarily to nonpolar compounds, which require high processing pressure (Valisakkagari et al., 2024). The reuse of CO_2 improves the sustainability of the process and reduces environmental waste (Arumugham et al., 2021). This technique provides pure extracts free of solvent residues, which are suitable for cosmetic and pharmaceutical applications (Arumugham et al., 2021). Overall, SFE is an effective and environmentally friendly method for bioactive phytochemical recovery (Luca et al., 2022).

5 Applications of vegetables in cosmetics

Vegetarian diets are an important factor in the prevention of photoaging, as they contain bioactive compounds with proven ultraviolet protection. Notably, luteolin (3′,4′,5,7-tetrahydroxyflavone), a flavonoid found in vegetables such as broccoli, carrots, and celery, as well as other plant-based foods, has been the subject of much research (Miean and Mohamed, 2001).

Luteolin has a wide range of biological effects, including antioxidant, anticancer, antiinflammatory, and antiallergic effects (Lim et al., 2013). These properties are essential for skin protection, since UV light causes increased oxidative stress and activation of signaling pathways, leading to the destruction of the basic substance in the extracellular matrix (Lim et al., 2013).

Recent studies have shown that luteolin consumed in vegetables may inhibit the excessive activation of metalloproteinases, which break down collagen in the skin and cause loss of elasticity and wrinkles (Lim et al., 2013). Specifically, UVB light activates the transcription factor AP-1, which leads to MMP-1 expression. This effect is significantly inhibited by luteolin (Angel et al., 1987; Angel and Karin, 1991). At the molecular level, luteolin interacts directly with JNK1 and p90RSK2, inhibiting the phosphorylation of key proteins such as c-Jun and c-Fos, which are involved in activating AP-1 (Angel and Karin, 1991).

This inhibitory effect is of particular relevance since the excessive activity of MMPs is associated with the occurrence of severe photoaging (Lim et al., 2013). Therefore eating a diet rich in luteolin not only offers general antioxidant and antiinflammatory benefits but also seems to act specifically against the molecular mechanisms that are activated by UVB exposure (Lim et al., 2013). These findings support the view that plant foods, particularly vegetables, can act as a natural sunscreen against exposure to radiation, reducing the appearance of blemishes and discoloration (Lim et al., 2013).

Overall, available data suggest that a simple but very effective strategy to prevent photoaging is to systematically consume vegetables rich in luteolin, which strengthens the natural skin defenses against UV radiation (Lim et al., 2013).

Carotenoids are important biological substances that accumulate in the skin following topical application and consumption of food. They have potent antiinflammatory, antioxidant, and photoprotective properties (Flieger et al., 2024) Clinical studies have shown that they improve minimum erythema dose and minimum pigment persistence dose by increasing the UV resistance of the skin (Flieger et al., 2024). Carotenoids present in foods such as carrots, sweet potatoes, and tomatoes—such as astaxanthin, lycopene, beta-carotene, and lutein—can be used topically to improve hydration and elasticity, enhance antioxidant protection, and inhibit the breakdown of the extracellular matrix by suppressing cytokines that promote inflammation (Stanescu et al., 2025).

Diet, metabolism, sun exposure, and physiological status all influence skin carotenoid pigmentation concentrations. Studies have shown that lower body fat and greater fitness are associated with higher carotenoid levels (De Souza Guedes et al., 2021). Specialized delivery systems have been developed, including hydrogels, solid lipid nanoparticles, liposomes, nanoemulsions, and nanostructured lipid reagents (Zandi and Schnug, 2022), to increase bioavailability, stability, and penetration into the skin. In addition, the photoprotective and antiaging properties of carotenoids are enhanced when combined with other antioxidants such as vitamin C, vitamin E, coenzyme Q10, and flavonoids (Darvin et al., 2011). Finally, Raman spectroscopy shows that their long-term storage in the epidermis provides a durable defense against UV light, pollutants, and aging, making them a promising substance for dermatological prevention and antiaging protocols (Darvin et al., 2011).

Unlike the widely used hyaluronic acid, a recent study evaluated pumpkin-derived polysaccharides as a cosmetic ingredient for hydration. To measure transdermal water loss and hydration, volunteers were tested with specialized instruments called Tewameters and Corneometers. The concentrations of hyaluronic acid and pumpkin polysaccharide were compared. The findings showed that pumpkin polysaccharide significantly improves the function of the skin barrier by reducing water loss and providing a more potent hydration effect than hyaluronic acid. Hyaluronic acid was more effective than pumpkin polysaccharide in the short-term retention of moisture in the skin, but the pumpkin polysaccharide appeared to be generally safe. Therefore the pumpkin polysaccharide is a promising natural alternative for creams and lotions intended to increase skin hydration (Chanpirom et al., 2022).

6 Conclusions

In recent years, demand for biofunctional cosmetics has grown rapidly, driven by consumers' desire for natural, health-friendly ingredients. Within the beauty and wellness sector, cosmeceuticals—pharmaceutical-like products combined with cosmetic benefits—represent a fast growing segment. Broccoli, cabbage, carrots, tomatoes, and other cruciferous vegetables are among the most promising sources of naturally biologically active substances. The beneficial effects of these active substances on the skin make their inclusion in the diet essential, especially in the summer when exposure to sunlight is higher. Bioactive compounds found in vegetables, such as lutein, carotene, SF, and lycopene, have antioxidant properties that reduce the effects of ROS, which are the main cause of premature aging of the skin.

Therefore eating a healthy diet rich in these vegetables may help prevent skin photosensitivity and reduce the risk of sunburn, discoloration, and even skin cancer. Plant-derived bioactives are incorporated into cosmetics to help create safer and more environmentally friendly cosmetic products that improve long-term dermatological health beyond their appearance.

References

Abbaoui, B., Lucas, C.R., Riedl, K.M., Clinton, S.K., Mortazavi, A., 2018. Cruciferous vegetables, isothiocyanates, and bladder cancer prevention. Mol. Nutr. Food Res. 62 (18), 1–14. doi:10.1002/mnfr.201800079.

Aghajanzadeh, T.A., Prajapati, D.H., Burow, M., 2019. Copper toxicity affects indolic glucosinolates and gene expression of key enzymes for their biosynthesis in Chinese cabbage. Arch. Agron. Soil Sci. 66 (9), 1288–1301. doi:10.1080/03650340.2019.1666208.

Ahmed, F.A., Ali, R.F.M., 2013. Bioactive compounds and antioxidant activity of fresh and processed white cauliflower. Biomed Res. Int. 2013, 1–9. doi:10.1155/2013/367819.

Akbari, E., Namazian, M., 2020. Sulforaphane: a natural product against reactive oxygen species. Comput. Theor. Chem. 1183, 1–6. doi:10.1016/j.comptc.2020.112850.

Ali, M.Y., Sina, A.A.I., Khandker, S.S., Neesa, L., Tanvir, E.M., Kabir, A., Khalil, M.I., Gan, S.H., 2020. Nutritional composition and bioactive compounds in tomatoes and their impact on human health and disease: a review. Foods 10 (1), 1–31. doi:10.3390/foods10010045.

Angel, P., Imagawa, M., Chiu, R., Stein, B., Imbra, R.J., Rahmsdorf, H.J., Jonat, C., Herrlich, P., Karin, M., 1987. Phorbol ester-inducible genes contain a common cis element recognized by a TPA-modulated trans-acting factor. Cell 49 (6), 729–739. doi:10.1016/0092-8674(87)90611-8.

Angel, P., Karin, M., 1991. The role of Jun, Fos and the AP-1 complex in cell-proliferation and transformation. Biochim. Biophys. Acta Rev. Cancer 1072 (2–3), 129–157. doi:10.1016/0304-419x(91)90011-9.

Arumugham, T., Rambabu, K., Hasan, S.W., Show, P.L., Rinklebe, J., Banat, F., 2021. Supercritical carbon dioxide extraction of plant phytochemicals for biological and environmental applications – a review. Chemosphere 271, 1–19. doi:10.1016/j.chemosphere.2020.129525.

Azeredo, H.M., 2008. Betalains: properties, sources, applications, and stability – a review. Int. J. Food Sci. Technol. 44 (12), 2365–2376. doi:10.1111/j.1365-2621.2007.01668.x.

Bagade, S.B., Patil, M., 2019. Recent advances in microwave assisted extraction of bioactive compounds from complex herbal samples: a review. Crit. Rev. Anal. Chem. 51 (2), 138–149. doi:10.1080/10408347.2019.1686966.

Balupillai, A., Nagarajan, R.P., Ramasamy, K., Govindasamy, K., Muthusamy, G., 2018. Caffeic acid prevents UVB radiation induced photocarcinogenesis through regulation of PTEN signaling in human dermal fibroblasts and mouse skin. Toxicol. Appl. Pharmacol. 352, 87–96. doi:10.1016/j.taap.2018.05.030.

Barba, F.J., Nikmaram, N., Roohinejad, S., Khelfa, A., Zhu, Z., Koubaa, M., 2016. Bioavailability of glucosinolates and their breakdown products: impact of processing. Front. Nutr. 3, 1–12. doi:10.3389/fnut.2016.00024.

Barbulova, A., Colucci, G., Apone, F., 2015. New trends in cosmetics: by-Products of plant origin and their potential use as cosmetic active ingredients. Cosmetics 2 (2), 82–92. doi:10.3390/cosmetics2020082.

Bechara, N., Flood, V.M., Gunton, J.E., 2022. A Systematic review on the role of Vitamin C in tissue healing. Antioxidants 11 (8), 1605. doi:10.3390/antiox11081605.

Bianconi, M., Ceriotti, L., Cuzzocrea, S., Esposito, E., Pressi, G., Sgaravatti, E., Bertaiola, O., Guarnerio, C., Barbieri, E., Semenzato, A., Negri, S., Commisso, M., Avesani, L., Guzzo, F., 2020. Red carrot cells cultured in vitro are effective, stable, and safe ingredients for skin care, nutraceutical, and food applications. Front. Bioeng. Biotechnol. 8, 1–14. doi:10.3389/fbioe.2020.575079.

Bravo, L., 2009. Polyphenols: chemistry, dietary sources, metabolism, and nutritional significance. Nutr. Rev. 56 (11), 317–333. doi:10.1111/j.1753-4887.1998.tb01670.x.

Cabello-Hurtado, F., Gicquel, M., Esnault, M., 2011. Evaluation of the antioxidant potential of cauliflower (*Brassica oleracea*) from a glucosinolate content perspective. Food Chem. 132 (2), 1003–1009. doi:10.1016/j.foodchem.2011.11.086.

Chanpirom, S., Saewan, N., Sripisut, T., 2022. Alternative utilization of vegetable crop: pumpkin polysaccharide extract and their efficacy on skin hydration. Cosmetics 9 (6), 113. doi:10.3390/cosmetics9060113.

Chemat, F., Rombaut, N., Sicaire, A., Meullemiestre, A., Fabiano-Tixier, A., Abert-Vian, M., 2016. Ultrasound assisted extraction of food and natural products. Mechanisms, techniques, combinations, protocols and applications. A review. Ultrason. Sonochem. 34, 540–560. doi:10.1016/j.ultsonch.2016.06.035.

Connolly, E.L., Sim, M., Travica, N., Marx, W., Beasy, G., Lynch, G.S., Bondonno, C.P., Lewis, J.R., Hodgson, J.M., Blekkenhorst, L.C., 2021. Glucosinolates from cruciferous vegetables and their potential role in chronic disease: investigating the preclinical and clinical evidence. Front. Pharmacol. 12, 1–12. doi:10.3389/fphar.2021.767975.

Cuellar-Núñez, M.L., Loarca-Piña, G., Berhow, M., De Mejia, E.G., 2020. Glucosinolate-rich hydrolyzed extract from *Moringa oleifera* leaves decreased the production of TNF-α and IL-1β cytokines and induced ROS and apoptosis in human colon cancer cells. J. Funct. Foods 75, 104270. doi:10.1016/j.jff.2020.104270.

Darvin, M.E., Sterry, W., Lademann, J., Vergou, T., 2011. The role of carotenoids in human skin. Molecules 16 (12), 10491–10506. doi:10.3390/molecules161210491.

De Souza Guedes, L., Martinez, R.M., Bou-Chacra, N.A., Velasco, M.V.R., Rosado, C., Baby, A.R., 2021. An overview on topical administration of carotenoids and coenzyme Q10 loaded in lipid nanoparticles. Antioxidants 10 (7), 1034. doi:10.3390/antiox10071034.

Di Mascio, P., Kaiser, S., Sies, H., 1989. Lycopene as the most efficient biological carotenoid singlet oxygen quencher. Arch. Biochem. Biophys. 274 (2), 532–538. doi:10.1016/0003-9861(89)90467-0.

Esteve, M., 2020. Mechanisms underlying biological effects of cruciferous Glucosinolate-Derived Isothiocyanates/Indoles: a focus on metabolic syndrome. Front. Nutr. 7, 1–22. doi:10.3389/fnut.2020.00111.

Fazekas, Z., Gao, D., Saladi, R.N., Lu, Y., Lebwohl, M., Wei, H., 2003. Protective effects of lycopene against ultraviolet B-Induced photodamage. Nutr. Cancer 47 (2), 181–187. doi:10.1207/s15327914nc4702_11.

Finley, J.W., Ip, C., Lisk, D.J., Davis, C.D., Hintze, K.J., Whanger, P.D., 2001. Cancer-protective properties of high-selenium broccoli. J. Agric. Food Chem. 49 (5), 2679–2683. doi:10.1021/jf0014821.

Flieger, J., Raszewska-Famielec, M., Radzikowska-Büchner, E., Flieger, W., 2024. Skin protection by carotenoid pigments. Int. J. Mol. Sci. 25 (3), 1431. doi:10.3390/ijms25031431.

Gill, N., Garg, M., Bansal, R., Sood, S., Muthuraman, A., Bali, M., Sharma, P., 2009. Evaluation of antioxidant and antiulcer potential of *Cucumis sativum* L. seed extract in rats. Asian J. Clin. Nutr. 1 (3), 131–138. doi:10.3923/ajcn.2009.131.138.

Gurib-Fakim, A., 2005. Medicinal plants: traditions of yesterday and drugs of tomorrow. Mol. Aspects Med. 27 (1), 1–93. doi:10.1016/j.mam.2005.07.008.

Halkier, B.A., Gershenzon, J., 2006. Biology and biochemistry of glucosinolates. Annu. Rev. Plant Biol. 57 (1), 303–333. doi:10.1146/annurev.arplant.57.032905.105228.

Heo, H., Madhavan, J., Eun, S., Jung, H., Lee, H., 2021. Pre-Clinical evaluation of proprietary lutein, zeaxanthin, and rosemary formulation for its dermal protective activity in male *Swiss albino* mice. Prev. Nutr. Food Sci. 26 (4), 425–433. doi:10.3746/pnf.2021.26.4.425.

Ignat, I., Volf, I., Popa, V.I., 2010. A critical review of methods for characterisation of polyphenolic compounds in fruits and vegetables. Food Chem. 126 (4), 1821–1835. doi:10.1016/j.foodchem.2010.12.026.

Jeffery, E., Brown, A., Kurilich, A., Keck, A., Matusheski, N., Klein, B., Juvik, J., 2003. Variation in content of bioactive components in broccoli. J. Food Compos. Anal. 16 (3), 323–330. doi:10.1016/s0889-1575(03)00045-0.

Jung, S.K., Lee, K.W., Kim, H.Y., Oh, M.H., Byun, S., Lim, S.H., Heo, Y., Kang, N.J., Bode, A.M., Dong, Z., Lee, H.J., 2010. Myricetin suppresses UVB-induced wrinkle formation and MMP-9 expression by inhibiting Raf. Biochem. Pharmacol. 79 (10), 1455–1461. doi:10.1016/j.bcp.2010.01.004.

Kai, H., Baba, M., Okuyama, T., 2008. Inhibitory effect of *Cucumis sativus* on melanin production in melanoma B16 cells by downregulation of tyrosinase expression. Planta Med. 74 (15), 1785–1788. doi:10.1055/s-0028-1088338.

Kaur, S., Das, M., 2011. Functional foods: an overview. Food Sci. Biotechnol. 20 (4), 861–875. doi:10.1007/s10068-011-0121-7.

Kaur, S., Panghal, A., Garg, M., Mann, S., Khatkar, S.K., Sharma, P., Chhikara, N., 2019. Functional and nutraceutical properties of pumpkin – a review. Nutr. Food Sci. 50 (2), 384–401. doi:10.1108/nfs-05-2019-0143.

Kerns, M.L., Chien, A.L., Kang, S., 2021. A role for NRF2-signaling in the treatment and prevention of solar lentigines. Plast. Reconstr. Surg. 148 (6S), 27S–31S. doi:10.1097/prs.0000000000008783.

Khoo, H., Prasad, K.N., Kong, K., Jiang, Y., Ismail, A., 2011. Carotenoids and their isomers: color pigments in fruits and vegetables. Molecules 16 (2), 1710–1738. doi:10.3390/molecules16021710.

Korkina, L., Kostyuk, V., Potapovich, A., Mayer, W., Talib, N., De Luca, C., 2018. Secondary plant metabolites for sun protective cosmetics: from Pre-Selection to product formulation. Cosmetics 5 (2), 32. doi:10.3390/cosmetics5020032.

Krinsky, N.I., Johnson, E.J., 2005. Carotenoid actions and their relation to health and disease. Mol. Aspects Med. 26 (6), 459–516. doi:10.1016/j.mam.2005.10.001.

Kurina, A.B., Solovieva, A.E., Khrapalova, I.A., Artemyeva, A.M., 2021. Biochemical composition of tomato fruits of various colors. Vavilov J. Genet. Breed. 25 (5), 514–527. doi:10.18699/vj21.058.

Lim, S.H., Jung, S.K., Byun, S., Lee, E.J., Hwang, J.A., Seo, S.G., Kim, Y.A., Yu, J.G., Lee, K.W., Lee, H.J., 2013. Luteolin suppresses UVB-induced photoageing by targeting JNK1 and p90RSK2. J. Cell. Mol. Med. 17 (5), 672–680. doi:10.1111/jcmm.12050.

Liu, J., Mu, T., Sun, H., Fauconnier, M.L., 2019. Optimization of ultrasonic–microwave synergistic extraction of flavonoids from sweet potato leaves by response surface methodology. J. Food Process. Preserv. 43 (5), e13928. doi:10.1111/jfpp.13928.

Llompart, M., Celeiro, M., Dagnac, T., 2019. Microwave-assisted extraction of pharmaceuticals, personal care products and industrial contaminants in the environment. TrAC Trends Anal. Chem. 116, 136–150. doi:10.1016/j.trac.2019.04.029.

Lm, K., Ib, P., Ki, E., 2020. Carrot juice nutritional profile. Probl. Nutr. 89 (1), 86–95. doi:10.24411/0042-8833-2020-10010.

Luca, S.V., Kittl, T., Minceva, M., 2022. Supercritical CO_2 extraction of spices: a systematic study with focus on terpenes and piperamides from black pepper (*Piper nigrum* L.). Food Chem. 406, 135090. doi:10.1016/j.foodchem.2022.135090.

Lutz, M., Fuentes, E., Ávila, F., Alarcón, M., Palomo, I., 2019. Roles of phenolic compounds in the reduction of risk factors of cardiovascular diseases. Molecules 24 (2), 366. doi:10.3390/molecules24020366.

Marić, M., Grassino, A.N., Zhu, Z., Barba, F.J., Brnčić, M., Brnčić, S.R., 2018. An overview of the traditional and innovative approaches for pectin extraction from plant food wastes and by-products: ultrasound-, microwaves-, and enzyme-assisted extraction. Trends Food Sci. Technol. 76, 28–37. doi:10.1016/j.tifs.2018.03.022.

Miao, H., Zeng, W., Wang, J., Zhang, F., Sun, B., Wang, Q., 2021. Improvement of glucosinolates by metabolic engineering in Brassica crops. aBIOTECH 2 (3), 314–329. doi:10.1007/s42994-021-00057-y.

Miean, K.H., Mohamed, S., 2001. Flavonoid (Myricetin, quercetin, kaempferol, luteolin, and apigenin) content of edible tropical plants. J. Agric. Food Chem. 49 (6), 3106–3112. doi:10.1021/jf000892m.

Moreno, D., Carvajal, M., López-Berenguer, C., García-Viguera, C., 2006. Chemical and biological characterisation of nutraceutical compounds of broccoli. J. Pharm. Biomed. Anal. 41 (5), 1508–1522. doi:10.1016/j.jpba.2006.04.003.

Moskwa, J., Bronikowska, M., Socha, K., Markiewicz-Żukowska, R., 2023. Vegetable as a source of bioactive compounds with photoprotective properties: implication in the aging process. Nutrients 15 (16), 3594. doi:10.3390/nu15163594.

Mu, J., Ma, H., Chen, H., Zhang, X., Ye, M., 2021. Luteolin prevents UVB-induced skin photoaging damage by modulating SIRT3/ROS/MAPK signaling: an in vitro and in vivo studies. Front. Pharmacol. 12. doi:10.3389/fphar.2021.728261.

Mukherjee, P.K., Maity, N., Nema, N.K., Sarkar, B.K., 2011. Bioactive compounds from natural resources against skin aging. Phytomedicine 19 (1), 64–73. doi:10.1016/j.phymed.2011.10.003.

Mukherjee, P.K., Nema, N.K., Maity, N., Sarkar, B.K., 2012. Phytochemical and therapeutic potential of cucumber. Fitoterapia 84, 227–236. doi:10.1016/j.fitote.2012.10.003.

Muntafiah, L., Shabrina, B.A., Sulistyowati, D., Asshagab, M.R.N., Jenie, R.I., 2017. Anti-aging activity of *Cucurbita moschata* ethanolic extract towards NIH3T3 fibroblast cells induced by doxorubicin. Indonesian J. Cancer Chemoprevent. 7 (2), 49. doi:10.14499/indonesianjcanchemoprev7iss2pp49-53.

Narbad, A., Rossiter, J.T., 2018. Gut glucosinolate metabolism and isothiocyanate production. Mol. Nutr. Food Res. 62 (18), 1–10. doi:10.1002/mnfr.201700991.

Naureen, Z., Dhuli, K., Donato, K., Aquilanti, B., Velluti, V., Matera, G., Iaconelli, A., Bertelli, M., 2022. Foods of the Mediterranean diet: citrus, cucumber and grape. PubMed 63 (2 Suppl 3), E21–E27. doi:10.15167/2421-4248/jpmh2022.63.2s3.2743.

Nishikimi, M., Fukuyama, R., Minoshima, S., Shimizu, N., Yagi, K., 1994. Cloning and chromosomal mapping of the human nonfunctional gene for L-gulono-gamma-lactone oxidase, the enzyme for L-ascorbic acid biosynthesis missing in man. J. Biol. Chem. 269 (18), 13685–13688. doi:10.1016/s0021-9258(17)36884-9.

Özyürek, M., Bektaşoğlu, B., Güçlü, K., Apak, R., 2009. Measurement of xanthine oxidase inhibition activity of phenolics and flavonoids with a modified cupric reducing antioxidant capacity (CUPRAC) method. Anal. Chim. Acta 636 (1), 42–50. doi:10.1016/j.aca.2009.01.037.

Panja, P., 2017. Green extraction methods of food polyphenols from vegetable materials. Curr. Opin. Food Sci. 23, 173–182. doi:10.1016/j.cofs.2017.11.012.

Pinto, T., Aires, A., Cosme, F., Bacelar, E., Morais, M.C., Oliveira, I., Ferreira-Cardoso, J., Anjos, R., Vilela, A., Gonçalves, B., 2021. Bioactive (poly) phenols, volatile compounds from vegetables, medicinal and aromatic plants. Foods 10 (1), 106. doi:10.3390/foods10010106.

Pullar, J., Carr, A., Vissers, M., 2017. The roles of vitamin C in skin health. Nutrients 9 (8), 866. doi:10.3390/nu9080866.

Redha, A.A., Torquati, L., Langston, F., Nash, G.R., Gidley, M.J., Cozzolino, D., 2023. Determination of glucosinolates and isothiocyanates in glucosinolate-rich vegetables and oilseeds using infrared spectroscopy: a systematic review. Crit. Rev. Food Sci. Nutr. 64 (23), 8248–8264. doi:10.1080/10408398.2023.2198015.

Rifna, E.J., Misra, N.N., Dwivedi, M., 2021. Recent advances in extraction technologies for recovery of bioactive compounds derived from fruit and vegetable waste peels: a review. Crit. Rev. Food Sci. Nutr. 63 (6), 719–752. doi:10.1080/10408398.2021.1952923.

Rovetto, L.J., Aieta, N.V., 2017. Supercritical carbon dioxide extraction of cannabinoids from *Cannabis sativa* L. J. Supercrit. Fluids 129, 16–27. doi:10.1016/j.supflu.2017.03.014.

Ruiz-Alcaraz, A.J., Martínez-Sánchez, M.A., García-Peñarrubia, P., Martinez-Esparza, M., Ramos-Molina, B., Moreno, D.A., 2022. Analysis of the anti-inflammatory potential of Brassica bioactive compounds in a human macrophage-like cell model derived from HL-60 cells. Biomed. Pharmacother. 149, 112804. doi:10.1016/j.biopha.2022.112804.

Sánchez-Moreno, C., 2002. Polyphenolic compounds: structure and classification. Presence in food and consumption. Bioavailability and metabolism. http://pascal-francis.inist.fr/vibad/index.php?action=getRecordDetail&idt=13459879.

Scalbert, A., Johnson, I.T., Saltmarsh, M., 2005. Polyphenols: antioxidants and beyond. Am. J. Clin. Nutr. 81 (1), 215S–217S. doi:10.1093/ajcn/81.1.215s.

Shin, E.J., Lee, J.S., Hong, S., Lim, T., Byun, S., 2019. Quercetin directly targets JAK2 and PKCΔ and prevents UV-Induced photoaging in human skin. Int. J. Mol. Sci. 20 (21), 5262. doi:10.3390/ijms20215262.

Singh, S., Lohani, A., Mishra, A.K., Verma, A., 2018. Formulation and evaluation of carrot seed oil-based cosmetic emulsions. J. Cosmet. Laser Ther. 21 (2), 99–107. doi:10.1080/14764172.2018.14697694.

Sotiroudis, G., Melliou, E., Sotiroudis, T.G., Chinou, I., 2010. Chemical analysis, antioxidant and antimicrobial activity of three Greek cucumber (*Cucumis sativus*) cultivars. J. Food Biochem. 34, 61–78. doi:10.1111/j.1745-4514.2009.00296.x.

Stahl, W., Heinrich, U., Aust, O., Tronnier, H., Sies, H., 2005. Lycopene-rich products and dietary photoprotection. Photochem. Photobiol. Sci. 5 (2), 238–242. doi:10.1039/b505312a.

Stahl, W., Sies, H., 2012. β-Carotene and other carotenoids in protection from sunlight. Am. J. Clin. Nutr. 96 (5), 1179S–1184S. doi:10.3945/ajcn.112.034819.

Stanescu, C., Chiscop, I., Mihalache, D., Popa, F., Tamas, C., Stoleriu, G., 2025. Skin aging and carotenoids: a Systematic review of their multifaceted protective mechanisms. Nutrients 17 (16), 2596. doi:10.3390/nu17162596.

Sun, G., Wang, J., Xu, X., Zhai, L., Li, Z., Liu, J., Zhao, D., Jiang, R., Sun, L., 2022. Panax ginseng Meyer cv. silvatica phenolic acids protect DNA from oxidative damage by activating Nrf2 to protect HFF-1 cells from UVA-induced photoaging. J. Ethnopharmacol. 302, 115883. doi:10.1016/j.jep.2022.115883.

Talalay, P., Fahey, J.W., Healy, Z.R., Wehage, S.L., Benedict, A.L., Min, C., Dinkova-Kostova, A.T., 2007. Sulforaphane mobilizes cellular defenses that protect skin against damage by UV radiation. Proc. Natl. Acad. Sci. U. S. A. 104 (44), 17500–17505. doi:10.1073/pnas.0708710104.

Teixeira, J., Gaspar, A., Garrido, E.M., Garrido, J., Borges, F., 2013. Hydroxycinnamic acid antioxidants: an electrochemical overview. Biomed Res. Int. 2013, 1–11. doi:10.1155/2013/251754.

Valisakkagari, H., Chaturvedi, C., Rupasinghe, H.P.V., 2024. Green extraction of phytochemicals from fresh vegetable waste and their potential application as cosmeceuticals for skin health. Processes 12 (4), 742. doi:10.3390/pr12040742.

Vinatoru, M., Mason, T., Calinescu, I., 2017. Ultrasonically assisted extraction (UAE) and microwave assisted extraction (MAE) of functional compounds from plant materials. TrAC Trends Anal. Chem. 97, 159–178. doi:10.1016/j.trac.2017.09.002.

Wertz, K., Seifert, N., Hunziker, P.B., Riss, G., Wyss, A., Lankin, C., Goralczyk, R., 2004. β-carotene inhibits UVA-induced matrix metalloprotease 1 and 10 expression in keratinocytes by a singlet oxygen-dependent mechanism. Free Radic. Biol. Med. 37 (5), 654–670. doi:10.1016/j.freeradbiomed.2004.05.018.

Zandi, P., Schnug, E., 2022. Reactive oxygen species, antioxidant responses and implications from a microbial modulation perspective. Biology 11 (2), 155. doi:10.3390/biology11020155.

Zhi, Q., Lei, L., Li, F., Zhao, J., Yin, R., Ming, J., 2019. The anthocyanin extracts from purple-fleshed sweet potato exhibited anti-photoaging effects on ultraviolent B-irradiated BALB/c-nu mouse skin. J. Funct. Foods 64, 103640. doi:10.1016/j.jff.2019.103640.

Zin, M.M., Anucha, C.B., Bánvölgyi, S., 2020. Recovery of phytochemicals via electromagnetic irradiation (microwave-assisted-extraction): betalain and phenolic compounds in perspective. Foods 9 (7), 918. doi:10.3390/foods9070918.

Chapter 11

Fruits and fruit by-products

Stefanos Michailidis, Theodora Adamantidi, Eleni Kourmazou, Anna Ofrydopoulou, and Alexandros Tsoupras
Hephaestus Laboratory, School of Chemistry, Faculty of Sciences, Democritus University of Thrace, Kavala University Campus, Kavala, Greece

1 Introduction

Since the latter half of the 20th century, the overexploitation of natural resources has become a critical environmental and social challenge, driven by industrial growth, population expansion, consumerism, and the pursuit of continuous economic growth. In response, the rising demand for sustainable, naturally derived cosmetic ingredients presents an opportunity to valorize fruit by-products, readily available resources often discarded by both the food and agricultural industries. Their utilization not only supports the development of innovative, functional products but also reduces industrial waste and generates significant economic and environmental benefits. Rich in enzymes and bioactive compounds, these by-products represent valuable alternatives for cosmetic applications, fully aligned with the principles of green chemistry and the circular economy (Lee and Hyun, 2023; Bom et al., 2019).

One of the sectors characterized by both high waste generation and strong valorization potential is the fruit juice industry, as it holds a pivotal role in the global economy, yet comes with significant environmental complications. Fruit processing for juice production generates substantial amounts of organic residues such as peels, seeds, fibers, pomace, pulp, and wastewater, which are often discarded, accounting for an estimated 0.5 billion tons of waste annually (Argun et al., 2025; Kandemir et al., 2022).

Apples naturally stand out as one of the most widely consumed fruits worldwide, since they are highly adaptable and easily accessible (Oyenihi et al., 2022; Perussello et al., 2017). Their popularity has grown rapidly, and global apple cultivation now represents an industry valued at over $10 billion (Zabetakis et al., 2023; Oyenihi et al., 2022; Tsoupras et al., 2024b). Although apple pomace is often regarded as waste, it constitutes a valuable reservoir of bioactives. Several studies have explored its use as a functional ingredient or substrate in food products, while recently, attention has shifted toward its application within the cosmeceutical industry due to its richness in skin-beneficial polyphenols, vitamins, and natural acids (Zabetakis et al., 2023; Vandorou et al., 2024; Gumul et al., 2023; Gorjanović et al., 2020; Zlatanović et al., 2019).

Avocados (*Persea americana*) and their by-products are rich in bioactive agents, offering significant potential for the development of cosmetic formulations with diverse functional benefits. Notably, the peel and seed contain higher concentrations of phenolic compounds compared to the pulp, with avocado peel extracts exceeding the phenolic levels of seed extracts (Marra et al., 2024, 2025). Over 3 million tons of avocados are produced annually, with only the pulp typically consumed, leaving seeds and peel (21%–30% of the raw material) as waste. Exploiting these phytochemical-rich by-products could enhance the value of the avocado industry and promote the development of more sustainable, high-value cosmetic ingredients (Bhuyan et al., 2019; Segovia et al., 2018; Mora-Sandí et al., 2021). In addition, the pineapple plant (*Ananas comosus*) is another promising bioactive source, particularly the enzyme bromelain, found in the fruit, stem, leaves, core, crown, root, and peel (Lau et al., 2021; Ali et al., 2020; Abbas et al., 2021). Similarly, the fig (*Ficus carica* L.) produces a milky latex containing ficin, an enzyme present in the unripe fruit, leaves, stem, bark, root, and peels (Venetikidou et al., 2025; Gagaoua et al., 2014; Ayuso et al., 2022). Furthermore, papaya (*Carica papaya*) latex contains papain, obtained from unripe fruit, peels, and leaves. In both fig and papaya, the latex exhibits the highest proteolytic activity, making these enzymes particularly valuable in exfoliating and regenerative cosmetic formulations (Venetikidou et al., 2025; Choudhary et al., 2025).

Grapes are another key fruit crop, with an annual production exceeding 70 million tons, generating around 20 million tons of winemaking by-products (~30% of the total vinified grapes) (Bordiga et al., 2019). Grape pomace and seed oil offer sustainable, eco-friendly resources rich in phenolics, proteins, and lipids such as unsaturated fatty acids

Biofunctional Cosmetics for Health. https://doi.org/10.1016/B978-0-443-27500-5.00011-3

(UFAs), polar lipids (PLs), and carotenoids (Tsiapali et al., 2025b). The valorization of enological by-products is crucial, especially considering the seven million tons of grape pomace discarded annually (Bordiga et al., 2019; Tsiapali et al., 2025b). In addition, kiwi (*Actinidiaceae* family) production has also increased globally, leading to large amounts of biowaste, including leaves, peels, and seeds, nutrient-dense materials often combined as kiwi pomace (Lau et al., 2021). Importantly, industrial kiwi processing generates roughly one million tons of by-products annually, representing a significant opportunity for extracting antioxidants and vitamins for skincare applications (Moysidou et al., 2024, 2025; Chamorro et al., 2022; Dias et al., 2020). Tomato (*Solanum lycopersicum*) extracts are a valuable natural source due to their high lycopene content, which is a potent antioxidant with photoprotective properties. Their incorporation into sunscreens and antiaging products aligns with circular economy practices and supports sustainable innovation in the cosmetic industry (Kontaxi et al., 2024; Butnariu and Giuchici, 2011). Similarly, pomegranate (*Punica granatum*) by-products, such as peels, seeds, and membranes, are rich in punicalagins, ellagic acid, and anthocyanins, offering strong antioxidant, antiinflammatory, and antiaging effects that make them ideal for skin-rejuvenating cosmetics (Sarkar et al., 2024; Siddiqui et al., 2024).

Recent research has focused on developing green extraction technologies to efficiently recover these high-value agents while maintaining environmental and economic sustainability. Techniques such as subcritical water extraction (SWE), ultrasound-assisted extraction (UAE), microwave-assisted extraction (MAE), and enzyme-assisted extraction (EAE) have exhibited superior yields and selectivity compared to conventional solvent extraction, enabling the recovery of thermolabile phenolics, carotenoids, vitamins, and proteolytic enzymes with minimal degradation (Ganjeh et al., 2025; Bitwell et al., 2023). For example, ethanol and SWE from apple pomace efficiently isolate polyphenols (Yilmaz-Turan et al., 2023; da Silva et al., 2021), while pressurized liquid extraction (PLE) and biphasic systems from avocado by-products may yield phenolics, carotenoids, and phospholipid bioactives with remarkable antiinflammatory and antioxidant potential (Muhammad et al., 2024). Similarly, enzymes such as bromelain, ficin, and papain, extracted via aqueous two-phase or chromatographic methods, exemplify the shift toward more sustainable bioprocesses in cosmeceutical development (Venetikidou et al., 2025), while grape and other winemaking by-products have also been investigated as valuable sources of bioactives (Bordiga et al., 2019; Tsiapali et al., 2025b). Kiwi by-products, including peels and seeds, are rich in vitamin C, polyphenols, and essential fatty acids that promote collagen synthesis and skin elasticity (Wang et al., 2021b), whereas tomato extracts, abundant in lycopene and β-carotene, exhibit exceptional antioxidant and photoprotective effects, making them suitable for antiaging and ultraviolet (UV)-protection formulations (Szabo et al., 2025). Moreover, pomegranate extracts obtained from peel and seed oils and residues demonstrate remarkable free-radical scavenging capacity and natural pigmentation potential, leading to the creation of antioxidant-rich, complexion-enhancing cosmetic formulations (Sarkar et al., 2024; Siddiqui et al., 2024).

Fruit-derived compounds, such as resveratrol, flavanols, lycopene, vitamins C and E, and ursolic acid (UA), as well as nutrients like dietary fibers, proteins, and polyphenols, exhibit notable antioxidant, antiaging, antiinflammatory, photoprotective, and antimicrobial properties, making them ideal for cosmetic products that enhance skin hydration, elasticity, and regeneration, often alleviating skin-related conditions. Despite formulation challenges related to stability and bioavailability, fruit-derived bioactives are widely recognized for their nutritional value and capacity to enhance both skin health and appearance. Their multifunctionality makes them ideal candidates for the creation of next-generation natural, eco-conscious formulations that combine efficacy with sustainability (Kandemir et al., 2022; Oyenihi et al., 2022; Marra et al., 2024; Venetikidou et al., 2025; Moysidou et al., 2024; Kontaxi et al., 2024; Szabo et al., 2025). This review focuses on the extraction methods, bioactive profiles, cosmetic effects, and applications of apple, avocado, pineapple, fig, papain, grape, kiwi, tomato, and pomegranate fruit-derived bioactives, also discussing their suitability and limitations toward future cosmetic product formulations like creams, serums, shampoos, natural exfoliants, sunscreens, and masks. The main key points of this research are presented in Fig. 11.1.

2 Extraction methods for bioactives from fruit by-products and factors affecting the extraction yield

The extraction of bioactives from fruit by-products has become an essential step in creating natural and sustainable cosmetic ingredients. Instead of relying on harsh chemical solvents, researchers and cosmetic formulators are increasingly turning to green extraction technologies such as UAE, MAE, EAE, PLE, supercritical fluid extraction (SFE), and SWE. These modern approaches help preserve delicate molecules like polyphenols, carotenoids, vitamins, and natural pigments that are easily degraded by heat or chemicals. For instance, UAE and MAE offer shorter extraction times and improved efficiency, while EAE gently releases antioxidant and moisturizing agents from fruit peels, pomace, and seeds, compounds highly valued for their skin-repairing and antiaging properties (Vandorou et al., 2024; Marra et al., 2024; Ali et al., 2020; Venetikidou et al., 2025; Ayuso et al., 2022; Moysidou et al., 2024; Szabo et al., 2025; García et al., 2021; Cejudo-Bastante et al., 2021).

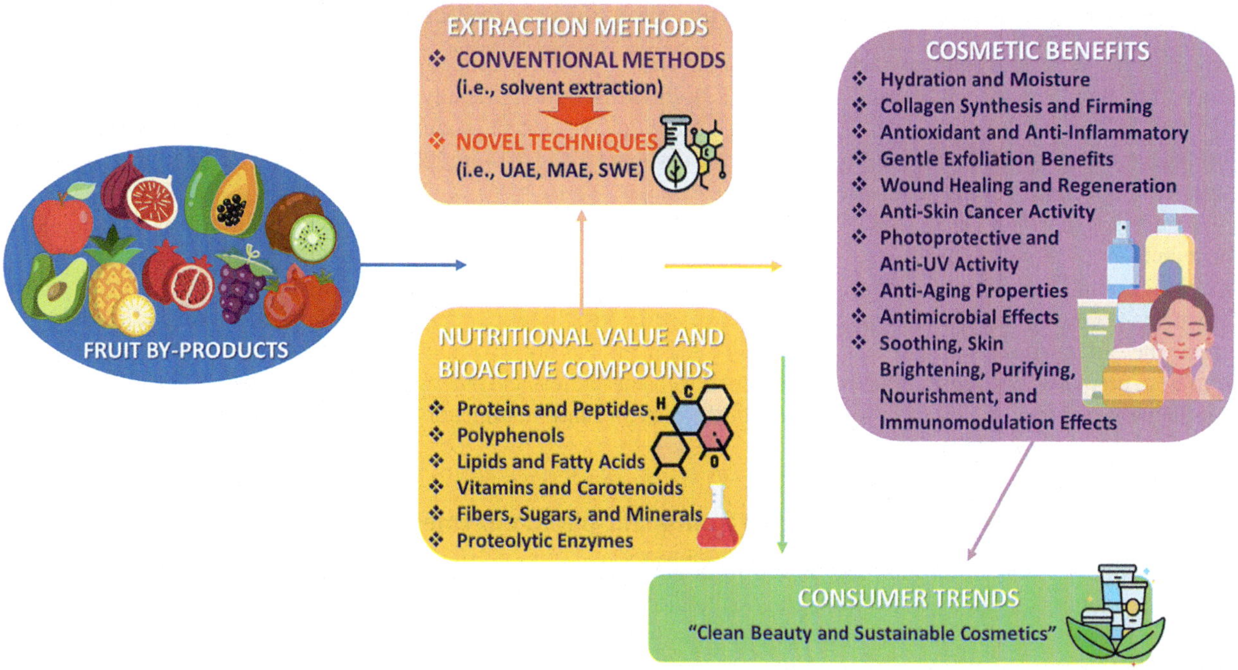

FIG. 11.1 Fruit bioactive extraction methods, pharmacological properties, and cosmetic applications. *(Parts of this figure were obtained from the open access free online platform https://www.flaticon.com/ (Accessed on September 23, 2025).)*

The success of these extraction processes depends on several factors. The type of solvent, temperature, extraction time, particle size, and even the ratio of solid material to solvent can greatly affect both the yield and quality of the recovered compounds (Singh et al., 2025; Mungwari et al., 2025). Equally important is the structure of the fruit matrix itself. Fibrous peels or dense seeds may require more intense or tailored methods to efficiently release bioactives. By fine-tuning these conditions and using eco-friendly solvents, such as ethanol or water, it becomes possible to obtain extracts rich in antioxidants, vitamins, and natural emollients that support skin hydration, protection, and rejuvenation. The move toward greener, more efficient extraction not only enhances the value of fruit by-products but also supports a circular approach to cosmetic innovation (Singh et al., 2025; Mungwari et al., 2025).

2.1 Extraction of bioactive compounds from apple by-products

Apple pomace contains numerous polar phenolics that can be effectively extracted using organic solvents like ethanol and methanol. However, several green and sustainable extraction methods, including EAE, MAE, and UAE, as well as conventional maceration, have also been successfully applied. To ensure safety and applicability in cosmetic formulations, food-grade solvents (ethanol and water) are preferred for extracting such microconstituents (Perussello et al., 2017; da Silva et al., 2021; Zhang et al., 2018).

Recent studies have compared ethanol solvent extraction and SWE for recovering apple pomace polyphenols, evaluating different apple parts such as the core, pulp, peel, seed, and stem. These findings highlight apple pomace as an abundant reservoir of polyphenolics with significant biomedical and cosmetic potential. Among the extracted fractions, apple pomace SWE extracts exhibited antioxidant activity comparable to ascorbic acid and ethanolic extracts and showed excellent biocompatibility with human fibroblast (3T3-L1) and salivary gland acinar cells (NS-SV-AC) (Perussello et al., 2017; da Silva et al., 2021; Zhang et al., 2018).

Nevertheless, further research is required to optimize eco-friendly extraction approaches directly on pomace, ensuring high yield and reduced environmental risk (Martins et al., 2023). Notably, the extraction solvent plays a crucial role: ethanol extracts from Arisoo apples yielded higher phenolic content and stronger bioactivity compared to water extracts, demonstrating superior antiwrinkle efficacy over Fuji apples. This suggests that Arisoo extracts may serve as highly promising antiaging cosmetic functional additives (Cho et al., 2019). Likewise, water and ethanol extracts of "Summer King" apples significantly inhibited elastase and collagenase, key enzymes in skin aging. Water extracts achieved 14.55% and 67.73% inhibition, while ethanol extracts reached 56.50% and 77.81%, respectively, confirming their value as natural antiwrinkle agents (Lee et al., 2020).

2.2 Extraction of bioactive compounds from avocado by-products

Avocado oil and bioactives are extracted from the pulp and by-products through various methods, though results often vary depending on processing conditions (Liu et al., 2023). Environmentally friendly extraction approaches have proven highly effective. In a recent study, a PLE extraction using a green solvent system produced phenolic-rich extracts with remarkable antioxidant capacity [3350 μmol Trolox equivalent/g dry extract and 0.14 μg/mL in ABTS and oxygen radical absorbance capacity (ORAC) assays] (Grisales-Mejía et al., 2024).

Tsoupras et al. (Marra et al., 2024, 2025) developed a sustainable lipid extraction protocol using a single-phase chloroform/methanol/water (1:2:0.8 v/v/v) system, followed by biphasic fractionation, yielding total amphiphilic compounds and lipophilic compounds. These fractions, rich in amphiphilic polar lipids (PLs), monounsaturated fatty acids, polyunsaturated fatty acids (PUFAs), carotenoids, and phenolics, exhibited potent antiinflammatory, antithrombotic, and antioxidant properties. The synergistic presence of PLs, carotenoids, and phenolics not only inhibits oxidative stress but also protects UFAs from lipid peroxidation. These findings underscore the cosmeceutical and pharmaceutical potential of avocado by-products as sustainable sources of bioactives with strong antioxidant and antiinflammatory activities, aligning with circular economy principles (Marra et al., 2024, 2025).

2.3 Extraction of bioactive compounds from plant-based enzymes

The extraction of bromelain, ficin, and papain from pineapple, fig, and papaya by-products, respectively, illustrates the circular economy concept by transforming agricultural residues into valuable bioactives through eco-friendly extraction methods. Bromelain, derived from pineapple fruit and stem, can be purified using various conventional and advanced methods to maintain high enzymatic activity. Conventional techniques include homogenization, ultrafiltration, and centrifugation, while innovative green techniques, such as aqueous two-phase systems (ATPS), reverse micellar extraction (RME), and ion exchange chromatography, have demonstrated enhanced selectivity, yield, and enzyme stability. Additional sustainable approaches, like polysaccharide precipitation (e.g., with carrageenan), membrane filtration, and MAE or UAE, are increasingly adopted to improve enzyme recovery and purity. However, issues such as salt accumulation, high cost, enzyme instability, and membrane fouling remain key limitations, requiring optimization for industrial scalability (Abbas et al., 2021; Venetikidou et al., 2025; Varilla et al., 2021; Colletti et al., 2021; Chakraborty et al., 2021; Krishna et al., 2002; Mala et al., 2021; Kaushal et al., 2024; Alara et al., 2021; Masbagusdanta et al., 2020).

Ficin, found in the latex, stem, roots, leaves, unripe fruit residues, and bark of *F. carica*, exhibits potent proteolytic activity (up to 209,000 units/mg) (Gagaoua et al., 2014; Ayuso et al., 2022; Milošević et al., 2020). Extraction typically involves latex collection, mechanical homogenization, and ultrafiltration (Gagaoua et al., 2014; Raskovic et al., 2014). Three-phase partitioning (TPP) using ammonium sulfate and tert-butanol is favored for its simplicity, cost-effectiveness, and high-enzyme recovery (Gagaoua et al., 2014; Raskovic et al., 2014; Homaei et al., 2017; Qurashi and Jabbar, 2022; Łubek-Nguyen et al., 2022). Chromatographic and membrane-based methods, like ion exchange chromatography [sulfopropyl (SP)-Sepharose] and ultrafiltration, are also used for high-purity recovery. Nevertheless, challenges such as enzyme oxidation, environmental sensitivity, and concentration variability persist (Homaei et al., 2017; Yang et al., 2017; Zare et al., 2013; Dini et al., 2021). Furthermore, papain, the main protease from *C. papaya*, is primarily extracted from unripe fruit latex or leaves (Venetikidou et al., 2025; Di Giacomo et al., 2022). Extraction involves latex collection, drying, homogenization, and filtration, whereas purification methods include ATPS, TPP, precipitation (using salts or organic solvents), and chromatographic separation, each offering varying levels of purity and yield (Di Giacomo et al., 2022; Babalola et al., 2023; Ayodipupo Babalola et al., 2024; Hafid et al., 2020; Lei et al., 2019). Emerging green techniques, including micellar systems with biodegradable surfactants, MAE, EAE, UAE, RME, and SFE, have shown promise in improving enzyme activity recovery while minimizing environmental impact (Alara et al., 2021; Yulirohyami and Wijaya, 2022; Biswas et al., 2023; Lin et al., 2017; Chai et al., 2020). Despite these advancements, challenges related to enzyme instability, seasonal variability, and limited clinical data persist, highlighting the need for improved standardization and comparative studies (Di Giacomo et al., 2022; Arshad et al., 2014).

2.4 Extraction of bioactive compounds from winemaking and grape by-products

Grape and winemaking residues represent rich, underutilized sources of polyphenols, flavonoids, and fatty acids. Optimizing extraction parameters is key to maximizing bioactive recovery. Among available technologies, SFE has shown superior efficacy compared to traditional solvent-based techniques, requiring fewer solvents, reducing processing time, and aligning with sustainability goals (Cejudo-Bastante et al., 2021; Otero-Pareja et al., 2015; Ferri et al., 2020; Oliveira et al., 2013).

Other advanced approaches, such as MAE, UAE, and EAE, are widely adopted for their high extraction efficacy, lower energy consumption, and ability to preserve thermolabile compounds (Biswas et al., 2023; Marinaccio et al., 2025; Bruno Romanini et al., 2021; Poblete et al., 2025).

Solid–liquid extraction remains the most established and scalable method. However, its long processing time and high solvent use limit sustainability. In contrast, UAE and MAE offer rapid extraction, though they demand careful control of parameters such as solvent polarity, temperature, and ultrasound intensity to ensure reproducibility and yield (Tsiapali et al., 2025b; Biswas et al., 2023; Otero-Pareja et al., 2015; Bruno Romanini et al., 2021). Finally, the need for environmentally friendly extractions has led to the increased study of EAE techniques (Sopyan et al., 2017). EAE represents a particularly promising green technology, enabling selective extraction of phenolics under mild conditions, while minimizing solvent requirements. Yet, its higher cost and limited scalability remain significant barriers (Poblete et al., 2025). Combining multiple eco-friendly extraction methods can enhance efficiency and promote the sustainable recovery of grape bioactives for cosmetic and dermatological applications (Da Porto et al., 2015).

2.5 Extraction of bioactive compounds from kiwi by-products

Kiwi (*Actinidia deliciosa*) pomace, peels, and seeds contain vitamin C, phenolic acids, flavonoids, and essential fatty acids, all contributing to strong antioxidant and regenerative properties. Extraction methods such as UAE, often optimized with RSM, MAE, and PLE, have been the most widely reported green techniques, delivering high total phenolic content (TPC) and strong antioxidant action in short processing times compared with studies on extracts derived by conventional maceration or ultrasound assisted extraction (UAE) on kiwi peel that have demonstrated improved yield and antioxidant capacity when tuning parameters (time: 14.8 min, power: 94.4 W, and ethanol concentration: 68.4%) via RSM, making UAE a time-saving, nonthermal, and scalable option for cosmetic ingredients and resulting in a maximum of 1.51 ± 0.04 mg of flavonoids (pre/g extract) (Giordano et al., 2021). PLE, including SWE and deep eutectic solvents (DES)/UAE hybrid methods, has also revealed promise for selective recovery of thermolabile vitamins and lipophilic seed oils (Silva et al., 2023; Guthrie et al., 2020; Wu et al., 2023).

2.6 Extraction of bioactive compounds from tomato by-products

Tomato (*S. lycopersicum*) industrial by-products (peels and seeds) are principally exploited for lycopene, β-carotene, tocopherols, and phenolics. Supercritical CO_2 (SC-CO_2) extraction is the leading green technology for carotenoid recovery (Trombino et al., 2021), providing high-purity lycopene oleoresins with extraction yields reported in the literature in the range of ~30%–60% (process-dependent) and excellent stability for cosmetic use. Maximum lycopene yield was obtained at 80°C, 50 MPa, and a 70/30 peel/seeds ratio (Hatami et al., 2019). UAE and pulsed-UAE, often with food-grade ethanol, natural deep eutectic solvents (NADES), or edible cosolvents, have also been shown to substantially increase lycopene and pectin yields versus conventional stirring, while preserving antioxidant activity (Marinaccio et al., 2024). Recent comparative studies confirm UAE and SC-CO_2 as complementary routes, as UAE may offer fast and lower-cost recovery, while SC-CO_2 can be exploited for its high-purity, solvent-free extract profile, suitable for topical formulations (Aniceto et al., 2022). Microencapsulation of SC-CO_2 lycopene extracts further improves stability and skin delivery in cosmetic matrices (Marinaccio et al., 2024; Mihalcea et al., 2021).

2.7 Extraction of bioactive compounds from pomegranate by-products

Pomegranate (*P. granatum*) peel, inner carpellar membrane, and seed by-products are the primary sources of pomegranate polyphenols (e.g., punicalagin, ellagic acid), anthocyanins, and tannins. Green extraction approaches, including UAE, MAE, EAE (Cano-Lamadrid et al., 2022), pressurized hot water extraction (PHWE) (Çam and Hışıl, 2010), and NADES use (usually applied in combination with UAE or PLE) (Bertolo et al., 2021; Oliveira et al., 2024), consistently outperform traditional solvent extraction in TPC, antioxidant capacity, yield, and extraction speed. Systematic reviews and experimental assays report that optimized UAE/MAE protocols (with aqueous-ethanol or DES solvent mixtures) deliver notably higher punicalagin and TPC recovery with lower solvent consumption (Bertolo et al., 2021; Ballistreri et al., 2024; Patil et al., 2024). Moreover, under the optimal conditions of 200°C and 77% ethanol, dry powdered pomegranate peel and seeds revealed effective release of polyphenols and decreased extraction times (García et al., 2021).

EAE technique may selectively enhance the release of bound peptides, antioxidant activity, and extraction yield when applied to pomegranate peel and seeds (40°C–55°C) (Patil et al., 2024; Kumar et al., 2020). Scale-up and techno-economic studies remain limited, but the available evidence supports UAE/MAE and PHWE/SFE as the most promising green strategies for cosmetic applications (Ballistreri et al., 2024; Patil et al., 2024). Finally, PLE and SWE have been pointed out as great green alternative methods for the extraction of polyphenols from pomegranate waste (García et al., 2021). Table 11.1 presents indicative examples of several extraction methods used for each fruit analyzed in this research, highlighting the main research outcomes and the efficacy of the methods.

3 Bioactive and health-promoting constituents in fruit by-products: Main bioactives found in fruits and their beneficial properties

3.1 Bioactive and health-promoting constituents in apple by-products

Apples contain several essential macro- and micronutrients, namely, carbohydrates, minerals, and vitamins. Among apple-derived waste materials, apple pomace represents the primary by-product of apple processing, consisting of the calyx, core, peel, seeds, and stem, as well as processed soft tissue such as the mesocarp. This composition makes it a diverse mixture of apple constituents. It is a high-value fraction of the food industry, exhibiting numerous health-promoting effects that should be recovered and valorized rather than treated as waste. Although factors such as apple cultivar, pedoclimatic conditions, maturity stage, and processing methods may influence the physicochemical composition of apple pomace, it remains a rich source of macronutrients and bioactive compounds. Apple pomace encompasses bioactives like fibers, minerals, polysaccharides, lipid bioactives, polyphenols, vitamins, triterpenes, and pigments, well-known for their antioxidant and antiinflammatory benefits (Perussello et al., 2017; Tsoupras et al., 2024b; Vandorou et al., 2024, 2025).

Apple pomace contains simple soluble sugars, including fructose, glucose, and galactose (~23%, 22%, and 6%–15%, respectively), accounting for approximately 45.1%–83.8% of total carbohydrates on a dry basis (Lyu et al., 2020). It also provides significant amounts of dietary fibers (up to 65% on a dry basis), most of which are insoluble, namely, cellulose, hemicellulose, and lignin. Among these, cellulose predominates (~43%), followed by hemicellulose (~20%–32%) (Lyu et al., 2020; Szabo et al., 2022). The presence of apple seeds in pomace further contributes to its high nutritional value, as they contain remarkable amounts of proteins and lipids (~49% and 24%, respectively) (Lyu et al., 2020; Szabo et al., 2022). Moreover, apple pomace is also a vital source of microconstituents, such as polyphenols, carotenoids, and phytosterols, containing several lipid bioactives, polar phenols, and tocopherols. These macro- and microconstituents play crucial roles in human metabolism and have been associated with numerous health-promoting properties, including anticancer, antihistaminic, antiinflammatory, antioxidant, antitumor, and antithrombotic benefits. The concentration of bioactives varies depending on the apple variety, growing conditions, maturity stage, and the applied production or extraction method (Vandorou et al., 2024, 2025; Feng et al., 2021; Tsoupras et al., 2021).

Importantly, apple pomace is rich in polar phenolic compounds, mainly tannins (Lyu et al., 2020; Szabo et al., 2022). The peels are the main source of these phenolics, meaning that apple pomace often contains higher amounts of such compounds compared to the whole fruit (Barreira et al., 2019). The principal polyphenols found in apple pomace, namely, flavanols, dihydrochalcones, quercetin glycosides, and phloridzin, exhibit potent antioxidant activity and effectively inhibit reactive oxygen species (ROS), thereby interrupting free radical chain reactions, particularly those involved in lipid peroxidation (Zabetakis et al., 2023; Lyu et al., 2020). Some of the main bioactives detected in apple by-products, namely, caffeic acid, quercetin-3-glucoside, gallic acid, rutin, quercetin-3-*O*-galactoside, epicatechin, cyanidin-3-galactoside, and chlorogenic acid, have shown vital antidiabetic, antimicrobial, antiinflammatory, antioxidant, antitumor, and cardioprotective effects by scavenging ROS, inhibiting oxidative DNA damage, and blocking platelet-activating factor (PAF)- and thrombin-mediated signaling. By such mechanisms, apple phenolics modulate key molecular targets, including the nuclear factor κB (NF-κB), nuclear factor erythroid 2-related factor 2, and aryl hydrocarbon receptor factors, promoting the upregulation of antioxidant defense mechanisms (Vandorou et al., 2024, 2025; Feng et al., 2021; Tsoupras et al., 2021).

Consequently, the polyphenolic profile of apple pomace highlights its vast potential for incorporation into cosmeceutical and dermatological formulations, where its bioactives can contribute to oxidative protection, skin repair, and antiaging value (Lyu et al., 2020; Szabo et al., 2022). Fig. 11.2 presents the antioxidant and antiinflammatory actions of phenolic bioactives from apple by-products against oxidative stress and thromboinflammatory signaling linked to aging and chronic disorders.

3.2 Bioactive and health-promoting constituents in avocado by-products

Avocados demonstrate strong antioxidant properties due to their rich composition of secondary metabolites and other active molecules, including flavonoids, phenolics, tannins, tocopherols, fatty alcohols, carotenoids, and anthocyanins. The avocado's by-products (e.g., seed and peel) are concentrated sources of valuable bioactives, often surpassing the levels found

TABLE 11.1 Indicative examples of each extraction method used for fruit by-product bioactive extraction.

Extraction method	Extractant and yield[a]	Conditions	Analysis method	Analytes[a] and method efficacy	References
Sequential UAE of pectin and phenolic compounds from "Granny Smith" apple peel waste	• Acetone 80% in a two-step extraction (phenolic compounds extraction followed by pectin extraction) produces the highest phenolic compound yield (TPC: 3.47 g gallic acid equivalents (GAE)/kg)	• Acetone 80% (0% formic acid concentration) • Pectin was obtained before (BE) and after (AE) phenolic compound extraction, either by conventional (TR) or UAE extraction	• The effect of solvent, formic acid concentration, and the number of extraction steps on individual phenolics, TPC, total flavonoids, and antioxidant capacity was measured using a two-step extraction technique	• Phenolic compounds and pectin recovery are enhanced by UAE in apple peel waste • Procyanidin B2 (0.03–0.77 g/kg) is the main phenolic compound extracted from apple peel waste • AE pectin extraction yield (6.38% for UAE and 4.92% for conventional extraction) was notably higher than BE • Pectin revealed a 57%–60% degree of esterification, 9.3%–10.3% methoxyl content, and 436–460 equivalent weight	(Villamil-Galindo and Piagentini, 2022)
Process optimization of the MAE of bioactives from avocado seeds	• Two experimental designs: one with acetone 70% (TPC: 307.09 ± 14.16 mg GAE/g) and one with ethanol (0%–100%, TPC: 254.40 ± 16.36 mg GAE/g)	• Optimal extraction conditions in the two experimental designs were: 72.18°C for 19.01 min and 71.64°C for 14.69 min, using 70% acetone and 58.51% ethanol, respectively • Two variables were used: temperature and time variables	• Optimal conditions using a central composite design (CCD) for acetone and a Box–Behnken design (BBD) for TPC content, 2,2-diphenyl-1-picrylhydrazyl (DPPH), 2,2′-azino-bis (3-ethylbenzothiazoline-6-sulfonic acid) (ABTS), oxygen radical absorbance capacity (ORAC), and bound phenolic evaluation assays were conducted	• 20 different compounds were identified • Procyanidins (dimer B and trimer A), phenolic acids, catechin, epicatechin, and perseitol are the main compounds found • Higher combinations of bioactives were obtained after method optimization • High antioxidant activity was recorded in both extracts (mainly acetone extracts) • Fiber residues obtained after MAE had bonded phenolics	(Araújo et al., 2020)
UAE of compounds from pineapple peels	• Water, ethanol, or an acid solution of 1 mol/L HCl was tested in different proportions • Ethanol (50%) and acid solution (50%) mixture led to the highest TPC content: 405.06 mg GAE/100 g	• Optimal extraction conditions for the extract with the highest TPC and antioxidant activity were obtained at 60°C, 50 W of ultrasonic power, and 30 min of extraction time	• UAE was carried out under a simplex-centroid design, with different types of solvents, operating conditions (time, temperature, and ultrasonic power), and extract characterizations for the TPC, antioxidant activity, and bioactivity of the peels were conducted	• TPC contents ranged from 219.75 to 405.06 mg GAE/100 g • Under the optimal conditions, the extract revealed high fructose (7.17 g/100 g) and glucose (8.29 g/100 g) as major sugars • Caffeic acid (217.65 mg/100 g) was the major phenolic acid	(Zampar and Zampar, 2022)
Sequential UAE-MAE (UMAE) of pectin from fig skin	• Ethanol (96%) was used as the solvent • Yield: 13.967% of pectin with an average molecular mass of 6.89×10^3 kDa	• Optimal conditions were: 21.35 min sonication time, 580.9 W microwave power, 11.67 min irradiation time, and 24.66 mL/g liquid-to-solid ratio	• The process was based on a second-order polynomial model with a high level of significanceAn acidic hot water extraction method was utilized, along with UMAE, and response surface methodology (RSM) was employed	• Field emission scanning electron microscopy (FE-SEM) and Fourier transform-infrared (FTIR) analysis of the extracted pectin under the optimal conditions revealed a structurally disintegrated network • The low-methoxy pectin (DE: 33.65%), with high lightness, contained notable amounts of uronic acids and glucose, fucose, arabinose, galactose, rhamnose, and mannose neutral monosaccharides • Dose-dependent antioxidant activity and cytotoxic inhibition of pectin were observed against HepG2 and A549 cells	(Gharibzahedi et al., 2019)

Continued

TABLE 11.1 Indicative examples of each extraction method used for fruit by-product bioactive extraction—cont'd

Extraction method	Extractant and yield[a]	Conditions	Analysis method	Analytes[a] and method efficacy	References
SWE compared to Soxhlet extraction of bioactive phenolics from papaya seeds	• Water solvent (green) • SWE revealed the highest yield of 26.3% ± 0.6% (150°C), in contrast to Soxhlet's 15.03% ± 0.01% • TPC: 34.7% ± 0.4% (70°C)—91.6 ± 3.0 mg/GAE g (150°C) for SWE (2.6×), while similar TPC values were reported for Soxhlet at 70°C–90°C	• SWE at 150°C revealed 22 compounds, followed by SWE at 70°C (21) and 110°C (21) • Soxhlet revealed 25 compounds	• The SWE was compared to Soxhlet extraction in terms of total yield, TPC, Maillard reaction products (MRPs), and antioxidant activity efficacy (DPPH and β-carotene bleaching)	• TPC and MRP values were maximized by SWE at 150°C for 5 min (best antioxidant activity, DPPH method)30 compounds were identified within the tested samples, among them ferulic, mandelic, and vanillic acids, utilizing liquid chromatography (LC) • Several phenolic acids, flavonoids, phenolic aldehydes, a stilbene (resveratrol), coumarins, and phenolic diterpenes were primarily found in the extracts	(Gonçalves Rodrigues et al., 2019)
PLE of bioactives from grape peel and application in pH-sensing in carboxymethyl cellulose films	• A hydroethanolic solution (70:30, v/v) was used as the solvent • Nd specific yield or TPC	• Semi-continuous PLE was conducted using this hydroethanolic solution (70:30) at a flow rate of 5 mL/min, 15 MPa, and 60°C	• Semi-continuous PLE was conducted, followed by a casting technique for the CMC films (2.5% w/v), made with glycerol (1% v/v) and functionalized with 10%, 30%, and 50% (v/v) grape peel extract • LC-mass spectroscopy (LC-MS/MS) was also used	• LC-MS/MS revealed that PLE extracted 27 phenolic compounds • Kaempferol-3-glucoside (367.23 ± 25.88 μg/mL), prunin (270.23 ± 3.62 μg/mL), *p*-coumaric acid (236.43 ± 26.02 μg/mL), and procyanidin (117.17 ± 7.29 μg/mL) • CMC films had a color and mechanical profile suitable for packaging applications • Grape peel extract promoted the pH-sensing properties, demonstrating the sensitivity of anthocyanins to pH changes, presented great bioactive release, and exhibited vast color changes linked to the pH of stored food	(Francisco et al., 2024)
UAE-assisted enzymatic extraction (UAEE) of kiwi starch, optimized by the RSM method	• 85% ethanol and several enzymes, including porcine pancreatic α-amylase and lipase, invertase, glucosidase, pectinase, cellulase, and papain, were utilized • Kiwi starch yield was about 4.25%	• Optimal conditions: pectinase-to-cellulase-to-papain ratio of 1:2:1 g/kg, solid-to-liquid ratio of 873.23 mg/g, pH of 5.23, ultrasound power of 300 W, and an extraction temperature of 52°C	• Enzymatic hydrolysis contrast test, single-factor experiment, BBD, SEM, particle size distribution (PSD), X-ray diffraction (XRD), FTIR, pH, transparency, water solubility index (WSI), swelling power (SP), differential scanning calorimetry (DSC), pasting, rheological, gel texture, nutritive content, antioxidant action, and in vitro digestibility evaluation were conducted	• The starch content of kiwi starch was 873.23 mg/g (high UAEE-achieved yield) • UAEE could obtain kiwi starch with high yield and purity under shorter extraction times, using less solvent and enzyme • Low gelatinization enthalpy (8.02 J/g) and high peak viscosity (7933 cP) were found • Kiwi starch is rich in polyphenols, has a high antioxidant action, and encompasses higher amylose starch (30.74%) and resistant starch (60.18%) content	(Wang et al., 2021a)

Supercritical CO_2 extraction (SFE-CO_2) of lycopene and β-carotene, extracted as oleoresins from tomato peels	• Supercritical CO_2 was utilized as the solvent • Relative extraction yields: 32.02%–60.85% for lycopene and 28.38%–58.80% for β-carotene	• Ground (300 μm) and unground tomato peels (1 mm) were subjected to SFE-CO_2 at 50°C, 400 bar, and a 4 g/min flow rate for 105 min (10 g batch)	• The effects of particle size, temperature (50°C, 70°C, and 80°C), pressure (300, 400, and 500 bar), CO_2 flow rate (3, 4, and 6 g/min), and their influence on the antioxidant activity of the extract were the tested parameters	• Recovered oleoresin: 4.86% ± 0.23% was extracted after 10 min of SFE-CO_2 from ground peels, while 3.97% ± 0.45% was extracted after 10 min of SFE-CO_2 from unground tomato peels • Temperature: 4.86% ± 0.23% at 50°C and 6.31% ± 0.13% (higher oleoresins were recovered at 80°C in ground samples) • Pressure: 5.5% ± 0.16% at 500 bar, 4.86% ± 0.23% at 400 bar, and 4.58% ± 0.18% (higher oleoresins at 500 bar, ground samples) • Oleoresins increased with the increase in the flow rate [5.62% ± 0.14% (6 g/min), 4.86% ± 0.23% (4 g/min), and 4.72% ± 0.27% (3 g/min)]	(Kehili et al., 2017)
SFE and preformulation process of pomegranate pericarp polar agents (ellagic acid and punicalagins)	• A hydroalcoholic mixture was used as the solventHigher bioactive agent recovery: 19.59 mg/g	• Optimal conditions: 40°C, 20% ethanol/water (80:20 v/v), for 60 min, 15 MPa, and 3 mL/min (1 g plant)	• The effects of temperature, modifier percentage, and water additive percentage added to the modifier were explored through BBD and extraction kinetics	• SFE is a comparable extraction technique to UAE, offering similar yieldsA screening of alternative solvents using glycine/water (80:20, v/v) allowed the development of an integrated SFE and preformulation of the extract with cosmetic potential, avoiding full evaporation	(Atwi-Ghaddar et al., 2023)

[a]Nd stands for "Not defined." Yield: % and analytes: % of the total content or concentration, if retrievable. The yield is mainly expressed as TPC.

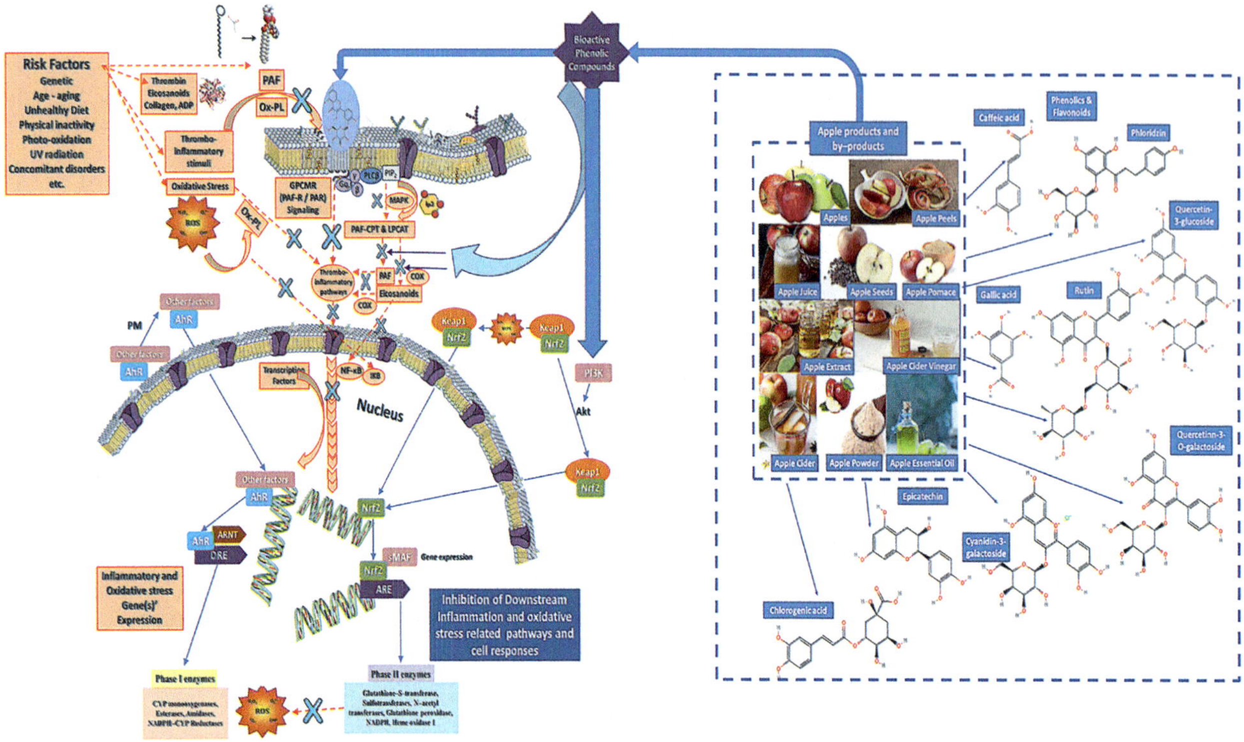

FIG. 11.2 Antioxidant and antiinflammatory mechanisms of phenolic bioactives from apple by-products. Red-labeled elements indicate oxidative stress and thromboinflammatory signaling triggered by aging-related factors (mainly ROS, PAF, and thrombin), while blue-labeled elements denote the inhibitory effects of apple pomace phenolics on ROS generation, oxidative damage, and PAF/thrombin receptor pathways (inhibitory effects are denoted by the blue "X" symbols). These interactions collectively attenuate oxidative stress, inflammation, and thromboinflammatory responses associated with aging and chronic disorders. Ahr, aryl hydrocarbon receptor; *ALA*, α-linolenic acid; *ARE*, antioxidant response element; *ARNT*, aryl hydrocarbon receptor nuclear translocator; *COX*, cyclooxygenase; *cPLA2*, cytoplasmic phospholipase A2; *DRE*, dioxin response element; *GPCMR*, G-protein-coupled membrane receptors; *IKB*, NF-κB inhibitor; *IP*$_3$, inositol trisphosphate; *Keap1*, Kelch-like ECH-associated protein 1; *MAPK*, mitogen-activated protein kinase; *NF-κB*, nuclear factor κB; *OA*, oleic acid; *Ox-PLs*, oxidized polar lipids; *PAF*, platelet-activating factor; *PAF-CPT* and *LPCAT*, PAF-cholinephosphotransferase and lyso-phosphatidylcholine acetyltransferase 2, respectively; *PAF-R*, PAF-receptor; *PAR*, protease-activated receptors for thrombin; *PIP2*, phosphatidylinositol 4,5-bisphosphate; *PLCβ*, phospholipase C β; *ROS*, reactive oxygen species. *(From Vandorou, M., Plakidis, C., Tsompanidou, I.M., Adamantidi, T., Panagopoulou, E.A., Tsoupras, A., 2024. A review on apple pomace bioactives for natural functional food and cosmetic products with therapeutic health-promoting properties. Int. J. Mol. Sci. 1422-0067. 25 (19), 10856. doi:10.3390/ijms251910856.)*

in the edible fruit pulp. These by-products are particularly rich in polyphenols that can be utilized for diverse biological activities, mainly because of their antibacterial, antimicrobial, antiinflammatory, anticarcinogenic, epigenetic, and chemopreventive properties (Marra et al., 2024, 2025; Weremfo et al., 2020).

Avocado by-products (mainly the seed and peel) are exceptionally rich in valuable bioactives, often at higher concentrations than in the edible pulp. They contain several polyphenols, flavonoids, tannins, tocopherols, carotenoids, anthocyanins, and UFAs, all contributing to their remarkable antioxidant, antimicrobial, antiinflammatory, and anticarcinogenic properties (Marra et al., 2024, 2025; Weremfo et al., 2020). Among the key compounds identified are ferulic acid, gallic acid, epicatechin, quercetin, chlorogenic acid, *p*-coumaric acid, β-carotene, lutein, and β-sitosterol, which act synergistically to neutralize free radicals, inhibit lipid peroxidation, and enhance skin barrier integrity. This composition provides notable UV-protective, antiaging, and regenerative benefits, making avocado by-products highly suitable for use in cosmetic and cosmeceutical formulations (Marra et al., 2024, 2025; Siol and Sadowska, 2023; Gonçalves et al., 2024). Fig. 11.3 illustrates the main avocado parts and the associated health benefits of avocado bioactives. Table 11.2 represents their nutritional composition, Table 11.3 includes their proximate phenolic and flavonoid content, and Table 11.4 refers to their antioxidant capacity, resulting from an extended compositional analysis of the constituents of avocado by-products (Marra et al., 2024, 2025; Siol and Sadowska, 2023; Gonçalves et al., 2024).

As demonstrated, avocado by-products hold great value across many key domains. They represent a high-fiber and nutrient-dense resource, particularly rich in insoluble dietary fiber, making them promising candidates for both nutritional and cosmetic formulations. Moreover, they serve as a phytochemical powerhouse, characterized by an abundant and diverse profile of phenolics and flavonoids. The exceptionally high levels of compounds such as benzoic acid, catechins,

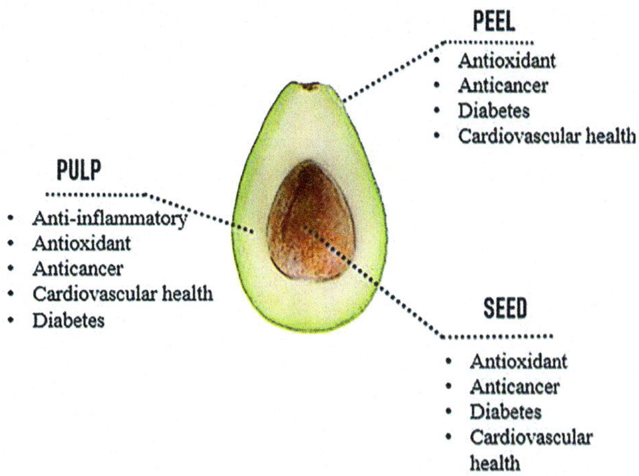

FIG. 11.3 Avocado parts and their associated health-promoting properties. *(From Marra, A., Manousakis, V., Zervas, G.P., Koutis, N., Finos, M.A., Adamantidi, T., Panoutsopoulou, E., Ofrydopoulou, A., Tsoupras, A., 2024. Avocado and its by-products as natural sources of valuable anti-inflammatory and antioxidant bioactives for functional foods and cosmetics with health-promoting properties. Appl. Sci. 2076-3417. 14 (14), 5978. doi:10.3390/app14145978.)*

TABLE 11.2 Proximate nutritional composition of avocado by-products.

Nutrients	Avocado by-products[a]
Ash	1.6
Carbohydrates	67.5
Lipids	1.41–1.42
Protein	3.4
Total Dietary Fiber	21.6
Total Insoluble Fiber	18.7
Vitamins	1.3–1.6

[a]*Estimation of typical gross composition expressed as grams of total compound per 100 g of avocado weight (g 100/g).*
Data from Marra, A., Manousakis, V., Zervas, G.P., Koutis, N., Finos, M.A., Adamantidi, T., Panoutsopoulou, E., Ofrydopoulou, A., Tsoupras, A., 2024. Avocado and its by-products as natural sources of valuable anti-inflammatory and antioxidant bioactives for functional foods and cosmetics with health-promoting properties. Appl. Sci. 2076-3417. 14 (14), 5978. doi:10.3390/app14145978; Marra, A., Manousakis, V., Koutis, N., Zervas, G.P., Ofrydopoulou, A., Shiels, K., Saha, S.K., Tsoupras, A., 2025. In vitro antioxidant, antithrombotic and anti-inflammatory activities of the amphiphilic bioactives extracted from avocado and its by-products. Antioxidants. 2076-3921. 14 (2), 146. doi:10.3390/antiox14020146; Siol, M., Sadowska, A., 2023. Chemical composition, physicochemical and bioactive properties of avocado (*Persea americana*) seed and its potential use in functional food design. Agriculture. 2077-0472. 13 (2), 316. doi:10.3390/agriculture13020316; Gonçalves, D., Gouveia, C.S.S., Ferreira, M.J., Ganança, J.F.T., Pinto, D.C.G., de Carvalho, M.A.A.P., 2024. Comparative analysis of antioxidant and fatty acid composition in avocado (*Persea americana* Mill.) fruits: exploring regional and commercial varieties. Food Chem. 18737072. 442. Available from: https://www.sciencedirect.com/science/journal/03088146. doi:10.1016/j.foodchem.2024.138403.

and protocatechuic acid, alongside a broad range in TPC, underscore the need to standardize extraction and processing techniques to maximize the recovery of these bioactives. This potent phytochemical composition directly contributes to a strong antioxidant capacity, as consistently exhibited through multiple assays [2,2'-azino-bis(3-ethylbenzothiazoline-6-sulfonic acid) (ABTS), 2,2-diphenyl-1-picrylhydrazyl (DPPH), ferric-reducing antioxidant power assay (FRAP), and total antioxidant activity (TAAC)]. Such a robust antioxidant profile suggests their potential as active ingredients in skin-protective, antiaging, and regenerative cosmetic products, which not only support waste minimization and sustainability but also align with circular economy principles (Marra et al., 2024, 2025; Siol and Sadowska, 2023; Gonçalves et al., 2024).

3.3 Bioactive and health-promoting enzymes from fruits and their by-products

Pineapple, fig, and papaya by-products are of remarkable interest due to their rich content of naturally occurring proteolytic enzymes like bromelain, ficin, and papain, respectively, which serve as promising cosmetic and cosmeceutical ingredients with multifunctional biofunctional activities. These enzymes have attracted considerable attention for their roles in

TABLE 11.3 Proximate composition of phenolic and flavonoid compounds extracted from avocado by-products.

Phenolic and flavonoid compounds[a]	Avocado by-products
TPC	66.1–4.250
Chlorogenic acid	0–34.96
p-Hydrobenzoic acid	0–11.19
Caffeic acid	0–4.53
Benzoic acid	128.51–147.73
Catechin	2.58–2.62
Epigallocachetin	0.82
Rutinoside-3-*O*-quercetin	0.35–0.45
Glycoside-3-*O*-kaempferol	0.87–0.93
Quercetin	2.72–2.9
Gallic acid	0.004–9.22

[a]*Expressed in mg GAE/g of fresh weight (FW), measured in gallic acid equivalents (GAE).*
Data from Marra, A., Manousakis, V., Zervas, G.P., Koutis, N., Finos, M.A., Adamantidi, T., Panoutsopoulou, E., Ofrydopoulou, A., Tsoupras, A., 2024. Avocado and its by-products as natural sources of valuable anti-inflammatory and antioxidant bioactives for functional foods and cosmetics with health-promoting properties. Appl. Sci. 2076-3417. 14 (14), 5978. doi:10.3390/app14145978; Marra, A., Manousakis, V., Koutis, N., Zervas, G.P., Ofrydopoulou, A., Shiels, K., Saha, S.K., Tsoupras, A., 2025. In vitro antioxidant, antithrombotic and anti-inflammatory activities of the amphiphilic bioactives extracted from avocado and its by-products. Antioxidants. 2076-3921. 14 (2), 146. doi:10.3390/antiox14020146; Siol, M., Sadowska, A., 2023. Chemical composition, physicochemical and bioactive properties of avocado (*Persea americana*) seed and its potential use in functional food design. Agriculture. 2077-0472. 13 (2), 316. doi:10.3390/agriculture13020316; Gonçalves, D., Gouveia, C.S.S., Ferreira, M.J., Ganança, J.F.T., Pinto, D.C.G., de Carvalho, M.A.A.P., 2024. Comparative analysis of antioxidant and fatty acid composition in avocado (*Persea americana* Mill.) fruits: exploring regional and commercial varieties. Food Chem. 18737072. 442. Available from: https://www.sciencedirect.com/science/journal/03088146. doi:10.1016/j.foodchem.2024.138403.

TABLE 11.4 Antioxidant capacity of avocado by-products.

Antioxidant capacity	Avocado by-products
TAAC[a]	22.01–63.54
ABTS[b]	63.67–155.04
DPPH[c]	94.56–182.66
FRAP[c]	1.74–4.38

FRAP, ferric-reducing antioxidant power assay; *TAAC*, total antioxidant activity.
[a]*Expressed as mg of ascorbic acid equivalents per g (AA/g) of FW.*
[b]*Expressed as ABTS values.*
[c]*Expressed as Trolox equivalent values.*
Data from Marra, A., Manousakis, V., Zervas, G.P., Koutis, N., Finos, M.A., Adamantidi, T., Panoutsopoulou, E., Ofrydopoulou, A., Tsoupras, A., 2024. Avocado and its by-products as natural sources of valuable anti-inflammatory and antioxidant bioactives for functional foods and cosmetics with health-promoting properties. Appl. Sci. 2076-3417. 14 (14), 5978. doi:10.3390/app14145978; Marra, A., Manousakis, V., Koutis, N., Zervas, G.P., Ofrydopoulou, A., Shiels, K., Saha, S.K., Tsoupras, A., 2025. In vitro antioxidant, antithrombotic and anti-inflammatory activities of the amphiphilic bioactives extracted from avocado and its by-products. Antioxidants. 2076-3921. 14 (2), 146. doi:10.3390/antiox14020146; Siol, M., Sadowska, A., 2023. Chemical composition, physicochemical and bioactive properties of avocado (*Persea americana*) seed and its potential use in functional food design. Agriculture. 2077-0472. 13 (2), 316. doi:10.3390/agriculture13020316; Gonçalves, D., Gouveia, C.S.S., Ferreira, M.J., Ganança, J.F.T., Pinto, D.C.G., de Carvalho, M.A.A.P., 2024. Comparative analysis of antioxidant and fatty acid composition in avocado (*Persea americana* Mill.) fruits: exploring regional and commercial varieties. Food Chem. 18737072. 442. Available from: https://www.sciencedirect.com/science/journal/03088146. doi:10.1016/j.foodchem.2024.138403.

skin regeneration, exfoliation, and antiinflammatory processes, making them vital natural alternatives to synthetic agents (Venetikidou et al., 2025).

Bromelain, a complex of several thiol endopeptidases, phosphatases, glucosidases, and glycoproteins, is abundant in pineapples, particularly in the fruit but also in the peels, leaves, cores, crowns, and roots (Venetikidou et al., 2025; Varilla et al., 2021). Pineapple waste, such as peels (30%–42% w/w), cores (9%–10% w/w), stems (2%–5% w/w), crowns (2%–4% w/w), and leaves, contains bromelain, though in lesser quantities compared to the fruit (~51%). Other studies have claimed that the crown may possess the highest proteolytic activity (173,000 and 322,000 units for Nang Lae and Phu Lae, respectively) (Abbas et al., 2021; Trevisol et al., 2022; Misran et al., 2019). Bromelain demonstrates powerful antiinflammatory, fibrinolytic, and immunomodulatory effects, helping reduce edema, promote wound healing, and alleviate skin irritation. It also supports tissue regeneration and collagen remodeling, making it an exceptional ingredient for antiaging and postinflammatory care (Abbas et al., 2021; Venetikidou et al., 2025; Trevisol et al., 2022; Misran et al., 2019). Factors such as cultivar, ripeness, and extraction conditions significantly influence enzyme yield and activity, underlining the importance of standardized extraction protocols (Abbas et al., 2021; Trevisol et al., 2022; Misran et al., 2019).

Ficin, a cysteine protease obtained from fig latex (*Ficus* spp.), consists of thiol-based endopeptidases, peroxidases, phosphatases, amylases, and glycoproteins, with the highest activity reported in unripe fig latex (Gagaoua et al., 2014; Ayuso et al., 2022; Milošević et al., 2020). It exhibits notable antiinflammatory, antioxidant, antibacterial, and keratinolytic properties, aiding in exfoliation by breaking down keratinized proteins, promotes smoother skin texture, and helps manage acne-prone or hyperpigmented skin without causing irritation, making it ideal for sensitive skin products. However, the variability of ficin content due to factors like fig variety, climate, and collection methods has posed challenges in standardizing its commercial cosmetic, medicinal, and food processing applications (Gagaoua et al., 2014; Ayuso et al., 2022; Milošević et al., 2020).

Papain, mainly derived from *C. papaya* latex, is a single proteolytic enzyme with many important catalytic functions (amidase, esterase, transamidase, transesterase, and thiolesterase), present in fruits, peels, and leaves (Choudhary et al., 2025; Babalola et al., 2023; Ayodipupo Babalola et al., 2024; Amri and Mamboya, 2012). Papain is distributed throughout different papaya tissues, including the latex (16.76% w/w) (Manosroi et al., 2014), fruit, peel, seeds, and leaves, with concentrations varying significantly between ripe and unripe fruit (Iordănescu et al., 2021). Traditionally, unripe papaya fruit latex has been the primary commercial source of papain, as it contains high proteolytic activity (1834–4293 units/mg), although these values vary among studies (Benito-Vázquez et al., 2024). Recently, efforts to recover papain from papaya by-products, such as peels and seeds, have gained attention, aligning with green extraction principles and waste valorization. However, the enzyme's activity is highly sensitive to parameters such as fruit maturity, processing techniques, and geographic origin (Ayodipupo Babalola et al., 2024; Amri and Mamboya, 2012; Feijoo-Siota and Villa, 2011). Papain exhibits potent antioxidant, antiinflammatory, antimicrobial, wound healing, and depigmenting properties, notably facilitating skin renewal via gentle enzymatic exfoliation, accelerating tissue repair, and assisting in scar reduction and melanin regulation (Banchhor and Saraf, 2008; Ayodipupo Babalola et al., 2024; Amri and Mamboya, 2012; Feijoo-Siota and Villa, 2011).

Bromelain, ficin, papain, and their peel-derived or other fruit by-products modulate cellular signaling pathways associated with oxidative stress, inflammation, immune response, and tissue regeneration. Genetic, epigenetic, or environmental factors can trigger oxidative stress, leading to excessive production of ROS. This redox imbalance activates phospholipase A_2 (PLA_2) and the PAF/PAF receptor (PAF-R) pathway, resulting in proinflammatory eicosanoid formation (thromboxanes, prostaglandins, and leukotrienes) and cytokines such as tumor necrosis factor-α (TNF-α), interleukins 6 and 1β (IL-6 and IL-1β). These mediators further activate NF-κB and activator protein-1 (AP-1) transcription factors within the nucleus, contributing to chronic inflammatory manifestations. Proteolytic bromelain, ficin, and papain intervene by inhibiting both PAF-R and NF-κB activation, thereby reducing proinflammatory mediator synthesis. They also exert antioxidant effects by mitigating oxidative stress and preventing lipid peroxidation. Moreover, they influence immune modulation by regulating T-regulatory cells, dendritic cells, and macrophage polarization, enhancing immune tolerance and antiinflammatory balance. Beyond their antiinflammatory role, these proteolytic enzymes also contribute to wound healing and tissue repair by promoting fibroblast proliferation, collagen synthesis, and cellular differentiation, accelerating necrotic tissue removal, and supporting regeneration. Finally, they reveal vast antiskin cancer activity, attributed to the inhibition of inflammatory transcriptional signaling and induction of apoptosis in malignant cells (Fig. 11.4) (Venetikidou et al., 2025; Varilla et al., 2021; Trevisol et al., 2022; Benito-Vázquez et al., 2024).

Bromelain is relatively cost-effective and widely available due to the extensive cultivation of pineapples and the utilization of by-products like stems. Its strong exfoliating, antiinflammatory, and antimicrobial benefits make it a popular ingredient in skincare products (Trevisol et al., 2022). Ficin, although slightly more expensive and less readily available because of limited fig cultivation and labor-intensive extraction, is valued in niche skincare products for its gentle exfoliating properties and compatibility with sensitive skin types (Isa et al., 2020). Papain, on the contrary, is highly abundant, easy to extract, and cost-effective, making it one of the most widely used natural proteolytic agents across the cosmetic, pharmaceutical, and food industries (Choudhary et al., 2025).

The shift toward utilizing bromelain, ficin, or papain supports biodiversity conservation and circular economy principles by promoting the recovery of useful by-products, such as fiber-rich fruit peels that can be converted into compost, while residual biomass can be repurposed for animal feed or bioenergy formation (Castillo-González et al., 2019; Rabinovich et al., 2024). Furthermore, the application of these enzymes contributes to improved skin health by exerting

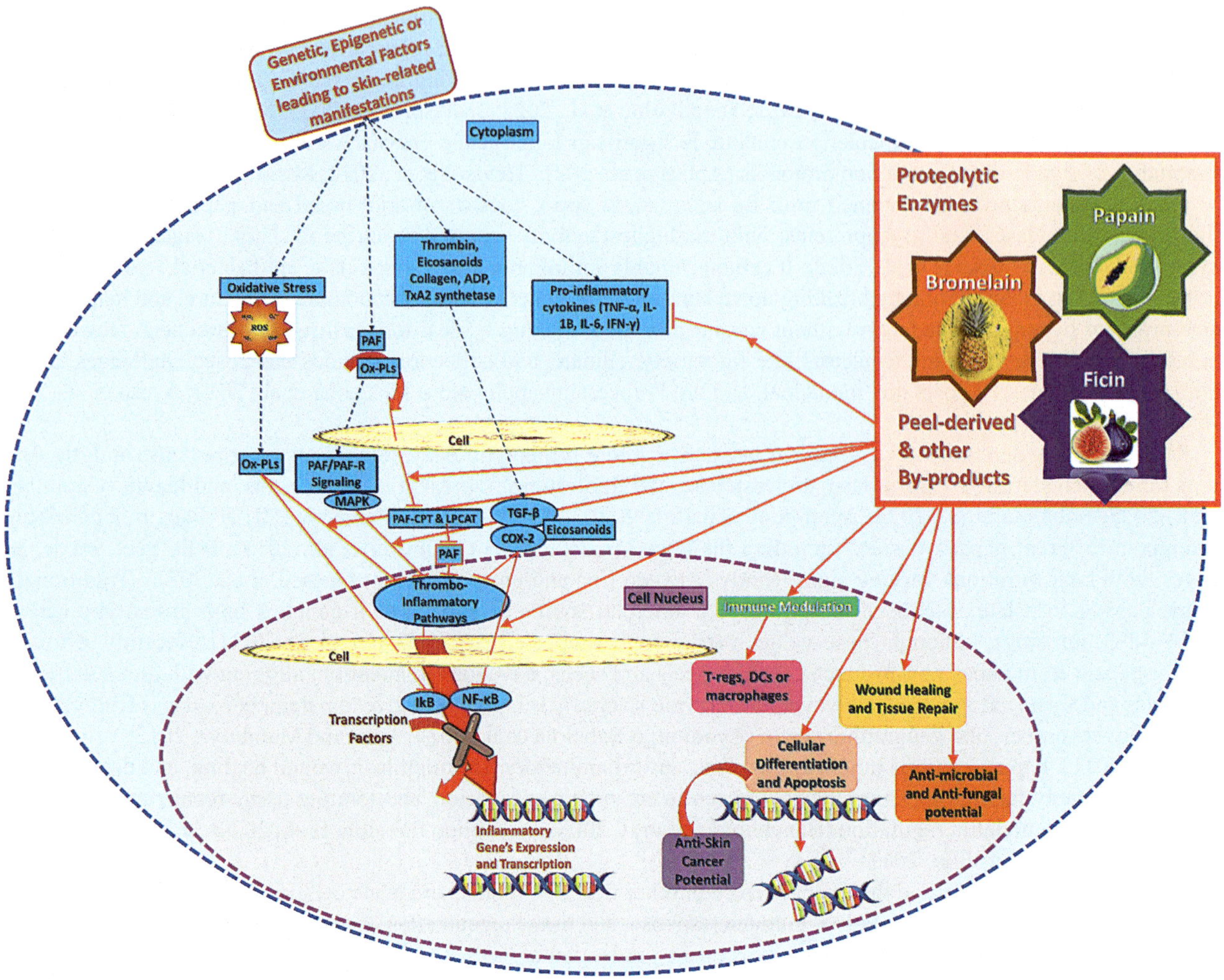

FIG. 11.4 Biochemical pathways and health-promoting properties of bromelain, ficin, and papain. *(From Venetikidou, M., Lykartsi, E., Adamantidi, T., Prokopiou, V., Ofrydopoulou, A., Letsiou, S., Tsoupras, A., 2025. Proteolytic enzyme activities of bromelain, ficin, and papain from fruit by-products and potential applications in sustainable and functional cosmetics for skincare. Appl. Sci. 2076-3417. 15 (5), 2637. doi:10.3390/app15052637.)*

antiinflammatory, wound healing, antioxidant, and rejuvenating properties, reinforcing their potential in sustainable skincare and dermatological solutions. Overall, the utilization of proteolytic enzymes from fruit by-products not only enhances economic and environmental sustainability but also drives innovation and product development in the natural cosmetics and cosmeceuticals sector (Machado et al., 2024; Nhani et al., 2024).

3.4 Bioactive and health-promoting constituents in winemaking and grape by-products

As far as grapes are concerned, different varieties are cultivated depending on the geographical location, climate, temperature, and soil type, resulting in variations in bioactive molecule content between red and white grapes. However, studies have shown that many of these bioactives remain in the by-products after vinification, especially in grape seeds. Thus grape pomace, a mixture of seeds, stems, and skins, represents a rich source of valuable compounds like fatty acids, proteins, carbohydrates, and polyphenols. Increasing interest has focused on their phenolic content for many industrial and biomedical applications (Marinaccio et al., 2025; Salem et al., 2022; Karastergiou et al., 2024). Recent research suggests that grape stem extracts hold vast potential in cosmetics, particularly in sunscreens and antiaging products. These extracts combat skin aging by reducing wrinkles, fine lines, and age spots, primarily via neutralization of free radicals, enhancement of skin elasticity and firmness, and attenuation of photoaging effects. In addition, grape pomace phenolics exhibit notable antiinflammatory and soothing actions, beneficial for sensitive or reactive skin, while contributing to a more even skin tone and hyperpigmentation protection (Serra et al., 2023).

According to Ribeiro et al. (2015), the highest phenolic content is found in grape seeds (60%–70%), followed by peels (28%–35%) and pulp (10%). Grape seeds are rich in fiber, proteins, essential oils, and phenolic substances such as tannins (e.g., gallic and ellagic acid), whereas grape skins contain anthocyanins such as cyanidin-3-glucoside, which possess potent antimutagenic and antioxidant properties (García-Lomillo et al., 2014). Specifically, hydroxybenzoic acids (e.g., protocatechuic, hydroxybenzoic, benzoic, vanillic, and syringic acid) and hydroxycinnamic acids (e.g., hydroxycinnamic, caffeic, cinnamic, and ferulic acid), volatile phenols (e.g., 4-ethylphenol, 4-vinyl-phenol, and vanillin), phenolic aldehydes (e.g., benzaldehyde and cinnamaldehyde), tyrosols (e.g., tyrosol and hydroxytyrosol), stilbenes (e.g., resveratrol and astringin), flavonols (e.g., quercetin), flavan-3-ols (e.g., catechin, epigallocatechin, and proanthocyanidins), and anthocyanins are the most common phenolic compounds identified in grape pomace (Fig. 11.5) (Mattos et al., 2017).

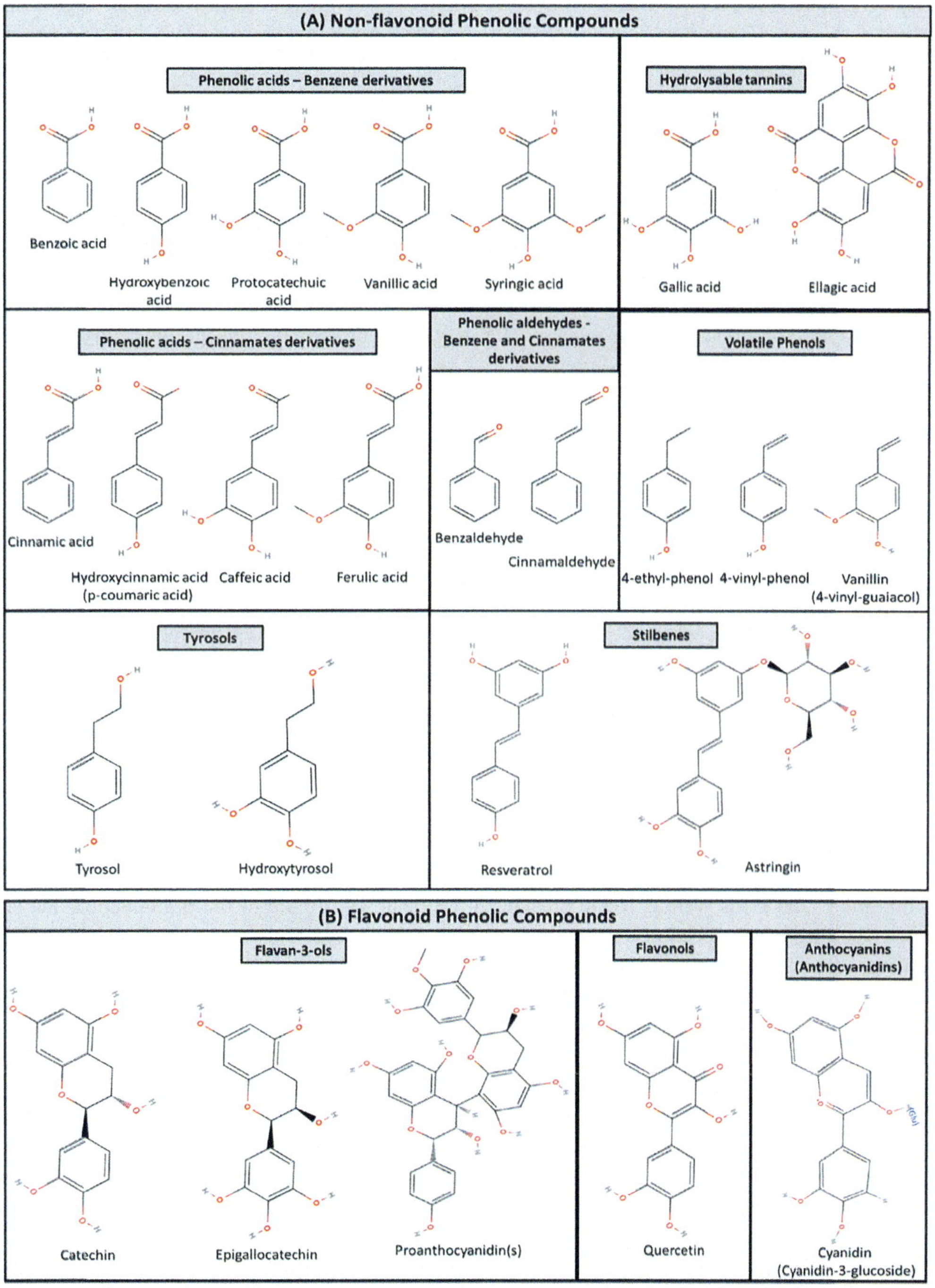

FIG. 11.5 Biofunctional agents in grapes and grape by-products (Tsiapali et al., 2025b; Tsoupras et al., 2023). *(Some figures (Structures) were derived from the open access free online platform MolView.Org).*

Proanthocyanidins (~90%) in grape seed, flesh, and bark extracts constitute the predominant phenolic fraction and, alongside flavanols, anthocyanins, and hydroxycinnamates, enhance the antioxidant, antiinflammatory, and photoprotective action of grape by-products (Nunes et al., 2017). Furthermore, anthocyanins protect cell membrane lipids from oxidative damage and display an antioxidant capacity up to four times greater than vitamin E, neutralizing enzymes that degrade connective tissue and repairing vascular proteins (Křížová, 2015). Flavonols and phenolic acids in grape skins and seeds further augment the overall antioxidant potential (Kontaxi et al., 2024; Křížová, 2015). The antioxidant hierarchy in grape bioactives typically follows: resveratrol > catechin > epicatechin = gallocatechin > gallic acid = ellagic acid (Yilmaz and Toledo, 2004).

Resveratrol, a stilbene found in grape pomace, exhibits multiple health-promoting effects, including antioxidant, antiinflammatory, and anticancer properties. Although grape pomace is an excellent source of resveratrol, its extraction can be costly and environmentally demanding (Kontaxi et al., 2024; Křížová, 2015; Yahia, 2018). In addition, gallic catechin and epigallocatechin gallate confer UV-protective and antiaging properties by preventing collagen degradation and oxidative stress. Furthermore, quercetin, a key flavonol, protects human keratinocytes from UVA-induced oxidative stress by enhancing intracellular antioxidant defenses. It prevents endogenous antioxidant depletion and lipid peroxidation during UV exposure, boosting skin hydration and elasticity by modulating lipid biosynthesis (Tsiapali et al., 2025b; Kontaxi et al., 2024; Tsoupras et al., 2023; Křížová, 2015; Yahia, 2018).

Grape seed oil is another valuable derivative, rich in vitamin E (10–530 mg/kg), primarily as α-tocopherol (Tsiapali et al., 2025b; Kontaxi et al., 2024; Tsoupras et al., 2023). It is composed mainly of UFAs, especially linolenic acid, and is widely used as a moisturizing and emollient cosmetic ingredient (Da Porto et al., 2013). According to Ferreira and Santos (Ferreira and Santos, 2022), grape pomace or seed oils and extracts reveal antioxidant effects comparable to synthetic agents, such as butylated hydroxytoluene (BHT), making them natural, sustainable alternatives (Tsiapali et al., 2025b; Kontaxi et al., 2024; Tsoupras et al., 2023). Most grape bioactives are amphiphilic, allowing them to penetrate the skin barrier when incorporated into ointments or sunscreens, where they exert antioxidant, antiinflammatory, and photoprotective effects against UV-induced oxidative stress and premature aging (Serra et al., 2023; Tsoupras et al., 2023; Křížová, 2015; Choleva et al., 2019). Moreover, grape pomace and seeds contain biofunctional lipids like UFAs and PUFAs (oleic, linoleic, and α-linolenic acids), bioactive PLs, and lipid-soluble vitamins (A, D, and E). Given their bioactivity, abundance, and sustainability, grape-derived agents are economically and ecologically feasible molecules for the cosmetic and pharmaceutical industries. Their wound healing, antioxidant, and photoprotective effects make them promising candidates for natural sunscreen formulations and skin repair products (Serra et al., 2023; Tsoupras et al., 2023; Křížová, 2015; Choleva et al., 2019).

3.5 Bioactive and health-promoting constituents in kiwi by-products

Kiwi is a major source of beneficial substances for human health, including vitamins, phenolics, minerals, pigments, and plant fibers. It is particularly rich in polar compounds (e.g., ascorbic, folic, citric, and glutamic acids), as well as amphiphilic bioactives, including phenolics (mainly hydroxybenzoic acids like *p*-coumaric, caffeic, chlorogenic, and protocatechuic acid), flavan-3-ols (catechin and epicatechin), and flavonol glycosides (e.g., quercetin-3-rhamnoside, quercetin-3-rutinoside, quercetin-3-glucoside, kaempferol-3-rhamnoside, and kaempferol-3-rutinoside), while sharing a low lipid content and containing no cholesterol (Moysidou et al., 2024; Wang et al., 2021b; Drummond, 2013; Richardson et al., 2018).

For many years, it was assumed that the seeds were the primary source of vitamin E due to their high lipid content. However, their resistance to digestion limits their bioavailability. Recently, α-tocopherol, the main vitamin E form in kiwi flesh, has been associated with cellular membranes, offering greater bioavailability compared to that in the seeds. Furthermore, vitamins C and E, as well as folate present in the flesh, contribute to the organization and stabilization of membrane lipids, resulting in enhanced cell membrane integrity and successful protection from oxidative stress. Kiwi pigments, including chlorophylls α and β, carotenoids like lutein, violaxanthin, β-carotene, and 9'-*cis*-neoxanthin, and anthocyanin 3-*O*-glucoside cyanidin, are primarily vital for the fruit's external appearance. Finally, fiber, the actinidin protein important for digestion, small amounts of lipids, including α-linoleic acid, and minerals like calcium, iron, potassium, magnesium, manganese, phosphorus, copper, zinc, and selenium are also of great importance as kiwi bioactives (Fig. 11.6) (Moysidou et al., 2024; Wang et al., 2021b; Drummond, 2013; Richardson et al., 2018).

Kiwi by-products, including peels, residual pulp or pomace, seeds, and leaves, represent nearly 30% of total kiwi fruit production and are currently regarded as sustainable natural resources rather than waste. These by-products retain high levels of phenolics, vitamins, and pigments, comparable to or exceeding those in edible portions (Sanz et al., 2021; Ilie et al., 2022). Among them, kiwi seeds stand out due to their oil content (28.3%–35%), rich in PUFAs such as linoleic and linolenic acids, which show potent antioxidant and antiinflammatory action. Importantly, the favorable ω-3/ω-6 ratio enhances their nutritional and cardioprotective value. In addition, the seeds (33–46 g/kg kiwi) contain 12.72%–14.94% protein, positioning them as a potential alternative plant-based source. Their antioxidant capacity, measured through FRAP (107 mg Trolox equivalents

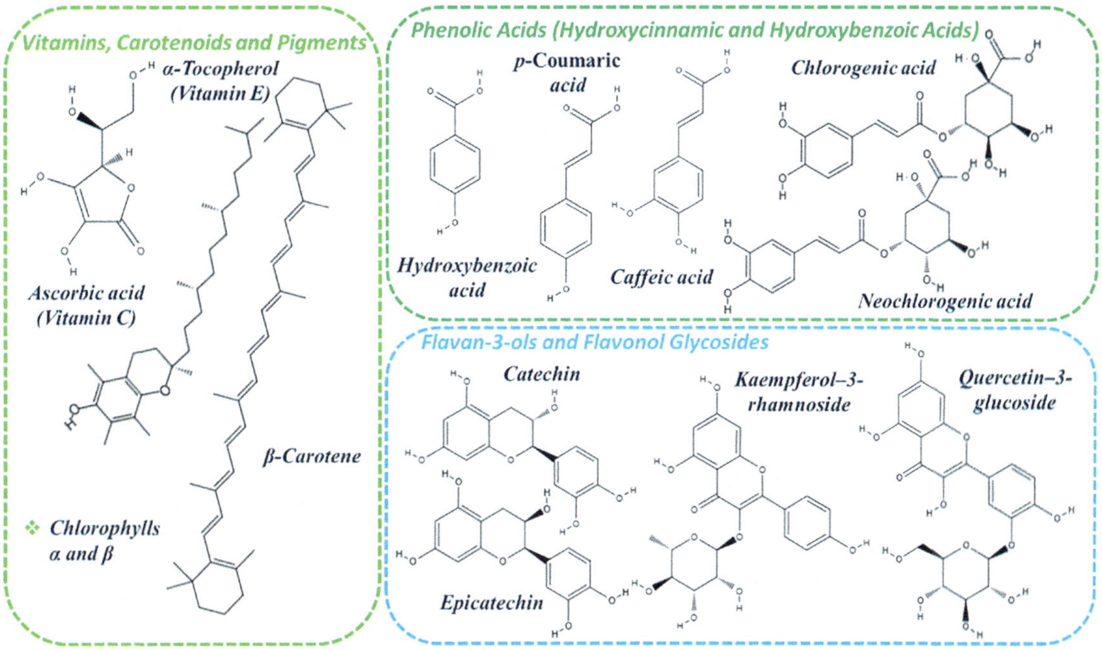

FIG. 11.6 Main kiwi by-products' bioactives. Nutrients and key bioactives present in kiwi and its by-products. *(Some structures were retrieved from the open access free online platform of MolView.Org.)*

(TE)/kg), ORAC (2 mg TE/kg), and DPPH [half-maximal inhibitory concentration (IC_{50}) of 35 mg/mL] assays, highlights their role in mitigating oxidative stress. The variation in bioactive content depends on cultivar, origin, and growing conditions (Moysidou et al., 2024; Wang et al., 2021b; Drummond, 2013; Richardson et al., 2018; Deng et al., 2018).

Kiwi leaves, which constitute a naturally renewable biomass due to annual shedding, have attracted considerable attention for their phenolic and organic acid composition. Representative phenolics include neochlorogenic, chlorogenic, cryptochlorogenic, and caffeic acid, as well as flavonoids such as quercetin, kaempferol, catechin, and procyanidin B-type dimers, reaching up to 200 mg/g leaf. *Actinidia arguta* leaves have demonstrated antioxidant, antiradical, antimicrobial, and antiinflammatory activities, with methanolic and ethanolic extracts providing protection against UVB- and UVC-induced oxidative damage in red blood cells. These effects are attributed to flavonoids, hydroxycinnamic derivatives, and flavan-3-ols, which also reduce erythrocyte fragility and promote membrane stabilization (Moysidou et al., 2024; Richardson et al., 2018; Sanz et al., 2021; Deng et al., 2018).

The peel and skin of kiwi are also rich in phenolics and demonstrate notably high antioxidant capacity. For *A. deliciosa*, TPC was reported as 13 mg GAE/g DW and 0.91 mg GAE/g FW, with protocatechuic, chlorogenic, caffeic, and p-hydroxybenzoic acids, as well as rutin and quercetin, being the key bioactives found (Moysidou et al., 2024; Sanz et al., 2021). Epicatechin (163 μg/g) is the most abundant polyphenol, conferring antioxidant, antibacterial, and anticancer potential. Ethanolic extracts revealed the highest antioxidant potential, with DPPH and ABTS values of 107 and 258 μg/mL, respectively. In addition, kiwi peels are mineral-rich, with significant levels of manganese (820 mg/100 g), potassium (230 mg/100 g), calcium (230 mg/100 g), and sodium (90 mg/100 g) (Moysidou et al., 2024; Sanz et al., 2021). They also contain carotenoids (~5.70 mg/g DW), primarily β-carotene, which enhances skin photoprotection and antioxidant defenses (Moysidou et al., 2024; Sanz et al., 2021; Ilie et al., 2022).

Kiwi's fiber content derives mainly from its skin rather than the pulp, composed mostly of polysaccharides that form both soluble and insoluble fibers, promoting gastrointestinal health (Richardson et al., 2018). In addition, vitamin E, which reveals a DPPH rate of 24%–25% and an α-tocopherol content of 2.4 mg/100 g FW, contributes significantly to the fruit's antioxidant profile. Specifically, its three isomers, α-, γ-, and δ-tocopherol, and the newly identified δ-tocomonoenol exhibit high bioavailability and strong lipid-protective properties (Moysidou et al., 2024, 2025; Chamorro et al., 2022; Dias et al., 2020). Finally, kiwi pomace, composed of condensed peels, leaves, and seeds, retains a wide range of phenolics, including chlorogenic acid, *p*-coumaric acid, catechin, protocatechuic acid, and caffeic acid derivatives, confirming its high antioxidant, antiinflammatory, and cosmeceutical potential (Moysidou et al., 2024, 2025; Chamorro et al., 2022; Dias et al., 2020). Table 11.5 contains quantitative and qualitative data on the composition of bioactives in kiwi by-products.

TABLE 11.5 Nutritional and bioactive composition of kiwi by-products.

Composition	Identified amount	Kiwi by-products
Total phenolics	329 mg/g	Seeds
	12.62%	Peels
Total proteins	12.72%–14.94%	Seeds
	3.7%	Peels
Total lipids	28.3%–35%	Seeds
	5.70 ± 0.033 mg/g DW	Peels
Total carotenoids	1.55 ± 0.093 mg/g DW	Pomace
Phenolic profile		
Total phenolics	14.3–24.6 mg GAE/g 9.71 ± 0.28 mg GAE/g DW	Peels
	3.79 ± 0.15 mg GAE/g DW	Pomace
	200 mg/g	Leaf
Chlorogenic acid	0.40 mg/g	Peels
	45 mg/g	Seeds
Catechin	0.36 mg/g	Peels
p-Coumaric acid	53 mg/g	Seeds
Hydroxybenzoic acid	63 mg/g	Seeds
Caffeic acid	0.15 mg/g	Peels
Epicatechin	0.32 mg/g	Peels

From Moysidou, A.M., Cheimpeloglou, K., Koutra, S.I., Finos, M.A., Ofrydopoulou, A., Tsoupras, A., 2024. A comprehensive review on the antioxidant and anti-inflammatory bioactives of kiwi and its by-products for functional foods and cosmetics with health-promoting properties. Appl. Sci. 2076-3417. 14 (14), 5990. doi:10.3390/app14145990.

3.6 Bioactive and health-promoting constituents in tomato by-products

Tomatoes exist in several varieties, round, oval, and cherry, all sharing similar nutritional characteristics. They are an important source of essential minerals like potassium, phosphorus, magnesium, and iron, which are crucial for the normal functioning of nerves and muscles, as well as vitamins A, B, C, and E. Notably, tomatoes rank as the third most significant dietary source of vitamin C and the fourth for vitamin A, primarily due to their β-carotene content. They also contain phytosterols, which regulate blood cholesterol levels, and folic acid, which supports homocysteine metabolism, contributing to cardiovascular protection (Trombino et al., 2021; Ali et al., 2021).

Beyond these nutrients, tomatoes are rich in bioactives such as carotenoids (lycopene, β-carotene, and lutein), ascorbic acid, and polyphenols, including phenolics (e.g., hydroxybenzoic, ferulic, gallic, caffeic, chlorogenic, and protocatechuic acid), anthocyanidins, flavones, and flavonols (e.g., quercetin, naringenin, rutin, and kaempferol-3-rhamnoside), saponins, and terpenoids, all of which exhibit potent antioxidant, antiinflammatory, and anticancer properties. Lycopene, the predominant tomato carotenoid, is a nonprovitamin A carotenoid and one of the most powerful natural antioxidants, displaying twice the free-radical antioxidant capacity of β-carotene (Trombino et al., 2021; Ali et al., 2021). Lycopene protects cellular membranes and lipoproteins from oxidative damage and reduces the risk of prostate, lung, and gastric cancers, as well as the occurrence of cardiovascular disorders (CVD). Moreover, it may act as a natural sunscreen and cosmetic ingredient, enhancing skin photoprotection against UV-induced oxidative stress, while concurrently accelerating both skin moisture and suppleness (Sjahjadi et al., 2021; Elbrolesy et al., 2023; Sopyan et al., 2017).

The synergistic interaction of lycopene with ascorbic acid (vitamin C), α-tocopherol (vitamin E), and phenolic acids further enhances its overall antioxidant and radical scavenging efficacy, neutralizing free radicals and preventing DNA oxidation. Both vitamins revealed UV photoprotection, antiwrinkle, antierythema, and skin-protective effects. Tomatoes comprise polyphenols and flavonoids, including chlorogenic acid, quercetin, rutin, and naringenin, which contribute to antiinflammatory, antioxidant, and antithrombotic benefits, while also supporting immune modulation and vascular health. Finally, monoterpenoids and sesquiterpenes enhance the aromatic and therapeutic potential of tomatoes, while saponins contribute to their cholesterol-lowering and hepatoprotective properties (Fig. 11.7) (Sjahjadi et al., 2021; Kontaxi et al., 2024; Trombino et al., 2021; Elbrolesy et al., 2023; Sopyan et al., 2017).

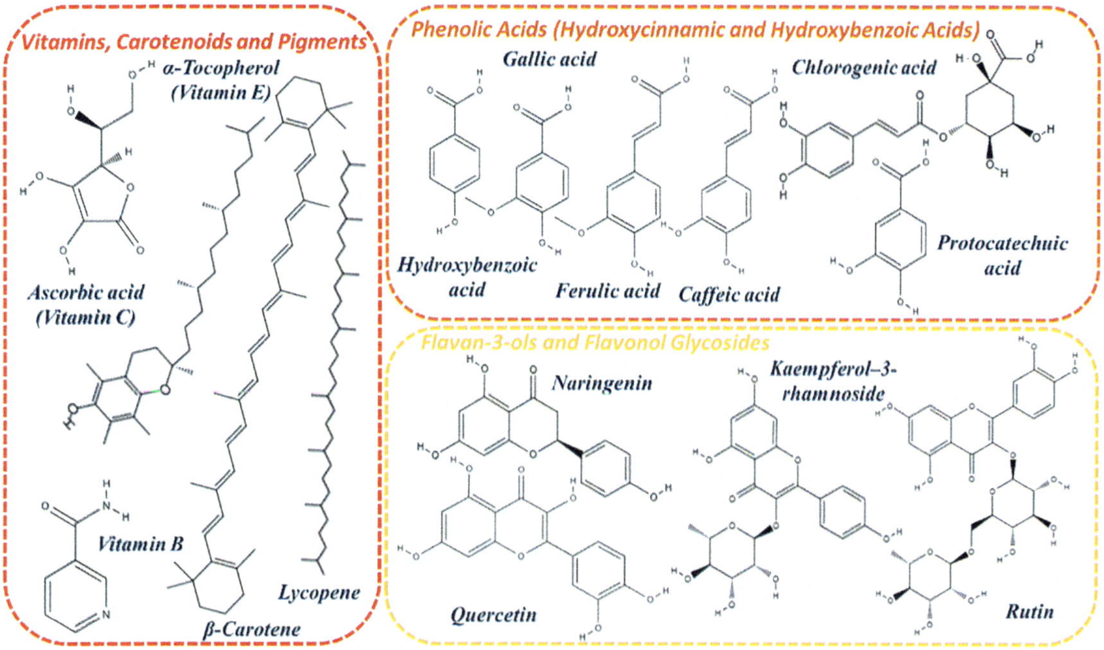

FIG. 11.7 Tomato and its by-products' main bioactives. Nutrients and key bioactives present in tomato and its by-products. *(Structures were retrieved from the open access free online platform of MolView.Org.)*

3.7 Bioactive and health-promoting constituents in pomegranate by-products

Pomegranates are widely recognized as an essential component of a health-promoting diet, offering numerous benefits due to their antioxidant, antimutagenic, antihypertensive, antiinflammatory, and antiatherosclerotic properties. Such activities contribute to their protective effects against chronic diseases such as osteoarthritis, prostate cancer, CVDs, and viral infections, including human immunodeficiency virus 1 (Nazir et al., 2025; Rajha et al., 2019; Caleb et al., 2013). Because the juice yield of pomegranates accounts for less than half of the fruit's total weight, significant quantities of by-products, particularly peels, are generated each year. Historically, this material was used as animal feed, but modern research has shown that pomegranate peels are a vibrant source of bioactives and antioxidants, especially phenolics, flavonoids, tannins, carotenoids, and organic acids, making them a valuable natural resource rather than waste (Nazir et al., 2025; Rajha et al., 2019; Caleb et al., 2013; Goula et al., 2017).

Carotenoids, characterized by their conjugated double bonds, not only give the fruit its vibrant color but also exhibit potent antioxidant, antiinflammatory, and anticancer effects, contributing to oxidative stress reduction and degenerative disease prevention. Phenolics, such as punicalagin and punicalin, are ellagitannins that represent the main polyphenols responsible for the high antioxidant, cardioprotective, and antibacterial capacity of pomegranate juice and peel (Benchagra et al., 2021). Upon hydrolysis, these ellagitannins release ellagic acid, which is subsequently metabolized by gut microbiota into urolithins, mainly urolithin A, a potent health-promoting agent. The metabolic conversion into urolithins depends on the individual's gut microbiome type, influencing the overall bioavailability and systemic effects of pomegranate polyphenols. Despite the limited absorption of native polyphenols, these gut-derived metabolites are largely responsible for the in vivo antioxidant and cytoprotective activities (Caballero et al., 2022; García-Mantrana et al., 2019).

Pomegranate anthocyanins, notably delphinidin, cyanidin, and pelargonidin glycosides, impart the deep red color of pomegranate juice and exert powerful antioxidant, vasoprotective, and antiaging effects, supporting endothelial function and microcirculation (Türkyılmaz et al., 2023). The peel, rich in flavonoids like quercetin and kaempferol, hydroxybenzoic acids (e.g., gallic, vanillic, and protocatechuic acid), hydroxycinnamic acids (e.g., caffeic, ferulic, and coumaric acid), ash, carbohydrates like pectin, and complex tannins (e.g., gallotannins and ellagitannins), exhibits strong antimicrobial, antiobesity, and hepatoprotective potential (Alexandre et al., 2019). Meanwhile, the seeds contain higher levels of proteins and lipids, especially the seed oil, abundant in UFAs and conjugated PUFAs like punicic acid (a rare ω-5 fatty acid), linoleic, and oleic acids (Alexandre et al., 2019; Faria and Silva, 2025; El-Shamy and Farag, 2021; Kandylis and Kokkinomagoulos, 2020).

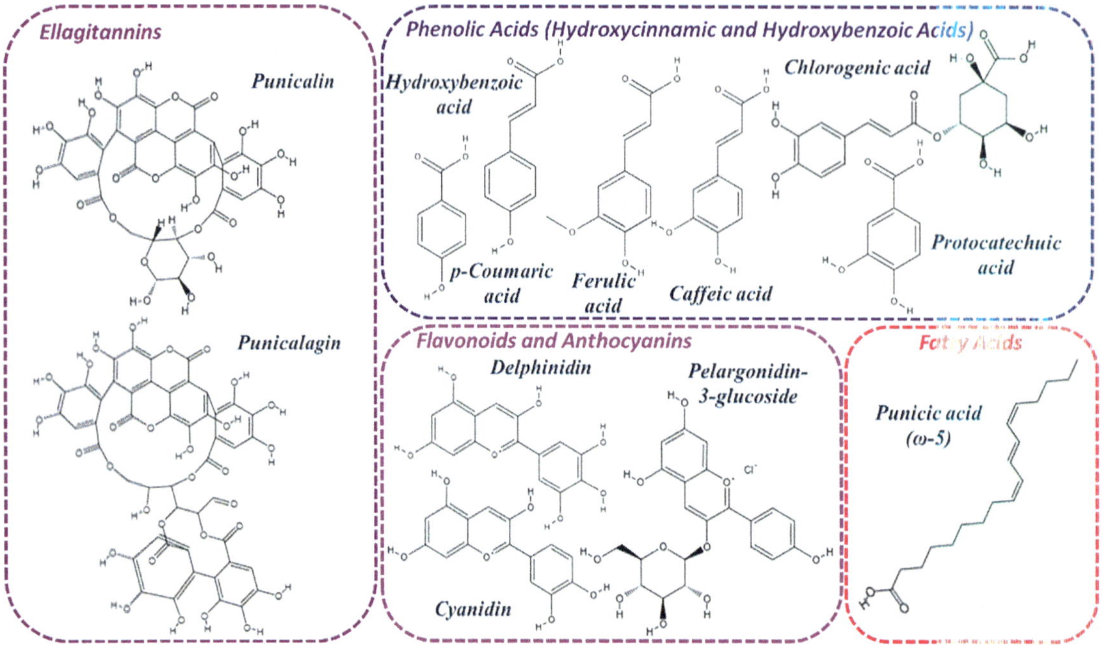

FIG. 11.8 Pomegranate and its by-products' main bioactives. Nutrients and key bioactives present in pomegranate by-products. *(Structures were retrieved from the open access free online platform MolView.Org.)*

From a nutritional standpoint, the peel is enriched with minerals such as calcium and sodium, while the kernel contains significant levels of zinc and magnesium, and the whole fruit provides high potassium content, supporting electrolyte balance and protection against CVDs. Plus, the kernel's structural carbohydrates, including cellulose, hemicellulose, and lignin, offer dietary fiber benefits and potential for biopolymer applications. Interestingly, the inedible parts of the pomegranate peel, seeds, and/or kernel constitute nearly 50% of the total fruit mass. These fruit parts represent a highly valuable and unexploited source of bioactives, particularly punicalagin, ellagic acid, anthocyanins, and punicic acid, which, in turn, exert strong antioxidant, anticancer, antiinflammatory, cardioprotective, antimicrobial, and antiaging vital attributes, reinforcing pomegranate's reputation as a multifunctional fruit (Fig. 11.8) (Alexandre et al., 2019; Faria and Silva, 2025; El-Shamy and Farag, 2021; Kandylis and Kokkinomagoulos, 2020; Gosset-Erard et al., 2021).

4 Applications in research and development for the cosmetic industry

So-called "green cosmetics" or "biocosmetics" represent a revolutionary and ecologically driven concept, emphasizing sustainability and consumer health benefits. These formulations utilize plant-derived extracts rich in bioactive compounds, such as polyphenols, flavonoids, vitamins, carotenoids, terpenes, and essential oils, which are naturally found in fruits and their by-products. Naturally, factors such as the extraction method, solvent polarity, temperature, and extraction duration significantly influence the recovery efficiency and chemical profile of these bioactives, leading to compositional variation among extracts. However, all such products share a common feature: the integration of naturally sourced agents from fruits, flowers, herbs, and other botanical materials that contribute to skin protection and rejuvenation (Lee and Hyun, 2023; Cejudo-Bastante et al., 2021; Zhang et al., 2018; Szabo et al., 2022).

Particular attention in modern cosmetic science is directed toward antiaging, antioxidant, and photoprotective effects, including efforts to slow the formation of wrinkles, discolorations, and other visible signs of aging. These actions are primarily mediated by neutralizing free radicals, stimulating collagen synthesis, and inhibiting matrix metalloproteinases (MMPs), which collectively maintain skin elasticity and firmness. Moreover, fruit-based bioactives like vitamin C, resveratrol, lycopene, and ellagic acid have been widely recognized for their UV-protective, antiinflammatory, and skin-brightening properties, positioning them as cornerstone ingredients in sustainable dermocosmetics (Lee and Hyun, 2023; Cejudo-Bastante et al., 2021; Zhang et al., 2018; Szabo et al., 2022).

Current research on bioactives for cosmetic applications involves numerous studies that have evaluated the functional properties of cosmetic formulations enriched with natural compounds from fruits and their by-products. Specifically, the incorporation of bioactives extracted from kiwi residues, avocado peels and seeds, apple pomace, olive pomace and other fruit by-products has been shown to enhance product stability, antioxidant capacity, and antiinflammatory activity. Hence, such products exhibit improved photoprotective, antiinflammatory, anti-melanoma and antiaging activities, and overall skin health-promoting properties (Tsoupras et al., 2009, 2023, 2024a; Vandorou et al., 2024, 2025; Marra et al., 2024, 2025; Venetikidou et al., 2025; Tsiapali et al., 2025b; Moysidou et al., 2024, 2025; Ferreira and Santos, 2022; Nazir et al., 2025; Tsiapali et al., 2025a; Di Lorenzo et al., 2024; Naeimifar et al., 2020; Lourenço et al., 2016; Hamouda and Felemban, 2023; Zhang et al., 2024).

In a recent research article, Annurca apple oleolite (AAO) (extract in sunflower oil containing 784.40 ± 7.579 μg/mL of UA) was declared a potential functional ingredient for antiaging cosmeceuticals. It effectively inhibited the elastase enzyme with an IC_{50} of 212.76 μg/mL, compared to the positive controls UA (IC_{50}: 135.24 μg/mL), pure molecules, and quercetin (IC_{50}: 72.47 μg/mL). Moreover, its topical application (2.5% w/w) in 40 volunteers revealed that after 28 treatment days, there was a significant reduction in the nasolabial fold (−7.2 vs. baseline) and forehead wrinkles (−5.3 vs. baseline), as well as a notable improvement in the viscoelastic skin parameters, ameliorating skin pliability/firmness (−13% vs. baseline), gross elasticity (+12% vs. baseline), and overall skin hydration (Di Lorenzo et al., 2024). Beyond apple by-products' cosmetic efficacy, pomegranate oil and residues have also revealed cosmetic potency in research and development pilot studies. A comparative analysis of two commercial products, namely, Avocom-M and TROSYD cream, and natural pomegranate seed oil extract (PSOE) was conducted against phenobarbital- and formaldehyde-induced skin biochemical changes in rats. A 21-day treatment with Avocom-M, TROSYD, or PSOE decreased collagenase, elastase, hyaluronidase, tyrosinase, cyclooxygenase-2, lipid peroxidation, and nitric oxide (NO) levels in rats, compared with those in rats treated with phenobarbital and formaldehyde, revealing a vast improvement in the rats' biochemical status. On the contrary, treatment with TROSYD and PSOE demonstrated remarkable amelioration of skin inflammation, suggesting that PSOE could be successfully used as a local treatment for skin issues (Hamouda and Felemban, 2023).

An antiaging cream containing avocado, apple, and kiwi by-products was extensively studied for its cosmetic potential, with nanobubbles (NB) and without NBs (S), compared to a control cream (X). A notably higher antioxidant capacity (FRAP assay), reflecting a ~250% improvement, was found in S (at production: 710.4 ± 344.3 and at 1 month: 631.7 ± 277.8 μmol TE/g DW) and NB (at production: 566.3 ± 185.0 and at 1 month: 1019.3 ± 574.0 μmol TE/g DW), in contrast to X (at production: 202.8 ± 145.6 and at 1 month: 449.8 ± 43.9 μmol TE/g DW). Moreover, the SPF increased after storage (from 8.7 ± 0.8 to 9.5 ± 0.6), while attenuated total reflectance–Fourier transform infrared (FTIR) with Strat-M membranes revealed enhanced penetration of bioactives in S creams, with NBs not significantly altering the absorption profiles. Finally, platelet aggregation demonstrated markedly lower IC50 values in S and NB creams than X ones for the PAF (μmol TE/g DW: S at production: 300.0 ± 42.0 and at 1 month: 325.0 ± 50.0; NB at production: 258.0 ± 31.0 and at 1 month: 275.0 ± 4; and X at production: 685.0 ± 35.0 and at 1 month: 885.0 ± 112.0) and the adenosine diphosphate (ADP) pathways (S at production: 450.0 ± 65.0 and at 1 month: 470.0 ± 52.0; NB at production: 400.0 ± 31.0 and at 1 month: 412.0 ± 42.0; and X at production: 880.0 ± 58.0 and at 1 month: 1102.0 ± 125.0), showcasing these fruit by-product extracts' potency as sustainable cosmetic agents (Tsiapali et al., 2025a).

In addition, several commercial cosmetic formulations already contain bioactives from these natural sources, demonstrating verified functional and health-related benefits. More specifically, Table 11.6 includes selected commercial and research-backed cosmetic agents or products from natural bioactives derived from fruits.

4.1 Applications of the bioactive and health-promoting constituents in apple by-products

Apple pomace is a highly promising by-product, with applications in functional foods, pharmaceuticals, and cosmeceuticals (Tsoupras et al., 2024b; Vandorou et al., 2024, 2025). Recent studies revealed the potential of UA from Annurca apples in cosmetics, demonstrating safety for topical use, wrinkle reduction, and improved skin hydration (Di Lorenzo et al., 2024). Phenolic compounds from Arisoo apples have exhibited stronger antiwrinkle effects than those from Fuji apples. Apple-derived nanovesicles (ADNVs) downregulate NF-κB and promote collagen synthesis, reducing extracellular matrix degradation and modulating gene expression related to skin aging. ADNVs incorporated into hyaluronic-acid-based hydrogels and patches showed promising antiwrinkle effects in clinical trials (Di Lorenzo et al., 2024).

A cosmetic cream containing wild apple fruit water extract, α-hydroxy acids (AHAs), and polyphenols displayed stable physicochemical properties, high antioxidant action, improved hydration, reduced melanin index, and no irritation in in vivo tests (Stojiljković et al., 2018). *Malus* sp. extract combined with rutin reduced apoptotic and caspase-3-positive cells in UVB-exposed human skin, confirming their potential against skin aging and UV-induced damage (Martins et al., 2020). ADNVs also inhibit toll-like receptor 4, affecting NF-κB pathways, and can be formulated as gels or patches for cosmetic and medical applications (Lourenço et al., 2016). Cosmetic creams with 6% wild apple extract showed stable physicochemical and antioxidant properties over 180 days, increased hydration, and decreased melanin index, suggesting

TABLE 11.6 Selected commercial and research-backed cosmetic agents or products from natural bioactives derived from fruits.

Cosmetic product	Cosmetic use	Fruit ingredient	Beneficial impact	Reference
ORIGINS—Youthtopia Peptide Plumping Apple Cream	Face cream	Apple stem cell extract, apple ferment, apple seed oil, peptides	Anti-aging, skin elasticity-improving, hydrating, plumping, and antioxidant-protective	(Origins, n.d.)
Annurca Apple Oleolite (AAO)	Active oil/extract	Ursolic acid from Annurca apple peel	Improves skin elasticity, reduces wrinkles, and enhances moisturizing	(Di Lorenzo et al., 2024)
Q + A—Apple AHA Exfoliating Gel	Exfoliating gel	Apple-derived apple α-hydroxy acids (AHAs, mainly malic acid)	Brightening, resurfacing, skin softening, and strengthening	(Q+A Skincare, n.d.)
TONYMOLY—I'm Avocado Nutrition Mask Sheet	Sheet mask	Avocado extract/oil	Nourishing, moisturizing, and skin softening	(TONYMOLY USA, n.d.)
Farmstay—Real Avocado Nutrition Eye Cream	Eye cream/ moisturizer	Avocado oil, fruit extracts, and vitamins E and C	Moisturizing, nourishing, improving skin elasticity, wrinkle-reducing, and skin brightening	(Farmstay, n.d.)
Densilab—Bromelain Enzymatic Peeling	Enzyme exfoliating cream	Bromelain (pineapple enzyme)	Gentle resurfacing removes dead cells and brightens	(Densi Lab, n.d.)
APIS Professional—Depigmenting Peeling (Ficin-based variant)	Face peeling	Ficin (fig enzyme) and 1% Tranexamic Acid	Anti-dark spots, cleansing, anti-aging, photoprotective, and discoloration combating	(MAKEUPTM, n.d.)
Alba Botanica—Hawaiian Papaya Enzyme Mask	Enzyme mask	Papain (papaya enzyme)	Exfoliation, rejuvenation, and radiance	(Living Cruelty Free, n.d.)
Caudalie—Vinoperfect Radiance Serum	Dark spot brightening serum	Viniferine (grapevine sap) and polyphenols	Vitamin C alternative—dark spot-brightening, offering a brighter complexion	(Caudalie, n.d.)
The Body Shop—Grapeseed Glossing Serum	Serum/hair and skin oil	Grape seed oil (*Vitis vinifera*)	Antioxidant, emollient, hydrating, and protection from oxidative stress	(The Body Shop, n.d.)
100% PURE Tomato Lycopene SPF 20	Natural sunscreen and SPF protection	Lycopene-based natural sunscreen	UVA/UVB protection, moisturizing, and sun damage minimizing	(100% PURE, n.d.)
Evterpa—Tomato Face Cream	Face cream	Tomato extract (lycopene)	Brightening, antioxidant protection, and pigmentation reducing	(Evterpa, n.d.)
Huda Beauty—Kiwi Facial Mask Sheet	Sheet mask	Kiwi extract (vitamins A and C, and polyphenols)	Brightening, collagen boosting, antiaging, nourishing, and revitalizing	(Pharmeden.gr, n.d.)
Garden—Revitalizing Pomegranate Scrub	Face scrub	Pomegranate polyphenols	Antioxidant, pore refining, skin soothing, and firming	(GARDEN, n.d.)

protection against oxidative damage and hyperpigmentation (Stojiljković et al., 2018). Apple polyphenols in sunscreens mitigated UV penetration, protected against sunburn cells, caspase-3 activation, cyclobutane pyrimidine dimer formation, lipid peroxidation, and metalloproteinase induction (Martins et al., 2020; Opriş et al., 2022). In vivo, apple stem cell (ASC) extract reduced UVB-induced inflammatory cell infiltration, improved collagen regulation, epidermal or dermal thickness, skin moisture, and lowered TNF-α expression (Khayatan et al., 2022).

AAO, rich in UA, inhibited porcine elastase, reduced nasolabial and forehead wrinkles, enhanced viscoelastic parameters, and improved skin hydration in clinical trials (Di Lorenzo et al., 2024; Maisto et al., 2023). Extracts from Aomori Hiba and apple polyphenols were identified as eco-friendly cosmetic ingredients. Heating apple lees powder increased polyphenol content, further enhancing skin protection (Kitayama et al., 2006). Moreover, hydroalcoholic apple extracts in emulsions displayed antioxidant activity and SPF improvement (highest SPF: 1.01), remaining stable after UV exposure (Opriş et al., 2022). Apple extracts, such as UFP, PF-III, and PF-IV, protected human fibroblasts from UV-induced DNA damage and exhibited antiproliferative effects on melanoma cells (de Oliveira Raphaelli et al., 2021). Interestingly, UA extraction from Annurca apples using sunflower oil produced potent antioxidant and skin-protective formulations (Zhang et al., 2024).

Formosan apple components, 3-hydroxyphloretin and catechol, inhibited tyrosinase activity and reduced melanin formation in human epidermal melanocytes, suggesting skin whitening potential (Lin et al., 2007). Apple procyanidins prevented UV-induced pigmentation, protected melanocytes, improved gut barrier function, reduced hepatic inflammation, and contributed to skin lightness maintenance (Shoji et al., 2020). Furthermore, apple polyphenols consistently demonstrated antioxidant properties, particularly quercetin, isoquercetin, and rutin, making them suitable for cosmetic sunscreens (Opriş et al., 2022). Importantly, gel and emulgel formulations containing several apple phenolic complexes exhibited robust antioxidant activity in vitro (Butkeviciute et al., 2022; Bonarska-Kujawa et al., 2011). Apple pomace also exhibited antimicrobial activity, attributed to compounds like phloridzin. Modified phloridzin derivatives (F2) are stable and suitable for creams, lotions, masks, and serums, as well as dermocosmetic products of high cosmetic significance (Arraibi et al., 2021; Baldisserotto et al., 2012). ASC extracts downregulated UVB-induced inflammation and dermal/epidermal thickness, improved collagen regulation and hydration, and reduced TNF-α, showcasing strong antiinflammatory potential in topical therapy (Khayatan et al., 2022).

Despite its benefits, apple pomace may alter textural and sensory properties in foods (Di Lorenzo et al., 2024). Using bioactive-rich extracts instead of pomace minimizes these effects without compromising functionality. Evidently, apple seed oil is safe within toxicity limits (Szabo et al., 2022), and Environmental Protection Agency guidelines confirm its safety as a functional food agent (Skinner et al., 2018).

4.2 Applications of the bioactive and health-promoting constituents in avocado by-products

Avocado extract provides multiple skincare benefits, including enhanced skin hydration, epithelial regeneration, and reinforcement of the epidermal barrier, thereby improving overall skin appearance. It also exhibits antibacterial and antiinflammatory properties, supporting the treatment of infections and wounds while accelerating healing by reducing bleeding, stimulating collagen synthesis, and aiding scar maturation (2% avocado oil) (Naeimifar et al., 2020; Ferreira et al., 2022; Sichani et al., 2021; Moldovan, 2021). These effects are largely attributed to its high fatty acid content, which facilitates energy storage, lipid bilayer synthesis, and epidermal homeostasis. Reportedly, fatty acids maintain barrier integrity, regulate sebum formation, and mediate keratinocyte signaling through peroxisome proliferator-activated receptors, which enhance barrier function and follicular development via protein palmitoylation, offering important cosmetic benefits (Vandorou et al., 2024, 2025; Lin and Khnykin, 2014).

Beyond its nutritive components, avocado also demonstrates notable antioxidant, antiinflammatory, and antibacterial activities, contributing to both skin protection and product preservation, even at low concentrations (0.5% avocado oil) (Ferreira et al., 2022; Nasri et al., 2022). Its efficacy has been further supported by preclinical research showing significant acceleration of wound closure and epithelialization in rat models treated with *P. americana* fruit extract (Sichani et al., 2021; Deuschle et al., 2019). Similarly, a semisolid formulation repair containing avocado oil enhanced collagen deposition and reduced inflammatory infiltration, confirming its tissue repair and antiinflammatory potential (Sichani et al., 2021; Deuschle et al., 2019; De Oliveira et al., 2013). Peel extracts show strong antioxidant and antibacterial properties and are compatible with both oil-in-water and water-in-oil emulsions, serving as natural alternatives to synthetic preservatives in moisturizing creams (Ferreira et al., 2022). Leaf essential oils also exhibit moderate antibacterial and antioxidant activity, supported by their rich phytochemical profile, while seed oil, marked by a high UFA content, enhances skin hydration and barrier repair, properties that have encouraged its incorporation into lip balm products (Ferreira et al., 2022; Nasri et al., 2022).

Interestingly, avocado leaf extract also displays therapeutic potential beyond conventional cosmetics. A 3% gel formulation effectively alleviated UVB-induced mechanical allodynia, providing significant postsunburn pain relief within 48–72 h after irradiation (Deuschle et al., 2019).

4.3 Applications of the bioactive and health-promoting enzymes from fruits and their by-products

Bromelain, ficin, and papain, three plant-derived cysteine proteinases belonging to the peptidase family C1 (papain family), are widely utilized in the cosmetic and dermatological sectors. The growing preference for eco-conscious and sustainable formulations in the cosmetic industry has enhanced interest in these “green beauty” enzymes. Although all three share a similar catalytic mechanism, they differ slightly in their optimal functional conditions, stability, and substrate specificity (Venetikidou et al., 2025; Bonarska-Kujawa et al., 2011; Lyu et al., 2023; Michalak, 2023; Boonkerd and Wantha, 2024). These enzymes are capable of hydrolyzing proteins, promoting gentle exfoliation, and accelerating epidermal renewal. They serve as effective, nonabrasive alternatives to traditional mechanical or chemical exfoliants, making them suitable for diverse skincare, haircare, and therapeutic products. Bromelain is often included in exfoliating masks, cleansers, and antiinflammatory creams, while ficin is preferred in mild exfoliants for sensitive skin, and papain is commonly used in deep exfoliators (Diogo Gonçalves, 2021; Arshad et al., 2014; Sharma and Vimal, 2023; Bhogal et al., 2014; Smith et al., 2007).

All three enzymes effectively degrade keratin and stratum corneum proteins, facilitating the removal of dead cells without irritation. Due to their nonabrasive nature, they are ideal for acne- or rosacea-prone skin and reduce the risk of overexfoliation, thus offering compatibility with sensitive skin types (Diogo Gonçalves, 2021; Trevisol et al., 2022; Bialkowski, 2022; Patra et al., 2024). In addition, bromelain, ficin, and papain exhibit antiinflammatory properties by suppressing proinflammatory cytokines and degrading inflammatory mediators, which, in turn, reduces edema, irritation, and fluid accumulation. Their proteolytic activity promotes collagen synthesis and enhances the skin barrier while preserving its natural defense system mechanisms (Kim et al., 2024; Kansakar et al., 2024).

Regular use of products containing these enzymes leads to a more even skin tone and a smoother texture. By removing melanin-rich keratinocytes and inhibiting tyrosinase-mediated melanin synthesis, they prevent hyperpigmentation, fade age spots, and improve overall complexion (Diogo Gonçalves, 2021; Trevisol et al., 2022; Bialkowski, 2022; Patra et al., 2024). In addition, enzymatic exfoliation enhances the skin's permeability, improving the absorption and bioavailability of other active ingredients, thereby optimizing the performance of skincare and haircare products. In hair and scalp care, proteolytic enzymes help dissolve excess keratin buildup, reduce scalp flakiness, dandruff, and scalp irritation, and prevent follicular blockage. Their gentle exfoliating action supports hair growth, strengthens strands, and maintains follicular health (Chakraborty et al., 2021; Trevisol et al., 2022; Nascimento et al., 2024). Moreover, bromelain, ficin, and papain have been studied for their wound healing potential due to their capacity to debride necrotic tissue, stimulate collagen formation, and promote new tissue regeneration. Their inclusion in postsurgical ointments and after-burn creams demonstrates their ability to reduce redness, pain, and scarring, thereby accelerating recovery (Baidamshina et al., 2020; Barbulova et al., 2015; da Silva Melo et al., 2023; Mendes et al., 2019).

Solubility is a key parameter influencing their cosmetic incorporation. Bromelain and papain are water-soluble (Chakraborty et al., 2021; Michalak, 2023), whereas ficin, though less soluble, remains stable in buffered or aqueous media. Conversely, organic solvents reduce the solubility of all three enzymes (Morellon-Sterling et al., 2020). It is important to note that AHAs or β-hydroxy acids and certain surfactants in cleansers or emulsifiers can denature these enzymes and diminish their activity (Tang and Yang, 2018; Michalak, 2023; Sołdacka and Barańska-Rybak, 2024; Minich et al., 2021; Divakaran et al., 2023). To counteract this, pH buffering, enzyme encapsulation, and the use of stabilizers or optimized formulation types (e.g., leave-on masks and serums versus wash-off cleansers or powder exfoliants) are essential for preserving enzymatic activity. In addition, stabilizing agents such as trehalose, glycerol, ethylenediaminetetraacetic acid, or ascorbic acid can form protective microenvironments around enzyme molecules, enhancing their structural integrity and storage stability (Nascimento et al., 2024; Duskey et al., 2020; Kuo et al., 2024).

Despite their benefits, bromelain, ficin, and papain may cause hypersensitivity reactions in susceptible individuals. Bromelain has been linked to skin rashes, itching, swelling, and allergic reactions, particularly in those allergic to pineapple. It may interfere with diagnostic tests, as well as cross-react with latex, papain, or wheat flour allergens. Similarly, ficin can cause irritation and allergic reactions in individuals sensitive to fig latex, with documented cross-sensitization to birch pollen allergens. Finally, papain may induce rashes, itching, contact dermatitis, and hives due to its keratinolytic effect on tight junction proteins, leading to increased skin permeability. Consequently, these enzymes should be used cautiously in individuals with sensitive or compromised skin (Chakraborty et al., 2021; Kansakar et al., 2024; Tanabe et al., 1997; Leelakanok et al., 2023; Giangrieco et al., 2023).

4.4 Applications of the bioactive and health-promoting constituents in grape and winemaking by-products

Winemaking by-products, such as grape pomace and seed oil, exhibit notable antioxidant, antimicrobial, antiaging, and antiinflammatory properties. In vitro and in vivo studies on keratinocytes and fibroblasts confirm their capacity to enhance skin hydration, elasticity, and UV protection, while mitigating oxidative stress and inflammation through molecular pathways like sirtuin 1 (SIRT1) and heat shock protein 47 (HSP47). With appropriate processing, the bioactives concentrated in grape tissues contribute to a wide array of skin-protective effects, offering antioxidant, antifungal, and antimicrobial actions (Salem et al., 2022).

Polyphenols, particularly proanthocyanidins and resveratrol, modulate cellular pathways essential for skin health (Nascimento et al., 2024). In keratinocytes, they reduce reactive ROS, lower proinflammatory cytokines, and protect DNA from UV-induced damage. Similarly, in fibroblasts, polyphenols enhance the expression of genes like SIRT1 and HSP47, which are linked to antiaging processes, promoting skin elasticity and moisture retention (Afaq and Katiyar, 2011; Marabini et al., 2020). These bioactivities make grape-derived extracts valuable in antiaging and skin-whitening formulations, where they improve hydration, softness, and elasticity while reducing roughness, wrinkle depth, redness, and hyperpigmentation. Moreover, they provide photoprotective effects, inhibiting enzymes such as proteinase, tyrosinase, collagenase (MMP-1), and elastase, important for the degradation of collagen and elastin and, thus, the provision of skin firmness and elasticity. Interestingly, grape seeds are rich in vitamin E, which, in cosmetics, is commonly used in day and night creams for its antioxidant properties (Marabini et al., 2020; Matos et al., 2019; Leal et al., 2020; Maidin et al., 2018).

Extracts from wine lees, red grape pomace, and other by-products have displayed potent antioxidant and antihyperpigmentation activities. Wine lees extracts, rich in phenolics and anthocyanins (e.g., caftaric acid, malvidin, peonidin-3-*O*-glucoside, myricetin, quercetin), strongly inhibit elastase, MMP-1, and tyrosinase (Matos et al., 2019). In comparative assays, six grape by-product extracts showed greater elastase inhibition than tyrosinase, confirming their antiwrinkle potential (Leal et al., 2020). Grape extracts (*Vitis vinifera* L.) also enhance mitochondrial adenosine triphosphate production and protect fibroblasts against UVA-induced oxidative stress by modulating DNA methylation and promoting SIRT1/HSP47 expression (Alcendor et al., 2007; Letsiou et al., 2020; Ito and Nagata, 2017). Similarly, *V. vinifera* L. leaf extract protects keratinocytes from UVA-induced ROS and DNA damage (Comet assay, γ-H2AX), displaying strong antioxidant and antimutagenic activity (Marabini et al., 2020).

In antioxidant assays (DPPH, FRAP, ABTS, and ORAC), phenolic extracts consistently outperform oils, whose activity mainly derives from tocopherols and tocotrienols (Di Stefano et al., 2022). Grape pomace extracts show greater antioxidant capacity than seed ones due to the combined presence of skins and seeds (Szabó et al., 2021). These by-products were used in a facial moisturizer base and nine formulations (0.1%), which remained stable for 35 days and replaced synthetic antioxidants (Ferreira and Santos, 2022; Szabó et al., 2021). Another study confirmed ellagic acid's presence in grape pomace by HPLC and found its DPPH inhibition comparable to that of BHT, though not significantly higher, while proving noncytotoxic under oxidative stress, verified by scanning electron microscopy (SEM) (Maluf et al., 2018). Comparative profiling of five grape varieties (Marselan, Syrah, Obeidi, Asswad Karech, and Cabernet Franc) revealed high phenolic content, with gallic acid (883.05 ± 98.59 μg/g in Obeidi), catechins (abundant in Marselan), and other antioxidants (chlorogenic, caffeic, and p-coumaric acids), correlating strongly with their antioxidant activity (Salem et al., 2022).

Beyond their antioxidant properties, grape by-products enhance antimicrobial protection in cosmetic formulations. A moisturizing face cream containing grape seed phenolic extract and oils inhibited Gram-positive bacteria (Kirby–Bauer method) (Di Stefano et al., 2022), while other grape extracts showed broad-spectrum inhibition in disc diffusion and minimum inhibitory concentration assays (Leal et al., 2020). In vivo, in vitro, and clinical data confirm that *V. vinifera* L. extracts effectively inhibit *Staphylococcus aureus* and *Cutibacterium acnes*, reducing biofilm formation and inflammation while preserving beneficial microbiota (Armari et al., 2024). Recent research further emphasizes their antiinflammatory potential. A 2024 study on a single grape extract (GSE-Ov) and its microdispersion demonstrated a significant concentration-dependent reduction of IL-1α in keratinocytes exposed to urban air particles (Castro et al., 2024). Similarly, grape stem extracts (GSEs) from six varieties significantly inhibited NO release under both basal and lipopolysaccharide-induced inflammatory conditions (Leal et al., 2020). Together, these findings confirm that grape-based extracts can attenuate inflammation via multiple pathways, supporting their dermatological and pharmacological applications.

Despite their multiple advantages, stability challenges remain a key limitation. The phenolic and lipidic constituents in grape by-products are highly sensitive to light, oxygen, and heat, resulting in reduced product stability and shorter shelf life. Incorporation of nanocapsules, microparticles, or liposomes facilitates controlled release and protects bioactive integrity. In parallel, allergenic potential and regulatory compliance remain important challenges in product development. To ensure consumer safety, stronger global collaborations between researchers, legislators, and regulatory authorities are essential for establishing validated clinical, toxicological, and standardization frameworks. Currently, the use of grape by-products in cosmetics within the European Union remains limited due to regulatory gaps and the absence of standardized safety guidelines and permitted concentration limits. Addressing these issues will be critical for broader industrial adoption and consumer confidence in sustainable grape-based cosmetics (Nhani et al., 2024; Elbrolesy et al., 2023; Patra et al., 2024; Duskey et al., 2020; Konopko et al., 2020; Manca et al., 2020; Coderoni and Perito, 2020).

4.5 Applications of the bioactive and health-promoting constituents in kiwi by-products

Kiwi and its by-products, including peel, branches, and leaves, represent valuable resources for the cosmetic industry. Their bioactive constituents, mainly phenolics, vitamins, and carotenoids, exhibit potent antioxidant, photoprotective, and antiaging effects, enhancing skin density, elasticity, hydration, and wrinkle reduction. Phenolics, particularly chlorogenic acid, accelerate wound healing and protect against oxidative stress at the wound site (Bayat et al., 2023; Hafezi et al., 2010; Kooshiar et al., 2012; Goudarzi et al., 2015).

Among kiwi's vitamins, vitamin C plays a crucial role in antihyperpigmentation, wound repair, and scar healing due to its antioxidant and antiinflammatory potential (Bagdas et al., 2015). It shields against UV-induced oxidative stress, stimulates collagen synthesis, and improves skin microstructure and tone in aged skin. Similarly, vitamin E provides photoprotective, antitumorigenic, and moisturizing benefits, reducing DNA damage and keratinocyte death after UV exposure, stabilizing the skin barrier, and diminishing skin roughness. When vitamin C and E are combined in stabilized antiaging formulations, they enhance UV protection, prevent DNA damage and inflammation, and promote cell renewal (Bayat et al., 2023; Hafezi et al., 2010; Kooshiar et al., 2012; Goudarzi et al., 2015).

Kiwi carotenoids contribute via robust antioxidant and antiglycation action, preventing collagen degradation, stimulating cell proliferation, and reducing oxidative stress. Their photoprotective role improves microcirculation and provides defense against skin aging, UV damage, and cellular degeneration. Collectively, these bioactives underline the versatility of kiwi-derived ingredients in cosmetic products tailored for skin protection, regeneration, and rejuvenation, as supported by numerous studies (Vandorou et al., 2024, 2025; Rakha et al., 2025). In addition, kiwi extracts have been safely integrated into creams and cosmeceuticals. Following extraction by diverse methods (Silva et al., 2021), the bioactive-rich resulting concentrate was incorporated into standard cream formulations and adjusted for concentration balance (Teixeira et al., 2022). These extracts have proven to be promising candidates for safe, effective skincare products, aligning with the current demand for natural cosmeceuticals, although further studies are needed to fully assess their in vivo efficacy and potential for commercial development (Silva et al., 2022).

Valorizing kiwi by-products supports the principles of sustainability and the circular economy, promoting eco-friendly cosmetic innovation. However, kiwi fruit is allergenic for some individuals, and its bioactives (vitamins, antioxidants, enzymes) may degrade during processing and storage, compromising product stability and efficacy. In addition, kiwi allergens can cross-react with latex and birch pollen, making transparent labeling essential for consumer safety (especially for children). Diagnostic approaches such as skin prick tests, specific immunoglobulin E tests, and component-resolved diagnostics help identify major allergens like actinidin (Act d1) and thaumatin-like protein (Act d2). Children often experience mono-sensitization, whereas adults frequently exhibit multiple sensitizations, indicating demographic variability in allergy patterns (Bringheli et al., 2023). Despite isolated reports of kiwi-related allergic reactions, the underlying mechanisms remain unclear, and toxicological studies on kiwi bioactives are limited. Further research is required to evaluate formulation stability, ideally over 6 months, along with assessments of moisturizing capacity and consumer safety. Finally, comprehensive sustainability assessments, including carbon footprint, resource use, and end-of-life analysis, are needed to compare kiwi-based cosmetics with conventional products and confirm their environmental advantages (Moysidou et al., 2024, 2025).

4.6 Applications of the bioactive and health-promoting constituents in tomato by-products

Tomato is another noteworthy source of diverse bioactives, exhibiting potent antioxidant, antiinflammatory, and UV-protective properties that underscore its relevance in advanced cosmetic applications. Lycopene, the predominant carotenoid in tomatoes, acts as a powerful antioxidant that prevents oxidative DNA damage and the transformation of normal cells into cancerous ones by quenching singlet oxygen and neutralizing free radicals (Kontaxi et al., 2024; Szabo et al., 2022; Ali et al., 2021). Recent research demonstrated that lycopene can function as a nontoxic antioxidant, reducing agent, and stabilizer during the green synthesis of zinc oxide (ZnO) nanoparticles (NPs), hence supporting the development of multifunctional sunscreen formulations (Elbrolesy et al., 2023). In another study, a sunscreen lotion containing 1.5% tomato extract retained its physical and chemical stability for 28 days while maintaining a high SPF value of 22.24 (Sopyan et al., 2017). Lycopene also removes lipid radicals, limits lipid peroxidation, and prevents UV-induced erythema. Interestingly, its ROS-quenching capacity is twice that of β-carotene and ten times greater than α-tocopherol (Sjahjadi et al., 2021).

Topically, lycopene protects against UVB-related skin damage by inhibiting epidermal ornithine decarboxylase, thereby reducing inflammation and preventing DNA injury. Studies in human keratinocytes (HaCaT cell line) suggest that lycopene may exert a corrective effect on irradiated cells, enhancing skin defense mechanisms depending on photodamage levels (Sopyan et al., 2017; Caseiro et al., 2020). Moreover, its use attenuates both acute (sunburn) and chronic (photocarcinogenesis, photoaging, skin cancer) effects of UV exposure (Butnariu and Giuchici, 2011; Caseiro et al., 2020; Ascenso et al., 2014; Mansuri et al., 2021). Lycopene strengthens the synthesis of prostaglandins and phospholipids, key membrane components that bolster cellular resilience. Topical 0.05% lycopene application in mice significantly reduced anthralin-induced swelling and erythema, showing stronger antiinflammatory effects than a 1 mg/g betamethasone solution (Caseiro et al., 2020). Lycopene-based nanoemulsions further enhance skin hydration, suppleness, and photoprotection, offering a modern, effective alternative to conventional cosmetics (Butnariu and Giuchici, 2011).

Beyond lycopene, tomato-derived bioactives, such as vitamins E and C, also demonstrate substantial photoprotective effects. In vivo studies confirm that topical vitamin E and, to a lesser extent, vitamin C effectively reduce DNA damage, lipid peroxidation, UV-induced erythema, and wrinkle formation, while botanical antioxidants further enhance protection when integrated into sunscreen products. Vitamin E, found in grape by-products, safeguards cell membranes from oxidative stress and mitigates photoaging, lipid peroxidation, immunosuppression, and photocarcinogenesis (Butnariu and Giuchici, 2011; Caseiro et al., 2020; Ascenso et al., 2014; Mansuri et al., 2021). Pretreatment with vitamin E-containing formulations with vitamin A or base vehicles showed similar effects. The acetylated derivative, α-tocopheryl acetate, offers higher stability, lipophilicity, and shelf life, enabling deeper skin penetration and gradual conversion to active tocopherol within cells. Consequently, it ranks among the most widely utilized antioxidants in sunscreens. Ongoing research aims to optimize its bioactivation and controlled release for enhanced photoprotection (Butnariu and Giuchici, 2011; Caseiro et al., 2020; Ascenso et al., 2014; Mansuri et al., 2021; Jesus et al., 2023).

In parallel, L-ascorbic acid in tomatoes and its by-products plays a crucial role in UV protection, wound healing, and collagen synthesis. Topical application significantly reduces UVA/UVB-induced photodamage, histologically verified by lower counts of sunburn cells. Unlike sunscreens, it does not absorb UV rays but neutralizes UV-generated ROS, reducing inflammation and even alleviating sunburn. Its antiinflammatory and antioxidant profile makes it an effective additive in postlaser or antiaging treatments, improving skin tone and resilience. Remarkably, vitamin C adheres firmly to the skin, resisting removal by rubbing, washing, or sweating, offering persistent protection for several days. It also prevents UV-linked immunosuppression, reducing the risk of nonmelanoma skin cancers. However, despite its proven efficacy, vitamin C products face challenges in stability and dermal penetration, which remain active fields of cosmetic research (Zhang et al., 2024; Al-Niaimi and Chiang, 2017; Motlhalamme et al., 2025).

4.7 Applications of the bioactive and health-promoting constituents in pomegranate by-products

Pomegranate processing generates abundant by-products (e.g., peels, seeds, pomace) that are exceptionally rich in polyphenols, tannins (punicalagins, ellagitannins), anthocyanins, and lipophilic actives (e.g., punicic acid, tocopherols). These compounds confer strong radical scavenging, metal-chelating, and antiinflammatory capacities, making peel and seed fractions attractive as natural antioxidant and cosmeceutical ingredients (Singh et al., 2023). Detailed phytochemical profiling confirms that peel extracts contain the highest total phenolic loads, while seed oil supplies unique conjugated fatty acids that support emollience and barrier repair (Eid et al., 2024).

Pomegranate peel extracts inhibit photodamage signaling and matrix-degrading enzymes that underlie skin aging. In vitro and ex vivo studies show that punicalagin and related tannins protect dermal fibroblasts from UVA-induced oxidative injury, reduce MMP-1/elastase activity, and preserve collagen integrity, mechanisms compatible with lower wrinkle formation and improved elasticity when formulated into antiaging creams or serums (Singh et al., 2023; Bianchetti et al., 2024). Moreover, the fruit's seed oil (PSO) contributes complementary, lipid-mediated benefits, including its high punicic acid and vitamin E content, which confer emollient, antioxidant, and antiinflammatory effects that improve skin hydration, reduce transepidermal water loss, and support barrier recovery. Recent formulation research studies demonstrate that pomegranate seed oil loaded into nano- or self-nanoemulsifying systems markedly increases its antioxidant potency and bioavailability, making this seed oil a promising ingredient for topical moisturizers, antiinflammatory balms, and potentially photoprotective oil-in-water systems (Eid et al., 2024; Hassanein et al., 2024; Baccarin et al., 2015; Sahafi et al., 2021).

Beyond antioxidant and antiaging actions, pomegranate by-products show robust antimicrobial and preservative-adjunct activity. Comparative studies on multiple peel extracts report inhibitory effects against Gram-positive and Gram-negative skin-relevant strains, supporting their use as natural preservatives or as bioactives in microbiome-modulating cosmetics, with strong antimicrobial properties, together with robust radical scavenging effects verified by DPPH, FRAP, or ABTS assays (Abu-Niaaj et al., 2024). *P. granatum* L. exhibits a notable cytotoxic effect on HeLa cells (IC_{50} of 49.51–91.54 μg/mL) and normal MRC-5 and EA.hy926 cells (IC_{50} of > 200 μg/mL), exerting its best antioxidant effect on the cervix adenocarcinoma cell line, while no cytotoxicity was found for normal cells, pointing out PSO's safety (Đurđević et al., 2018).

Crucially, emerging clinical and translational evidence supports the topical and cosmetic benefits in humans utilizing pomegranate cosmetic formulations. Pilot and controlled study data report major improvements in wrinkle metrics, tactile roughness, skin radiance, erythema, and pigmentation after the topical application of standardized extracts or PSO-enriched creams (Chakkalakal et al., 2022; Chan et al., 2022). Observational trials also indicate direct reductions in neurologically mediated hand dermatitis parameters following topical PSO application (Hamouda and Felemban, 2023). However, larger randomized trials with standardized extracts are needed to quantify effect sizes across skin types.

Formulation stability and regulatory factors play a crucial role in the large-scale application of pomegranate-based ingredients. Specifically, pomegranate phenolics are mainly sensitive to environmental conditions such as light, oxygen, and heat, which can reduce their activity over time. Interestingly, to overcome this, advanced formulation strategies like micro-/nano-encapsulation, liposomal systems, or NP-structured delivery are increasingly used to protect these compounds and ensure a gradual, controlled release in emulsions (Hassanein et al., 2024; Sahafi et al., 2021; Chakkalakal et al., 2022). Although pomegranate derivatives are generally considered safe at typical cosmetic concentrations, comprehensive safety documentation remains essential. This includes allergen testing, stability and photostability studies, and compliance with international cosmetic regulations, such as the International Nomenclature of Cosmetic Ingredients (INCI) listing and established concentration limits, before products reach the market (Singh et al., 2023; Eid et al., 2024; Abu-Niaaj et al., 2024).

5 Limitations, challenges, and future perspectives

Despite the growing success of fruit by-products in cosmetics, many important challenges still limit their widespread adoption. One of the biggest issues is the variability in bioactive content among raw materials. Environmental factors, cultivar differences, harvesting time, and extraction conditions can all influence the yield and composition of key compounds such as phenolics, flavonoids, and carotenoids (Ganjeh et al., 2025; Yahia, 2018; Rahaman et al., 2023). For instance, the concentration of punicalagin in pomegranate peel or lycopene in tomato skin can vary drastically between batches, making standardization and reproducibility difficult for large-scale production. Therefore developing reliable quality control systems and unified reference standards is essential to guarantee efficacy and consumer safety (Yahia, 2018; Bonarska-Kujawa et al., 2011; Singh et al., 2023; Eid et al., 2024). Challenges also arise in raw material supply and seasonal availability, as fruit waste is often generated at dispersed sites and is prone to rapid microbial spoilage, making it difficult to collect and process. Establishing a mini-biorefinery unit near such juice or canning factories could minimize transportation costs and ensure fresher inputs for extraction (Błaszczyk et al., 2024; Alexandri et al., 2021; Ariwaodo and Olaniyan, 2024).

Another critical limitation concerns formulation stability and bioavailability. Many fruit-derived bioactives, including vitamin C, phenolics, flavonoids, carotenoids, and enzymes, are highly sensitive to light, oxygen, pH, and temperature conditions, leading to degradation or decreased bioactivity over time. This instability shortens their shelf life and may alter their final color, texture, or fragrance. Advanced formulation techniques, such as microencapsulation, liposomal or NP delivery, and hydrogel-based matrices, have shown great promise in protecting these fragile molecules and ensuring a controlled release on the skin. Nevertheless, implementing these methods on an industrial scale still requires cost-effective optimization and strict process validation (Mihalcea et al., 2021; Baidamshina et al., 2020; Bayat et al., 2023; Motlhalamme et al., 2025; Bianchetti et al., 2024; Chuacharoen et al., 2024; Ahmed et al., 2020; Ataide et al., 2021; Fazolin et al., 2020).

Extraction and purification processes pose several technological and economic challenges. While green extraction methods such as UAE, MAE, and SFE reduce solvent consumption and environmental impact, they can be expensive and require advanced infrastructure. Matrix complexity, especially in fiber-abundant by-products such as kiwi, tomato, and apple pomace, can further lower their efficiency or complicate their downstream purification. Integrating green solvents, biorefinery, and circular-economy models could improve their cost-effectiveness and enable the use of multiple by-products within one production line (Ganjeh et al., 2025; Wu et al., 2023; El-Shamy and Farag, 2021; Abu-Niaaj et al., 2024). Moreover, safety and allergenicity are also key considerations. Although most fruit-derived ingredients are generally recognized as safe, certain proteolytic enzymes like bromelain, ficin, and papain, or phenolic-rich extracts may trigger skin irritation or allergic reactions, especially in sensitive individuals. Kiwi or papaya components, for instance, are well-documented allergens, sometimes cross-reacting with latex or birch pollen proteins. For this reason, comprehensive toxicological testing, patch studies, and in vivo evaluations remain essential before market approval. Adherence to frameworks such as the EU Cosmetic Regulation (EC No. 1223/2009) or INCI listing ensures transparency and consumer protection (Giangrieco et al., 2023; Bringheli et al., 2023; Ebo et al., 2024).

Looking forward, the integration of omics technologies and artificial intelligence can help identify novel bioactives and also predict their stability, dermal absorption, and, therefore, cosmetic value. Combining metabolomics with nanotechnology could revolutionize global skincare, allowing precise targeting of skin layers, improved antioxidant performance, and multi-targeting "smart" product development (Hamouda and Felemban, 2023; Abu-Niaaj et al., 2024; Gómez-Godínez et al., 2025; Akhter Bhat et al., 2025). In essence, the valorization of fruit by-products such as apple pomace, avocado peel, grape seeds, pomegranate rind, tomato skin, kiwi leaves, and/or proteolytic bromelain, ficin, and papain represents a significant step toward sustainable cosmetic innovation. Overcoming the remaining technological, economic, and regulatory barriers will require cross-disciplinary collaboration and continued investment in green chemistry principles and advanced formulation research. If addressed, these challenges could transform agrifood waste into a reliable source of bioactives for next-generation, sustainable cosmetics and dermocosmetics (Hamouda and Felemban, 2023; Abu-Niaaj et al., 2024; Gómez-Godínez et al., 2025; Akhter Bhat et al., 2025).

6 Conclusions

The increasing demand for sustainable and multifunctional cosmetic ingredients has brought fruit by-products to the forefront of green innovation. Rich in polyphenols, carotenoids, flavonoids, vitamins, and natural enzymes, these materials exhibit potent antioxidant, antiaging, antiinflammatory, and photoprotective effects, offering a natural and eco-friendly alternative to synthetic agents. Beyond efficacy, their valorization leads to high-performance skincare products while contributing to waste minimization and circular economy principles.

Although a few limitations persist, particularly in extraction scalability, formulation stability, and regulatory harmonization, fruit by-product-based cosmetics are highly promising in terms of their health-promoting profile and bioactivity. Ongoing advances in bioengineering, nanotechnology, and green extraction will further enhance the efficacy and safety of fruit-derived actives. As consumer awareness increasingly aligns with principles of transparency and sustainability, the use of fruit by-products in cosmetics is emerging not merely as a passing trend but as a lasting model that unites environmental responsibility, human health, and scientific and technological progress.

Acknowledgments

The authors would like to thank the School of Chemistry in the Faculty of Sciences at Democritus University of Thrace for their continuous support.

Conflicts of interest

The authors declare no conflicts of interest.

Funding

This research received no external funding.

Author contributions

A.T. was involved in conceptualization, methodology, validation, visualization, supervision, and project administration. A.T., S.M., E.K., and T.A. were involved in investigation. S.M., T.A., A.T., and E.K. were involved in writing—original draft preparation. A.T., A.O., and T.A. were involved in writing—review and editing. All authors contributed to software and have read and agreed to the published version of the manuscript.

References

100% PURE, n.d. All About Natural Sunscreen. https://www.100percentpure.com/blogs/feed/all-about-natural-sunscreen.

Abbas, S., Shanbhag, T., Kothare, A., 2021. Applications of bromelain from pineapple waste towards acne. Saudi J. Biol. Sci. 1319562X. 28 (1), 1001–1009. doi:10.1016/j.sjbs.2020.11.032.

Abu-Niaaj, L.F., Al-Daghistani, H.I., Katampe, I., Abu-Irmaileh, B., Bustanji, Y.K., 2024. Pomegranate peel: bioactivities as antimicrobial and cytotoxic agents. Food Sci. Nutr. 20487177. 12 (4), 2818–2832. Available from: https://onlinelibrary.wiley.com/journal/10.1002/%28ISSN%292048-7177. doi:10.1002/fsn3.3963.

Afaq, F., Katiyar, S.K., 2011. Polyphenols: skin photoprotection and inhibition of photocarcinogenesis. Mini-Rev. Med. Chem. 18755607. 11 (14), 1200–1215. Available from: http://www.eurekaselect.com/633/journal/mini-reviews-medicinal-chemistry. doi:10.2174/138955751111091200.

Ahmed, G.H.G., Fernández-González, A., Elena Díaz García, M., 2020. Nano-encapsulation of grape and apple pomace phenolic extract in chitosan and soy protein via nanoemulsification. Food Hydrocoll. 0268005X. 108, 105806. doi:10.1016/j.foodhyd.2020.105806.

Akhter Bhat, T., Rather, R.A., Bashir, S., Mishra, N.-S., John, R., 2025. Nanoparticles in plant systems: omics-based perspectives on stress adaptation and toxicological implications. Plant Nano Biol. 27731111. 13, 100181. doi:10.1016/j.plana.2025.100181.

Al-Niaimi, F., Chiang, N.Y.Z., 2017. Topical Vitamin C and the skin: mechanisms of action and clinical applications. J. Clin. Aesthet. Dermatol. 19412789. 10 (7), 14–17. Available from: http://jcadonline.epubxp.com/t/9606-journal-of-clinical-And-Aesthetic-dermatology.

Alara, O.R., Abdurahman, N.H., Ali, H.A., Zain, N.M., 2021. Microwave-assisted extraction of phenolic compounds from Carica papaya leaves: an optimization study and LC-QTOF-MS analysis. Future Foods. 26668335. 3, 100035. doi:10.1016/j.fufo.2021.100035.

Alcendor, R.R., Gao, S., Zhai, P., Zablocki, D., Holle, E., Yu, X., Tian, B., Wagner, T., Vatner, S.F., Sadoshima, J., 2007. Sirt1 regulates aging and resistance to oxidative stress in the heart. Circ. Res. 00097330. 100 (10), 1512–1521. doi:10.1161/01.RES.0000267723.65696.4a.

Alexandre, E.M.C., Silva, S., Santos, S.A.O., Silvestre, A.J.D., Duarte, M.F., Saraiva, J.A., Pintado, M., 2019. Antimicrobial activity of pomegranate peel extracts performed by high pressure and enzymatic assisted extraction. Food Res. Int. 18737145. 115, 167–176. Available from: https://www.elsevier.com/inca/publications/store/4/2/2/9/7/0. doi:10.1016/j.foodres.2018.08.044.

Alexandri, M., Maina, S., Tsouko, E., Papapostolou, H., Koutinas, A., Kourmentza, K., 2021. Valorization of fruit processing by-product streams into integrated biorefinery concepts: extraction of value-added compounds and bioconversion to chemicals. In: Bhat, R. (Ed.), Valorization of Agri-Food Wastes and By-Products: Recent Trends, Innovations and Sustainability Challenges. Elsevier, Greece, pp. 927–945. Available from: https://www.sciencedirect.com/book/9780128240441. doi:10.1016/B978-0-12-824044-1.00014-3.

Ali, M.M., Hashim, N., Aziz, S.A., Lasekan, O., 2020. Pineapple (*Ananas comosus*): a comprehensive review of nutritional values, volatile compounds, health benefits, and potential food products. Food Res. Int. 09639969. 137, 109675. doi:10.1016/j.foodres.2020.109675.

Ali, M.Y., Sina, A.A.I., Khandker, S.S., Neesa, L., Tanvir, E.M., Kabir, A., Khalil, M.I., Gan, S.H., 2021. Nutritional composition and bioactive compounds in tomatoes and their impact on human health and disease: a review. Foods 23048158. 10 (1). Available from: https://www.mdpi.com/2304-8158/10/1/45/pdf. doi:10.3390/foods10010045.

Amri, E., Mamboya, F., 2012. Papain, a plant enzyme of biological importance: a review. Am. J. Biochem. Biotechnol. 15533468. 8 (2), 99–104. Available from: http://thescipub.com/pdf/10.3844/ajbbsp.2012.99.104. doi:10.3844/ajbbsp.2012.99.104Tanzania.

Aniceto, J.P.S., Rodrigues, V.H., Portugal, I., Silva, C.M., 2022. Valorization of tomato residues by supercritical fluid extraction. Processes 22279717. 10 (1). Available from: https://www.mdpi.com/2227-9717/10/1/28/pdf. doi:10.3390/pr10010028.

Araújo, R.G., Rodriguez-Jasso, R.M., Ruiz, H.A., Govea-Salas, M., Pintado, M.E., Aguilar, C.N., 2020. Process optimization of microwave-assisted extraction of bioactive molecules from avocado seeds. Ind. Crops Prod. 09266690. 154. Available from: https://www.elsevier.com/inca/publications/store/5/2/2/8/2/5. doi:10.1016/j.indcrop.2020.112623.

Argun, M.E., Şamil Argun, M., Ates, H., 2025. Zero waste principle for the fruit processing industry: recovery, advanced conversion and revalorization approaches. J. Water Process Eng. 22147144. 71, 107243. doi:10.1016/j.jwpe.2025.107243.

Ariwaodo, C.A., Olaniyan, O.F., 2024. Fleshy fruit waste and the green chemistry of its conversion to valuable products for humans and animals. Food Chem. Adv. 2772753X. 4, 100634. doi:10.1016/j.focha.2024.100634.

Armari, M., Zavattaro, E., Trejo, C.F., Galeazzi, A., Grossetti, A., Veronese, F., Savoia, P., Azzimonti, B., Vitis Vinifera, L., 2024. Leaf extract, a microbiota green ally against infectious and inflammatory skin and scalp diseases: an in-depth update. Antibiotics. 2079-6382. 13 (8), 697. doi:10.3390/antibiotics13080697.

Arraibi, A.A., Liberal, Â., Dias, M.I., Alves, M.J., Ferreira, I.C.F.R., Barros, L., Barreira, J.C.M., 2021. Chemical and bioactive characterization of spanish and Belgian apple pomace for its potential use as a novel dermocosmetic formulation. Foods 23048158. 10 (8). Available from: https://www.mdpi.com/2304-8158/10/8/1949/pdf. doi:10.3390/foods10081949.

Arshad, Z.I.M., Amid, A., Yusof, F., Jaswir, I., Ahmad, K., Loke, S.P., 2014. Bromelain: an overview of industrial application and purification strategies. Appl. Microbiol. Biotechnol. 14320614. 98 (17), 7283–7297. Available from: https://link.springer.de/link/service/journals/00253/index.htm. doi:10.1007/s00253-014-5889-y.

Ascenso, A., Ribeiro, H., Marques, H.C., Oliveira, H., Santos, C., Simões, S., 2014. Chemoprevention of photocarcinogenesis by lycopene. Exp. Dermatol. 16000625. 23 (12), 874–878. Available from: http://onlinelibrary.wiley.com/journal/10.1111/(ISSN)1600-0625. doi:10.1111/exd.12491Portugal.

Ataide, J.A., Geraldes, D.C., Gérios, E.F., Bissaco, F.M., Cefali, L.C., Oliveira-Nascimento, L., Mazzola, P.G., 2021. Freeze-dried chitosan nanoparticles to stabilize and deliver bromelain. J. Drug Deliv. Sci. Technol. 17732247. 61. Available from: http://www.editionsdesante.fr/category.php?id_category=48. doi:10.1016/j.jddst.2020.102225.

Atwi-Ghaddar, S., Destandau, E., Lesellier, E., 2023. Integrated supercritical fluid extraction and pre-formulation process of *Punica granatum* L. pericarp polar compounds. Molecules. 1420-3049. 28 (24), 8110. doi:10.3390/molecules28248110.

Ayodipupo Babalola, B., Ifeolu Akinwande, A., Otunba, A.A., Ebenezer Adebami, G., Babalola, O., Nwufo, C., 2024. Therapeutic benefits of *Carica papaya*: a review on its pharmacological activities and characterization of papain. Arab. J. Chem. 18785352. 17 (1), 105369. doi:10.1016/j.arabjc.2023.105369.

Ayuso, M., Carpena, M., Taofiq, O., Albuquerque, T.G., Simal-Gandara, J., Oliveira, M.B.P.P., Prieto, M.A., Ferreira, I.C.F.R., Barros, L., 2022. Fig "*Ficus carica* L." and its by-products: a decade evidence of their health-promoting benefits towards the development of novel food formulations. Trends Food Sci. Technol. 09242244. 127, 1–13. Available from: http://www.elsevier.com/wps/find/journaldescription.cws_home/601278/description#description. doi:10.1016/j.tifs.2022.06.010.

Babalola, B.A., Akinwande, A.I., Gboyega, A.E., Otunba, A.A., 2023. Extraction, purification and characterization of papain cysteine-proteases from the leaves of Carica papaya. Sci. Afr. 24682276. 19, e01538. doi:10.1016/j.sciaf.2022.e01538.

Baccarin, T., Mitjans, M., Ramos, D., Lemos-Senna, E., Vinardell, M.P., 2015. Photoprotection by *Punica granatum* seed oil nanoemulsion entrapping polyphenol-rich ethyl acetate fraction against UVB-induced DNA damage in human keratinocyte (HaCaT) cell line. J. Photochem. Photobiol. B 18732682. 153, 127–136. Available from: https://www.elsevier.com/locate/jphotobiol. doi:10.1016/j.jphotobiol.2015.09.005.

Bagdas, D., Etoz, B.C., Gul, Z., Ziyanok, S., Inan, S., Turacozen, O., Gul, N.Y., Topal, A., Cinkilic, N., Tas, S., Ozyigit, M.O., Gurun, M.S., 2015. In vivo systemic chlorogenic acid therapy under diabetic conditions: wound healing effects and cytotoxicity/genotoxicity profile. Food Chem. Toxicol. 18736351. 81, 54–61. Available from: https://www.elsevier.com/locate/foodchemtox. doi:10.1016/j.fct.2015.04.001.

Baidamshina, D.R., Koroleva, V.A., Trizna, E.Y., Pankova, S.M., Agafonova, M.N., Chirkova, M.N., Vasileva, O.S., Akhmetov, N., Shubina, V.V., Porfiryev, A.G., Semenova, E.V., Sachenkov, O.A., Bogachev, M.I., Artyukhov, V.G., Baltina, T.V., Holyavka, M.G., Kayumov, A.R., 2020. Anti-biofilm and wound-healing activity of chitosan-immobilized Ficin. Federation Int. J. Biol. Macromol. 18790003. 164, 4205–4217. Available from: https://www.elsevier.com/locate/ijbiomac. doi:10.1016/j.ijbiomac.2020.09.030.

Baldisserotto, A., Malisardi, G., Scalambra, E., Andreotti, E., Romagnoli, C., Vicentini, C.B., Manfredini, S., Vertuani, S., 2012. Synthesis, antioxidant and antimicrobial activity of a new phloridzin derivative for dermo-cosmetic applications. Molecules 14203049. 17 (11), 13275–13289. Available from: http://www.mdpi.com/1420-3049/17/11/13275/pdf. doi:10.3390/molecules171113275Italy.

Ballistreri, G., Amenta, M., Fabroni, S., Timpanaro, N., Platania, G.M., 2024. Sustainable extraction protocols for the recovery of bioactive compounds from by-products of pomegranate fruit processing. Foods. 2304-8158. 13 (12), 1793. doi:10.3390/foods13121793.

Banchhor, M., Saraf, S., 2008. Potentiality of papain as an antiaging agent in cosmetic formulation. Pharmacogn. Rev. 2, 266–270.

Barbulova, A., Colucci, G., Apone, F., 2015. New trends in cosmetics: by-products of plant origin and their potential use as cosmetic active ingredients. Cosmetics. 2079-9284. 2 (2), 82–92. doi:10.3390/cosmetics2020082.

Barreira, J.C.M., Arraibi, A.A., Ferreira, I.C.F.R., 2019. Bioactive and functional compounds in apple pomace from juice and cider manufacturing: potential use in dermal formulations. Trends Food Sci. Technol. 09242244. 90, 76–87. Available from: http://www.elsevier.com/wps/find/journaldescription.cws_home/601278/description#description. doi:10.1016/j.tifs.2019.05.014.

Bayat, G., Fallah-Darrehchi, M., Zahedi, P., Moghaddam, A.B., Ghaffari-Bohlouli, P., Jafari, H., 2023. Kiwi extract-incorporated poly(ε-caprolactone)/cellulose acetate blend nanofibers for healing acceleration of burn wounds. J. Biomater. Sci. Polym. Ed. 15685624. 34 (1), 72–88. Available from: http://www.tandfonline.com/loi/tbsp20. doi:10.1080/09205063.2022.2110483.

Benchagra, L., Berrougui, H., Islam, M.O., Ramchoun, M., Boulbaroud, S., Hajjaji, A., Fulop, T., Ferretti, G., Khalil, A., 2021. Antioxidant Effect of Moroccan Pomegranate (Punica granatum L. Sefri Variety) Extracts Rich in Punicalagin against the Oxidative Stress Process. Foods. 2304-8158. 10 (9), 2219. doi:10.3390/foods10092219.

Benito-Vázquez, I., Muñoz-Labrador, A., Garrido-Romero, M., Hontoria-Caballo, G., García-García, C., Marina Diez-Municio, F.J.M., 2024. New pipeline for analysing fruit proteolytic products used as digestive health nutraceuticals. Int. J. Mol. Sci. 1422-0067. 25 (19), 10315. doi:10.3390/ijms251910315.

Bertolo, M.R.V., Martins, V.C.A., Plepis, A.M.G., Bogusz, S., 2021. Utilization of pomegranate peel waste: natural deep eutectic solvents as a green strategy to recover valuable phenolic compounds. J. Clean. Prod. 09596526. 327. Available from: https://www.journals.elsevier.com/journal-of-cleaner-production. doi:10.1016/j.jclepro.2021.129471.

Bhogal, R.K., Mouser, P.E., Higgins, C.A., Turner, G.A., 2014. Protease activity, localization and inhibition in the human hair follicle. Int. J. Cosmet. Sci. 14682494. 36 (1), 46–53. doi:10.1111/ics.12091.

Bhuyan, D.J., Alsherbiny, M.A., Perera, S., Low, M., Basu, A., Devi, O.A., Barooah, M.S., Li, C.G., Papoutsis, K., 2019. The odyssey of bioactive compounds in avocado (*Persea americana*) and their health benefits. Antioxidants 20763921. 8 (10). Available from: https://www.mdpi.com/2076-3921/8/10/426/pdf. doi:10.3390/antiox8100426.

Bialkowski, K., 2022. Proteolytic activity of cosmetic enzyme peel products. Acta Biochim. Pol. 69, 895. doi:10.18388/abp.2020_6485.

Bianchetti, G., Bottoni, P., Tringali, G., Maulucci, G., Tabolacci, E., Clementi, M.E., 2024. The polyphenolic compound punicalagin protects skin fibroblasts from UVA radiation oxidative damage. Curr. Res. Pharmacol. Drug Discov. 25902571. 6, 100186. doi:10.1016/j.crphar.2024.100186.

Biswas, R., Sarkar, A., Alam, M., Mukta Roy, M.M.M.H., 2023. Microwave and ultrasound-assisted extraction of bioactive compounds from Papaya: a sustainable green process. Ultrason. Sonochem. 13504177. 101, 106677. doi:10.1016/j.ultsonch.2023.106677.

Bitwell, C., Indra, S.S., Luke, C., Kakoma, M.K., 2023. A review of modern and conventional extraction techniques and their applications for extracting phytochemicals from plants. Sci. Afr. 24682276. 19, e01585. doi:10.1016/j.sciaf.2023.e01585.

Błaszczyk, A., Sady, S., Pachołek, B., Jakubowska, D., Grzybowska-Brzezińska, M., Krzywonos, M., Popek, S., 2024. Sustainable management strategies for fruit processing byproducts for biorefineries: a review. Sustainability. 2071-1050. 16 (5), 1717. doi:10.3390/su16051717.

Bom, S., Jorge, J., Ribeiro, H.M., Marto, J., 2019. A step forward on sustainability in the cosmetics industry: a review. J. Clean. Prod. 09596526. 225, 270–290. doi:10.1016/j.jclepro.2019.03.255.

Bonarska-Kujawa, D., Cyboran, S., Oszmiański, J., Kleszczyńska, H., 2011. Antioxidant properties of apple leaves and fruits extracts from apple leaves and fruits as effective antioxidants. J. Med. Plants Res. 19960875. 5 (11), 2339–2347. Available from: http://www.academicjournals.org/JMPR/PDF/pdf2011/4June/Bonarska-Kujawa%20et%20al.pdf.

Boonkerd, S., Wantha, L., 2024. Antisolvent crystallization of papain. ChemEngineering. 2305-7084. 8 (1), 4. doi:10.3390/chemengineering8010004.

Bordiga, M., Travaglia, F., Locatelli, M., 2019. Valorisation of grape pomace: an approach that is increasingly reaching its maturity – a review. Int. J. Food Sci. Technol. 0950-5423. 54 (4), 933–942. doi:10.1111/ijfs.14118.

Bringheli, I., Brindisi, G., Morelli, R., Marchetti, L., Cela, L., Gravina, A., Pastore, F., Semeraro, A., Cinicola, B., Capponi, M., Gori, A., Pignataro, E., Piccioni, M.G., Zicari, A.M., Anania, C., 2023. Kiwifruit's allergy in children: what do we know? Nutrients. 2072-6643. 15 (13), 3030. doi:10.3390/nu15133030.

Bruno Romanini, E., Rodrigues, L.M., Finger, A., Perez Cantuaria Chierrito, T., Regina da Silva Scapim, M., Madrona, G.S., 2021. Ultrasound assisted extraction of bioactive compounds from BRS Violet grape pomace followed by alginate-Ca^{2+} encapsulation. Food Chem. 03088146. 338, 128101. doi:10.1016/j.foodchem.2020.128101.

Butkeviciute, A., Ramanauskiene, K., Valdimaras, J., 2022. Release of apple extract and phenolic compounds from five semi-solid formulations. InterConf. 2709-4685. 15 (117), 209–214. doi:10.51582/interconf.19-20.07.2022.021.

Butnariu, M.V., Giuchici, C.V., 2011. The use of some nanoemulsions based on aqueous propolis and lycopene extract in the skin's protective mechanisms against UVA radiation. J. Nanobiotechnol. 1477-3155. 9 (1), 3. doi:10.1186/1477-3155-9-3.

Caballero, V., Estévez, M., Tomás-Barberán, F.A., Morcuende, D., Martín, I., Delgado, J., 2022. Biodegradation of *Punica granatum* punicalagin into ellagic acid by selected probiotic bacteria: a study of the underlying mechanisms by MS-based proteomics. J. Agric. Food Chem. 15205118. 70 (51), 16273–16285. Available from: http://pubs.acs.org/journal/jafcau. doi:10.1021/acs.jafc.2c06585.

Caleb, O.J., Fahad, P.V.M., Al-Said, A., Opara, U.L., 2013. Transpiration rate and quality of pomegranate arils as affected by storage conditions. CyTA J. Food. 1947-6337. 11 (3), 199–207. doi:10.1080/19476337.2012.721807.

Çam, M., Hışıl, Y., 2010. Pressurised water extraction of polyphenols from pomegranate peels. Food Chem. 03088146. 123 (3), 878–885. doi:10.1016/j.foodchem.2010.05.011.

Cano-Lamadrid, M., Martínez-Zamora, L., Castillejo, N., Artés-Hernández, F., 2022. From pomegranate by-products waste to worth: a review of extraction techniques and potential applications for their revalorization. Foods. 2304-8158. 11 (17), 2596. doi:10.3390/foods11172596.

Caseiro, M., Ascenso, A., Costa, A., Creagh-Flynn, J., Johnson, M., Simões, S., 2020. Lycopene in human health. LWT. 00236438. 127, 109323. doi:10.1016/j.lwt.2020.109323.

Castillo-González, E., Giraldi-Díaz, M.R., De Medina-Salas, L., Sánchez-Castillo, M.P., 2019. Pre-composting and vermicomposting of pineapple (*Ananas comosus*) and vegetable waste. Appl. Sci. 2076-3417. 9 (17), 3564. doi:10.3390/app9173564.

Castro, M.L., Azevedo-Silva, J., Valente, D., Machado, A., Ribeiro, T., Paulo Ferreira, J., Pintado, M., Ramos, O.L., Borges, S., Baptista-Silva, S., 2024. Elevating skincare science: grape seed extract encapsulation for dermatological care. Molecules. 1420-3049. 29 (16), 3717. doi:10.3390/molecules29163717.

Caudalie, n.d. Dark Spot Serum for Radiance - Vinoperfect | caudalie®. https://en.caudalie.com/p/432C/vinoperfect-radiance-serum-complexion-correcting-432c.html.

Cejudo-Bastante, C., Arjona-Mudarra, P., Fernández-Ponce, M.T., Casas, L., Mantell, C., de la Ossa, E.J.M., Pereyra, C., 2021. Application of a natural antioxidant from grape pomace extract in the development of bioactive jute fibers for food packaging. Antioxidants 20763921. 10 (2), 1–15. Available from: https://www.mdpi.com/2076-3921/10/2/216. doi:10.3390/antiox10020216.

Chai, Y.H., Yusup, S., Ruslan, M.S.H., Chin, B.L.F., 2020. Supercritical fluid extraction and solubilization of *Carica papaya* L. leaves in ternary system with CO_2 + ethanol solvents. Chem. Eng. Res. Des. 02638762. 156, 31–42. doi:10.1016/j.cherd.2020.01.025.

Chakkalakal, M., Nadora, D., Gahoonia, N., Dumont, A., Burney, W., Pan, A., Chambers, C.J., Sivamani, R.K., 2022. Prospective randomized double-blind placebo-controlled study of oral pomegranate extract on skin wrinkles, biophysical features, and the gut-skin axis. J. Clin. Med. 2077-0383. 11 (22), 6724. doi:10.3390/jcm11226724.

Chakraborty, A.J., Mitra, S., Tallei, T.E., Tareq, A.M., Nainu, F., Cicia, D., Dhama, K., Emran, T.B., Simal-Gandara, J., Capasso, R., 2021. Bromelain a potential bioactive compound: a comprehensive overview from a pharmacological perspective. Life 20751729. 11 (4). Available from: https://www.mdpi.com/2075-1729/11/4/317/pdf. doi:10.3390/life11040317.

Chamorro, F., Carpena, M., Fraga-Corral, M., Echave, J., Riaz Rajoka, M.S., Barba, F.J., Cao, H., Jianbo Xiao, M.A.P., Simal-Gandara, J., 2022. Valorization of kiwi agricultural waste and industry by-products by recovering bioactive compounds and applications as food additives: a circular economy model. Food Chem. 03088146. 370, 131315. doi:10.1016/j.foodchem.2021.131315.

Chan, L.P., Tseng, Y.P., Liu, C., Liang, C.H., 2022. Fermented pomegranate extracts protect against oxidative stress and aging of skin. J. Cosmet. Dermatol. 14732165. 21 (5), 2236–2245. Available from: http://onlinelibrary.wiley.com/journal/10.1111/(ISSN)1473-2165. doi:10.1111/jocd.14379.

Cho, Y.J., Lee, E.H., Yoo, J., Kwon, S.I., Choi, H.W., Kang, I.K., 2019. Analysis of functional properties in the new Korean apple cultivar Arisoo. Hortic. Environ. Biotechnol. 22113460. 60 (5), 787–795. Available from: http://www.springer.com/life+sciences/journal/13580. doi:10.1007/s13580-019-00167-z.

Choleva, M., Boulougouri, V., Panara, A., Panagopoulou, E., Chiou, A., Thomaidis, N.S., Antonopoulou, S., Fragopoulou, E., 2019. Evaluation of anti-platelet activity of grape pomace extracts. Food Funct. 2042650X. 10 (12), 8069–8080. Available from: http://pubs.rsc.org/en/journals/journal/fo. doi:10.1039/c9fo02138h.

Choudhary, R., Kaushik, R., Chawla, P., Manna, S., 2025. Exploring the extraction, functional properties, and industrial applications of papain from *Carica papaya*. J. Sci. Food Agric. 0022-5142. 105 (3), 1533–1545. doi:10.1002/jsfa.13776.

Chuacharoen, T., Polprasert, C., Sabliov, C.M., 2024. Avocado seed extract encapsulated in zein nanoparticles as a functional ingredient. J. Agric. Food Res. 26661543. 18, 101332. doi:10.1016/j.jafr.2024.101332.

Coderoni, S., Perito, M.A., 2020. Sustainable consumption in the circular economy. An analysis of consumers' purchase intentions for waste-to-value food. J. Clean. Prod. 09596526. 252, 119870. doi:10.1016/j.jclepro.2019.119870.

Colletti, A., Shuyi, L., Marengo, M., Adinolfi, S., Cravotto, G., 2021. Recent advances and insights into bromelain processing, pharmacokinetics and therapeutic uses. Appl. Sci. 2076-3417. 11 (18), 8428. doi:10.3390/app11188428.

Da Porto, C., Natolino, A., Decorti, D., 2015. The combined extraction of polyphenols from grape marc: ultrasound assisted extraction followed by supercritical CO_2 extraction of ultrasound-raffinate. LWT Food Sci. Technol. 00236438. 61 (1), 98–104. doi:10.1016/j.lwt.2014.11.027.

da Silva Melo, A.E.C., de Sousa, F.S.R., Dos Santos-silva, A.M., Do Nascimento, E.G., Fernandes-Pedrosa, M.F., de Medeiros, C.A.C.X., da Silva-junior, A.A., 2023. Immobilization of papain in chitosan membranes as a potential alternative for skin wounds. Pharmaceutics 19994923. 15 (12). Available from: http://www.mdpi.com/journal/pharmaceutics. doi:10.3390/pharmaceutics15122649.

da Silva, L.C., Viganó, J., de Souza Mesquita, L.M., Dias, A.L.B., de Souzade Souza, M.C., Sanches, V.L., Chaves, J.O., Pizani, R.S., Contieri, L.S., Rostagno, M.A., 2021. Recent advances and trends in extraction techniques to recover polyphenols compounds from apple by-products. Food Chem. X 25901575. 12. Available from: https://www.journals.elsevier.com/food-chemistry-x. doi:10.1016/j.fochx.2021.100133.

de Oliveira Raphaelli, C., Gonçalves Azevedo, J., Dos Santos Pereira, E., Vinholes, J.R., Camargo, T.M., Hoffmann, J.F., Araújo Ribeiro, J., Vizzotto, M., Valmor Rombaldi, C., Rosângela Wink, M., Braganhol, E., Nora, L., 2021. Phenolic-rich apple extracts have photoprotective and anti-cancer effect in dermal cells. Phytomedicine Plus. 26670313. 1 (4), 100112. doi:10.1016/j.phyplu.2021.100112.

De Oliveira, A.P., Franco, E.D.S., Barreto, R.R., Cordeiro, D.P., De Melo, R.G., De Aquino, C.M.F., Silva, A.A.R.E., De Medeiros, P.L., Silva, T.G.D., Góes, A.J.D.S., Maia, M.B.D.S., 2013. Effect of semisolid formulation of persea americana mill (Avocado) oil on wound healing in rats. Evid. Based Complement. Alternat. Med. 17414288. 2013. doi:10.1155/2013/472382.

Deng, J., Liu, Q., Zhang, Q., Zhang, C., Liu, D., Fan, D., Yang, H., 2018. Comparative study on composition, physicochemical and antioxidant characteristics of different varieties of kiwifruit seed oil in China. Food Chem. 03088146. 264, 411–418. doi:10.1016/j.foodchem.2018.05.063.

Densi Lab, n.d. Bromelain Enzymatic Peeling (Pineapple Extract). https://densilab.com/en/product/bromelain-enzymatic-peeling-pineapple-extract/.

Deuschle, V.C.K.N., Brusco, I., Piana, M., Faccin, H., de Carvalho, L.M., Oliveira, S.M., Viana, C., 2019. Persea americana Mill. crude extract exhibits antinociceptive effect on UVB radiation-induced skin injury in mice. Inflammopharmacology 15685608. 27 (2), 323–338. Available from: https://rd.springer.com/journal/10787. doi:10.1007/s10787-018-0441-9.

Di Giacomo, M., Bertoni, F.A., Victoria Rocha, M., Nerli, B.B., Rodríguez, F., 2022. Cloud point extraction based on non-ionic surfactants: an ecofriendly tool for recovering papain from papaya latex. J. Environ. Chem. Eng. 22133437. 10 (6), 108762. doi:10.1016/j.jece.2022.108762.

Di Lorenzo, R., Maisto, M., Ricci, L., Piccolo, V., Marzocchi, A., Greco, G., Tenore, G.C., Laneri, S., 2024. Annurca apple oleolite as functional ingredient for the formulation of cosmetics with skin-antiaging activity. Int. J. Mol. Sci. 1422-0067. 25 (3), 1677. doi:10.3390/ijms25031677.

Di Stefano, V., Buzzanca, C., Melilli, M.G., Indelicato, S., Mauro, M., Vazzana, M., Arizza, V., Lucarini, M., Durazzo, A., Bongiorno, D., 2022. Polyphenol characterization and antioxidant activity of grape seeds and skins from Sicily: a preliminary study. Sustainability. 2071-1050. 14 (11), 6702. doi:10.3390/su14116702.

Dias, M., Caleja, C., Pereira, C., Calhelha, R.C., Kostic, M., Sokovic, M., Tavares, D., José Baraldi, I., Barros, L., Ferreira, I.C.F.R., 2020. Chemical composition and bioactive properties of byproducts from two different kiwi varieties. Food Res. Int. 09639969. 127, 108753. doi:10.1016/j.foodres.2019.108753.

Dini, I., Falanga, D., Di Lorenzo, R., Tito, A., Carotenuto, G., Zappelli, C., Grumetto, L., Sacchi, A., Laneri, S., Apone, F., 2021. An extract from *Ficus carica* cell cultures works as an anti-stress ingredient for the skin. Antioxidants. 2076-3921. 10 (4), 515. doi:10.3390/antiox10040515.

Diogo Gonçalves, S., 2021. Use of enzymes in cosmetics: proposed enzymatic peel procedure. Cos ACTIVE J. 1, 27–33.

Divakaran, D., Sriariyanun, M., Suyambulingam, I., Rangappa, S.M., Siengchin, S., 2023. Exfoliation and physico-chemical characterization of novel bioplasticizers from Nelumbo nucifera leaf for biofilm application. Heliyon. 24058440. 9 (12), e22550. doi:10.1016/j.heliyon.2023.e22550.

Drummond, L., 2013. The composition and nutritional value of kiwifruit. Adv. Food Nutr. Res. 68, 33–57. Available from: http://www.elsevier.com/wps/find/bookdescription.cws_home/704624/description#description. doi:10.1016/B978-0-12-394294-4.00003-1.

Đurđević, S., Šavikin, K., Živković, J., Böhm, V., Stanojković, T., Damjanović, A., Petrović, S., 2018. Antioxidant and cytotoxic activity of fatty oil isolated by supercritical fluid extraction from microwave pretreated seeds of wild growing Punica granatum L. J. Supercrit. Fluids. 08968446. 133, 225–232. doi:10.1016/j.supflu.2017.10.021.

Duskey, J.T., da Ros, F., Ottonelli, I., Zambelli, B., Vandelli, M.A., Tosi, G., Ruozi, B., 2020. Enzyme stability in nanoparticle preparations part 1: bovine serum albumin improves enzyme function. Molecules. 1420-3049. 25 (20), 4593. doi:10.3390/molecules25204593.

Ebo, D.G., Toscano, A., Rihs, H.P., Mertens, C., Sabato, V., Elst, J., Beyens, M., Hagendorens, M.M., Van Houdt, M., Van Gasse, A.L., 2024. IgE-mediated cannabis allergy and cross-reactivity syndromes: a roadmap for correct diagnosis and management. Curr. Allergy Asthma Rep. 15346315. 24 (8), 407–414. Available from: https://www.springer.com/journal/11882. doi:10.1007/s11882-024-01159-5.

Eid, A.M., Issa, L., Arar, K., Abu-Zant, A., Makhloof, M., Masarweh, Y., 2024. Phytochemical screening, antioxidant, anti-diabetic, and anti-obesity activities, formulation, and characterization of a self-nanoemulsion system loaded with pomegranate (Punica granatum) seed oil. Sci. Rep. 20452322. 14 (1). Available from: https://www.nature.com/srep/. doi:10.1038/s41598-024-68476-7.

El-Shamy, S., Farag, M.A., 2021. Novel trends in extraction and optimization methods of bioactives recovery from pomegranate fruit biowastes: valorization purposes for industrial applications. Food Chem. 03088146. 365, 130465. doi:10.1016/j.foodchem.2021.130465.

Elbrolesy, A., Abdou, Y., Elhussiny, F.A., Morsy, R., 2023. Novel green synthesis of UV-sunscreen ZnO nanoparticles using *Solanum lycopersicum* fruit extract and evaluation of their antibacterial and anticancer activity. J. Inorg. Organomet. Polym. Mater. 15741451. 33 (12), 3750–3759. Available from: https://www.springer.com/journal/10904. doi:10.1007/s10904-023-02744-3.

Evterpa, n.d. Tomato Face Cream. http://evterpa.eu/en/tomato-face-cream-542.html.

Faria, G.M.L., Silva, E.K., 2025. Towards zero waste in pomegranate juice by-products: biomass valorization beyond phenolic compound recovery and development of bioactive pectin-based edible coatings. J. Clean. Prod. 09596526. 524, 146480. doi:10.1016/j.jclepro.2025.146480.

Farmstay, n.d. Farmstay Real Avocado Nutrition Eye Cream. https://en.fscos.com/product/farmstay-real-avocado-nutrition-eye-cream/411.

Fazolin, G.N., Varca, G.H.C., de Freitas, L.F., Rokita, B., Kadlubowski, S., Lugão, A.B., 2020. Simultaneous intramolecular crosslinking and sterilization of papain nanoparticles by gamma radiation. Radiat. Phys. Chem. 18790895. 171. Available from: https://www.elsevier.com/locate/radphyschem. doi:10.1016/j.radphyschem.2020.108697.

Feijoo-Siota, L., Villa, T.G., 2011. Native and biotechnologically engineered plant proteases with industrial applications. Food Bioproc. Technol. 19355149. 4 (6), 1066–1088. doi:10.1007/s11947-010-0431-4.

Feng, S., Jianyong, Y., Xuan, L., Xinye, W., Zhao, Y., Youchuan, M., Jinfeng, B., 2021. Systematic review of phenolic compounds in apple fruits: compositions, distribution, absorption, metabolism, and processing stability. J. Agric. Food Chem. 0021-8561. 69 (1), 7–27. doi:10.1021/acs.jafc.0c05481.

Ferreira, S.M., Falé, Z., Santos, L., 2022. Sustainability in skin care: incorporation of avocado peel extracts in topical formulations. Molecules. 1420-3049. 27 (6), 1782. doi:10.3390/molecules27061782.

Ferreira, S.M., Santos, L., 2022. A potential valorization strategy of wine industry by-products and their application in cosmetics—case study: grape pomace and grapeseed. Molecules. 1420-3049. 27 (3), 969. doi:10.3390/molecules27030969.

Ferri, M., Vannini, M., Ehrnell, M., Eliasson, L., Xanthakis, E., Monari, S., Sisti, L., Marchese, P., Celli, A., Tassoni, A., 2020. From winery waste to bioactive compounds and new polymeric biocomposites: a contribution to the circular economy concept. J. Adv. Res. 20901232. 24, 1–11. doi:10.1016/j.jare.2020.02.015.

Francisco, A.P., Sganzerla, W.G., Castro, L.E.N., Barroso, T.L.C.T., da Silva, A.P.G., da Rosa, C.G., Nunes, M.R., Forster-Carneiro, T., Rostagno, M.A., 2024. Pressurized liquid extraction of bioactive compounds from grape peel and application in pH-sensing carboxymethyl cellulose films: a promising material to monitor the freshness of pork and milk. Food Res. Int. 18737145. 179. Available from: https://www.sciencedirect.com/science/journal/09639969. doi:10.1016/j.foodres.2024.114017.

Gagaoua, M., Boucherba, N., Bouanane-Darenfed, A., Ziane, F., Nait-Rabah, S., Hafid, K., Boudechicha, H.-R., 2014. Three-phase partitioning as an efficient method for the purification and recovery of ficin from Mediterranean fig (*Ficus carica* L.) latex. Sep. Purif. Technol. 13835866. 132, 461–467. doi:10.1016/j.seppur.2014.05.050.

Ganjeh, A.M., Pinto, C.A., Casal, S., Habanova, M., Holovicova, M., Saraiva, J.A., 2025. Novel methods for extraction of monomeric phenols from plants and fruits with potential anti-obesity activity. J. Food Compos. Anal. 08891575. 141, 107383. doi:10.1016/j.jfca.2025.107383.

García-Lomillo, J., González-SanJosé, M.L., Pino-García, R.D., Rivero-Pérez, M.D., Muñiz-Rodríguez, P., 2014. Antioxidant and antimicrobial properties of wine byproducts and their potential uses in the food industry. J. Agric. Food Chem. 15205118. 62 (52), 12595–12602. Available from: http://pubs.acs.org/journal/jafcau. doi:10.1021/jf5042678.

García-Mantrana, I., Calatayud, M., Romo-Vaquero, M., Espín, J.C., Selma, M.V., Carmen Collado, M., 2019. Urolithin metabotypes can determine the modulation of gut microbiota in healthy individuals by tracking walnut consumption over three days. Nutrients. 2072-6643. 11 (10), 2483. doi:10.3390/nu11102483.

García, P., Fredes, C., Cea, I., Lozano-Sánchez, J., Leyva-Jiménez, F.J., Robert, P., Vergara, C., Jimenez, P., 2021. Recovery of bioactive compounds from pomegranate (*Punica granatum* L.) peel using pressurized liquid extraction. Foods. 2304-8158. 10 (2), 203. doi:10.3390/foods10020203.

GARDEN, n.d. Face Scrub with Pomegranate 50ml. https://gardenofficial.com/en/product/face-scrub-revitalizing-pomegranate-50ml/.

Gharibzahedi, S.M.T., Smith, B., Guo, Y., 2019. Ultrasound-microwave assisted extraction of pectin from fig (*Ficus carica* L.) skin: optimization, characterization and bioactivity. Carbohydr. Polym. 01448617. 222, 114992. doi:10.1016/j.carbpol.2019.114992.

Giangrieco, I., Ciardiello, M.A., Tamburrini, M., Tuppo, L., Rafaiani, C., Mari, A., Alessandri, C., 2023. Comparative analysis of the immune response and the clinical allergic reaction to papain-like cysteine proteases from fig, kiwifruit, papaya, pineapple and mites in an Italian population. Foods. 2304-8158. 12 (15), 2852. doi:10.3390/foods12152852.

Giordano, M., Pinela, J., Inês Dias, M., Calhelha, R.C., Stojković, D., Soković, M., Tavares, D., Laura Cánepa, A., Ferreira, I.C.F.R., Caleja, C., Barros, L., 2021. Ultrasound-assisted extraction of flavonoids from kiwi peel: process optimization and bioactivity assessment. Appl. Sci. 2076-3417. 11 (14), 6416. doi:10.3390/app11146416.

Gómez-Godínez, L.J., Cadena-Zamudio, J.D., Hernández-Cruz, E., Ruvalcaba-Gómez, J.M., Arteaga-Garibay, R.I. , 2025. Latest omics and approaches to elucidate fruit microbiome and their application as biocontrol agent. In: Kumar, A., de los Santos Villalobos, S., Solanki, M.K. (Eds.), Fruit Microbiome: Emerging Aspects in Postharvest Disease Management. Elsevier, Mexico, pp. 111–134. Available from: https://www.sciencedirect.com/book/9780443339639. doi:10.1016/B978-0-443-33963-9.00009-0.

Gonçalves Rodrigues, L.G., Mazzutti, S., Vitali, L., Micke, G.A., Ferreira, S.R.S., 2019. Recovery of bioactive phenolic compounds from papaya seeds agroindustrial residue using subcritical water extraction. Biocatal. Agric. Biotechnol. 18788181. 22. Available from: http://www.journals.elsevier.com/biocatalysis-and-agricultural-biotechnology/. doi:10.1016/j.bcab.2019.101367.

Gonçalves, D., Gouveia, C.S.S., Ferreira, M.J., Ganança, J.F.T., Pinto, D.C.G., de Carvalho, M.A.A.P., 2024. Comparative analysis of antioxidant and fatty acid composition in avocado (*Persea americana* Mill.) fruits: exploring regional and commercial varieties. Food Chem. 18737072. 442. Available from: https://www.sciencedirect.com/science/journal/03088146. doi:10.1016/j.foodchem.2024.138403.

Gorjanović, S., Micić, D., Pastor, F., Tosti, T., Kalušević, A., Ristić, S., Zlatanović, S., 2020. Evaluation of apple pomace flour obtained industrially by dehydration as a source of biomolecules with antioxidant, antidiabetic and antiobesity effects. Antioxidants. 2076-3921. 9 (5), 413. doi:10.3390/antiox9050413.

Gosset-Erard, C., Zhao, M., Lordel-Madeleine, S., Ennahar, S., 2021. Identification of punicalagin as the bioactive compound behind the antimicrobial activity of pomegranate (*Punica granatum* L.) peels. Food Chem. 03088146. 352, 129396. doi:10.1016/j.foodchem.2021.129396.

Goudarzi, I., Lashkarbolouki, T., Khorshidi, M., Ghorbanian, M.T., 2015. Effect of wound dressing with fresh kiwifruit on healing of cutaneous wound in rats. Zahedan J. Res. Med. Sci. 2008-7977. 17 (3). doi:10.5812/zjrms.1274.

Goula, A.M., Ververi, M., Adamopoulou, A., Kaderides, K., 2017. Green ultrasound-assisted extraction of carotenoids from pomegranate wastes using vegetable oils. Ultrason. Sonochem. 18732828. 34, 821–830. Available from: https://www.elsevier.com/inca/publications/store/5/2/5/4/5/1. doi:10.1016/j.ultsonch.2016.07.022.

Grisales-Mejía, J.F., Álvarez-Rivera, G., Andrade-Mahecha, M.M., Martínez-Correa, H.A., Mendiola, J.A., Cifuentes, A., Ibañez, E., 2024. Antioxidant and neuroprotective potential of extracts from Hass avocado peel obtained through a biorefinery process: a sustainable strategy for the valorization of agro-food waste. LWT 00236438. 214. Available from: https://www.sciencedirect.com/science/journal/00236438. doi:10.1016/j.lwt.2024.117119.

Gumul, D., Kruczek, M., Ivanišová, E., Słupski, J., Kowalski, S., 2023. Apple pomace as an ingredient enriching wheat pasta with health-promoting compounds. Foods. 2304-8158. 12 (4), 804. doi:10.3390/foods12040804.

Guthrie, F., Wang, Y., Neeve, N., Quek, S.Y., Mohammadi, K., Baroutian, S., 2020. Recovery of phenolic antioxidants from green kiwifruit peel using subcritical water extraction. Food Bioprod. Process. 09603085. 122, 136–144. Available from: http://www.elsevier.com/wps/find/journaldescription.cws_home/713883/description#description. doi:10.1016/j.fbp.2020.05.002.

Hafezi, F., Rad, H.E., Naghibzadeh, B., Nouhi, A.H., Naghibzadeh, G., 2010. Actinidia deliciosa (kiwifruit), a new drug for enzymatic debridement of acute burn wounds. Burns 03054179. 36 (3), 352–355. Available from: https://www.sciencedirect.com/science/journal/03054179. doi:10.1016/j.burns.2009.04.021.

Hafid, K., John, J., Sayah, T.M., Domínguez, R., Becila, S., Lamri, M., Dib, A.L., Lorenzo, J.M., Gagaoua, M., 2020. One-step recovery of latex papain from *Carica papaya* using three phase partitioning and its use as milk-clotting and meat-tenderizing agent. Int. J. Biol. Macromol. 18790003. 146, 798–810. Available from: https://www.elsevier.com/locate/ijbiomac. doi:10.1016/j.ijbiomac.2019.10.048.

Hamouda, A.F., Felemban, S., 2023. Biochemical pilot study on effects of pomegranate seed oil extract and cosmetic cream on neurologically mediated skin inflammation in animals and humans: a comparative observational study. Molecules. 1420-3049. 28 (2), 903. doi:10.3390/molecules28020903.

Hassanein, W.S., Meral, R., Ceylan, Z., Ahmed, M.M., Yilmaz, M.T., 2024. Use of encapsulated pomegranate seed oil in novel coarse and nanosized materials for improving the storage life of strawberry. Food Chem. 03088146. 441, 138251. doi:10.1016/j.foodchem.2023.138251.

Hatami, T., Meireles, M.A.A., Ciftci, O.N., 2019. Supercritical carbon dioxide extraction of lycopene from tomato processing by-products: mathematical modeling and optimization. J. Food Eng. 02608774. 241, 18–25. Available from: http://www.sciencedirect.com/science/journal/02608774. doi:10.1016/j.jfoodeng.2018.07.036.

Homaei, A., Stevanato, R., Etemadipour, R., Hemmati, R., 2017. Purification, catalytic, kinetic and thermodynamic characteristics of a novel ficin from Ficus johannis. Biocatal. Agric. Biotechnol. 18788181. 10, 360–366. doi:10.1016/j.bcab.2017.04.008.

Ilie, G.-I., Milea, Ş.-A., Râpeanu, G., Cîrciumaru, A., Stănciuc, N., 2022. Sustainable design of innovative kiwi byproducts-based ingredients containing probiotics. Foods. 2304-8158. 11 (15), 2334. doi:10.3390/foods11152334.

Iordănescu, O.A., Băla, M., Gligor (Pane), D., Zippenfening, S.E., Cugerean, M.I., Ionuţ Petroman, M., Hădărugă, D.I., Hădărugă, N.G., Riviş, M., 2021. A DPPH· kinetic approach on the antioxidant activity of various parts and ripening levels of papaya (*Carica papaya* L.) ethanolic extracts. Plants. 2223-7747. 10 (8), 1679. doi:10.3390/plants10081679.

Isa, M.M., Jaafar, M.N., Kasim, K.F., Mutalib, M.F.A., 2020. Cultivation of fig (*Ficus carica* L.) as an alternative high value crop in Malaysia: a brief review. IOP Conf. Ser. Mater. Sci. Eng. 1757-8981. 864 (1), 012134. doi:10.1088/1757-899x/864/1/012134.

Ito, S., Nagata, K., 2017. Biology of Hsp47 (Serpin H1), a collagen-specific molecular chaperone. Semin. Cell Dev. Biol. 10849521. 62, 142–151. doi:10.1016/j.semcdb.2016.11.005.

Jesus, A., Mota, S., Torres, A., Cruz, M.T., Sousa, E., Almeida, I.F., Cidade, H., 2023. Antioxidants in sunscreens: which and what for? Antioxidants. 2076-3921. 12 (1), 138. doi:10.3390/antiox12010138.

Kandemir, K., Piskin, E., Xiao, J., Tomas, M., Capanoglu, E., 2022. Fruit juice industry wastes as a source of bioactives. J. Agric. Food Chem. 0021-8561. 70 (23), 6805–6832. doi:10.1021/acs.jafc.2c00756.

Kandylis, P., Kokkinomagoulos, E., 2020. Food applications and potential health benefits of pomegranate and its derivatives. Foods. 2304-8158. 9 (2), 122. doi:10.3390/foods9020122.

Kansakar, U., Trimarco, V., Manzi, M.V., Cervi, E., Mone, P., Santulli, G., 2024. Exploring the therapeutic potential of bromelain: applications, benefits, and mechanisms. Nutrients. 2072-6643. 16 (13), 2060. doi:10.3390/nu16132060.

Karastergiou, A., Gancel, A.-L., Jourdes, M., Teissedre, P.-L., 2024. Valorization of grape pomace: a review of phenolic composition, bioactivity, and therapeutic potential. Antioxidants. 2076-3921. 13 (9), 1131. doi:10.3390/antiox13091131.

Kaushal, R., Kaur, B., Panesar, P.S., Anal, A.K., Chu-Ky, S., 2024. Valorization of pineapple rind for bromelain extraction using microwave assisted technique: optimization, purification, and structural characterization. J. Food Sci. Technol. 09758402. 61 (3), 551–562. Available from: https://www.springer.com/journal/13197. doi:10.1007/s13197-023-05863-4.

Kehili, M., Kammlott, M., Choura, S., Zammel, A., Zetzl, C., Smirnova, I., Allouche, N., Sayadi, S., 2017. Supercritical CO_2 extraction and antioxidant activity of lycopene and β-carotene-enriched oleoresin from tomato (*Lycopersicum esculentum* L.) peels by-product of a Tunisian industry. Food Bioprod. Process. 09603085. 102, 340–349. doi:10.1016/j.fbp.2017.02.002.

Khayatan, D., Nilforoushzadeh, M.A., Ashtiani, H.R.A., Hashemian, F., 2022. Effect of apple (*Malus domestica*) stem cells on UVB-induced damaged skin with anti-inflammatory properties: an in vivo study. Adv. Mater. Sci. Eng. 16878442. 2022. Available from: http://www.hindawi.com/journals/amse/. doi:10.1155/2022/2417766.

Kim, H.M., Kang, Y.M., Lee, M., An, H.J., 2024. Papain suppresses atopic skin inflammation through anti-inflammatory activities using in vitro and in vivo models. Antioxidants 20763921. 13 (8). Available from: https://www.mdpi.com/journal/antioxidants. doi:10.3390/antiox13080928.

Kitayama, Y., Kanazawa, T., Okabe, T., Morita, Y., Fukui, T., Yamamoto, T., et al., 2006. Development of extracts from Aomori hiba and apple polyphenols as cosmetic materials. Trans. Mater. Res. Soc. Jpn. 31, 965.

Konopko, A., Kusio, J., Litwinienko, G., 2020. Antioxidant activity of metal nanoparticles coated with tocopherol-like residues—the importance of studies in homo- and heterogeneous systems. Antioxidants. 2076-3921. 9 (1), 5. doi:10.3390/antiox9010005.

Kontaxi, N.-I., Panoutsopoulou, E., Ofrydopolou, A., Tsoupras, A., 2024. Anti-inflammatory benefits of grape pomace and tomato bioactives as ingredients in sun oils against UV radiation for skin protection. Appl. Sci. 2076-3417. 14 (14), 6236. doi:10.3390/app14146236.

Kooshiar, H., Abbaspour, H., Shariati, S.M.M.A., Rakhshandeh, H., Rad, A.K., Esmaily, H., Nia, B.V., 2012. Topical effectiveness of kiwifruit versus fibrinolysin ointment on removal of necrotic tissue of full-thickness burns in male rats. Dermatol. Ther. 15298019. 25 (6), 621–625. doi:10.1111/j.1529-8019.2012.01541.x.

Krishna, S.H., Srinivas, N.D., Raghavarao, K.S., Karanth, N.G., 2002. Reverse micellar extraction for downstream processing of proteins/enzymes. Adv. Biochem. Eng. Biotechnol. 07246145. 75, 119–183. doi:10.1007/3-540-44604-4_5.

Křížová, H., 2015. Changes in the antioxidant activity of polyphenols from grape pomace after interaction with UV radiation. ACC J. 18039782. 21 (1), 70–76. doi:10.15240/tul/004/2015-1-008.

Kumar, M., Tomar, M., Punia, S., Amarowicz, R., Kaur, C., 2020. Evaluation of cellulolytic enzyme-assisted microwave extraction of *Punica granatum* peel phenolics and antioxidant activity. Plant Foods Hum. Nutr. 0921-9668. 75 (4), 614–620. doi:10.1007/s11130-020-00859-3.

Kuo, C.H., Wang, H.M.D., Shieh, C.J., 2024. Enzymes in biomedical, cosmetic and food application. Catalysts 20734344. 14 (3). Available from: https://www.mdpi.com/journal/catalysts. doi:10.3390/catal14030162.

Lau, K.Q., Sabran, M.R., Shafie, S.R., 2021. Utilization of vegetable and fruit by-products as functional ingredient and food. Front. Nutr. 2296-861X. 8. doi:10.3389/fnut.2021.661693.

Leal, C., Gouvinhas, I., Santos, R.A., Rosa, E., Silva, A.M., Saavedra, M.J., Barros, A.I.R.N.A., 2020. Potential application of grape (*Vitis vinifera* L.) stem extracts in the cosmetic and pharmaceutical industries: valorization of a by-product. Ind. Crops Prod. 09266690. 154, 112675. doi:10.1016/j.indcrop.2020.112675.

Lee, E.H., Cho, E.B., Kim, B.O., Jung, H.Y., Lee, S.Y., Yoo, J., Kang, I.K., Cho, Y.J., 2020. Functional properties of newly-bred 'summer king' apples. Hortic. Sci. Technol. 24658588. 38 (3), 405–417. Available from: http://www.hst-j.org/articles/pdf/KadO/kshs-2020-038-03-11.pdf. doi:10.7235/HORT.20200039.

Lee, J., Hyun, C.-G., 2023. Natural products for cosmetic applications. Molecules. 1420-3049. 28 (2), 534. doi:10.3390/molecules28020534.

Leelakanok, N., Petchsomrit, A., Janurai, T., Saechan, C., Sunsandee, N., 2023. Efficacy and safety of bromelain: a systematic review and meta-analysis. Nutr. Health. 0260-1060. 29 (3), 479–503. doi:10.1177/02601060231173732.

Lei, Y., Zhang, H., Yang, L., Tian, K., 2019. Optimization of purification conditions for papain in a polyethylene glycol-phosphate aqueous two-phase system using quaternary ammonium ionic liquids as adjuvants by BBD-RSM. Protein Expr. Purif. 10465928. 156, 8–16. doi:10.1016/j.pep.2018.12.005.

Letsiou, S., Kapazoglou, A., Tsaftaris, A., Spanidi, E., Gardikis, K., 2020. Transcriptional and epigenetic effects of *Vitis vinifera* L. leaf extract on UV-stressed human dermal fibroblasts. Mol. Biol. Rep. 0301-4851. 47 (8), 5763–5772. doi:10.1007/s11033-020-05645-7.

Lin, M.H., Khnykin, D., 2014. Fatty acid transporters in skin development, function and disease. Biochim. Biophys. Acta Mol. Cell Biol. Lipids. 18792618. 1841 (3), 362–368. doi:10.1016/j.bbalip.2013.09.016.

Lin, M., Tingting, Y., Wan, J., Cao, X., 2017. Prediction of the reverse micellar extraction of papain using dissipative particle dynamics simulation. Appl. Biochem. Biotechnol. 0273-2289. 181 (4), 1338–1346. doi:10.1007/s12010-016-2287-1.

Lin, Y.P., Hsu, F.L., Chen, C.S., Chern, J.W., Lee, M.H., 2007. Constituents from the Formosan apple reduce tyrosinase activity in human epidermal melanocytes. Phytochemistry 00319422. 68 (8), 1189–1199. Available from: http://www.journals.elsevier.com/phytochemistry/. doi:10.1016/j.phytochem.2007.02.001.

Liu, Y., Xia, Q., Qian, Y., Kuang, Y., Liu, J., Lin, L., 2023. Effects of three extraction methods on avocado oil lipid compounds analyzed via UPLC-TOF-MS/MS with OPLS-DA. Foods. 2304-8158. 12 (6), 1174. doi:10.3390/foods12061174.

Living Cruelty Free, n.d. Alba Botanica Hawaiian Facial Mask - Papaya Enzyme 85g. https://livingcrueltyfree.gr/en/προϊόν/alba-botanica-hawaiian-facial-mask-papaya-enzyme-85g/.

Lourenço, C.B., Ataide, J.A., Cefali, L.C., Novaes, L.C.D.L., Moriel, P., Silveira, E., Tambourgi, E.B., Mazzola, P.G., 2016. Evaluation of the enzymatic activity and stability of commercial bromelain incorporated in topical formulations. Int. J. Cosmet. Sci. 14682494. 38 (5), 535–540. Available from: http://onlinelibrary.wiley.com/journal/10.1111/(ISSN)1468-2494. doi:10.1111/ics.12308.

Łubek-Nguyen, A., Ziemichód, W., Olech, M., 2022. Application of enzyme-assisted extraction for the recovery of natural bioactive compounds for nutraceutical and pharmaceutical applications. Appl. Sci. 2076-3417. 12 (7), 3232. doi:10.3390/app12073232.

Lyu, F., Luiz, S.F., Azeredo, D.R.P., Cruz, A.G., Ajlouni, S., Ranadheera, C.S., 2020. Apple pomace as a functional and healthy ingredient in food products: a review. Processes 22279717. 8 (3). Available from: https://res.mdpi.com/d_attachment/processes/processes-08-00319/article_deploy/processes-08-00319.pdf. doi:10.3390/pr8030319.

Lyu, X., Agar, O.T., Barrow, C.J., Dunshea, F.R., Suleria, H.A.R., 2023. Phenolic compounds profiling and their antioxidant capacity in the peel, pulp, and seed of Australian grown avocado. Antioxidants 20763921. 12 (1). Available from: https://www.mdpi.com/journal/antioxidants. doi:10.3390/antiox12010185.

Machado, M., Silva, S., Costa, E.M., 2024. Byproducts as a sustainable source of cosmetic ingredients. Appl. Sci. 2076-3417. 14 (22), 10241. doi:10.3390/app142210241.

Maidin, N.M., Michael, N., Oruna-Concha, M.J., Jauregi, P., 2018. Polyphenols extracted from red grape pomace by a surfactant based method show enhanced collagenase and elastase inhibitory activity. J. Chem. Technol. Biotechnol. 10974660. 93 (7), 1916–1924. Available from: http://onlinelibrary.wiley.com/journal/10.1002/(ISSN)1097-4660. doi:10.1002/jctb.5459.

Maisto, M., Piccolo, V., Novellino, E., Schiano, E., Iannuzzo, F., Ciampaglia, R., Summa, V., Tenore, G.C., 2023. Optimization of ursolic acid extraction in oil from Annurca apple to obtain oleolytes with potential cosmeceutical application. Antioxidants. 2076-3921. 12 (2), 224. doi:10.3390/antiox12020224.

MAKEUPTM, n.d. Depigmenting peeling with 1% tranexamic acid and ficin – Apis Depiq Pro system depigmenting peeling. https://makeup.ie/product/789812/.

Mala, T., Sadiq, M.B., Anal, A.K., 2021. Comparative extraction of bromelain and bioactive peptides from pineapple byproducts by ultrasonic- and microwave-assisted extractions. J. Food Process Eng. 0145-8876. 44 (6). doi:10.1111/jfpe.13709.

Maluf, D.F., Gonçalves, M.M., D'Angelo, R.W.O., Girassol, A.B., Tulio, A.P., Pupo, Y.M., Farago, P.V., 2018. Cytoprotection of antioxidant biocompounds from grape pomace: further exfoliant phytoactive ingredients for cosmetic products. Cosmetics 20799284. 5 (3). Available from: https://res.mdpi.com/cosmetics/cosmetics-05-00046/article_deploy/cosmetics-05-00046.pdf?filename=&attachment=1. doi:10.3390/COSMETICS5030046.

Manca, M.L., Casula, E., Marongiu, F., Bacchetta, G., Sarais, G., Zaru, M., Escribano-Ferrer, E., Peris, J.E., Usach, I., Fais, S., Scano, A., Orrù, G., Maroun, R.G., Fadda, A.M., Manconi, M., 2020. From waste to health: sustainable exploitation of grape pomace seed extract to manufacture antioxidant, regenerative and prebiotic nanovesicles within circular economy. Sci. Rep. 20452322. 10 (1). Available from: https://www.nature.com/srep/index.html. doi:10.1038/s41598-020-71191-8.

Manosroi, A., Chankhampan, C., Pattamapun, K., Manosroi, W., Manosroi, J., 2014. Antioxidant and gelatinolytic activities of papain from papaya latex and bromelain from pineapple fruits. Chiang Mai J. Sci. 01252526. 41 (3), 635–648. Available from: http://it.science.cmu.ac.th/ejournal/dl.php?journal_id=5033.

Mansuri, R., Diwan, A., Kumar, H., Dangwal, K., Yadav, D., 2021. Potential of natural compounds as sunscreen agents. Pharmacogn. Rev. 09737847. 15 (29), 47–56. doi:10.5530/phrev.2021.15.5.

Marabini, L., Melzi, G., Lolli, F., Dell'Agli, M., Piazza, S., Sangiovanni, E., Marinovich, M., 2020. Effects of *Vitis vinifera* L. leaves extract on UV radiation damage in human keratinocytes (HaCaT). J. Photochem. Photobiol. B. 10111344. 204, 111810. doi:10.1016/j.jphotobiol.2020.111810.

Marinaccio, L., Gentile, G., Llorent-Martínez, E.J., Zengin, G., Masci, D., Flamminii, F., Stefanucci, A., Mollica, A., 2025. Valorization of grape pomace extracts against cranberry, elderberry, rose Hip berry, goji berry and raisin extracts: phytochemical profile and in vitro biological activity. Food Chem. 03088146. 463 (Pt 2), 141323. doi:10.1016/j.foodchem.2024.141323.

Marinaccio, L., Zengin, G., Bender, O., Cichelli, A., Novellino, E., Stefanucci, A., Mollica, A., 2024. Ultrasound assisted lycopene extraction from tomato skin waste by volatile natural deep eutectic solvent. Food Chem. Adv. 2772753X. 4, 100656. doi:10.1016/j.focha.2024.100656.

Marra, A., Manousakis, V., Koutis, N., Zervas, G.P., Ofrydopoulou, A., Shiels, K., Saha, S.K., Tsoupras, A., 2025. In vitro antioxidant, antithrombotic and anti-inflammatory activities of the amphiphilic bioactives extracted from avocado and its by-products. Antioxidants. 2076-3921. 14 (2), 146. doi:10.3390/antiox14020146.

Marra, A., Manousakis, V., Zervas, G.P., Koutis, N., Finos, M.A., Adamantidi, T., Panoutsopoulou, E., Ofrydopoulou, A., Tsoupras, A., 2024. Avocado and its by-products as natural sources of valuable anti-inflammatory and antioxidant bioactives for functional foods and cosmetics with health-promoting properties. Appl. Sci. 2076-3417. 14 (14), 5978. doi:10.3390/app14145978.

Martins, R.M., Alves, G.D.A.D., Martins, S.D.S., De Freitas, L.A.P., Rochette, P.J., Moulin, V.J., Fonseca, M.J.V., 2020. Apple extract (*Malus* sp.) and rutin as photochemopreventive agents: evaluation of ultraviolet B-induced alterations on skin biopsies and tissue-engineered skin. Rejuvenation Res. 15578577. 23 (6), 465–475. Available from: https://www.liebertonline.com/rej. doi:10.1089/rej.2019.2219.

Martins, R., Sales, H., Pontes, R., Nunes, J., Gouveia, I., 2023. Food wastes and microalgae as sources of bioactive compounds and pigments in a modern biorefinery: a review. Antioxidants. 2076-3921. 12 (2), 328. doi:10.3390/antiox12020328.

Masbagusdanta, K., Setiasih, S., Handayani, S., Hudiyono, S., 2020. Partial purification and evaluation of bromelain from pineapple stem (*Ananas comosus*) in cream based preparation and its in vitro anti-inflammatory activity. AIP Conf. Proc. 15517616, 2243. http://scitation.aip.org/content/aip/proceeding/aipcp. doi:10.1063/5.0001345.

Matos, M.S., Romero-Díez, R., Álvarez, A., Bronze, M.R., Rodríguez-Rojo, S., Mato, R.B., Cocero, M.J., Matias, A.A., 2019. Polyphenol-rich extracts obtained from winemakingwaste streams as natural ingredients with cosmeceutical potential. Antioxidants 20763921. 8 (9). Available from: https://www.mdpi.com/2076-3921/8/9/355/pdf. doi:10.3390/antiox8090355.

Mattos, G.N., Tonon, R.V., Furtado, A.A.L., Cabral, L.M.C., 2017. Grape by-product extracts against microbial proliferation and lipid oxidation: a review. J. Sci. Food Agric. 10970010. 97 (4), 1055–1064. Available from: http://onlinelibrary.wiley.com/journal/10.1002/(ISSN)1097-0010. doi:10.1002/jsfa.8062.

Mendes, M.L.T., Nascimento-Júnior, E.M.D., Reinheimer, D.M., Martins-Filho, P.R.S., 2019. Efficacy of proteolytic enzyme bromelain on health outcomes after third molar surgery. Systematic review and meta-analysis of randomized clinical trials. Med. Oral Patol. Oral Cir. Bucal 16986946. 24 (1), e61. Available from: http://www.medicinaoral.com/pubmed/medoralv24_i1_p61.pdf. doi:10.4317/medoral.22731.

Michalak, M., 2023. Plant extracts as skin care and therapeutic agents. Int. J. Mol. Sci. 1422-0067. 24 (20), 15444. doi:10.3390/ijms242015444.

Mihalcea, L., Crăciunescu, O., Gheonea (Dima), I., Prelipcean, A.-M., Enachi, E., Barbu, V., Bahrim, G.E., Râpeanu, G., Oancea, A., Stănciuc, N., 2021. Supercritical CO_2 extraction and microencapsulation of lycopene-enriched oleoresins from tomato peels: evidence on antiproliferative and cytocompatibility activities. Antioxidants. 2076-3921. 10 (2), 222. doi:10.3390/antiox10020222.

Milošević, J., Vrhovac, L., Đurković, F., Janković, B., Malkov, S., Lah, J., Polović, N.Đ., 2020. Isolation, identification, and stability of Ficin 1c isoform from fig latex. New J. Chem. 1144-0546. 44 (36), 15716–15723. doi:10.1039/d0nj02938f.

Minich, I.A., Silyukov, O.I., Kurnosenko, S.A., Gak, V.V., Kalganov, V.D., Kolonitskiy, P.D., Zvereva, I.A., 2021. Physical–chemical exfoliation of n-alkylamine derivatives of layered perovskite-like oxide h2k0.5bi2.5ti4o13 into nanosheets. Fed. Nanomater. 20794991. 11 (10). Available from: https://www.mdpi.com/2079-4991/11/10/2708/pdf. doi:10.3390/nano11102708.

Misran, E., Idris, A., Sarip, S.H.M., Ya'akob, H., 2019. Properties of bromelain extract from different parts of the pineapple variety Morris. Biocatal. Agric. Biotechnol. 18788181. 18, 101095. doi:10.1016/j.bcab.2019.101095.

Moldovan, M.L., 2021. Cosmetic products containing natural-based emollients for restoring impaired skin barrier: formulation and in vivo evaluation. Farmacia. 00148237. 69 (1), 129–134. doi:10.31925/farmacia.2021.1.17.

Mora-Sandí, A., Ramírez-González, A., Castillo-Henríquez, L., Lopretti-Correa, M., Roberto Vega-Baudrit, J., 2021. Persea americana agro-industrial waste biorefinery for sustainable high-value-added products. Polymers. 2073-4360. 13 (11), 1727. doi:10.3390/polym13111727.

Morellon-Sterling, R., El-Siar, H., Tavano, O.L., Berenguer-Murcia, Á., Fernández-Lafuente, R., 2020. Ficin: a protease extract with relevance in biotechnology and biocatalysis. Int. J. Biol. Macromol. 01418130. 162, 394–404. doi:10.1016/j.ijbiomac.2020.06.144.

Motlhalamme, T., Kaningini, A.G., Maropeng, R., Thema, F.T., Mohale, K.C., Maaza, M., 2025. Tomato lycopene, total flavonoids, vitamin C content and mineral composition as affected by biosynthesized calcium carbonate nanoparticles foliar application. J. Food Compos. Anal. 08891575. 139. Available from: https://www.sciencedirect.com/science/journal/08891575. doi:10.1016/j.jfca.2024.107173.

Moysidou, A.M., Cheimpeloglou, K., Koutra, S.I., Finos, M.A., Ofrydopoulou, A., Tsoupras, A., 2024. A comprehensive review on the antioxidant and anti-inflammatory bioactives of kiwi and its by-products for functional foods and cosmetics with health-promoting properties. Appl. Sci. 2076-3417. 14 (14), 5990. doi:10.3390/app14145990.

Moysidou, A.M., Cheimpeloglou, K., Koutra, S.I., Manousakis, V., Ofrydopoulou, A., Shiels, K., Saha, S.K., Tsoupras, A., 2025. In vitro antioxidant, antithrombotic and anti-inflammatory activities of bioactive metabolites extracted from kiwi and its by-products. Metabolites. 2218-1989. 15 (6), 400. doi:10.3390/metabo15060400.

Muhammad, D.R.A., Ayouaz, S., Rachmawati, A.N., Madani, K., Fibri, D.L.N., Rafi, M., Julianti, E., Fahmy, K., 2024. Advanced and potential methods for extraction of bioactive compounds from avocado peel—a review. Appl. Sci. 2076-3417. 14 (14), 6018. doi:10.3390/app14146018.

Mungwari, C.P., King'ondu, C.K., Sigauke, P., Obadele, B.A., 2025. Conventional and modern techniques for bioactive compounds recovery from plants: review. Sci. Afr. 24682276. 27. Available from: https://www.sciencedirect.com/science/journal/24682276. doi:10.1016/j.sciaf.2024.e02509.

Naeimifar, A., Nasrollahi, S.A., Samadi, A., Talari, R., Ale-nabi, S.S., Hossini, A.M., Firooz, A., 2020. Preparation and evaluation of anti-wrinkle cream containing saffron extract and avocado oil. J. Cosmet. Dermatol. 1473-2130. 19 (9), 2366–2373. doi:10.1111/jocd.13284.

Nascimento, N.S., Torres-Obreque, K.M., Oliveira, C.A., Rabelo, J., Baby, A.R., Long, P.F., Young, A.R., Rangel-Yagui, C.D.O., 2024. Enzymes for dermatological use. Exp. Dermatol. 16000625. 33 (1). Available from: http://onlinelibrary.wiley.com/journal/10.1111/(ISSN)1600-0625. doi:10.1111/exd.15008.

Nasri, C., Halabi, Y., Aghzaf, S., Nounah, I., Brunel, M., Oubihi, A., El-Guorrami, O., Harhar, H., Costa, J., Tabyaoui, M., 2022. Seven Persea americana varieties essential oils comparison: chemical composition, toxicity, antibacterial, and antioxidant activities. Biocatal. Agric. Biotechnol. 18788181. 44, 102468. doi:10.1016/j.bcab.2022.102468.

Nazir, M., Haq, M.A., Sherazi, S.M.B., Naz, S., Mobin, L., Tsoupras, A., 2025. Effects of polyphenolic extracts from sumac, pomegranate peel, Indian almond leaves, falsa, and banana bracts on calcium oxalate and brushite crystallization in vitro. Chem. Biodivers. 1612-1872. 22 (7). doi:10.1002/cbdv.202500023.

Nhani, G.B.B., Di Filippo, L.D., de Paula, G.A., Mantovanelli, V.R., da Fonseca, P.P., Tashiro, F.M., Monteiro, D.C., Fonseca-Santos, B., Duarte, J.L., Chorilli, M., 2024. High-tech sustainable beauty: exploring nanotechnology for the development of cosmetics using plant and animal by-products. Cosmetics 20799284. 11 (4). Available from: https://www.mdpi.com/journal/cosmetics. doi:10.3390/cosmetics11040112.

Nunes, M.A., Rodrigues, F., Oliveira, M.B.P.P., 2017. Grape Processing By-Products as Active Ingredients for Cosmetic Proposes Handbook of Grape Processing By-Products: Sustainable Solutions. Elsevier Inc, Portugal, pp. 267–292. Available from: http://www.sciencedirect.com/science/book/9780128098707. doi:10.1016/B978-0-12-809870-7.00011-9.

Oliveira, D.A., Salvador, A.A., Smânia, A., Smânia, E.F.A., Maraschin, M., Ferreira, S.R.S., 2013. Antimicrobial activity and composition profile of grape (*Vitis vinifera*) pomace extracts obtained by supercritical fluids. J. Biotechnol. 18734863. 164 (3), 423–432. doi:10.1016/j.jbiotec.2012.09.014.

Oliveira, I.L.D., Domínguez-Rodríguez, G., Montero, L., Viganó, J., Cifuentes, A., Rostagno, M.A., Ibáñez, E., 2024. Advanced extraction techniques combined with natural deep eutectic solvents for extracting phenolic compounds from pomegranate (*Punica granatum* L.) peels. Int. J. Mol. Sci. 14220067. 25 (18). Available from: http://www.mdpi.com/journal/ijms. doi:10.3390/ijms25189992.

Opriş, O., Lung, I., Soran, M.-L., Stegarescu, A., Cesco, T., Ghendov-Mosanu, A., Podea, P., Sturza, R., 2022. Efficient extraction of total polyphenols from apple and investigation of its SPF properties. Molecules. 1420-3049. 27 (5), 1679. doi:10.3390/molecules27051679.

Origins, n.d. Youthtopia™ Plumping Apple Face Moisturizer With Peptides. https://www.origins.com/product/15352/128043/skincare/moisturize/moisturizers/youthtopiatm/plumping-apple-face-moisturizer-with-peptides.

Otero-Pareja, M.J., Casas, L., Fernández-Ponce, M.T., Mantell, C., Ossa, E.J.M.D.L., 2015. Green extraction of antioxidants from different varieties of red grape pomace. Molecules 14203049. 20 (6), 9686–9702. Available from: http://www.mdpi.com/journal/molecules. doi:10.3390/molecules20069686.

Oyenihi, A.B., Belay, Z.A., Mditshwa, A., Caleb, O.J., 2022. "An apple a day keeps the doctor away": the potentials of apple bioactive constituents for chronic disease prevention. J. Food Sci. 17503841. 87 (6), 2291–2309. Available from: http://onlinelibrary.wiley.com/journal/10.1111/(ISSN)1750-3841. doi:10.1111/1750-3841.16155.

Patil, N., Yadav, P., Gogate, P.R., 2024. Ultrasound assisted intensified enzymatic extraction of total phenolic compounds from pomegranate peels. Sep. Purif. Technol. 13835866. 350, 127967. doi:10.1016/j.seppur.2024.127967.

Patra, J.K., Shin, H.S., Yang, I.J., Nguyen, L.T.H., Das, G., 2024. Sustainable utilization of food biowaste (papaya peel) extract for gold nanoparticle biosynthesis and investigation of its multi-functional potentials. Antioxidants 20763921. 13 (5). Available from: https://www.mdpi.com/journal/antioxidants. doi:10.3390/antiox13050581.

Perussello, C.A., Zhang, Z., Marzocchella, A., Tiwari, B.K., 2017. Valorization of apple pomace by extraction of valuable compounds. Compr. Rev. Food Sci. Food Saf. 15414337. 16 (5), 776–796. Available from: http://www.interscience.wiley.com/jpages/1541-4337. doi:10.1111/1541-4337.12290.

Pharmeden.gr, n.d. Huda Beauty Kiwi Facial Mask Sheet Whitening & Anti Aging Mask 30gr - Μάσκες Προσώπου στο Pharmeden. https://pharmeden.gr/huda-beauty-kiwi-facial-mask-sheet-whitening-and-anti-aging-mask-30gr/.

Poblete, J., Aranda, M., Quispe-Fuentes, I., 2025. Efficient conditions of enzyme-assisted extractions and pressurized liquids for recovering polyphenols with antioxidant capacity from pisco grape pomace as a sustainable strategy. Molecules. 1420-3049. 30 (14), 2977. doi:10.3390/molecules30142977.

Porto, C.D., Porretto, E., Decorti, D., 2013. Comparison of ultrasound-assisted extraction with conventional extraction methods of oil and polyphenols from grape (Vitis vinifera L.) seeds. Ultrason. Sonochem. 13504177. 20 (4), 1076–1080. doi:10.1016/j.ultsonch.2012.12.002.

Q+A Skincare, n.d. Apple AHA Exfoliating Gel. https://www.qandaskin.com/products/apple-aha-exfoliating-gel.

Qurashi, A.A.F., Jabbar, A.D., 2022. Isolation, purification and partial characterization of ficin from *Ficus carica* latex. J. Wasit Sci. Med. 2791-3864. 2 (2), 55–66. doi:10.31185/jwsm.57.

Rabinovich, V.A., Linnenberg, C., Theilen, U., Weigand, H., 2024. Biogas production potential of mixed banana and pineapple waste as assessed by long-term laboratory-scale anaerobic digestion. Fermentation. 2311-5637. 10 (5), 261. doi:10.3390/fermentation10050261.

Rahaman, M.M., Hossain, R., Herrera-Bravo, J., Islam, M.T., Atolani, O., Adeyemi, O.S., Owolodun, O.A., Kambizi, L., Daştan, S.D., Calina, D., Sharifi-Rad, J., 2023. Natural antioxidants from some fruits, seeds, foods, natural products, and associated health benefits: an update. Food Sci. Nutr. 20487177. 11 (4), 1657–1670. Available from: https://onlinelibrary.wiley.com/journal/10.1002/%28ISSN%292048-7177. doi:10.1002/fsn3.3217.

Rajha, H.N., Abi-Khattar, A.-M., Kantar, S.E., Boussetta, N., Lebovka, N., Maroun, R.G., Louka, N., Vorobiev, E., 2019. Comparison of aqueous extraction efficiency and biological activities of polyphenols from pomegranate peels assisted by infrared, ultrasound, pulsed electric fields and high-voltage electrical discharges. Innov. Food Sci. Emerg. Technol. 14668564. 58, 102212. doi:10.1016/j.ifset.2019.102212.

Rakha, A., Rehman, N., Anwar, R., Rasheed, H., Rabail, R., Bhat, Z.F., Khaneghah, A.M., Aadil, R.M., 2025. *Actinidia* spp. (kiwifruit): a comprehensive review of its nutraceutical potential in disease mitigation and health enhancement. Food Front. 26438429. 6 (4), 1765–1788. Available from: https://onlinelibrary.wiley.com/journal/26438429. doi:10.1002/fft2.70041.

Raskovic, B., Bozovic, O., Prodanovic, R., Niketic, V., Polovic, N., 2014. Identification, purification and characterization of a novel collagenolytic serine protease from fig (*Ficus carica* var. Brown Turkey) latex. J. Biosci. Bioeng. 13891723. 118 (6), 622–627. doi:10.1016/j.jbiosc.2014.05.020.

Ribeiro, L.F., Ribani, R.H., Francisco, T.M.G., Soares, A.A., Pontarolo, R., Haminiuk, C.W.I., 2015. Profile of bioactive compounds from grape pomace (*Vitis vinifera* and *Vitis labrusca*) by spectrophotometric, chromatographic and spectral analyses. J. Chromatogr. B. 15700232. 1007, 72–80. doi:10.1016/j.jchromb.2015.11.005.

Richardson, D.P., Ansell, J., Drummond, L.N., 2018. The nutritional and health attributes of kiwifruit: a review. Eur. J. Nutr. 14366215. 57 (8), 2659–2676. Available from: http://www.springerlink.com/content/1436-6207. doi:10.1007/s00394-018-1627-z.

Sahafi, S.M., Goli, S.A.H., Kadivar, M., Varshosaz, J., Shirvani, A., 2021. Pomegranate seed oil nanoemulsion enriched by α-tocopherol; the effect of environmental stresses and long-term storage on its physicochemical properties and oxidation stability. Food Chem. 03088146. 345, 128759. doi:10.1016/j.foodchem.2020.128759.

Salem, Y., Rajha, H.N., Franjieh, D., Hoss, I., Manca, M.L., Manconi, M., Castangia, I., Perra, M., Maroun, R.G., Louka, N., 2022. Stability and antioxidant activity of hydro-glyceric extracts obtained from different grape seed varieties incorporated in cosmetic creams. Antioxidants. 2076-3921. 11 (7), 1348. doi:10.3390/antiox11071348.

Sanz, V., López-Hortas, L., Torres, M.D., Domínguez, H., 2021. Trends in kiwifruit and byproducts valorization. Trends Food Sci. Technol. 09242244. 107, 401–414. doi:10.1016/j.tifs.2020.11.010.

Sarkar, A., Haque, M.A., Alam, M., 2024. Unlocking the potential of pomegranate peels as a valuable source of bioactive compounds through effective drying strategies. Food Chem. Adv. 2772753X. 4, 100622. doi:10.1016/j.focha.2024.100622.

Segovia, F.J., Indra Hidalgo, G., Villasante, J., Ramis, X., Pilar Almajano, M., 2018. Avocado seed: a comparative study of antioxidant content and capacity in protecting oil models from oxidation. Molecules. 1420-3049. 23 (10), 2421. doi:10.3390/molecules23102421.

Serra, M., Casas, A., António Teixeira, J., Barros, A.N., 2023. Revealing the beauty potential of grape stems: harnessing phenolic compounds for cosmetics. Int. J. Mol. Sci. 1422-0067. 24 (14), 11751. doi:10.3390/ijms241411751.

Sharma, G., Vimal, A., 2023. Bromelain: an enzyme expanding its horizon from food to pharmaceutical industry. Curr. Pharm. Biotechnol. 13892010. 24 (14), 1715–1726. doi:10.2174/1389201024666230331115338.

Shoji, T., Masumoto, S., Moriichi, N., Ohtake, Y., Kanda, T., 2020. Administration of apple polyphenol supplements for skin conditions in healthy women: a randomized, double-blind, placebo-controlled clinical trial. Nutrients. 2072-6643. 12 (4), 1071. doi:10.3390/nu12041071.

Sichani, M.R., Farid, M., Moghtadaei Khorasgani, E., 2021. Histomorphological examination of skin wound healing under the effect of avocado oil in Wistar rats. Acta Vet. Eurasia 47 (3), 121–128. doi:10.5152/actavet.2021.20096.

Siddiqui, S.A., Singh, S., Nayik, G.A., 2024. Bioactive compounds from pomegranate peels - Biological properties, structure–function relationships, health benefits and food applications – a comprehensive review. J. Funct. Foods. 17564646. 116, 106132. doi:10.1016/j.jff.2024.106132.

Silva, A.M., Costa, P.C., Delerue-Matos, C., Latocha, P., Rodrigues, F., 2021. Extraordinary composition of *Actinidia arguta* by-products as skin ingredients: a new challenge for cosmetic and medical skincare industries. Trends Food Sci. Technol. 09242244. 116, 842–853. doi:10.1016/j.tifs.2021.08.031.

Silva, A.M., Pinto, D., Moreira, M.M., Costa, P.C., Delerue-Matos, C., Rodrigues, F., 2022. Valorization of kiwiberry leaves recovered by ultrasound-assisted extraction for skin application: a response surface methodology approach. Antioxidants 20763921. 11 (4). Available from: https://www.mdpi.com/2076-3921/11/4/763/pdf. doi:10.3390/antiox11040763.

Silva, S.S., Justi, M., Chagnoleau, J.B., Papaiconomou, N., Fernandez, X., Santos, S.A.O., Passos, H., Ferreira, A.M., Coutinho, J.A.P., 2023. Using bio-based solvents for the extraction of phenolic compounds from kiwifruit industry waste. Sep. Purif. Technol. 18733794. 304. Available from: http://www.journals.elsevier.com/separation-and-purification-technology/. doi:10.1016/j.seppur.2022.122344.

Singh, J., Kaur, H.P., Verma, A., Chahal, A.S., Jajoria, K., Rasane, P., Kaur, S., Kaur, J., Gunjal, M., Ercisli, S., Choudhary, R., Bozhuyuk, M.R., Sakar, E., Karatas, N., Durul, M.S., 2023. Pomegranate peel phytochemistry, pharmacological properties, methods of extraction, and its application: a comprehensive review. ACS Omega 24701343. 8 (39), 35452–35469. Available from: https://pubs.acs.org/journal/acsodf. doi:10.1021/acsomega.3c02586.

Singh, N., Kumar, S., Patle, D.S., 2025. Intensification of extraction of bioactive compounds from pomegranate peel using an ultrasound-microwave assisted extraction approach: parametric optimization, kinetics and thermodynamics. Sep. Purif. Technol. 13835866. 359, 130681. doi:10.1016/j.seppur.2024.130681.

Siol, M., Sadowska, A., 2023. Chemical composition, physicochemical and bioactive properties of avocado (*Persea americana*) seed and its potential use in functional food design. Agriculture. 2077-0472. 13 (2), 316. doi:10.3390/agriculture13020316.

Sjahjadi, F., Febriyenti, F., Lucida, H., 2021. Formula optimization of a sunscreen cream of tomato's purified extract. Proceedings series Advances in Health Sciences Research. doi:10.2991/ahsr.k.211105.007.

Skinner, R.C., Gigliotti, J.C., Ku, K.M., Tou, J.C., 2018. A comprehensive analysis of the composition, health benefits, and safety of apple pomace. Nutr. Rev. 17534887. 76 (12), 893–909. doi:10.1093/nutrit/nuy033.

Smith, W.P., Bishop, M., Gillis, G., Maibach, H., 2007. Topical proteolytic enzymes affect epidermal and dermal properties. Int. J. Cosmet. Sci. 0142-5463. 29 (1), 15–21. doi:10.1111/j.1467-2494.2007.00354.x.

Sołdacka, D., Barańska-Rybak, W., 2024. Evaluation of Safety and Efficacy of Chemical Peels With and Without Sonophoresis on Selected Skin Parameters—A Prospective Comparative Study. Cosmetics. 2079-9284. 11 (6), 185. doi:10.3390/cosmetics11060185.

Sopyan, I., Gozali, D., Tiassetiana, S., 2017. Formulation of tomato extracts (Solanum lycopersicum L.) as a sunscreen lotion. Natl. J. Physiol. Pharm. Pharmacol. 1, 2320–4672. doi:10.5455/njppp.2017.7.1039921112017.

Stojiljković, D., Tadić, V., Stanković, M., Roganović, S., Arsić, I., 2018. Standardized extract of wild apple fruit in alkyl-polyglucoside-based cosmetic cream – estimation of stability, safety, antioxidant activity and efficiency. Int. J. Cosmet. Sci. 0142-5463. 40 (3), 285–294. doi:10.1111/ics.12462.

Szabó, É., Marosvölgyi, T., Szilágyi, G., Kőrösi, L., Schmidt, J., Csepregi, K., Márk, L., Bóna, Á., 2021. Correlations between total antioxidant capacity, polyphenol and fatty acid content of native grape seed and pomace of four different grape varieties in Hungary. Antioxidants. 2076-3921. 10 (7), 1101. doi:10.3390/antiox10071101.

Szabo, K., Mitrea, L., Călinoiu, L.F., Teleky, B.E., Martău, G.A., Plamada, D., Pascuta, M.S., Nemeş, S.A., Varvara, R.A., Vodnar, D.C., 2022. Natural polyphenol recovery from apple-, cereal-, and tomato-processing by-products and related health-promoting properties. Molecules 14203049. 27 (22). Available from: http://www.mdpi.com/journal/molecules. doi:10.3390/molecules27227977.

Szabo, K., Varvara, R.A., Ciont, C., Macri, A.M., Vodnar, D.C., 2025. An updated overview on the revalorization of bioactive compounds derived from tomato production and processing by-products. J. Clean. Prod. 09596526. 497. Available from: https://www.sciencedirect.com/science/journal/09596526. doi:10.1016/j.jclepro.2025.145151.

Tanabe, S., Tesaki, S., Watanabe, M., Yanagihara, Y., 1997. Cross-reactivity between bromelain and soluble fraction from wheat flour. Arerugī = [Allergy]. 00214884. 46 (11), 1170–1173.

Tang, S.-C., Yang, J.-H., 2018. Dual effects of alpha-hydroxy acids on the skin. Molecules 23 (4). doi:10.3390/molecules23040863.

Teixeira, A.P., Coutinho, B., Cancela, J., Cullen, L., Brito, M., 2022. Valorisation of kiwifruit residues and their application in an anti-ageing facial cream. U.Porto J. Eng. 2183-6493. 8 (5), 68–85. doi:10.24840/2183-6493_008.005_0008.

The Body Shop, n.d. Grapeseed glossing serum https://www.thebodyshop.gr/grapeseed-glossing-serum.html.

TONYMOLY USA, n.d. I Am Sheet Mask (Set of 2). https://tonymoly.us/products/im-real-mask.

Trevisol, T.C., Henriques, R.O., Souza, A.J.A., Furigo, A., 2022. An overview of the use of proteolytic enzymes as exfoliating agents. J. Cosmet. Dermatol. 14732165. 21 (8), 3300–3307. Available from: http://onlinelibrary.wiley.com/journal/10.1111/(ISSN)1473-2165. doi:10.1111/jocd.14673.

Trombino, S., Cassano, R., Procopio, D., Di Gioia, M.L., Barone, E., 2021. Valorization of tomato waste as a source of carotenoids. Molecules. 1420-3049. 26 (16), 5062. doi:10.3390/molecules26165062.

Tsiapali, O.I., Ayfantopoulou, E., Tzourouni, A., Ofrydopoulou, A., Letsiou, S., Tsoupras, A., 2025b. Unveiling the utilization of grape and winery by-products in cosmetics with health-promoting properties. Appl. Sci. 2076-3417. 15 (3), 1007. doi:10.3390/app15031007.

Tsiapali, O.I., Kontaxi, N.I., Pavlidis, K., Ofrydopoulou, A., Prokopiou, V., Letsiou, S., Kosheleva, R.I., Mitropoulos, A., Tsoupras, A., 2025a. Anti-inflammatory and antioxidant properties of anti-UV creams enriched with natural extracts from avocado, apple, and kiwi by-products, with and without nanobubbles. Cosmetics 20799284. 12 (5). Available from: https://www.mdpi.com/journal/cosmetics. doi:10.3390/cosmetics12050231.

Tsoupras, A., Adamantidi, T., Finos, M.A., Philippopoulos, A., Detopoulou, P., Tsopoki, I., Kynatidou, M., Demopoulos, C.A., 2024a. Re-assessing the role of platelet activating factor and its inflammatory signaling and inhibitors in cancer and anti-cancer strategies. Front. Biosci. (Landmark Ed.) 29 (10), 345. doi:10.31083/j.fbl2910345. PMID: 39473406.

Tsoupras, A.B., Iatrou, C., Frangia, C., Demopoulos, C.A., 2009. The implication of platelet activating factor in cancer growth and metastasis: potent beneficial role of PAF-inhibitors and antioxidants. Infect. Disord. Drug Targets 9 (4), 390–399. doi:10.2174/187152609788922555. PMID: 19689381.

Tsoupras, A., Gkika, D.A., Markopoulos, T., Curran, R., Scallon, C., Karali, M., Kyzas, G.Z., 2024b. Apple Products (Apple Juice and Cider) and By-Products (Apple Pomace): Bioactive Compounds and Biological Properties, Vol. 3607. Springer Science and Business Media LLC, pp. 1–42. doi:10.1007/978-3-031-04195-2_214-1.

Tsoupras, A., Moran, D., Byrne, T., Ryan, J., Barrett, L., Traas, C., Zabetakis, I., 2021. Anti-inflammatory and anti-platelet properties of lipid bioactives from apple cider by-products. Molecules. 1420-3049. 26 (10), 2869. doi:10.3390/molecules26102869.

Tsoupras, A., Ni, V.L.J., O'Mahony, É., Karali, M., 2023. Winemaking: "with one stone, two birds"? A holistic review of the bio-functional compounds, applications and health benefits of wine and wineries' by-products. Fermentation. 2311-5637. 9 (9), 838. doi:10.3390/fermentation9090838.

Türkyılmaz, M., Hamzaoğlu, F., Çiftci, R.B.A., Özkan, M., 2023. Increase in colour stability of pomegranate juice against 5-hydroxymethylfurfural (HMF) through copigmentation with phenolic acids. J. Sci. Food Agric. 10970010. 103 (15), 7836–7848. Available from: http://onlinelibrary.wiley.com/journal/10.1002/(ISSN)1097-0010. doi:10.1002/jsfa.12866.

Vandorou, M., Plakidis, C., Tsompanidou, I.M., Adamantidi, T., Panagopoulou, E.A., Tsoupras, A., 2024. A review on apple pomace bioactives for natural functional food and cosmetic products with therapeutic health-promoting properties. Int. J. Mol. Sci. 1422-0067. 25 (19), 10856. doi:10.3390/ijms251910856.

Vandorou, M., Plakidis, C., Tsompanidou, I.M., Ofrydopoulou, A., Shiels, K., Saha, S.K., Tsoupras, A., 2025. In vitro antioxidant, antithrombotic and anti-inflammatory properties of the amphiphilic bioactives from Greek organic Starking apple juice and its by-products (apple pomace). Appl. Sci. 2076-3417. 15 (5), 2807. doi:10.3390/app15052807.

Varilla, C., Marcone, M., Paiva, L., Baptista, J., 2021. Bromelain, a group of pineapple proteolytic complex enzymes (*Ananas comosus*) and their possible therapeutic and clinical effects: a summary. Foods. 2304-8158. 10 (10), 2249. doi:10.3390/foods10102249.

Venetikidou, M., Lykartsi, E., Adamantidi, T., Prokopiou, V., Ofrydopoulou, A., Letsiou, S., Tsoupras, A., 2025. Proteolytic enzyme activities of bromelain, ficin, and papain from fruit by-products and potential applications in sustainable and functional cosmetics for skincare. Appl. Sci. 2076-3417. 15 (5), 2637. doi:10.3390/app15052637.

Villamil-Galindo, E., Piagentini, A.M., 2022. Sequential ultrasound-assisted extraction of pectin and phenolic compounds for the valorisation of 'Granny Smith' apple peel. Food Biosci. 22124292. 49, 101958. doi:10.1016/j.fbio.2022.101958.

Wang, J., Lan, T., Lei, Y., Suo, J., Zhao, Q., Wang, H., Lei, J., Sun, X., Tingting, M., 2021a. Optimization of ultrasonic-assisted enzymatic extraction of kiwi starch and evaluation of its structural, physicochemical, and functional characteristics. Ultrason. Sonochem. 13504177. 81, 105866. doi:10.1016/j.ultsonch.2021.105866.

Wang, K., Li, M., Wang, Y., Liu, Z., Yuanying, N., 2021b. Effects of extraction methods on the structural characteristics and functional properties of dietary fiber extracted from kiwifruit (Actinidia deliciosa). Food Hydrocoll. 0268005X. 110, 106162. doi:10.1016/j.foodhyd.2020.106162.

Weremfo, A., Adulley, F., Adarkwah-Yiadom, M., 2020. Simultaneous optimization of microwave-assisted extraction of phenolic compounds and antioxidant activity of avocado (*Persea americana* Mill.) seeds using response surface methodology. J. Anal. Methods Chem. 2090-8865. 2020, 1–11. doi:10.1155/2020/7541927.

Wu, D.T., Deng, W., Li, J., Geng, J.L., Hu, Y.C., Zou, L., Liu, Y., Liu, H.Y., Gan, R.Y., 2023. Ultrasound-assisted deep eutectic solvent extraction of phenolic compounds from thinned young kiwifruits and their beneficial effects. Antioxidants 20763921. 12 (7). Available from: https://www.mdpi.com/journal/antioxidants. doi:10.3390/antiox12071475.

Yahia, E.M. (Ed.), 2018. Postharvest physiology and biochemistry of fruits and vegetables. In: Postharvest Physiology and Biochemistry of Fruits and Vegetable. Elsevier, Mexico, pp. 1–476. Available from: https://www.sciencedirect.com/science/book/9780128132784. doi:10.1016/C2016-0-04653-3.

Yang, Y., Shen, D., Long, Y., Xie, Z., Zheng, H., 2017. Intrinsic peroxidase-like activity of ficin. Sci. Rep. 2045-2322. 7 (1). doi:10.1038/srep43141.

Yilmaz-Turan, S., Gál, T., Lopez-Sanchez, P., Martinez, M.M., Menzel, C., Vilaplana, F., 2023. Modulating temperature and pH during subcritical water extraction tunes the molecular properties of apple pomace pectin as food gels and emulsifiers. Food Hydrocoll. 0268005X. 145, 109148. doi:10.1016/j.foodhyd.2023.109148.

Yilmaz, Y., Toledo, R.T., 2004. Major flavonoids in grape seeds and skins: antioxidant capacity of catechin, epicatechin, and gallic acid. J. Agric. Food Chem. 00218561. 52 (2), 255–260. doi:10.1021/jf030117h.

Yulirohyami, H.H., Wijaya, A.R., 2022. Is Fatimah, papain enzyme-assisted extraction of virgin coconut oil as candidate in-house reference material. Processes. 2227-9717. 10 (2), 315. doi:10.3390/pr10020315.

Zabetakis, I., Tsoupras, A., Lordan, R., Ramji, D. (Eds.), 2023. Functional Foods and Their Implications for Health Promotion. Academic Press.

Zampar, G.G., Zampar, I.C., Beserra da Silva de Souza, S., da Silva, C., & Bolanho Barros, B.C., 2022. Effect of solvent mixtures on the ultrasound-assisted extraction of compounds from pineapple by-product. Food Biosci. 22124292. 50, 102098. doi:10.1016/j.fbio.2022.102098.

Zare, H., Moosavi-Movahedi, A.A., Salami, M., Mirzaei, M., Saboury, A.A., Sheibani, N., 2013. Purification and autolysis of the ficin isoforms from fig (*Ficus carica* cv. *Sabz*) latex. Phytochemistry. 00319422. 87, 16–22. doi:10.1016/j.phytochem.2012.12.006.

Zhang, Q.-W., Lin, L.-G., Wen-Cai, Y., 2018. Techniques for extraction and isolation of natural products: a comprehensive review. Chin. Med. 1749-8546. 13 (1). doi:10.1186/s13020-018-0177-x.

Zhang, S., Shan, L., Wang, Y., Jiayi, N., Xiao, G., 2024. The efficacy of a novel tomato extracts formulation on skin aging and pigmentation: a randomized, double-blind, parallel-controlled trial. J. Dermatol. Sci. Cosmet. Technol. 2950306X. 1 (1), 100005. doi:10.1016/j.jdsct.2024.100005.

Zlatanović, S., Kalušević, A., Micić, D., Laličić-Petronijević, J., Tomić, N., Ostojić, S., Gorjanović, S., 2019. Functionality and storability of cookies fortified at the industrial scale with up to 75% of apple pomace flour produced by dehydration. Foods. 2304-8158. 8 (11), 561. doi:10.3390/foods8110561.

Chapter 12

Plant-derived fermented beverages (wine, beer, cider) and their by-products

Stefanos Michailidis, Theodora Adamantidi and Alexandros Tsoupras

Hephaestus Laboratory, School of Chemistry, Faculty of Sciences, Democritus University of Thrace, Kavala University Campus, Kavala, Greece

1 Introduction

Fermented beverages such as wine, beer, and cider represent not only cultural and economic cornerstones of the global food industry but also reservoirs of valuable biofunctional compounds. In recent years, growing attention has been directed toward the valorization of winery and brewery by-products, including grape pomace, seeds, brewers' spent grain (BSG), yeast (BSY), and hops (BSH), as promising sources of natural bioactives for sustainable and innovative applications in the food, health, and cosmetic sectors (Tsoupras et al., 2022; Baptista et al., 2023).

The alcoholic beverage industry is a major contributor to global food waste, accounting for approximately 26% of total food waste worldwide (around 416 million tons in 2019), with beer being the most widely consumed alcoholic drink (Belardi et al., 2025). During brewing, large quantities of valuable by-products are generated, including 37.8 million tons of BSG, 44.2 thousand tons of BSY, and 2.6 million tons of BSH (2021). Despite their rich content of proteins, fibers, polyphenols, and minerals, these materials remain largely underutilized, often used as low-value feed, compost, or landfill material. Among them, BSH residues are particularly rich in expensive bioactives, while BSY is already used in cosmetics for its antioxidant, antiinflammatory, and dermo-conditioning properties (Tsoupras et al., 2022; Baptista et al., 2023; Belardi et al., 2025).

Wine is the second most consumed alcoholic beverage globally, with nearly 70% of grape production dedicated to winemaking (Llavata et al., 2022; Tsiapali et al., 2025b). The by-products of this process, grape pomace, skins, seeds, and stems, contain abundant polyphenols, lipids, and dietary fibers with notable antioxidant, antiinflammatory, and antiaging potential. Similarly, apple-based beverages such as juice and cider also contribute substantially to global production and waste streams. Apple pomace, the major by-product of these processes, represents a rich source of polyphenols, dietary fibers, and other bioactives that can be recovered and repurposed for functional food, nutraceutical, cosmetic, and cosmeceutical applications (Tsoupras et al., 2022; Llavata et al., 2022; Tsiapali et al., 2025b).

Fermentation has long been a time-honored preservation technique, extending the shelf life of perishable foods while improving their sensory qualities, such as taste, aroma, and texture (Xiang et al., 2019). In the case of apple juice fermentation, *Lactobacillus* species have been shown to enhance the phytochemical and antioxidant profile of the beverage, increasing phenolic content and promoting biological activities such as hypoglycemic effects and gut microbiota modulation. These attributes position apple pomace and fermented apple juice as promising sources of functional compounds for both health-promoting and cosmetic formulations (Llavata et al., 2022; Xiang et al., 2019; Vandorou et al., 2024; Tsoupras et al., 2024a).

The winemaking process, while historically and economically significant, generates large quantities of grape by-products, markedly rich in polyphenols, organic acids, and lipids. Efficient recovery of these bioactives is essential, yet conventional extraction methods often require high solvent volumes and energy inputs, leading to the potential degradation of thermolabile compounds. Consequently, green extraction technologies, like supercritical fluid (SFE), microwave-assisted (MAE), ultrasound-assisted (UAE), and pulsed electric field (PEF) extraction, have emerged as sustainable alternatives

Biofunctional Cosmetics for Health. https://doi.org/10.1016/B978-0-443-27500-5.00023-X

that improve efficiency, reduce solvent use, and preserve bioactivity. Optimizing these methods is critical for maximizing both the yield and stability of grape-derived bioactives for cosmetic applications (Tsiapali et al., 2025b; Xiang et al., 2019; Ferreira and Santos, 2022; Fragopoulou et al., 2018; Tsoupras et al., 2024a).

BSG, the main by-product of the brewing industry, is also a rich source of phenolic acids, mainly ferulic and p-coumaric acids, which contribute significantly to its antioxidant activity. Extraction efficiency depends on both the technique used, ranging from conventional solvent and hydrolysis methods to advanced green technologies like MAE and supercritical fluid CO_2 extraction (SFE-CO_2), and on the malt type, with lighter malts (e.g., Pilsen) generally yielding higher phenolic contents than darker varieties. Due to the complexity of BSG's lignocellulosic matrix, innovative approaches, including enzymatic hydrolysis and microencapsulation, are being developed to enhance recovery, improve compound stability, and expand potential applications of BSG phenolics in various products (Tsoupras et al., 2022; Censi et al., 2021; Almendinger et al., 2020; Postigo et al., 2025).

Apples rank among the most consumed fruits globally and are naturally rich in essential macro- and micronutrients, including carbohydrates, vitamins, and minerals. The well-known saying "an apple a day keeps the doctor away" reflects apples' recognized health benefits. Apple-based products and their by-products contain diverse bioactive constituents, including probiotics, phenolics, functional lipids, dietary fiber, vitamins, and minerals. Fermentation and extraction of these compounds yield valuable materials for diverse uses (Llavata et al., 2022; Vandorou et al., 2024; Tsoupras et al., 2024a; Oyenihi et al., 2022).

Grape pomace, a major by-product of winemaking, primarily comprises flavan-3-ols, procyanidins, anthocyanins, flavonols, and stilbenes, compounds which exhibit antioxidant, antiinflammatory, antielastase, and antityrosinase activities. These properties contribute to the skin-whitening, antiaging, antimicrobial, and antiinflammatory effects observed in cosmetics. In addition, grape seed extracts contain biofunctional lipids and vitamins that further enhance their protective and reparative capacities in skincare applications (Ferreira and Santos, 2022; Bordiga et al., 2019; Kontaxi et al., 2024).

Beer and its brewing by-products also serve as remarkable sources of bioactive compounds originating from malt, hops, and fermentation. These mainly include polyphenols, flavonoids, prenylated metabolites, bitter acids, and polar lipids (PLs), many of which possess antioxidant, antiinflammatory, neuroprotective, and chemopreventive effects. Although present in relatively low concentrations in beer due to its high-water content, these compounds still contribute to its overall health-promoting potential when consumed moderately. Brewing by-products such as BSC, BSY, and BSH are packed with dietary fibers, proteins, phenolic acids, and minerals, making them valuable for food, cosmetic, and nutraceutical applications (Tsoupras et al., 2022, 2024c; Almendinger et al., 2020; Postigo et al., 2025; Lordan et al., 2019b).

While studies on apple cider remain limited and primarily in vitro, emerging evidence highlights its potential in cosmetic science, especially concerning antiinflammatory pathways. Clinical investigations have reported the effectiveness of apple pomace bioactives, such as ursolic acid and apple-based nanovesicles, in decreasing wrinkles, enhancing skin hydration, and modulating inflammation, supporting their vital role in advanced cosmeceuticals (Vandorou et al., 2024; Tsoupras et al., 2024a; Maisto et al., 2023). Similarly, grape pomace and seed oils provide notable antioxidant, antiinflammatory, and antiaging benefits valuable for cosmetic use. However, their high water content and heat sensitivity reduce their stability, necessitating dehydration methods such as vacuum drying to preserve polyphenols. The inclusion of surfactants can further enhance phenolic stability, although sensory attributes and potential contaminants must be carefully monitored to ensure quality and consumer safety (Ferreira and Santos, 2022; Kontaxi et al., 2024; Di Stefano et al., 2022). Finally, utilizing beer and brewery by-products in cosmetics remains at an early developmental stage. Preliminary studies have identified various compounds with promising antioxidant and antiinflammatory potential. Nevertheless, further research is needed to evaluate their efficacy, safety, stability, and scalability within cosmetic products. Addressing challenges related to extraction methods, compound standardization, and large-scale production will be crucial to the successful integration of brewery-derived bioactives into commercial cosmetics. Continued interdisciplinary research and technological innovation will be vital in unlocking their full potential within the modern cosmetic industry (Tsoupras et al., 2022, 2024b, 2024c; Almendinger et al., 2020; Postigo et al., 2025). This review examines the extraction techniques, bioactive profile, health-promoting efficacy, and cosmetic applications of apple, cider, grape, wine, beer, and brewery by-product bioactives, also delving into their suitability and limitations toward potential cosmetic product creation. The main key points of this chapter are illustrated in Fig. 12.1.

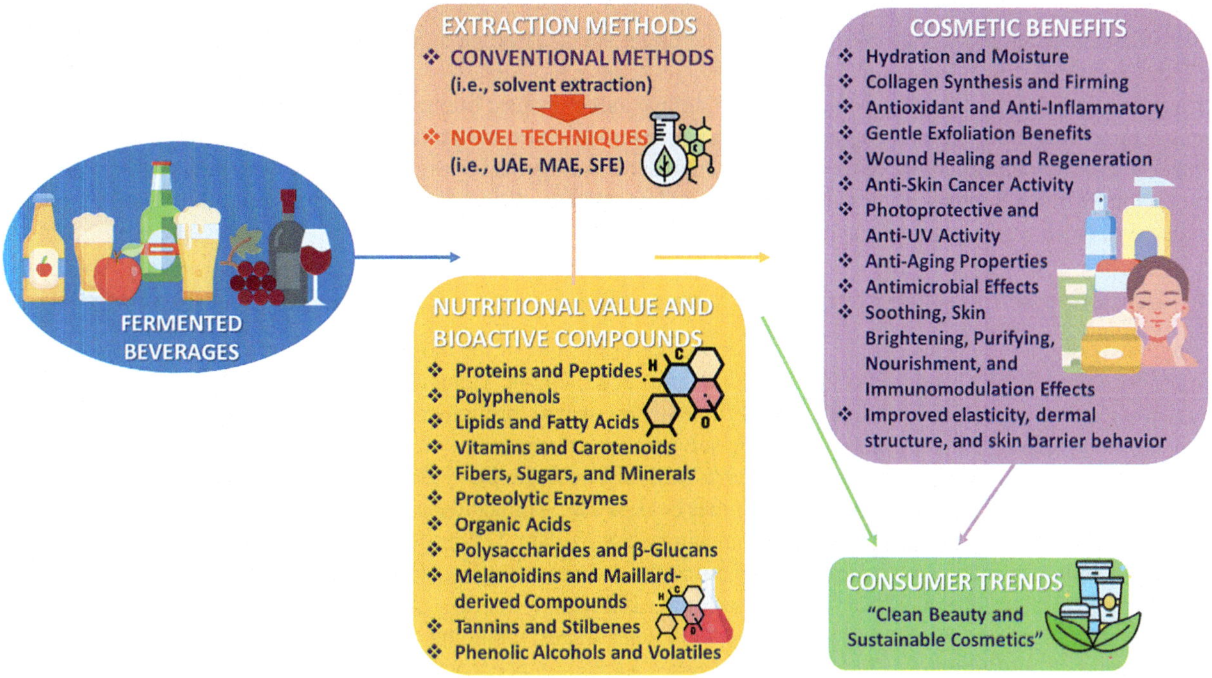

FIG. 12.1 Fermented beverage bioactives extraction techniques, pharmacological properties, and cosmetic applications. *(Parts of this figure were obtained from the open access free platform https://www.flaticon.com/ (Accessed 4 October 2025).)*

2 Extraction methods for bioactives from fermented beverages and factors affecting the extraction yield

The extraction of bioactive compounds from fermented beverage by-products poses a crucial challenge, particularly when aiming to employ eco-friendly, economically sustainable methods. These matrices, derived from apples, grapes, and brewery residues, contain a plethora of thermolabile and oxidation-sensitive compounds that can easily degrade under inappropriate processing conditions. High temperature, pH fluctuations, and exposure to oxygen are among the main factors that compromise the integrity and biological activity of the desired substances (Pedro et al., 2024). Therefore the development of green, low-energy, and solvent-efficient extraction methods has become a central focus in the valorization of winery, cidery, and brewery wastes for cosmeceutical applications (Lordan et al., 2019b; Maisto et al., 2023; Opriş et al., 2022; da Silva et al., 2021; Romanini et al., 2021; Bucić-Kojić et al., 2007; Duba et al., 2015).

Initially, mechanical pretreatments such as milling, sieving, and filtration are applied to break down the matrix and facilitate the release of intracellular compounds (Krbečková and Plachá, 2024). Conventional extraction techniques, such as Soxhlet extraction, maceration, and solid–liquid extraction, remain widely used due to their simplicity and accessibility in most laboratories. However, these methods are often associated with long extraction times, high solvent consumption, and thermal degradation of thermolabile compounds. To overcome these limitations, novel green extraction approaches have emerged, offering improved efficacy and selectivity without compromising compound stability. These include SFE, PLE, liquefied gas technology, MAE, UAE, enzyme-assisted extraction, and PEF. In addition, biological extraction methods like enzymatic hydrolysis and microbial-assisted fermentation have shown great potential for selectively releasing bound phenolics and peptides with higher recovery efficiency (Lordan et al., 2019b; Maisto et al., 2023; Opriş et al., 2022; da Silva et al., 2021; Romanini et al., 2021; Bucić-Kojić et al., 2007; Duba et al., 2015; Chakka and Babu, 2022; Areti et al., 2024). While most of these processes are noncatalytic, catalytic systems that involve metal-based, carbon-supported, or acid catalysts can also be employed to enhance both yield and target compound selectivity and specificity (Krbečková and Plachá, 2024).

The efficacy of extraction and the yield of bioactive recovery depend on multiple factors related to both the raw material and the extraction conditions. Key influencing parameters include the particle size of the substrate, solvent type and polarity, solid-to-liquid ratio, extraction temperature and time, pH, and agitation rate. In addition, the moisture content, matrix composition (comprising lignin, cellulose, protein, and lipid content), and storage conditions of the by-products significantly affect the availability and extractability of the target agents (Lordan et al., 2019b; Maisto et al., 2023; Opriş et al., 2022; da Silva et al., 2021; Romanini et al., 2021; Bucić-Kojić et al., 2007; Duba et al., 2015; Chakka and Babu, 2022). For thermolabile molecules, including polyphenols, vitamins, and enzymes, minimizing heat exposure and oxygen contact is essential to prevent oxidation and degradation. The use of antioxidant stabilizers, inert gas atmospheres, and closed-system extraction units can further improve the preservation of sensitive agents (Censi et al., 2021; Areti et al., 2024). Optimizing these factors, while aligning with sustainability principles, remains critical for maximizing yield, purity, and functionality of bioactives destined for cosmetics and cosmeceuticals.

2.1 Extraction of bioactive compounds from apple juice and/or cider and their by-products

As previously discussed in **Chapter 11**, apple pomace represents one of the most abundant and valuable by-products of the fruit processing industry (Vandorou et al., 2024; Tsoupras et al., 2024a; Vandorou et al., 2025). It is a rich source of fibers, polyphenolics, and organic acids, which can be efficiently recovered through both conventional and green extraction methods. Traditional techniques often employ organic solvents such as methanol or acetone, whereas eco-friendly alternatives, including ethanol and subcritical water extraction (SWE), offer comparable yields while minimizing environmental impact (Massias et al., 2015; Gil-Martín et al., 2022; Somat et al., 2025; Yilmaz-Turan et al., 2023). Extracts derived from apple pomace have demonstrated remarkable antiinflammatory, antioxidant, UV-protective, and antiaging bioactivities, supporting their potential for incorporation into natural cosmetic and cosmeceutical formulations (Massias et al., 2015; Yilmaz-Turan et al., 2023; Arraibi et al., 2021; Di Lorenzo et al., 2024).

The production of apple cider and juice involves several stages, including fruit washing, crushing, pressing, clarification, fermentation, and filtration. During these processes, apple pomace, composed of peel, core, seeds, and residual pulp, is generated in large quantities as a by-product (Vandorou et al., 2024; Perussello et al., 2017; Karantonis et al., 2023). The growing global consumption of apple-based beverages has led to apple pomace becoming one of the most produced fruit-processing residues worldwide (Barreira et al., 2019). The characteristics of apple juice and cider, including aroma, flavor, nutrient composition, and bioactive composition, are strongly influenced by apple cultivar, maturity stage, ripeness, climatic conditions, fermentation parameters, additives, and yeast strain selection. While apple cider contains a lower alcohol content than wine, it remains an alcoholic beverage. Therefore its consumption should be moderate and incorporated within a balanced diet (Tsoupras et al., 2022, 2023b; Moran et al., 2021; Tsoupras et al., 2021a).

Fermentation plays a pivotal role in modifying the bioactive composition of apple juice. When fermented by *Lactobacillus* species, apple juice exhibits enhanced phytochemical content, antioxidant potential, and stability during both storage and simulated gastrointestinal digestion. Postfermentation studies have reported a notable increase in phenolics, particularly chlorogenic acid, alongside substantially improved 2,2-diphenyl-1-picrylhydrazyl (DPPH) radical scavenging and ferric reducing antioxidant power (FRAP) values (Llavata et al., 2022; Vandorou et al., 2025; Massias et al., 2015; Karantonis et al., 2023; Caiyun et al., 2023). Beyond antioxidant effects, *Lactobacillus*-fermented apple juice demonstrates additional biological benefits, including hypoglycemic and lipid-regulating effects, attributed to the enrichment of functional metabolites. Experimental models in diabetic animals revealed improvements in fasting blood glucose, insulin sensitivity, and lipid metabolism, as well as a reduction in oxidative stress and restoration of pancreatic islet cell integrity. These effects were associated with favorable shifts in gut microbiota composition, namely, an increased relative abundance of Actinobacteria, Bifidobacteria, and Faecalibaculum, highlighting the systemic potential of fermented apple products in promoting metabolic and dermal health (Wang et al., 2022).

2.2 Extraction of bioactive compounds from wine and its by-products

The vinification process is one of the most culturally significant traditions, especially within Mediterranean civilizations such as the Greek and Roman societies, where wine held ritualistic and social importance. With industrialization, winemaking evolved from small-scale craftsmanship into a globalized process, resulting in a wide diversity of wine types and production scales. Most wines contain roughly 12%–14% v/v ethanol, though nonalcoholic wine variants have gained market presence in recent decades. Interestingly, the vinification process is based on the alcoholic fermentation of grape juice in the presence of yeast strains, mainly *Saccharomyces cerevisiae,* and the specific methods applied depend on grape variety, maturity, and the type of wine produced (Zabetakis et al., 2022; Tsiapali et al., 2025b; Ferreira and Santos, 2022; Fragopoulou et al., 2018; Tsoupras et al., 2024a; Postigo et al., 2025; Chakka and Babu, 2022).

To utilize the vast amounts of winery by-products for applications in the food, health, and cosmetic sectors, attention must be directed toward efficient and sustainable extraction methods capable of preserving the integrity of bioactives (Beres et al., 2017; Panzella et al., 2020; Ilyas et al., 2021; Chowdhary et al., 2021; Drevelegka and Goula, 2020; Barba et al., 2016). The selection of raw materials, such as grape pomace, is essential and should involve a careful preliminary assessment of functional compound composition to ensure optimal quality for further processing. In typical extraction protocols, bioactive compounds are separated from inert components using targeted solvents (Panzella et al., 2020). Conventional techniques such as Soxhlet extraction, maceration, and reflux extraction have been employed for decades. However, their reliance on large volumes of potentially toxic solvents, high temperatures, and extended extraction times renders them unsuitable for modern sustainable applications. These methods, which are also usually associated with toxicity issues, are not suitable for commercial use. These conditions often lead to oxidation or thermal degradation of sensitive molecules such as polyphenols and unsaturated fatty acids (UFAs), while also increasing energy demand and operational costs. Furthermore, mechanical disruption of grape tissues can activate oxidative enzymes like polyphenol oxidase and peroxidase, accelerating polyphenol degradation. For grape seed oil production, cold pressing and controlled mechanical extraction are preferred to maximize yield and preserve thermolabile agents (Rombaut et al., 2015). Consequently, green and nonconventional extraction methods have been developed to achieve high recovery efficiency with reduced environmental impact and minimal bioactive loss (Beres et al., 2017; Panzella et al., 2020; Ilyas et al., 2021; Chowdhary et al., 2021; Drevelegka and Goula, 2020; Barba et al., 2016).

Among the most utilized procedures, solid–liquid extraction with agitation or Soxhlet extraction using ethanolic or methanolic solvents remains common for recovering polyphenols, lipids, and dietary fibers from grape pomace. The extraction yield is influenced by parameters such as solvent polarity, type, temperature, extraction duration, and solid-to-liquid ratio, all of which determine the recovery and antioxidant potential of the final extracts. For example, while anthocyanins and low-molecular-weight phenolics are best recovered using hydroalcoholic solvents, dietary fibers and grape seed oils require distinct conditions for optimal yield. Despite a few standardized procedures for polyphenol extraction, ongoing research is required to establish reproducible, high-yield methods that preserve compound integrity (Beres et al., 2017; Panzella et al., 2020; Drevelegka and Goula, 2020; Barba et al., 2016).

Driven by the demand for cleaner processes, several green extraction technologies have been introduced. Nanofiltration and SFE are emerging as efficient separation and purification tools for valuable compounds from grape pomace. In SFE, fluids are maintained above their critical temperature and pressure, where liquid and gas phases merge into a single supercritical state with exceptional solvent properties (Panzella et al., 2020). Supercritical CO_2, due to its low toxicity and cost, has been widely adopted for extracting antioxidants, pigments, and fatty acids from grape seeds (Yang et al., 2021). When modified with ethanol as a co-solvent, SFE drastically improves polyphenol recovery and reduces extraction time compared to Soxhlet or solid–liquid methods (Panzella et al., 2020; Pinelo et al., 2007). Experimental studies show that 66% ethanol-modified SFE enhances polyphenol and anthocyanin yields, boosting the antioxidant, antiproliferative, and antiinflammatory potential of wine extracts (Jeong et al., 2010). Similarly, the combined use of CO_2 and ethanol markedly increases resveratrol recovery compared to CO_2 alone (Casas et al., 2010).

Additional advanced methods, including MAE and UAE, have proven highly effective in valorizing grape pomace (Tsiapali et al., 2025b; Li et al., 2011, 2025). MAE enables the rapid release of polyphenols through internal heating, leading to higher yields and reduced solvent use compared to conventional approaches (Al Bittar et al., 2013). Likewise, UAE utilizes ultrasonic waves to disrupt cell walls and enhance solvent penetration, reducing extraction time and solvent usage while preserving thermo-sensitive compounds. For grape seed oil, UAE has shown superior efficacy relative to Soxhlet extraction, providing higher yields in less time (Tsiapali et al., 2025b; Da Porto et al., 2013; Drosou et al., 2015). Moreover, another promising nonthermal technique is PEF treatment, which uses high-voltage pulses to cause electroporation of cell membranes, facilitating polyphenol extraction without heating. PEF is energy-efficient, rapid, and scalable, resulting in high-quality extracts with extended shelf life due to microbial inactivation (Brianceau et al., 2015; Carpentieri et al., 2023). Studies indicate that PEF treatment can increase total anthocyanin yield by up to 45% from grape pomace and other by-products (Barba et al., 2015; Arcena et al., 2021).

Although traditional methods, such as Soxhlet and maceration, remain widespread due to their accessibility, they are increasingly being replaced by innovative, green extraction technologies that deliver high yields, reduced environmental impact, and better preservation of thermolabile agents. The integration of technologies like SFE, MAE, UAE, and PEF represents the future of sustainable grape by-product valorization, providing natural, high-quality extracts.

2.3 Extraction of bioactive compounds from beer and brewery by-products

Beer is produced through the fermentation of sugar wort, comprising water, hops (*Humulus lupulus*), malted barley (*Hordeum vulgare*), and BSY, mainly *S. cerevisiae* and *Saccharomyces pastorianus* strains (de Gaetano et al., 2016; Humia et al., 2019). Unlike other fermented alcoholic beverages, brewing involves several prefermentation steps that influence not only the quality and sensory characteristics of the beer but also its nutritional composition and the formation of valuable by-products (Humia et al., 2019; Bamforth, 2017; Steenackers et al., 2015). By-products arise throughout the six main stages of beer production. During mashing, barley is combined with hot water to hydrolyze starches into fermentable sugars.

Lautering separates the liquid wort from solid residues, generating BSG as a primary by-product. During boiling, hops are added to impart flavor and bitterness, followed by cooling and fermentation, where yeast converts sugars into ethanol and CO_2. Finally, conditioning and maturation yield BSH and BSY, valuable residues rich in bioactives such as polyphenols, proteins, and fibers (Humia et al., 2019; Bamforth, 2017; Steenackers et al., 2015).

Numerous studies have examined the extraction of phenolic acids from BSG using liquid-liquid and liquid-solid methods with solvents like methanol or ethyl acetate, as well as acid hydrolysis and alkaline saponification. Innovative techniques, including microwave-assisted derivatization, have also been tested to enhance recovery. For instance, alkaline hydrolysis efficiently liberates ferulic acid from BSG, achieving yields of around 0.3%. The addition of esterases (e.g., xylanase, *Aspergillus niger*, *Trichoderma viride*) or β-glucanase (*Humicola insolens*) further enhances phenolic release by enzymatically degrading ester linkages within the lignocellulosic matrix. Fungal enzymes such as *Fusarium oxysporum* have likewise increased ferulic acid yield by improving accessibility within the cell wall (Zago et al., 2022; McCarthy et al., 2013)

The use of MAE has also been proven effective for BSG, significantly increasing the total phenolic content (TPC) and associated antioxidant capacity (Hejna et al., 2024; Yang and Gao, 2021). The phenolic profile of BSG extracts is dominated by ferulic acid and p-coumaric acid, though the concentration varies depending on the malt type and kilning temperature. The results indicated that light malt BSG contained a higher concentration of phenolic compounds, with antioxidant activity decreasing as kilning temperatures increased. Comparative analyses indicate that light malt varieties (e.g., pilsen, melano) yield nearly double the phenolic content of darker malts (e.g., chocolate, black). For example, light malt BSG extracts contained 149.7 mg ferulic acid/100 g dry weight (DW) and 47.7 mg p-coumaric acid/100 g DW (Pilsen type), whereas dark malt extracts contained 77.3 mg ferulic acid/100 g DW and 21.1 mg p-coumaric acid/100 g DW (black type), respectively. Correspondingly, TPC levels, measured as gallic acid equivalents (GAE), reached 19.5 mg GAE/g DW for light malt and 16.2 mg GAE/g DW for dark malt (Lynch et al., 2016; Shopska et al., 2021; Osei et al., 2025). Such differences highlight the significance of raw material selection and thermal processing conditions in determining extraction yield and phenolic stability (Chowdhary et al., 2021).

Supercritical CO_2 extraction has also been applied for the recovery of polyphenols and flavonoids from BSG. In addition to improving yield, this method allows the production of extracts suitable for food or cosmetic applications by avoiding residual solvents. When combined with microencapsulation, SFE-CO_2 enhances stability, sensory quality, and bioactive preservation by protecting phenolics from oxidation and masking bitterness. This approach facilitates the integration of BSG-derived extracts into functional foods and natural cosmetic products, aligning with the principles of sustainability and the circular economy (Rachwał et al., 2020; Ferreira et al., 2022).

Overall, the recovery of bioactives from apple and cider, grape and wine, and beer and brewery by-products (BSG, BSY, and BSH) is increasingly viewed as a promising route for obtaining high-value natural ingredients. These extracts, once considered waste, are now recognized as renewable resources capable of delivering antioxidant, antiinflammatory, and dermo-conditioning compounds that can be integrated into innovative cosmeceutical and cosmetic products. Continued advancements in green extraction methods, enzyme-assisted processing, and material valorization are expected to further enhance their potential in both the food and beauty industries. Table 12.1 presents indicative examples of several extraction methods used for each fermented beverage or by-product analyzed, showcasing the main research outcomes and method efficacy.

3 Bioactive and health-promoting constituents in fermented beverages: Main bioactives found in fermented beverages and by-products and their beneficial properties

3.1 Bioactive and health-promoting constituents in apple juice, cider, and their by-products

From a cosmetic perspective, the bioactives extracted from apple pomace and fermented apple juice, particularly chlorogenic acid, quercetin, ursolic acid, and natural α-hydroxy acids (such as malic acid), exhibit potent antioxidant, exfoliating, and collagen-stimulating properties that enhance skin brightness, elasticity, and hydration. Incorporating these extracts into cosmetic formulations not only supports skin rejuvenation but also aligns with circular and sustainable cosmetic economy principles, valorizing materials once considered waste into high-value, biologically active raw materials (Vandorou et al., 2024; Di Lorenzo et al., 2024; Tsoupras et al., 2021a; Gonçalves Bortolini et al., 2020).

Apples are rich in a broad range of vitamins (e.g., C, E, and B6), organic acids (e.g., malic acid), minerals (e.g., potassium, calcium, nitrogen, and magnesium), and trace elements (e.g., zinc, iron, copper, and manganese). Apples and their by-products also contain abundant micronutrients and phytochemicals, including triterpenoids (e.g., ursolic acid) and diverse phenolics like flavanols, hydroxycinnamic acids, flavonols, dihydrochalcones, anthocyanins, and other antioxidants (no date). Compared to their juice or cider derivatives, apples and apple pomace provide higher levels of dietary fiber, of which ~70% is insoluble and the remainder soluble, primarily in the form of pectin. Interestingly, apple pectin plays a crucial role in regulating gut microbiota composition, promoting gastrointestinal health, and reducing the risk of cardiovascular disease (CVD), cancer, and other chronic conditions (Shinohara et al., 2010).

TABLE 12.1 Indicative examples of each extraction method used for fermented beverage and by-product bioactive extraction.

Extraction method	Extractant and yield[a]	Conditions	Analysis method	Analytes[a] and method efficacy	References
MAE recovery of pectin from apple pomace as a potential bioactive agent for apple cider production.	• Citric acid solutions of different pH values, following the Box–Behnken design • Highest phenolic yield: 10.6 ± 0.3%	• Optimal conditions: a 5-min extraction with a solid-to-liquid ratio of 1:10 was sufficient to provide the highest extraction yield of 10.6 ± 0.3% • Conventional extraction (CE) needed 90 min for a 9.5 ± 0.3% yield	• CE heating and MAE were compared to extract pectin from apple pomace • Citric acid concentrations were 0.135, 0.0135, and 0.00135 M for the pH values of 2.0, 2.5, and 3.0 (1:10, 5 min, 20 mL citric acid) • Galacturonic acid content, thermogravimetric analysis, ζ-potential, characterization methods, and hydrogel preparation were also conducted	• A pectin yield of 10.6 ± 0.3% was obtained by MAE with the 5-min extraction, in contrast to CE (9.5 ± 0.3%, 2 h) • The pectin extracted by both methods had a low methoxyl content, indicating a low degree of esterification • The galacturonic acid content was greater than 60% for most samples • ζ-Potential revealed the ability of pectin to form stable hydrogels, while X-ray diffraction (XRD) revealed that increasing the temperature reduced pectin crystallinity	(Costa et al., 2025)
Comparative analysis of UAE, CE, and SFE extraction of apple seed oil for potential cider production	• Hexane was utilized as the UAE solvent • Yield: 17.2 ± 2.3%	• UAE was optimized using response surface methodology (RSM) with 56 W of power (64% amplitude) for 30 min, at 30°C	• UAE-RSM was conducted using 33 g of sample mixed with 500 mL of hexane, under 56 W of power (64% amplitude) for 30 min, at 30°C • A 1:15 solid-to-liquid ratio was utilized	• The obtained oil presented a fatty acid profile rich in linoleic acid (35.5 ± 2.8 g/100 g), with an antioxidant activity of 0.22 ± 0.1 mg Trolox/g oil • TPC was equal to 0.16 ± 0.1 mg GAE/g oil • UAE gave a similar yield (17.2 ± 2.3%) compared to SFE (19.3 ± 2.1%) and Soxhlet extraction (19.1 ± 1.5%) • The UAE oil was richer in phloretin and phloridzin, while amygdalin was detected in UAE and SE but not in SFE oils • UAE was more efficient and time-saving than SFE and SE, whereas SFE provided an amygdalin-free oil	(Gasparini et al., 2023)
Apple pomace utilization in cider making for the recovery of phenolic compounds	• Alcoholic fermentation of ciders • Nd-specific extraction yield	• Solids immersed in the liquid in the proportion of 47.3 g/L and centrifuged at 10,200 g, 5°C	• The must of the apple was added to ferment and inoculated with 1.7×10^6 cells/mL of *Saccharomyces cerevisiae* • The must of the apple was divided into two groups: Cider I (control) and Cider II (with added dried apple pomace, 47.3%, 15-day monitoring) • Cider processing was followed by fermentation monitoring and cider characterization	• The use of apple pomace in ciders results in the extraction of phenolics • The majority of flavonoids found in apple pomace were recovered in the ciders • The main sensory properties were positively modified by the added apple pomace • During fermentation, Cider II produced increased phenolic levels and antioxidant capacity, while being lighter than Cider I • Sensory analysis revealed that Cider II had lower sourness and higher bitterness levels, with astringency and odor being similar for both Cider I and Cider II	(Bortolini et al., 2020)

(*Continued*)

Table 12.1 Indicative examples of each extraction method used for fermented beverage and by-product bioactive extraction—cont'd

Extraction method	Extractant and yield[a]	Conditions	Analysis method	Analytes[a] and method efficacy	References
UAE (alkaline-assisted, UAAE) was utilized to extract sustainable proteins from grape seeds from a wine industrial by-product	• Hexane was utilized as the extraction solvent • The extraction yield was 14.3%, while the protein content was 55.1%	• The optimal UAE-RSM conditions were pH 11, at 33°C for 37 min, and a liquid-to-solid ratio of 16 mL/g	• UAAE of grape seed flour proteins was conducted using 20 g of grape seed under 40 kHz and 200 W • RSM design, protein fractionation, amino acid profile, and several characterization methods • The structural and functional attributes of grape seed protein and its major fractions (albumins and glutelins) were compared as well	• The extraction yield/protein content of the UAAE protein was 14.3%/55.1%, while it was 4.7%/68.2% for albumin and 15.3%/40.0% for gluteli • nThe albumin fraction had higher emulsifying properties, solubility, and in vitro digestibility, but lower fluid-binding capacity and thermal stability than the UAAE proteins and the glutelin fraction • UAAE showed better water and oil-binding capacity, glutelin revealed better emulsion formation and solubility, and albumin exhibited better emulsion formation and solubility	(Garcia et al., 2024)
SFE-CO_2 extraction of policosanols from grape marc as a sustainable biorefinery approach for the wine industry	• SFE-CO_2 was utilized as the extraction solvent • Policosanol (PC) ranged between 3922–4083 mg/kg (~8% of the total extraction yield)	• Optimal operating conditions were 280 bar pressure, 70°C, and a flow rate of 10 kg CO_2/h	• SFE-CO_2 extraction, with the optimal conditions of 280 bar pressure at 70°C and a flow rate of 10 kg CO_2/h, was followed by a comparison with Soxhlet extraction	• PC ranged between 3922–4083 mg/kg (~8% of the total extraction yield) • PC was of the same order of magnitude detected in beeswax yellow (a natural policosanol source) • Primary aliphatic alcohols found in PC from grape marc were hexacosanol, octacosanol, and triacontanol • SFE-CO_2 extraction ensures a faster and solvent-free process	(Da Porto and Natolino, 2024)
PLE of BSG from beer industry by-products for the isolation of compounds with vast biological activity	• Ethanol and water were used as the solvents • Highest extraction yield: 20.1 wt. %	• Optimal PLE conditions were 10 MPa at 120°C, with a 2 mL/min flow rate and an ethanol/water ratio of 0.5	• BSG using PLE was investigated and compared with Soxhlet extraction results, while TPC, total flavonoid content (TFC), antioxidant capacity, reducing sugars (RS), and total reducing sugars (TRS)	• The highest extraction yield of 20.1 wt.% was achieved under the optimal conditions • The highest antioxidant capacity was obtained with water at 120°C and 4 mL/min, achieving 9944, 4769, and 4096 μmol TE/100 g of BSG extract, respectively • PLE presented high extraction yields, maintaining RS and TRS in the BSG matrix • BSG, being defatted with compressed propane, was proven highly efficient in recovering the needed lipid fraction	(Herbst et al., 2021)
BSG's pretreatment with PEF revealed an enhanced biological profile	• Pulsed electric fields were utilize • dHighest extraction yield: 71.4%	• Optimal conditions: 3 kV/cm, 2 Hz • No significant difference was observed between the 30 and 120 extracts (protein content: 1.5 times increase) • pH notably affected the functional traits (varied between 3 and 7)	• Before PEF treatment, BSG was mixed with NaOH (0.11 M) to achieve a pH of 11.5 in a 1:20 (w/w) ratio • Compositional analysis, protein characterization, free sulfhydryl group and surface hydrophobicity determination, and functional properties were evaluated	• The protein extraction yield with the best PEF pretreatment condition of 120 pulses (71.4%) was not significantly improved compared to the unpretreated extraction (74.0%) • PEF, however, led to extracts with better structural integrity compared to conventional ones • Protein solubility was improved by ~ 81%, foaming capacity by 104%, stability by 21%, and water-holding capacity by ~ 11.5 g/g (vs. conventional extract: 3.9 g/g)	(Rouissi et al., 2025)

[a]*Nd stands for "Not defined." Yield: % and analytes: % of the total content or concentration, if retrievable. The yield is mainly expressed as TPC.*

Cider, an alcoholic beverage produced from fermented apple juice, typically contains 1%–7% alcohol by volume, distinguishing it into soft cider (1%–5%) and hard cider (6%–7%). Cider production is particularly prominent in Western and Northwestern Europe, where favorable climates allow for the cultivation of cider apple varieties. Today, cider represents a multibillion-euro industry, with the United Kingdom leading global production, followed by Spain, France, Ireland, and Germany (Tsoupras et al., 2022). Cider retains most of the bioactive compounds of apples and apple juice, while fermentation introduces additional bioactive metabolites, augmenting its nutritional and functional profile (Moran et al., 2021; Tsoupras et al., 2021a, 2021b). As a result, cider is now recognized as a functional beverage with significant probiotic, antiinflammatory, anticancer, cardioprotective, and antioxidant effects, potentially reducing the risk of all-cause mortality (Barreira et al., 2019; Kunzmann et al., 2018). Distinct yeast strains, fermentation techniques, and apple cultivars (sweet, sharp, bittersweet, bittersharp) produce a wide spectrum of flavors, aromas, and bioactive compositions (Laaksonen et al., 2017).

Apple juices are similarly rich in minerals, vitamins, antioxidants, and antiinflammatory phenolic and lipid compounds, and when consumed in moderation, they provide multiple health benefits despite their naturally high sugar content. Apples stand out among fruits for their high abundance of free compounds, which are readily available and efficiently absorbed in the human body (Tsoupras et al., 2021b; Kalinowska et al., 2014). Notably, not-from-concentrate clarified apple juices, which undergo minimal processing and contain no additives or pectin, exhibit higher phenolic contents compared to from-concentrate juices (Lei et al., 2022). Thus lower processing intensity appears to preserve bioactivity and nutritional quality, supporting better health outcomes.

3.1.1 Phenolic bioactives in apple juice, cider, and their by-products and associated health benefits

Phytochemicals, including flavonoids and diverse polyphenolic compounds, are abundant in apples, apple juice, cider, and apple pomace. Apple and apple-based by-products' phenolic bioactives include flavan-3-ols (e.g., catechin, epigallocatechin, procyanidin B_2), flavonols (e.g., rutin, quercetin, quercetin-3-galactoside), hydroxycinnamic acids (e.g., 5-*O*-caffeoylquinic acid, 4-p-coumaroylquinic acid), dihydrochalcones (e.g., phloridzin), and anthocyanidins (e.g., cyanidin-3-*O*-galactoside, cyanidin-3-*O*-glucoside), as well as several other simple phenolics, flavonoids, and polyphenols (Fig. 12.2).

Several of these phenolic bioactives are linked to numerous health-promoting effects, extending beyond antioxidation to include antiinflammatory, antiproliferative, and anticarcinogenic effects (Fig. 12.3). Interestingly, apple phytochemicals

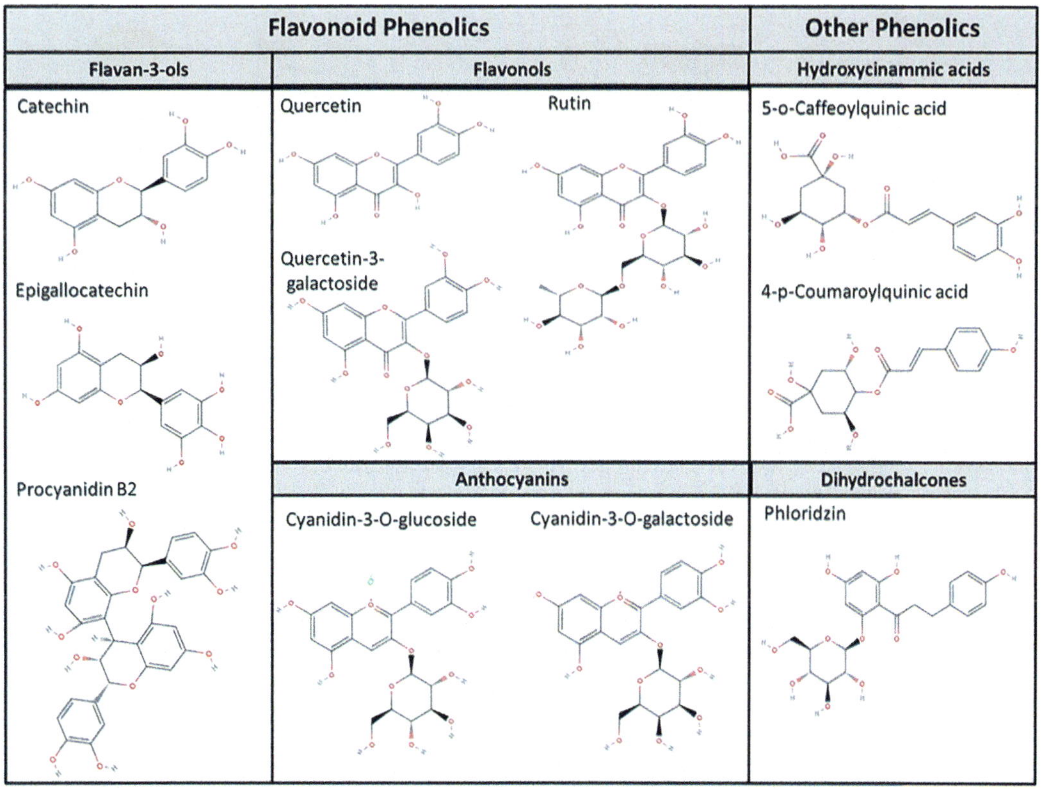

FIG. 12.2 The molecular compositions of the most characteristic phenolic bioactives (simple phenolics, flavonoids, and polyphenols) associated with the multifaceted bioactive properties of apple-based products (including apple fruit, juice, and cider) and their by-products (such as apple pomace). *(The structures for each individual phenolic bioactive were obtained from the open access free platform https://molview.org (Accessed at 17/11/2025).)*

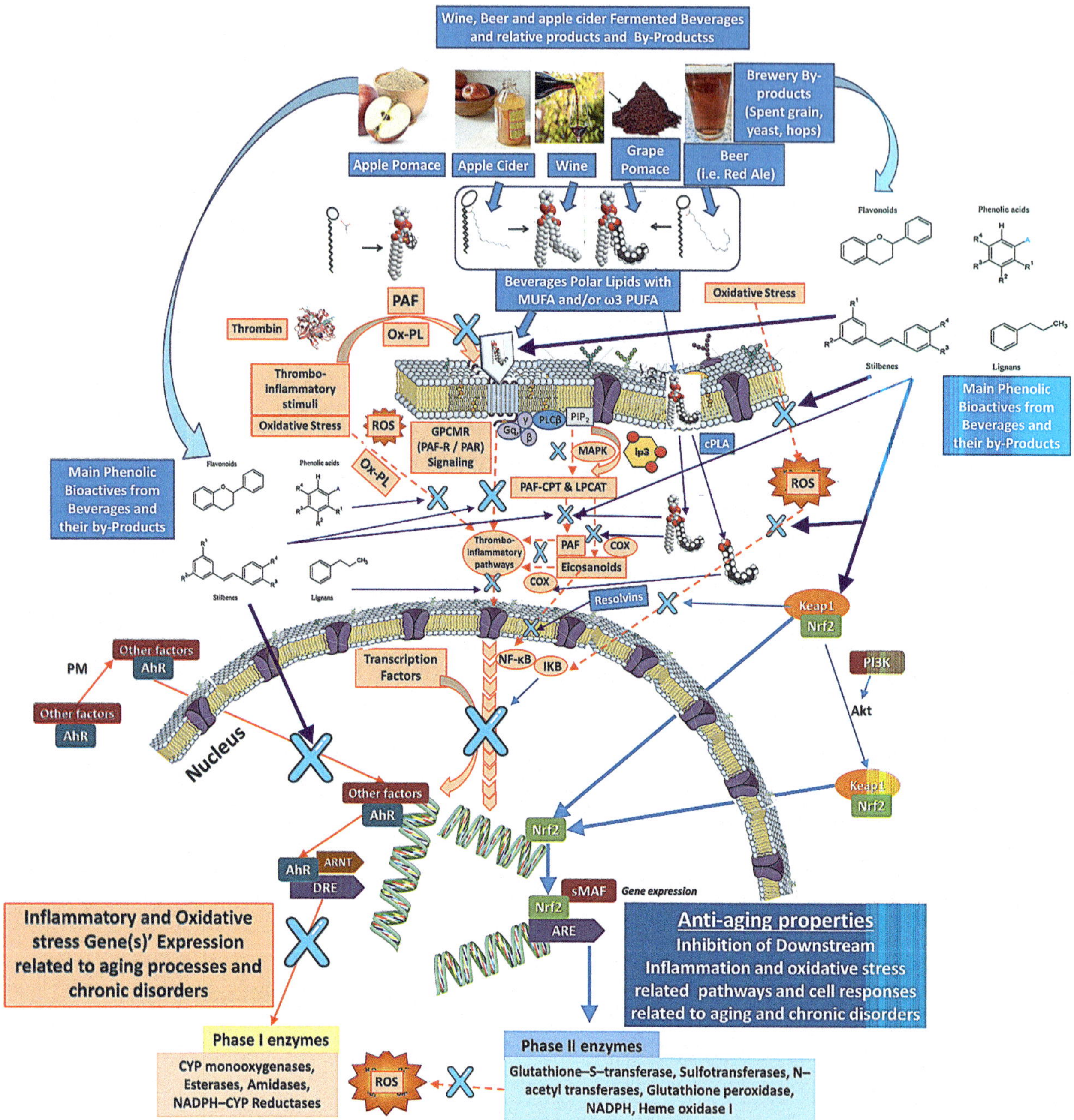

FIG. 12.3 Biochemical mechanisms of action of amphiphilic bioactives from fermented alcoholic beverages. The most representative amphiphilic bioactives (PLs rich in monounsaturated fatty acids (MUFA) and omega-3 (ω3) polyunsaturated fatty acids (PUFA) and main classes of bioactive phenolics from the primary fermented apple beverage product (apple cider) and by-product (apple pomace), grape fermented beverage product (wine) and by-product (grape pomace), and barley fermented beverage product (beer) and by-products (spent grain, yeast, and hops) are shown, along with representative biochemical mechanisms of antiinflammatory, antithrombotic, and antioxidant health-promoting properties against oxidative stress and thromboinflammatory signaling associated with aging and chronic disorders. Red colors: the signaling of oxidative stress and thromboinflammatory stimuli induced by aging-related risk factors, such as the induction of oxidative stress and the thrombotic and inflammatory pathways of PAF, thrombin, and arachidonic-eicosanoids–cyclooxygenase (COX), which are associated with aging processes and chronic disorders. Blue colors: amphiphilic bioactives (PLs and phenolic bioactives) from these sources affect all these signaling pathways related to oxidative stress, inflammation, aging, and associated chronic disorders. Bioactive phenolics act through the deactivation of ROS, the inhibition of oxidative damage to DNA, proteins, and lipid molecules (especially to the PLs in cellular and intracellular membranes), and downregulate oxidative stress and inflammation gene expression by inhibiting the NFkb transcription factor signaling, while upregulating antioxidant and antiinflammatory gene expression through signal amplification in the KEAP1-NRF2-ARE antioxidant response pathway. Most importantly, both bioactive phenolics and PLs (especially those bearing MUFA or PUFA in their structures) present strong antiinflammatory and antithrombotic activities through the inhibition of oxidized PLs, PAF-/thrombin-/eicosanoids (arachidonic acid and its eicosanoids) binding on their receptors, and thus through the reduction of their thrombo-inflammatory signaling and their aging-associated manifestations. They also

inhibit inflammatory enzymes (COX, PAF-CPT, Lyso-PAF-AT, etc.) and downregulate the expression of thrombo-inflammatory signaling by reducing the NFkB transcription factor pathways. (The blue X represents an inhibitory effect on a pathway and/or an enzyme and/or a receptor and/or a transcription factor and/or an expression of a gene related to oxidative stress and inflammation by apple pomace bioactive phenolics, as indicated by the blue arrows). 5'-TATCGATA-binding factor; *ADP*, adenosine diphosphate; *AhR*, aryl hydrocarbon receptor; *Akt*, protein kinase B; *ALA*, alpha-linolenic acid; *ARE*, antioxidant response elements; *ARNT*, aryl hydrocarbon receptor nuclear translocator; *COX*, cyclooxygenase; *cPLA*, cytoplasmic phospholipase A2; *DREF/DRE*, DNA replication-related element (DRE; 5'-TATCGATA) binding factor; *GPCMR*, G-protein-coupled membrane receptors; *IKB*, inhibitor of NF-kB; *IP3*, inositol trisphosphate; *Keap1*, Kelch-like ECH-associated protein 1; *MAPK*, mitogen-activated protein kinase; *NF-kB*, nuclear factor kappa beta; *OA*, oleic acid; *Ox-PL*, oxidized phospholipids; *PAF*, platelet-activating factor; *PAF-CPT* and *LPCAT*, the basic biosynthetic enzymes of the two distinct pathways of PAF synthesis, PAF-cholinephosphotransferase and lyso-phosphatidylcholine acetyltransferase 2, respectively; *PAF-R*, PAF receptor; *PAR*, protease-activated receptors for thrombin; *PI3K*, phosphatidylinositol 3-kinase; *PL*, polar lipids; *PLC*, phospholipase C; *Nrf2*, nuclear factor E2-related factor 2; *ROS*, reactive oxygen species; *sMAF*, small musculoaponeurotic fibrosarcoma. *(Some structures of molecules were obtained from the open access free platform MolView.Org).*

have displayed vast anticancer activity, influencing both nuclear factor κB [NF-κB, by downregulating tumor necrosis factor α (TNF-α), interferon γ, and interleukins 1β and 6 (IL-1β and IL-6)] and nuclear factor erythroid 2-related factor 2 (Nrf2) signaling, as well as the existing crosstalk between these pathways, potentially alleviating cancer symptoms and proliferation (Fig. 12.3) (Koseoğlu and Al-Taie, 2022; Gado et al., 2023).

The presence of vitamins C and E further amplifies all the aforementioned effects by supporting radical and reactive oxygen species (ROS) scavenging, as well as cellular protection (Oyenihi et al., 2022). The synergy between apple-derived polyphenols and vitamins has also been proven beneficial in mitigating liver damage induced by carbon tetrachloride (CCl_4), downregulating microvascular damage resulting from cerebral hyperperfusion and reperfusion injury, and enhancing metabolic hormone balance. However, storage duration, temperature, and pasteurization can lead to the degradation of key nutrients such as vitamin C, chlorogenic acid, and total polyphenols, as well as color changes, potentially reducing overall bioavailability and bioactivity (Suárez-Jacobo et al., 2012, 2011). Importantly, apple phytochemicals play a critical role in maintaining redox and inflammatory homeostasis, thus mitigating oxidative stress and chronic disease development, including various forms of cancer. Certain apple varieties and phytochemical subgroups have even demonstrated efficacy in protecting against radiation-induced cellular damage (Lyu et al., 2020).

Comprehensive analyses of cider polyphenols reveal that, across diverse cultivars, the total polyphenol concentration averages ~ 33 mg/100 mL, primarily composed of hydroxycinnamic acids (HCAs), flavonols, procyanidins, and dihydrochalcones. HCAs and their derivatives (HCADs) (mean content of ~ 7.5 and 0.3 mg/100 mL, respectively), notably chlorogenic, caffeic, p-coumaric, and ferulic acid, exhibit strong antioxidant and antiinflammatory actions by scavenging ROS, inhibiting NF-κB activation, and reducing oxidative tissue damage (Tsoupras et al., 2021b; Laaksonen et al., 2017; Riekstina-Dolge et al., 2014; Kim et al., 2012; Mathew et al., 2015). The molecular structure of HCAs determines their potency. Specifically, the number and arrangement of electron-donating groups enhance antioxidant stability and phenoxy radical neutralization (no date; Chen et al., 2020). Interestingly, cider generally contains higher phenolic levels than apple juice, suggesting that fermentation enhances both the phenolic content and biofunctionality of the final product or by-product (Barreira et al., 2019; Tsoupras et al., 2021a, 2021b).

3.1.2 Lipid bioactives in apple juice, cider, and their by-products and associated health benefits

Recent studies have also characterized the lipid composition of fresh apple juices, ciders, and commercial equivalents, revealing small yet functionally significant amounts of bioactive PLs, with recently proven remarkable bioactivity against adenosine diphosphate (ADP) and platelet-activating factor (PAF) signaling. These amphipathic lipids, predominantly phosphatidylcholines and phosphatidylethanolamines, constitute 80%–95% of total lipids (TLs) in apple juices, while neutral lipids account for the remaining 5%–20%. Even though they are present in apple juice and cider in trace amounts (0.05–0.5 g/100 mL), PLs possess notable antiinflammatory, antithrombotic, and platelet-modulating activities. An estimated 0.5 L serving of cider provides ~ 200 mg of bioactive PLs, suggesting that moderate consumption (1–2 pints weekly) may offer cardioprotective and antiinflammatory benefits (Tsoupras et al., 2021a, no date, 2021b). Gas chromatography–mass spectrometry analyses of these extracts confirm a predominance of UFAs, including monounsaturated UFAs (MUFAs) such as ω-9 oleic acid (OA; 18:1, ω-9) and polyunsaturated UFAs (PUFAs) like the ω-3 α-linolenic acid (ALA; 18:3, ω-3), linoleic acid (LA), and γ-linolenic acid, which contribute to their biological activity, presenting consistent results with those observed in grape juice and wine studies (Tsoupras et al., 2024a, 2021b). Expectedly, their high UFA content likely underpins the biomultifunctional potency of apple-derived lipid bioactives (Fig. 12.3) (Tsoupras et al., 2021a, 2021b).

Complementary studies examining the influence of yeast strains on cider lipid profiles revealed that fermentation microbiota play a crucial role in determining TL yield and composition. Yeast isolated from apple surfaces and musts of cultivars such as Jonagold, Dabinett, and Aston Bitter exhibited strain-dependent differences in PL productivity and bioactivity. Ciders produced with these selected strains displayed lipid yields and bioactivities comparable to those achieved using *S. cerevisiae* inoculation (Moran et al., 2021; Tsoupras et al., 2021b).

Apple-based fermented beverages, such as cider, have recently gained attention as nondairy probiotic carriers, offering vegan-friendly, cholesterol-free alternatives to traditional dairy products. During malolactic fermentation, lactic acid bacteria (LAB), especially *Lactobacillus, Pediococcus, Oenococcus,* and *Leuconostoc*, convert malic acid into lactic acid, improving cider's stability and sensory qualities while enriching it with bioactive metabolites. LABs can produce exopolysaccharides (EPSs), complex biopolymers with antioxidant, antiinflammatory, anticancer, antidiabetic, and cardioprotective activities (no date; Tsoupras et al., 2021b). EPSs neutralize ROS, prevent cells from lipid peroxidation, and enhance antioxidant enzyme activity. EPSs may act as prebiotic and immunomodulatory agents, promoting beneficial gut microbiota such as *Bifidobacterium* and inhibiting pathogens like *Staphylococcus aureus*. Their biological action depends on composition, as mannose-rich EPSs show strong anticancer potential, while (1,3)-β-D-glucan EPSs from cider-derived *Pediococcus parvulus* exhibit immunomodulatory and gut-protective effects. Together, these findings highlight cider's dual role as a probiotic and prebiotic beverage, supporting gut health, immune function, and metabolic disorders associated with inflammation, such as diabetes and inflammatory bowel diseases (IBDs) (Tsoupras et al., 2021b).

Finally, as discussed in **Chapter 11**, apple pomace remains one of the most nutrient-dense by-products of apple processing, containing substantial levels of fiber, sugars, proteins, lipids, polyphenols, carotenoids, and phytosterols (Moran et al., 2021; Tsoupras et al., 2021b). These compounds are associated with antioxidant, antiinflammatory, antimicrobial, and cardioprotective properties, underscoring the potential of apple pomace as a multifunctional raw material for cosmetic and cosmeceutical formulations that promote skin health and overall well-being.

3.2 Bioactive and health-promoting constituents in wine and its by-products

Grape pomace, composed of seeds, stems, and skins, retains a substantial concentration of bioactive compounds following vinification, including polyphenols, fatty acids, proteins, and carbohydrates. These constituents exhibit strong antioxidant, antiinflammatory, antimicrobial, and skin-protective effects, making winery by-products valuable for cosmeceutical applications such as antiaging and photoprotective formulations. Improper disposal of grape pomace as industrial waste can lead to environmental and economic burdens, yet its high content of dietary fiber, lipid bioactives, flavonoids, flavonoid derivatives, and phenolic antioxidants supports its valorization within circular economy strategies (Karantonis et al., 2023; Beres et al., 2017; Ilyas et al., 2021; Sabra et al., 2021).

Wine is particularly distinguished among alcoholic beverages for its rich polyphenolic profile, which varies according to grape variety, terroir, climate, and vinification methods (Zabetakis et al., 2022; Tsoupras et al., 2024a). Polyphenols, including resveratrol, phenolic acids, anthocyanins, flavonoids, and their microbiota-derived metabolites, exhibit potent antioxidant, antiinflammatory, antiatherogenic, and cardioprotective properties (Zabetakis et al., 2022; Tsoupras et al., 2024a; Calabriso et al., 2016; Fernandes et al., 2017; Tsoupras et al., 2007, 2009). Lipid bioactives, particularly PLs and UFAs, also contribute to the health benefits of wine and its by-products. These lipids originate from both grape tissues and fermenting yeasts, undergoing beneficial modifications during fermentation that enhance their antiinflammatory and antithrombotic effects (Tsoupras et al., 2024a, 2018; Fragopoulou et al., 2007; Choleva et al., 2019, 2020; Fragopoulou et al., 2002).

3.2.1 *Phenolic bioactives in wine and winery by-products and associated health benefits*

The phenolic compounds in wine are primarily divided into flavonoids, including flavan-3-ols (e.g., catechin, epigallocatechin, and proanthocyanidins), flavonols (e.g., quercetin), and anthocyanins/anthocyanidins (e.g., cyanidin-3-glucoside), and nonflavonoids, such as phenolic benzene derivatives (e.g., benzoic, hydroxybenzoic, protocatechuic, vanillic, and syringic acid), hydrolysable tannins (e.g., gallic and ellagic acid), cinnamate derivatives (e.g., cinnamic, hydroxycinnamic, caffeic, and ferulic acid), benzene and cinnamate derivatives (e.g., benzaldehyde, cinnamaldehyde), volatile phenols (e.g., 4-ethyl-phenol, 4-vinyl-phenol, vanillin), tyrosols (e.g., tyrosol and hydroxytyrosol), and stilbenes (e.g., resveratrol and astringin), with flavonoids accounting for approximately 85% of total phenolics in red wine (Fig. 12.4) (Zabetakis et al., 2022; Calabriso et al., 2016; Fernandes et al., 2017; Visioli et al., 2020). Phenolics are predominantly found in grape seeds and skins, except for hydroxycinnamic acids, which are located in lesser amounts in the flesh. Flavonoids such as flavan-3-ols, anthocyanins, and flavonols are concentrated in grape seeds and skins, whereas nonflavonoid compounds, including phenolic acids, stilbenes (e.g., resveratrol), tannins, and coumarins, occur mainly in the pulp and wine must (Lingua et al., 2016; Kupe et al., 2021; Chedea et al., 2022). The phenolic content of red wines typically ranges from 1531 to 3192 mg of GAE/L, while white wines contain 210–402 mg GAE/L, depending on grape variety and processing methods (Zabetakis et al., 2022; Tsoupras et al., 2024a). Red grape varieties and extended maceration increase the polyphenolic yield, antioxidant, and antiinflammatory potential of the product (Lago-Vanzela et al., 2014; Zabetakis et al., 2022; Tsoupras et al., 2024a; Sabra et al., 2021; Choleva et al., 2019; Lingua et al., 2016; Chedea et al., 2022; Rockenbach et al., 2011; Onache et al., 2022; Szabó et al., 2021; van Bussel et al., 2018).

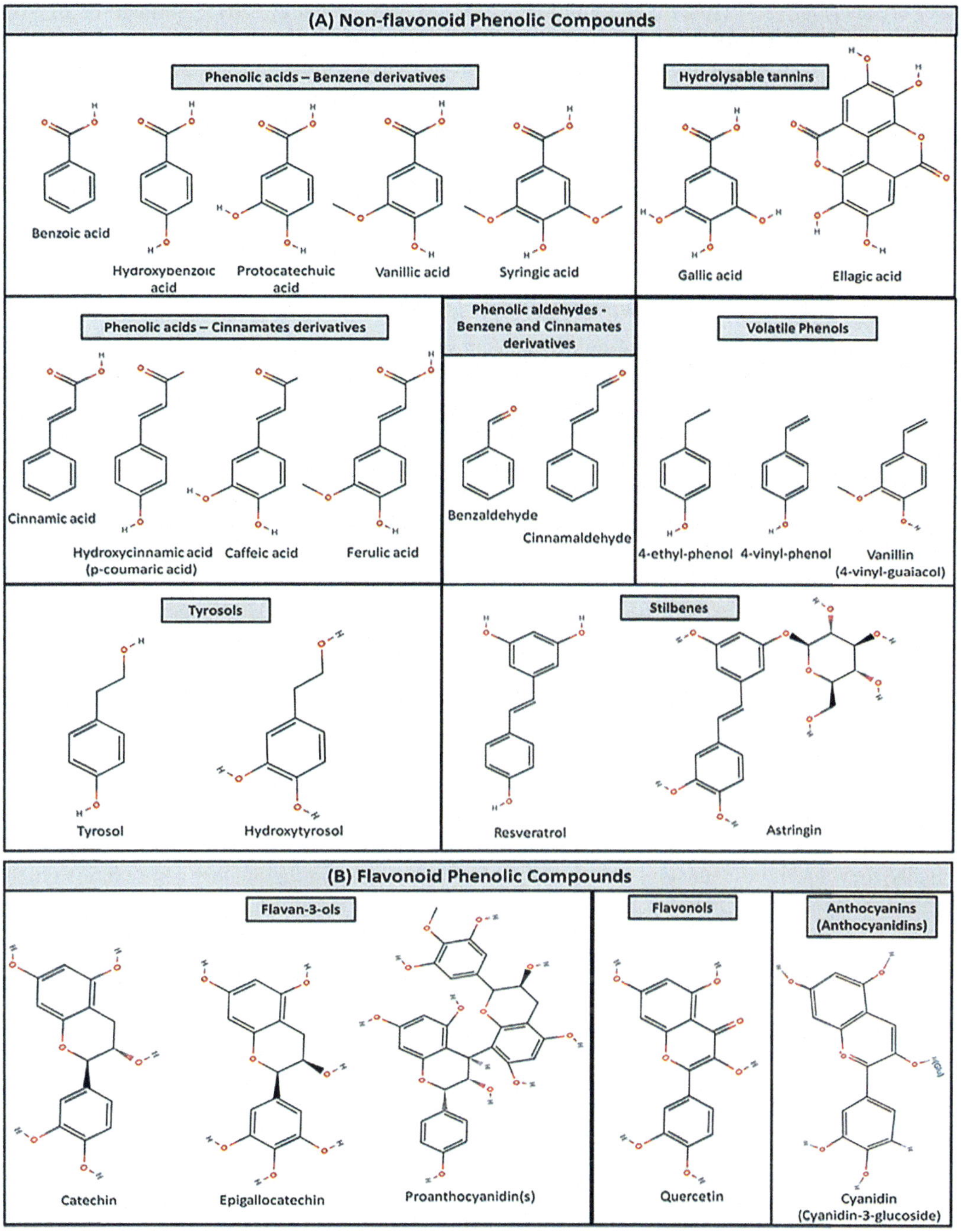

FIG. 12.4 The structure of the most characteristic nonflavonoid (A) and flavonoid (B) phenolic compounds present in wine and/or grape pomace. *(From the open-access published article of Tsoupras, A., Gkika, D.A., Markopoulos, T., Curran, R., Scallon, C., Karali, M., Kyzas, G., 2023a. Apple products (apple juice and cider) and by-products (apple pomace): bioactive compounds and biological properties. In: Mérillon, J.-M., Riviere, C., Lefèvre, G., Eds., Botany, Phytochemistry, Pharmacology and Processing. Springer International Publishing, Cham, pp. 1–42.)*

Polyphenols exert their antioxidant effects by scavenging ROS and inhibiting the oxidation of low-density lipoproteins, thereby mitigating endothelial dysfunction and atherosclerosis. Moderate wine consumption with meals enhances plasma total antioxidant capacity and suppresses NF-κB signaling (by suppressing proinflammatory cytokines TNF-α and interleukins IL-1β and IL-6), supporting the so-called French Paradox, the cardioprotective effects of moderate wine intake despite dietary fat consumption. Furthermore, grape pomace polyphenols have been shown to combat thrombotic and inflammatory mediators, including PAF [mainly via downregulating the expression of its receptor (PAF-R)], thromboxane A_2 (T_XA_2) and B_2 (T_XB_2), thrombin, collagen, fibrinogen, arachidonic acid (AA), and ADP, offering antiinflammatory, antithrombotic, and anticancer effects (Fig. 12.3) (Aviram and Fuhrman, 2002; Apostolidou et al., 2015; Stranieri et al., 2022; Schrieks et al., 2013; Chiva-Blanch et al., 2013; Fragopoulou et al., 2009).

Resveratrol's great health-promoting profile has been proven remarkably useful toward the inhibition of thrombin-induced platelet aggregation through decreasing stored Ca^{2+} release, inhibiting store-operated Ca^{2+} influx into platelets, reducing platelet aggregation induced by epinephrine, and increasing NO production. Moreover, it activates the AMP-activated protein kinase, decreasing fat accumulation (antiobesity profile), cholesterol synthesis, and inflammatory cytokine release, while stimulating sirtuin 1 (SIRT1), and consequently reducing the risk of atherosclerosis, coronary diseases, and CVDs (Aviram and Fuhrman, 2002; Apostolidou et al., 2015; Stranieri et al., 2022; Schrieks et al., 2013; Chiva-Blanch et al., 2013; Fragopoulou et al., 2009).

3.2.2 Lipid bioactives in wine and winery by-products and associated health benefits

In addition to phenolics, wine and winery by-products contain several functional lipid bioactives that play crucial roles in regulating inflammation and protecting the cardiovascular system. Over the past two decades, studies led by Prof. C.A. Demopoulos and collaborators (Prof. Antonopoulou S.A., Dr. Fragopoulou E., Dr. Nomikos T., Dr. Tsoupras A., et al.) have shown that amphiphilic PLs, including phospholipids and glycolipids derived from grapes, yeasts, and wine must, demonstrate antiinflammatory, antithrombotic, and antiatherogenic cardioprotection. Moreover, grape seed oil, another high-value product, is rich in ω-6 LA and other UFAs, offering dermo-protective and emollient properties that are relevant for cosmetic formulations. Although its hydrophilic polyphenol content is relatively low, grape seed oil contains phenol–lipid conjugates that contribute to skin barrier support and oxidative stress reduction (Zabetakis et al., 2022; Fragopoulou et al., 2018; Tsoupras et al., 2024a, 2009, 2018; Choleva et al., 2019, 2020; Fragopoulou et al., 2002, 2009; Xanthopoulou et al., 2017; Argyrou et al., 2017; Fragopoulou et al., 2018; Fragopoulou and Antonopoulou, 2020; Fragopoulou et al., 2021; Choleva et al., 2022, 2023; Zabetakis et al., 2019).

Not only ω-6 LA, but also other UFAs, such as ω-3 ALA, and PL UFAs, such as OA, can reduce thromboxane and PAF activity, as well as the synthesis of proinflammatory cytokines, serving as neuroprotective, antiinflammatory, antiatherosclerotic, cardioprotective (anti-CVD), and anticancer agents. Being present in the lipid membrane microenvironment, they bind to G-protein-coupled membrane receptors, inhibiting the inflammatory manifestations of the upstream thrombo-inflammatory stimuli (e.g., IL-1β, IL-6, TNF-α, endothelin, oxidative stress, PAF, thrombin, ADP, collagen, and AA). Specifically, regarding PAF inhibition, they suppress both PAF synthesis and catabolism by releasing biofunctional fatty acids (OA and/or ALA), prostaglandins, and resolvins, which, in turn, modulate eicosanoid pathways and cyclooxygenase activities. Finally, they inhibit inflammatory gene expression by inducing antiinflammatory gene expression, thereby being beneficial against thrombo-inflammatory signaling (Tsoupras et al., 2024a) (Fig. 12.3).

3.3 Bioactive and health-promoting constituents in beer and brewery by-products

Beer, one of the world's oldest and most widely consumed fermented beverages, is produced from malted cereals, hops, water, and yeast. Beyond its cultural and economic importance, beer represents a complex biochemical system rich in bioactives, such as phenolics, flavonoids, iso-α-acids, and PLs, that arise from both raw materials and fermentation. Increasing scientific interest has focused on the health-promoting and cosmetic potential of beer and its brewing by-products, such as BSG, BSH, and BSY, all of which are abundant in valuable bioactive agents. These by-products, traditionally considered industrial waste, are currently recognized as sustainable sources of natural antioxidants, antimicrobial molecules, and skin-beneficial agents, aligning with modern circular economy and green chemistry principles (Tsoupras et al., 2022, 2024b, 2024c; Lordan et al., 2019a, 2019b; Humia et al., 2019; Yang and Gao, 2021; Bonatto, 2022; Gordon et al., 2018; Neto et al., 2017; Samuels et al., 2018; Nardini, 2023; Kao, 2018; Ano et al., 2017; Arranz et al., 2012; Roldán-López et al., 2024). Fig. 12.5 highlights the structures of the most important phenolic bioactives present in both beer (1–44) and its brewery by-products, and more specifically, BSG, BSH, and BSY (Tsoupras et al., 2024b).

3.3.1 Nutrients and biofunctional compounds in beer and brewery by-products

Beer and its by-products are valuable sources of bioactive compounds derived from malt, hops, and yeast fermentation. These include lipids, polyphenols, iso-α acids, prenyl-flavonoids, and their metabolic derivatives (Tsoupras et al., 2022, 2021b, 2018). Key examples, such as xanthohumol and humulone, demonstrate potent antioxidant, antiinflammatory, neuroprotective, insulin-resistance, and chemopreventive effects. However, due to beer's high-water content, the concentration of these compounds present in the final beverage remains relatively low (Tsoupras et al., 2022; de Gaetano et al., 2016; Humia et al., 2019; Arranz et al., 2012; Fukizawa et al., 2020; Saito et al., 2018; Salanţă et al., 2020; Tomita et al., 2017; Chen et al., 2021; Yao et al., 2015; Yen et al., 2012).

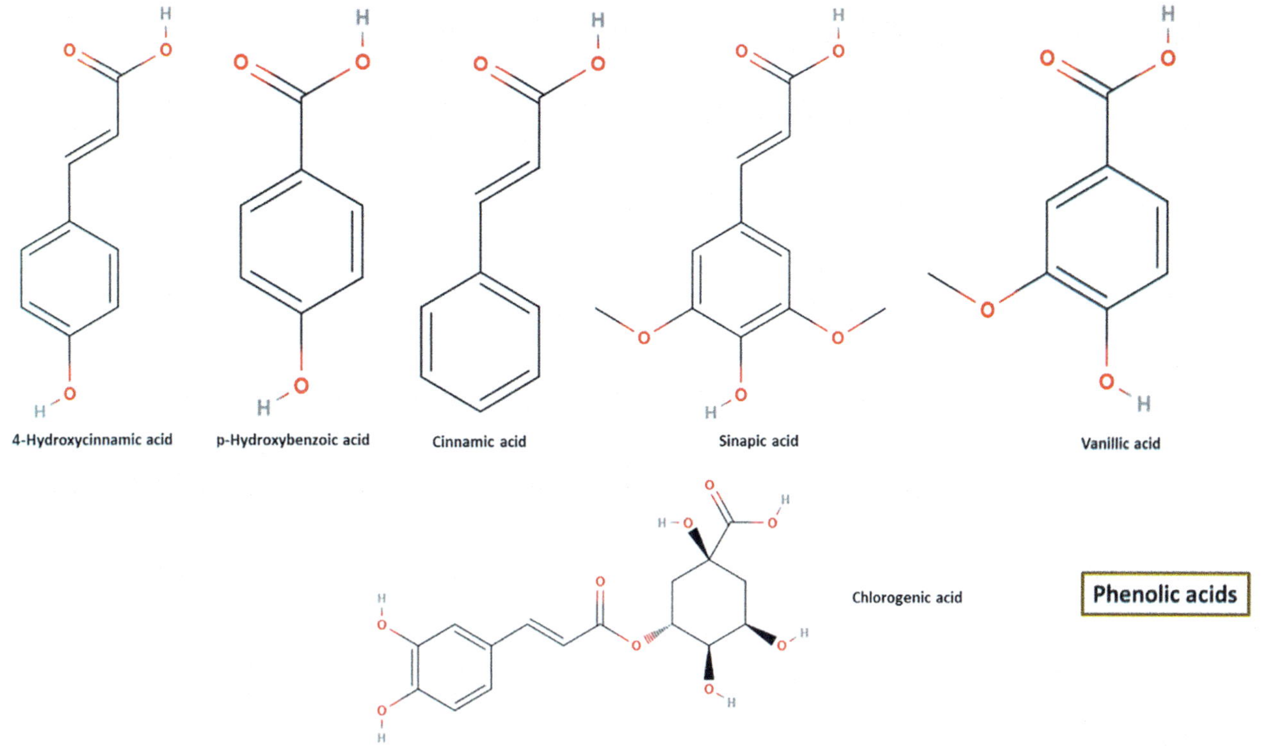

FIG. 12.5 Structures of the most important phenolic bioactives in beer and brewery by-products. *Structures were obtained from the open-access, free platform MolView.Org.)*

Beer primarily consists of water (90%–96%), ethanol [4%–6% alcohol by volume (ABV)], and smaller fractions of carbohydrates, proteins, lipids, polyphenols, vitamins, minerals, carbon dioxide, alcohol, hop-derived bitter acids, and pre/probiotics (Tsoupras et al., 2022, 2023b, 2024b; Lordan et al., 2019b; Salanță et al., 2020). Its energy value derives mainly from carbohydrates (4 kcal/g), amino acids (4 kcal/g), total organic acids (4 kcal/g), and alcohol (7 kcal/g) (Salanță et al., 2020). When it comes to macronutrients, beer contains a relatively small quantity of protein because it is frequently eliminated during beer production, which involves steps such as maturation, clarification, and pasteurization. On average, 5% ABV beer contains ~ 0.5 g of protein/100 mL and ~ 3.3–4.4 g of carbohydrates/100 mL (dextrins, monosaccharides, oligosaccharides, arabinoxylans, and β-glucans (Salanță et al., 2020)). Moreover, the lipid concentrations are low (<0.1%), influenced by the choice of raw ingredients and processing conditions, and mainly ascribed to barley (2%–4%) and malt (3.4%). The brewing process results in diverse lipid classes, including triacylglycerols, phospholipids, glycolipids, sterols, and free fatty acids originating from barley and yeast metabolism (Tsoupras et al., 2022, 2023b, 2024b; Lordan et al., 2019b; Salanță et al., 2020).

Beer also contains various micronutrient components, such as esters, higher alcohols, flavonoids, polyphenols, carbonyl compounds, aldehydes, and ketones, varying based on the raw ingredients and processing methods employed (Tsoupras et al., 2022; Humia et al., 2019; Karabín et al., 2016). Hops contribute bitter acids (α acids like humulone and adhumulone, as well as other β acids like colupulone, lupulone, adlupulone, postlupulone, and prelupulone) and volatile terpenes, which not only define beer's flavor and stability but also impart antioxidant, antimicrobial, and potential chemopreventive activities (Steenackers et al., 2015; Ano et al., 2017; Karabín et al., 2016). Furthermore, yeast strains enhance beer's nutritional and functional properties by generating bioactives such as melatonin and hydroxytyrosol, as well as acting as probiotic drivers in unfiltered beers (Steenackers et al., 2015; Ano et al., 2017; Roldán-López et al., 2024; Karabín et al., 2016).

Nutrients and biofunctional compounds in brewery by-products

Beer production generates several nutrient-rich by-products, primarily brewer's BSG, BSH, and BSY. BSG, which accounts for ~ 85% of the total by-products, consists mainly of barley husks and endosperm starch granule residues. It is rich in dietary fiber (60%–71%), especially soluble pectic polysaccharides, arabinogalactans, β-glucans, branched arabinoxylan, and xyloglucans, as well as insoluble dietary cellulose, several monosaccharides (e.g., glucose, xylose, arabinose, and traces of rhamnose and galactose), lignin (22%–28%), arabinoxylan, galactomannans, and xyloglucans (Lynch et al., 2016; Merten et al., 2022; Wang et al., 2018; Fărcaş et al., 2017). Moreover, BSG contains proteins, several essential amino acids, vitamins, minerals, and notable amounts of phenolics. Therefore its lignocellulosic structure makes it a valuable raw material for cosmetic, cosmeceutical, nutraceutical, and bioeconomic valorization (Fărcaş et al., 2017; Aliyu and Bala, 2011).

Interestingly, only ~ 15% of the hops used in the brewing process actually make it into the final beer, leaving the remaining 85% as BSH. BSH, representing unutilized hop residues, retains fibers, proteins, and bitter acids, though its intense bitterness limits its use in food. It contains several mono- and disaccharides, including xylose, mannose, galactose, and glucose, while pectin, arabinose, rhamnose, and uronic acid are also present alongside bitter α-acids (e.g., humulone) and β-acids (e.g., lupulone), contributing to BSH's antioxidant and antimicrobial activity (Fărcaş et al., 2017). In addition, the brewery's hot trub, the insoluble residue that comprises colloidal proteins, may vary among brewers, generally falling within the range of 40%–70% (Kao, 2018).

BSY, constituting ~ 10% of brewery residues (based on variations in cell physiology and the number of cell cycles), is composed predominantly of proteins (45%–55%) (Rachwał et al., 2020), free amino acids (including glutamine, glutamic acid, and alanine), carbohydrates (32%), and moisture (74%–86%), along with B vitamins, minerals (sodium and potassium), fat (6%), and ash (7%). Furthermore, young yeast, which has not been extensively utilized, tends to have higher phosphate levels and, consequently, a higher ash content (Rachwał et al., 2020; Kao, 2018; Carvalheira et al., 2022).

3.3.2 Phenolic compounds of beer

Beer's phenolic profile arises mainly from malt (~70%) and hops (~30%) (Zabetakis et al., 2022; Boronat et al., 2020). These compounds, including tannins, phenolic acids, flavonoids (flavones, flavanols, isoflavones, flavanones, flavanolol, flavanol, and anthocyanidins), and simple phenolic alcohols such as tyrosol, contribute to its antioxidant activity, stability, and flavor (Zabetakis et al., 2022; Salanţă et al., 2020; Boronat et al., 2020; Shahidi and Ambigaipalan, 2015). Hops used in beer production provide diverse prenylflavonoids, notably xanthohumol, isoxanthohumol, and 6-/8-prenylnaringenin, as well as iso-α-acids formed during boiling (Boronat et al., 2020; Fukuda et al., 2020; Morimoto-Kobayashi et al., 2016).

Xanthohumol, a prenylated chalcone unique to hops, is the most studied beer bioactive, typically ranging from 0.2% to 1.1% (predominantly influenced by the hop variety and the environmental conditions in which it is grown) (Morimoto-Kobayashi et al., 2016; Magalhães et al., 2009). It exhibits broad antiinflammatory, antitumor, and antiobesity effects, regulates glucose and lipid metabolisms, and shows neuroprotective and hepatoprotective potential (Nardini, 2023; Neumann et al., 2022). Following this, iso-α-acids, also known as isohumulones, are also present in beer (3.3–64.0 and 19.1–210 mg/L) (Samuels et al., 2018; Morimoto-Kobayashi et al., 2016; Vesaghhamedani et al., 2022; Ambrož et al., 2019). During brewing, xanthohumol partially converts to isoxanthohumol, a more stable compound with similar antioxidant, antimicrobial, cardioprotective, anticancer, and antidiabetic properties (Neto et al., 2017; Ambrož et al., 2019; Silva et al., 2022; Chiva-Blanch et al., 2015). Moreover, phenolic compounds like tyrosol may also transform into hydroxytyrosol during digestion, enhancing beer's antioxidant value (Soldevila-Domenech et al., 2019). Craft beers, which typically have a higher TPC (343.8–2,172.5 mg GAE/L), show greater antioxidant capacity and metal-chelating activity compared to industrial beers (Neto et al., 2017; Ambrož et al., 2019; Silva et al., 2022; Chiva-Blanch et al., 2015). Overall, beer bioactive phenolics show simultaneous antioxidant and antiinflammatory activities against specific thromboinflammatory and oxidative stress stimuli, in a similar synergistic way to that of similar phenolic bioactives from other sources and beverages (i.e., wine, apple cider, and their by-products) (Fig. 12.3).

Bioactive phenolic compounds of brewery by-products

BSG and BSH brewery by-products retain significant phenolic acids, such as ferulic acid and p-coumaric acid (2.1–9.9 mg GAE/g), primarily derived from barley (~70%–80%) and hops (~20%–30%) (Kao, 2018; Fărcaş et al., 2017), recognized for their remarkable anticarcinogenic, antiinflammatory, DNA-protective, and antioxidant attributes. However, depending on their concentration and the presence of metal ions, certain phenolics, like caffeic, ferulic, and p-coumaric acid, may exert prooxidant behavior, emphasizing the need for further mechanistic studies (McCarthy et al., 2013; Ikram et al., 2017).

BSY contains hop- and malt-derived phenolics, offering antioxidant and anticarcinogenic effects (Rachwał et al., 2020), whereas BSH includes tannins, glycosylated flavonoids, and trace amounts of resveratrol (Magalhães et al., 2009). BSH and BSY also retain bitter acids (~8017 and ~1130 μg/g, respectively) and volatile oils, with notable antimicrobial and antiinflammatory potential. Furthermore, Vieira et al. identified 13 classic phenolic compounds in BSY using HPLC, including gallic, protocatechuic, p-coumaric, caffeic, vanillic, chlorogenic, syringic, ferulic, and cinnamic acids, as well as rutin, isoquercetin, (+-)-catechin, and (−)-epicatechin (Tsoupras et al., 2024c; Vieira et al., 2016).

3.3.3 Lipid bioactives of beer and brewery by-products

Although beer contains <0.1% lipids, its PL fraction possesses high biological relevance. Derived primarily from barley (2%–4% lipids) and yeast metabolism, these include phospholipids and glycolipids rich in MUFAs and UFAs, mainly influenced by the barley variety, malting conditions, and process conditions (Zabetakis et al., 2022; Bonatto, 2022; Gordon et al., 2018).

During brewing, lipid hydrolysis releases fatty acids that crucially influence yeast viability, proteostasis, autophagy, ethanol tolerance, and general foam stability (Bonatto, 2022; Gordon et al., 2018). While lipids are present in minimal quantities in the final beer product, their presence is mostly undesirable due to their impact on its sensory characteristics (primarily "off-flavors"), whereas foam stability ("krausen") is a critical quality parameter that can be affected by the presence of fatty acids (Zabetakis et al., 2022; Bonatto, 2022; Gordon et al., 2018). Certain PLs, notably in stouts, ales, and lagers, exhibit antithrombotic and antiinflammatory activities, complementing the bioactive profile of beer phenolics (Fig. 12.3), in a similar way and through biochemical mechanisms akin to those of other beverages like wine and apple cider, where phenolics and PLs act synergistically. Though present in small amounts, these lipids may contribute to the health-promoting effects of moderate beer consumption, yet they warrant further in vivo validation (Lordan et al., 2019a, 2019b; Tsoupras et al., 2020).

4 Fermented beverages and their by-products: Cosmetic applications and research and development potential

Fermented beverages and their by-products represent an emerging frontier in sustainable innovation, offering a dual benefit of environmental protection and bioeconomic growth. Apple juice, cider, wine, and beer, long valued for their sensory and nutritional appeal, also serve as rich reservoirs of bioactives such as polyphenols, organic acids, triterpenoids, and biofunctional lipids. Their respective by-products, including apple pomace, grape pomace, BSG, BSH, and BSY, contain high-value constituents like phenolics, flavonoids, vitamins, dietary fibers, and PLs. These molecules exhibit a wide range of antioxidant, antiinflammatory, antimicrobial, and antiaging properties, supporting applications in cosmetic and cosmeceutical formulations. Valorizing this waste transforms it from an environmental burden into an efficient bioresource, fully aligned with circular economy and green extraction principles (Tsoupras et al., 2024a, 2024b, 2024c).

Ongoing research and industrial development are increasingly focusing on optimizing the extraction and purification techniques (e.g., SWE, UAE, MAE, and green solvents) utilized to recover and stabilize these bioactives for advanced formulation formation. The cosmetic and dermatological potential of fermented beverage derivatives is particularly promising, as their phenolic and lipid fractions can protect against oxidative stress, improve skin hydration and elasticity, and support collagen synthesis. Furthermore, the incorporation of fermented extracts or probiotic metabolites from cider and beer into topical products introduces new avenues for skin microbiome modulation and natural preservation. Future research and development (R&D) efforts should focus on scaling up the "green extraction" approach, enhancing compound bioavailability, and developing formulations that integrate these natural bioactives to create eco-friendly, multifunctional cosmetics and therapeutics (Tsoupras et al., 2022, 2024a, 2024c; Tsiapali et al., 2025b; Vandorou et al., 2024; Ferreira and Santos, 2022; Almendinger et al., 2020; Arraibi et al., 2021; Di Lorenzo et al., 2024; Barreira et al., 2019). Several commercial cosmetic formulations already contain bioactives from these natural sources, revealing confirmed functional and health-related properties. Table 12.2 includes selected commercial and research-backed cosmetic agents or products derived from natural bioactives in the aforementioned fermented beverages.

4.1 Apple juice, cider, and their by-products: Indicative cosmetic applications and R&D potential

Apple, white grape, and orange juice functional drinks containing hydrolyzed fish collagen (1%–3%) and other natural acids, such as citric and ascorbic acid, with a natural mint flavor, were produced as potent functional foods with cosmeceutical potential. Adding preferably 2.5% hydrolyzed collagen increased the protein content (0.56 to 2.22–2.48 g/100 mL), with the orange (95.73%) and apple (90.71%) juice drinks revealing higher bioavailability (5%–14%) than the white grape juice blends. The remarkable vitamin C (ascorbic acid) content (81.39–113.5 mg/100 mL), TPC (86.93–117.43 mg GAE/100 mL), and antioxidant capacity (2,2'-azino-bis (3-ethylbenzothiazoline-6-sulfonic acid): 104–127 μmol TEAC/100 mL) further supported the potential of these collagen drinks to aid in relieving joint pain and improving important skin properties and parameters (Bilek and Bayram, 2015; Kandemir et al., 2022).

The efficacy of a formulation comprising *Kalonji* (*Nigella sativa*) seed powder and cane Sirka, an apple cider vinegar (Unani group), was compared to benzoyl peroxide 5% (control group) for the treatment of acne *vulgaris*. This formulation was applied topically at night, and the primary outcomes encompassed changes in the Global Acne Grading System

TABLE 12.2 Commercial and research-backed cosmetic agents or products from natural bioactives derived from fermented beverages and their by-products.

Cosmetic product	Cosmetic use	Fruit ingredient	Beneficial impact	References
Annurca Apple Oleolite (AAO)	Active oil/ extract	Ursolic acid from Annurca apple peel	Improves skin elasticity, antiwrinkle, and moisturizing	(Maisto et al., 2023; Di Lorenzo et al., 2024)
Ariul—Apple Cider Deep Cleansing Oil	Deep cleansing oil	Apple cider vinegar and apple seed oil [+ *Vitis vinifera* (grape) seed oil]	Deep cleansing, dirt and sebum removing, smoothing, emollient, emulsifying, moisturizing, antioxidant, and nonirritating properties	(Ariul Apple Cider Deep Cleansing Oil Ingredients (Explained), n.d.)
Juice Beauty—Green Apple Protein Conditioner	Conditioner	*Pyrus malus* green apple juice	Antioxidant, radiance boosting, deep conditioning, strengthening, smoothing, and stress-protective effects	(Juice Beauty, n.d.)
Plantnery—Hydra-Rich Lip Serum (SOP/PA++++ 50 +)	Lip serum	Apple Cider Vinegar [+ *Vitis vinifera* (grape seed oil)]	Anti-UV, photoprotective, soothing, and deeply moisturizing effects	(Plantnery, n.d.)
Caudalie—Vinoperfect Radiance Serum	Dark spot brightening serum	Viniferine (grapevine sap) and polyphenols	Vitamin C alternative—dark spot brightening, offering a brighter complexion	(Caudalie, n.d.)
Apivita—Face Mask Grape	Face mask	*Vitis vinifera* (grape) seed extract	Nourishing, antioxidant, firmness-boosting, antiaging, revitalizing, and skin elasticity-enhancing effects	(APIVITA, n.d.b)
Apivita—Wine Elixir Renewing Lift Night Cream	Night lift cream	*Vitis vinifera* (grape), leaf, fruit, and seed oil extract, and three Santorini vine varieties (Athiri, Aidani, and Assyrtiko)	Nourishing, face-lifting, revitalizing, rejuvenating, firmness-enhancing, antioxidant, youthful complexion-offering, exfoliating, and skin elasticity-enhancing effects	(APIVITA, n.d.a; Team MW, n.d.)
Neogen—Bio-Peel Gauze Peeling Wine	Gauze peeling pads	*Vitis vinifera* (grape) seed and wine extract	Deep exfoliation, smoothing, antioxidant, and soothing properties	(NEOGENLAB Global, n.d.)
ORZENE—Beer Shampoo for Dry Damaged Hair	Hair shampoo	Beer malting barley (beer malt)	Nourishing, moisturizing, strengthening, revitalizing, elasticity-repairing, and glowing properties	(ORZENE, n.d.)
Kundal—Beer Yeast Scalp Shampoo	Hair loss relief shampoo	Brewer's Yeast Extract (BSY)	Hair strengthening, exfoliating, volumizing, and cooling care properties	(KUNDAL, n.d.)
BLEACH London—Beer Conditioner	Hair conditioner	Brewer's yeast extract (BSY)	Hair strengthening, exfoliating, nourishing, and elasticity-repairing effects	(Bleach London, n.d.)

(GAGS) and Cook's Acne Grading Scale using photographic standards for acne grading (PSAG) scores, whereas the secondary outcome was the change in "Quality of Life" assessed via the Cardiff Acne Disability Index (CADI). GAGS scores revealed a mean difference of −2.600 (95% CI: −5.770–0.570, d = 0.57, p = 0.105), PSAG showed a mean difference of −0.600 (95% CI: −1.793–0.593, d = 0.49, p = 0.315), and CADI scores exhibited a mean difference of −1.500 (95% CI: −3.470–0.470, d = 0.32, p = 0.132) at the trial inclusion. All the above results suggest that the formulation may exert therapeutic effects as an alternative acne treatment method. However, further studies involving larger sample sizes and extended follow-up periods are also recommended (Abbas et al., 2025).

Recently, research conducted by Tsiapali et al. (2025a) revealed that an antiaging cream enriched with apple-derived bioactives, in combination with avocado and kiwi by-products, provided vast cosmetic benefits. This cream was extensively studied in formulations containing nanobubbles (NB) and without them (S), compared to a control cream (X). The inclusion of apple pomace-based extracts, rich in phenolic antioxidants and natural α-hydroxy acids, significantly enhanced the product's antioxidant performance (FRAP assay), achieving up to a ~ 250% improvement over the control. Specifically, S (at production: 710.4 ± 344.3 and at 1 month: 631.7 ± 277.8 μmol TE/g DW) and NB formulations (at production: 566.3 ± 185.0 and at 1 month: 1019.3 ± 574.0 μmol TE/g DW) exhibited markedly higher antioxidant capacities in contrast to X (at production: 202.8 ± 145.6 and at 1 month: 449.8 ± 43.9 μmol TE/g DW). Beyond antioxidant improvement, the sun protection factor increased following storage (from 8.7 ± 0.8 to 9.5 ± 0.6), suggesting the stability and photoprotective contribution of apple polyphenols. Attenuated total reflectance–FTIR using Strat-M membranes confirmed enhanced skin penetration of apple-derived bioactives in S creams, while NBs did not notably alter absorption profiles. Moreover, platelet aggregation assays demonstrated markedly lower IC_{50} values in S and NB creams than in the X ones for both PAF (μmol TE/g DW: S at production: 300.0 ± 42.0 and at 1 month: 325.0 ± 50.0; NB at production: 258.0 ± 31.0 and at 1 month: 275.0 ± 4, and X at production: 685.0 ± 35.0 and at 1 month: 885.0 ± 112.0) and ADP signaling (S at production: 450.0 ± 65.0 and at 1 month: 470.0 ± 52.0; NB at production: 400.0 ± 31.0 and at 1 month: 412.0 ± 42.0; and X at production: 880.0 ± 58.0 and at 1 month: 1102.0 ± 125.0), thus indicating superior antiinflammatory and antithrombotic effects attributed to the bioactive apple constituents (Tsiapali et al., 2025a). Additional clinical studies underscore the efficacy of apple pomace bioactives, such as ursolic acid from Annurca apples and apple-derived nanovesicles, in reducing wrinkles, improving skin hydration, and modulating inflammatory pathways. Topical formulations containing these compounds have shown promising antiwrinkle, antioxidant, UV-protective, and antiinflammatory effects in both in vivo and clinical settings, supporting their valuable role in advanced cosmeceutical products (Maisto et al., 2023; Di Lorenzo et al., 2024, no date; Ahmed et al., 2020).

Given the increasing demand for apple juice, cider, and vinegar, the co-production of apple pomace in substantial quantities globally highlights its potential as a sustainable natural source of valuable biofunctional compounds. It is crucial, though, to note that studies on apple cider have been primarily conducted in vitro and remain limited. Further research, including in vitro and in vivo studies, is necessary to explore the benefits of cider and its cosmetic potential, as well as its effects on inflammation-related signaling and disorders (Di Lorenzo et al., 2024; Lyu et al., 2020; Tsiapali et al., 2025a).

4.2 Applications of the bioactive and health-promoting constituents in wine and winery by-products

Wine-making by-products of the Mediterranean area, specifically grape pomace skin, were utilized to extract phytochemicals and bioactives via maceration in a hydroethanolic solution, where catechin, quercetin, fisetin, and gallic acid antioxidants were the predominant compounds of the extract. The study's liposomes and phospholipid vehicles, modified using glycerol and/or Montanov 82 as carrier vesicles, were small (~183 nm), slightly polydispersed (PI ≥ 0.28), and highly negatively charged (~−50 mV), while the extract was loaded in high amounts in all vesicles (~100%). The antioxidant activity of the extract, measured by the DPPH assay, was 84 ± 1% and slightly elevated to ~89% ($P < 0.05$) when loaded into the vesicles. Grape pomace-loaded vesicles were highly biocompatible and able to protect fibroblasts (3T3) from oxidative stress induced by hydrogen peroxide (Perra et al., 2021). Moreover, liquid chromatography–electrospray ionization–mass spectrometry identified 26 anthocyanins in the selected chokeberry and red grape extracts. Red grape anthocyanins, specifically, contained glycosylated derivatives of five different aglycones and were selected to be tested on normal and melanoma cell lines. These anthocyanins markedly reduced cancer proliferation, increased oxidative stress biomarkers, and finally diminished mitochondrial membrane potential in melanoma cells, having no negative influence on normal cells, showcasing their value as active ingredients for cosmetics and nutraceuticals (Diaconeasa et al., 2017).

Recently, white and red wines were used as raw materials for the formulation of an antiaging cosmetic product, where their alcoholic fraction was removed and analyzed by LC-MS. The cytotoxic effects of the wines were tested on fibroblasts using the 3-(4,5-dimethylthiazol-2-yl)-2,5-diphenyltetrazolium assay, whereas the antioxidant capacity and antiaging potential were studied through the catalase activity test (under stressing conditions) and the β-galactosidase colorimetric assay. Wine extracts revealed remarkable antioxidant and antiaging properties, especially on cells exposed to a marked stressful event, highlighting their promising application as cosmetic products aiding in skin regeneration and revitalization (Cruciani et al., 2021).

Interestingly, extracts derived from wine lees, red grape pomace, and other vinification by-products exhibit strong antioxidant and antihyperpigmentation properties. Wine lees extracts, rich in phenolics and anthocyanins such as caftaric acid, malvidin, peonidin-3-*O*-glucoside, myricetin, and quercetin, effectively inhibit elastase, matrix metalloproteinase-1 (MMP-1), and tyrosinase activity (Matos et al., 2019). Comparative studies show that six different grape by-product extracts suppress elastase more than tyrosinase, highlighting their antiaging and antiwrinkle potential (Leal et al., 2020). In addition, grape extracts (*Vitis vinifera* L.) enhance mitochondrial adenosine triphosphate production and protect fibroblasts from UV_A-induced oxidative stress by influencing DNA methylation and increasing sirtuin 1/heat shock protein 47 expression (Alcendor et al., 2007; Letsiou et al., 2020; Ito and Nagata, 2017). Likewise, *V. vinifera* L. leaf extract shields keratinocytes from UV_A-triggered ROS and DNA damage (as displayed by the Comet and γ-H2AX assays), demonstrating potent antioxidant and antimutagenic effects (Marabini et al., 2020)

Winemaking by-products, such as grape pomace and seed oil, contain high levels of polyphenols, flavonoids, anthocyanins, and UFAs, all of which exhibit strong antioxidant, antiinflammatory, photoprotective, and antiaging effects. These bioactives improve skin hydration, elasticity, and barrier function, making grape-derived ingredients valuable for cosmeceutical formulations. Their multipurpose roles, ranging from ROS scavenging to MMP inhibitory agents, further support their utilization in antiaging creams, sunscreens, and skin repair products (Tsoupras et al., 2024a; Onache et al., 2022; Cruciani et al., 2021; Leal et al., 2020). Nevertheless, a major challenge to their broader industrial use is the poor stability of fresh grape pomace due to its high moisture content, which accelerates microbial growth and the degradation of sensitive molecules. To preserve bioactivity, drying is essential, with methods such as vacuum drying at 70°C being able to retain polyphenols more efficiently than conventional techniques. Although advanced extraction technologies like UAE, MAE, or PEF yield high-quality extracts, they remain highly expensive. Therefore traditional drying and solvent extraction remain the most common industrial choices (Tseng and Zhao, 2012; Ageyeva et al., 2021; Sokač et al., 2022). In addition, further processing using surfactants could also increase polyphenol stability. For instance, in a study aimed at slowing the degradation and color change of anthocyanins, Polysorbate 20 and sorbic acid, used as surfactants, proved to be successful in processing these substances (MohdMaidin et al., 2019).

Safety and quality control are critical, as pomace may contain trace contaminants, although vinification steps and drying substantially reduce pesticide and fungicide residues. Occasional findings of sodium or trace heavy metals remain below legal limits but still require monitoring. Despite minor sensory defects due to phenolic bitterness, grape pomace extracts have already been incorporated into numerous cosmetic products, further supporting their role as sustainable, high-value ingredients within circular, cosmetic-focused economy principles (Čuš et al., 2010; Hou et al., 2020; Moncalvo et al., 2016).

4.3 Applications of the bioactive and health-promoting constituents in beer and brewery by-products

Different types of handcrafted beers (EGO, Alter, Fiat Lux, Triplo Malto, Ubi, and Maior), as well as the starting materials (malts, hops, and yeast), intermediate materials, and waste materials (spent malt, hops, and yeast), were tested for their total phenol content, antioxidant activity, and potential use in cosmetic formulations. Extractions from starting and spent samples were performed using water or 70% v/v alcohol, while the Folin–Ciocalteu assay was employed to evaluate the TPC yield. The highest TPC values were found in starting hops (93–155 mg GAE/g), intermediate values in starting malt and starting yeast, whereas the lowest values were recorded in wort. Moreover, nonnegligible amounts were found in spent products, suggesting that starting products are enriched with bioactives, but spent products contain nonnegligible amounts of phenols as well. Interestingly, BSY often revealed higher TPC values than the starting material; thus it is capable of absorbing beer phenols during brewing. Furthermore, "Alter" brewery products (spent malt, BSH, and BSY) were evaluated on a keratinocyte cell culture (HaCaT cells). BSH and BSY notably improved mitochondrial activity and prevented oxidative stress, showcasing potent bioactive agents for use in skin antiaging cosmetics (Censi et al., 2021).

In a recent comparative study, malt and beer-related by-products, including caramalt, aromatic and roasted malt, malt sprouts, dark beer BSGs, and wheat beer BSGs, were extracted using water under moderate experimental conditions. All extracts were characterized for their carbohydrate, amino acid, and phenolic content, as well as for their in vitro antioxidant potential using keratinocyte cell cultures. Malt sprouts provided a high amino acid content (57.6 mg/g) and the highest yields of glucose (50.1 mg/g) and fructose (38.4 mg/g), while other malt and beer by-products reached a maximum of ~ 13.5 mg/g. Caramalt and roasted malt recorded the highest TPC yields (12.9 mg GAE/g), whereas dark and wheat BSGs revealed the lowest TPC yields (5.1 and 1.8 mg GAE/g, respectively). In addition, caramalt phenolic extracts inhibited tyrosinase activity by 78% and 87% when applying 0.5% and 1% extracts, respectively, while, similarly, dark malt, roasted malt, and malt sprout extracts achieved 86% and 80% inhibition when using a 1% extract. Dark and wheat BSGs exhibited low inhibitory effects. Collectively, all these results showcase the potential of malt and beer-related by-products as biological sources of ingredients for cosmeceuticals such as skin-whitening products (Almendinger et al., 2020).

Recent scientific data confirm that beer and brewery by-products, especially hop extracts, could be effective cosmetic agents in treating acne, loose skin, stretch marks, sagging, antiaging, and hair-associated conditions. BSHs contain high levels of antioxidant, antiinflammatory, antiaging, antihyperpigmentation, and antimicrobial bioactives, capable of preventing ROS and oxidative stress, combating *Propionibacteriumacnes* and *taphylococcus aureus* acne-related strains, downregulating proinflammatory cytokine (e.g., IL-6) production, and, finally, inhibiting tyrosinase, intracellular melanin, and melanogenesis activity (Pereira et al., 2022).

Researchers are actively developing methods to extract high-value bioactive components from brewing waste, aiming to transform these abundant by-products into functional, health-promoting ingredients. To achieve this, a wide range of extraction techniques, physical, chemical, biological, and increasingly green and sustainable technologies, are being explored to isolate specific molecules with commercial potential. A major factor guiding these efforts is the economic feasibility of recovering valuable molecules at scale. Among brewery residues, BSG, BSH, and BSY are the most extensively studied, each containing a diverse array of valorizable bioactive constituents (Tsoupras et al., 2024b, 2024c; Kao, 2018; Silva et al., 2022; McCarthy et al., 2013; Vieira et al., 2016).

Despite the well-recognized bioactive potential of beer and brewery by-products, their integration into cosmetic formulations remains limited. Most applications are still at the niche or experimental-product level, constrained by gaps in formulation compatibility, stability data, and comprehensive safety assessments. As a result, the cosmetic utilization of beer-derived bioactives is still in an emerging phase. Continued research is needed to optimize extraction efficiency, improve ingredient stability, and address regulatory considerations to enable broader industrial adoption and large-scale implementation (Tsoupras et al., 2024b, 2024c; Kao, 2018; Silva et al., 2022; McCarthy et al., 2013; Vieira et al., 2016).

5 Limitations, challenges, and future perspectives

Despite the promising biological activities of bioactives derived from apples, grapes, wine, beer, and brewery by-products, several limitations hinder their wider integration into cosmetic and cosmeceutical formulations. One of the predominant challenges lies in the high variability of raw materials, driven by cultivar, soil, climate, and fermentation conditions, as well as by their processing intensity and storage conditions. This recorded variability directly affects their polyphenol, lipid, and macro- and micronutrient profiles, frequently leading to inconsistent extract compositions. As a consequence, their standardization remains difficult, and reproducible efficacy in formulations is not always guaranteed (Chakka and Babu, 2022; Somat et al., 2025; Caiyun et al., 2023; Wang et al., 2022; Bamforth, 2017; Shopska et al., 2021; Karabín et al., 2016; Ageyeva et al., 2021; Pereira et al., 2022).

Another major limitation concerns the stability issues of bioactives, including phenolics, triterpenoids, vitamins, and biofunctional lipids. Many of these compounds are sensitive to heat, oxygen, UV radiation, soil, and pH fluctuations, leading to rapid degradation during extraction, storage, or formulation. Brewery and winery by-products, specifically, possess high moisture content and enzymatic systems that accelerate oxidation and microbial spoilage, requiring immediate stabilization. While drying techniques like vacuum or freeze-drying help preserve sensitive molecules, they increase production costs and energy demand (Tseng and Zhao, 2012; Ageyeva et al., 2021; Sokač et al., 2022). Technical and economy-related barriers also persist in adopting green extraction technologies for apples, grapes, wine, beer, and brewery by-products. Although methods such as SFE, MAE, UAE, and PEF improve extraction yields and preserve thermolabile compounds from degradation, their implementation requires high capital investment, specialized equipment, and trained personnel. Unfortunately, for many small- or medium-scale producers, these factors limit their scalability, along with the lack of sufficient industrial infrastructure (Krbečková and Plachá, 2024; Gil-Martín et al., 2022; Panzella et al., 2020; Ilyas et al., 2021; Barba et al., 2016; Aliyu and Bala, 2011).

From a regulatory and safety perspective, the introduction of bioactives derived from waste streams raises concerns about contaminants, including heavy metals, pesticides, mycotoxins, and fermentation-derived residues. Although cider and juice-making, winemaking, and brewing processes tend to reduce such contaminants, direct monitoring and rapid quality control are essential. In addition, the cosmetic industry practices require detailed toxicological data, skin compatibility studies, and long-term stability assessments, many of which are still limited or incomplete for emerging fermented-beverage-derived extracts (Bamforth, 2017; Gonçalves Bortolini et al., 2020; Nardini, 2023; Čuš et al., 2010; Hou et al., 2020; Moncalvo et al., 2016). Consumer perception presents another major challenge. While the cosmetic and cosmeceutical market is currently embracing sustainability, formulations derived from beer or winery waste may be overlooked without strong evidence of their safety, efficacy, and sensory acceptability. For instance, polyphenols may impart undesirable color, odor, or astringency, requiring advanced encapsulation or formulation strategies to overcome sensory limitations (Bamforth, 2017; Gonçalves Bortolini et al., 2020; Nardini, 2023; Moncalvo et al., 2016).

Future research must prioritize the standardization of extraction protocols, the development of fingerprinting tools, and the establishment of analytical frameworks to ensure consistency across batches. Encapsulation technologies, including the biobased formation of liposomes, micelles, nanoemulsions, and biopolymer nanoparticles, may offer several promising solutions for successfully improving the stability, penetration, and targeted delivery of phenolics, triterpenoids, lipids, and probiotics. Therefore integrating skin microbiome science with fermented-beverage bioactives could open new avenues for pro- and postbiotic cosmetics (Krbečková and Plachá, 2024; Tsiapali et al., 2025a; Perra et al., 2021; Trentini et al., 2022; Castro et al., 2024; Zheng et al., 2024).

6 Conclusions

Fermented beverages and their by-products represent a rich and underutilized reservoir of bioactive compounds with significant antioxidant, antiinflammatory, antiaging, and dermo-protective potential. Through the valorization of apple and grape pomace, as well as BSG, BSH, and BSY, the cosmetic sector can access a diverse spectrum of natural phenolics, flavonoids, organic acids, triterpenoids, and biofunctional lipids that support skin health while aligning with sustainability and circular economy principles. At the same time, advances in green extraction methods have further enabled the recovery of high-quality, albeit thermolabile, bioactives suitable for modern cosmetic and cosmeceutical formulation strategies.

Even though technical, economic, and regulatory challenges remain unsolved, emerging clinical and in vitro evidence highlights the strong promise of fermented beverage-derived compounds for future cosmeceutical innovation. With ongoing research focusing on effective standardization, stability, formulation compatibility, quality control, and safety evaluation, such natural resources can be effectively harnessed to produce next-generation, eco-conscious cosmetics. Fermented beverages and their by-products, thus, lie at the crossroads of science, sustainability, and biotechnology, offering a powerful platform for the development of high-value, multifunctional natural cosmetics and cosmeceuticals.

Acknowledgments

The authors would like to thank the School of Chemistry in the Faculty of Sciences at Democritus University of Thrace for their continuous support.

Conflicts of interest

The authors declare no conflicts of interest.

Funding

This research received no external funding.

Author contributions

A.T. was involved in conceptualization, methodology, validation, visualization, supervision, and project administration. A.T., S.M., and T.A. were involved in investigation and writing—original draft preparation. A.T. and T.A. were involved in writing—review and editing. All authors contributed to software and have read and agreed to the published version of the manuscript.

References

Abbas, S.N.A., Horti, A., Allapat, M.R., Razzaq, M.S.A., Parveen, F.S., Husain, N., 2025. Evaluation of the efficacy of topical *Nigella sativa* L. with vinegar in the treatment of acne vulgaris: a randomized controlled trial. J. Dermatol. Sci. Cosmet. Technol. 2950306X. 2 (1), 100069. doi:10.1016/j.jdsct.2025.100069.

Ageyeva, N., Tikhonova, A., Burtsev, B., Biryukova, S., Globa, E., 2021. Grape pomace treatment methods and their effects on storage. Foods Raw Mater. 2308-4057. 9 (2), 215–223. doi:10.21603/2308-4057-2021-2-215-223.

Ahmed, G.H.G., Fernández-González, A., Díaz García, M.E., 2020. Nano-encapsulation of grape and apple pomace phenolic extract in chitosan and soy protein via nanoemulsification. Food Hydrocoll. 0268005X. 108, 105806. doi:10.1016/j.foodhyd.2020.105806.

Al Bittar, S., Périno-Issartier, S., Dangles, O., 2013. Farid Chemat, An innovative grape juice enriched in polyphenols by microwave-assisted extraction. Food Chem. 03088146. 141 (3), 3268–3272. doi:10.1016/j.foodchem.2013.05.134.

Alcendor, R.R., Gao, S., Zhai, P., Zablocki, D., Holle, E., Yu, X., Tian, B., Wagner, T., Vatner, S.F., Sadoshima, J., 2007. Sirt1 regulates aging and resistance to oxidative stress in the heart. Circ. Res. 00097330. 100 (10), 1512–1521. doi:10.1161/01.RES.0000267723.65696.4a.

Aliyu, S., Bala, M., 2011. Brewer's spent grain: a review of its potentials and applications. Afr. J. Biotechnol. 16845315. 10 (3), 324–331. Available from: http://www.academicjournals.org/AJB/PDF/pdf2011/17Jan/Aliyu%20and%20%20Bala.pdf.

Almendinger, M., Rohn, S., Pleissner, D., 2020. Malt and beer-related by-products as potential antioxidant skin-lightening agents for cosmetics. Sustain. Chem. Pharm. 23525541. 17, 100282. doi:10.1016/j.scp.2020.100282.

Ambrož, M., Lněničková, K., Matoušková, P., Skálová, L., Boušová, I., 2019. Antiproliferative effects of hop-derived prenylflavonoids and their influence on the efficacy of oxaliplatine, 5-fluorouracil and irinotecan in human colorectalC cells. Nutrients. 2072-6643. 11 (4), 879. doi:10.3390/nu11040879.

Ano, Y., Dohata, A., Taniguchi, Y., Hoshi, A., Uchida, K., Takashima, A., Nakayama, H., 2017. Iso-α-acids, bitter components of beer, prevent inflammation and cognitive decline induced in a mouse model of Alzheimer's disease. J. Biol. Chem. 00219258. 292 (9), 3720–3728. doi:10.1074/jbc.m116.763813.

APIVITA, n.d.b. Face Mask Grape Line Smoothing & Firming 10-22-45-063. https://www.apivita.com/en/face-mask-grape-line-smoothing-firming-10-22-45-063.html.

APIVITA, n.d.a. Natural Cosmetics | natural Beauty Skincare, Hair & Body. https://www.apivita.com.

Apostolidou, C., Adamopoulos, K., Lymperaki, E., Iliadis, S., Papapreponis, P., Kourtidou-Papadeli, C., 2015. Cardiovascular risk and benefits from antioxidant dietary intervention with red wine in asymptomatic hypercholesterolemics. Clin. Nutr. ESPEN. 24054577. 10 (6), e224. doi:10.1016/j.clnesp.2015.08.001.

Arcena, M.R., Leong, S.Y., Then, S., Hochberg, M., Sack, M., Mueller, G., Sigler, J., Kebede, B., Silcock, P., Oey, I., 2021. The effect of pulsed electric fields pre-treatment on the volatile and phenolic profiles of Merlot grape musts at different winemaking stages and the sensory characteristics of the finished wines. Innov. Food Sci. Emerg. Technol. 14668564. 70, 102698. doi:10.1016/j.ifset.2021.102698.

Areti, H.A., Muleta, M.D., Abo, L.D., Hamda, A.S., Adugna, A.A., Edae, I.T., Daba, B.J., Gudeta, R.L., 2024. Innovative uses of agricultural by-products in the food and beverage sector: a review. Food Chem. Adv. 2772753X. 5, 100838. doi:10.1016/j.focha.2024.100838.

Argyrou, C., Vlachogianni, I., Stamatakis, G., Demopoulos, C.A., Antonopoulou, S., Fragopoulou, E., 2017. Postprandial effects of wine consumption on Platelet Activating Factor metabolic enzymes. Prostaglandins Other Lipid Mediat. 10988823. 130, 23–29. doi:10.1016/j.prostaglandins.2017.03.002.

Ariul Apple Cider Deep Cleansing Oil ingredients (Explained), n.d. https://incidecoder.com/products/ariul-apple-cider-deep-cleansing-oil.

Arraibi, A.A., Liberal, Â., Dias, M.I., Alves, M.J., Ferreira, I.C.F.R., Barros, L., Barreira, J.C.M., 2021. Chemical and bioactive characterization of spanish and Belgian apple pomace for its potential use as a novel dermocosmetic formulation. Foods 23048158. 10 (8). Available from: https://www.mdpi.com/2304-8158/10/8/1949/pdf. doi:10.3390/foods10081949.

Arranz, S., Chiva-Blanch, G., Valderas-Martínez, P., Medina-Remón, A., Lamuela-Raventós, R.M., Estruch, R., Wine, B., 2012. Alcohol and polyphenols on cardiovascular disease and cancer. Nutrients. 2072-6643. 4 (7), 759–781. doi:10.3390/nu4070759.

Aviram, M., Fuhrman, B., 2002. Wine flavonoids protect against LDL oxidation and atherosclerosis. Ann. N. Y. Acad. Sci. 0077-8923. 957 (1), 146–161. doi:10.1111/j.1749-6632.2002.tb02913.x.

Bamforth, C.W., 2017. Progress in brewing science and beer production. Annu. Rev. Chem. Biomol. Eng. 1947-5438. 8 (1), 161–176. doi:10.1146/annurev-chembioeng-060816-101450.

Baptista, F., Almeida, M., Paié-Ribeiro, J., Barros, A.N., Rodrigues, M., 2023. Unlocking the potential of spent mushroom substrate (SMS) for enhanced agricultural sustainability: from environmental benefits to poultry nutrition. Life. 2075-1729. 13 (10), 1948. doi:10.3390/life13101948.

Barba, F.J., Brianceau, S., Turk, M., Boussetta, N., Vorobiev, E., 2015. Effect of alternative physical treatments (ultrasounds, pulsed electric fields, and high-voltage electrical discharges) on selective recovery of bio-compounds from fermented grape pomace. Food Bioprocess Technol. 1935-5130. 8 (5), 1139–1148. doi:10.1007/s11947-015-1482-3.

Barba, F.J., Zhu, Z., Koubaa, M., Sant'Ana, A.S., Orlien, V., 2016. Green alternative methods for the extraction of antioxidant bioactive compounds from winery wastes and by-products: a review. Trends Food Sci. Technol. 09242244. 49, 96–109. Available from: http://www.elsevier.com/wps/find/journaldescription.cws_home/601278/description#description. doi:10.1016/j.tifs.2016.01.006.

Barreira, J.C.M., Arraibi, A.A., Ferreira, I.C.F.R., 2019. Bioactive and functional compounds in apple pomace from juice and cider manufacturing: potential use in dermal formulations. Trends Food Sci. Technol. 09242244. 90, 76–87. doi:10.1016/j.tifs.2019.05.014.

Belardi, I., De Francesco, G., Alfeo, V., Bravi, E., Sileoni, V., Marconi, O., Marrocchi, A., 2025. Advances in the valorization of brewing by-products. Food Chem. 03088146. 465 (Pt 1), 141882. doi:10.1016/j.foodchem.2024.141882.

Beres, C., Costa, G.N.S., Cabezudo, I., da Silva-james, N.K., Teles, A.S.C., Cruz, A.P.G., Mellinger-Silva, C., Tonon, R.V., Cabral, L.M.C., Freitas, S.P., 2017. Towards integral utilization of grape pomace from winemaking process: a review. Waste Manag. 18792456. 68, 581–594. Available from: https://www.elsevier.com/locate/wasman. doi:10.1016/j.wasman.2017.07.017.

Bilek, S.E., Bayram, S.K., 2015. Fruit juice drink production containing hydrolyzed collagen. J. Funct. Foods 17564646. 14, 562–569. Available from: http://www.elsevier.com/wps/find/journaldescription.cws_home/717426/description#description. doi:10.1016/j.jff.2015.02.024.

Bleach London, n.d. Beer Conditioner 250ml. https://bleachlondon.com/us/products/beer-conditioner-250ml.

Bonatto, D., 2022. The multiple roles of lipid metabolism in yeast physiology during beer fermentation. Genet. Mol. Biol. 16784685. 45 (3). Available from: https://www.scielo.br/j/gmb/a/dy7wTDfxYVkX94bwVys8Xdb/?format=pdf&lang=en. doi:10.1590/1678-4685-GMB-2021-0325.

Bordiga, M., Travaglia, F., Locatelli, M., 2019. Valorisation of grape pomace: an approach that is increasingly reaching its maturity – a review. Int. J. Food Sci. Technol. 0950-5423. 54 (4), 933–942. doi:10.1111/ijfs.14118.

Boronat, A., Soldevila-Domenech, N., Rodríguez-Morató, J., Martínez-Huélamo, M., Lamuela-Raventós, R.M., de la Torre, R., 2020. Beer phenolic composition of simple phenols, prenylated flavonoids and alkylresorcinols. Molecules. 1420-3049. 25 (11), 2582. doi:10.3390/molecules25112582.

Bortolini, D.G., Benvenutti, L., Demiate, I.M., Nogueira, A., Alberti, A., Antonio Ferreira Zielinski, A., 2020. A new approach to the use of apple pomace in cider making for the recovery of phenolic compounds. LWT. 00236438. 126, 109316. doi:10.1016/j.lwt.2020.109316.

Brianceau, S., Turk, M., Vitrac, X., Vorobiev, E., 2015. Combined densification and pulsed electric field treatment for selective polyphenols recovery from fermented grape pomace. Innov. Food Sci. Emerg. Technol. 14668564. 29, 2–8. doi:10.1016/j.ifset.2014.07.010.

Bucić-Kojić, A., Planinić, M., Tomas, S., Bilić, M., Velić, D., 2007. Study of solid–liquid extraction kinetics of total polyphenols from grape seeds. J. Food Eng. 02608774. 81 (1), 236–242. doi:10.1016/j.jfoodeng.2006.10.027.

Caiyun, W., Wang, J., Liu, N., Chen, X., Huaide, X., Lei, H., 2023. Phytochemical properties and antioxidant capacities of apple juice fermented by probiotics during refrigerated storage and simulated gastrointestinal digestion. Appl. Biochem. Biotechnol. 0273-2289. 195 (10), 6032–6049. doi:10.1007/s12010-022-04255-2.

Calabriso, N., Scoditti, E., Massaro, M., Pellegrino, M., Storelli, C., Ingrosso, I., Giovinazzo, G., Carluccio, M.A., 2016. Multiple anti-inflammatory and anti-atherosclerotic properties of red wine polyphenolic extracts: differential role of hydroxycinnamic acids, flavonols and stilbenes on endothelial inflammatory gene expression. Eur. J. Nutr. 1436-6207. 55 (2), 477–489. doi:10.1007/s00394-015-0865-6.

Carpentieri, S., Ferrari, G., Pataro, G., 2023. Pulsed electric fields-assisted extraction of valuable compounds from red grape pomace: process optimization using response surface methodology. Front. Nutr. 2296-861X. 10. doi:10.3389/fnut.2023.1158019.

Carvalheira, M., Amorim, C.L., Oliveira, A.C., Guarda, E.C., Costa, E., Teixeira, M.R., Castro, P.M.L., Duque, A.F., Reis, M.A.M., 2022. Valorization of brewery waste through polyhydroxyalkanoates production supported by a metabolic specialized microbiome. Life. 2075-1729. 12 (9), 1347. doi:10.3390/life12091347.

Casas, L., Mantell, C., Rodríguez, M., de la Ossa, E.J.M., Roldán, A., Ory, I.D., Caro, I., Blandino, A., 2010. Extraction of resveratrol from the pomace of *Palomino fino* grapes by supercritical carbon dioxide. J. Food Eng. 02608774. 96 (2), 304–308. doi:10.1016/j.jfoodeng.2009.08.002.

Castro, M.L., Azevedo-Silva, J., Valente, D., Machado, A., Ribeiro, T., Paulo Ferreira, J., Pintado, M., Ramos, O.L., Borges, S., Baptista-Silva, S., 2024. Elevating skincare science: grape seed extract encapsulation for dermatological care. Molecules. 1420-3049. 29 (16), 3717. doi:10.3390/molecules29163717.

Caudalie, n.d. Dark Spot Serum for Radiance – vinoperfect. https://en.caudalie.com/p/432C/vinoperfect-radiance-serum-complexion-correcting-432c.html.

Censi, R., Peregrina, D.V., Gigliobianco, M.R., Lupidi, G., Angeloni, C., Pruccoli, L., Tarozzi, A., Di Martino, P., 2021. New antioxidant ingredients from brewery by-products for cosmetic formulations. Cosmetics. 2079-9284. 8 (4), 96. doi:10.3390/cosmetics8040096.

Chakka, A.K., Babu, A.S., 2022. Bioactive compounds of winery by-products: extraction techniques and their potential health benefits. Appl. Food Res. 27725022. 2 (1), 100058. doi:10.1016/j.afres.2022.100058.

Chedea, V.S., Octavian Macovei, Ş., Bocşan, I.C., Măgureanu, D.C., Levai, A.M., Buzoianu, A.D., Pop, R.M., 2022. Grape pomace polyphenols as a source of compounds for management of oxidative stress and inflammation—A possible alternative for non-steroidal anti-inflammatory drugs? Molecules. 1420-3049. 27 (20), 6826. doi:10.3390/molecules27206826.

Chen, J., Yang, J., Ma, L., Li, J., Shahzad, N., Kim, C.K., 2020. Structure-antioxidant activity relationship of methoxy, phenolic hydroxyl, and carboxylic acid groups of phenolic acids. Sci. Rep. 20452322. 10 (1). Available from: https://www.nature.com/srep/index.html. doi:10.1038/s41598-020-59451-z.

Chen, X., Zhengli, L., Hong, H., Wang, N., Chen, J., Sisi, L., Zhang, H., Zhang, X., Bei, C., 2021. Xanthohumol suppresses inflammation in chondrocytes and ameliorates osteoarthritis in mice. Biomed. Pharmacother. 07533322. 137, 111238. doi:10.1016/j.biopha.2021.111238.

Chiva-Blanch, G., Arranz, S., Lamuela-Raventos, R.M., Estruch, R., 2013. Effects of wine, alcohol and polyphenols on cardiovascular disease risk factors: evidences from human studies. Alcohol Alcohol. 1464-3502. 48 (3), 270–277. doi:10.1093/alcalc/agt007.

Chiva-Blanch, G., Magraner, E., Condines, X., Valderas-Martínez, P., Roth, I., Arranz, S., Casas, R., Navarro, M., Hervas, A., Sisó, A., Martínez-Huélamo, M., Vallverdú-Queralt, A., Quifer-Rada, P., Lamuela-Raventos, R.M., Estruch, R., 2015. Effects of alcohol and polyphenols from beer on atherosclerotic biomarkers in high cardiovascular risk men: a randomized feeding trial. Nutr. Metab. Cardiovasc. Dis. 09394753. 25 (1), 36–45. doi:10.1016/j.numecd.2014.07.008.

Choleva, M., Argyrou, C., Detopoulou, M., Donta, M.-E., Gerogianni, A., Moustou, E., Papaemmanouil, A., Skitsa, C., Kolovou, G., Kalogeropoulos, P., Fragopoulou, E., 2022. Effect of moderate wine consumption on oxidative stress markers in coronary heart disease patients. Nutrients. 2072-6643. 14 (7), 1377. doi:10.3390/nu14071377.

Choleva, M., Boulougouri, V., Panara, A., Panagopoulou, E., Chiou, A., Thomaidis, N.S., Antonopoulou, S., Fragopoulou, E., 2019. Evaluation of anti-platelet activity of grape pomace extracts. Food Funct. 2042650X. 10 (12), 8069–8080. Available from: http://pubs.rsc.org/en/journals/journal/fo. doi:10.1039/c9fo02138h.

Choleva, M., Matalliotaki, E., Antoniou, S., Asimomyti, E., Drouka, A., Stefani, M., Yannakoulia, M., Fragopoulou, E., 2023. Postprandial metabolic and oxidative stress responses to grape pomace extract in healthy normal and overweight/obese women: a randomized, double-blind, placebo-controlled crossover study. Nutrients. 2072-6643. 15 (1), 156. doi:10.3390/nu15010156.

Choleva, M., Tsota, M., Boulougouri, V., Panara, A., Thomaidis, N.S., Antonopoulou, S., Fragopoulou, E., 2020. Anti-platelet and anti-inflammatory properties of an ethanol-water red grape pomace extract. Proc. Nutr. Soc. 0029-6651. 79 (OCE2). doi:10.1017/s0029665120003183.

Chowdhary, P., Gupta, A., Gnansounou, E., Pandey, A., Chaturvedi, P., 2021. Current trends and possibilities for exploitation of Grape pomace as a potential source for value addition. Environ. Pollut. 02697491. 278, 116796. doi:10.1016/j.envpol.2021.116796.

Costa, J.M., Wang, W., Nakasu, P.Y.S., Changwei, H., Forster-Carneiro, T., Hallett, J.P., 2025. Impacts of microwaves on the pectin extraction from apple pomace: technological properties in structuring of hydrogels. Food Hydrocoll. 0268005X. 160, 110766. doi:10.1016/j.foodhyd.2024.110766.

Cruciani, S., Trenta, M., Rassu, G., Garroni, G., Petretto, G.L., Ventura, C., Maioli, M., Pintore, G., 2021. Identifying a role of red and white wine extracts in counteracting skin aging: effects of antioxidants on fibroblast behavior. Antioxidants. 2076-3921. 10 (2), 227. doi:10.3390/antiox10020227.

Čuš, F., Baša Česnik, H., Velikonja Bolta, Š., Gregorčič, A., 2010. Pesticide residues in grapes and during vinification process. Food Control. 09567135. 21 (11), 1512–1518. doi:10.1016/j.foodcont.2010.04.024.

Da Porto, C., Natolino, A., 2024. Policosanols from grape marc: a new step towards a sustainable biorefinery for the wine industry by SC-CO2 extraction. J. CO2 Util. 22129820. 82, 102762. doi:10.1016/j.jcou.2024.102762.

Da Porto, C., Porretto, E., Decorti, D., 2013. Comparison of ultrasound-assisted extraction with conventional extraction methods of oil and polyphenols from grape (*Vitis vinifera* L.) seeds. Ultrason. Sonochem. 13504177. 20 (4), 1076–1080. doi:10.1016/j.ultsonch.2012.12.002.

da Silva, L.C., Viganó, J., de Souza Mesquita, L.M., Dias, A.L.B., de Souzade Souza, M.C., Sanches, V.L., Chaves, J.O., Pizani, R.S., Contieri, L.S., Rostagno, M.A., 2021. Recent advances and trends in extraction techniques to recover polyphenols compounds from apple by-products. Food Chem. X. 25901575. 12. Available from: https://www.journals.elsevier.com/food-chemistry-x. doi:10.1016/j.fochx.2021.100133.

de Gaetano, G., Costanzo, S., Di Castelnuovo, A., Badimon, L., Bejko, D., Alkerwi, A., Chiva-Blanch, G., Estruch, R., Vecchia, C.L., Panico, S., Pounis, G., Sofi, F., Stranges, S., Trevisan, M., Ursini, F., Cerletti, C., Donati, M.B., Iacoviello, L., 2016. Effects of moderate beer consumption on health and disease: a consensus document. Nutr. Metab. Cardiovasc. Dis.. 09394753. 26 (6), 443–467. doi:10.1016/j.numecd.2016.03.007.

Di Lorenzo, R., Maisto, M., Ricci, L., Piccolo, V., Marzocchi, A., Greco, G., Tenore, G.C., Laneri, S., 2024. Annurca apple oleolite as functional ingredient for the formulation of cosmetics with skin-antiaging activity. Int. J. Mol. Sci. 1422-0067. 25 (3), 1677. doi:10.3390/ijms25031677.

Di Stefano, V., Buzzanca, C., Melilli, M.G., Indelicato, S., Mauro, M., Vazzana, M., Arizza, V., Lucarini, M., Durazzo, A., Bongiorno, D., 2022. Polyphenol characterization and antioxidant activity of grape seeds and skins from Sicily: a preliminary study. Sustainability. 2071-1050. 14 (11), 6702. doi:10.3390/su14116702.

Diaconeasa, Z., Ayvaz, H., Rugină, D., Leopold, L., Stănilă, A., Socaciu, C., Tăbăran, F., Luput, L., Mada, D.C., Pintea, A., Jefferson, A., 2017. Melanoma inhibition by anthocyanins is associated with the reduction of oxidative stress biomarkers and changes in mitochondrial membrane potential. Plant Foods Hum. Nutr. 0921-9668. 72 (4), 404–410. doi:10.1007/s11130-017-0638-x.

Drevelegka, I., Goula, A.M., 2020. Recovery of grape pomace phenolic compounds through optimized extraction and adsorption processes. Chem. Eng. Process. 02552701. 149, 107845. doi:10.1016/j.cep.2020.107845.

Drosou, C., Kyriakopoulou, K., Bimpilas, A., Tsimogiannis, D., Krokida, M., 2015. A comparative study on different extraction techniques to recover red grape pomace polyphenols from vinification byproducts. Ind. Crops Prod. 09266690. 75, 141–149. doi:10.1016/j.indcrop.2015.05.063.

Duba, K.S., Casazza, A.A., Mohamed, H.B., Perego, P., Fiori, L., 2015. Extraction of polyphenols from grape skins and defatted grape seeds using subcritical water: experiments and modeling. Food Bioprod. Process. 09603085. 94, 29–38. Available from: http://www.elsevier.com/wps/find/journaldescription.cws_home/713883/description#description. doi:10.1016/j.fbp.2015.01.001.

Fărcaş, A.C., Ancuţa Socaci, S., Mudura, E., Dulf, F.V., Vodnar, D.C., Tofană, M., Salanţă, L.C., 2017. Exploitation of Brewing Industry Wastes to Produce Functional Ingredients. InTech. doi:10.5772/intechopen.69231.

Fernandes, I., Pérez-Gregorio, R., Soares, S., Mateus, N., De Freitas, V., 2017. Wine flavonoids in health and disease prevention. Molecules. 1420-3049. 22 (2), 292. doi:10.3390/molecules22020292.

Ferreira, M.R., Garzón, A.G., Oliva, M.E., Cian, R.E., Drago, S.R., D'Alessandro, M.E., 2022. Lipid-lowering effect of microencapsulated peptides from brewer's spent grain in high-sucrose diet-fed rats. Food Biosci. 22124292. 49, 101981. doi:10.1016/j.fbio.2022.101981.

Ferreira, S.M., Santos, L., 2022. A potential valorization strategy of wine industry by-products and their application in cosmetics—case study: grape pomace and grapeseed. Molecules. 1420-3049. 27 (3), 969. doi:10.3390/molecules27030969.

Fragopoulou, E., Antonopoulou, S., 2020. The French paradox three decades later: role of inflammation and thrombosis. Clin. Chim. Acta. 00098981. 510, 160–169. doi:10.1016/j.cca.2020.07.013.

Fragopoulou, E., Antonopoulou, S., Demopoulos, C.A., 2002. Biologically active lipids with antiatherogenic properties from white wine and must. J. Agric. Food Chem. 00218561. 50 (9), 2684–2694. doi:10.1021/jf011288u.

Fragopoulou, E., Argyrou, C., Detopoulou, M., Tsitsou, S., Seremeti, S., Yannakoulia, M., Antonopoulou, S., Kolovou, G., Kalogeropoulos, P., 2021. The effect of moderate wine consumption on cytokine secretion by peripheral blood mononuclear cells: a randomized clinical study in coronary heart disease patients. Cytokine. 10434666. 146, 155629. doi:10.1016/j.cyto.2021.155629.

Fragopoulou, E., Choleva, M., Antonopoulou, S., Demopoulos, C.A., 2018. Wine and its metabolic effects. A comprehensive review of clinical trials. Metabolism. 00260495. 83, 102–119. doi:10.1016/j.metabol.2018.01.024.

Fragopoulou, E., Demopoulos, C.A., Antonopoulou, S., 2009. Lipid minor constituents in wines. A biochemical approach in the French paradox. Int. J. Wine Res. 11791403. 1 (1), 131–143. Available from: http://www.dovepress.com/getfile.php?fileID=4644. doi:10.2147/IJWR.S4587Greece.

Fragopoulou, E., Nomikos, T., Karantonis, H.C., Apostolakis, C., Pliakis, E., Samiotaki, M., Panayotou, G., Antonopoulou, S., 2007. Biological activity of acetylated phenolic compounds. J. Agric. Food Chem. 00218561. 55 (1), 80–89. doi:10.1021/jf0627221.

Fukizawa, S., Yamashita, M., Wakabayashi, K.-I., Fujisaka, S., Tobe, K., Nonaka, Y., Murayama, N., 2020. Anti-obesity effect of a hop-derived prenylflavonoid isoxanthohumol in a high-fat diet-induced obese mouse model. Biosci. Microbiota Food Health. 2186-3342. 39 (3), 175–182. doi:10.12938/bmfh.2019-040.

Fukuda, T., Obara, K., Saito, J., Umeda, S., Ano, Y., 2020. Effects of hop bitter acids, bitter components in beer, on cognition in healthy adults: a randomized controlled trial. J. Agric. Food Chem. 0021-8561. 68 (1), 206–212. doi:10.1021/acs.jafc.9b06660.

Gado, F., Ferrario, G., Vedova, L.D., Zoanni, B., Altomare, A., Carini, M., Aldini, G., D'Amato, A., Baron, G., 2023. Targeting Nrf2 and NF-κB signaling pathways in cancer prevention: the role of apple phytochemicals. Molecules. 1420-3049. 28 (3), 1356. doi:10.3390/molecules28031356.

Garcia, S.R., Orellana-Palacios, J.C., McClements, D.J., Moreno, A., Hadidi, M., 2024. Sustainable proteins from wine industrial by-product: ultrasound-assisted extraction, fractionation, and characterization. Food Chem. 03088146. 455, 139743. doi:10.1016/j.foodchem.2024.139743.

Gasparini, A., Ferrentino, G., Angeli, L., Morozova, K., Zatelli, D., Scampicchio, M., 2023. Ultrasound assisted extraction of oils from apple seeds: a comparative study with supercritical fluid and conventional solvent extraction. Innov. Food Sci. Emerg. Technol. 14668564. 86, 103370. doi:10.1016/j.ifset.2023.103370.

Gil-Martín, E., Forbes-Hernández, T., Romero, A., Cianciosi, D., Giampieri, F., Battino, M., 2022. Influence of the extraction method on the recovery of bioactive phenolic compounds from food industry by-products. Food Chem. 03088146. 378, 131918. doi:10.1016/j.foodchem.2021.131918.

Gordon, R., Power, A., Chapman, J., Chandra, S., Cozzolino, D., 2018. A review on the source of lipids and their interactions during beer fermentation that affect beer quality. Fermentation. 2311-5637. 4 (4), 89. doi:10.3390/fermentation4040089.

Hejna, A., Aniśko, J., Skórczewska, K., Barczewski, M., Sulima, P., Przyborowski, J.A., Cieśliński, H., Marć, M., 2024. Brewers' spent grain from different types of malt: a comprehensive evaluation of appearance, structure, chemical composition, antimicrobial activity, and volatile emissions. SSRN 15565068. Available from: https://www.ssrn.com/index.cfm/en/. doi:10.2139/ssrn.4907864.

Herbst, G., Hamerski, F., Errico, M., Corazza, M.L., 2021. Pressurized liquid extraction of brewer's spent grain: kinetics and crude extracts characterization. J. Ind. Eng. Chem. 1226086X. 102, 370–383. doi:10.1016/j.jiec.2021.07.020.

Hou, X., Zhiyi, X., Zhao, Y., Liu, D., 2020. Rapid analysis and residue evaluation of six fungicides in grape wine-making and drying. J. Food Compos. Anal. 08891575. 89, 103465. doi:10.1016/j.jfca.2020.103465.

Humia, B.V., Santos, K.S., Barbosa, A.M., Sawata, M., Mendonça, M.D.C., Padilha, F.F., 2019. Beer molecules and its sensory and biological properties: a review. Molecules 14203049. 24 (8). Available from: https://www.mdpi.com/1420-3049/24/8/1568/pdf. doi:10.3390/molecules24081568.

Ikram, S., Huang, L., Zhang, H., Wang, J., Yin, M., 2017. Composition and nutrient value proposition of brewers' spent grain. J. Food Sci. 0022-1147. 82 (10), 2232–2242. doi:10.1111/1750-3841.13794.

Ilyas, T., Chowdhary, P., Chaurasia, D., Gnansounou, E., Pandey, A., Chaturvedi, P., 2021. Sustainable green processing of grape pomace for the production of value-added products: an overview. Environ. Technol. Innov. 23521864. 23, 101592. doi:10.1016/j.eti.2021.101592.

Ito, S., Nagata, K., 2017. Biology of Hsp47 (Serpin H1), a collagen-specific molecular chaperone. Semin. Cell Dev. Biol. 10849521. 62, 142–151. doi:10.1016/j.semcdb.2016.11.005.

Jeong, J.H., Jung, H., Lee, S.R., Lee, H.J., Hwang, K.T., Kim, T.Y., 2010. Anti-oxidant, anti-proliferative and anti-inflammatory activities of the extracts from black raspberry fruits and wine. Food Chem. 03088146. 123 (2), 338–344. doi:10.1016/j.foodchem.2010.04.040.

Juice Beauty, n.d. Green Apple Protein Conditioner. https://juicebeauty.com/products/green-apple-conditioner

Kalinowska, M., Bielawska, A., Lewandowska-Siwkiewicz, H., Priebe, W., Lewandowski, W., 2014. Apples: content of phenolic compounds vs. variety, part of apple and cultivation model, extraction of phenolic compounds, biological properties. Plant Physiol. Biochem. 09819428. 84, 169–188. doi:10.1016/j.plaphy.2014.09.006.

Kandemir, K., Piskin, E., Xiao, J., Tomas, M., Capanoglu, E., 2022. Fruit juice industry wastes as a source of bioactives. J. Agric. Food Chem. 0021-8561. 70 (23), 6805–6832. doi:10.1021/acs.jafc.2c00756.

Kao, T.-H., 2018. Health Potential for Beer Brewing Byproducts. IntechOpen. doi:10.5772/intechopen.76126.

Karabín, M., Hudcová, T., Jelínek, L., Dostálek, P., 2016. Biologically active compounds from hops and prospects for their use. Compr. Rev. Food Sci. Food Saf. 1541-4337. 15 (3), 542–567. doi:10.1111/1541-4337.12201.

Karantonis, H.C., Tsoupras, A., Moran, D., Zabetakis, I., Nasopoulou, C., 2023. Olive, Apple, and Grape Pomaces with Antioxidant and Anti-inflammatory Bioactivities for Functional Foods. Elsevier BV, pp. 131–159. doi:10.1016/b978-0-12-823811-0.00007-9.

Kim, E.O., Min, K.J., Kwon, T.K., Um, B.H., Moreau, R.A., Choi, S.W., 2012. Anti-inflammatory activity of hydroxycinnamic acid derivatives isolated from corn bran in lipopolysaccharide-stimulated Raw 264.7 macrophages. Food Chem. Toxicol. 18736351. 50 (5), 1309–1316. doi:10.1016/j.fct.2012.02.011.

Kontaxi, N.-I., Panoutsopoulou, E., Ofrydopolou, A., Tsoupras, A., 2024. Anti-inflammatory benefits of grape pomace and tomato bioactives as ingredients in sun oils against UV radiation for skin protection. Appl. Sci. 2076-3417. 14 (14), 6236. doi:10.3390/app14146236.

Koseoğlu, A., Al-Taie, A., 2022. The potential chemo-preventive roles of Malus domestica against the risk of colorectal cancer: a suggestive insight into clinical application. Clin. Nutr. ESPEN. 24054577. 52, 360–364. doi:10.1016/j.clnesp.2022.09.017.

Krbečková, V., Plachá, D., 2024. Raw biowaste conversion to high-value compounds for food, cosmetic and pharmaceutical industries. Environ. Res. 00139351. 263 (Pt 2), 120134. doi:10.1016/j.envres.2024.120134.

KUNDAL, n.d. Beer Yeast Hair Loss Relief Shampoo 300ml * 2EA. https://kundal.us/products/beer-yeast-hair-loss-relief-shampoo-300ml-herb-mint.

Kunzmann, A.T., Coleman, H.G., Huang, W.Y., Berndt, S.I., 2018. The association of lifetime alcohol use with mortality and cancer risk in older adults: a cohort study. PLoS Med. 15491676. 15 (6). Available from: http://medicine.plosjournals.org/perlserv/?request=index-html&issn=1549-1676. doi:10.1371/journal.pmed.1002585.

Kupe, M., Karatas, N., Unal, M.S., Ercisli, S., Baron, M., Sochor, J., 2021. Phenolic composition and antioxidant activity of peel, pulp and seed extracts of different clones of the Turkish grape cultivar 'Karaerik'. Plants. 2223-7747. 10 (10), 2154. doi:10.3390/plants10102154.

Laaksonen, O., Kuldjärv, R., Paalme, T., Virkki, M., Yang, B., 2017. Impact of apple cultivar, ripening stage, fermentation type and yeast strain on phenolic composition of apple ciders. Food Chem. 03088146. 233, 29–37. doi:10.1016/j.foodchem.2017.04.067.

Lago-Vanzela, E., Alves Baffi, M., Castilhos, M., Ribeiro-Pinto, M., Del Bianchi, V., Ramos, A., et al., 2014. Phenolic compounds in grapes and wines: chemical and biochemical characteristics and technological quality. In: Câmara, J.S. (Ed.), Grapes: Production, Phenolic Composition and Potential Biomedical Effects, first ed. Nova Science Publishers Inc., pp. 47–106 (Chapter 3).

Leal, C., Gouvinhas, I., Santos, R.A., Rosa, E., Silva, A.M., José Saavedra, M., Barros, A.I.R.N.A., 2020. Potential application of grape (*Vitis vinifera* L.) stem extracts in the cosmetic and pharmaceutical industries: valorization of a by-product. Ind. Crops Prod. 09266690. 154, 112675. doi:10.1016/j.indcrop.2020.112675.

Lei, X., Yang, S., Wang, K., Anjing, L., Wang, X., Zhenzhen, X., 2022. Impact of clarified apple juices with different processing methods on gut microbiota and metabolomics of rats. Nutrients. 2072-6643. 14 (17), 3488. doi:10.3390/nu14173488.

Letsiou, S., Kapazoglou, A., Tsaftaris, A., Spanidi, E., Gardikis, K., 2020. Transcriptional and epigenetic effects of *Vitis vinifera* L. leaf extract on UV-stressed human dermal fibroblasts. Mol. Biol. Rep. 0301-4851. 47 (8), 5763–5772. doi:10.1007/s11033-020-05645-7.

Li, Y., Skouroumounis, G.K., Elsey, G.M., Taylor, D.K., 2011. Microwave-assistance provides very rapid and efficient extraction of grape seed polyphenols. Food Chem. 18737072. 129 (2), 570–576. doi:10.1016/j.foodchem.2011.04.068.

Lingua, M.S., Fabani, M.P., Wunderlin, D.A., Baroni, M.V., 2016. From grape to wine: changes in phenolic composition and its influence on antioxidant activity. Food Chem. 18737072. 208, 228–238. Available from: https://www.elsevier.com/locate/foodchem. doi:10.1016/j.foodchem.2016.04.009.

Llavata, B., Picinelli, A., Simal, S., Cárcel, J.A., 2022. Cider apple pomace as a source of nutrients: evaluation of the polyphenolic profile, antioxidant and fiber properties after drying process at different temperatures. Food Chem. X. 25901575. 15, 100403. doi:10.1016/j.fochx.2022.100403.

Lordan, R., O'Keeffe, E., Dowling, D., Mullally, M., Heffernan, H., Tsoupras, A., Zabetakis, I., 2019a. The in vitro antithrombotic properties of ale, lager, and stout beers. Food Biosci. 22124292. 28, 83–88. doi:10.1016/j.fbio.2019.01.012.

Lordan, R., O'Keeffe, E., Tsoupras, A., Zabetakis, I., 2019b. Total, neutral, and polar lipids of brewing ingredients, by-products and beer: evaluation of antithrombotic activities. Foods. 2304-8158. 8 (5), 171. doi:10.3390/foods8050171.

Lynch, K.M., Steffen, E.J., Arendt, E.K., 2016. Brewers' spent grain: a review with an emphasis on food and health. J. Inst. Brew. 20500416. 122 (4), 553–568. Available from: http://onlinelibrary.wiley.com/journal/10.1002/(ISSN)2050-0416. doi:10.1002/jib.363.

Lyu, F., Luiz, S.F., Azeredo, D.R.P., Cruz, A.G., Ajlouni, S., Ranadheera, C.S., 2020. Apple pomace as a functional and healthy ingredient in food products: a review. Processes 22279717. 8 (3). Available from: https://res.mdpi.com/d_attachment/processes/processes-08-00319/article_deploy/processes-08-00319.pdf. doi:10.3390/pr8030319.

Magalhães, P.J., Carvalho, D.O., Cruz, J.M., Guido, L.F., Barros, A.A., 2009. Fundamentals and health benefits of xanthohumol, a natural product derived from hops and beer. Nat. Prod. Commun. 15559475. 4 (5), 591–610. Available from: http://members.naturalproduct.us/Secure/ViewDoc.aspx?docId=1952. doi:10.1177/1934578x0900400501.

Maisto, M., Piccolo, V., Novellino, E., Schiano, E., Iannuzzo, F., Ciampaglia, R., Summa, V., Tenore, G.C., 2023. Optimization of ursolic acid extraction in oil from Annurca apple to obtain oleolytes with potential cosmeceutical application. Antioxidants. 2076-3921. 12 (2), 224. doi:10.3390/antiox12020224.

Marabini, L., Melzi, G., Lolli, F., Dell'Agli, M., Piazza, S., Sangiovanni, E., Marinovich, M., 2020. Effects of *Vitis vinifera* L. leaves extract on UV radiation damage in human keratinocytes (HaCaT). J. Photochem. Photobiol. B. 10111344. 204, 111810. doi:10.1016/j.jphotobiol.2020.111810.

Massias, A., Boisard, S., Baccaunaud, M., F.L. Calderon, Subra-Paternault, P., 2015. Recovery of phenolics from apple peels using CO2+ethanol extraction: kinetics and antioxidant activity of extracts. J. Supercrit. Fluids. 08968446. 98, 172–182. doi:10.1016/j.supflu.2014.12.007.

Mathew, S., Abraham, T.E., Zakaria, Z.A., 2015. Reactivity of phenolic compounds towards free radicals under in vitro conditions. J. Food Sci. Technol. 09758402. 52 (9), 5790–5798. Available from: http://www.springerlink.com/content/121580/. doi:10.1007/s13197-014-1704-0.

Matos, M.S., Romero-Díez, R., Álvarez, A., Bronze, M.R., Rodríguez-Rojo, S., Mato, R.B., Cocero, M.J., Matias, A.A., 2019. Polyphenol-rich extracts obtained from winemakingwaste streams as natural ingredients with cosmeceutical potential. Antioxidants 20763921. 8 (9). Available from: https://www.mdpi.com/2076-3921/8/9/355/pdf. doi:10.3390/antiox8090355.

McCarthy, A.L., O'Callaghan, Y.C., Piggott, C.O., FitzGerald, R.J., O'Brien, N.M., 2013. Brewers' spent grain; Bioactivity of phenolic component, its role in animal nutrition and potential for incorporation in functional foods: a review. Proc. Nutr. Soc. 14752719. 72 (1), 117–125. doi:10.1017/S0029665112002820.

Merten, D., Erman, L., Marabelli, G.P., Leners, B., Ney, Y., Nasim, M.J., Jacob, C., Tchoumtchoua, J., Cajot, S., Bohn, T., 2022. Potential health effects of brewers' spent grain as a functional food ingredient assessed by markers of oxidative stress and inflammation following gastro-intestinal digestion and in a cell model of the small intestine. Food Funct. 2042650X. 13 (9), 5327–5342. Available from: http://pubs.rsc.org/en/journals/journal/fo. doi:10.1039/d1fo03090f.

MohdMaidin, N., Oruna-Concha, M.J., Jauregi, P., 2019. Surfactant TWEEN20 provides stabilisation effect on anthocyanins extracted from red grape pomace. Food Chem. 18737072. 271, 224–231. Available from: https://www.elsevier.com/locate/foodchem. doi:10.1016/j.foodchem.2018.07.083.

Moncalvo, A., Marinoni, L., Dordoni, R., Garrido, G.D., Lavelli, V., Spigno, G., 2016. Waste grape skins: evaluation of safety aspects for the production of functional powders and extracts for the food sector. Food Addit. Contam. Part A. 1944-0049. 33 (7), 1116–1126. doi:10.1080/19440049.2016.1191320.

Moran, D., Fleming, M., Daly, E., Gaughan, N., Zabetakis, I., Traas, C., Tsoupras, A., 2021. Anti-platelet properties of apple must/skin yeasts and of their fermented apple cider products. Beverages. 2306-5710. 7 (3), 54. doi:10.3390/beverages7030054.

Morimoto-Kobayashi, Y., Ohara, K., Ashigai, H., Kanaya, T., Koizumi, K., Manabe, F., Kaneko, Y., Taniguchi, Y., Katayama, M., Kowatari, Y., Kondo, S., 2016. Matured hop extract reduces body fat in healthy overweight humans: a randomized, double-blind, placebo-controlled parallel group study. Nutr. J. 14752891. 15 (1). Available from: http://www.nutritionj.com/home/. doi:10.1186/s12937-016-0144-2.

Nardini, M., 2023. An overview of bioactive phenolic molecules and antioxidant properties of beer: emerging trends. Molecules. 1420-3049. 28 (7), 3221. doi:10.3390/molecules28073221.

NEOGENLAB Global, n.d. NEOGEN Dermalogy Bio-Peel Gauze Peeling Wine 200ml (30 Pads). https://neogenlab.co/products/neogen-bio-peel-gauze-peeling-wine.

Neto, J.R.O., de Oliveira, T.S., Ghedini, P.C., Vaz, B.G., Gil, E.D.S., 2017. Antioxidant and vasodilatory activity of commercial beers. J. Funct. Foods 17564646. 34, 130–138. Available from: http://www.elsevier.com/wps/find/journaldescription.cws_home/717426/description#description. doi:10.1016/j.jff.2017.04.019.

Neumann, H.F., Frank, J., Venturelli, S., Egert, S., 2022. Bioavailability and cardiometabolic effects of xanthohumol: evidence from animal and human studies. Mol. Nutr. Food Res. 1613-4125. 66 (6). doi:10.1002/mnfr.202100831.

Onache, P.A., Geana, E.I., Ciucure, C.T., Florea, A., Sumedrea, D.I., Ionete, R.E., Tița, O., 2022. Bioactive phytochemical composition of grape pomace resulted from different white and red grape cultivars. Separations 22978739. 9 (12). Available from: https://www.mdpi.com/journal/separations. doi:10.3390/separations9120395.

Opriş, O., Lung, I., Soran, M.-L., Stegarescu, A., Cesco, T., Ghendov-Mosanu, A., Podea, P., Sturza, R., 2022. Efficient extraction of total polyphenols from apple and investigation of its SPF properties. Molecules. 1420-3049. 27 (5), 1679. doi:10.3390/molecules27051679.

ORZENE, n.d. Beer Shampoo For Dry and Damaged Hair - Overstressed Series. Orzene Beer. https://www.orzenebeer.com/el/προϊόντα/katallilo-gia-talaiporimena-kai-ftharmena-mallia.

Osei, E.D., Naik, A.S., Kinsella, G., Delaney, T., Kirwan, S., 2025. Potential of Brewer's spent grain bioactive fractions as functional ingredients for companion and farm animal foods – a review. Appl. Food Res. 27725022. 5 (2), 101138. doi:10.1016/j.afres.2025.101138.

Oyenihi, A.B., Belay, Z.A., Mditshwa, A., Caleb, O.J., 2022. "An apple a day keeps the doctor away": the potentials of apple bioactive constituents for chronic disease prevention. Africa J. Food Sci. 17503841. 87 (6), 2291–2309. Available from: http://onlinelibrary.wiley.com/journal/10.1111/(ISSN)1750-3841. doi:10.1111/1750-3841.16155.

Panzella, L., Moccia, F., Nasti, R., Marzorati, S., Verotta, L., Napolitano, A., 2020. Bioactive phenolic compounds from agri-food wastes: an update on green and sustainable extraction methodologies. Front. Nutr. 2296-861X. 7. doi:10.3389/fnut.2020.00060.

Pedro, A.C., Maciel, G.M., Lima, N.P., Lima, N.F., Ribeiro, I.S., Fernandes Pinheiro, D., Haminiuk, C.W.I., 2024. Valorization of bioactive compounds from juice industry waste: applications, challenges, and future prospects. Trends Food Sci. Technol. 09242244. 152, 104693. doi:10.1016/j.tifs.2024.104693.

Pereira, O.R., Santos, G., João Sousa, M., 2022. Hop by-products: pharmacological activities and potential application as cosmetics. Cosmetics. 2079-9284. 9 (6), 139. doi:10.3390/cosmetics9060139.

Perra, M., Lozano-Sánchez, J., Leyva-Jiménez, F.-J., Segura-Carretero, A., Luis Pedraz, J., Bacchetta, G., Muntoni, A., De Gioannis, G., Manca, M.L., Manconi, M., 2021. Extraction of the antioxidant phytocomplex from wine-making by-products and sustainable loading in phospholipid vesicles specifically tailored for skin protection. Biomed. Pharmacother. 07533322. 142, 111959. doi:10.1016/j.biopha.2021.111959.

Perussello, C.A., Zhang, Z., Marzocchella, A., Tiwari, B.K., 2017. Valorization of apple pomace by extraction of valuable compounds. Compr. Rev. Food Sci. Food Saf. 15414337. 16 (5), 776–796. Available from: http://www.interscience.wiley.com/jpages/1541-4337. doi:10.1111/1541-4337.12290.

Pinelo, M., Ruiz-Rodríguez, A., Sineiro, J., Señoráns, F.J., Reglero, G., Núñez, M.J., 2007. Supercritical fluid and solid–liquid extraction of phenolic antioxidants from grape pomace: a comparative study. Eur. Food Res. Technol. 1438-2377. 226 (1-2), 199–205. doi:10.1007/s00217-006-0526-3.

Plantnery, n.d. Plantnery Blue Ceramide Deep Moist UV Vegan Lip Serum 10g. https://en.plantnery.com/product/plantnery-blue-ceramide-deep-moist-uv-vegan-lip-serum-10g/.

Postigo, V., García, M., Crespo, J., Canonico, L., Comitini, F., Ciani, M., 2025. Bioactive properties of fermented beverages: wine and beer. Fermentation. 2311-5637. 11 (5), 234. doi:10.3390/fermentation11050234.

Rachwał, K., Waśko, A., Gustaw, K., Polak-Berecka, M., 2020. Utilization of brewery wastes in food industry. PeerJ. 2167-8359. 8, e9427. doi:10.7717/peerj.9427.

Riekstina-Dolge, R., Kruma, Z., Dimins, F., Straumite, E., Karklina, D., 2014. Phenolic composition and sensory properties of ciders produced from latvian apples. Proc. Latv. Univ. Agric.. 2255-8535. 31 (1), 39–45. doi:10.2478/plua-2014-0005.

Rockenbach, I.I., Rodrigues, E., Gonzaga, L.V., Caliari, V., Genovese, M.I., Gonçalves, A.E.D.S.S., Fett, R., 2011. Phenolic compounds content and antioxidant activity in pomace from selected red grapes (*Vitis vinifera* L. and *Vitis labrusca* L.) widely produced in Brazil. Food Chem. 03088146. 127 (1), 174–179. doi:10.1016/j.foodchem.2010.12.137.

Roldán-López, D., Muñiz-Calvo, S., Daroqui, N., Knez, M., Guillamón, J.M., Pérez-Torrado, R., 2024. The potential role of yeasts in the mitigation of health issues related to beer consumption. Crit. Rev. Food Sci. Nutr. 15497852. 64 (10), 3059–3074. Available from: https://www.tandfonline.com/loi/bfsn20. doi:10.1080/10408398.2022.2129584.

Romanini, E.B., Rodrigues, L.M., Finger, A., Perez Cantuaria Chierrito, T., Regina da Silva Scapim, M., Madrona, G.S., 2021. Ultrasound assisted extraction of bioactive compounds from BRS Violet grape pomace followed by alginate-Ca2+ encapsulation. Food Chem. 03088146. 338, 128101. doi:10.1016/j.foodchem.2020.128101.

Rombaut, N., Savoire, R., Thomasset, B., Castello, J., Van Hecke, E., Lanoisellé, J.L., 2015. Optimization of oil yield and oil total phenolic content during grape seed cold screw pressing. Ind. Crops Prod. 09266690. 63, 26–33. Available from: https://www.elsevier.com/inca/publications/store/5/2/2/8/2/5. doi:10.1016/j.indcrop.2014.10.001.

Rouissi, E., Faucher, M., Turgeon, S.L., Ravallec, R., Mikhaylin, S., 2025. Enhancing the potential of brewer's spent grain utilization in human nutrition through pulsed electric field-assisted protein extraction. Innov. Food Sci. Emerg. Technol. 14668564. 104, 104082. doi:10.1016/j.ifset.2025.104082.

Sabra, A., Netticadan, T., Wijekoon, C., 2021. Grape bioactive molecules, and the potential health benefits in reducing the risk of heart diseases. Food Chem. X. 25901575. 12, 100149. doi:10.1016/j.fochx.2021.100149.

Saito, K., Matsuo, Y., Imafuji, H., Okubo, T., Maeda, Y., Sato, T., Shamoto, T., Tsuboi, K., Morimoto, M., Takahashi, H., Ishiguro, H., Takiguchi, S., 2018. Xanthohumol inhibits angiogenesis by suppressing nuclear factor-κB activation in pancreatic cancer. Cancer Sci. 1347-9032. 109 (1), 132–140. doi:10.1111/cas.13441.

Salanţă, L.C., Coldea, T.E., Ignat, M.V., Pop, C.R., Tofană, M., Mudura, E., Borşa, A., Pasqualone, A., Anjos, O., Zhao, H., 2020. Functionality of special beer processes and potential health benefits. Processes 22279717. 8 (12), 1–21. Available from: https://www.mdpi.com/2227-9717/8/12/1613. doi:10.3390/pr8121613.

Samuels, J.S., Shashidharamurthy, R., Rayalam, S., 2018. Novel anti-obesity effects of beer hops compound xanthohumol: role of AMPK signaling pathway. Nutr. Metab. 1743-7075. 15 (1). doi:10.1186/s12986-018-0277-8.

Schrieks, I.C., van den Berg, R., Sierksma, A., Beulens, J.W.J., Vaes, W.H.J., Hendriks, H.F.J., 2013. Effect of red wine consumption on biomarkers of oxidative stress. Alcohol Alcohol. 14643502. 48 (2), 153–159. doi:10.1093/alcalc/ags086.

Shahidi, F., Ambigaipalan, P., 2015. Phenolics and polyphenolics in foods, beverages and spices: antioxidant activity and health effects – a review. J. Funct. Foods. 17564646. 18, 820–897. doi:10.1016/j.jff.2015.06.018.

Shinohara, K., Ohashi, Y., Kawasumi, K., Terada, A., Fujisawa, T., 2010. Effect of apple intake on fecal microbiota and metabolites in humans. Anaerobe. 10759964. 16 (5), 510–515. doi:10.1016/j.anaerobe.2010.03.005.

Shopska, V., Denkova-Kostova, R., Dzhivoderova-Zarcheva, M., Teneva, D., Denev, P., Kostov, G., 2021. Comparative study on phenolic content and antioxidant activity of different malt types. Antioxidants. 2076-3921. 10 (7), 1124. doi:10.3390/antiox10071124.

Silva, S., Oliveira, A.I., Cruz, A., Oliveira, R.F., Almeida, R., Pinho, C., 2022. Physicochemical properties and antioxidant activity of portuguese craft beers and raw materials. Molecules. 1420-3049. 27 (22), 8007. doi:10.3390/molecules27228007.

Sokač, T., Gunjević, V., Pušek, A., Tušek, A.J., Dujmić, F., Brnčić, M., Ganić, K.K., Jakovljević, T., Uher, D., Mitrić, G., Redovniković, I.R., 2022. Comparison of drying methods and their effect on the stability of graševina grape pomace biologically active compounds. Foods 23048158. 11 (1). Available from: https://www.mdpi.com/2304-8158/11/1/112/pdf. doi:10.3390/foods11010112.

Soldevila-Domenech, N., Boronat, A., Mateus, J., Diaz-Pellicer, P., Matilla, I., Pérez-Otero, M., Aldea-Perona, A., de la Torre, R., 2019. Generation of the antioxidant hydroxytyrosol from tyrosol present in beer and red wine in a randomized clinical trial. Nutrients. 2072-6643. 11 (9), 2241. doi:10.3390/nu11092241.

Somat, H.A., Thani, N.M., Mustapha, W.A.W., Lim, S.J., Seng, N.S.S., Rahman, H.A., Razali, N.S.M., Ali, M.M., Kamal, S.M.M., 2025. Subcritical water extraction of bioactive compounds from plant materials: recent advances. J. Future Foods. 27725669. doi:10.1016/j.jfutfo.2024.10.005.

Steenackers, B., De Cooman, L., De Vos, D., 2015. Chemical transformations of characteristic hop secondary metabolites in relation to beer properties and the brewing process: a review. Food Chem. 03088146. 172, 742–756. doi:10.1016/j.foodchem.2014.09.139.

Stranieri, C., Guzzo, F., Gambini, S., Cominacini, L., Fratta Pasini, A.M., 2022. Intracellular polyphenol wine metabolites oppose oxidative stress and upregulate Nrf2/ARE pathway. Antioxidants. 2076-3921. 11 (10), 2055. doi:10.3390/antiox11102055.

Suárez-Jacobo, A., Rüfer, C.E., Gervilla, R., Guamis, B., Roig-Sagués, A.X., Saldo, J., 2011. Influence of ultra-high pressure homogenisation on antioxidant capacity, polyphenol and vitamin content of clear apple juice. Food Chem. 03088146. 127 (2), 447–454. doi:10.1016/j.foodchem.2010.12.152.

Suárez-Jacobo, A., Saldo, J., Rüfer, C.E., Guamis, B., Roig-Sagués, A.X., Gervilla, R., 2012. Aseptically packaged UHPH-Treated apple juice: safety and quality parameters during storage. J. Food Eng. 02608774. 109 (2), 291–300. Available from: http://www.sciencedirect.com/science/journal/02608774. doi:10.1016/j.jfoodeng.2011.09.007.

Szabó, É., Marosvölgyi, T., Szilágyi, G., Kőrösi, L., Schmidt, J., Csepregi, K., Márk, L., Bóna, Á., 2021. Correlations between total antioxidant capacity, polyphenol and fatty acid content of native grape seed and pomace of four different grape varieties in Hungary. Antioxidants. 2076-3921. 10 (7), 1101. doi:10.3390/antiox10071101.

Team MW, n.d. Apivita Wine Elixir Renewing Lift Night Cream, Κρέμα Νύχτας για Ανανέωση & Lifting 50ml | myPharmacy.gr Online Φαρμακείο. https://www.mypharmacy.gr/apivita-wine-elixir-renewing-lift-night-cream-krema-nykhtas-ghia-anancosi-lifting-50ml-p-15071.

Tomita, J., Mochizuki, S., Fujimoto, S., Kashihara, N., Akasaka, T., Tanimoto, M., Yoshida, K., 2017. Acute improvement of endothelial functions after oral ingestion of isohumulones, bitter components of beer. Biochem. Biophys. Res. Commun. 0006291X. 484 (4), 740–745. doi:10.1016/j.bbrc.2017.01.133.

Trentini, M., Zanolla, I., Zanotti, F., Tiengo, E., Licastro, D., Monego, S.D., Lovatti, L., Zavan, B., 2022. Apple-derived exosomes improve collagen type I production and decrease MMPs during aging of the skin through downregulation of the NF-κB pathway as mode of action. Cells. 2073-4409. 11 (24), 3950. doi:10.3390/cells11243950.

Tseng, A., Zhao, Y., 2012. Effect of different drying methods and storage time on the retention of bioactive compounds and antibacterial activity of wine grape pomace (Pinot Noir and Merlot). J. Food Sci. 17503841. 77 (9), H192. doi:10.1111/j.1750-3841.2012.02840.x.

Tsiapali, O.I., Ayfantopoulou, E., Tzourouni, A., Ofrydopoulou, A., Letsiou, S., Tsoupras, A., 2025b. Unveiling the utilization of grape and winery by-products in cosmetics with health-promoting properties. Appl. Sci. 2076-3417. 15 (3), 1007. doi:10.3390/app15031007.

Tsiapali, O.I., Kontaxi, N.I., Pavlidis, K., Ofrydopoulou, A., Prokopiou, V., Letsiou, S., Kosheleva, R.I., Mitropoulos, A., Tsoupras, A., 2025a. Anti-inflammatory and antioxidant properties of anti-UV creams enriched with natural extracts from avocado, apple, and kiwi by-products, with and without nanobubbles. Cosmetics 20799284. 12 (5). Available from: https://www.mdpi.com/journal/cosmetics. doi:10.3390/cosmetics12050231.

Tsoupras, A.B., Fragopoulou, E., Nomikos, T., Iatrou, C., Antonopoulou, S., Demopoulos, C.A., 2007. Characterization of the de novo biosynthetic enzyme of platelet activating factor, DDT-insensitive cholinephosphotransferase, of human mesangial cells. Mediators Inflamm. 14661861. 2007, 27683. doi:10.1155/2007/27683.

Tsoupras, A., Gkika, D.A., Markopoulos, T., Curran, R., Scallon, C., Karali, M., Kyzas, G.Z., 2024a. Apple products (apple juice and cider) and by-products (apple pomace): bioactive compounds and biological properties. In: Mérillon, J.-M., Riviere, C., Lefèvre, G. (Eds.), Natural Products in Beverages: Botany, Phytochemistry, Pharmacology and Processing. Springer International Publishing, Cham, pp. 1–42. doi:10.1007/978-3-031-04195-2_214-1.

Tsoupras, A., Gkika, D., Markopoulos, T., Voorhout, A., Gurnee, K., Meghwar, P., Kyzas, G., 2024b. Beneficial effects of beer, brewery by-products and their bioactives: potential applications in novel health-promoting products. In: Mérillon, J.M., Riviere, C., Lefèvre, G. (Eds.), Natural Products in Beverages. In: Reference Series in Phytochemistry. Springer Cham, pp. 1–61. doi:10.1007/978-3-031-04195-2_215-1.

Tsoupras, A., Iatrou, C., Frangia, C., Demopoulos, C., 2009. implication of platelet-activating factor in cancer growth and metastasis: potent beneficial role of PAF inhibitors and antioxidants. Infect. Disord. Drug Targets. 18715265. 9 (4), 390–399. doi:10.2174/187152609788922555.

Tsoupras, A., Lordan, R., O'keefe, E., Shiels, K., Saha, S.K., Zabetakis, I., 2020. Structural elucidation of Irish ale bioactive polar lipids with antithrombotic properties. Biomolecules 2218273X. 10 (7), 1–17. Available from: https://www.mdpi.com/2218-273X/10/7/1075/pdf. doi:10.3390/biom10071075.

Tsoupras, A., Lordan, R., Zabetakis, I., 2018. Inflammation, not cholesterol, is a cause of chronic disease. Nutrients. 2072-6643. 10 (5), 604. doi:10.3390/nu10050604.

Tsoupras, A., Moran, D., Byrne, T., Ryan, J., Barrett, L., Traas, C., Zabetakis, I., 2021a. Anti-inflammatory and anti-platelet properties of lipid bioactives from apple cider by-products. Molecules. 1420-3049. 26 (10), 2869. doi:10.3390/molecules26102869.

Tsoupras, A., Moran, D., Lordan, R., Zabetakis, I., 2022. Functional Properties of the Fermented Alcoholic Beverages: Apple Cider and Beer Functional Foods and Their Implications for Health Promotion. Elsevier, Ireland, pp. 319–339. Available from: https://www.sciencedirect.com/book/9780128238110. doi:10.1016/B978-0-12-823811-0.00013-4.

Tsoupras, A., Moran, D., Pleskach, H., Durkin, M., Traas, C., Zabetakis, I., 2021b. Beneficial anti-platelet and anti-inflammatory properties of Irish apple juice and cider bioactives. Foods. 2304-8158. 10 (2), 412. doi:10.3390/foods10020412.

Tsoupras, A., Ni, V.L.J., O'Mahony, É., Karali, M., 2023b. Winemaking: "with one stone, two birds"? A holistic review of the bio-functional compounds, applications and health benefits of wine and wineries' by-products. Fermentation. 2311-5637. 9 (9), 838. doi:10.3390/fermentation9090838.

Tsoupras, A., Panagopoulou, E.A., Kyzas, G.Z., 2024c. Anti-inflammatory, antithrombotic and anti-oxidant bioactives of beer and brewery by-products, as ingredients of bio-functional foods, nutraceuticals, cosmetics, cosmeceuticals and pharmaceuticals with health promoting properties. AIMS Agric. Food. 2471-2086. 9 (2), 568–606. doi:10.3934/agrfood.2024032.

van Bussel, B.C.T., Henry, R.M.A., Schalkwijk, C.G., Dekker, J.M., Nijpels, G., Feskens, E.J.M., Stehouwer, C.D.A., 2018. Alcohol and red wine consumption, but not fruit, vegetables, fish or dairy products, are associated with less endothelial dysfunction and less low-grade inflammation: the Hoorn Study. Eur. J. Nutr. 14366215. 57 (4), 1409–1419. Available from: http://www.springerlink.com/content/1436-6207. doi:10.1007/s00394-017-1420-4.

Vandorou, M., Plakidis, C., Tsompanidou, I.M., Adamantidi, T., Panagopoulou, E.A., Tsoupras, A., 2024. A review on apple pomace bioactives for natural functional food and cosmetic products with therapeutic health-promoting properties. Int. J. Mol. Sci. 1422-0067. 25 (19), 10856. doi:10.3390/ijms251910856.

Vandorou, M., Plakidis, C., Tsompanidou, I.M., Ofrydopoulou, A., Shiels, K., Saha, S.K., Tsoupras, A., 2025. In vitro antioxidant, antithrombotic and anti-inflammatory properties of the amphiphilic bioactives from Greek organic Starking apple juice and its by-products (apple pomace). Appl. Sci. 2076-3417. 15 (5), 2807. doi:10.3390/app15052807.

Vesaghhamedani, S., Ebrahimzadeh, F., Najafi, E., Shabgah, O.G., Askari, E., Shabgah, A.G., Mohammadi, H., Jadidi-Niaragh, F., Navashenaq, J.G., 2022. Xanthohumol: an underestimated, while potent and promising chemotherapeutic agent in cancer treatment. Prog. Biophys. Mol. Biol. 00796107. 172, 3–14. Available from: https://www.elsevier.com/inca/publications/store/4/0/8. doi:10.1016/j.pbiomolbio.2022.04.002.

Vieira, E.F., Carvalho, J., Pinto, E., Cunha, S., Almeida, A.A., Ferreira, I.M.P.L.V.O., 2016. Nutritive value, antioxidant activity and phenolic compounds profile of brewer's spent yeast extract. J. Food Compos. Anal. 08891575. 52, 44–51. Available from: http://www.elsevier.com/inca/publications/store/6/2/2/8/7/8/index.htt. doi:10.1016/j.jfca.2016.07.006.

Visioli, F., Panaite, S.-A., Tomé-Carneiro, J., 2020. Wine's phenolic compounds and health: a pythagorean view. Molecules. 1420-3049. 25 (18), 4105. doi:10.3390/molecules25184105.

Wang, J., Mengqi, L., Zheng, F., Niu, C., Liu, C., Li, Q., Sun, J., 2018. Cell wall polysaccharides: before and after autolysis of brewer's yeast. World J. Microbiol. Biotechnol. 0959-3993. 34 (9). doi:10.1007/s11274-018-2508-6.

Wang, X., Wang, Y., Han, M., Liang, J., Zhang, M., Bai, X., Yue, T., Gao, Z., 2022. Evaluating the changes in phytochemical composition, hypoglycemic effect, and influence on mice intestinal microbiota of fermented apple juice. Food Res. Int. 09639969. 155, 110998. doi:10.1016/j.foodres.2022.110998.

Xanthopoulou, M.N., Kalathara, K., Melachroinou, S., Arampatzi-Menenakou, K., Antonopoulou, S., Yannakoulia, M., Fragopoulou, E., 2017. Wine consumption reduced postprandial platelet sensitivity against platelet activating factor in healthy men. Eur. J. Nutr. 1436-6207. 56 (4), 1485–1492. doi:10.1007/s00394-016-1194-0.

Xiang, H., Sun-Waterhouse, D., Waterhouse, G.I.N., Cui, C., Ruan, Z., 2019. Fermentation-enabled wellness foods: a fresh perspective. Food Sci. Hum. Wellness 22134530. 8 (3), 203–243. Available from: https://www.keaipublishing.com/en/journals/food-science-and-human-wellness/. doi:10.1016/j.fshw.2019.08.003.

Yang, C., Shang, K., Lin, C., Wang, C., Shi, X., Wang, H., Hua, L., 2021. Processing technologies, phytochemical constituents, and biological activities of grape seed oil (GSO): a review. Trends Food Sci. Technol. 09242244. 116, 1074–1083. doi:10.1016/j.tifs.2021.09.011.

Yang, D., Gao, X., 2021. Research progress on the antioxidant biological activity of beer and strategy for applications. Trends Food Sci. Technol. 09242244. 110, 754–764. doi:10.1016/j.tifs.2021.02.048.

Yao, J., Zhang, B., Chunpo, G., Peng, S., Fang, J., 2015. Xanthohumol, a polyphenol chalcone present in hops, activating Nrf2 enzymes to confer protection against oxidative damage in PC12 cells. J. Agric. Food Chem. 0021-8561. 63 (5), 1521–1531. doi:10.1021/jf505075n.

Yen, T.L., Hsu, C.K., Lu, W.J., Hsieh, C.Y., Hsiao, G., Chou, D.S., Wu, G.J., Sheu, J.R., 2012. Neuroprotective effects of xanthohumol, a prenylated flavonoid from hops (humulus lupulus), in ischemic stroke of rats. J. Agric. Food Chem. 15205118. 60 (8), 1937–1944. doi:10.1021/jf204909p.

Yilmaz-Turan, S., Gál, T., Lopez-Sanchez, P., Martinez, M.M., Menzel, C., Vilaplana, F., 2023. Modulating temperature and pH during subcritical water extraction tunes the molecular properties of apple pomace pectin as food gels and emulsifiers. Food Hydrocoll. 0268005X. 145, 109148. doi:10.1016/j.foodhyd.2023.109148.

Zabetakis, I., Lordan, R., Tsoupras, A., 2019. The Impact of Nutrition and Statins on Cardiovascular Diseases the Impact of Nutrition and Statins on Cardiovascular Diseases. Elsevier, Ireland, pp. 1–348. Available from: http://www.sciencedirect.com/science/book/9780128137925. doi:10.1016/C2017-0-00506-2.

Zabetakis, I., Tsoupras, A., Lordan, R., Ramji, D., 2022. Functional Foods and Their Implications for Health Promotion Functional Foods and Their Implications for Health Promotion. Academic Press, pp.1–386. doi:10.1016/C2020-0-00556-6.

Zago, E., Tillier, C., De Leener, G., Nandasiri, R., Delporte, C., Bernaerts, K.V., Shavandi, A., 2022. Sustainable production of low molecular weight phenolic compounds from Belgian Brewers' spent grain. Bioresour. Technol. Rep. 2589014X. 17, 100964. doi:10.1016/j.biteb.2022.100964.

Zheng, Y., Wang, Z., Huang, Y., Wang, H., Xiao, Q., Hui, Y., Huang, X., 2024. Extraction and preparation of cellulose nanocrystal from Brewer's spent grain and application in pickering emulsions. Bioact. Carbohydr. Diet. Fibre. 22126198. 31, 100418. doi:10.1016/j.bcdf.2024.100418.

Further reading

Rongfang, L., Zhu, H., Wenjie, D., Gaopo, L., Zhao, Y., Song, K., Qiu, J., Liu, J., Fang, S., 2025. Effect of ultrasound-assisted extraction combined with enzymatic pretreatment on bioactive compounds, antioxidant capacity and flavor characteristics of grape pulp extracts. Ultrason. Sonochem. 13504177. 121, 107572. doi:10.1016/j.ultsonch.2025.107572.

Chapter 13

Nuts

Theodora Adamantidi[a], Gkentsidis Georgios[a], Evangelia Baltzi[b], and Alexandros Tsoupras[a]
[a]*Hephaestus Laboratory, School of Chemistry, Faculty of Sciences, Democritus University of Thrace, Kavala University Campus, Kavala, Greece*
[b]*Department of Food Science & Technology, School of Agricultural Sciences, University of Patras, Agrinio, Greece*

1 Introduction

Global nut production during the 2022/2023 season reached approximately 56.1 million metric tons, with peanuts dominating, while tree nuts such as almonds, pistachios, cashews, Brazil nuts, hazelnuts, and walnuts contributed a smaller, but economically significant fraction (Alasalvar et al., 2025). Traditionally, nuts have been mainly consumed as raw or processed food ingredients. Nevertheless, their industrial processing generates substantial quantities of by-products. These side streams, such as husks, hulls, shells, skins, septa, and press cakes, are currently recognized as valuable sources of bioactive compounds, including vitamins, minerals, fibers, lignin, proteins, peptides, phenolics, and polysaccharides, rather than low-value waste (Alasalvar et al., 2025; Alara et al., 2021; Lama-Muñoz and Contreras, 2022; Bodoira and Maestri, 2020).

Recent studies highlight that nut constituents exhibit great antioxidant, antimicrobial, and preservative properties, supporting their promising valorization in functional food, cosmetic, cosmeceutical, and pharmaceutical formulations. Beyond their functional activity, these compounds also contribute to product stability, safety, and shelf-life extension, which is particularly relevant for cosmetic and cosmeceutical formulations (Alara et al., 2021; Lama-Muñoz and Contreras, 2022).

To enhance the recovery of valuable constituents, green extraction technologies, such as ultrasound-assisted extraction (UAE) or microwave-assisted extraction (MAE) methods, have been successfully applied to improve the extraction efficiency of phenolics and proteins from walnut husks, hazelnut skins, and/or pistachio shells (Alasalvar et al., 2025; Alara et al., 2021; Lama-Muñoz and Contreras, 2022; Bodoira and Maestri, 2020). In particular, walnut septa and cashew nut shells have emerged as promising sources of polyphenols and bioactive lipids with demonstrated antimicrobial effects. Nut by-products generally represent valuable sources of bioactives, yet their content and stability can be influenced by processing conditions. Certain chemical and thermal treatments, like roasting and skin removal, have notably altered their phytochemical composition, as they, for example, have markedly reduced the phenolic content of nuts, highlighting the urgent need for optimized and mild processing strategies (Taş and Gökmen, 2017).

Nuts are rich in compounds with established health-promoting effects, including vitamin E (α-tocopherol), vitamin K, vitamin B_3 (niacin), ω-3 and ω-6 polyunsaturated fatty acids (PUFAs), phenolic acids (e.g., gallic, vanillic, and chlorogenic acid), and essential minerals such as copper (Rui et al., 2022). Such compounds, which are associated with several health-promoting properties, have attracted vast interest beyond plain nutrition, particularly in the development of cosmetic and cosmeceutical products, as well as nutricosmetics, which involve the oral intake of nutrients to improve skin, hair, and nail health. Research has highlighted their potential roles in antiaging effects, regulation of skin pigmentation, ultraviolet (UV) protection, wound healing, and the management of dermatological conditions such as xerosis and rosacea (Faria-Silva et al., 2020).

Most bioactive compounds present in nuts are concentrated in their oils. For instance, peanut oil contains high levels of essential minerals such as calcium, phosphorus, magnesium, zinc, and iron, alongside its diverse fatty acid profile comprising at least 12 different fatty acids, predominantly oleic and linoleic acid (Alara et al., 2021; Lama-Muñoz and Contreras, 2022). In addition, starch represents another important nut-derived constituent with applications in gel formation and

Biofunctional Cosmetics for Health. https://doi.org/10.1016/B978-0-443-27500-5.00001-0

delivery systems. However, its native form often exhibits instability during storage. To address this limitation, physicochemical and chemical modifications have been employed, while recent advances in nanoparticle-based formulations have further expanded the functional applications of nut and water chestnut starches, particularly in controlled-release cosmetic delivery systems (Kaur et al., 2023).

An alternative approach involves utilizing nut-derived agents for the shelf-life proliferation of many edible products or as natural additives, including their use as colorants, stabilizers, biofilms, antioxidants, and carriers of active compounds (Taş and Gökmen, 2017; Faria-Silva et al., 2020; Echegaray et al., 2018). More recently, attention has shifted toward the incorporation of nut bioactives into active and smart packaging systems, where they can function as deterioration-protective agents, freshness indicators, or sustained-release carriers, and potentially constitute future cosmetic packaging technologies (Matthes and Schmid, 2024).

Despite their nutritional and functional value, the use of nuts is limited due to their well-documented allergenic effects, which affect approximately 1%–3% of the population in Western countries. Another major concern is the contamination of nuts with aflatoxins, secondary metabolites of *Aspergillus* species, which are associated with severe adverse health effects and are recognized as potent carcinogens in both humans and animals (Machado et al., 2025). Furthermore, the processing and refining of nut oils may further introduce hazardous contaminants, including polycyclic aromatic hydrocarbons (PAHs), as well as 3-monochloropropane-1,2-diol esters and glycidyl esters, all of which raise significant food and consumer safety concerns (Zhang and Sun, 2023).

Historically, nut by-products have been primarily utilized as low-value materials, such as natural fertilizers, fuel sources, or animal feed for poultry and livestock. With the growing importance of the circular economy, however, these residues are now being examined as potential renewable raw materials for the production of high-value edible pharmaceuticals, nutraceuticals, and cosmeceuticals, thereby reducing waste and promoting resource efficiency (Çiftçi and Suna, 2022). The most promising fractions include the hulls, shells, skins, and powders of almonds, pistachios, cashews, and walnuts, rich in bioactive compounds (Lama-Muñoz and Contreras, 2022). In parallel, new regulations introduced by the European Union aim to minimize agricultural waste and encourage its reuse as a source of energy and functional nutrients, emphasizing waste management strategies, environmental protection, and human health (Zhang and Sun, 2023).

Among tree nuts, almonds (*Prunus amygdalus*) are the most widely produced globally and contain numerous compounds of cosmetic interest, such as flavonoids and phenolic acids like catechin, vanillic acid, and p-hydroxybenzoic acid. Bioactive fractions are distributed across multiple almond components, including the kernel, hull, brown skin, blanch water, green shell cover, and shell (Dias et al., 2023). Chestnuts (*Fagaceae*) are also produced on a large scale, with China being the leading global producer. Their composition is dominated by starch, followed by proteins, lipids, and phenolics. Although primarily used as food, chestnut-derived agents have demonstrated promising potential in medicinal, material, and cosmetic science (Rui et al., 2022).

The extraction of nut bioactives can be achieved through both conventional and nonconventional methods. Conventional approaches, such as mechanical pressing and solvent extraction, often rely on organic solvents and may raise environmental and safety concerns. In contrast, nonconventional techniques, such as supercritical fluid extraction, enzyme-assisted extraction, carbon dioxide extraction, and ultrasound- or microwave-assisted methods, offer more sustainable alternatives by improving extraction efficacy, preserving bioactivity, and reducing solvent consumption and environmental impact. All afore-mentioned challenges underline the importance of implementing strict quality control, optimized processing technologies, traceability, and risk assessment to ensure the safety of nut-derived products while maximizing their nutritional and functional cosmetic benefits within the principles of clean beauty and sustainable cosmetics (Çiftçi and Suna, 2022; Roselló-Soto et al., 2018).

The aim of this study is to systematically present a comprehensive discussion of major edible nuts and their by-products. Particular emphasis is placed on their nutritional composition and bioactive profiles, followed by an analysis of the most utilized extraction technologies and the factors influencing extraction efficacy. The mechanisms through which these constituents contribute to skin health and biofunctional cosmetic performance are further examined, alongside current commercial cosmetic and cosmeceutical applications based on nut-derived ingredients. Finally, safety concerns, limitations, challenges, and future perspectives are also outlined within the framework of sustainability and circular economy principles. Fig. 13.1 highlights the main key points of this comprehensive review.

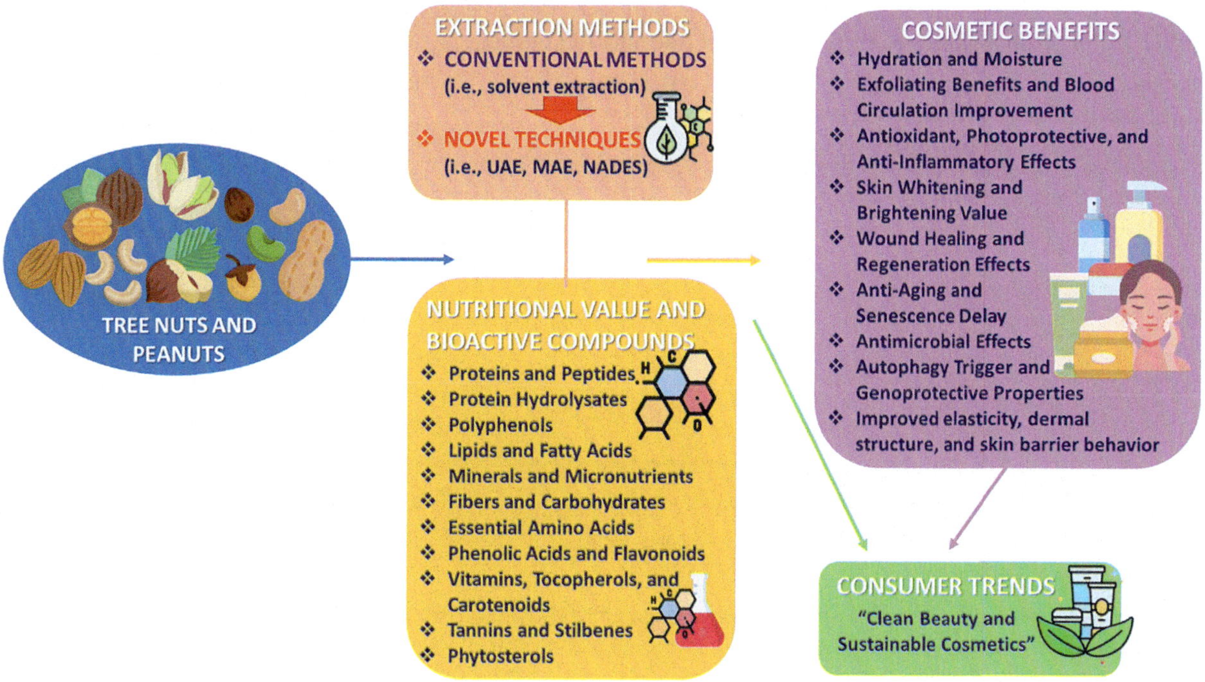

FIG. 13.1 Nut bioactive extraction techniques, pharmacological properties, and cosmetic benefits. *(Parts of this figure were obtained from the open access free platform: https://www.flaticon.com/ (Accessed on January 24, 2026).)*

2 Nutritional composition and bioactive profile of the selected nut extracts

Edible nuts are widely recognized for their high nutritional value and dense energy content. Nuts are an abundant source of a plethora of lipids, proteins, dietary fiber, vitamins, minerals, and various phytochemicals that contribute to their biological activity. Although the exact nut composition mainly varies depending on species, cultivar, geographical origin, and processing conditions, most nuts exhibit relatively similar macronutrient distributions. From a nutritional and culinary standpoint, nuts are divided into two main categories: tree nuts, which grow on trees and include almonds, hazelnuts, chestnuts, cashews, pistachios, Brazil nuts, macadamias, pecans, pine nuts, walnuts, and peanuts (Runner, Spanish, Valencia, and Virginia) (Rui et al., 2022; King et al., 2008; Rico et al., 2016; Polmann et al., 2021). The typical proximate nutritional composition of nuts, regarding their moisture, protein, lipid, ash, carbohydrate, and dietary fiber content of tree nuts and peanuts, is presented in Table 13.1.

Nuts are also significant sources of micronutrients, including vitamin E (particularly α-tocopherol), B-complex vitamins, carotenoids, and minerals such as potassium, magnesium, calcium, zinc, copper, selenium, and iron, compounds mainly concentrated in the skins, shells, and other processing residues. In addition to these nutritional components, nuts contain a wide range of phytochemicals, such as phenolic acids (e.g., hydroxybenzoic and hydroxycinnamic acids), naphthoquinones, lignans, phenolic aldehydes, alkyl phenols, tannins, proanthocyanidins, hydrolysable tannins (e.g., gallotannins, ellagitannins), flavonoids (e.g., flavones, flavonols, flavan-3-ols, flavanones, isoflavones, dihydroflavonols, anthocyanins, anthocyanidins), sterols, fatty acids, stilbenes, amino acids, and terpenoids, which contribute to antioxidant, antiinflammatory, and antimicrobial activities relevant to nutritional, cosmetic, and cosmeceutical applications (Taş and Gökmen, 2017). The main bioactive compounds present in nuts and nut by-products are presented in both Table 13.2 and Fig. 13.2, while a representation of each type of nut rich in bioactives analyzed in this review is presented in Fig. 13.3 (King et al., 2008; Polmann et al., 2021; Bonku and Jianmei, 2020).

TABLE 13.1 Proximate nutritional composition of tree nuts and peanuts.

Nutrient	Tree nut[a]	Peanuts[a]	References
Moisture	1.9–11.4% (~2–10%[a])	~5–10%[a]	(Polmann et al., 2021; Bonku and Jianmei, 2020)
Protein[a]	6.28 (~6–30%[a])	10.07 (~22–34%[a])	(King et al., 2008; Polmann et al., 2021; Bonku and Jianmei, 2020)
Total lipid/fat[a]	26.06 (~45–70%[a])	21.12 (~44–56%[a])	(King et al., 2008; Polmann et al., 2021; Bonku and Jianmei, 2020)
Monounsaturated fatty acids (MUFAs)[a]	13.301 (~20–68%[a])	10.478 (~54%[a])	(King et al., 2008; Polmann et al., 2021)
Polyunsaturated fatty acids (PUFAs)[a]	7.877 (~17–70%[a])	6.674 (~27%[a])	(King et al., 2008; Polmann et al., 2021)
Carbohydrate[a]	7.68 (~7–30%[a])	9.15 (~21–37%[a])	(King et al., 2008; Polmann et al., 2021; Bonku and Jianmei, 2020)
Fiber[a]	3.3 (~3–11%[a])	3.4 (~1.4–3.9%[a])	(King et al., 2008; Polmann et al., 2021; Bonku and Jianmei, 2020)
Ash[a]	~2.0–3.0%[a]	~1.2–2.3%[a]	(Polmann et al., 2021; Bonku and Jianmei, 2020)
Energy[a]	271 (1.14)	249 (1.05)	(King et al., 2008; Polmann et al., 2021)

Nutritional content (g) of 1.5 oz (42 g) of tree nuts or peanuts (mean value of the selected ones).*Kcal (MJ).
[a]*Proximate composition for tree nuts and peanuts in general.*

TABLE 13.2 Bioactive compounds in nuts with potential cosmetic and cosmeceutical applications.

Bioactive compounds	Indicative nut source	Cosmetic and cosmeceutical function	References
Minerals (e.g., iron, magnesium, phosphorus, potassium, sodium, zinc, selenium, copper)	Almonds, Brazil nuts, pecans, cashews, hazelnuts, pine nuts, macadamias, pistachios, walnuts, and peanuts	Skin renewal, antifatigue, cellular metabolism support, soothing, and immunomodulatory effects	(King et al., 2008; Polmann et al., 2021; Bonku and Jianmei, 2020)
Vitamins (e.g., A, B_1, B_2, B_3, B_5, B_6, B_9, B_{12}, C, and E)	Almonds, Brazil nuts, pecans, cashews, hazelnuts, pine nuts, macadamias, pistachios, walnuts, and peanuts	Natural UV filters, antiphotoaging, and antioxidant agents	(King et al., 2008; Polmann et al., 2021; Bonku and Jianmei, 2020)
Carotenoids and pigments (e.g., β-carotene, lycopene, lutein, zeaxanthin, astaxanthin)	Almonds, Brazil nuts, pecans, cashews, hazelnuts, pine nuts, macadamias, pistachios, walnuts, and peanuts	Antiaging, antioxidant, UV protection, skin-protective, colorant, and antipigmentation benefits	(King et al., 2008; Polmann et al., 2021)
Fatty acids (e.g., myristic, palmitic, palmitoleic, stearic, oleic, margaric, linoleic, linolenic, arachidic, gondoic, behenic, paullinic, docosanoic, and lignoceric acids)	Peanuts, grains, nonconventional tree nuts (e.g., Baru, Gurgueia), and tree nuts like almonds, walnuts, pine nuts, pecans, pistachios, Brazil nuts, cashews, and hazelnuts	Moisturizing, skin barrier restoration, antioxidant, antiaging, and antiinflammatory agents	(Polmann et al., 2021; Bonku and Jianmei, 2020)
Essential amino acids (e.g., isoleucine, leucine, valine)	Tree nuts and peanuts	Antiaging, antioxidant, and skin hydration properties	(Polmann et al., 2021)
Phytosterols (e.g., β-sitosterol, brassicasterol, stigmasterol, campesterol, sitostanol, δ5-avenasterol, and δ7-stigmasterol)	Tree nuts and peanuts	Barrier repair, antiinflammatory, antioxidant, immunomodulatory, and antiaging ingredients	(Polmann et al., 2021)

Bioactive compounds	Indicative nut source	Cosmetic and cosmeceutical function	References
Phenolic acids (e.g., *p*-coumaric, ellagic, caffeic, gallic, *p*-hydroxybenzoic, ferulic, salicylic, vanillic, rosmarinic, protocatechuic, gentisic, chlorogenic)	Tree nuts and peanuts	Antioxidant, antiglycation, antiaging, barrier repair, moisturizing, and antiinflammatory properties	(Polmann et al., 2021)
Flavonoids (e.g., total anthocyanins, catechin, epicatechin, gallocatechin, quercetin, myricetin)	Tree nuts and peanuts	Antioxidant, antiglycation, antiaging, barrier repair, moisturizing, and antiinflammatory properties	(Polmann et al., 2021)
Stilbenes (e.g., resveratrol) and tannins	Almonds, Brazil nuts, pecans, cashews, hazelnuts, pine nuts, macadamias, pistachios, walnuts, and peanuts	Moisturizing, barrier repair, antioxidant action, and antiinflammatory effects	(King et al., 2008; Polmann et al., 2021; Bonku and Jianmei, 2020)
Terpenes (e.g., squalene, β-bourbonene, α-calacorene, *p*-cymene, β-pinene, α-terpinene) and terpenoids	Groundnuts (e.g., peanuts) and tree nuts (e.g., walnuts, hickory nuts)	Wound healing, antiinflammatory, structural support, biomimetic emollient, sebum regulation, and moisturizing properties	(King et al., 2008; Polmann et al., 2021; Bonku and Jianmei, 2020; Maestri, 2024; Yan et al., 2024)
Peanut protein hydrolysates	Peanuts	Antihypertensive and antioxidant activities	(Bonku and Jianmei, 2020)

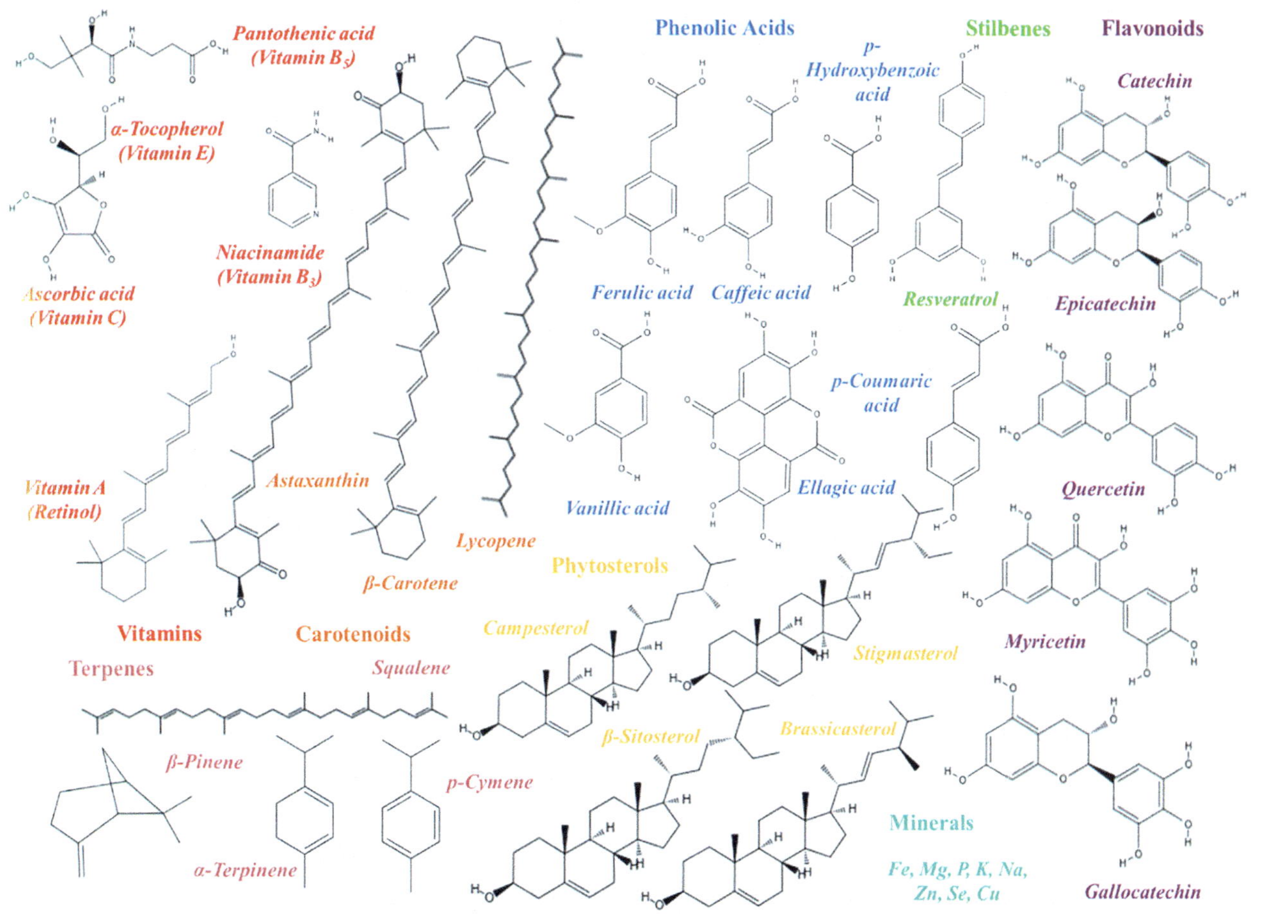

FIG. 13.2 Main representatives of each bioactive class present in nuts and nut by-products. *(Parts of this figure were obtained from the open access free platform: https://www.molview.org/ (Accessed on January 24, 2026).)*

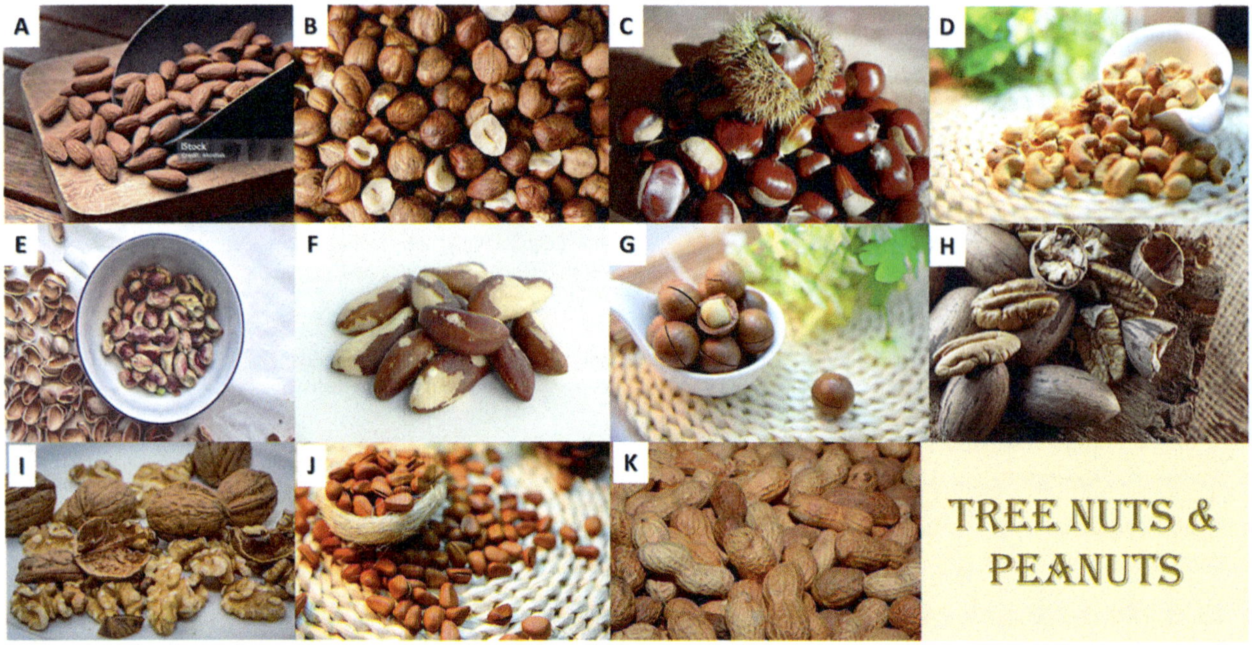

FIG. 13.3 Visual representation of the analyzed nuts: A) almonds, B) hazelnuts, C) sweet chestnuts, D) cashews, E) pistachios, F) Brazil nuts, G) macadamias, H) pecans, I) pine nuts, J) walnuts, and K) peanuts. *(Parts of this figure were obtained from the open access free platform: https://pixabay.com/ (Accessed on January 26, 2026).)*

2.1 Tree nuts bioactive profile and extraction methods

2.1.1 *Almonds (Prunus dulcis and Prunus amygdalus) bioactive profile and extraction methods*

Almond trees are among the most widely cultivated tree nuts worldwide. Almond kernels are rich in lipids, proteins, vitamins, minerals, and polyphenolic compounds, making them nutritionally valuable and attractive for cosmetic and pharmaceutical applications. The almond fruit consists of several anatomical components, including the kernel (meat), middle shell, outer hull, and brown skin, all of which may contain bioactive constituents (Dias et al., 2023; Freitas et al., 2023).

Almonds' chemical composition can vary significantly depending on the geographical origin and cultivar. For example, Kalogiouri et al. (2021) reported that almonds cultivated in Greece exhibited higher total phenolic content (TPC) than those produced in the United States, whereas flavonoid concentrations were higher in American cultivars. Using reversed-phase high-performance liquid chromatography with UV detection, fourteen different phenolic compounds were identified in almond samples (Kalogiouri et al., 2021).

Almonds also contain numerous water-soluble vitamins, including pantothenic acid (B_5), riboflavin (B_2), biotin (B_7), thiamine (B_1), cyanocobalamin (B_{12}), nicotinamide and nicotinic acid (B_3), pyridoxine (B_6), and folic acid (B_9). A rapid, robust liquid chromatography–mass spectrometry method has been developed for the simultaneous quantification of these vitamins and has also been successfully applied to walnuts, hazelnuts, and pistachios (Yilmaz et al., 2023).

Almonds are typically classified into sweet and bitter varieties. Sweet almonds generally exhibit higher antioxidant activity due to their elevated phenolic and flavonoid contents. The kernel also contains essential minerals like iron, manganese, and zinc (El Bernoussi et al., 2024). Storage conditions can notably influence almond quality. For instance, storage at elevated temperatures (60°C) for 4 weeks has been shown to reduce chlorophyll and carotenoid levels by approximately 80%, while tocopherols, sterols, and free fatty acids undergo slower degradation (El Bernoussi et al., 2020).

Proteins and peptides represent an important fraction of almond flour. The major storage proteins, prunin-1 and prunin-2, are components of amandin, the principal almond protein, which is also associated with allergenic responses in sensitive individuals. Protein extraction is commonly achieved using aqueous or enzymatic methods, although enzymatic treatments may lead to protein fragmentation (Dias et al., 2023). Almonds are also widely used for the production of plant-based beverages such as almond milk, which is rich in lipids and proteins. Residual almond cake generated during milk production can be further processed using supercritical extraction with CO_2 to recover valuable compounds. Extracts obtained using this technique have shown low cytotoxicity in human keratinocyte (HaCaT) cell lines, indicating potential suitability for a plethora of cosmetic and cosmeceutical applications (Strieder et al., 2025).

Almond by-products represent between 35% and 75% of the total fruit mass, making them promising sources of bioactive compounds. Almond skin, although often discarded, contains considerable amounts of lipids and phenolic compounds. Its lipid fraction is dominated by oleic acid [monounsaturated fatty acids (MUFAs), ~ 56%], linoleic acid (PUFAs, 34%), and palmitic acid [saturated fatty acids (SFAs), 10%]. In addition, almond skin contains high concentrations of vitamin E, primarily in the form of α-tocopherol (Freitas et al., 2023). Subcritical water extraction (SWE) has been successfully applied to recover phenolic compounds from almond skin, with TPC reaching ~ 3 g gallic acid equivalents (GAE)/100 g of material, demonstrating strong antioxidant capacity (Freitas et al., 2023). Optimal extraction conditions reported include temperatures around 80°C, ethanol concentrations of 70% (v/v), pH 8, and extraction times of ~ 57 min (Olbińska et al., 2023). Under these conditions, extracts showed high antioxidant activity as measured by ferric reducing antioxidant power and 2,2-diphenyl-1-picrylhydrazyl (DPPH) assays (Olbińska et al., 2023).

Supercritical CO_2 extraction can produce high-quality almond oil with strong antioxidant potential, although it may not preserve certain heat-sensitive compounds as effectively as cold-press extraction (Valdés et al., 2022). Conversely, cold-press methods generally produce oils with slightly lower antioxidant activity but better preservation of delicate bioactive molecules. The presence of almond skin during extraction has also been shown to increase overall oil yield (Sayah et al., 2025).

Almond husks are rich in cellulose (~38.48%), hemicellulose (~28.82%), and lignin (~29.54%). MAE has been explored for the production of cellulose nanocrystals from almond husks, offering a faster and more environmentally-friendly alternative to conventional extraction processes (Xuemin et al., 2018; Valdés et al., 2023). Finally, genetic factors appear to influence the fatty acid composition and tocopherol content of almonds more strongly than cultivation conditions. Understanding these genetic variations may enable the development of cultivars optimized for higher antioxidant content and improved suitability for cosmetic and cosmeceutical ingredient production (Zhu et al., 2015).

2.1.2 Hazelnuts (*Corylus avellana*) bioactive profile and extraction methods

Hazelnut is one of the most commercially important and widely available nuts, with Turkey representing the largest global producer. The fruit consists of three main components: the kernel, the skin (testa), and the hard shell. Hazelnuts are particularly valued for their high lipid content and rich phenolic profile (Yilmaz et al., 2023; Bener et al., 2022; Capaldi et al., 2025). Hazelnut kernels contain approximately 60% oil, predominantly composed of MUFAs, particularly oleic acid, along with smaller amounts of linoleic and palmitic acids, lipid fractions that contribute to oxidative stability and moisturizing properties. The kernel also contains several phenolic compounds, including D-(-)-quinic acid, quercetin-3-*O*-glucoside, and gallic acid, which represent some of the most abundant bioactive constituents identified in hazelnut extracts (Bener et al., 2022).

Hazelnuts (*Corylus avellana*) are among the most commercially important tree nuts worldwide, with major production recorded in Turkey, Italy, and the United States. Hazelnut kernels possess a high nutritional value, typically composed of 62% fat, mostly in the form of oleic (78.1%–84.7%) and linoleic acid (5.35%–14%), 16% protein, 11% carbohydrates, 8.7% fiber, several amino acids (e.g., arginine, alanine), 40.6 mg/100 g vitamin E, and 291–875 mg/100 g polyphenols. Meanwhile, the hazelnut skin contains 67.7% fiber, 14.5% fat, 8% protein, 7.5% moisture, 1.7% ash, and ~27% polyphenols (Mohammed et al., 2023; Kurt and Karakaya, 2025).

Hazelnuts and their by-products contain a variety of bioactives, including phenolic acids (e.g., gallic, ferulic, *p*-coumaric, and ellagic acid), flavonoids (e.g., catechin, epicatechin, and rutin), tannins, lignans, phytosterols like campesterol and stigmasterol, squalene, tocopherols, and several vitamins such as B_1, B_2, B_3, B_5, B_6, B_9, and B_{12}, bioactive compounds that play a major role in their antioxidant, antiinflammatory, and skin-protective properties (Zhao et al., 2023).

Green extraction, including MAE, UAE, EAE, pressurized liquid extraction (PLE), green solvent extraction, and other sustainable methods, has been proven to be a really promising technique for the effective isolation of antioxidants from hazelnut by-products. Specifically, UAE and NADES extraction have been successfully applied for the extraction of several tannins, phenolic acids, and flavonoids (e.g., gallic, chlorogenic, and caffeic acid, as well as catechin and kaempferol), which are bioactive agents with remarkable antimicrobial, antioxidant, and skin-protective activity (Zhao et al., 2023).

The recovery of phenolic compounds from hazelnut matrices can be influenced by the complexity of the food matrix, which may hinder solvent penetration and compound release. Therefore the extraction method, operating conditions, and cultivar selection play critical roles in determining extraction efficacy and bioactive yield (Fanali et al., 2018). Moreover, environmental factors may also influence phenolic composition. For instance, flavanol concentrations have been reported to correlate with high solar irradiation during the nuts' growth phase, whereas gallic acid, the most abundant phenolic acid in hazelnut kernels, appears relatively stable across different cultivation conditions (Solar et al., 2022).

Recent studies have highlighted the application of natural deep eutectic solvents (NADES) for the extraction of hazelnut bioactives. NADES are composed of hydrogen bond donors and hydrogen bond acceptors that form eutectic mixtures with melting points lower than those of their individual components. These solvents are considered low-cost, biodegradable, and biocompatible, making them promising alternatives to conventional organic solvents for eco-friendly extraction processes. Hazelnut pomace extracts obtained with NADES have revealed higher antioxidant capacity compared to extracts obtained from hazelnut flour, suggesting that processing residues represent valuable sources (Bener et al., 2022).

Recently, the green extraction of antioxidants from hazelnut by-products using MAE, UAE, and PLE revealed interesting results. The extracts were characterized for their total antioxidant capacity (TAC), free radical scavenging capacity, 2,2'-azino-bis-(3-ethylbenzothiazoline-6-sulfonic acid) (ABTS), and TPC, with gallic acid, catechin, and protocatechuic acid being the predominant isolated phenolics. UAE was the most effective method for hazelnut meal, achieving a TAC of 53.1 μmol trolox (TR)/g, while MAE was the most effective for hazelnut skins, achieving a TAC of 3.12 mmol TR/g (Elmas et al., 2025).

At this point, it must be noted that hazelnut oil is generally considered safe for consumption and topical application; however, large doses of hazelnut oil have been reported to reduce mitochondrial succinate dehydrogenase activity in cellular assays, suggesting potential cytotoxic effects at excessive doses (Ramezan et al., 2023). To date, although numerous bioactive compounds have been identified in hazelnuts, the complete phytochemical profile is still not fully characterized. Recent investigations have isolated two novel acetophenone glycosides from hazelnut kernels with less antioxidant activity in DPPH assays than the control sample (Uchikura et al., 2023).

From a circular economy perspective, the efficient utilization of hazelnut by-products is of increasing interest. Hazelnut processing generates two major by-products: the skin (testa) and the shell. The skin contains high concentrations of tannins and other phenolic compounds that contribute to strong antioxidant activity. Semiindustrial scale SWE of hazelnut skins has demonstrated notable antimicrobial activity against Gram-positive bacteria. Furthermore, the tannin content of these extracts has been positively correlated with antioxidant capacity measured using DPPH, oxygen radical absorbance capacity using fluorescein (ORAC-FL), and iron-chelating assays (Capaldi et al., 2025). Further optimization studies using NADES have exhibited that under optimal conditions (80°C, solid-to-liquid ratio of 35%), up to 18 phenolic acids and flavan-3-ols could be extracted with concentrations ~ 39% higher than those obtained using conventional organic solvents (Fanali et al., 2021).

Beyond the kernel and processing residues, hazelnut leaves have also been investigated as potential sources of bioactive agents. Methanolic extracts of hazelnut leaves have displayed antimicrobial activity, particularly against Gram-positive bacteria. In addition, these extracts have shown potential as photoprotective agents when incorporated into formulations containing benzophenone-3, a commonly used UV filter. The addition of hazelnut leaf extracts has been reported to increase the sun protection factor (SPF) of such formulations (Saglam and Asan-Ozusaglam, 2023). Finally, agricultural waste management practices, like composting of hazelnut leaves, may contribute to improving soil quality and potentially enhancing the phenolic content of subsequent plant growth, highlighting an additional sustainability aspect in hazelnut production systems (Medic et al., 2023).

2.1.3 Sweet chestnut (*Castanea sativa*) bioactive profile and extraction methods

Sweet chestnut (*Castanea sativa*) is widely cultivated in Southern Europe, particularly in Portugal, where it represents an economically important agricultural product. Chestnut processing generates substantial quantities of by-products, mainly shells, burs, fruits, and inner skins, as well as flowers, bark, and leaves, which are increasingly recognized as valuable sources of bioactives. Among these, chestnut shells are particularly rich in polyphenols and other phytochemicals with potential applications in medicine, food, and cosmetics (Echegaray et al., 2018).

Several extraction techniques have been investigated for the recovery of bioactives from chestnut by-products, including SWE, UAE, and supercritical CO_2 extraction. Studies have shown that SWE and UAE produce extracts with significant antiaging activity, mainly due to their ability to inhibit enzymes associated with skin aging, such as elastase and hyaluronidase. In contrast, supercritical extraction produced extracts with comparatively lower biological activity under the evaluated conditions (Pinto et al., 2021).

The obtained extracts also demonstrated notable antimicrobial activity, particularly against Gram-positive bacteria, highlighting their potential as natural preservatives or active agents in cosmetic formulations. Cytotoxicity and biocompatibility assessments were conducted using HaCaT and human foreskin fibroblast (HFF-1) cell lines, and the results indicated good cellular viability, supporting the potential use of chestnut extracts in topical formulations. Moreover, skin compatibility was further evaluated using reconstructed human epidermis models, including Episkin and SkinEthic, which showed no significant irritation effects. These findings suggest that chestnut-derived extracts are compatible with human skin and suitable for dermal applications. In addition, studies evaluating the skin permeation of phenolic agents revealed that ellagic acid exhibited the highest permeation capacity, indicating its potential effectiveness as a bioactive compound in topical cosmetic formulations (Pinto et al., 2021).

Chestnut processing produces large quantities of by-products, particularly shells, which represent a promising source of phenolic compounds. Extracts obtained from chestnut shells have shown high total phenolic and flavonoid content, with extraction efficacy strongly influenced by the extraction technique and operating conditions. Elevated temperatures may lead to the degradation of thermolabile compounds. One study reported optimal extraction conditions using 40% ethanol at 50°C, which resulted in high recovery of major phenolic acids such as ellagic, gallic, and tannic acids. Further purification and concentration of the bioactive compounds can be achieved using nanofiltration, which allows the selective concentration of water-soluble polyphenols, significantly enhancing the phenolic content and antioxidant activity of the resulting extracts (Conidi et al., 2022).

Beyond the recovery of phenolic compounds, chestnut shells can also serve as a source of cellulose nanocrystals. These nanomaterials can be produced through chemical treatments followed by acidic hydrolysis of lignocellulosic components. The resulting nanocellulose particles exhibit high surface area, thermal stability, and good dispersibility. Chestnut shell nanocellulose has also been investigated as a stabilizing agent in Pickering emulsions, mostly spherical or square shaped, revealing potential as an agent in cosmetic formulations, controlled delivery systems, and environmentally friendly packaging materials (Tiwari and Sanjog, 2025).

2.1.4 Cashews (Anacardium occidentale) bioactive profile and extraction methods

The cashew tree (*Anacardium occidentale*) is widely cultivated in tropical regions, with Brazil, India, and Vietnam among the largest producers worldwide. The plant produces two main components: the cashew nut (seed) and the cashew apple, a fleshy pseudofruit that is often processed into juices, beverages, and other fermented products. Both the nut and its by-products are currently viewed as valuable sources of several health-promoting bioactives (Gutiérrez-Paz et al., 2024).

The polyphenolic composition of cashew apple juice and fiber has been extensively investigated using advanced analytical techniques like ultra-performance liquid chromatography coupled with quadrupole time-of-flight mass spectrometry. Notably, the phytochemical profile varies significantly during the maturation stages of the fruit. In a recent study, 12 phenolic compounds were identified, including gallic acid, quercetin, myricetin, and flavonol glucosides, all of which are well known for their antioxidant, antiinflammatory, and skin-protective abilities (Cunha et al., 2017).

In addition to the edible fruit, cashew processing generates large quantities of agro-industrial by-products, particularly shells and shell liquids. The cashew nut shell contains cashew nut shell liquid, a complex mixture rich in phenolic lipids such as anacardic acid, cardanol, cardol, and 2-methylcardol, which exhibit antimicrobial, antioxidant, and antiinflammatory activities (León et al., 2025). Extraction of bioactive compounds from cashew shells has been explored using environmentally friendly techniques, including SWE. SWE enabled the efficient recovery of phenolic compounds without the use of toxic organic solvents. Studies have shown that cashew shells contain a high proportion of lignocellulosic materials, with lignin representing the dominant solid fraction (de Paiva et al., 2024). Although the fatty acid content of shell extracts is relatively low, the TPC can be substantial, depending on the extraction parameters such as temperature, pressure, and extraction time (Valdés et al., 2022).

Interestingly, a recent synergistic extraction approach combining Viscozyme L enzymatic treatment with enzyme-assisted UAE (E-UAE) was demonstrated to be superior to single-method techniques (EAE or UAE) for the recovery of high-value bioactives from cashew nut testa. The E-UAE process, characterized by a 60-minute enzymatic incubation followed by 40 min of sonication, yielded significantly higher concentrations of total phenolics, flavonoids, catechins, and epigallocatechin gallate (EGCG). Moreover, the extracts exhibited superior α-amylase inhibitory activity, robust antioxidant capacity, and remarkable selective cytotoxicity. At a concentration of 100 μg/mL, the extract reduced the cell viability of MCF-7 breast cancer cells to 22%, outperforming commercial doxorubicin (39% viability), while maintaining a safe profile for healthy bovine aortic endothelial cells (91% viability) (Van Thanh et al., 2023).

2.1.5 Pistachio (Pistacia vera) bioactive profile and extraction methods

Pistachio (*Pistacia vera*) is an economically vital tree nut belonging to the *Anacardiaceae* family, which also includes cashew and mango species. Pistachio cultivation is widespread in countries such as Iran, the United States, Turkey, and Greece, where pistachio is a significant agricultural product. Its kernels are highly valued for their ample bioactive profile, including phenolic compounds, tocopherols, carotenoids, and terpenoids (Alalwan et al., 2022; Mandalari et al., 2022).

Pistachio oil is primarily extracted from the kernel (meat) and contains several volatile and nonvolatile compounds. Among the volatile agents identified in pistachio oil are α-pinene, octane, and decane, which contribute to the characteristic aroma and biological activity of the oil. However, extraction conditions may significantly influence the chemical composition of the oil. High temperatures associated with conventional extraction processes, such as Soxhlet extraction, as well as other novel methods like UAE, have been reported to downregulate the concentration of volatile terpenes due to thermal degradation (Valasi et al., 2023).

More recently, MAE has been investigated as an alternative technique for the recovery of phenolic compounds from pistachio kernels and by-products. MAE has demonstrated high extraction efficiency due to rapid heating and enhanced solvent penetration into plant matrices. Using this method, thirteen phenolic compounds were identified, with gallic acid, epicatechin, and catechin being the most abundant compounds. Furthermore, among the tocopherol isoforms detected, the β + γ-tocopherol fraction was present at the highest concentration. These agents are known for their antioxidant ability, which contributes to the oxidative stability of pistachio oil and its potential benefits toward skin health. Interestingly, MAE seemed to be the best method for the highest extraction yields, mainly because of the low temperatures needed (Kalogiouri et al., 2022).

2.2 Brazil nuts bioactive profile and extraction methods

Brazil nuts (*Bertholletia excelsa*) are native to the Amazon rainforest and are primarily produced in Brazil, Bolivia, and Peru. The nuts are well known for their exceptional nutritional value, particularly their high lipid content (~60%–70%), moderate protein levels (~14%–18%), and significant dietary fiber, minerals, and vitamins. Especially regarding their lipid content, Brazil nuts are composed of 23.9% MUFAs, 24.4% PUFAs, and 16.134% SFAs, where α-linolenic acid (ω-3) constitutes up to 7% of the total fats within the nut (Takeda et al., 2025). Among their mineral constituents, selenium is present at comparatively high concentrations, playing important roles in antioxidant defense mechanisms through its role in selenoproteins such as glutathione peroxidase, which protects skin cells from oxidative damage (Cardoso et al., 2017).

Brazil nuts, apart from selenium and lipid agents, contain a variety of bioactives, such as phenolic acids (e.g., gallic, ellagic, vanillic, ferulic, coumaric, *p*-hydroxybenzoic, sinapinic, and protocatechuic acid), flavonoids (e.g., catechin, catechin gallate, epicatechin, epicatechin gallate, epigallocatechin 3-*O*-gallate, myricetin-3-*O*-rhamnoside, quercetin, and taxifolin), ascorbic acid, tocopherols, phytosterols, and unsaturated fatty acids (UFAs) (Takeda et al., 2025; Cardoso et al., 2017).

Conventional extraction techniques are nowadays more used in the industry for isolating Brazil nut oil, predominantly due to their better yield and stable chemical characteristics, while the use of green solvents, supercritical, and ultrasound conditions is still less applied because of difficulties in the feasibility of large-scale use (Carvalho et al., 2022). For example, semidefatted Brazilian flour oil (BNSDFO) obtained using pressurized fluids (*n*-propane at 40°C and 2, 4, and 8 MPa or a CO_2/*n*-propane mixture at 40°C and 12 MPa) revealed higher linoleic acid, β-sitosterol, and PUFAs than the Brazilian nut kernel oil obtained by a conventional cold-pressing method. The use of pressurized *n*-propane resulted in a 13.7% yield at 4 MPa, with myricetin 3-*O*-rhamnoside and higher oxidative stability achieved at the intermediate pressure of 4 MPa than 2 MPa. Moreover, the CO_2/*n*-propane mixture increased squalene yields by 4.5 times, phenolic compound recovery, and oxidative stability (12 h), but concurrently reduced the overall yield (2.2%) (Abrantes et al., 2024). Other methods like UAE (de Oliveira et al., 2025) and PLE with isopropyl alcohol and ethyl alcohol (EtOH) (Cornelio-Santiago et al., 2019) are also simple, fast, and low-cost alternative techniques that offer both high recovery of bioactives and quality of final products.

2.3 Macadamia's bioactive profile and extraction methods

Macadamia nuts (*Macadamia integrifolia* and *Macadamia tetraphylla*) originate from Australia but are currently cultivated in several tropical and subtropical regions worldwide. Macadamia kernels are highly valued for their rich lipid composition, containing ~ 70%–80% oil, which is one of the highest oil contents among edible nuts (Xing-Hao et al., 2021; Shi et al., 2021). The oil fraction is mainly comprised of MUFAs, particularly oleic (~40%–51%), palmitoleic (~24%–36%), palmitic acid (~8.4%–13.1%), and PUFAs, while macadamia nuts also contain proteins, dietary fiber, and micronutrients like magnesium, potassium, vitamin E, and phytosterols (Shuai et al., 2021; Aquino-Bolaños et al., 2017).

The bioactive profile of macadamia nuts includes phenolic compounds (e.g., chlorogenic, vanillic, gallic, caffeic, protocatechuic, and *p*-hydroxybenzoic acid) in its husk and leaves, flavonoids (e.g., catechin, rutin, quercetin, and kaempferol) in its leaves, flowers, and husk, tannins, carotenoids, vitamin E, minerals, and fatty acids in its leaves, flowers, and husk, while its shell is composed of cellulose, hemicellulose, lignin, phenolic acids, and flavonoids (Ahmed et al., 2024).

Macadamia oil is primarily extracted via conventional mechanical cold pressing or solvent extraction using, for instance, *n*-hexane, or advanced techniques like supercritical CO_2 and UAE extraction methods. In a related research study, the highest extraction rate was 74.63% via Soxhlet extraction, 70.53% via supercritical CO_2 extraction, 57.19% via UAE, and 50.37% through solvent extraction, whereas the relative extraction rates of UFAs were 36.53%, 44.21%, 60.62%, and 56.81%, respectively, mainly yielding *Z*-9-hexadecenoic acid, E-11-hexadecenoic acid, 9,12-octadecadienoic acid, 9-octadecenoic acid, E-9-octadecenoic acid, and 9-eicosenoate by gas chromatography–mass spectrometry. Although the extraction rate was the highest via Soxhlet extraction, the relative content of *Z*-9-hexadecenoic acid and 9,12-octadecadienoic acid was higher using supercritical CO_2 extraction (Zhu et al., 2013).

2.4 Pecans bioactive profile and extraction methods

Pecans (*Carya illinoinensis*) are native to North America and are widely cultivated in the United States and Mexico. They are characterized by a high nutritional value, containing ~ 53%–70% lipids, ~ 7%–9% proteins, ~ 5%–17% carbohydrates, ash ~ 1.1%–1.7%, and significant amounts of dietary fiber (~5.5%–16%), phytosterols, and micronutrients (Sandhu, 2025). The lipid fraction mainly comprises MUFAs, particularly oleic acid (~49%–76.5%), along with smaller amounts of PUFAs such as linoleic acid (~13%–40%) and SFAs (~6%–17%) (Scapinello et al., 2017).

Pecans are also rich in phenolic compounds and other phytochemicals with remarkable antioxidant and cytoprotective activity. Phenolic acids (e.g., gallic, ellagic, and chlorogenic acid), flavonoids (e.g., EGCG, catechin, and proanthocyanidins), α/γ-tocopherols and tocotrienols like vitamin E, and phytosterols like β-sitosterol, campesterol, stigmasterol, sitostanol, campestanol, and Δ^5-avenasterol (Atanasov et al., 2018).

The extraction of bioactives from pecans has traditionally been performed using organic solvent extraction techniques, such as ethanol or methanol extraction (Yemmireddy et al., 2020; Cason et al., 2021). Interestingly, the conventional cold pressing method yielded 58.9%, while pressurized *n*-butane yielded from 53% to 65% being the highest yield at 55°C and 40 bar pressure (Scapinello et al., 2017). Similarly, more sustainable techniques like UAE have successfully improved the recovery of phenolic compounds, mainly polyphenols and proteins, under the optimal conditions of 400 W and 55°C, using water or aqueous ethanol mixtures to maximize the yield in under 15 min (Garcia-Larez et al., 2025).

2.5 Pine nuts bioactive profile and extraction methods

Pine nuts are edible seeds obtained from several species of the genus *Pinus*, including *Pinus pinea, Pinus koraiensis,* and *Pinus sibirica*. These nuts are mainly consumed in the Asian and Mediterranean regions and are valued for their high nutritional value. Pine nuts typically contain 50%–60% lipids (~64% fat, including 10%–45% SFAs, mainly palmitic and stearic acid, and predominantly UFAs: ~ 35% MUFAs, mainly oleic acid, and ~ 20% PUFAs, mainly linoleic acid), 13%–20% proteins, and moderate amounts of carbohydrates (56.2%), fiber (27.5%), and micronutrients like magnesium, potassium, and vitamin E (primarily present as γ-tocopherol). Interestingly, Korean and Siberian pine nuts are abundant sources of pinolenic acid (PNLA), which forms up to 20% and 27% of their total bioactive content, respectively (Teneva et al., 2024; Nolasco et al., 2024; Takala et al., 2023).

The bioactive composition of pine nuts includes several tocopherols (α/γ-tocopherol), phytosterols (e.g., stigmasterol, β-sitosterol), PAHs (e.g., fluorene, phenanthrene), polyphenols (phenolic acids like gallic and protocatechuic acid, and flavonoids like catechin), and carotenoids (Nolasco et al., 2024; Lutz et al., 2016). In addition, pinolenic acid, a characteristic fatty acid found in pine nut oil, has demonstrated strong antiinflammatory and lipid-regulating properties (Teneva et al., 2024; Nolasco et al., 2024; Takala et al., 2023).

Extraction of pine nut oil is commonly performed using cold pressing, Soxhlet extraction, or solvent extraction methods. In a recent study, solvent extraction using *n*-hexane resulted in high yields during pine nut oil extraction under the optimal conditions of 39.3°C, 33.4 min, and a solvent-to-solid extraction ratio of 10.8:1 (mL/g) (Kemerli-Kalbaran and Ozdemir, 2019). Advanced extraction techniques, including supercritical CO_2 extraction or UAE, have been investigated to improve efficacy and maintain the integrity of bioactives. UAE, followed by thermal degradation for a zero-waste process, led to a high yield of phytochemicals, enhancing the volatile matter content of the pinecones, while the char residue could be further used for soil enhancement (Kumar and Bhaduri, 2025).

2.6 Walnuts bioactive profile and extraction methods

Walnuts (*Juglans regia*) are among the most widely consumed tree nuts globally and are cultivated extensively in regions such as China, the United States, Iran, and several European countries. Walnut kernels are nutritionally rich, containing ~ 52%–70% lipids, 15%–20% proteins and protein hydrolysates (e.g., albumin, globulin, protoprotein, and gluten), bioactive peptides, polysaccharides, and significant amounts of dietary fiber, vitamins, and minerals (Dai et al., 2024; Fan et al., 2023). More specifically, walnuts are abundant in PUFAs (~69%–72.8% of the total fatty acids, especially ω-3 PUFAs), including linoleic acid, α-linolenic acid (10%–18%), 5,11-eicosadienoic acid, and arachidonic acid, as well as ω-9 MUFAs like oleic acid (11.26%–25.09%) (Dai et al., 2024).

Walnuts' health-promoting properties are further clarified by their phytochemical profile, which includes phenolic acids (e.g., ellagic, cinnamic, tannic, and gallic acid), flavonoids (e.g., apigenin, eugenol, 7-hydroxymethylcoumarin, and catechin), tannins, juglone, tocopherols (e.g., α-, β-, γ-, and δ-tocopherol), phytosterols (e.g., β-sitosterol, campesterol, stigmasterol), and sphingolipids (e.g., ceramides, glycosphingolipids, and hexosylceramides) (Dai et al., 2024; Fan et al., 2023; Rusu et al., 2020).

Reflux extraction with 60% ethanol for 60 min has been identified as a highly efficient extraction method for isolating phenolics from walnut septa compared to maceration, UAE, and other solvents tested (Luksiene et al., 2025). Recently, the highest TPC [5625 mg GAE/100 g dry weight (d.w.)] was obtained using UAE combined with EAE (US-EAE), where ultrasound pretreatment (200 W, 10 min) was followed by enzymatic extraction using 0.06 mL/g Viscozyme L (pH 3.5, 45°C), whereas UAE alone yielded the second-highest TPC of 4129 mg GAE/100 g d.w. Moreover, US-EAE extracts demonstrated an ABTS scavenging activity of 14,478 mg TE/100 g d.w. and enhanced DPPH activity of 45.38 mg TE/100 g d.w. (Celik et al., 2025).

2.7 Peanuts bioactive profile and extraction methods

Peanuts (*Arachis hypogaea*) are one of the most widely cultivated legume crops globally and represent an important source of nutrients and bioactive agents. Although commonly classified as nuts due to their culinary use and nutritional profile, peanuts are botanically classified as legumes belonging to the *Fabaceae* family. Major peanut-producing countries include China, India, the United States, and several African nations (King et al., 2008; Bonku and Jianmei, 2020). Peanuts contain multiple natural micronutrients, including vitamins, minerals, and stilbenes like resveratrol, alongside lignans, phytosterols, tocopherols, and isoflavonoids (Arya et al., 2016; Çiftçi and Suna, 2022).

Peanuts are classified into four market types: Runners, Spanish, Virginia, and Valencia. Isorhamnetin was present in Valencia cultivars, whereas its glucoside, isorhamnetin-3-*O*-glucoside, as well as genistein, daidzein, rutin, quercetin, and trans-resveratrol, were identified in both Valencia and Runner market types (Chukwumah et al., 2012). Using temperatures from 90°C to 180°C, peanut skins (PSs), including Runner, Virginia, and Spanish, were extracted using 70% ethanol in water solutions. Runner peanuts displayed 280 mg/g TPC, whereas Virginia and Spanish peanuts did not show any significant change in TPC, revealing 149 and 137 mg/g, respectively (Dean, 2020).

3 Health-promoting properties of nut and nut by-product extracts

Nut-derived extracts and oils have received significant attention recently due to their rich composition of health-promoting bioactives, such as phenolic acids, flavonoids, tocopherols, phytosterols, carotenoids, fatty acids, and other secondary metabolites. These compounds, present in nut and nut by-product extracts, exhibit antioxidant, antiinflammatory, antimicrobial, photoprotective, and skin-repairing properties ideal for cosmetic formulations (King et al., 2008; Dean, 2020). Several commonly consumed nuts, including almonds, hazelnuts, sweet chestnuts, cashews, pistachios, Brazil nuts, macadamias, pecans, pine nuts, walnuts, and peanuts, have been investigated using modern extraction techniques and explored for their cosmetic value (King et al., 2008; Dean, 2020). A preview of nuts' health-promoting properties is depicted in Fig. 13.4.

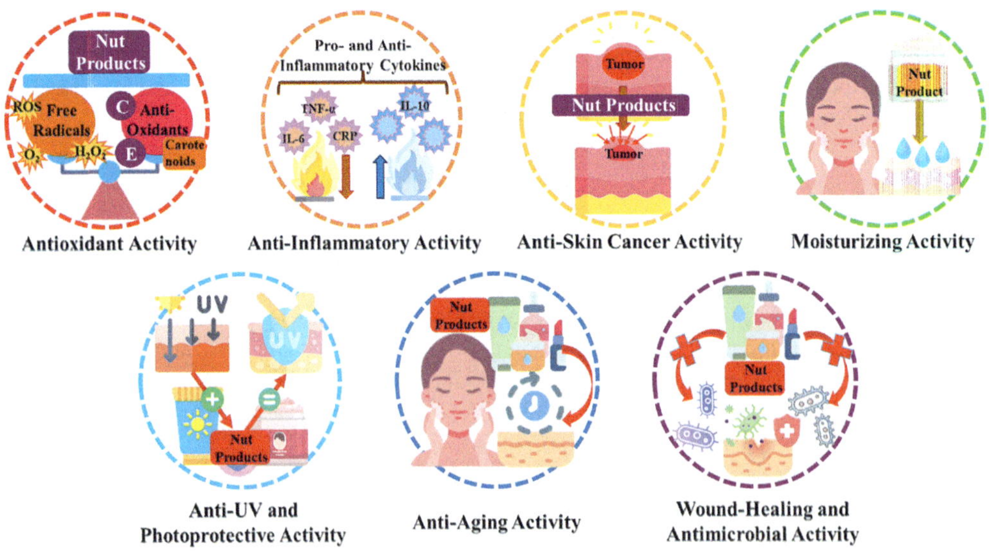

FIG. 13.4 Health-promoting effects of nut bioactives. *(Parts and icons of this figure were obtained from the open access free platform: https://www.flaticon.com/ (Accessed on January 26, 2026).)*

3.1 Antioxidant activity

Antioxidant activity is one of the most extensively studied biological properties of nut-derived extracts, where oxidative stress, mainly via reactive oxygen species (ROS), plays a vital role in premature aging, skin inflammation, and the development of dermatological disorders (King et al., 2008; Dean, 2020). A comparative study involving several nut types revealed that walnuts possess the highest TPC, followed by pecans, peanuts, pistachios, cashews, almonds, Brazil nuts, pine nuts, macadamia nuts, and hazelnuts, whereas macadamia nuts had the highest bound phenolics. Regarding the soluble free flavonoid content, pecans exhibited the highest values, followed by walnuts, peanuts, pistachios, cashews, almonds, Brazil nuts, hazelnuts, pine nuts, and macadamia nuts, while walnuts had the highest bound flavonoids. Among the nuts, walnuts demonstrated the greatest antioxidant activity (458.1 ± 14.0 μmol/g, 8067 mg of vitamin C/100 g), followed by pecans (427.0 ± 21.6 μmol/g), peanuts (81.3 ± 3.2 μmol/g), pistachios (75.9 ± 1.2 μmol/g), cashews (29.5 ± 2.7 μmol/g), almonds (25.4 ± 2.0 μmol/g), Brazil nuts (16.0 ± 1.2 μmol/g), pine nuts (14.6 ± 1.1 μmol/g), macadamia nuts (13.4 ± 0.4 μmol/g), and hazelnuts (7.1 ± 0.9 μmol/g). Nuts, as nutritional powerhouses, are rich in phytochemicals like polyphenols, flavonoids, selenium, and tocopherols, which directly quench free radicals and reduce oxidative stress (Yang et al., 2009).

Similar studies also supported that raw and roasted walnuts had the highest free and total polyphenols among several types of nuts. As a result, walnut polyphenols, including catechin, had the best lipoprotein-bound antioxidant activity capable of inhibiting oxidative processes that lead to atherosclerosis in vivo. Walnuts had a fivefold longer lag time than both almonds and peanuts, a negative effect of lag time versus the control sample; therefore a high prooxidant activity, and increased the lag time twofold and eightfold compared to almonds and peanuts, respectively. Moreover, in human supplementation studies, nuts have been shown to improve the lipid profile, accelerate endothelial function, and downregulate inflammation, without leading to weight gain, thereby being a great nutritional option or food additive (Vinson and Cai, 2012).

3.2 Antiinflammatory activity

Inflammation is a natural biological response to tissue injury, infection, or environmental stressors. However, chronic or excessive inflammatory responses are associated with several skin disorders, including dermatitis, psoriasis, acne, and premature skin aging. Nut-derived extracts contain numerous bioactives with proven antiinflammatory action. Current evidence from several randomized controlled trials and research gaps indicated that almonds were not associated with any changes in tumor necrosis factor α (TNF-α), adhesion molecules, and oxidized metabolites, but they downregulated C-reactive protein (CRP), interleukin-6 (IL-6), and oxidized low-density lipoprotein (Ox-LDL). Brazil nuts, on the contrary, were not related to any changes in Ox-LDL, CRP, or oxidized metabolites, while they upregulated antioxidant enzymes. In addition, walnuts were not associated with any alterations in CRP, Ox-LDL, and oxidized metabolites, whereas they downregulated IL-6, TNF-α, and adhesion molecules (Vinson and Cai, 2012; Rajaram et al., 2023; Hariri et al., 2023). In addition to phenolic compounds, the nut lipid fraction also contributes to their antiinflammatory properties. Nut oils, like macadamia and almond oils, rich in oleic, linoleic, and palmitoleic acids, reduce inflammatory responses and promote skin barrier recovery (Mohammed et al., 2023; Shi et al., 2021).

Recently, a study on a walnut-derived peptide, leucine–proline–leucine–leucine–arginine (LP-5), in oxidative stress-induced Caco-2 cells and model mice demonstrated that LP-5 significantly upregulated catalase and superoxide dismutase (SOD), while decreasing malondialdehyde (MDA) both in vivo and in vitro. Oxidative stress indices were suppressed by LP-5, promoting the nuclear factor erythroid-2-related factor 2 (Nrf2), elevating heme oxygenase-1 expression, and reducing Keap1 expression by effectively binding to this stressor. Furthermore, LP-5 notably inhibited the NOD-like receptor family pyrin domain-containing 3 inflammasome by downregulating its expression, apoptosis-associated speck-like protein containing a CARD (ASC), and caspase-1, ideally reducing inflammatory cytokine release, including IL-18, IL-1β, and TNF-α, decreasing inflammatory biomarkers like inducible nitric oxide synthase and cyclooxygenase-2, and increasing the levels of antiinflammatory markers like IL-10 (Yuan et al., 2023).

3.3 Antiskin cancer activity

Bioactive compounds present in nut extracts have attracted considerable interest due to their potential chemopreventive properties, which may help protect skin cells from carcinogenic processes. Nut consumption has been widely associated with the risk of total cancer and five specific cancers, as evidence indicates from three large prospective cohort studies. Compared with nonconsumers, the pooled multivariable HRs of total nut consumption for ≥ 5 times/week were 0.99 for total cancer, 0.88 for lung cancer, 1.07 for colorectal cancer, 0.90 for bladder cancer, 0.96 for breast cancer, and 1.18 for aggressive prostate cancer. Therefore frequent nut consumption was not correlated with total cancer risk or other common individual cancers (Fang et al., 2021).

Polyphenols from PSs, including catechin, syringic acid, and vanillic acid, increased the oxidative stability of sunflower oil by four times its initial levels, while possessing high inhibitory activity against MCF-7, HepG-2, HCT-116, and PC-3 cancer cell lines, with half-maximal inhibitory concentration (IC_{50}) ranging from 1.85 ± 0.13 to 6.1 ± 0.43 μg/mL. Moreover, the UAE-derived PS extract examined in HFB4 human normal melanocytes showed promising antioxidant and anticancer properties (Hammad et al., 2023). Furthermore, the antitumor potential of the cashew gum (CG) structure was investigated using the MTT assay in a B16–F10 melanoma model. CG did not exhibit any cytotoxicity in vitro but demonstrated significant tumor inhibition in vivo, leading to a 36.9%–43% tumor mass reduction, without any toxicity to organs. In addition, CG induced tumor inhibition in the presence of apoptotic morphotype cells, without any alterations in the levels of antioxidant components, while it suppressed the expression of phosphorylated histone H2AX and did not alter the expression of caspase-3, highlighting its potential as an anticancer agent and/or as a suppressor of side effects associated with standard drugs (Barros et al., 2020).

3.4 Moisturizing properties

Maintaining adequate skin hydration is essential for preserving skin barrier integrity and preventing dryness, irritation, and premature aging. Nut oils are widely recognized for their excellent emollient and moisturizing properties, which are largely attributed to their remarkable content of UFAs and lipid-soluble vitamins. Hazelnut oil moisturizes the skin, is rich in vitamin E, helps to thicken hair, and, topically, can be used as a sunscreen, a hair mask, and a moisturizer. Moreover, its niacin content prevents water loss and increases skin moisture content, while vitamin E smooths the skin and maintains moisture in the outer skin layer (Ur Rehman and Ahmad, 2025).

Almond oil contains fatty acids that aid in clearing the pores of excess oil and dirt, calming skin inflammation and irritation, deteriorating skin conditions, and preventing transepidermal water loss (TEWL). It is an effective moisturizer, capable of calming and hydrating the lips, lessening the appearance of fine wrinkles, and minimizing the appearance of dark circles around the eyes. For instance, a beeswax, borax, and almond oil-based cream moisturized the skin and can be used in the winter to prevent skin dryness, including cracks on the lips and cheeks during the cold season (Selwyn and Govindaraj, 2023). Similarly, macadamia nut oil, as an abundant source of oleic acid, is great for softening the skin, regenerating skin cells, and offering deep moisturization, while its high linoleic acid content aids in restoring the skin barrier and reducing TEWL (Hanum et al., 2019).

3.5 Anti-UV and photoprotective properties

Skin damage is highly correlated with UV radiation exposure, contributing to skin damage, photoaging, and skin cancer development. Nut bioactives are responsible for neutralizing ROS and reducing oxidative damage to skin cells, being also capable of enhancing the SPF of cosmetic sunscreen formulations when combined with conventional UV filters (Yeh et al., 2025; Zhou et al., 2026). Two polyphenol-rich extracts from skins (TP) and decorticated seeds (SP) of Bronte pistachios contained high levels of phenolics (TP being ~ 10 times richer than SP), with anthocyanins being the most abundant compound in the TP extract. Interestingly, TP, more than the SP extract, revealed great radical scavenger/antioxidant activities, photoprotective potential, and, when topically applied, reduced UV_B-induced skin erythema (Martorana et al., 2013).

A hydroalcoholic extract of roasted hazelnut skins, abundant in polyphenols (308.4 ± 4.6 mg GAE/g) and proanthocyanidins (169.3 ± 10 mg CE/g), demonstrated significant antioxidant activity (DPPH half maximal effective concentration (EC_{50}) of 5.08 ± 1.08 μg/mL, TAC of 2.82 ± 0.03 mM Trolox/mg), while showing a strong UV absorbance of synthetic UV filters, enhancing the SPF by 9.4%, and increasing the radical scavenging from 52% to 80%, compared to the blank sample (Mencherini et al., 2025). In addition, the methanolic extract of walnuts exhibited major antioxidant and photoprotective effects on human epidermal keratinocytes against inflammatory responses induced by UV_B radiation (Rahbardar et al., 2025).

3.6 Antiaging activity

Skin aging is a complex biological process influenced by both intrinsic factors, such as genetic and metabolic processes, and extrinsic factors, including UV radiation, pollution, and oxidative stress. One of the primary mechanisms involved in skin aging is the degradation of structural proteins such as collagen and elastin, which leads to wrinkle formation and loss of skin elasticity. Nut-derived extracts contain several bioactive compounds that can effectively delay aging-promoting processes by inhibiting collagenase, elastase, and hyaluronidase, enzymes responsible for the breakdown of the extracellular matrix (Yajing et al., 2025; Rusu et al., 2019). Interestingly, bioactive agents from tree nuts delay both aging and aging-related diseases by upregulating the Nrf2/electrophile-responsive elements (EpRE) pathway and downregulating the nuclear factor κB (NF-κB) cascade, which play a major role in cell protection (Yajing et al., 2025; Rusu et al., 2019).

Macadamia nut oil nanocream dosage form revealed great skin antiaging activity when compared to a conventional cream, positively altering skin parameters such as water content, pore size, melanin, and wrinkles. Macadamia oil's oleic acid content softened the skin, offered deep moisturization, protected against UV-induced lipid peroxidation, and enhanced antioxidant capacity and cell regeneration (Hanum et al., 2019). Similarly, nanoemulsions containing macadamia seed oil promoted deep skin hydration and wrinkle reduction, exhibiting significant potency as an ABTS radical scavenger, as well as a lipid peroxidation and hyaluronidase inhibitor (Somwongin and Chaiyana, 2024).

Procyanidin A1 (PCA1), derived from PS, exerts antiaging effects and attenuates senescence via antioxidative stress and autophagy induction. PCA1 reduced ROS, MDA, and SOD levels, decreased the percentage of senescent cells, and induced autophagy (Yajing et al., 2025). At the same time, according to a study based on UAE-based extraction of bioactives from peanut shells, a reverse transcription polymerase chain reaction revealed that their extract decreased mRNA levels of tyrosinase-related protein-1 and metalloproteinase-3 genes, offering remarkable skin-whitening, antiwrinkle, and thereby antiaging effects (Gam et al., 2021).

3.7 Wound healing and antimicrobial activity

The wound healing procedure involves a series of standard biological events, including inflammation, tissue proliferation, and tissue remodeling, where nuts have demonstrated the ability to support these processes by promoting tissue repair, enhancing barrier restoration, and preventing microbial infections against various bacterial and fungal strains (e.g., Gram-positive and Gram-negative microorganisms) (Zhou et al., 2026). Walnut root provided accelerated healing through its antioxidant, antimicrobial, and antiinflammatory activity. It showed a significant decrease in the percent inhibition of paw edema (0.63 ± 0.03 to 0.33 ± 0.02 after 24 h) with an increase in root concentration, while also increasing antioxidant and antimicrobial properties (Huo et al., 2020).

PS and meal from dry-blanched peanuts (MDBP) were demonstrated to be major sources of phenolic compounds such as phenolic acids (both PS and MDBP), proanthocyanidins (PS), and monomeric flavonoids (PS), which were responsible for their vast antimicrobial activity against several bacteria tested, including *Escherichia coli*, *Bacillus cereus*, and *Staphylococcus aureus* (de Camargo et al., 2017). A walnut green husk extract, one of the main waste products from walnut processing, could be used as a natural source of dyeing compounds such as juglone. When the extract was mixed with ascorbic acid (vitamin C, developer), ferrous sulfate (mordant agent), and an Aloe vera extract (secondary mordant), it resulted in a dark brown color on hair samples. The dyed hair was associated with appropriate color strength, excellent morphology for a hair surface coated with dye molecules, and great resistance to washing and daylight fastness, without inducing any irritation or other side effects (Beiki et al., 2018). On a similar basis, cashew nuts (Campos et al., 2012), almonds (Silva et al., 2025), hazelnuts (Zhao et al., 2023), and chestnuts (Pinto et al., 2021) have also been indicated as efficient sources of antimicrobial constituents.

4 Applications of nut and nut by-product extracts in cosmetic and cosmeceutical products

4.1 Skincare, haircare, and barrier-protective applications of nut extracts

Nut-derived oils and extracts are currently widely employed in commercial cosmetic and cosmeceutical products, especially for their emollient, antioxidant, and barrier repair properties. Nut oils from almonds, hazelnuts, sweet chestnuts, cashews, pistachios, macadamias, pine nuts, pecans, Brazil nuts, walnuts, and peanuts are rich in several lipid constituents, such as oleic, linoleic, and palmitoleic acids, which help restore the lipid matrix of the *stratum corneum*, improve hydration, and reduce TEWL (Pinto et al., 2021; Vinson and Cai, 2012; Selwyn and Govindaraj, 2023; Mungwari et al., 2025). Consequently, nut ingredients are commonly incorporated into creams, serums, lotions, lip balms, and hydrogels, where they enhance skin softness, elasticity, and overall barrier function. Concurrently, their content in tocopherols and phenolics provides protection against oxidative stress and environmental damage, whereas their polyphenol-rich extracts from nut skins and shells exhibit antiaging activity through the inhibition of collagenase, elastase, and hyaluronidase (Michalak and Kieltyka-Dadasiewicz, 2019; Srisuksomwong et al., 2023; Qingyang et al., 2022; Lin et al., 2018).

In haircare applications, nut oils are highly valued for their ability to penetrate the hair shaft, reduce protein loss, and improve hair strength and shine. Nut-based components such as tocopherols, phytosterols, and flavonoids in almonds, Brazil nuts, macadamias, and walnut oils are frequently included in shampoos, hair conditioners, and masks, where they smooth the hair cuticle, support scalp health, downregulate inflammation, and reduce breakage (Ballistreri et al., 2011; Lipan et al., 2025; Gavazzoni Dias, 2015; Mir et al., 2016). Beyond hydration and nourishment, nut-derived bioactives play an important role in soothing, barrier repair, and photoprotective formulations, being suitable for sensitive, irritated, or atopic skin while supporting UV-induced oxidative damage protective activities as natural UV-boosting agents in sunscreen cosmetic formulations (Martorana et al., 2013; Somwongin and Chaiyana, 2024; Ballistreri et al., 2011; Ryczaj et al., 2023).

4.2 Examples of commercial products using nut extracts

Nut-derived ingredients are widely utilized in commercial cosmetic and cosmeceutical products due to their multifunctional properties. These ingredients can be found in a wide range of formulations, including moisturizers, facial oils, antiaging creams, hair conditioners, body care products, and sunscreens or other UV-protective formulations (Pinto et al., 2021; Vinson and Cai, 2012; Selwyn and Govindaraj, 2023; Mungwari et al., 2025). Table 13.3 includes commercial nut and nut by-product-based cosmetic and cosmeceutical products.

TABLE 13.3 Commercial nut and nut by-product-derived cosmetic and cosmeceutical products.

Cosmetic product	Cosmetic use	Nut ingredient	Beneficial impact	References
Garnier—Ultimate Blends Almond Crush Shampoo	Hair shampoo	*Prunus amygdalus dulcis* seed extract and sweet almond seed extract	Shampoo for hydrated, healthy hair with antiacne, exfoliating, and soothing properties	(Garnier, n.d.)
Nivea—Cleansing Milk Almond Oil	Cleansing milk	*Prunus amygdalus dulcis* oil	Gentle cleansing and makeup removal product without causing drying, suitable for dry skin	(Nivea, n.d.)
Nuxe Bio—Hazelnut Replenishing Nourishing Body Oil	Body oil	*Corylus avellana* seed oil	Nourishing, regenerating, and sublimating dry skin formulation, making it more supple and elastic	(Nuxe, n.d.)
Bodyfarm—Men's Care Hazelnut	Face cream	*Corylus americana* seed oil and *Prunus amygdalus dulcis* oil	Antiwrinkle face cream for men with high antioxidant activity due to its vitamin E, C, and F content	(Bodyfarm, n.d.)
Yves Rocher—Shea & Chestnut Milk Nourishing Body Milk	Body milk	*Castanea sativa* seed extract and *Macadamia ternifolia* seed oil	Moisturizing, restorative, comforting, nourishing, and antioxidant formula	(Yves Rocher, n.d.)
Clarins—Renew-plus Body Serum	Body serum	*Anacardium occidentale* seed and *Corylus avellana* seed oil	Appearance and youthfulness-boosting, radiance-enhancing, softening, and moisturizing effects	(Clarins, n.d.)
Pistache—Pistachio Body Butter	Body butter	*Pistacia vera* seed oil and extract, and hydrogenated *Pistacia vera* seed	Soothing, hydrating, and skin brightening formula	(Pistache, n.d.)
Irene Forte—Pistachio Face Mask	Face mask	*Pistacia vera* seed oil	Hydrating, face plumping, and soothing face mask	(Irene Forte, n.d.)
Angel Professional—Brazil Nut Hair Mask	Hair mask	Brazil nut drupe oil	Replenishing, antioxidant, and soothing formulation	(Angel Professional, n.d.)
Suncademy—Botanical Facial Sunscreen	Sunscreen	*Pinus pinea* kernel oil and *Prunus amygdalus dulcis* oil	SPF (50^+)-enhancing, antioxidant, antiacne, exfoliant, skin brightening, and soothing formula	(Suncademy, n.d.)
Savannah Bee Company—Beeswax Hand Cream	Hand cream	*Carya illinoinensis* seed oil and *Prunus amygdalus dulcis* oil	Replenishing, moisturizing, antioxidant, and soothing formulation	(Savannah Bee Company, n.d.)
Macadamia Professional—Weightless Moisture Masque	Moisture masque	*Macadamia ternifolia* nut oil and *Juglans regia* walnut seed oil	Nourishing, deep conditioning, antioxidant, emollient, and soothing formulation	(Macadamia Professional, n.d.)
Kundal—Macadamia & Sugar Body Scrub	Body scrub	*Macadamia ternifolia* seed extract	Exfoliating, nourishing, moisturizing, and soothing formula	(Kundal, n.d.)

Cosmetic product	Cosmetic use	Nut ingredient	Beneficial impact	References
Rossen—Carrot & Walnut Tanning Body Oil (with Shimmer)	Tanning body oil	*Juglans regia* flower extract	Antioxidant, emollient, tanning, and sunscreen formula	(Rossen, n.d.)
Revolution Skincare—Green Tea & Walnut Exfoliating Face Mask	Exfoliating face mask	*Juglans regia* shell powder	Exfoliating, skin smoothing, antioxidant, soothing, deep cleansing, and appearance-boosting formulation	(Revolution Skincare, n.d.)
Carroten—Protect & Care Suncare Milk SPF 30	Cream sunscreen	*Arachis hypogea* nut oil	UV-protective, water-resistant, antioxidant, and soothing sunscreen formula	(Carroten, n.d.)
Biodermal—Anti Age 60$^+$ Night Cream	Night face cream	*Arachis hypogaea* nut oil and *Macadamia ternifolia* seed oil	Antiaging, antiwrinkle, antioxidant, skin brightening, and soothing formula	(Biodermal, n.d.)

5 Limitations, challenges, and future perspectives

Despite the significant potential of nut-derived extracts in cosmetic and cosmeceutical formulations, major limitations and challenges associated with their widespread application in the cosmetic industry must be considered to ensure their safe, effective, and sustainable use. One of the primary concerns associated with nut-derived ingredients is allergenicity. Tree nuts and peanuts are among the most common food allergens. However, while the topical application of nut-based formulations generally poses a lower risk compared to ingestion, sensitive individuals may still experience allergic reactions. As a result, rigorous safety testing, proper allergen labeling, and more human-based clinical trials are vital to minimizing potential risks (Ryczaj et al., 2023).

Another important challenge involves the stability of nut bioactives in cosmetic products. Many phenolic compounds, flavonoids, proanthocyanidins, and UFAs present in nut and nut by-product extracts are highly susceptible to oxidation, photodegradation, and thermal decline, which may reduce their biological activity and enhance side effects. Advanced formulation strategies like microencapsulation, nanoemulsions, liposomes, and polymeric delivery systems (e.g., a system incorporating pine nut shell, peanut shell, and jujube leaf in chitosan films (Zhang et al., 2020)) are increasingly explored to improve the stability, protection, and controlled release of these bioactives in cosmetic and cosmeceutical products (Hanum et al., 2019; Zhang et al., 2020; Gupta et al., 2022; Okumus and Temiz, 2026; Ezeanolue et al., 2026). In addition, variability in raw material composition, geographical origin, cultivar differences, and processing conditions may affect the concentration and composition of bioactives present in nut extracts, mainly influencing the reproducibility associated with large-scale production of cosmetics (Bandyopadhyay et al., 2025).

From a future perspective, the valorization of nut-processing by-products/waste (e.g., shells, skins, and press cakes) represents a promising and sustainable approach aligned with circular economy principles (Bandyopadhyay et al., 2025). Future research is expected to focus on the identification, purification, and characterization of individual bioactives, alongside the development of green extraction technologies, including supercritical CO_2 extraction, MAE, UAE, and NADES, for improving the efficacy and sustainability of bioactive recovery from nuts. Furthermore, future research must focus on further improving the safety evaluation and standardization of nut-derived cosmetic ingredients, particularly as new extraction technologies and bioactive compound isolation methods continue to emerge (Luksiene et al., 2025; Mungwari et al., 2025; Zhang et al., 2020; Bandyopadhyay et al., 2025).

6 Conclusions

Nut-derived materials represent a valuable and sustainable source of bioactive agents for cosmetic and cosmeceutical applications. Nuts and their by-products are rich in phenolics, UFAs, and lipid-soluble vitamins, which contribute to their antioxidant, antiinflammatory, antiaging, and moisturizing properties. Recent advances in green extraction technologies have improved the recovery efficacy and environmental sustainability of these compounds, thereby enhancing their industrial applicability. Overall, the increasing interest in natural ingredients and green cosmetic strategies highlights the strong potential of nut-derived bioactives in the cosmetic industry. The valorization of nut by-products as natural preservatives and functional cosmetic actives in the manufacturing of nut-based cosmetic formulations is of high importance and is expected to play a major role in future cosmetic innovations.

Acknowledgments

The authors would like to thank the School of Chemistry in the Faculty of Sciences at Democritus University of Thrace for their continuous support.

Funding

This research received no external funding.

A.T. was involved in conceptualization, methodology, validation, visualization, supervision, and project administration. A.T., T.A., G.G., and E.B. were involved in investigation. A.T. and T.A. were involved in writing—review and editing. All authors contributed to software, were involved in writing—original draft preparation, and have read and agreed to the published version of the manuscript.

Conflicts of interest

The authors declare no conflicts of interest.

References

Abrantes, K.K.B., Pimentel, T.C., da Silva, C., de Oliveira Santos Junior, O., Barão, C.E., Cardozo-Filho, L., 2024. Brazil nut semi-defatted flour oil: impact of extraction using pressurized solvents on lipid profile, bioactive compounds composition, and oxidative stability. Plants. 2223-7747. 13 (19), 2678. doi:10.3390/plants13192678.

Ahmed, M.F., Popovich, D.G., Whitby, C.P., Rashidinejad, A., 2024. Phenolic compounds from macadamia husk: an updated focused review of extraction methodologies and antioxidant activities. Food Bioprod. Process. 09603085. 148, 165–175. Available from: https://www.sciencedirect.com/science/journal/09603085. doi:10.1016/j.fbp.2024.09.014.

Alalwan, T.A., Mohammed, D., Hasan, M., Sergi, D., Ferraris, C., Gasparri, C., Rondanelli, M., Perna, S., 2022. Almond, hazelnut, and pistachio skin: an opportunity for nutraceuticals. Nutraceuticals 16613821. 2 (4), 300–310. Available from: https://www.mdpi.com/journal/nutraceuticals. doi:10.3390/nutraceuticals2040023.

Alara, O.R., Abdurahman, N.H., Ukaegbu, C.I., 2021. Extraction of phenolic compounds: a review. Curr. Res. Food Sci. 26659271. 4, 200–214. Available from: https://www.journals.elsevier.com/current-research-in-food-science. doi:10.1016/j.crfs.2021.03.011.

Alasalvar, C., Huang, G., Bolling, B.W., Jantip, P., Pegg, R.B., Wong, X.K., Chang, S.K., Pelvan, E., de Camargo, A.C., Mandalari, G., Hossain, A., Shahidi, F., 2025. Upcycling commercial nut byproducts for food, nutraceutical, and pharmaceutical applications: a comprehensive review. Food Chem. 18737072. 467. Available from: https://www.sciencedirect.com/science/journal/03088146. doi:10.1016/j.foodchem.2024.142222.

Angel Professional, n.d. Brazil Nut Hair Mask. https://incidecoder.com/products/angel-professional-brazil-nut-hair-mask (Accessed March 31, 2026).

Aquino-Bolaños, E.N., Mapel-Velazco, L., Martín-del-Campo, S.T., Chávez-Servia, J.L., Martínez, A.J., Verdalet-Guzmán, I., 2017. Fatty acids profile of oil from nine varieties of Macadamia nut. Int. J. Food Prop. 15322386. 20 (6), 1262–1269. Available from: https://www.tandf.co.uk/journals/titles/10942912.asp. doi:10.1080/10942912.2016.1206125.

Arya, S.S., Salve, A.R., Chauhan, S., 2016. Peanuts as functional food: a review. J. Food Sci. Technol. 09758402. 53 (1), 31–41. Available from: https://www.springer.com/journal/13197. doi:10.1007/s13197-015-2007-9.

Atanasov, A.G., Sabharanjak, S.M., Zengin, G., Mollica, A., Szostak, A., Simirgiotis, M., Huminiecki, Ł., Horbanczuk, O.K., Nabavi, S.M., Mocan, A., 2018. Pecan nuts: a review of reported bioactivities and health effects. Trends Food Sci. Technol. 09242244. 71, 246–257. Available from: http://www.elsevier.com/wps/find/journaldescription.cws_home/601278/description#description. doi:10.1016/j.tifs.2017.10.019.

Ballistreri, G., Fallico, B., Arena, E., Tokusoglu, O., 2011. Nut bioactives: phytochemicals and lipid-based components of almonds, hazelnuts, peanuts, pistachios, and walnuts. In: Tokusoglu, Ö., Hall III, C.A. (Eds.), Fruit and Cereal Bioactives. CRC Press, pp. 185–212.

Bandyopadhyay, A., Selvan, S.A., Patial, P.K., Pal, T., 2025. Plant-based ingredients in cosmetic science: current applications, limitations, and prospects. Int. J. Cosmet. Sci. 0142–5463. doi:10.1111/ics.70034.

Barros, A.B., Moura, A.F., Silva, D.A., Oliveira, T.M., Barreto, F.S., Ribeiro, W.L.C., Alves, A.P.N.N., Araújo, A.J., Filho, M.O.M., Iles, B., Medeiros, J.V.R., Marinho-Filho, J.D.B., 2020. Evaluation of antitumor potential of cashew gum extracted from Anacardium occidentale Linn. Int. J. Biol. Macromol. 01418130. 154, 319–328. doi:10.1016/j.ijbiomac.2020.03.096.

Beiki, T., Najafpour, G.D., Hosseini, M., 2018. Evaluation of antimicrobial and dyeing properties of walnut (*Juglans regia* L.) green husk extract for cosmetics. Color. Technol. 1472-3581. 134 (1), 71–81. doi:10.1111/cote.12322.

Bener, M., Şen, F.B., Önem, A.N., Bekdeşer, B., Çelik, S.E., Lalikoglu, M., Aşçı, Y.S., Capanoglu, E., Apak, R., 2022. Microwave-assisted extraction of antioxidant compounds from by-products of Turkish hazelnut (*Corylus avellana* L.) using natural deep eutectic solvents: modeling, optimization and phenolic characterization. Food Chem. 18737072. 385. Available from: https://www.elsevier.com/locate/foodchem. doi:10.1016/j.foodchem.2022.132633.

Bernoussi, S.E., Boujemaa, I., Harhar, H., Belmaghraoui, W., Matthäus, B., Tabyaoui, M., 2020. Evaluation of oxidative stability of sweet and bitter almond oils under accelerated storage conditions. J. Stored Prod. Res. 0022474X. 88, 101662. doi:10.1016/j.jspr.2020.101662.

Biodermal, n.d. Anti Age 60+ Night Cream. https://incidecoder.com/products/biodermal-anti-age-60-night-cream (Accessed March 31, 2026).

Bodoira, R., Maestri, D., 2020. Phenolic compounds from nuts: extraction, chemical profiles, and bioactivity. J. Agric. Food Chem. 0021-8561. 68 (4), 927–942. doi:10.1021/acs.jafc.9b07160.

Bodyfarm, n.d. Men's Care Hazelnut. https://incidecoder.com/products/bodyfarm-mens-care-hazelnut (Accessed March 31, 2026).

Bonku, R., Jianmei, Y., 2020. Health aspects of peanuts as an outcome of its chemical composition. Food Sci. Hum. Wellness. 22134530. 9 (1), 21–30. doi:10.1016/j.fshw.2019.12.005.

Campos, D.A., Ribeiro, A.C., Costa, E.M., Fernandes, J.C., Tavaria, F.K., Araruna, F.B., Eiras, C., Eaton, P., Leite, J.R.S.A., Pintado, M.M., 2012. Study of antimicrobial activity and atomic force microscopy imaging of the action mechanism of cashew tree gum. Carbohydr. Polym. 01448617. 90 (1), 270–274. doi:10.1016/j.carbpol.2012.05.034.

Capaldi, G., Voss, M., Tabasso, S., Stefanetti, V., Branciari, R., Chaji, S., Grillo, G., Cravotto, C., Tagliazucchi, D., Fiego, D.P.L., Marinucci, M.T., Roila, R., Natalello, A., Pravettoni, D., Cravotto, G., Forte, C., 2025. Upgrading hazelnut skins: green extraction of polyphenols from lab to semi-industrial scale. Food Chem. 03088146. 463 (Pt 1), 140999. doi:10.1016/j.foodchem.2024.140999.

Cardoso, B.R., Duarte, G.B.S., Reis, B.Z., Cozzolino, S.M.F., 2017. Brazil nuts: nutritional composition, health benefits and safety aspects. Food Res. Int. 18737145. 100, 9–18. Available from: https://www.elsevier.com/inca/publications/store/4/2/2/9/7/0. doi:10.1016/j.foodres.2017.08.036.

Carroten, n.d. Protect & Care Suncare Milk SPF 30. https://incidecoder.com/products/carroten-protect-care-suncare-milk-30spf (Accessed March 31, 2026).

Carvalho, A.L.S., Martelli, M.C., Nascimento, S.C.C., Do Sb, B.D., 2022. Brazil Nut oil: extraction methods and industrial applications. Res. Soc. Dev. 11. e29511427256–e29511427256. doi:10.33448/rsd-v11i4.27256.

Cason, C., Yemmireddy, V.K., Moreira, J., Adhikari, A., 2021. Antioxidant properties of pecan shell bioactive components of different cultivars and extraction methods. Foods. 2304-8158. 10 (4), 713. doi:10.3390/foods10040713.

Celik, B.A., Celik, M.A., Jūrienė, L., Jovaišaitė, J., Kazernavičiūtė, R., Bekar, E., Omeroglu, P.Y., Venskutonis, P.R., Kamiloglu, S., 2025. Biorefining of walnut shells into polyphenol-rich extracts using ultrasound-assisted, enzyme-assisted, and pressurized liquid extraction coupled with chemometrics. Foods. 2304-8158. 14 (13), 2245. doi:10.3390/foods14132245.

Chukwumah, Y., Walker, L., Vogler, B., Verghese, M., 2012. Profiling of bioactive compounds in cultivars of Runner and Valencia peanut market-types using liquid chromatography/APCI mass spectrometry. Food Chem. 03088146. 132 (1), 525–531. doi:10.1016/j.foodchem.2011.10.050.

Çiftçi, S., Suna, G., 2022. Functional components of peanuts (*Arachis hypogaea* L.) and health benefits: a review. Future Foods. 26668335. 5, 100140. doi:10.1016/j.fufo.2022.100140.

Clarins, n.d. Renew-Plus Body Serum https://incidecoder.com/products/clarins-renew-plus-body-serum (Accessed March 31, 2026).

Conidi, C., Donato, L., Algieri, C., Cassano, A., 2022. Valorization of chestnut processing by-products: a membrane-assisted green strategy for purifying valuable compounds from shells. J. Clean. Prod. 09596526. 378, 134564. doi:10.1016/j.jclepro.2022.134564.

Cornelio-Santiago, H.P., Mazalli, M.R., Rodrigues, C.E.C., de Oliveira, A.L., 2019. Extraction of Brazil nut kernel oil using green solvents: effects of the process variables in the oil yield and composition. J. Food Process Eng. 17454530. 42 (7). Available from: http://onlinelibrary.wiley.com/journal/10.1111/(ISSN)1745-4530. doi:10.1111/jfpe.13271.

Cunha, A.G., Brito, E.S., Moura, C.F.H., Ribeiro, P.R.V., Miranda, M.R.A., 2017. UPLC–qTOF-MS/MS-based phenolic profile and their biosynthetic enzyme activity used to discriminate between cashew apple (*Anacardium occidentale* L.) maturation stages. J. Chromatogr. B. 15700232. 1051, 24–32. doi:10.1016/j.jchromb.2017.02.022.

Dai, K., Agarwal, N., Rodriguez-Palacios, A., Basson, A., 2024. Regulation of intestinal inflammation by walnut-derived bioactive compounds. Nutrients. 2072-6643. 16 (16), 2643. doi:10.3390/nu16162643.

de Camargo, A.C., Regitano-d'Arce, M.A.B., Rasera, G.B., Canniatti-Brazaca, S.G., Do Prado-silva, L., Alvarenga, V.O., Sant'Ana, A.S., Shahidi, F., 2017. Phenolic acids and flavonoids of peanut by-products: antioxidant capacity and antimicrobial effects. Food Chem. 18737072. 237, 538–544. Available from: https://www.elsevier.com/locate/foodchem. doi:10.1016/j.foodchem.2017.05.046.

de Oliveira, S.H., Dos Santos Rolim, C.S., Alves, T.C.L., Dos Santosdos Santos, C.L., Lotas, K.M., Do Do Nascimento, I.S., Do Do Nascimento Rolim, L., Pereira, A.M., Bonomo, R.C.F., 2025. Ultrasound-assisted extraction and characterization of Brazil nut oil (*Bertholletia excelsa*). Sustain. Chem. Environ. 29498392. 9, 100218. doi:10.1016/j.scenv.2025.100218.

de Paiva, E.M., Mattos, A.L.A., da Silva, G.S., Canuto, K.M., Leitão, R.C., Alves, J.L.F., de Brito, E.S., 2024. Valorizing cashew nutshell residue for sustainable lignocellulosic panels using a bio-based phenolic resin as a circular economy solution. Ind. Crops Prod. 09266690. 212. Available from: https://www.sciencedirect.com/science/journal/09266690. doi:10.1016/j.indcrop.2024.118379.

Dean, L.L., 2020. Extracts of peanut skins as a source of bioactive compounds: methodology and applications. Appl. Sci. 2076-3417. 10 (23), 8546. doi:10.3390/app10238546.

Dias, F.F.G., Huang, Y.-P., Schauer, J., Barile, D., Van de Water, J., Leite Nobrega de Moura Bell, J.M., 2023. Effects of protease-assisted aqueous extraction on almond protein profile, digestibility, and antigenicity. Curr. Res. Food Sci. 26659271. 6, 100488. doi:10.1016/j.crfs.2023.100488.

Echegaray, N., Gómez, B., Barba, F.J., Franco, D., Estévez, M., Carballo, J., Marszałek, K., Lorenzo, J.M., 2018. Chestnuts and by-products as source of natural antioxidants in meat and meat products: a review. Trends Food Sci. Technol. 09242244. 82, 110–121. Available from: http://www.elsevier.com/wps/find/journaldescription.cws_home/601278/description#description. doi:10.1016/j.tifs.2018.10.005.

El Bernoussi, S.E., Boujemaa, I., Guezzane, C.E., Bou-Ouzoukni, Y., Nounah, I., Bouyahya, A., Ullah, R., Iqbal, Z., Maggi, F., Caprioli, G., Harhar, H., Tabyaoui, M., 2024. Comparative analysis of nutritional value and antioxidant activity in sweet and bitter almonds. LWT. 00236438. 206, 116587. doi:10.1016/j.lwt.2024.116587.

Elmas, E., Şen, F.B., Kublay, İ.Z., Baş, Y., Tüfekci, F., Derman, H., Bekdeşer, B., Aşçı, Y.S., Capanoglu, E., Bener, M., Apak, R., 2025. Green extraction of antioxidants from hazelnut by-products using microwave-assisted extraction, ultrasound-assisted extraction, and pressurized liquid extraction. Food Bioprocess Technol. 19355149. 18 (6), 5388–5406. Available from: https://www.springer.com/journal/11947. doi:10.1007/s11947-025-03775-z.

Ezeanolue, G., Ohioze, O., Elechi, L., et al., 2026. Pecan (*Carya illinoinensis*) shells as a source of antioxidants: implications for oxidative stress-driven pathologies. Molecules (Basel, Switzerland) 31. doi:10.3390/molecules31060993.

Fan, N., Fusco, J.L., Rosenberg, D.W., 2023. Antioxidant and anti-inflammatory properties of walnut constituents: focus on personalized cancer prevention and the microbiome. Antioxidants 20763921. 12 (5). Available from: https://www.mdpi.com/journal/antioxidants. doi:10.3390/antiox12050982.

Fanali, C., Gallo, V., Posta, S.D., Dugo, L., Mazzeo, L., Cocchi, M., Piemonte, V., De Gara, L., 2021. Choline chloride–lactic acid-based NADES as an extraction medium in a response surface methodology-optimized method for the extraction of phenolic compounds from hazelnut skin. Molecules. 1420-3049. 26 (9), 2652. doi:10.3390/molecules26092652.

Fanali, C., Tripodo, G., Russo, M., Posta, S.D., Pasqualetti, V., De Gara, L., 2018. Effect of solvent on the extraction of phenolic compounds and antioxidant capacity of hazelnut kernel. ELECTROPHORESIS. 0173-0835. 39 (13), 1683–1691. doi:10.1002/elps.201800014.

Fang, Z., Wu, Y., Li, Y., Zhang, X., Willett, W.C., Eliassen, A.H., Rosner, B., Song, M., Mucci, L.A., Giovannucci, E.L., 2021. Association of nut consumption with risk of total cancer and 5 specific cancers: evidence from 3 large prospective cohort studies. Am. J. Clin. Nutr. 19383207. 114 (6), 1925–1935. Available from: http://www.ajcn.org/contents-by-date.2005.shtml. doi:10.1093/ajcn/nqab295.

Faria-Silva, C., Ascenso, A., Costa, A.M., Marto, J., Carvalheiro, M., Ribeiro, H.M., Simões, S., 2020. Feeding the skin: a new trend in food and cosmetics convergence. Trends Food Sci. Technol. 09242244. 95, 21–32. Available from: http://www.elsevier.com/wps/find/journaldescription.cws_home/601278/description#description. doi:10.1016/j.tifs.2019.11.015.

Freitas, P.A.V., Martín-Pérez, L., Gil-Guillén, I., González-Martínez, C., Chiralt, A., 2023. Subcritical water extraction for valorisation of almond skin from almond industrial processing. Foods. 2304-8158. 12 (20), 3759. doi:10.3390/foods12203759.

Gam, D.H., Hong, J.W., Kim, J.H., Kim, J.W., 2021. Skin-whitening and anti-wrinkle effects of bioactive compounds isolated from peanut shell using ultrasound-assisted extraction. Molecules. 1420-3049. 26 (5), 1231. doi:10.3390/molecules26051231.

Garcia-Larez, F.L., Esquer, J., Guzmán, H., Zepeda-Quintana, D.S., Jesús Moreno-Vásquez, M., Rodríguez-Félix, F., Del-Toro-Sánchez, C.L., López-Corona, B.E., Agustín Tapia-Hernández, J., 2025. Effect of Ultrasound-Assisted Extraction (UAE) parameters on the recovery of polyphenols from pecan nutshell waste biomass and its antioxidant activity. Biomass Convers. Biorefin. 2190-6815. 15 (7), 10977–10995. doi:10.1007/s13399-024-05901-x.

Garnier, n.d. Ultimate Blends Almond Crush Shampoo https://incidecoder.com/products/garnier-ultimate-blends-almond-crush-almond-milk-agave-sap (Accessed March 31, 2026).

Gavazzoni Dias, M.F.R., 2015. Hair cosmetics: an overview. Int. J. Trichology 7, 2–15. doi:10.4103/0974-7753.153450.

Gupta, V., Mohapatra, S., Mishra, H., Farooq, U., Kumar, K., Ansari, M., Aldawsari, M., Alalaiwe, A., Mirza, M., Iqbal, Z., 2022. Nanotechnology in cosmetics and cosmeceuticals—a review of latest advancements. Gels. 2310-2861. 8 (3), 173. doi:10.3390/gels8030173.

Gutiérrez-Paz, C., Rodríguez-Moreno, M.C., Hernández-Gómez, M.S., Fernández-Trujillo, J.P., 2024. The cashew pseudofruit (*Anacardium occidentale*): composition, processing effects on bioactive compounds and potential benefits for human health. Foods 23048158. 13 (15). Available from: https://www.mdpi.com/journal/foods. doi:10.3390/foods13152357.

Hammad, K.S.M., El-Roby, A.M., Galal, S.M., 2023. Antioxidant and anticancer activities of peanut (*Arachis hypogaea* L.) skin ultrasound extract. Grasas Y Aceites. 1988-4214. 74 (3), e517. doi:10.3989/gya.0990221.

Hanum, T.I., Laila, L., Sumaiyah, S., Syahrina, E., 2019. Macadamia nuts oil in nanocream and conventional cream as skin anti-aging: a comparative study. Open Access Maced. J. Med. Sci. 18579655. 7 (22), 3917–3920. Available from: https://www.id-press.eu/mjms/article/download/oamjms.2019.533/4335. doi:10.3889/oamjms.2019.533.

Hariri, M., Amirkalali, B., Baradaran, H.R., Gholami, A., 2023. A systematic review and meta-analysis of almond effect on C-reactive protein and interleukin-6 in adults. Complement. Ther. Med. 09652299. 72, 102911. doi:10.1016/j.ctim.2022.102911.

Huo, J., Zhao, Z., Hua, Z., Fan, J., Du, J., Guo, B., 2020. Evaluation of *Juglans regia* L. root for wound healing via antioxidant, antimicrobial and anti-inflammatory activity. Indian J. Biochem. Biophys. 09750959. 57 (3), 304–311. Available from: http://nopr.niscair.res.in/bitstream/123456789/54467/1/IJBB%2057(3)%20304-311.pdf.

Irene Forte, n.d. Pistachio Face Mask https://incidecoder.com/products/irene-forte-pistachio-face-mask (Accessed March 31, 2026).

Kalogiouri, N.P., Mitsikaris, P.D., Klaoudatos, D., Papadopoulos, A.N., Samanidou, V.F., 2021. A rapid hplc-uv protocol coupled to chemometric analysis for the determination of the major phenolic constituents and tocopherol content in almonds and the discrimination of the geographical origin. Molecules 14203049. 26 (18). Available from: https://www.mdpi.com/1420-3049/26/18/5433/pdf. doi:10.3390/molecules26185433.

Kalogiouri, N.P., Mitsikaris, P.D., Papadopoulos, A.N., Samanidou, V.F., 2022. Microwave-assisted extraction coupled to HPLC-UV combined with chemometrics for the determination of bioactive compounds in pistachio nuts and the guarantee of quality and authenticity. Molecules 14203049. 27 (4). Available from: https://www.mdpi.com/1420-3049/27/4/1435/pdf. doi:10.3390/molecules27041435.

Kaur, K., Kaur, G., Singh, A., 2023. Water chestnut starch: extraction, chemical composition, properties, modifications, and application concerns. Sustain. Food Technol. 2753-8095. 1 (2), 228–262. doi:10.1039/d2fb00041e.

Kemerli-Kalbaran, T., Ozdemir, M., 2019. Multi-response optimization of oil extraction from pine nut (*Pinus pinea* L.) by response surface methodology: extraction efficiency, physicochemical properties and antioxidant activity. LWT. 00236438. 103, 34–43. doi:10.1016/j.lwt.2018.12.067.

King, J.C., Blumberg, J., Ingwersen, L., Jenab, M., Tucker, K.L., 2008. Tree nuts and peanuts as components of a healthy diet. J. Nutr. 00223166. 138 (9), 1736S. doi:10.1093/jn/138.9.1736s.

Kumar, R., Bhaduri, G.A., 2025. Biorefining of pine cone forest waste: ultrasound assisted extraction followed with thermal degradation for a zero waste process. Ind. Crops Prod. 09266690. 224, 120278. doi:10.1016/j.indcrop.2024.120278.

Kundal, n.d. Macadamia & Sugar Body Scrub https://incidecoder.com/products/kundal-macadamia-sugar-body-scrub (Accessed March 31, 2026).

Kurt, H., Karakaya, O., 2025. Geographical origin affects the nut traits, bioactive compounds, and fatty acid composition of Turkish hazelnut cultivars (*Corylus avellana* L. cvs. Çakıldak, Palaz, and Tombul). Horticulturae. 2311-7524. 11 (8), 987. doi:10.3390/horticulturae11080987.

Lama-Muñoz, A., Contreras, M.D.M., 2022. Extraction systems and analytical techniques for food phenolic compounds: a review. Foods. 2304-8158. 11 (22), 3671. doi:10.3390/foods11223671.

León, J., Ortiz, G., Barrios, A.F.G., Álvarez, O., Maranon, A., Hernandez, C., Ayala-Garcia, C., Porras, A., 2025. Understanding the effects of pre-treatment and extraction methods on lipid fingerprint of cashew nut shell liquid (CNSL) by non-targeted lipidomics analysis. Sci. Rep. 20452322. 15 (1). Available from: https://www.nature.com/srep/. doi:10.1038/s41598-025-03071-y.

Lin, T.K., Zhong, L., Santiago, J.L., 2018. Anti-inflammatory and skin barrier repair effects of topical application of some plant oils. Int. J. Mol. Sci. 14220067. 19 (1). Available from: http://www.mdpi.com/1422-0067/19/1/70/pdf. doi:10.3390/ijms19010070.

Lipan, L., Miarnau, X., Calle, A., Carbonell, Á., Sendra, E., Batlle, I., Romero, A., 2025. Factors influencing the almond kernel breakage during shelling processes and the impact of water conditioning on kernel color and free acidity. LWT. 00236438. 215, 117250. doi:10.1016/j.lwt.2024.117250.

Luksiene, J., Zevzikoviene, A., Kazlauskaite, J.A., Marksa, M., Majiene, D., Zevzikovas, A., 2025. Extraction systems and analytical techniques for food phenolic compounds: a review. Plants. 2223-7747. 14 (16), 2524. doi:10.3390/plants14162524.

Lutz, M., Álvarez, K., Loewe, M.V., 2016. Chemical composition of pine nut (*Pinus pinea* L.) grown in three geographical macrozones in Chile. CyTA - J. Food 15, 1–7. doi:10.1080/19476337.2016.1250109.

Macadamia Professional, n.d. Macadamia Professional Weightless Moisture Masque https://incidecoder.com/products/macadamia-professional-macadamia-professional-weightless-moisture-masque (Accessed March 31, 2026).

Machado, N.M., Nunes, Y.C., de Lima, E.P., Chehadi, A.C., Otoboni, A.M.M.B., Miola, V.F.B., Nicolau, C.C.T., Fiorini, A.M.R., Oshiiwa, M., Laurindo, L.F., Barbalho, S.M., 2025. Peanuts (*Arachis hypogaea* L.) in food industry and their benefits for human health – a review of the current literature. J. Food Compos. Anal. 08891575. 143. Available from: https://www.sciencedirect.com/science/journal/08891575. doi:10.1016/j.jfca.2025.107574.

Maestri, D., 2024. Groundnut and tree nuts: a comprehensive review on their lipid components, phytochemicals, and nutraceutical properties. Crit. Rev. Food Sci. Nutr. 1040-8398. 64 (21), 7426–7450. doi:10.1080/10408398.2023.2185202.

Mandalari, G., Barreca, D., Gervasi, T., Roussell, M.A., Klein, B., Feeney, M.J., Carughi, A., 2022. Pistachio nuts (*Pistacia vera* L.): production, nutrients, bioactives and novel health effects. Plants 22237747. 11 (1). Available from: https://www.mdpi.com/2223-7747/11/1/18/pdf. doi:10.3390/plants11010018.

Martorana, M., Arcoraci, T., Rizza, L., Cristani, M., Bonina, F.P., Saija, A., Trombetta, D., Tomaino, A., 2013. In vitro antioxidant and in vivo photoprotective effect of pistachio (*Pistacia vera* L., variety Bronte) seed and skin extracts. Fitoterapia. 18736971. 85 (1), 41–48. doi:10.1016/j.fitote.2012.12.032.

Matthes, J., Schmid, M., 2024. Biogenic raw materials from food waste and by-products for smart packaging applications. Curr. Opin. Green Sustain. Chem. 24522236. 46, 100894. doi:10.1016/j.cogsc.2024.100894.

Medic, A., Solar, A., Hudina, M., Veberic, R., Zamljen, T., 2023. Effect of different walnut and hazelnut leaf compost treatments on yield and phenolic composition of *Lactuca sativa* L.. Foods. 2304-8158. 12 (14), 2738. doi:10.3390/foods12142738.

Mencherini, T., Esposito, T., Sansone, F., Eletto, D., Pannetta, M., Gordobil, O., Piccinelli, A.L., Ferniani, C., Auriemma, G., Rastrelli, L., Aquino, R.P., 2025. Valorization of hazelnut (*Corylus avellana* L.) skin by-product as a multifunctional ingredient for cosmetic emulsions. Antioxidants. 2076-3921. 14 (10), 1199. doi:10.3390/antiox14101199.

Michalak, M., Kieltyka-Dadasiewicz, A., 2019. Nut oils and their dietetic and cosmetic significance: a Review. J. Oleo Sci. 13473352. 68 (2), 111–120. Available from: https://www.jstage.jst.go.jp/article/jos/68/2/68_ess18216/_pdf. doi:10.5650/jos.ess18216.

Mir, G., Nisar, O., Iqbal, U., 2016. Scientific processing of walnuts necessary for amazing health benefits. J. Chem. Chem. Sci. 6, 783–793.

Mohammed, D., Freije, A., Abdulhussain, H., Khonji, A., Hasan, M., Ferraris, C., Gasparri, C., Aljar, M.A.A., Redha, A.A., Giacosa, A., Rondanelli, M., Perna, S., 2023. Analysis of the antioxidant activity, lipid profile, and minerals of the skin and seed of hazelnuts (*Corylus avellana* L.), pistachios (*Pistacia vera*), and almonds (*Prunus dulcis*)—a comparative analysis. AppliedChem. 2673-9623. 3 (1), 110–118. doi:10.3390/appliedchem3010008.

Mungwari, C.P., King'ondu, C.K., Sigauke, P., Obadele, B.A., 2025. Conventional and modern techniques for bioactive compounds recovery from plants: review. Sci. Afr. 24682276. 27. Available from: https://www.sciencedirect.com/science/journal/24682276. doi:10.1016/j.sciaf.2024.e02509.

Nivea, n.d. Cleansing Milk Almond Oil https://incidecoder.com/products/nivea-reinigingsmelk-amandelolie (Accessed March 31, 2026).

Nolasco, A., Squillante, J., Velotto, S., D'Auria, G., Ferranti, P., Mamone, G., Errico, M.E., Avolio, R., Castaldo, R., De Luca, L., Romano, R., Esposito, F., Cirillo, T., 2024. Exploring the untapped potential of pine nut skin by-products: a holistic characterization and recycling approach. Foods. 2304-8158. 13 (7), 1044. doi:10.3390/foods13071044.

Nuxe, n.d. Bio Hazelnut Replenishing Nourishing Body Oil. https://incidecoder.com/products/nuxe-bio-hazelnut-replenishing-nourishing-body-oil (Accessed March 31, 2026)

Okumus, E., Temiz, M.A., 2026. Use of hazelnut by-products as a sustainable source for nanoparticle synthesis: characterization, bioactive components and health effects of maltodextrin-coated nanocapsules. J. Food Meas. Charact. 21934134. 20 (3), 3346–3361. Available from: https://www.springer.com/journal/11694. doi:10.1007/s11694-025-03912-4.

Olbińska, E., Trela-Makowej, A., Larysz, W., Orzechowska, A., Szymańska, R., 2023. The effect of α-tocopherol incorporated into different carriers on the oxidative stability of oil in water (O/W) emulsions. Colloids Surf. B Biointerfaces. 09277765. 230, 113536. doi:10.1016/j.colsurfb.2023.113536.

Pinto, D., de la Luz Cádiz-gurrea, M., Garcia, J., José Saavedra, M., Freitas, V., Costa, P., Sarmento, B., Delerue-Matos, C., Rodrigues, F., 2021. From soil to cosmetic industry: validation of a new cosmetic ingredient extracted from chestnut shells. Sustain. Mater. Technol. 22149937. 29, e00309. doi:10.1016/j.susmat.2021.e00309.

Pistache, n.d. Pistachio Body Butter https://incidecoder.com/products/pistache-pistachio-body-butter (Accessed March 31, 2026).

Polmann, G., Badia, V., Danielski, R., Ferreira, S.R.S., Block, J.M., 2021. Non-conventional nuts: an overview of reported composition and bioactivity and new approaches for its consumption and valorization of co-products. Future Foods. 26668335. 4, 100099. doi:10.1016/j.fufo.2021.100099.

Qingyang, L., Runhong, M., Wang, R., Zhanglin, N., Zheng, Y., Han, Y., Shutian, W., Tang, F., Yuan, X., Liu, Y., 2022. Characterization and assessment of chemical components in walnuts with various appearances. J. Food Compos. Anal. 08891575. 107, 104361. doi:10.1016/j.jfca.2021.104361.

Rahbardar, M.G., Rashki, M., Boskabady, M.H., 2025. A review of antioxidant activity, anti-inflammatory properties, apoptosis-regulatory effects, and immune system modulation of *Juglans regia* L. (walnut). Food Sci. Nutr. 20487177. 13 (11). Available from: https://onlinelibrary.wiley.com/journal/10.1002/%28ISSN%292048-7177. doi:10.1002/fsn3.71081.

Rajaram, S., Damasceno, N.R.T., Braga, R.A.M., Martinez, R., Kris-Etherton, P., Sala-Vila, A., 2023. Effect of nuts on markers of inflammation and oxidative stress: a narrative review. Nutrients 20726643. 15 (5). Available from: http://www.mdpi.com/journal/nutrients/. doi:10.3390/nu15051099.

Ramezan, M., Hosseini, H.M., Salimi, A., Ramezan, Y., 2023. Study of the apoptotic impacts of hazelnut oil on the colorectal cancer cell line. Adv. Biomed. Res. 2277-9175. 12 (1). doi:10.4103/abr.abr_297_21.

Rehman, F.U., Ahmad, A., 2025. The potential of hazelnut (*Corylus avellana*) nutritive composition and its bioactive properties in cosmetics. J. Contemp. Pharm. 2521-0521. 9 (1), 39–43. doi:10.56770/jcp2025917.

Revolution Skincare, n.d. Green Tea & Walnut Exfoliating Face Mask https://incidecoder.com/products/revolution-skincare-green-tea-walnut-exfoliating-face-mask (Accessed March 31, 2026).

Rico, R., Bulló, M., Salas-Salvadó, J., 2016. Nutritional composition of raw fresh cashew (*Anacardium occidentale* L.) kernels from different origin. Food Sci. Nutr. 2048-7177. 4 (2), 329–338. doi:10.1002/fsn3.294.

Roselló-Soto, E., Poojary, M.M., Barba, F.J., Lorenzo, J.M., Mañes, J., Moltó, J.C., 2018. Tiger nut and its by-products valorization: from extraction of oil and valuable compounds to development of new healthy products. Innov. Food Sci. Emerg. Technol. 14668564. 45, 306–312. Available from: http://www.elsevier.com/locate/ifset. doi:10.1016/j.ifset.2017.11.016.

Rossen, n.d. Carrot & Walnut Tanning Body Oil (with Shimmer). https://incidecoder.com/products/rossen-carrot-walnut-tanning-body-oil-with-shimmer (Accessed March 31, 2026).

Rui, L., Sharma, A.K., Zhu, J., Zheng, B., Xiao, G., Chen, L., 2022. Nutritional biology of chestnuts: a perspective review. Food Chem. 03088146. 395, 133575. doi:10.1016/j.foodchem.2022.133575.

Rusu, M.E., Fizesan, I., Pop, A., Mocan, A., Gheldiu, A.M., Babota, M., Vodnar, D.C., Jurj, A., Berindan-Neagoe, I., Vlase, L., Popa, D.S., 2020. Walnut (*Juglans regia* L.) septum: assessment of bioactive molecules and in vitro biological effects. Molecules 14203049. 25 (9). Available from: https://www.mdpi.com/1420-3049/25/9/2187/pdf. doi:10.3390/molecules25092187.

Rusu, M.E., Simedrea, R., Gheldiu, A.M., Mocan, A., Vlase, L., Popa, D.S., Ferreira, I.C.F.R., 2019. Benefits of tree nut consumption on aging and age-related diseases: mechanisms of actions. Trends Food Sci. Technol. 09242244. 88, 104–120. Available from: http://www.elsevier.com/wps/find/journaldescription.cws_home/601278/description#description. doi:10.1016/j.tifs.2019.03.006.

Ryczaj, K., Chojnowska-Wójtowicz, M., Dumycz, K., Feleszko, W., Kulus, M., 2023. Prevalence of major food allergens in skincare products for atopic dermatitis. Adv. Dermatol. Allergol. 1642-395X. 40 (6), 762–765. doi:10.5114/ada.2023.133819.

Saglam, A., Asan-Ozusaglam, M., 2023. A natural additive alternative to the cosmetics industry: hazelnut and its waste products. J. Skin Stem Cell. 2423-7086. 10 (2). doi:10.5812/jssc-137580.

Sandhu, A.K., Edirisinghe, I., Burton-Freeman, B., 2025. Pecans and Human Health: distinctive Benefits of an American Nut. Nutrients. 2072-6643. 17 (23), 3686. doi:10.3390/nu17233686.

Savannah Bee Company, n.d. Beeswax Hand Cream. https://incidecoder.com/products/savannah-bee-company-beeswax-hand-cream (Accessed March 31, 2026).

Sayah, O., Taibi, S., Bouakline, H., Yousfi, R.E., Tayebi, A., Ziani, I., Tahani, A., Bachiri, A.E., 2025. Comparison of sweet and bitter almond oilquality: impact of kernel skin and green supercritical CO_2 extraction method. Food Chem. 03088146. 486, 144540. doi:10.1016/j.foodchem.2025.144540.

Scapinello, J., Magro, J.D., Block, J.M., Di Luccio, M., Tres, M.V., Oliveira, J.V., 2017. Fatty acid profile of pecan nut oils obtained from pressurized n-butane and cold pressing compared with commercial oils. J. Food Sci. Technol. 09758402. 54 (10), 3366–3369. Available from: http://www.springerlink.com/content/121580/. doi:10.1007/s13197-017-2771-9.

Selwyn, A., Govindaraj, S., 2023. Study of plant-based cosmeceuticals and skin care. S. Afr. J. Bot. 02546299. 158, 429–442. doi:10.1016/j.sajb.2023.05.039.

Shi, R., Bai, H., Biao, L., Liu, C., Ying, Z., Xiong, Z., Wang, W., 2021. Combined transcriptome and lipidomic analyses of lipid biosynthesis in *Macadamia ternifolia* nuts. Life. 2075-1729. 11 (12), 1431. doi:10.3390/life11121431.

Shuai, X., Dai, T., Chen, M., Liang, R., Liqing, D., Chen, J., Liu, C., 2021. Comparative study of chemical compositions and antioxidant capacities of oils obtained from 15 macadamia (*Macadamia integrifolia*) cultivars in China. Foods. 2304-8158. 10 (5), 1031. doi:10.3390/foods10051031.

Silva, V., Oliveira, I., Alberto Pereira, J., Gonçalves, B., 2025. Almond by-products: a comprehensive review of composition, bioactivities, and influencing factors. Foods. 2304-8158. 14 (6), 1042. doi:10.3390/foods14061042.

Solar, A., Medic, A., Slatnar, A., Mikulic-Petkovsek, M., Botta, R., Rovira, M., Sarraquigne, J.-P., Silva, A.P., Veberic, R., Stampar, F., Hudina, M., Bacchetta, L., 2022. The effects of the cultivar and environment on the phenolic contents of hazelnut kernels. Plants. 2223-7747. 11 (22), 3051. doi:10.3390/plants11223051.

Somwongin, S., Chaiyana, W., 2024. Clinical efficacy in skin hydration and reducing wrinkles of nanoemulsions containing *Macadamia integrifolia* seed oil. Nanomaterials. 2079-4991. 14 (8), 724. doi:10.3390/nano14080724.

Srisuksomwong, P., Kaenhin, L., Mungmai, L., 2023. Collagenase and tyrosinase inhibitory activities and stability of facial cream formulation containing cashew leaf extract. Cosmetics. 2079-9284. 10 (1), 17. doi:10.3390/cosmetics10010017.

Strieder, M.M., Mendiola, J., Cokdinleyen, M., Valdés, A., Bragagnolo, F.S., Filho, C.A.B., Lanza, M., Ferreira, S.R.S., Cifuentes, A., Rostagno, M.A., Ibáñez, E., 2025. Sustainable valorization of almond and peanut plant-based milk cakes: the use of terpenoid mixtures as ready-to-use solvents to enhance supercritical CO2 extraction. Food Chem. 18737072. 479. Available from: https://www.sciencedirect.com/science/journal/03088146. doi:10.1016/j.foodchem.2025.143796.

Suncademy, n.d. Botanical Facial Sunscreen. https://incidecoder.com/products/suncademy-botanical-facial-sunscreen (Accessed March 31, 2026).

Takala, R., Ramji, D.P., Choy, E., 2023. The beneficial effects of pine nuts and its major fatty acid, pinolenic acid, on inflammation and metabolic perturbations in inflammatory disorders. Int. J. Mol. Sci. 1422-0067. 24 (2), 1171. doi:10.3390/ijms24021171.

Takeda, L.N., Omine, A., Laurindo, L.F., Araújo, A.C., Machado, N.M., Dias, J.A., Kavalakatt, J., Banerjee, S., de Alvares Goulart, R., Atanasov, A.G., Bishayee, A., Barbalho, S.M., 2025. Brazil nut (*Bertholletia excelsa* Bonpl.) in health and disease: a narrative review. Food Chem. 18737072. 477. Available from: https://www.sciencedirect.com/science/journal/03088146. doi:10.1016/j.foodchem.2025.143425.

Taş, N.G., Gökmen, V., 2017. Phenolic compounds in natural and roasted nuts and their skins: a brief review. Curr. Opin. Food Sci. 22147993. 14, 103–109. Available from: http://www.journals.elsevier.com/current-opinion-in-food-science/. doi:10.1016/j.cofs.2017.03.001.

Teneva, O., Petkova, Z., Toshev, N., Solakov, N., Loginovska, K., Platov, Y., 2024. Effect of roasting on the chemical and lipid composition of pine nuts in two regions in Russia. Heliyon. 24058440. 10 (14), e34576. doi:10.1016/j.heliyon.2024.e34576.

Tiwari, A., Sanjog, J., 2025. Morphological, structural, and thermal properties of cellulose nanocrystals extracted from Indian water chestnut shells (agricultural waste). Next Mater. 29498228. 8, 100653. doi:10.1016/j.nxmate.2025.100653.

Uchikura, T., Kitano, T., Yoshimura, M., Amakura, Y., 2023. Characterization of phenolic constituents in hazelnut kernels. Biosci. Biotechnol. Biochem.. 1347-6947. 87 (7), 688–695. doi:10.1093/bbb/zbad043.

Valasi, L., Zafeiri, E.C., Thanou, I., Pappas, C.S., 2023. Study of volatile compounds in Greek pistachio (*Pistacia vera* L. 'Aegina' cultivar) oils using Soxhlet and ultrasound-assisted extraction. Heliyon. 24058440. 9 (5), e15623. doi:10.1016/j.heliyon.2023.e15623.

Valdés, A., Carmen Garrigós, M., Jiménez, A., 2022. Extraction and characterization of antioxidant compounds in almond (*Prunus amygdalus*) shell residues for food packaging applications. Membranes. 2077-0375. 12 (8), 806. doi:10.3390/membranes12080806.

Valdés, A., Mondragon, G., Garrigós, M.C., Eceiza, A., Jiménez, A., 2023. Microwave-assisted extraction of cellulose nanocrystals from almond (*Prunus amygdalus*) shell waste. Front. Nutr. 2296861X. 9. Available from: https://journal.frontiersin.org/journal/nutrition. doi:10.3389/fnut.2022.1071754.

Van Thanh, H., Phi, N.T.L., Khoi, N.T., Hoan, N.X., Van Hung, P., 2023. Green extraction and biological activity of phenolic extracts from cashew nut testa using a combination of enzyme and ultrasound-assisted treatments. J. Sci. Food Agric. 10970010. 103 (11), 5626–5633. Available from: http://onlinelibrary.wiley.com/journal/10.1002/(ISSN)1097-0010. doi:10.1002/jsfa.12641.

Vinson, J.A., Cai, Y., 2012. Nuts, especially walnuts, have both antioxidant quantity and efficacy and exhibit significant potential health benefits. Food Funct. 2042-6496. 3 (2), 134–140. doi:10.1039/c2fo10152a.

Xing-Hao, T., Bang-fu, W., Xie, Y., Shu-Ling, X., Zong-Yuan, W., Xin, L., Wei, F., Li-Qing, D., Chen, H., 2021. A comprehensive study of raw and roasted macadamia nuts: lipid profile, physicochemical, nutritional, and sensory properties. Food Sci. Nutr. 2048-7177. 9 (3), 1688–1697. doi:10.1002/fsn3.2143.

Xuemin, L., Liu, Y., Hao, J., Wang, W., 2018. Study of almond shell characteristics. Materials. 1996-1944. 11 (9), 1782. doi:10.3390/ma11091782.

Yajing, L., Xiang, L., Jianhua, Q., 2025. Procyanidin A1 from peanut skin exerts anti-aging effects and attenuates senescence via antioxidative stress and autophagy induction. Antioxidants. 2076-3921. 14 (3), 322. doi:10.3390/antiox14030322.

Yan, L., Lyu, S., Gao, C., Xiaolin, S., Wang, K., Huang, C., Chen, J., Huang, J., 2024. Comparative analysis of aroma profiles in walnut, pecan and hickory nuts during the roasting process using E-nose, HS-SPME-GC-MS, and HS-GC-IMS. LWT. 00236438. 210, 116810. doi:10.1016/j.lwt.2024.116810.

Yang, J., Liu, R.H., Halim, L., 2009. Antioxidant and antiproliferative activities of common edible nut seeds. LWT. 00236438. 42 (1), 1–8. doi:10.1016/j.lwt.2008.07.007.

Yeh, W.J., Yan, C., Wu, C.H., 2025. Photoprotective effects of phytochemicals on blue light-induced retinal damage: current evidence and future perspectives. Nutrients 20726643. 17 (2). Available from: http://www.mdpi.com/journal/nutrients/. doi:10.3390/nu17020331.

Yemmireddy, V.K., Cason, C., Moreira, J., Adhikari, A., 2020. Effect of pecan variety and the method of extraction on the antimicrobial activity of pecan shell extracts against different foodborne pathogens and their efficacy on food matrices. Food Control. 09567135. 112, 107098. doi:10.1016/j.foodcont.2020.107098.

Yilmaz, M.A., Cakir, O., Yener, I., 2023. A fast, accurate and comprehensive LC-MS/MS method validation for the sensitive quantification of water-soluble vitamins in walnut, almond, hazelnut and pistachio fruits. Int. J. Mass Spectrom. 13873806. 488, 117040. doi:10.1016/j.ijms.2023.117040.

Yuan, Q., Dan, W., Fang, L., Leng, Y., Wang, X., Liu, C., Liu, X., Wang, J., Min, W., 2023. Anti-inflammatory effect of walnut-derived peptide via the activation of Nrf2/Keap1 pathway against oxidative stress. J. Funct. Foods. 17564646. 110, 105839. doi:10.1016/j.jff.2023.105839.

Yves Rocher, n.d. Shea & Chestnut Milk Nourishing Body Milk. https://incidecoder.com/products/yves-rocher-shea-chestnut-milk-nourishing-body-milk (Accessed March 31, 2026).

Zhang, X., Lian, H., Shi, J., Meng, W., Peng, Y., 2020. Plant extracts such as pine nut shell, peanut shell and jujube leaf improved the antioxidant ability and gas permeability of chitosan films. Int. J. Biol. Macromol. 01418130. 148, 1242–1250. doi:10.1016/j.ijbiomac.2019.11.108.

Zhang, Y., Sun, S., 2023. Tiger nut (*Cyperus esculentus* L.) oil: a review of bioactive compounds, extraction technologies, potential hazards and applications. Food Chem. X. 25901575. 19, 100868. doi:10.1016/j.fochx.2023.100868.

Zhao, J., Wang, X., Lin, H., Lin, Z., 2023. Hazelnut and its by-products: a comprehensive review of nutrition, phytochemical profile, extraction, bioactivities and applications. Food Chem. 03088146. 413, 135576. doi:10.1016/j.foodchem.2023.135576.

Zhou, F., Yang, H., Liu, L., et al., 2026. The value-added challenge of nuts: antioxidant components, functions and applications in nut by-products. Front. Nutr. 13. doi:10.3389/fnut.2026.1789610.

Zhu, B., Lin, L., Li, J., Lv, G., Huang, M., 2013. Comparison of four different extraction methods of oil from macadamia integrifolia. Adv. Mater. Res. 10226680. 610-613, 3382–3386. doi:10.4028/www.scientific.net/AMR.610-613.3382.

Zhu, Y., Wilkinson, K.L., Wirthensohn, M.G., 2015. Lipophilic antioxidant content of almonds (*Prunus dulcis*): a regional and varietal study. J. Food Compos. Anal. 08891575. 39, 120–127. Available from: http://www.elsevier.com/inca/publications/store/6/2/2/8/7/8/index.htt. doi:10.1016/j.jfca.2014.12.003.

Chapter 14

Plant oils and their biowastes

Haralabos C. Karantonis and Constantina Nasopoulou
Laboratory of Food Chemistry – Technology and Quality of Food of Animal Origin, Department of Food Science and Nutrition, School of Environment, University of the Aegean, Lemnos, Greece

1 Introduction

Global production of edible plant oils has risen steadily over the past two decades, driven by growing demand in the food, cosmetic, and biofuel sectors (Alcock et al., 2022; Kastakova et al., 2023). According to FAO statistics, this expansion between 2000 and 2022 has been supported by both increased cultivation areas and intensified production practices (Alcock et al., 2022; FAO, 2023). Today, >85% of global vegetable oil output originates from just four crops: oil palm, soybean, rapeseed (canola), and sunflower (Alcock et al., 2022). Palm and soybean oils dominate worldwide production, followed by rapeseed and sunflower (Tamothran et al., 2022). Among herbaceous crops, soybean and rapeseed provide the highest yields (Zhou et al., 2020). Although olive oil represents a smaller share of total global output, it remains the cornerstone lipid of the Mediterranean diet and a key source of bioactive-rich by-products. The global vegetable oil market is projected to continue expanding, with strong growth expected in food, cosmetic, and energy applications (Sarpong, 2024).

Edible plant oils are increasingly valued in cosmetic science as multifunctional ingredients due to their content of fatty acids, tocopherols, carotenoids, phytosterols, squalene, and phenolic compounds (Abdalla et al., 2024; Rashid, 2024). Importantly, many of these bioactives are also abundant in processing by-products, reframing residues once regarded as waste into valuable sources of high-value cosmetic ingredients. Fatty acids and lipophilic minor compounds contribute to barrier reinforcement, moisturization, and protection against photodamage, while phenolics act as natural antioxidants and antiinflammatory agents (Chu and Nyam, 2021; Moore et al., 2020). Their affinity with cutaneous lipids facilitates penetration into the stratum corneum, improving barrier integrity and modulating repair responses. In addition, biodiversity-derived oils have been shown to regulate sebum production and influence skin physiology (Lozada et al., 2025).

Olive oil by-products—particularly olive mill wastewater (OMWW), pomace, and leaves—are notable for their very high concentrations of polyphenols such as hydroxytyrosol and oleuropein, which exhibit antioxidant, antiinflammatory, antimicrobial, and photoprotective activities (Albini et al., 2025b). These compounds inhibit elastase and collagenase, protect against oxidative stress, and promote wound healing, while maintaining excellent safety in dermatological use (Albini et al., 2025a). Traditional applications of olive-derived products in soap making reflect these regenerative qualities, while modern cosmeceutical formulations benefit from well-validated bioactivities (Albini et al., 2025b). Other oil-processing residues also provide valuable actives: for example, canola by-products enriched with aloe vera pulp yield sterols and aloin with antioxidant and wound healing effects (Itsarasook et al., 2025), soybean and sunflower residues supply lecithin for emulsification and barrier repair (Thy et al., 2025), and palm or corn by-products contribute tocopherols, carotenoids, and other lipophilic antioxidants (Foti et al., 2021; Itsarasook et al., 2025).

Despite these opportunities, large-scale oil production—particularly from palm and soybean—raises environmental concerns. The expansion of cultivation areas has been linked to deforestation, peatland occupation, and other land-use changes with significant climate impacts (Martinez et al., 2017). For instance, deforestation can increase the climate-change footprint of a cosmetic cream by approximately 9%, while peat soil occupation adds a further 16% (Martinez et al., 2017). Palm oil is often criticized for these impacts (Candellone et al., 2023), though its high yield per hectare complicates the debate, since substituting it with lower-yield crops could exacerbate land-use pressures (Beyer and Rademacher, 2021; Murphy et al., 2021).

Biofunctional Cosmetics for Health. https://doi.org/10.1016/B978-0-443-27500-5.00020-4

A major innovation trend in this sector is the valorization of oil-processing by-products, including olive pomace, OMWW, rapeseed press cake, soybean meal, sunflower residues, and palm oil mill effluents (POMEs). These side streams are rich in phenolics, proteins, lipids, and other bioactives with significant potential for cosmetics (Barbulova et al., 2015; Morganti et al., 2022; Rodrigues et al., 2023). Their valorization reduces environmental burdens, enhances sustainability, and supports the principles of the circular bioeconomy (Cádiz-Gurrea et al., 2021). The main challenge lies in balancing whole-extract synergies with the isolation of targeted bioactive fractions, while ensuring stability, safety, and consumer-acceptable sensory qualities.

Together, these insights demonstrate how edible plant oils and their by-products serve as renewable resources for eco-responsible and effective cosmetic formulations. By linking sustainability with dermatological efficacy, they provide a foundation for multifunctional biocosmetics that address skin aging, inflammation, and environmental stress while promoting the circular use of agricultural resources (Tsoupras et al., 2024).

2 Bioactives in edible plant oils and by-products for biocosmetics

Edible plant oils such as palm, soybean, rapeseed, sunflower, and olive are valuable sources of fatty acids and other bioactive minor components, many of which are widely incorporated into cosmetic and biocosmetic formulations. Their composition—particularly fatty acid distribution and the concentrations of phenolics, tocopherols, sterols, carotenoids, and squalene—dictates both their biological activity and formulation potential (Mohanty et al., 2024; Rodrigues et al., 2023).

The fatty acid fraction provides structural building blocks for skin lipids, supporting hydration, elasticity, and barrier integrity. Linoleic acid contributes to ceramide synthesis, oleic acid enhances emolliency and penetration, and saturated fatty acids such as palmitic and stearic confer occlusive protection (Franco, 2018; Kasmin et al., 2015). The minor bioactive fraction further strengthens cosmetic efficacy: phenolics provide antioxidant, antiinflammatory, and antimicrobial activity (Cádiz-Gurrea et al., 2021; Thiyam et al., 2004); tocopherols and tocotrienols act as radical scavengers against photoaging (Gotor and Rhazi, 2016; Japir et al., 2017); carotenoids such as β-carotene exert pigmentation and photoprotective effects (Imo, 2020); phytosterols reinforce the skin barrier and modulate inflammation (Percival et al., 2019); and squalene, a natural component of sebum, enhances moisturization and antioxidant protection (Rodrigues et al., 2015).

Beyond the oils themselves, processing by-products (press cakes, pomace, mill wastewater, deodorizer distillates) are increasingly recognized as concentrated reservoirs of bioactives. Valorizing these residues not only supplies cost-effective functional ingredients but also advances sustainability and circular economy goals (Barbulova et al., 2015; Morganti et al., 2022).

2.1 Palm oil and by-products

Palm oil consists mainly of triacylglycerols, with palmitic (~45%), oleic (~39%), and linoleic (~10%) acids (Kasmin et al., 2015). Its bioactives include α- and β-carotene (500–700 ppm), tocopherols and tocotrienols (600–1200 mg/kg), phytosterols (250–600 mg/kg), and aliphatic alcohols (Imo, 2020; Japir et al., 2017; Sundram et al., 2003). Palm oil by-products, such as POME, are rich in phenolic acids and flavonoids, with contents up to 40.5 mg gallic acid equivalent (GAE)/mL (Sundram et al., 2003). Catalytic hydrotreating of palm oil further yields biowaxes, renewable alternatives to petroleum waxes with film-forming and occlusive properties (Chaparro et al., 2023). Cosmetically, palm oil supports hydration and barrier function, while carotenoids and vitamin E confer antioxidant, photoprotective, and antiaging effects (Rashid, 2024).

2.2 Soybean oil and by-products

Soybean oil is notable for its high polyunsaturated fatty acid (PUFA) content: linoleic (~54%), oleic (~23%), palmitic (~11%), linolenic (~8%), and stearic (~4%) (Mohanty et al., 2024). Its minor compounds include phospholipids with emulsifying properties, phenolic acids, saponins, phytic acid, glyceollins, terpenes, and tocopherols (1000–2000 mg/kg, γ-tocopherol predominant) (Freitas et al., 2019; Pessoa et al., 2020; Torres et al., 2009). Isoflavones (genistein, daidzein) stand out for their antioxidant and estrogen-like effects (Bragagnolo et al., 2021; Kim et al., 2021). Processing by-products add further value: soybean meal contains genistin, daidzin, and malonylgenistin (up to 1.76 mg/g) (Freitas et al., 2019); soy residues provide soluble polysaccharides with prebiotic and antiinflammatory activity (Le et al., 2020); and deodorizer distillates concentrate phytosterol esters, tocopherols, and squalene (Torres et al., 2009). Cosmetically, soybean oil derivatives support barrier repair, prevent transepidermal water loss, and contribute antiaging, skin-brightening, antioxidant, and soothing effects (Mohanty et al., 2024).

2.3 Rapeseed oil and by-products

Rapeseed oil is rich in monounsaturated fatty acids (oleic 50%–65%) and balanced PUFAs (linoleic 18%–28%, α-linolenic 8%–15%), with low saturated content (<10%) (Tileuberdi et al., 2022). Minor compounds include tocopherols (~700 mg/kg), phytosterols, terpenes, and polyphenols such as sinapic acid and its ester sinapine, both of which are potent antioxidants (Shen et al., 2023; Thiyam et al., 2004; Yates et al., 2019). Rapeseed press cake and pomace are particularly rich in proteins (30%–40% dry weight) with emulsifying and film-forming properties, along with high sinapic acid content (up to 20 mg/g) (Cairone et al., 2023; Rivera et al., 2015). Hydrolyzed peptides exhibit antioxidant and antimicrobial effects (Beaubier et al., 2023; Duan et al., 2021; Östbring et al., 2020). Processing strategies reduce antinutritional compounds (glucosinolates, phytic acid, tannins) and improve compatibility with formulations (Zhu et al., 2023). Cosmetically, rapeseed derivatives provide hydration, emulsion stability, antioxidant defense, and antiaging benefits.

2.4 Sunflower oil and by-products

Sunflower oil occurs in high-oleic and high-linoleic types, with fatty acid profiles of linoleic (48%–74%), oleic (14%–39%), palmitic (3%–6%), and stearic (3%–6%) (Franco, 2018). Its main bioactives include tocopherols (400–1000 mg/kg, with α-tocopherol predominant), phytosterols, squalene, carotenoids, chlorophyll, and phenolics (Gotor and Rhazi, 2016; Rhazi et al., 2022). By-products such as press cakes retain fatty acids, proteins, and amino acids, while receptacles contain flavonoids, alkaloids, and chlorogenic acid (He et al., 2022; Perez et al., 2004; Petraru et al., 2021). These compounds together enhance antioxidant, antimicrobial, and skin-protective functions. Cosmetically, sunflower derivatives strengthen barrier function, support ceramide synthesis, reduce inflammation, and improve skin softness and smoothness (Abdalla et al., 2024; Kesarwani et al., 2024).

2.5 Olive oil and by-products

Olive oil is distinguished by its high MUFA content (oleic acid 55%–83%) and moderate linoleic (3.5%–21%), palmitic (7.5%–20%), and stearic (0.5%–5%) acids (Rodrigues et al., 2015). Its minor bioactives include phenolics such as hydroxytyrosol, tyrosol, and oleuropein; tocopherols (50–300 mg/kg); squalene (2000–7500 mg/kg); phospholipids; and triterpenes (Cádiz-Gurrea et al., 2021; Rodrigues et al., 2023). By-products are especially rich in phenolics: OMWW contains >10,000 mg/L of hydroxytyrosol and oleuropein (Albini et al., 2025a); pomace retains 98%–99% of fruit phenolics, including secoiridoids (Tsoupras et al., 2024); and olive leaves provide up to 100 mg/g of oleuropein, along with rutin and luteolin derivatives (Buzzi et al., 2023; Clodoveo et al., 2022). These compounds deliver antioxidant, photoprotective, depigmenting, antimicrobial, and wound healing benefits (Carrara et al., 2021; Rodrigues et al., 2023). Sustainable extraction techniques, such as deep eutectic solvents, enhance phenolic recovery and stability (Öztürk et al., 2025). Historically, residues such as amurca were used for microbial control, reflecting the long-recognized bioactivity of olive by-products (Albini et al., 2025a).

3 Applications in biofunctional cosmetics and mechanisms of bioactives

Effective cosmetic use of oil-derived bioactives depends on stability during storage, skin penetration, and nonirritancy. Plant oils and their by-products supply complementary hydrophilic and lipophilic actives, so formulations often pair aqueous phenolics with lipid carriers to cover both compartments. For example, OMWW fractions rich in hydroxytyrosol inhibit elastase and collagenase (Albini et al., 2025b); combining them with tocopherols from olive pomace yields dual-phase antioxidant protection (Loschi et al., 2024). Olive leaf extract maintains efficacy at modest concentrations (5%) without adverse effects and enhances photoprotection when combined with UV filters (Tsoupras et al., 2024).

Delivery systems can be leveraged to align actives with targets: soy-derived lecithin acts as an emulsifier and penetration enhancer, improving isoflavone delivery for collagen-supportive effects (Ferreira et al., 2025). Pairing lecithin with OMWW phenolics unites regenerative and protective actions. Sunflower residues, rich in linoleic acid, restore ceramide synthesis and complement OMWW polyphenols in after-sun repair (Kesarwani et al., 2024). Palm-based esters provide occlusivity, though their use must be weighed against sustainability concerns.

Stabilization and controlled release are central for phenolics and PUFAs: encapsulating OMWW phenolics in lipid microcapsules prolongs antioxidant activity (Tsoupras et al., 2024), while phytosterols from soybean deodorizer distillates reinforce barrier resilience in creams (Karim et al., 2025). Incorporating probiotics into phenolic-rich bases can further address acne or rosacea by modulating microbiota and inflammation (Biyimba et al., 2025).

Circular bioeconomy strategies add functional and sustainability value. Olive pomace extracts containing maslinic acid and α-tocopherol enrich lotions or serums while demonstrating waste valorization (Albini et al., 2025a). Pigment-rich fractions from rapeseed or cold-pressed oils contribute color with added antioxidant capacity, enabling tinted moisturizers with mild photoprotection (Loschi et al., 2024).

Key challenges include oxidative instability of PUFAs and phenolics; co-formulation with tocopherols and/or encapsulation mitigates degradation (Albini et al., 2025a). Synergistic blends are often superior to single actives: sunflower linoleic acid plus OMWW hydroxytyrosol balances hydration and defense, and soy lecithin–isoflavone systems combined with squalene-rich olive pomace lipids enhance emolliency and radical scavenging (Albini et al., 2025a). Aligning product design with physiology—ROS neutralization, NF-κB downregulation, collagen preservation—enables multifunctional, sustainable skincare. Advances in extraction and stabilization continue to expand opportunities against aging, inflammation, and environmental stress (Albini et al., 2025a).

Hair-care uses parallel skin-care logic but must consider follicular biology and scalp physiology. Hair protects against UV and thermal extremes and contributes to sensory function (Albini et al., 2025b); maintaining follicle health has physiological and psychological value. Oil-residue actives can target follicular cycling, sebaceous balance, and scalp inflammation.

OMWW extracts rich in hydroxytyrosol may counter dihydrotestosterone (DHT)-related oxidative stress and support insulin-like growth factor 1 (IGF-1) signaling in dermal papilla cells to sustain anagen (Albini et al., 2025a). Olive leaf polyphenols provide antioxidant and antimicrobial benefits that help regulate scalp microbiota and reduce dandruff, while emollients soothe irritation and protect keratin fibers (Tsoupras et al., 2024). Botanical starches act as gentle absorptive cleansers, reducing sebum without disturbing the barrier; combining them with soybean-derived phytosterols enables dual-action cleansing plus barrier reinforcement (Biyimba et al., 2025). Fermented plant biomasses (e.g., aloe vera or citrus bioferments) aid seboregulation, moisturization, and antiitch performance in hair-dye systems (Majchrzak et al., 2022). Essential oils add targeted effects: lemon controls dandruff via antisepsis, lavender may stimulate follicles with aromatherapeutic benefits, and neem supports keratinocyte turnover for thickness (Tripathy et al., 2024).

Antioxidant protection for UV-exposed scalps is critical. Pairing α-tocopherol with hydroxytyrosol provides two-phase defense across lipid and aqueous domains, ideal for leave-in sprays (Albini et al., 2025a). PUFAs from sunflower by-products (notably linoleic acid) promote ceramide biosynthesis and comfort, while rapeseed-derived sinapic acid adds antiinflammatory support (Kesarwani et al., 2024). Natural thickeners (plant starches, pomace mucilage) contribute humectancy and film-forming protection against friction, and phenolic-rich OMWW fractions can slow color fading by scavenging radicals during photobleaching, especially when combined with UV filters. Valorizing residues from olive, soy, sunflower, and rapeseed reduces environmental impact and appeals to eco-conscious consumers (Albini et al., 2025a), while layered strategies—polyphenolic antioxidants, sterol-mediated barrier repair, and seboregulation—improve scalp balance, shine, manageability, and color retention (Albini et al., 2025b).

4 Mechanistic basis of biocosmetic activities

Oil-derived actives act through overlapping antioxidant, antiinflammatory, antimicrobial, photoprotective, pigmentation-modulating, regenerative, and structural-preserving pathways, with efficacy shaped by molecular structure, polarity, and stability.

Antioxidant: Hydroxytyrosol/oleuropein neutralizes ROS via orthodiphenolic groups and upregulates endogenous defenses (superoxide dismutase, glutathione reductase) (Albini et al., 2025b; Waqas et al., 2014). Tocopherols act as chain-breaking antioxidants in lipophilic domains; pairing with aqueous phenolics achieves compartment-spanning protection (Albini et al., 2025b).

Antiinflammatory: Phenolics inhibit NF-κB and MAPK, reducing IL-1β, IL-8, and TNF-α (Albini et al., 2025b). Soy isoflavones modulate estrogen receptors in fibroblasts to curb mediator release and promote repair (Ferreira et al., 2025).

Photoprotection/extracellular matrix (ECM) preservation: Phenolics suppress UV-induced ROS and matrix metalloproteinases (MMPs) (collagenase, elastase), limiting connective tissue breakdown. Olive secoiridoids attenuate erythema via cytokine modulation. Carotenoids from palm/rapeseed quench singlet oxygen and mitigate photooxidation (Albini et al., 2025a, 2025b).

Pigmentation control: Hydroxytyrosol inhibits tyrosinase comparably to kojic acid, supporting tone evening with a low cytotoxic risk (Rodrigues et al., 2023); its antiinflammatory effects further reduce postinflammatory hyperpigmentation.

Follicular support: Olive polyphenols can increase IGF-1 in dermal papilla cells, supporting anagen and keratinocyte proliferation (Albini et al., 2025a, 2025b); antioxidant load reduction sustains cycling.

Antimicrobial: Oil-derived phenolics disrupt microbial cell walls or quorum sensing (e.g., *S. aureus*, *P. acnes*) and show antifungal activity against *Candida* spp. (Albini et al., 2025a).

Barrier and regeneration: Soy phytosterols integrate into membranes to improve resilience (Karim et al., 2025); linoleic acid from sunflower residues fuels ceramide biosynthesis (Kesarwani et al., 2024). Olive phenolics inhibit lipoxygenase (LOX), reducing leukotriene-driven inflammation and PUFA peroxidation (Marijan et al., 2022). Whole-extract synergies often exceed single compounds, e.g., crude OMWW outperforming pure oleuropein (Carrara et al., 2021).

Adjunct mechanisms and delivery: Vitamin K improves microcirculation and capillary stability (Sayanhika and Selvakumar, 2024). Carrier peptides can target bioactives to fibroblasts for collagen stimulation (Pintea et al., 2025). Encapsulation enhances the protection of unstable molecules and enables controlled release (Tsoupras et al., 2024).

5 Clinical data supporting cosmetic use of edible plant oils and by-products

Clinical evidence supporting edible plant oils in cosmetics is steadily expanding, though the depth of validation differs by oil type.

Palm oil and its by-products remain the least explored in clinical dermatology. A phase I single-blind trial confirmed the safety of oil palm phenolic supplementation in healthy volunteers, indicating the translational potential of palm-derived bioactives for future cosmetic applications (Fairus et al., 2018).

Soybean oil and its by-products show stronger emerging evidence, primarily linked to their isoflavone content. Systematic reviews report that topical and oral soy supplementation can reduce wrinkles and pigmentation while improving elasticity, hydration, and overall appearance (Lee et al., 2022; Natarelli et al., 2023). Additional studies reinforce this potential: fermented soybean extract-loaded niosomes enhanced dermal absorption without systemic toxicity in animal models (Rungseevijitprapa et al., 2021), and black soybean sprout extracts demonstrated antioxidant, whitening, and safety benefits in cosmetic formulations (Lai et al., 2012).

Rapeseed oil and by-products remain underexplored. While rapeseed phospholipids have been shown to optimize cosmetic formulation properties (Górecki et al., 2015), direct human trials assessing rapeseed oil or its by-products are lacking, highlighting a significant research gap.

Sunflower oil and its by-products have some of the strongest clinical evidence among edible plant oils. Randomized controlled trials demonstrate that topical sunflower oil improves stratum corneum hydration, reduces transepidermal water loss, and preserves barrier integrity in both preterm infants and adults, without inducing erythema (Danby et al., 2013; Kanti et al., 2014). Further studies show its safety and efficacy in managing mild-to-moderate plaque-type psoriasis (Ilagan et al., 2021). Sunflower oleodistillate also enhances epidermal lipid synthesis and reduces inflammation, with promising applications in pediatric dermatology (Eichenfield et al., 2009).

Olive oil and its by-products are supported by robust evidence across multiple modalities. Placebo-controlled trials in healthy volunteers reported improved collagen density, elasticity, and photoprotection following supplementation with olive leaf and wastewater extracts (Buzzi et al., 2023). Topical creams containing olive leaf extracts improved facial rejuvenation (Wanitphakdeedecha et al., 2020), while human repeat-insult patch tests confirmed their safety (Nunes et al., 2021). Oleocanthal extracts showed antiinflammatory potential after photodynamic therapy (Palacios et al., 2019), and fibroblast studies confirmed the protective effects of hydroxytyrosol, tyrosol, and oleocanthal (González-Acedo et al., 2023). A recent review synthesized evidence supporting olive mill waste extracts in skin health applications (Laveriano-Santos et al., 2024).

To facilitate comparison, this provides a consolidated overview of the five major oils—palm, soybean, rapeseed, sunflower, and olive—summarizing fatty acid profiles, key bioactives, processing by-products, cosmetic relevance, and clinical validation. It highlights shared functions (hydration, antioxidation), unique features (palm carotenoids, soy isoflavones, rapeseed sinapic acid, sunflower tocopherols, olive hydroxytyrosol), and differing levels of human evidence, identifying clear priorities for future research (Table 14.1).

6 Regulatory limits

The use of bioactive components derived from edible plant oils and their by-products in cosmetic and biocosmetic formulations is regulated to ensure consumer safety. In the European Union (EU), this framework is defined by Regulation No. 1223/2009, which applies across all member states (Basketter and White, 2016) with regular amendments to its Annexes (e.g., 2024/996, 2024/858) and related measures (e.g., 2023/1545 on fragrance allergen labeling and REACH 2023/2055 on microplastics) that update ingredient conditions and labeling over time. The regulation requires that products must be safe under normal or reasonably foreseeable conditions of use, and that manufacturers provide a Cosmetic Product Safety Report (Annex I), including full details of composition, function, and toxicological profile (Basketter and White, 2016).

EU law distinguishes between: (1) prohibited substances, which are not permitted in cosmetics at any concentration; (2) restricted substances, which are permitted only under conditions such as maximum concentration, purity standards, or

TABLE 14.1 Comparative overview of major edible plant oils, their by-products, cosmetic relevance, and clinical validation.

Ot	Main fatty acids	Key bioactives	By-products (bioactives)	Cosmetic relevance	Clinical evidence	LoE	Clinical endpoints tested
P	Palmitic (~45%), oleic (~39%), linoleic (~10%)	Carotenoids (α-, β-carotene), tocopherols, tocotrienols, phytosterols	Palm oil mill effluent (phenolic acids, flavonoids); biowaxes (structuring agents)	Barrier reinforcement, hydration, antioxidant/ photoprotection	Phase I trial: safety of palm phenolic supplementation (Fairus et al., 2018). No efficacy trials yet.	L	Safety only
Sb	Linoleic (~54%), oleic (~23%), palmitic (~11%), linolenic (~8%)	Isoflavones (genistein, daidzein), tocopherols (γ-tocopherol), phospholipids, saponins	Soybean meal (isoflavones), soy residues (polysaccharides), deodorizer distillates (phytosterols, squalene)	Wrinkle and pigmentation reduction, elasticity, hydration, antiaging	Systematic reviews: wrinkle/pigmentation reduction, improved elasticity/hydration (Lee et al., 2022; Natarelli et al., 2023). Fermented soy extract and black soybean sprout formulations support absorption and safety (Lai et al., 2012; Rungseevijitprapa et al., 2021).	E	Wrinkle reduction, pigmentation, elasticity, hydration
R	Oleic (50%–65%), linoleic (18%–28%), α-linolenic (8%–15%), saturated < 10%	Sinapic acid, sinapine, tocopherols, phytosterols	Press cake (proteins, phenolics), pomace (sinapine)	Antioxidant protection, barrier support, emulsification	No direct human dermatology trials. Evidence limited to formulation optimization with phospholipids (Górecki et al., 2015).	G	None
Sf	Linoleic (48%–74%), oleic (14%–39%), palmitic (3%–6%), stearic (3%–6%)	Tocopherols (α-tocopherol), phytosterols, carotenoids, chlorogenic acid	Press cakes (residual fatty acids, FAs, proteins), receptacles (flavonoids, chlorogenic acid)	Barrier integrity, hydration, antiinflammatory, psoriasis care	Randomized controlled trials (RCTs): improved hydration, reduced transepidermal water loss (TEWL), preserved barrier integrity in infants/ adults (Danby et al., 2013; Kanti et al., 2014). Effective in mild/moderate psoriasis (Ilagan et al., 2021). Oleodistillate supports lipid synthesis and reduces inflammation in children (Eichenfield et al., 2009).	S	Hydration, TEWL, barrier integrity, psoriasis, inflammation
O	Oleic (55%–83%), linoleic (3.5%–21%), palmitic (7.5%–20%), stearic (0.5%–5%)	Hydroxytyrosol, oleuropein, tyrosol, squalene, tocopherols	Pomace & OMWW (phenolics), olive leaves (oleuropein, flavonoids)	Moisturization, photoprotection, collagen support, antiinflammatory, antiaging.	Placebo-controlled trials: improved collagen density, elasticity, photoprotection (Buzzi et al., 2023). Topical creams improved rejuvenation (Wanitphakdeedecha et al., 2020). Patch tests confirm safety (Nunes et al., 2021). Oleocanthal extracts antiinflammatory post-PDT (Palacios et al., 2019). Fibroblast assays: hydroxytyrosol, tyrosol, oleocanthal protective (González-Acedo et al., 2023). A review confirms olive waste extracts potential (Laveriano-Santos et al., 2024).	S	Collagen density, elasticity, photoprotection, rejuvenation, antiinflammatory, safety.

E, emerging; *G*, gap; *L*, limited; *LoE*, level of evidence; *O*, olive; *Ot*, oil type; *P*, palm; *R*, rapeseed; *S*, strong; *Sb*, soybean; *Sf*, sunflower.

warning labels; and (3) allowed substances, which are permitted without specific restrictions, provided they meet general safety requirements.

Many natural compounds fall into the category of restricted substances due to sensitization or irritation risks (Klaschka, 2016). Importantly, natural origin does not guarantee safety. Several natural substances used in cosmetics have been classified as hazardous for skin or eyes under European labeling rules, underscoring the need for thorough risk assessment (Klaschka, 2016).

Regulations outside the EU vary widely and are not fully harmonized. While principles of ingredient control are broadly shared, lists of permitted, restricted, or prohibited substances differ, as do testing and labeling requirements (Ferreira et al., 2022). For example, in vivo animal testing remains mandatory in some countries, although it is banned in the EU (Knight et al., 2021).

For highly produced oils such as palm, soybean, rapeseed, sunflower, and olive, the oils themselves are generally recognized as safe due to their edibility. However, their cosmetic use is still subject to safety evaluation of the final product. Regulatory focus is therefore placed on isolated compounds and by-products, which may require additional scrutiny:

Soy isoflavones, rapeseed sinapine, and olive hydroxytyrosol are examples of bioactives evaluated for potential sensitization, irritation, or endocrine effects. The European Scientific Committee on Consumer Safety provides scientific opinions that guide usage limits (von der Ohe and Aalizadeh, 2020). Purity requirements apply universally. While the standard for mineral oils is compliance with pharmaceutical-grade specifications (Chuberre et al., 2019), the same principle applies to plant oils and their derivatives to ensure the absence of harmful contaminants. By-product valorization (e.g., olive pomace extracts, rapeseed press cake hydrolysates) introduces novel cosmetic ingredients. These must undergo toxicological evaluation and dermatological testing before approval for market use (Moore et al., 2020).

Although precise concentration limits for every plant-derived bioactive are not established, the regulatory approach prioritizes a case-by-case safety assessment. Substances shown to present risks may be prohibited or restricted, while others remain unrestricted if safety is demonstrated. Ultimately, the responsibility for ensuring compliance rests with the cosmetic manufacturer.

Although regulatory systems provide safeguards for current applications, the future development of edible plant oils in cosmetics will depend on innovation in sustainability, green technologies, and targeted formulations. At the same time, critical research gaps must be addressed to fully unlock their potential.

7 Future perspectives

The expanding vegetable oil market, driven by growing demand in the food, cosmetic, and biofuel industries, positions edible plant oils and their by-products as key resources for next-generation biocosmetics (Sarpong, 2024). The sector is increasingly shaped by consumer preferences for natural, safe, and effective ingredients, alongside sustainability goals (Furman et al., 2022; Goyal and Jerold, 2023). Future progress will rely on sustainable valorization, advanced extraction methods, and targeted formulations, while addressing critical research gaps in safety, efficacy, and supply balance.

7.1 Valorization of agroindustrial by-products

Future innovation will focus on upcycling residues such as olive pomace, mill wastewater, rapeseed press cake, soybean meal, and palm effluents into high-value cosmetic actives. This strategy supports the circular economy, reducing waste and environmental impact while generating cost-effective bioactive ingredients (Barbulova et al., 2015; Leyva-Jiménez et al., 2022; Puton et al., 2025). For example, phenolic-rich olive by-products already show antioxidant and antiaging effects in cosmetics (Buzzi et al., 2023), and rapeseed hydrolysates are being explored for skincare proteins and polyphenols (Rivera et al., 2015). More standardized methods are needed to ensure consistent quality and reproducibility of these by-product-derived ingredients.

7.2 Green and advanced extraction technologies

Sustainable extraction methods—including enzymatic hydrolysis, ultrasound-assisted extraction, microwave-assisted extraction, pressurized liquid extraction, and supercritical fluids—are expected to dominate the field due to their efficiency and lower environmental impact (Dauber et al., 2023; Gullón et al., 2020; Leyva-Jiménez et al., 2022). These technologies also help preserve the activity of sensitive bioactives. Further optimization is needed to maximize yields and maintain functional integrity, particularly by studying the effects of polarity, time, and temperature on compound stability (Gómez-Cruz et al., 2021).

7.3 Development of novel biobased ingredients

Replacing fossil-derived materials with plant-based alternatives remains a major trend. Novel lipids, wax esters, and phytosterol-based oleogels engineered from edible oils are emerging as sustainable substitutes for petrolatum and other synthetics (Bom et al., 2020; Chen et al., 2019; Duprat-De-Paule et al., 2018; Goyal and Jerold, 2023; Azmi et al., 2022) (Nooratiqah). More clinical validation is needed to confirm that these innovations perform as effectively as traditional synthetic ingredients in consumer formulations.

7.4 Tailored formulations for specific skin needs

Future research will emphasize customized oil blends designed to target specific dermatological needs, such as barrier repair, antiaging, pigmentation, or inflammation. This requires a deeper understanding of the biological and toxicological profiles of different oils and their compositional variability (Moore et al., 2020; Rivera et al., 2015). Limited mechanistic insight exists into how individual compounds (e.g., isoflavones, hydroxytyrosol, sinapic acid) interact with skin pathways at the molecular level (Rodrigues et al., 2015).

7.5 Balancing supply, demand, and ethical sourcing

The growing use of vegetable oils in cosmetics must be balanced against competing demands for food and energy, particularly for high-impact crops like palm oil (Hill, 2008). Sustainable sourcing, certification schemes, and transparency in supply chains will be critical to avoiding negative impacts on food security, land use, and biodiversity (Candellone et al., 2023; Schmidt, 2015). Studies are needed to evaluate how scaling cosmetic applications of edible oils might affect global resource allocation and sustainability targets.

The future of biocosmetics will be defined by the integration of sustainability, green extraction, novel biobased formulations, and personalized applications. At the same time, research must address gaps in process optimization, safety and efficacy validation, molecular mechanisms, and ethical sourcing, ensuring that edible plant oils and their by-products deliver on both consumer expectations and environmental responsibilities.

8 Conclusions

Edible plant oils—particularly palm, soybean, rapeseed, sunflower, and olive—and their processing by-products represent versatile and sustainable resources for the cosmetic and biocosmetic industries. Once regarded as waste, residues such as OMWW, olive pomace, olive leaves, soybean hulls, deodorizer distillates, and okara are now recognized as concentrated sources of valuable actives. These fractions provide fatty acids, phenolics, tocopherols, carotenoids, phytosterols, proteins, and squalene, which deliver hydration, barrier reinforcement, antioxidation, antiaging, antiinflammatory, antimicrobial, photoprotective, and regenerative effects (Albini et al., 2025a; Chu and Nyam, 2021; Nile et al., 2022; Rodrigues et al., 2023; Tsoupras et al., 2024). Their mechanisms include ROS scavenging (Albini et al., 2025a; Waqas et al., 2014), enzyme inhibition (Albini et al., 2025a; Rodrigues et al., 2023), modulation of NF-κB/MAPK signaling (Albini et al., 2025b), and reinforcement of barrier integrity via ceramide biosynthesis (Kesarwani et al., 2024).

Synergies between hydrophilic phenolics and lipophilic fractions provide complementary protection, while encapsulation technologies enhance stability and targeted delivery (Tsoupras et al., 2024). Examples include hydroxytyrosol with tocopherols (Albini et al., 2025a, 2025b) and soy lecithin with isoflavones (Ferreira et al., 2025), which support collagen preservation, hydration, and pigmentation control.

In hair care, olive phenolics sustain IGF-1 signaling in follicles (Albini et al., 2025b), while antimicrobial and antiinflammatory compounds regulate scalp balance (Tsoupras et al., 2024). Additives such as starches (Biyimba et al., 2025), essential oils (Tripathy et al., 2024), and fermented extracts (Majchrzak et al., 2022) further expand functionality.

Clinical evidence strongly supports the dermatological benefits of sunflower and olive oils, while soybean demonstrates promising outcomes, particularly linked to isoflavones. Palm and rapeseed oils remain underexplored in human trials, highlighting opportunities for further research (Buzzi et al., 2023; Danby et al., 2013; Kanti et al., 2014; Lee et al., 2022; Natarelli et al., 2023).

Overall, oil-processing by-products deliver multifunctional, safe, and sustainable cosmetic actives. Their future integration will depend on advances in green extraction technologies, rigorous safety evaluations, clinical validation, and ethically balanced sourcing, ensuring that edible plant oils and their residues remain at the forefront of biocosmetic innovation (Albini et al., 2025a, 2025b; Barbulova et al., 2015; Cádiz-Gurrea et al., 2021; Morganti et al., 2022).

References

Abdalla, S., Aroua, M.K., Gew, L.T., 2024. A comprehensive review of plant-based cosmetic oils (virgin coconut oil, olive oil, argan oil, and jojoba oil): chemical and biological properties and their cosmeceutical applications. ACS Omega. 24701343. Available from: https://www.pubs.acs.org/journal/acsodf. doi:10.1021/acsomega.4c04277.

Albini, A., Corradino, P., Morelli, D., Albini, F., Noonan, D., 2025a. Cosmeceutical and dermatological potential of olive mill wastewater: a sustainable and eco-friendly source of natural ingredients. Cosmetics 12 (4), 142. doi:10.3390/cosmetics12040142.

Albini, A., Corradino, P., Morelli, D., Albini, F., Noonan, D., 2025b. Cosmetic and Dermatological Properties of Olive Oil Byproduct-Supplemented Skin and Hair Care Products. MDPI AG. Available from. doi:10.20944/preprints202505.0906.v3.

Alcock, T.D., Salt, D.E., Wilson, P., Ramsden, S.J., 2022. More sustainable vegetable oil: balancing productivity with carbon storage opportunities. Sci. Total Environ. 18791026. 829. Available from: www.elsevier.com/locate/scitotenv. doi:10.1016/j.scitotenv.2022.154539.

Azmi, N., Radzi, S.M., Rehan, M.M., Amin, N.A.M., 2022. A review on cosmetic formulations and physicochemical characteristics of emollient and day cream using vegetable based-wax ester. Malaysian J. Sci. Health Technol. 2601-0003. 8 (2), 38–45. doi:10.33102/2022291.

Barbulova, A., Colucci, G., Apone, F., 2015. New trends in cosmetics: by-products of plant origin and their potential use as cosmetic active ingredients. Cosmetics. 2079-9284. 2 (2), 82–92. doi:10.3390/cosmetics2020082.

Basketter, D., White, I.R., 2016. Legislative aspects of cosmetic safety in the European Union: the case of contact allergy. Cosmetics. 20799284. 3 (2). Available from: https://www.mdpi.com/2079-9284/3/2/17/pdf. doi:10.3390/cosmetics3020017.

Beaubier, S., Durand, E., Lenclume, C., Fine, F., Aymes, A., Framboisier, X., Kapel, R., Villeneuve, P., 2023. Chelating peptides from rapeseed meal protein hydrolysates: identification and evaluation of their capacity to inhibit lipid oxidation. Food Chem. 03088146. 422, 136187. doi:10.1016/j.foodchem.2023.136187.

Beyer, R., Rademacher, T., 2021. Species richness and carbon footprints of vegetable oils: can high yields outweigh palm oil's environmental impact? Sustainability (Switz.). 20711050. 13 (4), 1–10. Available from: https://www.mdpi.com/2071-1050/13/4/1813/pdf. doi:10.3390/su13041813.

Biyimba, B.N., Ekaette, I., Cobbinah-Sam, E., 2025. Starch functionality in cosmetics and personal care products. Carbohydr. Polym. 01448617. 364. Available from: https://www.sciencedirect.com/science/journal/01448617. doi:10.1016/j.carbpol.2025.123597.

Bom, S., Fitas, M., Martins, A.M., Pinto, P., Ribeiro, H.M., Marto, J., 2020. Replacing synthetic ingredients by sustainable natural alternatives: a case study using topical O/W emulsions. Molecules. 14203049. 25 (21). Available from: https://www.mdpi.com/1420-3049/25/21/4887. doi:10.3390/MOLECULES25214887.

Bragagnolo, F.S., Funari, C.S., Ibáñez, E., Cifuentes, A., 2021. Metabolomics as a tool to study underused soy parts: in search of bioactive compounds. Foods. 23048158. 10 (6). Available from: https://www.mdpi.com/2304-8158/10/6/1308/pdf. doi:10.3390/foods10061308.

Buzzi, R., Gugel, I., Costa, S., Molesini, S., Boreale, S., Baldini, E., Marchetti, N., Vertuani, S., Pinelli, P., Urciuoli, S., Baldisserotto, A., Manfredini, S., 2023. Up-cycling of *Olea europaea* L. ancient cultivars side products: study of a combined cosmetic–food supplement treatment based on leaves and olive mill wastewater extracts. Life. 2075-1729. 13 (7), 1509. doi:10.3390/life13071509.

Cádiz-Gurrea, M.D.L.L., Pinto, D., Delerue-Matos, C., Rodrigues, F., 2021. Olive fruit and leaf wastes as bioactive ingredients for cosmetics—a preliminary study. Antioxidants. 20763921. 10 (2), 1–18. Available from: https://www.mdpi.com/2076-3921/10/2/245/pdf. doi:10.3390/antiox10020245.

Cairone, F., Allevi, D., Cesa, S., Fabrizi, G., Goggiamani, A., Masci, D., Iazzetti, A., 2023. Valorisation of side stream products through green approaches: the rapeseed meal case. Foods. 2304-8158. 12 (17), 3286. doi:10.3390/foods12173286.

Candellone, E., Aleta, A., de Arruda, H.F., Meijaard, E., Moreno, Y., 2023. Understanding the vegetable oil debate and its implications for sustainability through social media. arXiv. 23318422. Available from: https://arxiv.org. doi:10.48550/arXiv.2308.07108.

Carrara, M., Kelly, M.T., Roso, F., Larroque, M., Margout, D., 2021. Potential of olive oil mill wastewater as a source of polyphenols for the treatment of skin disorders: a review. J. Agric. Food Chem. 0021-8561. 69 (26), 7268–7284. doi:10.1021/acs.jafc.1c00296.

Chaparro, L.M., Neira, L.F., Molina, D., Rivera-Barrera, D., Castañeda, M., López-Giraldo, L.J., Escobar, P., 2023. Biowaxes from palm oil as promising candidates for cosmetic matrices and pharmaceuticals for human use. Materials. 19961944. 16 (12). Available from: http://www.mdpi.com/journal/materials. doi:10.3390/ma16124402.

Chen, X.W., Sun, S.D., Yang, G.L., Ma, C.G., 2019. Engineering phytosterol-based oleogels for potential application as sustainable petrolatum replacement. RSC Adv. 20462069. 10 (1), 244–252. Available from: http://pubs.rsc.org/en/journals/journal/ra. doi:10.1039/c9ra06950j.

Chu, C.C., Nyam, K.L., 2021. Application of seed oils and its bioactive compounds in sunscreen formulations. J. Am. Oil Chem. Soc. 15589331. 98 (7), 713–726. Available from: http://www.aocs.org/press. doi:10.1002/aocs.12491.

Chuberre, B., Araviiskaia, E., Bieber, T., Barbaud, A., 2019. Mineral oils and waxes in cosmetics: an overview mainly based on the current European regulations and the safety profile of these compounds. J. Eur. Acad. Dermatol. Venereol. 14683083. 33 (7), 5–14. Available from: http://onlinelibrary.wiley.com/journal/10.1111/(ISSN)1468-3083. doi:10.1111/jdv.15946.

Clodoveo, M.L., Crupi, P., Annunziato, A., Corbo, F., 2022. Innovative extraction technologies for development of functional ingredients based on polyphenols from olive leaves. Foods. 23048158. 11 (1). Available from: https://www.mdpi.com/2304-8158/11/1/103/pdf. doi:10.3390/foods11010103.

Danby, S.G., Alenezi, T., Sultan, A., Lavender, T., Chittock, J., Brown, K., Cork, M.J., 2013. Effect of olive and sunflower seed oil on the adult skin barrier: implications for neonatal skin care. Pediatr. Dermatol. 15251470. 30 (1), 42–50. doi:10.1111/j.1525-1470.2012.01865.x.

Dauber, C., Parente, E., Zucca, M.P., Gámbaro, A., Vieitez, I., 2023. *Olea europea* and by-products: extraction methods and cosmetic applications. Cosmetics. 20799284. 10 (4). Available from: www.mdpi.com/journal/cosmetics. doi:10.3390/cosmetics10040112.

Duan, X., Zhang, M., Chen, F., 2021. Prediction and analysis of antimicrobial peptides from rapeseed protein using in silico approach. J. Food Biochem. 0145-8884. 45 (4). doi:10.1111/jfbc.13598.

Duprat-De-Paule, S., Guilbot, J., Roso, A., Cambos, S., Pierre, A., 2018. Augmented bio-based lipids for cosmetics. Oilseeds Fats Crops Lipids. 22576614. 25 (5). Available from: http://www.ocl-journal.org/. doi:10.1051/ocl/2018036.

Eichenfield, L.F., McCollum, A., Msika, P., 2009. The benefits of sunflower oleodistillate (SOD) in pediatric dermatology. Pediatr. Dermatol. 15251470. 26 (6), 669–675. doi:10.1111/j.1525-1470.2009.01042.x.

Fairus, S., Leow, S.S., Mohamed, I.N., Tan, Y.A., Sundram, K., Sambanthamurthi, R., 2018. A phase i single-blind clinical trial to evaluate the safety of oil palm phenolics (OPP) supplementation in healthy volunteers. Sci. Rep. 20452322. 8 (1). Available from: www.nature.com/srep/index.html. doi:10.1038/s41598-018-26384-7.

FAO, 2023. Agricultural Production Statistics 2000–2022. doi:10.4060/cc9205en.

Ferreira, M., Matos, A., Couras, A., Marto, J., Ribeiro, H., 2022. Overview of cosmetic regulatory frameworks around the world. Cosmetics. 20799284. 9 (4). Available from: https://www.mdpi.com/2079-9284/9/4/72/pdf?version=1656597779. doi:10.3390/cosmetics9040072.

Ferreira, R.S.B., Ferreira, A.M., Almeida, M., Oliveira, M., Coutinho, J.A.P., Batista, E.A.C., 2025. Towards sustainable soybean waste management: bio-based solvent extraction of isoflavones for food and cosmetic applications. Sep. Purif. Technol. 18733794. 372. Available from: https://www.sciencedirect.com/science/journal/13835866. doi:10.1016/j.seppur.2025.133435.

Foti, P., Romeo, F.V., Russo, N., Pino, A., Vaccalluzzo, A., Caggia, C., Randazzo, C.L., 2021. Olive mill wastewater as renewable raw materials to generate high added-value ingredients for agro-food industries. Appl. Sci. (Switz.). 20763417. 11 (16). Available from: https://www.mdpi.com/2076-3417/11/16/7511/pdf. doi:10.3390/app11167511.

Franco, R., 2018. Sunflower oil functional properties for specialty food. Nutr. Food Sci. Int. J. 2474767X. 5 (4). doi:10.19080/nfsij.2018.05.555668.

Freitas, C.S., Silva, G.A.D., Perrone, D., Vericimo, M.A., Baião, D.D.S., Pereira, P.R., Paschoalin, V.M.F., Aguila, E.M.D., 2019. Recovery of antimicrobials and bioaccessible isoflavones and phenolics from soybean (glycine max) meal by aqueous extraction. Molecules. 14203049. 24 (1). Available from: https://www.mdpi.com/1420-3049/24/1/74/pdf. doi:10.3390/molecules24010074.

Furman, A.C., Teresinha Veit, M., Palácio, S.M., da Cunha Gonçalves, G., Caroline Zanette Barbieri, J., 2022. Sustentabilidade no processo produtivo da indústria cosmética: uma revisão da literatura. Res. Soc. Dev. 2525-3409. 11 (13), e586111335852. doi:10.33448/rsd-v11i13.35852.

Gómez-Cruz, I., Contreras, M.D.M., Carvalheiro, F., Duarte, L.C., Roseiro, L.B., Romero, I., Castro, E., 2021. Recovery of bioactive compounds from industrial exhausted olive pomace through ultrasound-assisted extraction. Biology. 20797737. 10 (6). Available from: https://www.mdpi.com/2079-7737/10/6/514/pdf. doi:10.3390/biology10060514.

González-Acedo, A., Ramos-Torrecillas, J., Illescas-Montes, R., Costela-Ruiz, V.J., Ruiz, C., Melguizo-Rodríguez, L., García-Martínez, O., 2023. The benefits of olive oil for skin health: study on the effect of hydroxytyrosol, tyrosol, and oleocanthal on human fibroblasts. Nutrients. 20726643. 15 (9). Available from: http://www.mdpi.com/journal/nutrients/. doi:10.3390/nu15092077.

Górecki, M., Kurek-Górecka, A., Sosada, M., Pasker, B., Pajak, M., Fraś, P., 2015. The optimization of the oiling bath cosmetic composition containing rapeseed phospholipids and grapeseed oil by the full factorial design. Cosmetics. 20799284. 2 (2), 127–135. Available from: https://res.mdpi.com/cosmetics/cosmetics-02-00127/article_deploy/cosmetics-02-00127.pdf?filename=&attachment=1. doi:10.3390/cosmetics2020127.

Gotor, A.A., Rhazi, L., 2016. Effects of refining process on sunflower oil minor components: a review. Oilseeds Fats Crops Lipids. 22576614. 23 (2). Available from: http://www.ocl-journal.org/. doi:10.1051/ocl/2016007.

Goyal, N., Jerold, F., 2023. Biocosmetics: technological advances and future outlook. Environ. Sci. Pollut. Res. 16147499. 30 (10), 25148–25169. Available from: https://www.springer.com/journal/11356. doi:10.1007/s11356-021-17567-3.

Gullón, P., Gullón, B., Astray, G., Carpena, M., Fraga-Corral, M., Prieto, M.A., Simal-Gandara, J., 2020. Valorization of by-products from olive oil industry and added-value applications for innovative functional foods. Food Res. Int. 18737145. 137. Available from: www.elsevier.com/inca/publications/store/4/2/2/9/7/0. doi:10.1016/j.foodres.2020.109683.

He, Y., Liu, K., Han, L., Han, W., 2022. Clustering analysis, structure fingerprint analysis, and quantum chemical calculations of compounds from essential oils of sunflower (*Helianthus annuus* L.) receptacles. Int. J. Mol. Sci. 1422-0067. 23 (17), 10169. doi:10.3390/ijms231710169.

Hill, K., 2008. Industrial development and application of biobased oleochemicals. In: Kamm, B., Gruber, P.R., Kamm, M. (Eds.), Biorefineries—Industrial Processes and Products: Status Quo and Future Directions, vol. 2. Wiley-VCH Verlag GmbH & Co. KGaA, Weinheim, pp. 291–314. Available from: http://onlinelibrary.wiley.com/book/10.1002/9783527619849. doi:10.1002/9783527619849.ch26.

Ilagan, F.M.D., Letran, E.L., Policarpio, B.O., 2021. Efficacy and safety of sunflower oil for mild to moderate plaque-type psoriasis: a double-blind, randomized controlled trial. J. Med. Univ. Santo Tomas. 25461621. 5 (2), 755–773. doi:10.35460/2546-1621.2019-0068.

Imo, C., 2020. Phytochemical constituents of palm oil. J. Biotechnol. Res. 2413-3256. 66, 57–61. doi:10.32861/jbr.66.57.61.

Itsarasook, K., Prompamorn, P., Tanghiranrat, J., Srisukong, A., Komutiban, O., Haritakun, W., Chantree, K., 2025. In vitro antioxidant, anti-inflammatory, and wound healing properties of aloe vera infused with canola oil for possible application in skin cosmetics. J. Food Health Bioenviron. Sci. 26300311. 18 (1), 27–38. Available from https://li01.tci-thaijo.org/index.php/sdust/article/download/265619/179997.

Japir, A.A.W., Salimon, J., Derawi, D., Bahadi, M., Al-Shuja'A, S., Yusop, M.R., 2017. Physicochemical characteristics of high free fatty acid crude palm oil. Oilseeds Fats Crops Lipids. 22576614. 24 (5). Available from: http://www.ocl-journal.org/. doi:10.1051/ocl/2017033.

Kanti, V., Grande, C., Stroux, A., Bührer, C., Blume-Peytavi, U., Bartels, N.G., 2014. Influence of sunflower seed oil on the skin barrier function of preterm infants: a randomized controlled trial. Dermatology. 1018-8665. 229 (3), 230–239. doi:10.1159/000363380.

Karim, A., Osse, E.F., Khalloufi, S., 2025. Innovative strategies for valorization of byproducts from soybean industry: a review on status, challenges, and sustainable approaches towards zero-waste processing systems. Heliyon. 24058440. 11 (3). Available from: https://www.sciencedirect.com/science/journal/24058440. doi:10.1016/j.heliyon.2025.e42118.

Kasmin, H., Lazim, A.M., Awang, R., 2015. Determination of fatty acid composition and quality characteristics of oils from palm fruits using solvent extraction. AIP Conf. Proc. 1678, 15517616. doi:10.1063/1.4931281. http://scitation.aip.org/content/aip/proceeding/aipcp.

Kastakova, E., Bato, V., Dubenova, D., 2023. Competitiveness on the global oilseeds market. J. Econ. Res. Bus. Adm. 2617-7161. 144 (2), 3–13. doi:10.26577/be.2023.v144.i2.01.

Kesarwani, S., Kumar, M., Tripathy, D.B., Gupta, A., Kumar, S., 2024. Oils and Fats as Raw Materials for Industry. Wiley, pp. 1–32. doi:10.1002/9781119910558.ch1.

Kim, I.S., Kim, C.H., Yang, W.S., 2021. Physiologically active molecules and functional properties of soybeans in human health—a current perspective. Int. J. Mol. Sci. 14220067. 22 (8). Available from: https://www.mdpi.com/1422-0067/22/8/4054/pdf. doi:10.3390/ijms22084054.

Klaschka, U., 2016. Natural personal care products—analysis of ingredient lists and legal situation. Environ. Sci. Eur. 2190-4707. 28 (1). doi:10.1186/s12302-016-0076-7.

Knight, J., Rovida, C., Kreiling, R., Zhu, C., Knudsen, M., Hartung, T., 2021. Continuing animal tests on cosmetic ingredients for REACH in the EU. Altex. 18688551. 38 (4), 653–668. Available from: https://www.altex.org/index.php/altex/article/view/2291. doi:10.14573/altex.2104221.

Lai, J., Xin, C., Zhao, Y., Feng, B., Congfen, H., Dong, Y., Fang, Y., Wei, S., 2012. Study of active ingredients in black soybean sprouts and their safety in cosmetic use. Molecules. 1420-3049. 17 (10), 11669–11679. doi:10.3390/molecules171011669.

Laveriano-Santos, E.P., Vallverdú-Queralt, A., Bhat, R., Tresserra-Rimbau, A., Gutiérrez-Alcalde, E., Campins-Machado, F.M., Lamuela-Raventós, R.M., Pérez, M., 2024. Unlocking the potential of olive residues for functional purposes: update on human intervention trials with health and cosmetic products. J. Sci. Food Agric. 10970010. 104 (7), 3816–3822. Available from: http://onlinelibrary.wiley.com/journal/10.1002/(ISSN)1097-0010. doi:10.1002/jsfa.13451.

Le, B., Pham, T.N.A., Yang, S.H., 2020. Prebiotic potential and anti-inflammatory activity of soluble polysaccharides obtained from soybean residue. Foods. 23048158. 9 (12). Available from: https://www.mdpi.com/2304-8158/9/12/1808/pdf. doi:10.3390/foods9121808.

Lee, J.W., Peng, L., Jegal, H., Park, N.J., Bong, S.K., Lee, J.W., Pyo, J.J., Choi, Y., Kim, S.N., 2022. The soybean cultivar SCEL-1 shows potent anti-photoaging effects in a UV-induced three-dimensional human skin and hairless mouse model. Appl. Biol. Chem. 24680842. 65 (1). Available from: https://www.springer.com/journal/13765. doi:10.1186/s13765-022-00677-y.

Leyva-Jiménez, F.J., Fernández-Ochoa, Á., Cádiz-Gurrea, M.D.L.L., Lozano-Sánchez, J., Oliver-Simancas, R., Alañón, M.E., Castangia, I., Segura-Carretero, A., Arráez-Román, D., 2022. Application of response surface methodologies to optimize high-added value products developments: cosmetic formulations as an example. Antioxidants. 20763921. 11 (8). Available from: www.mdpi.com/journal/antioxidants. doi:10.3390/antiox11081552.

Loschi, F., Zengin, G., Zancato, M., Ferrarese, I., De Zordi, N., Dall'Acqua, S., Sut, S., 2024. Valorisation of olive pomace from Veneto region: oven-dried material for food, nutraceutical, and cosmetic application of the OLIVARE project. Process Biochem. 13595113. 137, 153–163. doi:10.1016/j.procbio.2024.01.001.

Lozada, P., Victoria-Tinoco, L., Muñoz, A.M., Rojas, J., 2025. Evaluation of sebum control and safety for daily use of a cosmetic elastomer formulated with vegetable oils from peruvian biodiversity. Cosmetics. 20799284. 12 (2). Available from: www.mdpi.com/journal/cosmetics. doi:10.3390/cosmetics12020066.

Majchrzak, W., Motyl, I., Śmigielski, K., 2022. Biological and cosmetical importance of fermented raw materials: an overview. Molecules. 14203049. 27 (15). Available from: http://www.mdpi.com/journal/molecules. doi:10.3390/molecules27154845.

Marijan, M., Mitar, A., Jakupović, L., Kardum, J.P., Končić, M.Z., 2022. Optimization of bioactive phenolics extraction and cosmeceutical activity of eco-friendly polypropylene-glycol–lactic-acid-based extracts of olive leaf. Molecules. 14203049. 27 (2). Available from: https://www.mdpi.com/1420-3049/27/2/529/pdf. doi:10.3390/molecules27020529.

Martinez, S., Bessou, C., Hure, L., Guilbot, J., Hélias, A., 2017. The impact of palm oil feedstock within the LCA of a bio-sourced cosmetic cream. J. Clean. Prod. 09596526. 145, 348–360. doi:10.1016/j.jclepro.2017.01.042.

Mohanty, B., Behera, A., Shaw, T.K., Habibullah, S., Acharya, B., 2024. Soybean oil: a versatile asset in pharmaceutical drug delivery. In: Jimenez-Lopez, J.C., Escudero-Feliu, J. (Eds.), Soybean Crop—Physiological and Nutraceutical Aspects. IntechOpen. doi:10.5772/intechopen.115033.

Moore, E.M., Wagner, C., Komarnytsky, S., 2020. The enigma of bioactivity and toxicity of botanical oils for skin care. Front. Pharmacol. 16639812. 11. Available from: http://www.frontiersin.org/Pharmacology. doi:10.3389/fphar.2020.00785.

Morganti, P., Gao, X., Vukovic, N., Gagliardini, A., Lohani, A., Morganti, G., 2022. Food loss and food waste for green cosmetics and medical devices for a cleaner planet. Cosmetics. 2079-9284. 9 (1), 19. doi:10.3390/cosmetics9010019.

Murphy, D.J., Goggin, K., Paterson, R.R.M., 2021. Oil palm in the 2020s and beyond: challenges and solutions. CABI Agric. Biosci. 26624044. 2 (1). Available from: https://www.springer.com/journal/43170. doi:10.1186/s43170-021-00058-3.

Natarelli, N., Gahoonia, N., Maloh, J., Sivamani, R.K., 2023. Clinical efficacy of topical or oral soy supplementation in dermatology: a systematic review. J. Clin. Med. 20770383. 12 (12). Available from: https://www.mdpi.com/journal/jcm. doi:10.3390/jcm12124171.

Nile, S.H., Venkidasamy, B., Samynathan, R., Nile, A., Shao, K., Chen, T., Sun, M., Khan, M.U., Dutta, N., Thiruvengadam, M., Shariati, M.A., Rebezov, M., Kai, G., 2022. Soybean processing wastes: novel insights on their production, extraction of isoflavones, and their therapeutic properties. J. Agric. Food Chem. 15205118. 70 (23), 6849–6863. Available from: http://pubs.acs.org/journal/jafcau. doi:10.1021/acs.jafc.1c04927.

Nunes, A., Gonçalves, L., Marto, J., Martins, A.M., Silva, A.N., Pinto, P., Martins, M., Fraga, C., Ribeiro, H.M., 2021. Investigations of olive oil industry by-products extracts with potential skin benefits in topical formulations. Pharmaceutics. 19994923. 13 (4). Available from: https://www.mdpi.com/1999-4923/13/4/465/pdf. doi:10.3390/pharmaceutics13040465.

Östbring, K., Nilsson, K., Ahlström, C., Fridolfsson, A., Rayner, M., 2020. Emulsifying and anti-oxidative properties of proteins extracted from industrially cold-pressed rapeseed press-cake. Foods. 2304-8158. 9 (5), 678. doi:10.3390/foods9050678.

Öztürk, M., Ender, S., Kurtulbaş, E., Şahin, S., 2025. Olive leaf as a functional cosmetic ingredient and analysis of the principal component. Anal. Biochem. 00032697. 700, 115802. doi:10.1016/j.ab.2025.115802.

Palacios, J.M.S., Blázquez Sánchez, N., Ruiz, F.R., Bernier, M.A., Ramírez López, B., Sánchez, M.E.F., de Troya Martín, M., 2019. Topical treatment with oleocanthal extract in reducing inflammatory reactions after photodynamic therapy: a prospective quasi-experimental pilot study. Complement. Ther. Med. 18736963. 42, 298–301. Available from: http://www.elsevier.com/wps/find/journaldescription.cws_home/623020/authorinstructions. doi:10.1016/j.ctim.2018.12.003.

Percival, B., Savel, E., Ampem, G., Gibson, M., Edgar, M., Jafari, F., Woodason, K., Frederick, K., Wilson, P., Grootveld, M., Konuskan, D.B., 2019. Molecular composition of and potential health benefits offered by natural east african virgin sunflower oil products: a 400 MHz 1H NMR analysis study. Int. J. Nutr. 23797835. 3 (3), 22–43. doi:10.14302/issn.2379-7835.ijn-19-2677.

Perez, E.E., Carelli, A.A., Crapiste, G.H., 2004. Chemical characterization of oils and meals from wild sunflower (*Helianthus petiolaris* Nutt). J. Am. Oil Chem. Soc. 0003021X. 81 (3), 245–249. Available from: http://www.aocs.org/press. doi:10.1007/s11746-004-0890-y.

Pessoa, F.L.P., Villardi, H., da Silva Calixto, E.E., Durão Vieira, E., de Souza, A.L.B., Aparecida Souza Machado, B., 2020. Integrated soybean biorefinery. In: Beschkov, V. (Ed.), Biorefinery Concepts, Energy and Products. IntechOpen. doi:10.5772/intechopen.88111.

Petraru, A., Ursachi, F., Amariei, S., 2021. Nutritional characteristics assessment of sunflower seeds, oil and cake. Perspective of using sunflower oilcakes as a functional ingredient. Plants. 2223-7747. 10 (11), 2487. doi:10.3390/plants10112487.

Pintea, A., Manea, A., Pintea, C., Vlad, R.A., Bîrsan, M., Antonoaea, P., Rédai, E.M., Ciurba, A., 2025. Peptides: emerging candidates for the prevention and treatment of skin senescence: a review. Biomolecules. 2218273X. 15 (1). Available from: http://www.mdpi.com/journal/biomolecules. doi:10.3390/biom15010088.

Puton, B.M.S., Oro, C.E.D., Bernardi, J.L., Finkler, D.E., Venquiaruto, L.D., Dallago, R.M., Tres, M.V., 2025. Sustainable valorization of plant residues through enzymatic hydrolysis for the extraction of bioactive compounds: applications as functional ingredients in cosmetics. Processes. 22279717. 13 (5). Available from: http://www.mdpi.com/journal/processes. doi:10.3390/pr13051314.

Rashid, A., 2024. Nano Fullerenes with The Ability to Store Electrostatic Energy That can be Used as Nano Supercapacitors With Very High Capacity. ResearchHub Technologies, Inc. doi:10.55277/ResearchHub.vq5dnd6h.

Rhazi, L., Depeint, F., Gotor, A.A., 2022. Loss in the intrinsic quality and the antioxidant activity of sunflower (*Helianthus annuus* L.) oil during an industrial refining process. Molecules. 14203049. 27 (3). Available from: https://www.mdpi.com/1420-3049/27/3/916/pdf. doi:10.3390/molecules27030916.

Rivera, D., Rommi, K., Fernandes, M.M., Lantto, R., Tzanov, T., 2015. Biocompounds from rapeseed oil industry co-stream as active ingredients for skin care applications. Int. J. Cosmet. Sci. 0142-5463. 37 (5), 496–505. doi:10.1111/ics.12222.

Rodrigues, F., Pimentel, F.B., Oliveira, M.B.P.P., 2015. Olive by-products: challenge application in cosmetic industry. Ind. Crops Prod. 09266690. 70, 116–124. Available from: www.elsevier.com/inca/publications/store/5/2/2/8/2/5. doi:10.1016/j.indcrop.2015.03.027.

Rodrigues, R., Alves, R.C., Oliveira, M.B.P.P., 2023. Exploring olive pomace for skincare applications: a review. Cosmetics. 20799284. 10 (1). Available from: www.mdpi.com/journal/cosmetics. doi:10.3390/cosmetics10010035.

Rungseevijitprapa, W., Yingngam, B., Chaiyasut, C., 2021. Improvement of biophysical skin parameters of topically applied fermented soybean extract-loaded niosomes with no systemic toxicity in ovariectomized rats. Pharmaceutics. 1999-4923. 13 (7), 1068. doi:10.3390/pharmaceutics13071068.

Sarpong, P., 2024. Emerging trends in vegetable oil market: healthier oils, safety challenges, and sustainability. SSRN Electron. J. 1556–5068. doi:10.2139/ssrn.4813829.

Sayanhika, S., Selvakumar, P.M., 2024. An insight into the cosmetic and dermatologic applications of the molecules of palmyra palm. Cosmetics. 20799284. 11 (6). Available from: www.mdpi.com/journal/cosmetics. doi:10.3390/cosmetics11060196.

Schmidt, J.H., 2015. Life cycle assessment of five vegetable oils. J. Clean. Prod. 09596526. 87 (C), 130–138. doi:10.1016/j.jclepro.2014.10.011.

Shen, J., Liu, Y., Wang, X., Bai, J., Lin, L., Luo, F., Zhong, H., 2023. A comprehensive review of health-benefiting components in rapeseed oil. Nutrients. 20726643. 15 (4). Available from: http://www.mdpi.com/journal/nutrients/. doi:10.3390/nu15040999.

Sundram, K., Sambanthamurthi, R., Tan Y.-A., 2003. Palm fruit chemistry and nutrition. Asia Pac. J. Clin. Nutr. 12 (3), 355–362.

Tamothran, A.M., Bhubalan, K., Anuar, S.T., Curtis, J.M., 2022. The degradation and toxicity of commercially traded vegetable oils following spills in aquatic environment. Environ. Res. 10960953. 214. Available from: http://www.elsevier.com/inca/publications/store/6/2/2/8/2/1/index.htt. doi:10.1016/j.envres.2022.113985.

Thiyam, U., Kuhlmann, A., Stöckmann, H., Schwarz, K., 2004. Prospects of rapeseed oil by-products with respect to antioxidative potential. C. R. Chim. 1878-1543. 7 (6-7), 611–616. doi:10.1016/j.crci.2004.02.011.

Thy, L.T.M., Duy, H.K., Dat, N.M., 2025. Applications of lecithin in emulsion stabilization and advanced delivery systems in cosmetics: a mini-review. Results Surf. Interfaces. 26668459. 19. Available from: https://www.sciencedirect.com/science/journal/26668459. doi:10.1016/j.rsurfi.2025.100543.

Tileuberdi, N., Turgumbayeva, A., Yeskaliyeva, B., Sarsenova, L., Issayeva, R., 2022. Extraction, isolation of bioactive compounds and therapeutic potential of rapeseed (*Brassica napus* L.). Molecules. 14203049. 27 (24). Available from: http://www.mdpi.com/journal/molecules. doi:10.3390/molecules27248824.

Torres, C.F., Fornari, T., Torrelo, G., Señoráns, F.J., Reglero, G., 2009. Production of phytosterol esters from soybean oil deodorizer distillates. Eur. J. Lipid Sci. Technol. 14389312. 111 (5), 459–463. Available from: http://www3.interscience.wiley.com/cgi-bin/fulltext/122295432/PDFSTART. doi:10.1002/ejlt.200800141Spain.

Tripathy, D.B., Gupta, A., Agarwal, P., Mishra, A., Jain, A.K., 2024. Oils and Fats as Raw Materials for Cosmetics Oils and Fats as Raw Materials for Industry. Wiley, pp. 145–167. doi:10.1002/9781119910558.ch6.

Tsoupras, A., Panagopoulou, E., Kyzas, G.Z., 2024. Olive pomace bioactives for functional foods and cosmetics. AIMS Agric. Food. 24712086. 9 (3), 743–766. Available from: www.aimspress.com/journal/agriculture. doi:10.3934/agrfood.2024040.

von der Ohe, P., Aalizadeh, R., 2020. S13 EUCOSMETICS Combined Inventory of Ingredients Employed in Cosmetic Products (2000) and Revised Inventory (2006). doi:10.5281/ZENODO.3959386.

Wanitphakdeedecha, R., Ng, J.N.C., Junsuwan, N., Phaitoonwattanakij, S., Phothong, W., Eimpunth, S., Manuskiatti, W., 2020. Efficacy of olive leaf extract–containing cream for facial rejuvenation: a pilot study. J. Cosmet. Dermatol. 14732165. 19 (7), 1662–1666. Available from: http://onlinelibrary.wiley.com/journal/10.1111/(ISSN)1473-2165. doi:10.1111/jocd.13457.

Waqas, M.K., Akhtar, N., Rasul, A., Rashid, S.U., Mustafa, R., Khan, B.A., Murtaza, G., 2014. In vivo evaluation of a cosmetic emulsion containing soybean extract for anti-aging. Trop. J. Pharm. Res. 15969827. 13 (9), 1401–1406. Available from: http://www.tjpr.org/vol13_no9/2014_13_9_4.pdf. doi:10.4314/tjpr.v13i9.4.

Yates, K., Pohl, F., Busch, M., Mozer, A., Watters, L., Shiryaev, A., Lin, P.K.T., 2019. Determination of sinapine in rapeseed pomace extract: its antioxidant and acetylcholinesterase inhibition properties. Food Chem. 03088146. 276, 768–775. doi:10.1016/j.foodchem.2018.10.045.

Zhou, Y., Zhao, W., Lai, Y., Zhang, B., Zhang, D., 2020. Edible plant oil: global status, health issues, and perspectives. Front. Plant Sci. 1664-462X. 11. doi:10.3389/fpls.2020.01315.

Zhu, X., Chen, Y., Hao, S., Jin, S., Xiangqian, L., 2023. Improvement of the nutritional quality of rapeseed meal through solid-state fermentation with *B. subtilis*, *S. cerevisiae*, and *B. amyloliquefaciens*. Fermentation. 2311-5637. 9 (5), 492. doi:10.3390/fermentation9050492.

Chapter 15

Cereals

Vassiliki Chrysikopoulou, Konstantina Kyprou, and Alexandros Tsoupras
Hephaestus Laboratory, School of Chemistry, Faculty of Sciences, Democritus University of Thrace, Kavala University Campus, Kavala, Greece

1 Introduction

In recent years, the trend toward the use of natural and sustainable ingredients in the cosmetic industry has gained momentum, as consumers seek products that are environmentally friendly and, at the same time, effective for skin health. An important and thoroughly investigated field of research concerns the use of bioactive ingredients derived from cereals and their by-products. Cereals such as wheat, oats, corn, and barley, as well as their by-products, such as bran and germ, are rich in natural compounds that possess excellent biological activities, including antioxidant, antiinflammatory, antiaging, and moisturizing properties (Dykes, 2007; Soycan et al., 2019; Liu, 2007; Zieliński, 2000; Adamantidi et al., 2025; Ghosh and Scheepens, 2009; Zillich et al., 2015; Shahidi and Ambigaipalan, 2015; Mukherjee et al., 2011).

According to European agrifood data, there is a production of around 300 million tons of cereals per year, since they are a fundamental element in the diet of both humans and animals, as suggested by the balanced nutrition pyramid (Agridata, 2025). As reported, there are several sources of cereals, like rice, wheat, barley, oats, maize (Bansal et al., 2017), sorghum, rye, and millet (Van Hung, 2016), with a positive effect on human nutrition and health, providing 56% of the food energy and 50% of the protein consumed on Earth (Van Hung, 2016). Specifically, cereals contain macroconstituents and microconstituents, like carbohydrates, proteins, fats, vitamins, fiber, and bioactive compounds (Foligni et al., 2024).

Cereals are a rich source of natural bioactive compounds that have gained substantial attention in both dermatology and cosmetic science due to their multifunctional skin and health benefits. Phenolic bioactives, carotenoids, polyunsaturated lipids, and lipid (pro-) vitamins like tocopherols and carotenoid–vitaminoids A have shown antioxidant, antiinflammatory, and antiaging properties (Zillich et al., 2015; Adamantidi et al., 2025). β-Glucan, a structural polysaccharide present in oats, wheat, and barley, exhibits antioxidant, antiinflammatory, and wound healing properties, making it a valuable agent for moisturizing, barrier repair, and antiaging formulations (Sousa et al., 2023). Likewise, plant-derived ceramides and glucosyl ceramides, found in wheat, rice, and other cereals, can improve barrier integrity, increase skin moisturization, and restore the lipid matrix, leading to enhanced elasticity and the prevention of wrinkle formation (Kern et al., 2024; Bizot et al., 2017). Moreover, cereal extracts rich in polyphenols, such as barley, seem to provide potential antioxidant activities, with free radical scavenging and molecule regulation, thereby protecting collagen and promoting skin health (Yao and Xu, 2022; Di Michele et al., 2023).

Thus the use of such natural bioactive ingredients seems to offer many possibilities for the development of products that enhance skin barrier function, combat aging, and improve skin health. Besides their biological activity, bioactives derived from cereals can act as natural thickeners and agents for stability and formulation enhancement, while supporting a circular economy approach (Michalak et al., 2021; Morganti et al., 2023).

Therefore this chapter summarizes the origins and subclasses of cereal-derived bioactives, the appropriate extraction methods for their isolation, their chemical properties, biochemical mechanistic actions, and biofunctionality in skin care and health. Emphasis is given to current and emerging applications of natural bioactives from cereals and their by-products as ingredients in functional cosmetics and skin health, with a focus on their action regarding skin protection, hydration, photoprotection, antiaging, and connective tissue (collagen, hyaluronic acid, elastin, etc.) modulation and repair.

Nevertheless, challenges arise regarding the efficiency and sustainability of these raw materials, as well as their effective incorporation into cosmetic formulas. Thus limitations, future perspectives, and viability challenges regarding their use in the cosmetic industry are also discussed.

Biofunctional Cosmetics for Health. https://doi.org/10.1016/B978-0-443-27500-5.00015-0

Overall, this chapter provides a holistic review of the significance of cereals' bioactives in cosmetic chemistry and the biochemistry of skin health and highlights the future prospects of their use as biofunctional ingredients in the cosmetic industry for the development of innovative, natural cosmetic products.

2 Cereals: Definition, morphology, and nutritional composition

2.1 Origin of cereals and their historical review

Cereals are monocotyledonous plants of the family Poaceae (Gramineae), also known as the grass family (Kellogg, 2001). This is one of the largest families of monocotyledonous plants, comprising over 10,000 species, the most important of which are wheat (*Triticum* spp.), oats (*Avena sativa*), rice (*Oryza sativa*), maize (*Zea mays*), barley (*Hordeum vulgare*), and rye (*Secale cereale*). They are herbaceous, mainly annual plants, which produce dry, grain-like fruits (caryopsis), in which the endosperm is the main storage structure. They are characterized by linear leaves, a hollow stem (cane), and spikes or panicles as flowers. Their physiology and morphology make them highly adapted to different agroclimatic environments, which explains their wide geographical distribution and agricultural importance.

Cereal cultivation was "born" in the Neolithic Age, when the first human communities abandoned the nomadic lifestyle and adopted agriculture. Wheat and barley were among the first crops domesticated in the Fertile Crescent region (Mesopotamia, Levant, Egypt) (Nesbitt and Samuel, 1996). Shortly thereafter, cereals formed the basis of the Mesopotamian, Indian, and Chinese diets and were instrumental in the development of the first organized societies, providing storable and nutritious sources of energy.

From an agricultural point of view, cereals occupy >50% of the cultivated land worldwide, while at the same time they are the main source of calories for humans (e.g., rice covers up to 50% of caloric needs in some Asian countries) and have economic importance, both as food and as raw materials for animal feed, biofuels, and industrial products (FAO, 2021). Agrobiotechnology has contributed significantly to the improvement of varieties, their resistance to diseases and climatic stresses, and to the increase in their content of functional or bioactive components (Shewry and Hey, 2015; Zafar et al., 2026).

However, as far as their modern perspective is concerned, in addition to their nutritional importance, cereals are intensively studied for their biofunctional properties through their bioactive compounds, such as phenolic acids, beta-glucans, lignans, and tocopherols. These components are found in both the endosperm and the milling by-products, making them suitable candidates for use in the cosmetic and pharmaceutical industries (Bechtel et al., 1990; Awika et al., 2003; Shewry and Halford, 2002; Yu, 2001; Slavin, 2004).

2.2 Morphological and chemical structure of the grain

Cereal grains are multilayered biological structures, which include distinct morphological and functional parts, each of which has particular importance from both a nutritional and biotechnological perspective (Table 15.1) (Bechtel et al., 1990). Knowledge of the structure of these parts is crucial for the evaluation and utilization of bioactive ingredients, especially in the context of the development of cosmetic formulations with functional action. The bran is the outer covering of the grain and includes the pericarp, the seed coat of the seed, and the aleurone layer. It has a protective role, but it is also of high biochemical interest, due to its rich phenolic content, as it consists of polyphenolic acids (mainly ferulic and caffeic), tocopherols and tocotrienols (forms of vitamin E), alkylresorcinols, phytosterols, antioxidant enzymes, as well as dietary fiber (Liu, 2007; Zieliński, 2000; Awika et al., 2003).

TABLE 15.1 Structural and chemical characteristics of the main morphological parts of the cereal grain.

Structural part	Percentage (%)	Morphological description	Main compounds
Bran	14%	Outer covering of the grain, includes the pericarp, the seed coat, and the aleurone layer	Fiber, phenolics, tocopherols, alkylresorcinols, B vitamins
Endosperm	82%–85%	Internal storage tissue, contains most of the starch	Starch, storage proteins
Germ	2%–3%	Embryonic structure from which the new plant emerges	Unsaturated lipids, tocopherols, tocotrienols, B vitamins, phytosterols, proteins of high biological and nutritional value

The endosperm, on the contrary, is the main storage tissue of the grain, responsible for providing energy to the embryo during germination. It constitutes the main part of milled products, with its main components being starch, which is primarily composed of amylose and amylopectin, storage proteins such as gliadins and glutenins, as well as minor phenolics and lipids (Shewry and Halford, 2002).

Next, the germ constitutes approximately 2%–3% of the grain and is essentially the embryo of the seed, i.e., the part with the greatest nutritional and biochemical density. It is the biologically active part responsible for the germination process. It contains unsaturated fatty acids such as linoleic and oleic, fat-soluble vitamins such as vitamin E, phytosterols, and ferulic lipids, but also proteins of high biological value and enzyme systems (Zieliński, 2000; Yu, 2001; Slavin, 2004).

2.3 Representative cereals rich in natural bioactives

The cereal group includes species with different chemical and nutritional profiles, with a characteristic presence of carbohydrates (mainly starch), fiber, protein, as well as secondary metabolites such as polyphenols, tocopherols, phytosterols, and carotenoids. Below are briefly presented six main types of cereals:

2.3.1 Wheat (Triticum spp.)

It is the dominant crop worldwide, especially for flour production. From a chemical point of view, it consists of 60%–70% starch, 10%–15% protein, and 2%–3% lipids and fiber. Its by-products, the bran and the germ, are rich in phenolic acids, vitamins, and tocopherols (Dykes, 2007; Liu, 2007; Shewry and Hey, 2015)

2.3.2 Oat (Avena sativa)

It is rich in β-glucans and unsaturated lipids and contains unique polyphenolic molecules such as avenanthramides, and its by-products are the bran and oat husk (Zieliński, 2000; Shahidi and Ambigaipalan, 2015; Butt et al., 2008).

2.3.3 Rice (Oryza sativa): Key source of energy for the population of Asia

It is rich in γ-oryzanol, phytosterols, tocotrienols, and with by-products such as rice oil, rice bran, and germ extracts (Zieliński, 2000; Xu et al., n.d.).

2.3.4 Corn (Zea mays)

It is high in starch and carotenoids (lutein, zeaxanthin), with its by-products, the husk and bran, while in this variety, anthocyanins "bloom" in dark-seeded varieties (Awika et al., 2003; Kurilich and Juvik, 1999).

2.3.5 Barley (Hordeum vulgare)

It is rich in beta-glucans and bioactive phenolics and amphiphilic (polar) lipids, often used in malt form, with bran, malt, and germ as by-products (Bashir and Choi, 2017; Tsoupras et al., 2024b).

2.3.6 Rye (Secale cereale)

It is lower in gluten, high in fiber, and alkylresorcinols. It is also of interest for the antimicrobial activity of its extracts. Its by-products are the germ, the husk, and the bran (Ross et al., 2003).

3 Classes of bioactive compounds in cereals and their by-products and their valorization in cosmetics

3.1 Nature and categorization of bioactive components in cereals and their by-products

Bioactive compounds and phytochemicals are compounds found mainly in plant-based foods, such as cereals, which, although not classified as essential nutrients, have beneficial properties for human health (Shahidi and Ambigaipalan, 2015; Scalbert et al., 2005). These compounds affect metabolic functions, enhance defense mechanisms, and contribute to the prevention and/or treatment of various pathological conditions, including inflammatory, degenerative, and skin disorders.

Several such bioactive compounds are produced through secondary metabolism in plants in response to stressors, such as ultraviolet radiation, pathogen attack, or other forms of stress. Cereals and their by-products contain a rich spectrum of such compounds, which are of interest to both pharmacology and the dermocosmetic industry, due to their antioxidant, antiinflammatory, photoprotective, and healing effects (Zillich et al., 2015; Grether-Beck et al., 2014).

The main categories of bioactive compounds found in cereals are shown in Fig. 15.1 and include:

Phenolic compounds: Mainly simple phenolics like phenolic acids (e.g., ferulic, caffeic, etc.), flavonoids, and polyphenolic compounds like lignans, all of which exhibit strong antioxidant activity, while flavonoids specifically possess potent antiinflammatory, health-promoting properties. They are mainly found in the bran and germ of wheat (Agah et al., 2017; Huang and Xu, 2025).

Tocopherols and tocotrienols: Fat-soluble forms of vitamin E, which protect cell membranes from oxidative stress. They are mainly found in wheat germ, corn, and rice (Zieliński, 2000; Kurilich and Juvik, 1999; Bramley et al., 2000).

Phytosterols: Plant-derived sterols, structurally similar to cholesterol, with documented hypolipidemic and antiinflammatory effects (Ostlund, 2002).

Polysaccharides and β-glucans: Dietary fibers that contribute to hydration, elasticity, and protection of the skin, making cereals a source of natural polymers with applications in dermocosmetic technology (Butt et al., 2008; Brennan and Cleary, 2005).

Carotenoids: Antioxidant pigments and precursors of vitamin A, with photoprotective properties. Although less abundant in cereals, they are mainly found in various corn and red rice varieties (Adamantidi et al., 2025; Kurilich and Juvik, 1999).

Alkylamines and other secondary compounds: Compounds with immunomodulatory and possibly anticancer activity, which, although found at lower concentrations, are a field of intensive research (Matsumoto et al., 2001).

The diversity and richness of these components highlight cereals, and especially their by-products, as strategic raw materials for the development of natural, innovative cosmetic formulations, with the most well-established ones being examined in more detail in the following sections.

3.1.1 Phenolic compounds

Cereals contain a wide variety of phenolic compounds, depending on their type, which are the most extensively studied bioactives, as they play a leading role in various health-promoting effects. Phenolics are natural compounds, naturally derived as secondary metabolites of plants, occurring in free, bound, or conjugated forms, and are widely known for their biological activities, including their characteristic antioxidant activity and antiinflammatory properties (Chrysikopoulou et al., 2025). For example, some dominant simple phenolic compounds might include ferulic, p-coumaric, caffeic, syringic, and vanillic acids, which are commonly found in many cereal sources (Van Hung, 2016).

Ferulic acid is the most abundant phenolic compound found in cereals, accounting for over 75%, mainly located in the kernel husk (Horvat et al., 2020). Similarly, a research study investigating wheat antioxidants showed that the most dominant phenolic compound is ferulic acid, with the presence of other phenolics like sinapic acid, vanillic acid, 4-hydroxybenzoic acid, p-coumaric acid, syringic acid, and caffeic acid, detected in decreasing order using high pressure liquid

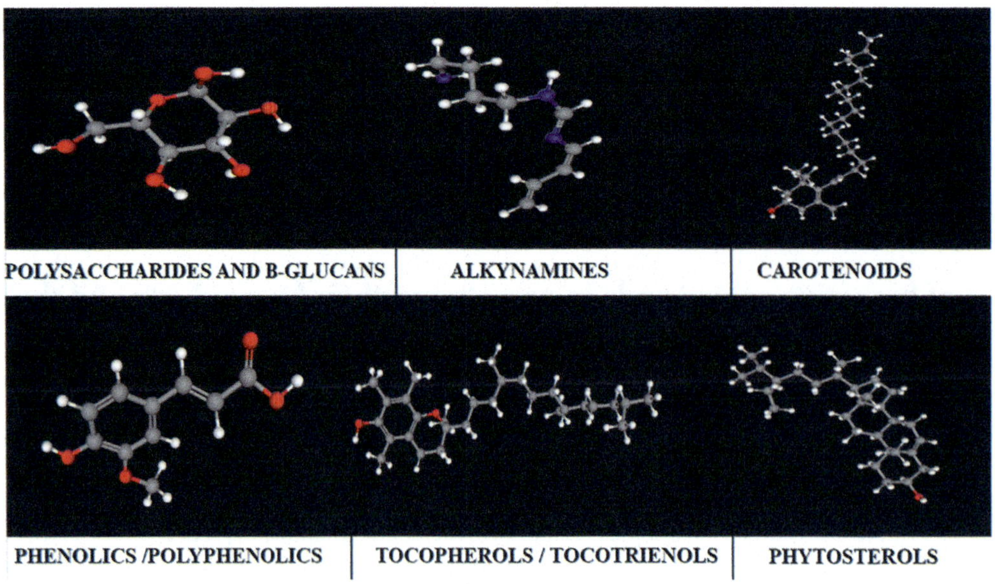

FIG. 15.1 Molecular view of the most important cereal-derived bioactives. *(Source: 3D structures were obtained from the free open-access platform MolView. https://molview.org/ (Accessed 24 November 2025).)*

chromatography (HPLC). In the same research, there were multiple examinations of several types of cereals, including corn, with ferulic acid as the dominant phenolic type; rice, with ferulic and p-coumaric acid; and barley, with p-hydroxybenzoic acid as the major phenolic compound (Van Hung, 2016).

These compounds can act as potential antioxidants in dermal formulations, donating hydrogen atoms or electrons, and are able to neutralize reactive oxygen species (ROS), enhancing their protective effects (Horvat et al., 2020). Also, recent studies on ferulic acid have shown its potential in the cosmetic industry, with photoprotective properties against UV, antioxidant support, skin-brightening, and antiaging activity, yielding very promising results (Jacobo-Velázquez, 2025).

Cereal flavonoids are the main bioactive phenolic compounds with notable antiinflammatory, photoprotective, and antiaging health-promoting properties for skin care and health (Chrysikopoulou et al., 2025). Many phenolics, and specifically flavonoids, are able to block the pathway of platelet activating factor (PAF), thus reducing the inflammation caused by PAF in the skin in certain conditions, like melanoma, while also having antitumor activity (Tsoupras et al., 2024a). Last but not least, as shown in Fig. 15.2, according to molecular docking techniques, phenolic components are able to enhance inflammation reduction, photoprotection, and reduction of melanoma risk (Tsiapali et al., 2025).

3.1.2 Tocopherols and tocotrienols

Tocopherols and tocotrienols are a vital group, derivatives of vitamin E analogs. These are found mainly in cereal germ oils, with α- and γ-tocopherols and tocotrienols being the dominant groups regarding lipid analysis (Ma et al., 2025). After quantitative analysis by HPLC, α- and β-homologs of tocopherols are mainly found in wheat and barley, while barley also contains the δ-homolog and α- and β-tocotrienols, with oats having a very low content (Nogala-Kałucka et al., 2020). These lipophilic compounds have enhanced antioxidant activity and can prevent lipid peroxidation, retinal damage, and muscle weakness, providing protection for barrier integrity, while also contributing to anticancer and neuroprotective effects with in vivo and in vitro results (Ma et al., 2025).

3.1.3 Phytosterols and squalene

Another group of bioactives naturally occurring in cereals, and specifically in cereal germ fractions, are phytosterols and squalene (Kaur et al., 2014; Soujanya and Jayadeep, 2022). The most common phytosterols found in cereals are stigmastanol, campestanol, and sitostanol, which are associated with a decrease in cholesterol levels (Soujanya and Jayadeep, 2022).

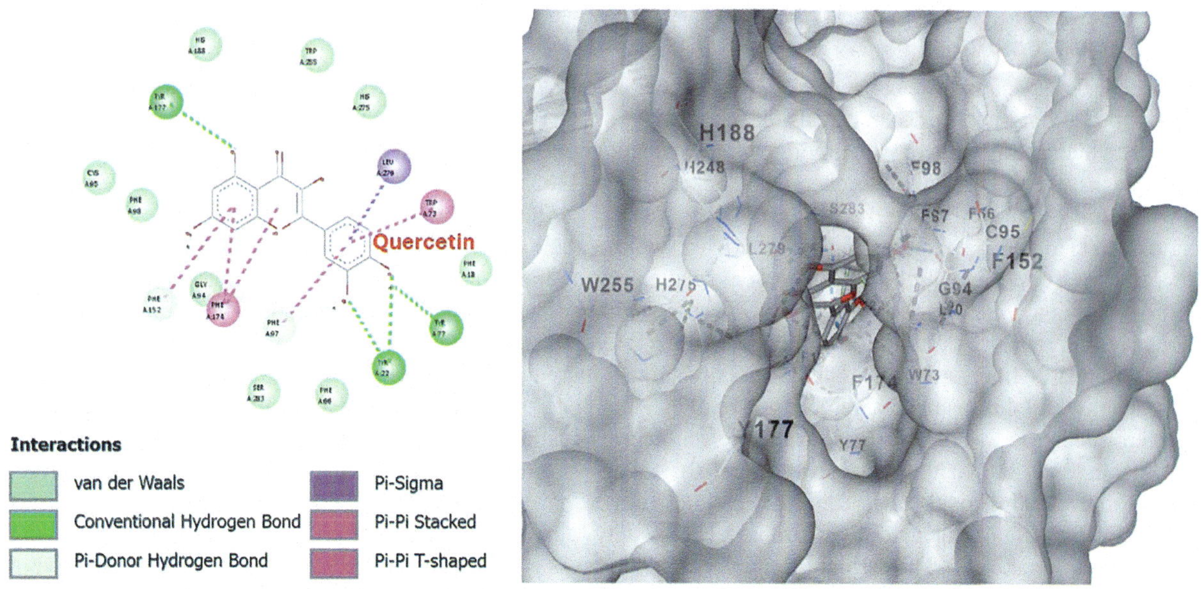

FIG. 15.2 Two-dimensional interaction diagram (left) and three-dimensional binding pose (right) of quercetin docked to the PAFR active site. The 2D diagram highlights hydrogen bonds (dashed green lines) between rutin and residues Arg115(A), Ala118(A), Glu225(A), and Lys298(A). Other interactions, such as pi–sigma, pi–pi stacking, and van der Waals, are also visible. The 3D structure shows rutin positioned within the PAFR binding pocket. *(Source: Figure was retrieved from the open access publication of Tsiapali, O.I., Kontaxi, N.I., Pavlidis, K., Ofrydopoulou, A., Prokopiou, V., Letsiou, S., Kosheleva, R.I., Mitropoulos, A., Tsoupras, A., 2025. Anti-inflammatory and antioxidant properties of anti-UV creams enriched with natural extracts from avocado, apple, and kiwi by-products, with and without nanobubbles. Cosmetics. 20799284. 12 (5). Available from: https://www.mdpi.com/journal/cosmetics. doi:10.3390/cosmetics12050231.)*

Specifically, phytosterols, after digestion, are solubilized and formed into micelles, and due to their common characteristic structure with cholesterol, they compete for absorption in the intestine, thus leading to lower serum or plasma cholesterol and low density lipoprotein (LDL) cholesterol (Soujanya and Jayadeep, 2022). There are several records where phytosterols from other sources are used as antiinflammatory agents to improve skin conditions, such as psoriasiform inflammation (Chang et al., 2023). Also, phytosterols can be used in the cosmetics field for lipstick or cream formulations, making them appealing natural-source bioactives for the cosmetic industry (Fernandes and Cabral, 2007).

3.1.4 Bioactive peptides

Bioactive peptides have gained attention for their multifunctional health-promoting effects, including cosmetic use. They are short chains liberated from wheat, oat, barley, millet, or rice, and they can be produced using various methods, with the most common being gastrointestinal digestion in vitro, fermentation, enzymatic hydrolysis, and malting (Aderinola and Duodu, 2022). There are several health-promoting effects they offer, including antihypertensive, antidiabetic, and anticancer activities. Also, they are strong antioxidants, as they can successfully prevent lipid peroxidation and scavenge free radicals, thereby decreasing ROS production (Aderinola and Duodu, 2022).

Wheat oligopeptides, produced through enzymatic hydrolysis of wheat, are rich in glutamic acid and proline residues that are easily absorbed and digested (Wang et al., 2025). Also, kernel proteins from oats can lead to multifunctional peptides that inhibit enzymes associated with hypertension and type 2 diabetes, displaying antioxidant activity after in silico or in vitro digestion (Darewicz et al., 2022). Grains like millet and pearl millet have also been studied for their novel peptide sequences through proteomics and bioinformatic screening (Fernández-Tomé et al., 2023).

Bioactive peptides can be incorporated into functional foods, beverages, and nutraceuticals, with several health-promoting effects and improvements in product quality (Sartagoda et al., 2024; Najafian, 2023). Moreover, peptide-rich hydrolysates can act as natural additives in active packaging, extending product life and providing antimicrobial protection (Najafian, 2023). Furthermore, studies have confirmed their antioxidant potential, scavenging free radicals and thus providing protection for cells against oxidative stress (Wang et al., 2025; Rafique et al., 2022). Several peptides can act as angiotensin-converting enzyme inhibitors, contributing to the reduction of blood pressure and showing antihypertensive effects (Nirmal et al., 2024; Darewicz et al., 2022). Likewise there are dipeptidyl peptidase-4 (DPP-IV) inhibitory peptides that can contribute to the improvement of glycemic control, thus exhibiting antidiabetic potential (FAO, 2021; Awika et al., 2003). Collectively, these bioactive peptides are promising candidates for the prevention of cardiometabolic syndromes and other diseases.

3.1.5 Polysaccharides

Polysaccharides are composites of cell walls, rich in fiber components, and thus very important in dietary intake. There are several types of polysaccharides in cereals like oat, barley, wheat, rye, or rice, including glucans, heteroxylans, and heteromannans, which are increasingly incorporated into cosmetic formulations (Palmer et al., 2015).

β-Glucans, are glucose polymers chemically linked with β-(1→3) and β-(1→4) bonds, mainly occurring in oats and barley, with a mostly linear chain and occasional linkages, structures that increase their solubility and enable gel formation in the gut (Edo et al., 2025a). Another polysaccharide group is arabinoxylans, which consist of a xylose backbone substituted with arabinose residues, with the cereal genotype and extraction method mainly affecting their characteristics (Yao et al., 2024; Zannini et al., 2022; Boukid, 2024). β-Glucans and arabinoxylans are present in the endosperm and aleurone layers, where they serve mostly as structural components and as storage forms of dietary fiber (Edo et al., 2024; Boukid, 2024).

These kinds of fibers are commonly used as functional ingredients in foods and nutraceuticals for their pronounced health benefits. β-Glucans have a soluble nature, thus are able to trap bile acids, reduce reabsorption, and lead to LDL-cholesterol decrease, while their viscous profile can decrease carbohydrate digestion and improve postprandial glucose control (Edo et al., 2024, 2025b; Mejía et al., 2020). According to clinical trials, cereal health-promoting effects include cholesterol level reduction, hypoglycemic effects, and immune enhancement for cereal β-glucans, leading to health claims approval from regulatory agencies like European Food Safety Authority (EFSA) and Food and Drug Administration (FDA) (Lante and Canazza, 2023). Furthermore, arabinoxylans can act as prebiotics, stimulating beneficial gut microbes, which in turn lead to short-chain fatty acid production, improving blood-glucose responses (Zannini et al., 2022).

3.1.6 Lipids and ceramides

Cereals such as rice, barley, wheat, and maize contain ceramides and glucosylceramides, which can be observed after their isolation from grains and the processing of their by-products like bran or husk (Takeda et al., 2023; Paosila et al., 2020). Glucosylceramides and ceramides from rice include a variety of fatty acids and sphingoid bases with C18-C26 (Paosila et al., 2020). They include lipids like triacylglycerols, rich in linoleic acid, tocopherols, phytosterols, and several polar lipids, including phospholipid bioactives such as diacyl and/or acyl-alkyl phosphatidylcholines and phosphatidylethanolamines with unsaturated fatty acids, especially at the *sn*-2 position of their glycerol backbones (Tsoupras et al., 2024b), as well as several subclasses of glycolipid bioactives like glucosylceramides and ceramides (Zargar et al., 2023). It is important to mention that, to preserve the unsaturation degree of these lipids and the sphingolipid structures, several green extraction techniques have been developed and applied to isolate these bioactives intact from cereals, their products, and/or by-products (Fărcaş et al., 2022). These kinds of lipid extracts are highly used as nutraceuticals and as functional food ingredients, improving the components in combination with other essential lipid bioactives (polyunsaturated fatty acids and lipid vitamins) for the cosmetic industry (Wang et al., 2021; Fărcaş et al., 2022).

Health benefits and modes of action have been reported for cereal lipids, which include antioxidant and antiinflammatory effects, modulation of lipid metabolic pathways, and anticancer properties, supporting their use in nutrition and therapeutic skin care formulations (Tsoupras et al., 2024b; Zargar et al., 2023; Fărcaş et al., 2022). For example, in cosmetics, cereal-derived ceramides and glucosylceramides can be incorporated into moisturizers and creams that focus on barrier restoration, since they can act like skin sphingolipids and improve water loss in the skin, with enhancement of protein expression in the barrier (Nicolaou and Kendall, 2024).

3.2 Bran as a source of bioactive compounds: Comparative advantages and potential for utilization

Bran, i.e., the outer shell of the cereal grain, has emerged in recent years as one of the most interesting sources of bioactive compounds for the development of functional cosmetic products. Its composition of polyphenols, tocopherols, phytosterols, and dietary fibers makes it a by-product with high added value for the dermocosmetic industry.

Bran includes, as we said, the pericarp, the seed coat of the seed, and the aleurone layer, with significant differences in composition between cereal species (e.g., wheat, oats, barley, rice). The presence of phenolic compounds, including bitter acids, flavonoids, and phenolic acids such as ferulic and caffeic acid, as well as humulone derivatives, confers strong antioxidant and antiinflammatory activity (Liu, 2007; Slavin, 2004; Tsoupras et al., 2024b). In addition, it contains tocopherols and tocotrienols (forms of vitamin E) with photoprotective and antiaging effects, as well as alkylresorcinols, which are being studied for their antimicrobial properties and their potential to inhibit cell proliferation.

Compared to other parts of the fruit, such as the endosperm and bran, it has a significantly higher content of polyphenols and fat-soluble vitamins. Furthermore, due to its structure, its bioactive elements are often found bound to cell walls, which requires more targeted extraction techniques, but also leads to more stable and functional extracts, with prolonged release in the skin (Cengiz et al., 2021).

The use of bran extracts in cosmetics has shown promise in several areas, such as antiaging through the neutralization of free radicals and enhancement of collagen synthesis; hydration, thanks to polysaccharide fibers and the action of β-glucans; photoprotection, due to the presence of phenolics and tocopherols; and a soothing effect, with emphasis on irritated or sensitive skin (Slavin, 2004). It is also worth mentioning that, compared to other agricultural by-products, bran offers high availability, low cost, and ease of integration into existing production lines, thus contributing to a more sustainable circular economy model in the cosmetics sector (Galanakis, 2013).

3.3 Methods for extracting bioactive components from cereals and their by-products

The extraction, separation, isolation, and recovery of bioactive components from cereals and their by-products, such as bran or germ, is a key step for their utilization in the production of biofunctional cosmetics and other cosmetic applications. Extraction techniques play a crucial role, as they affect the composition, stability, and bioavailability of the final extracts, as well as the effectiveness of the cosmetic formulations in which they are incorporated. The choice of method depends on the nature of the targeted compounds (polyphenols, tocopherols, phytosterols, β-glucans, etc.), the type of substrate, as well as the technological and environmental requirements. Subsequently, the choice of the appropriate methodology determines the chemical composition, bioavailability, and ultimately, the bioactivity of the extracts from these sources and their appropriate utilization in cosmetic applications. Extraction methods are distinguished into conventional and innovative, with the latter, and especially those named as "Green" ones, gaining ground due to the need for sustainable, environmentally friendly, and efficient processes.

3.3.1 Conventional solvent extraction

This is the most basic and most widespread method, which uses organic solvents (e.g., methanol, acetone, chloroform, hexane, petroleum ether, dichloromethane, ether, etc.) to extract polar and nonpolar compounds. Conventional extraction techniques include processes such as long-term extraction with several mixtures and combinations of the aforementioned organic solvents, Soxhlet extraction, and extraction with aqueous or alcoholic solutions under heat.

More specifically, the use of organic solvents for these extractions is one of the oldest and simplest methods. The aforementioned organic solvents, or several of their mixtures and combinations, are commonly used to extract lipid-soluble, amphiphilic, or polar compounds, depending on their chemical nature. However, this method carries risks of toxicity and environmental footprint and often requires significant time and high amounts of solvent. More importantly, although it is simple to apply, it has limitations in terms of sustainability and safety in cosmetic uses due to possible solvent residues (Mandal et al., 2007; Stalikas, 2007).

The Soxhlet method is based on repeated extraction cycles through heating and concentration of the solvent (Mandal et al., 2007). Although it achieves high extraction yields, it is energy-intensive, time-consuming, and unsuitable for heat-sensitive compounds such as many polyphenols. In addition, it usually requires a mixture of organic solvents, the residues of which, along with their environmental footprint in cosmetics, pose sustainability and safety issues.

3.3.2 Innovative "Green" extraction techniques

Modern techniques focus on reducing the use of toxic solvents and preserving the bioactivity of the ingredients. They offer advantages in terms of speed, efficiency, sustainability, and a green-ecological profile. Here, we present the most well-established methods for extracting natural bioactives from cereals for cosmetic applications, as also presented in Table 15.2.

Ultrasound-assisted extraction

The use of ultrasound enhances and causes cavitation phenomena that facilitate the penetration of the solvent into the plant tissues, thus disrupting the cell walls more efficiently and facilitating the release of bioactive compounds. This method is rapid, requires a smaller amount of solvent, and is thus more energy-efficient, while it also offers high yields, making it suitable for heat-sensitive compounds as it retains bioactivity better (Toma et al., 2001; Chemat et al., 2017).

Microwave-assisted extraction

The application of microwaves increases the extraction rate by thermally stimulating the liquid solvent medium and thus accelerating the diffusion of bioactive molecules. Consequently, this method is used highly efficiently for the targeted extraction of phenolics and tocopherols, mainly from bran and germ, while minimizing the use of solvents in a more environmentally friendly way (Chan et al., 2011).

Supercritical fluid extraction

This methodology utilizes CO_2 in a supercritical state as an extraction solvent medium, offering excellent selectivity and purity of extracts without toxic residues. It is a green and safe technique, applicable to sensitive bioactive substances intended for use in dermocosmetic products (Reverchon and De Marco, 2006; Herrero et al., 2010). For example, it is ideal for the extraction of fat-soluble compounds such as tocopherols, tocotrienols, and phytosterols (Herrero et al., 2006).

Enzyme-assisted extraction

This method utilizes enzymes (e.g., cellulases, proteases, xylanases) to facilitate the degradation of the cell wall and release trapped compounds like polysaccharides, β-glucans, and water-soluble phenolics. It is ideal for applications requiring mild conditions and natural character, with a high yield of hydrophilic components, such as the extraction of phenolics from bran (Puri et al., 2012; Rosell et al., 2002).

TABLE 15.2 Comparative evaluation of the main extraction methods applied in cereals.

Method	Advantages	Disadvantages
Conventional solvent extraction	Simplicity, applicability	High toxicity, low selectivity
Soxhlet	High yield	Time-consuming, energy-consuming, not for heat-sensitive
Ultrasound-assisted extraction	Fast, low cost, ecological	Partial destruction if times are exceeded
Microwave-assisted extraction	High speed, efficient	Limitations on sensitive compounds
Supercritical fluid extraction	Pure extracts, solvent-free	Expensive equipment
Enzyme-assisted extraction	Mild environment, biocompatible	Cost demanding and requires enzymatic specialization

Other green innovative technologies

Recent techniques, such as extraction with natural deep eutectic solvents (NADESs) and pulsed electric field, are also being promoted as environmentally friendly alternatives, enhancing the sustainable production of cosmetic raw materials from agricultural by-products (Paiva et al., 2014; Barba et al., 2015).

The application of extraction techniques to real cereal substrates allows for the evaluation of the practical effect, depending on the complexity of the plant substrate and the chemical nature of the targeted compounds. In the literature, many cases of the application of innovative methods to specific cereals are recorded, aiming at the recovery of valuable bioactive components. The case of wheat bran is characteristic, where the application of ultrasound-assisted extraction has led to a significant increase in the yield of ferulic acid compared to conventional methods. Ferulic acid is bound to the lignocellular structure of the bran through ester bonds, and the mechanical action of ultrasound facilitates its release. The optimization of parameters such as ultrasound power, temperature, and type of solvent has proven to be crucial for increasing the extraction yield (Cengiz et al., 2021). Similarly, microwave-assisted extraction has been successfully applied to corn bran for the recovery of tocopherols and other lipid-soluble compounds, where targeted heating of the material allows for the selective disruption of cellular structures, without extensive thermal degradation of the compounds (Chemat et al., 2017).

In rice bran, NADES has been utilized for the extraction of polyphenols, offering a green alternative without the use of organic solvents. NADES has demonstrated satisfactory efficiency in the recovery of water-soluble and moderately polar compounds, while maintaining the stability of the extracts (Paiva et al., 2014). In addition, enzyme-assisted extraction has been applied to oat bran, aiming to release bound phenolics through hydrolysis of cellular structures. The use of enzymes such as cellulase and xylanase has been shown to be effective, especially when combined with mild temperature conditions, minimizing the loss of bioactivity (Puri et al., 2012).

It is worth noting that each cereal substrate presents unique physicochemical characteristics (e.g., lignin content, proteins, lipids), which makes it necessary to adjust the extraction parameters and the combined use of techniques to achieve maximum yield and quality of the extract. In summary, the appropriate selection and optimization of the extraction methodology depend on the goal of the application (enhancing hydration, photoprotection, antiaging, etc.), as well as on the nature of the substrate.

4 Mechanisms of action of cereal bioactives in skin health

The use of natural raw materials in cosmetic chemistry is a rapidly growing field, with an emphasis on the safety, environmental sustainability, and biofunctionality of cosmetic formulations. Cereals and their by-products, such as bran, have emerged as excellent sources of bioactive compounds with multifaceted effects on the skin. These compounds, such as phenolic acids, phytosterols, β-glucans, tocopherols, and other lipid vitamins and bioactives, display a wide range of properties, including antioxidant, photoprotective, moisturizing, antiinflammatory, and antimicrobial activity, making them extremely useful in the development of cosmetic products of natural origin.

4.1 Antioxidant properties

Cereal bioactives, such as polyphenols, glucosylceramides, and protein-derived peptides, can be obtained from grains like barley or oats through aqueous/ethanolic extraction, enzymatic hydrolysis, or fermentation (Arezoumand et al., 2024; Aloo et al., 2023; Cho et al., 2024). These bioactive compounds can exhibit antioxidant effects by directly scavenging ROS, with phenolic groups donating electrons to eliminate lipid-peroxidation chains (Arezoumand et al., 2024; Cho et al., 2024). For example, the phenolic compounds found in bran, such as ferulic acid and caffeic acid, play a key role in protecting the skin from oxidative stress. Their mechanism of action lies in their ability to bind and neutralize free radicals, such as superoxide radicals (O_2-), hydroxyl radicals (OH), and nitrogen radicals. By binding these ROS, the oxidation of cell membrane lipids, proteins, and DNA is prevented, processes that are directly related to skin aging and inflammation (Shahidi and Ambigaipalan, 2015).

In addition, phenolic acids induce the activation of the antioxidant enzyme glutathione and regulate the expression of genes related to the antioxidant response by activating the Nrf2 signaling pathway, leading to the regulation of endogenous enzymes, enhancing cellular redox capacity (Liu et al., 2025), and thus providing cellular protection at a deeper molecular level (Tsoupras et al., 2024b; Zhang and Tsao, 2016).

In human skin fibroblasts exposed to UV radiation, barley polyphenol extracts reduce ROS levels and matrix metalloproteinase-1 (MMP-1) expression and increase sirtuin-1 production, thus preserving collagen integrity. Likewise, fermented oat extracts have the ability to mitigate oxidative stress and prevent melanin overproduction, supporting barrier function and cell viability (Cho et al., 2024). Last but not least, beyond their topical use, cereal peptides can be formulated in cosmetics for their antioxidant and antiinflammatory properties, improving skin hydration, elasticity, and photoprotection (Li et al., 2023; César et al., 2024; Liu et al., 2025).

4.2 Antiinflammatory and soothing effects

Antiinflammatory effects of cereal bioactives, and specifically polyphenols from barley or oat, have been studied and seem to suppress inflammation, with the inhibition of cytokine release. For example, an in vitro study showed that phenolic extracts from sorghum reduced IL-1β and IL-18 levels in human macrophages, modulating inflammatory pathways (Nguyen and Beta, 2024). Moreover, glucans and phenolic acids derived from barley can lead to TNF-α and resistin level reduction, modulation of gut microbiota, and thus having an antiinflammatory result (Ahmed et al., 2025). Furthermore, β-glucan extracts are widely used in cosmeceutical formulations for their antiinflammatory action, enhancing antioxidant defenses, promoting wound healing, and reducing oxidative stress caused in keratinocytes and fibroblasts (Sousa et al., 2023).

Glucosylceramides and ceramide bioactives isolated from oat can act as immunomodulatory agents, reinforcing barrier integrity with antiinflammatory effects. A study focused on oat bioactives for the allergic treatment of dermatitis resulted in MAPK signaling, to improve epidermal differentiation complex proteins and functions that soothe irritated skin (Kim et al., 2023). Other polar lipids from barley bran and by-products, as well as phenolic bioactives, have also shown strong anti-PAF antiinflammatory properties against the PAF/PAF receptor pathway through several biofunctionalities (Tsoupras et al., 2024b) and thus suggest potential applications for skin protection against skin inflammation, erythema, and melanoma, in which PAF is potently implicated (Tsoupras et al., 2024a).

Other antiinflammatory bioactives from cereals include several phytosterols, such as β-sitosterol, and compounds like alkylresorcinols and lignans, which exhibit antiinflammatory activity through the suppression of prostaglandin synthesis (especially prostaglandin E2, PGE2), inhibition of cyclooxygenase-2, and suppression of proinflammatory cytokines (IL-6, TNF-α). These mechanisms make these ingredients suitable for use in skin care products for sensitive, reactive, or skin prone to disorders. At the same time, their mild action does not cause irritation, which enhances their dermatological safety.

Last but not least, there are bioactive peptides from cereal proteins that can also enhance skin with soothing effects. These peptides are absorbed through gastrointestinal pathways, reach skin tissue, and modulate the gut and skin axis with antiinflammatory effects and skin tissue improvement (Liu et al., 2025). Recent research studies highlight that these kinds of peptides can inhibit pathways like NF-Kb, leading to a decrease in ROS-induced cytokine production and supporting the regeneration of the dermal barrier, offering a dual antiinflammatory and repairing activity for the skin (Liu et al., 2025).

4.3 Photoprotection in UV radiation

Photoprotection is also an evident result of cereal-derived bioactives, like polyphenols from rice, barley, or wheat, with the absorption of UV photons and the neutralization of ROS, thereby preventing oxidative damage to DNA and proteins (Zhang et al., 2025). Also, they can activate the Nrf2 pathway, upregulating antioxidant enzymes that restore balance after exposure to UV radiation (Navabhatra et al., 2025).

More specifically, some bioactive compounds, notably ferulic acid and tocopherols, exhibit UV absorption capacity, mainly in the ultraviolet B (UVB) (280–320 nm) and ultraviolet A (UVA) (320–400 nm) light range, acting as natural photoprotective filters. Ferulic acid exhibits an absorption spectrum that complements that of vitamin C and vitamin E, enhancing their photochemical stability in cosmetic formulas. As a result, ferulic acid can reduce the expression of the metalloproteinase MMP-1, which is activated by UV exposure and leads to the breakdown of collagen and elastin (Grether-Beck et al., 2014; Lin and Fisher, 2007). Likewise, extracts from wheat, rich in ferulic acid and tocopherols, are able to inhibit MMPs, MMP-1 and MMP-3, that are induced by UV ROS, protecting collagen and elastin, and preventing wrinkle formation (Kobayashi et al., 2025). In this way, cereal bioactives protect against photoaging, improving skin firmness and elasticity.

β-Glucans and glucosylceramides from oat and barley germ have been examined, and they can improve barrier function, limiting water loss triggered by UV-induced barrier disruption (Parisi et al., 2023). In addition, cereal nutraceuticals promote short-chain fatty acid production that downregulates NF-Kβ signaling and UV-induced inflammation in skin cells (Singh et al., 2025). Collectively, these mechanisms, along with UV-absorption, ROS scavenging, antioxidant activation, MMP inhibition, and antiinflammatory effects, contribute to the photoprotective potential of cereal bioactives in skin care strategies.

4.4 Moisturizing and skin-strengthening action

Cereal bioactives like glucosylceramides and ceramides can directly reinforce the stratum corneum lipid matrix. Specifically, glucosylceramides from purified rice led to increased keratohyalin granules, thus enhancing filaggrin and corneodesmosin (Takeda et al., 2023). As a result, these molecules promote further production of ceramides, reducing transepidermal water loss (Takeda et al., 2023). Likewise, there are similar effects with rice ceramides, as shown in a study where they improved skin hydration, reduced water loss, and increased firmness in 50 participants (Leo et al., 2022).

Also, oat sprout bioactive extracts, in lipopolysaccharides (LPS) -treated keratinocytes, resulted in the activation of the MAPK signaling pathway, leading to higher levels of profilaggrin and filaggrin protein levels (Kim et al., 2023). These compounds are very important since they are key contributors to natural moisturizing formation and barrier integrity (Kim et al., 2023). Moreover, polar lipids from wheat, containing 98% polar lipids in which dominant sphingolipids, ceramides, and diglycerides are present, led to an enhancement of skin hydration and a reduction of water loss after 14 days of oral intake, reflecting potential in barrier improvement and water-binding capacity (Kern et al., 2024). Another study investigating wheat ceramide powder supported barrier repair, with stimulation of hyaluronan synthase, ceramide synthase, and tumor growth factor beta (TGF-β) receptor expression, thus increasing ceramides and hyaluronic acid production, maintaining moisturization (Park et al., 2023).

The β-glucans, polysaccharides, and soluble dietary fibers of cereals also exhibit a remarkable water retention capacity through the formation of a hydrogel on the skin surface, providing immediate hydration. These compounds create a film on the epidermis that reduces transepidermal water loss, strengthening the epidermal barrier and contributing to the restoration of the stratum corneum. At the same time, the β-glucans interact with the toll-like-receptors of keratinocytes, inducing the secretion of growth factors (such as TGF-β) that enhance skin regeneration and epithelialization, resulting in accelerated healing of microwounds (Volz et al., 2019).

Collectively, cereal bioactives can successfully restore barrier lipids, boost structural proteins contributing to barrier integrity, activate signaling pathways, and elevate endogenous moisturizing agents, resulting in enhanced skin hydration and a reduction in water loss.

4.5 Antiaging effects and collagen modulation

Ceramides extracted from cereals can act as potent antiaging agents, protecting collagen from UV radiation that leads to degradation and promoting collagen synthesis. Research on wheat ceramide powder resulted in the suppression of UVB-triggered kinase pathways related to the activation of collagen proteolysis and led to the upregulation of synthetic factors for collagen deposition and extracellular matrix remodeling (Park et al., 2023).

Bioactives from rice extract, after examination, showed antiaging effects through collagen production enhancement. A research study with different skin models (two-dimensional and three-dimensional) demonstrated an increase in collagen expression, a boost in elastin content, and improved skin moisturization, leading to enhancements in wrinkle reduction and elasticity in an in vivo model.

Moreover, barley-derived bioactives, like polyphenols, resulted in the attenuation of collagen breakdown, supporting cellular longevity, with a reduction in MMP-1 levels and an increase in SIRT1 in UVB-exposed fibroblasts (Arezoumand et al., 2024). Another study on barley extracts, specifically procyanidins and prodelphinidin oligomers, demonstrated inhibition of collagenase and stimulation of collagen production, with potential antiwrinkle effects (Park et al., 2021). Likewise, barley supplements reduced MMP-1 levels, increasing antioxidant enzyme activities and protecting collagen from UV exposure (Gromkowska-Kępka et al., 2021). Last but not least, β-glucan from oats and barley has also been reviewed for its antiaging effects, with enhancements in antioxidant defenses, modulation of immune responses, and protection of collagen through the reduction of oxidative stress and inflammation, showing great potential in skin-health applications (Sousa et al., 2023).

4.6 Antimicrobial properties

Some cereal extracts have emerged as mild antimicrobial agents, with activity against Gram-positive bacteria (such as *Staphylococcus aureus*) and acne-associated bacteria such as *Cutibacterium acnes*. Simple phenolics, flavonoids, and polyphenols possess strong antimicrobial properties for skin health. For example, polyphenols and lignans are thought to act by disrupting the bacterial membrane and inhibiting microbial metabolic enzymes (Draelos, 2010; Borges et al., 2012). Although their activity is milder compared to synthetic antimicrobials, their combined use with other natural compounds (e.g., essential oils or trace elements) can provide significant results without the side effects of traditional preservatives.

5 Applications in functional cosmetics and skin health

As shown in Table 15.3, several bioactives from cereals are increasingly incorporated into the cosmetic industry and cosmeceutical products, since they provide both skin-health benefits with a sustainable source from natural products and grain by-products (Sousa et al., 2023; Nguyen and Beta, 2024; Nemes et al., 2022).

β-Glucans extracted from oats or barley have exhibited antioxidant, antiwrinkle, and wound healing activity, while their ability to regulate immune responses is also protective against oxidative stress factors (Sousa et al., 2023). Ceramide

TABLE 15.3 Overview of the most important cereal-derived bioactive compound activities, useful in functional cosmetics and skin health.

Cereal bioactive	Reported cosmetic effect	References
β-Glucans	Antioxidant, antiwrinkle, moisturizing, barrier repair, wound healing	(Sousa et al., 2023; Du et al., 2014)
Rice or wheat ceramides	Improvement of skin hydration, firmness, elasticity, reduction of water loss, and wrinkle depth	(Kern et al., 2024; Leo et al., 2022)
Polyphenols	Strong free radical scavenging, collagen preservation, antiinflammatory, antiaging, photoprotective	(Fărcaş et al., 2022; Michalak et al., 2021; Nguyen and Beta, 2024; Tsoupras et al., 2024b)
Young barley extracts	Enhancement of fibroblast survival, antioxidant, protection against UV-B, and support in barrier function	(Gromkowska-Kępka et al., 2021)
Lipid vitamins and other lipid bioactives (tocopherols, carotenoids, polar lipids, and unsaturated lipids)	Antiinflammatory, antiaging, antithrombotic	(Tsoupras et al., 2024b)

extracts from wheat or rice can restore the lipid matrix, improving skin barrier function and moisturization (Goyal et al., 2022). Last but not least, polyphenolic compounds like ferulic acid can contribute by scavenging free radicals, with antiinflammatory effects improving skin health (Nguyen and Beta, 2024).

In the cosmetic industry, these molecules can be useful in formulation science, serving multiple technological roles. Natural polysaccharides can act as thickeners, enhancing stability in the formulated texture (Yao and Xu, 2022). Their water-binding activity provides skin hydration and chemical functionalization that can enhance their solubility (Sousa et al., 2023; Yao and Xu, 2022). Polyphenol extracts from wheat can act as natural antioxidants to protect active ingredients from oxidation, extending product shelf-life (Kobayashi et al., 2025). Ceramide powders and glucosylceramide fractions are added as active moisturizers, reinforcing barrier lipids (Goyal et al., 2022). Likewise, rice-derived glucosylceramides can lead to a decrease in water loss and strengthen barrier function and hydration (Takeda et al., 2023).

Beyond topical use, cereal bioactives are gaining attention as oral nutraceuticals to support skin health, promoting beauty from within. Fermented barley extracts, rich in polyphenols, when taken as oral supplements, seem to decrease MMP-1 expression, thereby protecting collagen and reducing wrinkle formation (Arezoumand et al., 2024). Thus this approach takes advantage of the antioxidant and antiinflammatory activity of cereal-derived bioactives to improve nutraceuticals and cosmeceuticals.

The above properties have led to the widespread use of bioactive compounds from cereals in various types of cosmetic products (2012). Characteristic examples include:

- Antiaging products: Formulations with ferulic acid, tocopherols, and phytosterols that aim to reduce wrinkles and improve elasticity.
- Sunscreens: Enriched with phenolic acids to enhance UV protection.
- Cleansers and exfoliants: Products with bran microparticles for mild mechanical exfoliation and enzymatic action.
- Moisturizers: Enriched with β-glucans and polysaccharides for enhanced hydration and repair of the stratum corneum.
- Cosmetics for sensitive or inflamed skin: With phytosterols and alkylresorcinols that reduce reactivity and irritation (58).

6 Limitations and future perspectives

The utilization of bioactive components of cereals and their by-products (e.g., bran, germ) in cosmetic chemistry is of increasing scientific and industrial interest, as they have gained attention and seem to have significant potential for skin care and health. However, there are several limitations to their use, as the transition from the laboratory to commercial application is accompanied by a multitude of challenges, technological, regulatory, and economic.

The isolation and stabilization of bioactive components present various technical problems (Crascì et al., 2018; Galanakis, 2021). Many of these compounds are vulnerable to oxidation, photodegradation, or thermal degradation. Furthermore, their incorporation into cosmetic formulations requires studies of solubility, compatibility with other substances, and stability during storage (2018). For example, the water solubility of phenolics or fat-soluble tocopherols necessitates the use of carriers or dispersions.

Another obstacle is the diversity of the raw material. The content of bioactive compounds in cereals can be influenced by variety, geographical origin, growing conditions, and technological processing. The lack of standard isolation and quality control methods can lead to inconsistent results and variable yields in the final products (2021). Thus cereal-derived bioactives often have variability from batch to batch, even though their composition seems to be similar. Specifically, their composition depends on growth conditions, processing, and cultivar, making the process difficult for larger-scale production (Edo et al., 2024; Fărcaş et al., 2022).

Also, gluten contamination in oat extracts raises safety concerns for many patients and requires purification processes, which are rarely applied in the cosmetic industry (Frasier et al., 2025). Many studies remain confined to in vitro or animal models, while data and trials on human efficacy are still limited (Kobayashi et al., 2025). Furthermore, the high molecular weight and limited solubility of β-glucan may reduce its compatibility with oil-in-water emulsions; therefore further techniques are needed to achieve stable formulations (Sousa et al., 2023; Di Michele et al., 2023). Last but not least, the stability of polyphenols is compromised by oxidation and their sensitivity to pH, which can reduce their antioxidant activity over time (Nguyen and Beta, 2024).

Advances in extraction processes, whether enzymatic or ultrasonic, can improve the extraction yield, enhance the purity of bioactives, and produce reproducible results, supporting a new circular economy model that valorizes bran and germ waste (Di Michele et al., 2023; Fărcaş et al., 2022). At the same time, approaches such as spray-drying or freeze-drying enable the mass production of stable and active extracts. The effectiveness of bioactive components of cereals in cosmetic formulations depends largely on their stability, bioavailability, and ability to penetrate the skin, ultimately allowing them to exert their biological action. In this direction, in recent years, research has focused on the development of innovative delivery systems, aiming to maximize the biological performance of these compounds and overcome their physical limitations (Müller et al., 2000). Thus chemical functionalization or encapsulation are emerging strategies needed to enhance solubility, protect bioactives, and improve stability and bioavailability (Sousa et al., 2023; Badalkhani et al., 2023). Advances in nanotechnology and encapsulation methods offer solutions to many of the aforementioned challenges (Müller et al., 2000; Liu et al., 2016). Encapsulation in the form of nanoparticles, polymer microspheres, or biocompatible lipids contributes to the protection and prolonged action of the active ingredients, while increasing their bioavailability (Müller et al., 2000).

Other innovative forms of transport and optimization of the bioavailability of cereal compounds include the use of liposomes and nanoemulsions. Liposomes are phospholipid vesicles that form bilayers, capable of entrapping both hydrophilic and lipophilic substances. Their lipid nature favors transdermal penetration, making them particularly useful for the transport of phenolic compounds and tocopherols. Nanoemulsions, on the contrary, are two-phase systems (usually oil-in-water) with droplet sizes below 200 nm, which ensure stability, increased surface contact with the skin, and improved absorption of the encapsulated molecules.

In addition, modern applications of solid lipid nanoparticles (SLNs) and nanostructured lipid carriers (NLCs) are also useful tools for surpassing such limitations. SLNs are colloidal particles with a solid lipid core, suitable for protecting sensitive compounds from oxidation, photodegradation, or thermal destabilization. NLCs, a more advanced form, combine solid and liquid lipids, increasing loading capacity and stability. Phenolic compounds from wheat bran or germ, such as ferulic acid or tocotrienols, have been successfully tested in such systems, showing improved skin retention and prolonged release (Puglia and Bonina, 2012).

In addition to technological encapsulation forms, enhancement of transdermal absorption and synergistic effects are also utilized for increasing the bioefficacy and delivery of cereal bioactives. The improvement of transdermal absorption is also achieved through the use of absorption enhancers (penetration enhancers), such as essential oils or fatty acid esters, which modify the permeability of the stratum corneum (Touitou et al., 2000). At the same time, synergistic effects between phenolics and other natural components (e.g., vitamin C, resveratrol, hyaluronic acid) have been demonstrated, enhancing the overall antioxidant or antiinflammatory response (Chrysikopoulou et al., 2025). Such strategies increase the effectiveness of cosmetics and contribute to the development of new-generation complex and targeted cosmetic products (Touitou et al., 2000).

New cosmetic approaches combine oral cereal extracts with topical formulations to limit oxidation stress and improve collagen (Arezoumand et al., 2024; Park et al., 2023). Personalized cosmetics could match specific cereal-derived bioactives to skin profiles, and well-designed clinical trials will be essential to unlock the full potential of cereal bioactives in the next generation of functional cosmetics and skin-health products.

Regulatory framework and compliance also need to be considered for current and future research and applications of the use of these natural bioactives from cereals in cosmetic applications and products. For example, cosmetics legislation in Europe (Regulation EC 1223/2009) and globally requires strict controls for safety and substantiation of claims (Official Journal of the European Union, n.d.). Natural compounds derived from food or food residues must meet criteria of purity, stability, and nontoxicity. The European Union's CosIng list provides the acceptable categories and uses of natural ingredients (European Commission, n.d.). Furthermore, the trend toward "clean beauty" products requires full transparency on the origin, extraction, and use of natural compounds, reinforcing the importance of traceability.

Ecological and purchasing perspectives should also be considered. The global market for sustainable cosmetics and products from "upcycled" agricultural by-products is growing rapidly (Clark, 2017; Galanakis, 2012). Consumers are looking for clean, natural, and environmentally responsible solutions, which places cereal derivatives in a privileged position. The reuse of materials such as bran or germ, which were considered waste, is consistent with the principles of the circular economy and sustainable production.

Investment in innovative methods of utilizing these compounds, combined with growing consumer awareness, creates the right conditions for the integration of bioactive cereal ingredients into the new era of natural cosmetics (Rigoletto et al., 2022).

7 Conclusion

This work highlighted the value of bioactive components found in cereals, and mainly in the by-products of their milling and processing, such as bran and germ, as a source of functional compounds with significant interest for cosmetic chemistry. Cereals can constitute a reservoir of bioactive compounds to meet the growing demand for natural, multifunctional ingredients.

Cereals, and especially their by-products, can supply a diverse variety of skin-beneficial bioactives, including polysaccharides, ceramides, phenolic compounds, tocopherols, phytosterols, and carotenoids, among many others, each contributing complementary diverse biological activities and multifaceted mechanisms of action, such as antioxidant, antiinflammatory, photoprotective, moisturizing, and healing. These activities are documented by a multitude of research studies, supporting the possibility of utilizing these natural molecules in modern dermocosmetic formulas.

β-Glucan polysaccharides provide properties that improve barrier integrity, moisturization, and wound healing effects while delivering antioxidant protection. Grain-derived ceramides and glucosylceramides, as structural analogs of skin lipids, can enhance hydration, elasticity, and reduce transepidermal water loss. Polyphenol-rich extracts from barley, oat, and wheat can act as free radical scavengers and are associated with signaling pathways, thereby preserving collagen and exhibiting antiaging effects. The combination of these bioactives can address multiple facets of skin health, making cereals an attractive ingredient for next-generation functional cosmetics.

A central finding is the superiority of bran as an extractive source, due to its high concentration of phenolic compounds (especially ferulic acid), its accessibility as an industrial by-product, but also its association with circular and sustainable production models. The use of green extraction techniques, such as ultrasonic and microwave extraction, contributes to maintaining the activity of the compounds and improves the environmental footprint of their production.

Despite the significant prospects, the practical incorporation of these bioactive ingredients into cosmetic products is accompanied by technological challenges, such as low bioavailability, sensitivity to external factors, and difficulty in transdermal absorption. Also, issues related to production and composition, gluten contamination, formulation, and evident trials must also be overcome before these bioactives can achieve widespread use.

Future research should focus on developing scalable, green extraction technologies that deliver reproducible bioactive fractions from cereals and cereal by-products, supporting a circular economy model. The development of innovative delivery systems—such as liposomes, nanoemulsions, and SLNs—has offered functional solutions in this direction, preserving or even enhancing the activity of these compounds in the final product. Furthermore, the increasing consumption of sustainable and "clean" cosmetics, combined with the market shift toward natural, agroindustrial ingredients, makes cereals and their by-products a strategic tool in the design of innovative and environmentally friendly cosmetics.

Therefore the increasing data suggest that the systematic study and exploitation of bioactive compounds of cereals, through targeted technologies and scientific practices, can offer significant opportunities in the field of cosmetic chemistry. Further research, standardized production, data from clinical trials, and harmonization with regulatory frameworks are necessary to ensure customer safety for the full integration of these cereal-derived bioactive compounds in the next generation of sustainable, effective, and innovative functional cosmetic products of the skin-health industry.

References

Adamantidi, T., Lafara, M.-P., Venetikidou, M., Likartsi, E., Toganidou, I., Tsoupras, A., 2025. Utilization and bio-efficacy of carotenoids, vitamin a and its vitaminoids in nutricosmetics, cosmeceuticals, and cosmetics' applications with skin-health promoting properties. Appl. Sci. 2076-3417. 15 (3), 1657. doi:10.3390/app15031657.

Aderinola, T.A., Duodu, K.G., 2022. Production, health-promoting properties and characterization of bioactive peptides from cereal and legume grains. BioFactors. 18728081. 48 (5), 972–992. Available from: http://iubmb.onlinelibrary.wiley.com/hub/journal/10.1002/(ISSN)1872-8081/. doi:10.1002/biof.1889.

Agah, S., Kim, H., Mertens-Talcott, S.U., Awika, J.M., 2017. Complementary cereals and legumes for health: synergistic interaction of sorghum flavones and cowpea flavonols against LPS-induced inflammation in colonic myofibroblasts. Mol. Nutr. Food Res. 16134133. 61 (7). Available from: https://www.mnf-journal.de. doi:10.1002/mnfr.201600625.

Agridata, 2025. European Agri-Food data: cereals production, pp. 11–30. https://agridata.ec.europa.eu/extensions/DataPortal/cereals.html.

Ahmed, H.G.M.D., Shah, A.N., Mushtaq, M.A., Yang, X., Yang, J., Xia, L., Yang, L., Xiaoying, P., Zeng, Y., 2025. Antiinflammatory mechanisms of barley-based functional foods beyond diabetes management. Turk. J. Agric. For. 1300-011X. 49 (3), 468–484. doi:10.55730/1300-011x.3280.

Aloo, S.O., Ofosu, F.K., Muchiri, M.N., Vijayalakshmi, S., Pyo, C.G., Oh, D.H., 2023. In vitro bioactivities of commonly consumed cereal, vegetable, and legume seeds as related to their bioactive components: an untargeted metabolomics approach using UHPLC–QTOF-MS2. Antioxidants. 20763921. 12 (8). Available from: https://www.mdpi.com/journal/antioxidants. doi:10.3390/antiox12081501.

Arezoumand, E., Bagheri, K., Mazloum, S., Noh, G.M., Hamishehkar, H., Kosari-Nasab, M., Kim, K.H., 2024. B-Cyclodextrin as an elicitor of polyphenolic contents of barley (*Hurdeum vulgare*) callus with antioxidant and anti-aging properties on human skin fibroblast cells (Hff2). SSRN. 15565068. Available from: https://www.ssrn.com/index.cfm/en/. doi:10.2139/ssrn.4926738.

Awika, J.M., et al., 2003. Anthocyanin composition of colored wheat, maize, and sorghum. J. Agric. Food Chem. 51 (3), 715–720.

Badalkhani, O., Pires, P.C., Mohammadi, M., Babaie, S., Paiva-Santos, A.C., Hamishehkar, H., 2023. Nanogel containing gamma-oryzanol-loaded nanostructured lipid carriers and TiO_2/MBBT: a synergistic nanotechnological approach of potent natural antioxidants and nanosized UV filters for skin protection. Pharmaceuticals. 14248247. 16 (5). Available from: https://www.mdpi.com/journal/pharmaceuticals. doi:10.3390/ph16050670.

Bansal, M., Sharma, M., Kanwar, P., goyal, A., 2017. Recent advances in proteomics of cereals. Biotechnol. Genet. Eng. Rev. 20465556. 32 (1-2), 1–17. Available from: https://www.tandfonline.com/action/journalInformation?journalCode=tbgr20. doi:10.1080/02648725.2016.1272357.

Barba, F.J., et al., 2015. Pulsed electric field technology for extraction. Trends Food Sci. Technol. 42 (2), 128–141.

Bashir, K.M.I., Choi, J.S., 2017. Clinical and physiological perspectives of β-Glucans: the past, present, and future. Int. J. Mol. Sci. 18 (9), 1906. doi:10.3390/ijms18091906. PMID: 28872611. PMCID: PMC5618555.

Bechtel, D.B., et al., 1990. Cereal grains: properties, processing, and nutritional attributes. In: Structure and Composition of Cereal Grains. CRC Press, pp. 1–707.

Bizot, V., Cestone, E., Michelotti, A., Nobile, V., 2017. Improving skin hydration and age-related symptoms by oral administration of wheat glucosylceramides and digalactosyl diglycerides: a human clinical study. Cosmetics. 2079-9284. 4 (4), 37. doi:10.3390/cosmetics4040037.

Borges, A., Saavedra, M.J., Simões, M., 2012. The activity of ferulic and gallic acids in biofilm prevention and control of pathogenic bacteria. Biofouling. 10292454. 28 (7), 755–767. doi:10.1080/08927014.2012.706751.

Boukid, F., 2024. Comprehensive review of barley dietary fibers with Emphasis on arabinoxylans. Bioact. Carbohydr. Diet. Fibre. 22126198. 31, 100410. doi:10.1016/j.bcdf.2024.100410.

Bramley, P.M., Elmadfa, I., Kafatos, A., Kelly, F.J., Manios, Y., Roxborough, H.E., Schuch, W., Sheehy, P.J.A., Wagner, K.-.H., 2000. Vitamin E. J. Sci. Food Agric. 00225142. 80 (7), 913–938. doi:10.1002/(SICI)1097-0010(20000515)80:7<913::AID-JSFA600>3.3.CO;2-V.

Brennan, C.S., Cleary, L.J., 2005. The potential use of cereal (1→3,1→4)-β-d-glucans as functional food ingredients. J. Cereal Sci. 42 (1), 1–13. doi:10.1016/j.jcs.2005.01.002.

Butt, M.S., Tahir-Nadeem, M., Khan, M.K.I., Shabir, R., Butt, M.S., 2008. Oat: unique among the cereals. Eur. J. Nutr. 14366207. 47 (2), 68–79. doi:10.1007/s00394-008-0698-7.

Cengiz, M.F., Babacan, U., Akinci, E., Kesci, S.T., Kaba, A., 2021. Extraction of phenolic acids from ancient wheat bran samples by ultrasound application. J. Chem. Technol. Biotechnol. 96 (1), 134–141. doi:10.1002/jctb.6519.

César, A.P.C., Lopes, F.E.S., Azevedo, F.F.N., Pinto, Y.O., Andrade, C.R., Mesquita, F.P., Silva, G.O., Freitas, C.D.T., Souza, P.F.N., 2024. Antioxidant peptides from plants: a review. Phytochem. Rev. 1572980X. 23 (1), 95–104. Available from: https://www.springer.com/journal/11101. doi:10.1007/s11101-023-09875-y.

Chan, C.-H., et al., 2011. MAE of bioactive compounds. Chem. Eng. Process. 50, 11–12.

Chang, Z.-Y., Chen, C.-W., Tsai, M.-J., Chen, C.-C., Alshetaili, A., Hsiao, Y.-T., Fang, J.-Y., 2023. The elucidation of structure–activity and structure-permeation relationships for the cutaneous delivery of phytosterols to attenuate psoriasiform inflammation. Int. Immunopharmacol. 15675769. 119, 110202. doi:10.1016/j.intimp.2023.110202.

Chemat, F., Rombaut, N., Sicaire, A.G., Meullemiestre, A., Fabiano-Tixier, A.S., Abert-Vian, M., 2017. Ultrasound assisted extraction of food and natural products. Mechanisms, techniques, combinations, protocols and applications. a review. Ultrason. Sonochem. 18732828. 34, 540–560. Available from: https://www.elsevier.com/inca/publications/store/5/2/5/4/5/1. doi:10.1016/j.ultsonch.2016.06.035.

Cho, H., Yang, J., Kang, J.Y., Kim, K.E., 2024. Inhibitory effects of fermented sprouted oat extracts on oxidative stress and melanin overproduction. Antioxidants. 20763921. 13 (5). Available from: https://www.mdpi.com/journal/antioxidants. doi:10.3390/antiox13050544.

Chrysikopoulou, V., Rampaouni, A., Koutsia, E., Ofrydopoulou, A., Mittas, N., Tsoupras, A., 2025. Anti-inflammatory, antithrombotic and antioxidant efficacy and synergy of a high-dose vitamin C supplement enriched with a low dose of bioflavonoids. Nutrients. 20726643. 17 (16). Available from: http://www.mdpi.com/journal/nutrients/. doi:10.3390/nu17162643.

Clark, J.H., 2017. From waste to wealth using green chemistry: the way to long term stability. Curr. Opin. Green Sustain. Chem. 2452-2236. 8, 10–13.

Crascì, L., Panico, A.M., Puglisi, G., Bonina, F., 2018. Cosmetic and dermatological use of rice bran oil. Cosmetics 5 (3), 26.

Darewicz, M., Pliszka, M., Borawska-Dziadkiewicz, J., Minkiewicz, P., Iwaniak, A., 2022. Multi-bioactivity of protein digests and peptides from oat (*Avena sativa* L.) kernels in the prevention of the cardiometabolic syndrome. Molecules. 14203049. 27 (22). Available from: http://www.mdpi.com/journal/molecules. doi:10.3390/molecules27227907.

Di Michele, A., Laura Pérez Gutiérrez, C., Pagano, C., Beccari, T., Ceccarini, M.R., Luzi, F., Puglia, D., Tensi, L., D'Agosto, E., Antonio Viseras Iborra, C., Ricci, M., Perioli, L., 2023. Formulation and characterization of sustainable bioadhesive films for wound treatment based on barley β-glucan extract obtained using the high power ultrasonic technique. Int. J. Pharm. 03785173. 638, 122925. doi:10.1016/j.ijpharm.2023.122925.

Draelos, Z.D., 2010. Cosmetic Dermatology: Products and Procedures (Draelos, Z.D.). John Wiley & Sons.

Du, B., Bian, Z., Xu, B., 2014. Skin health promotion effects of natural beta-glucan derived from cereals and microorganisms: a review. Phytother. Res. 10991573. 28 (2), 159–166. doi:10.1002/ptr.4963.

Dykes, 2007. Phenolic compounds in cereal grains and their health benefits. Cereal Foods World 01466283 52 (3). doi:10.1094/CFW-52-3-0105.

Edo, G.I., Mafe, A.N., Ali, A.B.M., Akpoghelie, P.O., Yousif, E., Isoje, E.F., Igbuku, U.A., Zainulabdeen, K., Owheruo, J.O., Essaghah, A.E.A., Umar, H., Ahmed, D.S., Alamiery, A.A., 2025a. Mechanistic insights into β-glucans and gut microbiota interactions for enhancing human health. Discover Food. 27314286. 5 (1). Available from: https://www.springer.com/journal/44187. doi:10.1007/s44187-025-00503-6.

Edo, G.I., Mafe, A.N., Ali, A.B.M., Akpoghelie, P.O., Yousif, E., Isoje, E.F., Igbuku, U.A., Zainulabdeen, K., Owheruo, J.O., Essaghah, A.E.A., Umar, H., Ahmed, D.S., Alamiery, A.A., 2025b. A critical review on the impacts of β-glucans on gut microbiota and human health. Microbe. 29501946. 7, 100394. doi:10.1016/j.microb.2025.100394.

Edo, G.I., Ndudi, W., Makia, R.S., Ainyanbhor, I.E., Yousif, E., Gaaz, T.S., Zainulabdeen, K., Jikah, A.N., Opiti, R.A., Akpoghelie, P.O., Owheruo, J.O., Essaghah, A.E.A., Umar, H., 2024. Beta-glucan: an overview in biological activities, derivatives, properties, modifications and current advancements in food, health and industrial applications. Process Biochem. 13595113. 147, 347–370. Available from: https://www.sciencedirect.com/science/journal/13595113. doi:10.1016/j.procbio.2024.09.011.

European Commission, n.d. CosIng—Cosmetic Ingredients & Substances Database. https://ec.europa.eu/growth/sectors/cosmetics/cosing_en.

FAO, 2021. FAO Rice Market Monitor (RMM) https://www.fao.org/markets-and-trade/commodities/rice/rmm/en.

Fărcaş, A.C., Ancuţa Socaci, S., Nemeş, S.A., Pop, O.L., Coldea, T.E., Fogarasi, M., Biriş-Dorhoi, E.S., 2022. An update regarding the bioactive compound of cereal by-products: health benefits and potential applications. Nutrients. 2072-6643. 14 (17), 3470. doi:10.3390/nu14173470.

Fernandes, P., Cabral, J.M.S., 2007. Phytosterols: applications and recovery methods. Bioresour. Technol. 09608524. 98 (12), 2335–2350. doi:10.1016/j.biortech.2006.10.006.

Fernández-Tomé, S., Ashaolu, T.J., Hernández-Ledesma, B., 2023. Exploration of the nutritional and functional properties of underutilized grains as an alternative source for the research of food-derived bioactive peptides. Nutrients. 20726643. 15 (2). Available from: http://www.mdpi.com/journal/nutrients/. doi:10.3390/nu15020351.

Foligni, R., Glicerina, V.T., Orkusz, A., Mannozzi, C., 2024. Editorial: cereals and cereal products: nutritional and physicochemical characterization and novel foods. Front. Nutr. 2296861X. 11. Available from: https://www.journal.frontiersin.org/journal/nutrition. doi:10.3389/fnut.2024.1446657.

Frasier, K., Werpachowski, N., Dragovic, M., Forsyth, A., Podwojniak, A., Remé, B., 2025. Evaluating the potential impact of oat-based skincare on celiac disease patients with compromised skin integrity. J. Biosci. Med. 2327-5081. 13 (02), 129–147. doi:10.4236/jbm.2025.132011.

Galanakis, C.M., 2012. Recovery of high added-value components from food wastes: conventional, emerging technologies and commercialized applications. Trends Food Sci. Technol. 09242244. 26 (2), 68–87. doi:10.1016/j.tifs.2012.03.003.

Galanakis, C.M., 2013. Emerging technologies for the recovery of bioactive compounds from food waste and by-products. Trends Food Sci. Technol. 26 (2), 68–87.

Galanakis, C.M., 2021. Green Extraction of Natural Products: Theory and Practice. Elsevier.

Ghosh, D., Scheepens, A., 2009. Vascular action of polyphenols. Mol. Nutr. Food Res. 1613-4125. 53 (3), 322–331. doi:10.1002/mnfr.200800182.

Goyal, A., Sharma, A., Kaur, J., Kumari, S., Garg, M., Sindhu, R.K., Rahman, M.H., Akhtar, M.F., Tagde, P., Najda, A., Banach-Albińska, B., Masternak, K., Alanazi, I.S., Mohamed, H.R.H., El-kott, A.F., Shah, M., Germoush, M.O., Al-malky, H.S., Abukhuwayjah, S.H., Altyar, A.E., Bungau, S.G., Abdel-Daim, M.M., 2022. Bioactive-based cosmeceuticals: an update on emerging trends. Molecules. 1420-3049. 27 (3), 828. doi:10.3390/molecules27030828.

Grether-Beck, S., et al., 2014. Photoprotection by plant polyphenols. Photochem. Photobiol. 90 (6), 1416–1426.

Gromkowska-Kępka, K.J., Markiewicz-Żukowska, R., Nowakowski, P., Naliwajko, S.K., Moskwa, J., Puścion-Jakubik, A., Bielecka, J., Grabia, M., Mielcarek, K., Soroczyńska, J., Socha, K., 2021. Chemical composition and protective effect of young barley (*Hordeum vulgare* L. Antioxidants. 2076-3921. 10 (9), 1402. doi:10.3390/antiox10091402.

Herrero, M., et al., 2010. Supercritical fluid extraction: a review. J. Chromatogr. A 1217 (16), 2495–2511.

Herrero, M., Cifuentes, A., Ibañez, E., 2006. Sub- and supercritical fluid extraction of functional ingredients from different natural sources: plants, food-by-products, algae and microalgae—a review. Food Chem. 03088146. 98 (1), 136–148. Available from: https://www.elsevier.com/locate/foodchem. doi:10.1016/j.foodchem.2005.05.058.

Horvat, D., Šimić, G., Drezner, G., Lalić, A., Ledenčan, T., Tucak, M., Plavšić, H., Andrić, L., Zdunić, Z., 2020. Phenolic acid profiles and antioxidant activity of major cereal crops. Antioxidants. 20763921. 9 (6), 1–12. Available from: https://www.mdpi.com/2076-3921/9/6/527/pdf. doi:10.3390/antiox9060527.

Huang, Y., Xu, B., 2025. Critical review on the intervention effects of flavonoids from cereal grains and food legumes on lipid metabolism. Food Chem. 03088146. 464 (Pt 3), 141790. doi:10.1016/j.foodchem.2024.141790.

Jacobo-Velázquez, D.A., 2025. Ferulic acid: mechanistic insights and multifaceted applications in metabolic syndrome, food preservation, and cosmetics. Molecules. 14203049. 30 (18). Available from: http://www.mdpi.com/journal/molecules. doi:10.3390/molecules30183716.

Kaur, K.D., Jha, A., Sabikhi, L., Singh, A.K., 2014. Significance of coarse cereals in health and nutrition: a review. J. Food Sci. Technol. 09758402. 51 (8), 1429–1441. Available from: http://www.springerlink.com/content/121580/. doi:10.1007/s13197-011-0612-9.

Kellogg, E.A., 2001. Evolutionary history of the grasses. Plant Physiol. 00320889. 125 (3), 1198–1205. Available from: http://www.plantphysiol.org/. doi:10.1104/pp.125.3.1198.

Kern, C., Dudonné, S., Garcia, C., 2024. Dietary supplementation with a wheat polar lipid complex improves skin conditions in women with dry skin and mild-to-moderate skin aging. J. Cosmet. Dermatol. 14732165. 23 (4), 1320–1330. Available from: http://onlinelibrary.wiley.com/journal/10.1111/(ISSN)1473-2165. doi:10.1111/jocd.16130.

Kim, H.S., Hwang, H.J., Seo, W.D., Do, S.H., 2023. Oat (*Avena sativa* L.) sprouts restore skin barrier function by modulating the expression of the epidermal differentiation complex in models of skin irritation. Int. J. Mol. Sci. 14220067. 24 (24). Available from: http://www.mdpi.com/journal/ijms. doi:10.3390/ijms242417274.

Kobayashi, K., Suzauddula, M., Bender, R., Li, C., Li, Y., Sun, X.S., Wang, W., 2025. Functional properties and potential applications of wheat bran extracts in food and cosmetics: a review of antioxidant, enzyme-inhibitory, and anti-aging benefits. Foods. 23048158. 14 (3). Available from: https://www.mdpi.com/journal/foods. doi:10.3390/foods14030515.

Kurilich, A.C., Juvik, J.A., 1999. Quantification of carotenoid and tocopherol antioxidants in *Zea mays*. J. Agric. Food Chem. 00218561. 47 (5), 1948–1955. doi:10.1021/jf981029d.

Lante, A., Canazza, E., 2023. Insight on extraction and preservation of biological activity of cereal β-D-glucans. Appl. Sci. 2076-3417. 13 (19), 11080. doi:10.3390/app131911080.

Leo, T.K., Tan, E.S.S., Amini, F., Rehman, N., Ng, E.S.C., Tan, C.K., 2022. Effect of rice (*Oryza sativa* L.) ceramides supplementation on improving skin barrier functions and depigmentation: an open-label prospective study. Nutrients. 2072-6643. 14 (13), 2737. doi:10.3390/nu14132737.

Li, J., Wang, J., Zhang, N., Li, Y., Cai, Z., Li, G., Liu, Z., Liu, Z., Wang, Y., Shao, X., Chen, J., 2023. Anti-aging activity and their mechanisms of natural food-derived peptides: current advancements. Food Innov. Adv. 2836774X. 2 (4), 272–290. Available from: https://www.maxapress.com/article/doi/10.48130/FIA-2023-0028. doi:10.48130/FIA-2023-0028.

Lin, J.Y., Fisher, D.E., 2007. Melanocyte biology and skin pigmentation. Nature. 14764687. 445 (7130), 843–850. Available from: http://www.nature.com/nature/index.html. doi:10.1038/nature05660.

Liu, R.H., 2007. Whole grain phytochemicals and health. J. Cereal Sci. 10959963. 46 (3), 207–219. doi:10.1016/j.jcs.2007.06.010.

Liu, X., Bi, J., Xiao, H., McClements, D.J., 2016. Enhancement of nutraceutical bioavailability using excipient nanoemulsions: role of lipid digestion products on bioaccessibility of carotenoids and phenolics from mangoes. J. Food Sci. 81, N754–N761. doi:10.1111/1750-3841.13227.

Liu, Y., Xiong, L., Wang, L., Zhou, J., Wang, F., Luo, F., Shen, X., 2025. Targeting the gut–skin axis by food-derived active peptides ameliorates skin photoaging: a comprehensive review. Food Funct. 2042-6496. 16 (2), 366–388. doi:10.1039/d4fo04202f.

Ma, F., Dai, T., Guo, L., Wang, C., Li, C., Li, C., Chen, J., Ren, C., 2025. Comparative study of chemical compositions and antioxidant capacities of oils obtained from sixteen oat cultivars in China. Foods. 23048158. 14 (12). Available from: www.mdpi.com/journal/foods. doi:10.3390/foods14122007.

Mandal, V., et al., 2007. Solvent extraction of plant bioactives. Pharmacogn. Rev. 1 (1), 23–31.

Matsumoto, K., et al., 2001. Immunomodulatory effects of alkylamines. Int. J. Immunopharmacol. 23 (8), 625–632.

Mejía, S.M.V., de Francisco, A., Bohrer, B.M., 2020. A comprehensive review on cereal β-glucan: extraction, characterization, causes of degradation, and food application. Crit. Rev. Food Sci. Nutr. 15497852. 60 (21), 3693–3704. Available from: https://www.tandfonline.com/loi/bfsn20. doi:10.1080/10408398.2019.1706444.

Michalak, M., Pierzak, M., Kręcisz, B., Suliga, E., 2021. Bioactive compounds for skin health: a review. Nutrients. 20726643. 13 (1), 1–31. Available from: https://www.mdpi.com/2072-6643/13/1/203/pdf. doi:10.3390/nu13010203.

Morganti, P., Lohani, A., Gagliardini, A., Morganti, G., Coltelli, M.B., 2023. Active ingredients and carriers in nutritional eco-cosmetics. Compounds. 26736918. 3 (1), 122–141. Available from: https://www.mdpi.com/journal/compounds. doi:10.3390/compounds3010011.

Mukherjee, P.K., Maity, N., Nema, N.K., Sarkar, B.K., 2011. Bioactive compounds from natural resources against skin aging. Phytomedicine. 1618095X. 19 (1), 64–73. Available from: https://www.urbanfischer.de/journals/phytomed. doi:10.1016/j.phymed.2011.10.003.

Müller, R.H., Mäder, K., Gohla, S., 2000. Solid lipid nanoparticles (SLN) for controlled drug delivery—a review of the state of the art. Eur. J. Pharm. Biopharm. 09396411. 50 (1), 161–177. doi:10.1016/S0939-6411(00)00087-4.

Najafian, L., 2023. A review of bioactive peptides as functional food ingredients: mechanisms of action and their applications in active packaging and food quality improvement. Food Funct. 2042-6496. 14 (13), 5835–5857. doi:10.1039/d3fo00362k.

Navabhatra, A., Yangchaiya, C., Yangchaiya, A., Sermsutjarit, N., Sakanoue, T., 2025. Molecular mechanisms of skin photoaging and the therapeutic applications of plant-derived bioactive compounds. Interprof. J. Health Sci. 23 (1), IJHS-0685.

Nemes, S.A., Călinoiu, L.F., Dulf, F.V., Fărcas, A.C., Vodnar, D.C., 2022. Integrated technology for cereal bran valorization: perspectives for a sustainable industrial approach. Antioxidants. 20763921. 11 (11). Available from: https://www.mdpi.com/journal/antioxidants. doi:10.3390/antiox11112159.

Nesbitt, M., Samuel, D., 1996. From staple crop to extinction? The archaeology and history of the hulled wheats. Hulled Wheats 4, 41–100. doi:10.4236/as.2017.82014.

Nguyen, S.N., Beta, T., 2024. Cereal-derived polyphenols and their bioactive properties. Curr. Opin. Food Sci. 22147993. 56. Available from: https://www.sciencedirect.com/science/journal/22147993. doi:10.1016/j.cofs.2024.101136.

Nicolaou, A., Kendall, A.C., 2024. Bioactive lipids in the skin barrier mediate its functionality in health and disease. Pharmacol. Ther. 01637258. 260, 108681. doi:10.1016/j.pharmthera.2024.108681.

Nirmal, N., Khanashyam, A.C., Shah, K., Awasti, N., Babu, K.S., Ucak, İ., Afreen, M., Hassoun, A., Tuanthong, A., 2024. Plant protein-derived peptides: frontiers in sustainable food system and applications. Front. Sustain. Food Syst. 2571-581X. 8. doi:10.3389/fsufs.2024.1292297.

Nogala-Kałucka, M., Kawka, A., Dwiecki, K., Siger, A., 2020. Evaluation of bioactive compounds in cereals. Study of wheat, barley, oat and selected grain products. Acta Sci. Pol. Technol. Aliment 19 (4). doi:10.17306/J.AFS.0858.

Official Journal of the European Union, n.d. Regulation (EC) No 1223/2009 of the European Parliament and of the Council on cosmetic products.

Ostlund, R.E., 2002. Phytosterols and cholesterol metabolism. Curr. Opin. Lipidol. 15 (1), 37–41. doi:10.1097/00041433-200402000-00008. PMID: 15166807.

Paiva, A., Craveiro, R., Aroso, I., Martins, M., Reis, R.L., Duarte, A.R.C., 2014. Natural deep eutectic solvents—solvents for the 21st Century. ACS Sustain. Chem. Eng. 2168-0485. 2 (5), 1063–1071. doi:10.1021/sc500096j.

Palmer, R., Cornuault, V., Marcus, S.E., Knox, J.P., Shewry, P.R., Tosi, P., 2015. Comparative in situ analyses of cell wall matrix polysaccharide dynamics in developing rice and wheat grain. Planta. 14322048. 241 (3), 669–685. Available from: https://www.link.springer.de/link/service/journals/00425/index.htm. doi:10.1007/s00425-014-2201-4.

Paosila, C., Rumpagaporn, P., Jom, K.N., 2020. Investigation of hydrolyzed ceramide in Thai color rice (*Oryza sativa* L.) and byproducts. Food Res. 25502166. 4 (S4), 56–64. doi:10.26656/fr.2017.4(s4).009.

Parisi, M., Verrillo, M., Luciano, M.A., Caiazzo, G., Quaranta, M., Scognamiglio, F., Di Meo, V., Villani, A., Cantelli, M., Gallo, L., Altobelli, G.G., Poggi, S., Spaccini, R., Fabbrocini, G., 2023. Use of natural agents and agrifood wastes for the treatment of skin photoaging. Plants. 22237747. 12 (4). Available from: https://www.mdpi.com/journal/plants. doi:10.3390/plants12040840.

Park, S.C., Wu, Q., Ko, E.Y., Baek, J.H., Ryu, J., Kang, S., Sung, M.K., Cho, A.R., Jang, Y.P., 2021. Secondary metabolites changes in germinated barley and its relationship to anti-wrinkle activity. Sci. Rep. 20452322. 11 (1). Available from: https://www.nature.com/srep/index.html. doi:10.1038/s41598-020-80322-0.

Park, S.H., Park, J., Lee, M., Jun, W., Kim, J., Geum, J., Kim, O.K., Lee, J., 2023. Wheat ceramide powder mitigates ultraviolet B-induced oxidative stress and photoaging by inhibiting collagen proteolysis and promoting collagen synthesis in hairless mice. Prev. Nutr. Food Sci. 22878602. 28 (4), 418–426. Available from: https://www.pnfs.or.kr/journal/view.html?doi=10.3746/pnf.2023.28.4.418. doi:10.3746/pnf.2023.28.4.418.

Puglia, C., Bonina, F., 2012. Lipid nanoparticles as novel delivery systems for cosmetics and dermal pharmaceuticals. Expert Opin. Drug Deliv. 9 (4), 429–441. doi:10.1517/17425247.2012.666967.

Puri, M., Sharma, D., Barrow, C.J., 2012. Enzyme-assisted extraction of bioactives from plants. Trends Biotechnol. 18793096. 30 (1), 37–44. doi:10.1016/j.tibtech.2011.06.014.

Rafique, H., Dong, R., Wang, X., Alim, A., Aadil, R.M., Li, L., Zou, L., Hu, X., 2022. Dietary-nutraceutical properties of oat protein and peptides. Front. Nutr. 2296861X. 9. Available from: https://www.journal.frontiersin.org/journal/nutrition. doi:10.3389/fnut.2022.950400.

Reverchon, E., De Marco, I., 2006. Supercritical fluid extraction. J. Supercrit. Fluids 38 (2), 146–166. doi:10.1016/j.supflu.2006.03.020.

Rigoletto, R., Lorini, C., Montuori, A., Bonaccorsi, G., 2022. Sustainable cosmetics and consumer behavior: a systematic review. Sustainability 14 (4), 2351.

Rosell, C.M., et al., 2002. Enzymatic extraction from cereals. Trends Food Sci. Technol. 13 (11), 394–401.

Ross, A.B., et al., 2003. Alkylresorcinols in rye. Br. J. Nutr. 89 (3), 287–294.

Sartagoda, K.J.D., Tiozon, R.J.N., Sreenivasulu, N., 2024. Cereal-based proteins: bridging health, sustainability, and future innovations for food industries. J. Food Compos. Anal. 08891575. 136. Available from: https://www.sciencedirect.com/science/journal/08891575. doi:10.1016/j.jfca.2024.106720.

Scalbert, A., Manach, C., Morand, C., Rémésy, C., Jiménez, L., 2005. Dietary polyphenols and the prevention of diseases. Crit. Rev. Food Sci. Nutr. 1040-8398. 45 (4), 287–306. doi:10.1080/1040869059096.

Shahidi, F., Ambigaipalan, P., 2015. Phenolics and polyphenolics in foods, beverages and spices: antioxidant activity and health effects—a review. J. Funct. Foods 18, 820–897. doi:10.1016/j.jff.2015.06.018.

Shewry, P.R., Halford, N.G., 2002. Cereal seed storage proteins: structures, properties and role in grain utilization. J. Exp. Bot. 00220957. 53 (370), 947–958. http://jxb.oxfordjournals.org/. doi:10.1093/jexbot/53.370.947.

Shewry, P.R., Hey, S.J., 2015. The contribution of wheat to human diet and health. Food Energy Secur. 20483694. 4 (3), 178–202. Available from: http://onlinelibrary.wiley.com/journal/10.1002/(ISSN)2048-3694. doi:10.1002/FES3.64.

Singh, H., Kamal, Y.T., Pandohee, J., Mishra, A.K., Biswas, A., Mohanto, S., Kumar, A., Nag, S., Mishra, A., Singh, M., Gupta, H., Chopra, H., 2025. Dietary phytochemicals alleviate the premature skin aging: a comprehensive review. Exp. Gerontol. 05315565. 199, 112660. doi:10.1016/j.exger.2024.112660.

Slavin, J., 2004. Whole grains and human health. Nutr. Res. Rev. 0954-4224. 17 (1), 99–110. doi:10.1079/nrr200374.

Soujanya, K.V., Jayadeep, A.P., 2022. Obesity-associated biochemical markers of inflammation and the role of grain phytochemicals. J. Food Biochem. 17454514. 46 (9). Available from: http://onlinelibrary.wiley.com/journal/10.1111/(ISSN)1745-4514. doi:10.1111/jfbc.14257.

Sousa, P., Tavares-Valente, D., Amorim, M., Azevedo-Silva, J., Pintado, M., Fernandes, J., 2023. β-Glucan extracts as high-value multifunctional ingredients for skin health: a review. Carbohydr. Polym. 01448617. 322, 121329. doi:10.1016/j.carbpol.2023.121329.

Soycan, G., Schär, M.Y., Kristek, A., Boberska, J., Alsharif, S.N.S., Corona, G., Shewry, P.R., Spencer, J.P.E., 2019. Composition and content of phenolic acids and avenanthramides in commercial oat products: are oats an important polyphenol source for consumers? Food Chem. X 3. doi:10.1016/j.fochx.2019.100047.

Stalikas, C.D., 2007. Extraction, separation, and detection of phenolic acids. J. Sep. Sci. 30 (18), 3268–3295.

Takeda, S., Yoneda, A., Miyasaka, K., Manse, Y., Morikawa, T., Shimoda, H., 2023. Comparative study on epidermal moisturizing effects and hydration mechanisms of rice-derived glucosylceramides and ceramides. Int. J. Mol. Sci. 14220067. 24 (1). Available from: http://www.mdpi.com/journal/ijms. doi:10.3390/ijms24010083.

Toma, M., et al., 2001. Extraction of polyphenols using ultrasound. Ultrason. Sonochem. 8 (3), 303–307.

Tsiapali, O.I., Kontaxi, N.I., Pavlidis, K., Ofrydopoulou, A., Prokopiou, V., Letsiou, S., Kosheleva, R.I., Mitropoulos, A., Tsoupras, A., 2025. Anti-inflammatory and antioxidant properties of anti-UV creams enriched with natural extracts from avocado, apple, and kiwi by-products, with and without nanobubbles. Cosmetics. 20799284. 12 (5). Available from: https://www.mdpi.com/journal/cosmetics. doi:10.3390/cosmetics12050231.

Tsoupras, A., Adamantidi, T., Finos, M.A., Philippopoulos, A., Detopoulou, P., Tsopoki, I., Kynatidou, M., Demopoulos, C.A., 2024a. Re-assessing the role of platelet activating factor and its inflammatory signaling and inhibitors in cancer and anti-cancer strategies. Front. Biosci. Landmark. 27686698. 29 (10). Available from: https://www.imrpress.com/journal/FBL/29/10. doi:10.31083/j.fbl2910345.

Tsoupras, A., Panagopoulou, E.A., Kyzas, G.Z., 2024b. Anti-inflammatory, antithrombotic and anti-oxidant bioactives of beer and brewery by-products, as ingredients of bio-functional foods, nutraceuticals, cosmetics, cosmeceuticals and pharmaceuticals with health promoting properties. AIMS Agric. Food. 24712086. 9 (2), 568–606. Available from: https://www.aimspress.com/journal/agriculture. doi:10.3934/agrfood.2024032.

Van Hung, P., 2016. Phenolic compounds of cereals and their antioxidant capacity. Crit. Rev. Food Sci. Nutr. 15497852. 56 (1), 25–35. Available from: https://www.tandf.co.uk/journals/titles/10408398.asp. doi:10.1080/10408398.2012.708909.

Volz, T., Skabytska, Y., Guenova, E., Kolbinger, F., 2019. Interleukin-4 and interleukin-13 as critical drivers in atopic dermatitis. J. Invest. Dermatol. 139 (4), 819–826.

Wang, J., Tang, J., Ruan, S., Ruiling, L., Zhou, J., Tian, J., Cheng, H., Enbo, X., Liu, D., 2021. A comprehensive review of cereal germ and its lipids: chemical composition, multi-objective process and functional application. Food Chem. 03088146. 362, 130066. doi:10.1016/j.foodchem.2021.130066.

Wang, Z., Shen, Q., Wang, C., Zhao, Q., 2025. Research progress in function and processing of wheat oligopeptides. Food Sci. 10026630. 46 (7), 337–345. Available from: https://www.spkx.net.cn/EN/10.7506/spkx1002-6630-20240828-206. doi:10.7506/spkx1002-6630-20240828-206.

Xu, Z., et al., n.d. γ-Oryzanol: antioxidant and hypocholesterolemic activities in rice bran oil. *Food Rev. Int.* 17 (1).

Yao, H., Yin, J., Nie, S., 2024. Structural characteristics and biological activities of polysaccharides from barley: a review. Food Funct. 2042650X. 15 (7), 3246–3258. Available from: http://pubs.rsc.org/en/journals/journal/fo. doi:10.1039/d3fo05793c.

Yao, Y., Xu, B., 2022. Skin health promoting effects of natural polysaccharides and their potential application in the cosmetic industry. Polysaccharides. 26734176. 3 (4), 818–830. Available from: https://www.mdpi.com/journal/polysaccharides. doi:10.3390/polysaccharides3040048.

Yu, L., 2001. Antioxidant properties of cereal products. J. Agric. Food Chem. 49 (3), 1626–1634.

Zafar, H., Saeed, F., Niaz, B., Rasheed, A., Akhmedov, S., Jumaniyazova, I., Ahmed, F., Afzaal, M., Islam, F., Kinki, A.B., 2026. Biochemical and structural attributes of wheat & corn bran hydrolysates in relation to their end use-quality. Sci. Rep. 16 (1). doi:10.1038/s41598-025-30461-z.

Zannini, E., Núñez, Á.B., Sahin, A.W., Arendt, E.K., 2022. Arabinoxylans as functional food ingredients: a review. Foods. 23048158. 11 (7). Available from: https://www.mdpi.com/2304-8158/11/7/1026/pdf. doi:10.3390/foods11071026.

Zargar, S., Wani, T.A., Ahamad, S.R., 2023. An insight into wheat germ oil nutrition, identification of its bioactive constituents and computer-aided multidimensional data analysis of its potential anti-inflammatory effect via molecular connections. Life. 20751729. 13 (2). Available from: https://www.mdpi.com/journal/life/. doi:10.3390/life13020526.

Zhang, H., Tsao, R., 2016. Dietary polyphenols, oxidative stress and antioxidant and anti-inflammatory effects. Curr. Opin. Food Sci. 22147993. 8, 33–42. doi:10.1016/j.cofs.2016.02.002.

Zhang, T., Zuo, H.-L., Liu, Y., Huang, H.-Y., Shang-Fu, L., Jing, L., Li-Ping, L., Chen, Y.-G., Lin, T.-S., Huang, S.-H., Lin, Y.-C.-D., Huang, H.-D., 2025. Mechanistic insights into pigmented rice bran in mitigating UV-induced oxidative stress, inflammation, and pigmentation. Cosmetics. 2079-9284. 12 (2), 51. doi:10.3390/cosmetics12020051.

Zieliński, K., 2000. Antioxidant activity and total phenolics in selected cereal grains and their different morphological fractions. J. Agric. Food Chem. 48 (6), 2008–2016. doi:10.1021/jf990619o.

Zillich, O.V., Schweiggert-Weisz, U., Eisner, P., Kerscher, M., 2015. Polyphenols as active ingredients for cosmetic products. Int. J. Cosmet. Sci. 0142-5463. 37 (5), 455–464. doi:10.1111/ics.12218.

Touitou, E., Godin, B., Weiss, C., 2000. Enhanced delivery of drugs into and across the skin by ethosomal carriers. Drug Dev. Res. 50, 3–4. doi:10.1002/1098-2299.

Section III

Sustainable bioactive ingredients from microorganisms

Chapter 16

Healthy benefits of bacteria

Athina Velissaridou, Theodora Adamantidi, Antigoni Bourgani, and Alexandros Tsoupras
Hephaestus Laboratory, School of Chemistry, Faculty of Sciences, Democritus University of Thrace, Kavala University Campus, Kavala, Greece

1 Introduction

The history of human health, hygiene, and beauty practices has been quietly shaped by microorganisms, especially bacteria. Traditional skincare rituals in various cultures frequently incorporated fermented products such as yogurt, kefir, and rice water, which are naturally rich in lactic acid bacteria (LABs) and other beneficial microbes. These fermented agents were used to ease irritation and promote skin health long before the mechanisms were understood. For instance, Cleopatra reportedly bathed in sour donkey's milk, taking advantage of the lactic acid produced by bacterial fermentation to provide gentle exfoliation. Similarly, ancient Egyptian depictions of fermented dairy products suggest that the use of bacteria-containing substances dates back thousands of years. Modern research has revealed that bacterial derivatives, such as peptides, polysaccharides, and metabolites, can modulate inflammation, support the skin barrier, inhibit pathogens, and help maintain a balanced skin microbiome (McFarland, 2015; Lolou and Panayiotidis, 2019). Contemporary omics-based analyses (e.g., genomics, proteomics, metabolomics) have further clarified the molecular pathways through which these components exert their effects (Yuan et al., 2025; Kahraman Ilıkkan, 2025).

In cosmetic science, bacteria and their derivatives are broadly classified according to both their taxonomic origin and their functional role in skincare. Taxonomically, the most commonly utilized genera include *Lactobacillus, Bifidobacterium, Streptococcus, Bacillus,* and *Cutibacterium,* each selected for its characteristic metabolic pathways and safety profile (Kahraman Ilıkkan, 2025; Zhang et al., 2022; Zhou et al., 2021; Guéniche et al., 2010; Gao et al., 2023; Augello et al., 2025; Ganesan and Rangarajan, 2021; Rozas et al., 2021). Functionally, bacterial ingredients are classified into probiotics (live microorganisms that confer skin benefits), prebiotics (substrates that selectively stimulate beneficial skin microbes), postbiotics or metabiotics (nonviable microbial cells or fragments, lysates, and metabolites), paraprobiotics (inactivated microbial cells with retained bioactivity), and synbiotics, which represent synergistic combinations of probiotics and prebiotics designed to enhance microbial survival and functional efficacy (McFarland, 2015; Lolou and Panayiotidis, 2019; Li and Luo, 2025; Cuevas-González et al., 2020; Martyniak et al., 2021; Bulut et al., 2025; De Almeida et al., 2023; Puebla-Barragan and Reid, 2021; Shirkhan et al., 2024; Dou et al., 2023). Within postbiotics, additional subgroups include exopolysaccharides (EPSs), antimicrobial peptides, enzymes, organic acids, short-chain fatty acids (SCFAs), and biosurfactants, each contributing specific dermatological functions such as barrier reinforcement, pH modulation, antioxidation, hydration, and pathogen inhibition (McFarland, 2015; Lolou and Panayiotidis, 2019; Li and Luo, 2025; Cuevas-González et al., 2020; Martyniak et al., 2021; Bulut et al., 2025; De Almeida et al., 2023; Puebla-Barragan and Reid, 2021; Shirkhan et al., 2024; Dou et al., 2023).

Beyond taxonomic and functional classifications, bacteria used in cosmetic science can also be categorized according to their ecological origin and physiological adaptations, which significantly influence their metabolic profiles and cosmetic potential. Terrestrial bacteria, commonly isolated from soil or plant-associated environments, often produce polysaccharides, enzymes, peptides, and antimicrobial molecules that support skin barrier function and protection (Gupta et al., 2019; da Silva et al., 2025). Marine bacteria and extremophiles, including thermophiles, halophiles, and psychrophiles, are increasingly valued for their unique stress-resistant biomolecules, such as extremozymes, ultraviolet (UV)-protective pigments, and highly stable EPSs, which enhance hydration and environmental resilience in skincare formulations (Papadopoulou et al., 2025; Rotter et al., 2024). Cyanobacteria (blue-green algae), especially *Arthrospira* (Spirulina) and *Nostoc* species,

Biofunctional Cosmetics for Health. https://doi.org/10.1016/B978-0-443-27500-5.00028-9

contribute bioactive peptides, phycobiliproteins, vitamins, and antioxidant compounds with antiaging, antiinflammatory, and photoprotective properties (Koukouraki et al., 2020; Shiels et al., 2022; Favas et al., 2021; Lopes et al., 2020; Mourelle et al., 2017). Probiotic skin commensals, like *Staphylococcus epidermidis* and *Cutibacterium acnes* subgroups, are another emerging category due to their direct compatibility with the skin microbiome and their ability to modulate host immunity, promote barrier recovery, and suppress pathogens (Rozas et al., 2021; Puebla-Barragan and Reid, 2021; Dou et al., 2023; Fournière et al., 2020).

The transition from empirical, culture-based beauty practices to a science-driven approach to microbiome skincare marks a broader shift: specific strains and their derivatives are now selected, characterized, and incorporated into formulations to target skin health in controlled, reproducible ways. In an era where consumer demand for "clean beauty" is growing, driven by interest in formulations free of harsh synthetic chemicals and respectful of environmental and biological systems, bacteria-derived ingredients are particularly well-suited (Gupta et al., 2019; Atallah et al., 2025). These ingredients offer natural, biodegradable, multifunctional molecules that align with consumer values and support the move toward more sustainable, biologically integrated cosmetic formulations (Lolou and Panayiotidis, 2019; Dou et al., 2023; Gupta et al., 2019). Their low ecotoxicity, high cosmetic value, and potential for green bioprocessing further enhance their applicability in circular economy cosmetic models (Gupta et al., 2019; Atallah et al., 2025; Rušanac et al., 2025).

Bacteria's role in cosmetics has been transformed by scientific advancements in microbiology, biotechnology, and dermatology. While bacteria were previously regarded primarily as pathogens or contaminants, specific strains are now recognized for their bioactive potential and their ability to interact beneficially with the skin's microbiota (Zhou et al., 2021; Guéniche et al., 2010; Augello et al., 2025; Dou et al., 2023; Roca et al., 2015). The most commonly exploited bacteria and their derivatives in cosmetics include *Lactobacillus*, *Bifidobacterium*, *Streptococcus,* and *Bacillus* species. Their metabolites, such as peptides, EPSs, probiotics, and prebiotics, reveal diverse functions like moisturizing, antioxidant, and antiinflammatory effects, antimicrobial action, UV protection, and reduction of visible aging signs. These compounds support skin barrier integrity, microbiome balance, and resilience against environmental stressors (Zhou et al., 2021; Guéniche et al., 2010; Augello et al., 2025; Dou et al., 2023; Roca et al., 2015). Emerging bacterial genera such as *Cutibacterium* and *Nitrosomonas* are also being explored for targeted microbiome-modulating applications (Rozas et al., 2021; Rušanac et al., 2025).

Lactobacillus species, for example, are recognized for generating lactic acid, which decreases skin pH and restrains the proliferation of harmful bacteria, promoting a healthy skin microbiome (Kahraman Ilıkkan, 2025; Zhang et al., 2022; Zhou et al., 2021). *Bifidobacterium* strains have been associated with enhancing skin hydration and elasticity, as well as contributing to the maintenance of the skin's moisture barrier (Guéniche et al., 2010; Gao et al., 2023). *Streptococcus* species, commonly used in yogurt fermentation, produce peptides that protect the skin from oxidative stress (Augello et al., 2025; Allahkarami et al., 2021). *Bacillus* species demonstrate antimicrobial properties and can modulate the skin's immune responses, making them valuable in maintaining skin health. These bacterial species are increasingly being incorporated into cosmetic formulations, reflecting a broader trend toward microbiome-friendly skincare products (Ganesan and Rangarajan, 2021; Allahkarami et al., 2021). Including bacteria in cosmetic products not only aligns with consumer demand for natural and effective ingredients, but also highlights the increasing recognition of the critical role of the skin microbiome in dermatological health (Rušanac et al., 2025; Allahkarami et al., 2021).

The shift from traditional empirical practices to scientifically validated formulations has been driven by a deeper understanding of the skin microbiome and its vital role in maintaining skin health. Modern research has demonstrated that sustaining a balanced microbial ecosystem on the skin surface can modulate the immune system, prevent pathogenic colonization, and improve conditions such as acne, eczema, and premature aging. This shift led to a new generation of cosmetic products that contain ingredients such as probiotics and postbiotics (Lolou and Panayiotidis, 2019; Dou et al., 2023; Mazumder et al., 2024). Furthermore, the rise of the clean beauty movement has increased consumer demand for natural, safe, and sustainable cosmetic ingredients. Bacteria-derived compounds embody these principles by offering biodegradable, nontoxic, and multifunctional alternatives to synthetic chemicals. Their renewable nature and compatibility with eco-friendly production methods make them valuable assets for developing next-generation sustainable cosmetics. Therefore incorporating bacteria and their derivatives into skincare products represents both scientific innovation and a cultural return to natural, biologically inspired beauty (Puebla-Barragan and Reid, 2021; Shirkhan et al., 2024; Mazumder et al., 2024).

Despite these advancements, regulatory guidelines for microbiome-based cosmetics remain limited and vary across regions, necessitating standardization to ensure product safety, efficacy, and consumer transparency. As the field progresses, this review will examine the extraction and stabilization methods that enable their cosmetic use, the bioactive profiles of bacterial derivatives, their health-promoting properties, and their current and emerging applications. Future trends suggest high regulatory attention, standardization of microbiome-based testing methods, and the formation of strain-specific cosmetic claims supported by robust clinical data (Puebla-Barragan and Reid, 2021; Shirkhan et al., 2024; Mazumder et al., 2024). The evolution of bacterial use in cosmetics is presented in Fig. 16.1.

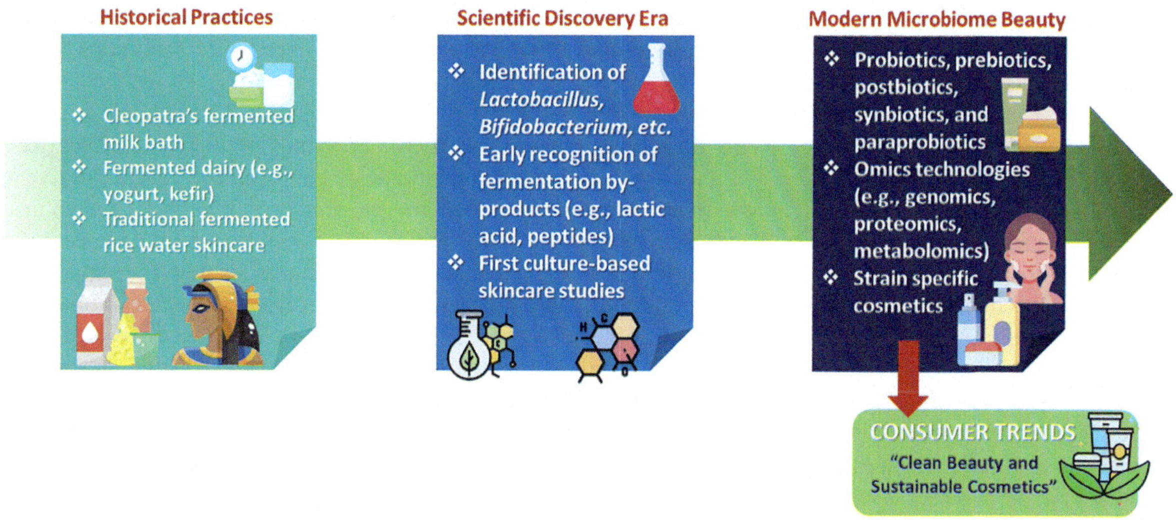

FIG. 16.1 Evolution of bacterial use in cosmetics and cosmeceuticals. *(Source: Parts of this figure were obtained from the open-access free platform: https://www.flaticon.com/ (Accessed 7 December 2025).)*

2 Extraction methods for bioactives from bacteria and factors affecting the extraction yield

2.1 Extraction methods for bioactives from bacteria and their derivatives

Extracting bioactive compounds from bacteria and their derivatives requires methods capable of disrupting robust cell envelopes, releasing intracellular components, and isolating sensitive metabolites while preserving their structural integrity. Extraction techniques are broadly divided into conventional and advanced (innovative) methods, each offering distinct advantages in terms of yield, selectivity, sustainability, and suitability for thermo- or pH-sensitive bacterial products such as peptides, EPSs, enzymes, lipids, biosurfactants, and SCFAs (Allahkarami et al., 2021; Khan et al., 2019; Jha and Sit, 2022; Xie et al., 2021; Abdel-Nasser et al., 2023).

Conventional extraction techniques include maceration, solid–liquid or solvent extraction, Soxhlet extraction, steam distillation or hydrodistillation, acid, solvent, or enzymatic precipitation, and membrane filtration and centrifugation (micro-, ultra-, or nanofiltration). Maceration, though a simple method where the bacterial biomass is soaked in a solvent (e.g., ethanol, methanol, water) for a usually 24-h time period at room temperature, has many drawbacks, such as long extraction times and lower efficacy (Sun et al., 2025). Polar and nonpolar solvents are selected based on the target metabolites. Polar solvents extract proteins, peptides, and polysaccharides, whereas nonpolar ones, such as hexane and chloroform, are used for extracting lipids and membrane constituents (Utami and Putri, 2020; Adebajo et al., 2020). Moreover, steam or hydrodistillation is applied mainly for volatile bacterial metabolites, such as low-molecular organic acids, ketones, esters, and aromatic agents produced during fermentation (Płaza et al., 2008). Following this, enzymatic (e.g., proteases), solvent (e.g., ethanol), or acid (e.g., HCl) precipitation facilitates cell wall disruption and protein, EPS, or cell wall fragment precipitation (Bajpai et al., 2016). Finally, membrane filtration (micro-, ultra-, and nanofiltration) with membrane-based fractionation allows the selective recovery of extracellular metabolites relying on molecular weight cut-offs. Notably, ultrafiltration is particularly useful for EPSs, peptides, and biosurfactants (D'ambrosio et al., 2024; Yadav et al., 2024).

Novel, advanced extraction methods for extracting bioactive compounds from bacterial species include ultrasound-assisted extraction (UAE), microwave-assisted extraction (MAE), enzyme-assisted extraction (EAE), supercritical fluid extraction (especially CO_2, SFE-CO_2), pressurized liquid extraction (PLE), pulsed electric field extraction (PEF), ionic liquid-assisted extraction, deep eutectic solvent extraction, cold plasma-assisted extraction, bioprospecting, genome mining, and metabolic engineering (Allahkarami et al., 2021; Khan et al., 2019; Jha and Sit, 2022; Xie et al., 2021; Abdel-Nasser et al., 2023). Ultrasonic cavitation used in UAE can disrupt bacterial cell walls, enhance solvent penetration, and accelerate the release of intracellular bioactives. UAE improves yields at lower temperatures, making it suitable for thermo-labile agents such as enzymes and peptides (Fu et al., 2024; Meena et al., 2024). Microwave irradiation in MAE rapidly heats intracellular water, causing ruptures in bacterial cells and improving mass transfer. MAE achieves high extraction efficacy in a short extraction duration (Pagels et al., 2021). In addition, enzyme-assisted extraction with specific enzymes (e.g., lysozyme, cellulase, proteases) is used to degrade bacterial cell walls or membranes under mild conditions, preserving thermo-labile agents (Pagels et al., 2021).

SFE-CO_2 extraction is a green method primarily applied for isolating lipids, carotenoids, hydrophobic peptides, and membrane-bound compounds, where co-solvents like ethanol enhance polarity to target amphiphilic biomolecules (Rakhuba et al., 2009; Zhou et al., 2022). Moreover, PLE, due to its high pressure and moderate temperatures, enhances solvent penetration and solubilization, enabling efficient extraction of EPS, peptides, and phenolic-rich microbial metabolites with minimal solvent usage (Pagels et al., 2021). High-intensity electric pulses in PEF induce electroporation, increasing membrane permeability and facilitating the rapid release of intracellular compounds with minimal heating (Carullo et al., 2020; Lytras et al., 2024). In addition, ionic liquids have enhanced carotenoid extraction from *Gordonia alkanivorans* biomass, remarkably reducing energy consumption, related costs, and emissions (Silva et al., 2024). Cold plasma-assisted extraction promotes bacterial cell wall and membrane disruption, inactivating microorganisms via physical disruption (intracellular content leakage and integrity loss) and biochemical damage (Mahmoud et al., 2025).

Interestingly, natural deep eutectic solvents have been widely applied to bacteria, leading to both efficient extraction of valuable intracellular molecules (e.g., carotenoid pigments such as astaxanthin, polysaccharides, proteins) and potent antimicrobial efficacy (Bedair et al., 2024; Mussagy et al., 2025). Recently, bioprospecting, genome mining, and metabolic engineering applied to bacteria act synergistically to discover and optimize the production of valuable natural compounds, such as novel antibiotics or biofuels, by identifying promising microbial genes and utilizing genetic tools to enhance their output, often targeting unculturable microbes or bacteria (Sekurova et al., 2019). Table 16.1 summarizes all extraction methods, targeting compounds, presenting the main pros and cons, and setting examples.

TABLE 16.1 Summary of extraction methods for bioactive compounds from bacteria: Targeted metabolites, advantages, limitations, and characteristic examples.

Extraction method	Target compounds	Advantages	Limitations	References
Conventional extraction methods				
Maceration/solid–liquid extraction	EPSs, organic acids, peptides, and hydrophilic molecules	Simple, low-cost, and little equipment requirement	Longer extraction times, lower efficacy, and possible contamination	(Sun et al., 2025)
Polar or nonpolar solvent extraction/ Soxhlet	Proteins, peptides, lipids, polysaccharides, glycolipids, hydrophilic metabolites, pigments, and biosurfactants	High selectivity primarily based on solvent polarity and high efficiency	Solvent toxicity, risk of protein denaturation by high temperatures, and impurities co-extraction	(Utami and Putri, 2020; Adebajo et al., 2020)
Steam or hydrodistillation	Volatile organic acids, esters, ketones, and aromatic fermentation by-products	Suitable for volatile compounds and solvent-free extraction	Limited to volatile metabolites, while thermolabile agents may degrade	(Płaza et al., 2008)
Acid/enzymatic or solvent precipitation	Proteins, EPSs, cell wall membrane fragments, and postbiotic components	Effective cell disruption, great for protein or EPS recovery	Acid may denature proteins, and such techniques require high optimization	(Bajpai et al., 2016)
Membrane filtration (micro-, ultra-, or nanofiltration)	EPSs, peptides, biosurfactants, and postbiotic fractions	High method selectivity and gentle processing (especially ultrafiltration)	Membrane fouling, high equipment costs, and partial loss of bioactives	(D'ambrosio et al., 2024; Yadav et al., 2024)
Novel and advanced extraction methods				
Ultrasound-assisted extraction (UAE)	EPSs, enzymes, peptides, and intracellular metabolites	Low temperature, rapid extraction, and enhanced cell wall disruption	Possible free radical formation [e.g., reactive oxygen species (ROS)]	(Fu et al., 2024; Meena et al., 2024)
Microwave-assisted extraction (MAE)	Pigments and carotenoids, enzymes, peptides, and intracellular metabolites	Rapid heating, high extraction yields, and short extraction duration	Risk of overheating being unsuitable for thermolabile components	(Pagels et al., 2021)
Enzyme-assisted extraction (EAE)	EPSs, proteins, and cell wall components	Mild conditions and high selectivity/bioactivity	Enzyme cost and the need for the specification of the enzyme–substrate match	(Pagels et al., 2021)

Extraction method	Target compounds	Advantages	Limitations	References
Supercritical fluid extraction with CO_2 (SFE-CO_2)	Lipids, carotenoids, hydrophobic peptides, and membrane-bound agents	Green, solvent-free, selective method that preserves bioactivity	High cost, offering limited extraction of hydrophilic agents without co-solvents	(Rakhuba et al., 2009; Zhou et al., 2022)
Pressurized liquid extraction (PLE)	EPSs, phenolic-like metabolites, and peptides	High solvent penetration, reduced solvent usage, and rapid extraction	Costly equipment and the risk of bioactivity loss	(Pagels et al., 2021)
Pulsed electric field (PEF)	Intracellular peptides, enzymes, and metabolites	Minimal heating needed and high-cell penetration	High energy requirements and equipment costs	(Carullo et al., 2020; Lytras et al., 2024)
Ionic-assisted extraction	Carotenoids, hydrophobic pigments, and lipids	Highly efficient and a method that reduces solvent usage	Toxicity concerns	(Silva et al., 2024)
Cold plasma-assisted extraction	Intracellular metabolites and cell wall fragments	Strong cell disruption with minimal solvent utilization at low temperatures	Limited industrial-scale established data	(Mahmoud et al., 2025)
Natural deep eutectic solvents (NADES)	Primarily, carotenoids, pigments, polysaccharides, and EPSs	Biodegradable, low toxicity, and efficient for polar and nonpolar agents	Possible oxidative degradation by free radical formation	(Bedair et al., 2024; Mussagy et al., 2025)
Bioprospecting, genome mining, and metabolic engineering	Novel metabolites, enzymes, antimicrobials, and other optimized constituents	Discovery, identification, and yield enhancement of new target compounds	Regulatory complexity, highly specialized personnel needs, and high costs	(Sekurova et al., 2019)

2.2 Factors affecting the extraction yield of bacteria and their derivatives

The extraction of bioactive compounds from bacteria presents unique challenges due to the complexity of their cellular structures and the biochemical diversity of microbial systems. Bacteria possess resistant, membrane-bound biomolecules, mostly proteins and lipids, which can limit the release of intracellular or surface-associated compounds. Consequently, efficacious extraction necessitates meticulous regulation of chemical, mechanical, or enzymatic degradation to ensure effective bacterial cell lysis while preserving the integrity of sensitive bioactive molecules such as peptides, EPSs, and lipopolysaccharides (LPSs). In addition, the heterogeneity in bacterial cell wall composition between Gram-positive and Gram-negative species introduces significant variability in extraction efficacy, making the optimization of the lysis procedure essential for achieving reproducible yields across different strains (Strahl and Errington, 2017; Wong and Amir, 2019; Liang et al., 2024; Lin et al., 2021).

Temperature is a critical factor influencing both extraction efficiency and compound stability, as many bacterial metabolites, particularly proteins, peptides, enzymes, and polysaccharides, are sensitive to thermal fluctuations. Excessive temperatures can accelerate oxidation, hydrolysis, and conformational changes, leading to functional loss. Conversely, extremely low temperatures restrict solvent diffusion and interpenetration, thereby reducing extraction rates. Maintaining mild thermal conditions is generally recommended to maximize the recovery of bioactives while avoiding the thermal degradation of compounds such as biosurfactants and antimicrobial peptides (Strahl and Errington, 2017; Wong and Amir, 2019; Liang et al., 2024; Lin et al., 2021).

The type of solvent used is also crucial in determining extraction yield, selectivity, and preservation of biochemical functionality. Polar solvents, such as water, ethanol, and methanol, are widely used for recovering hydrophilic metabolites, whereas nonpolar solvents or supercritical CO_2 (SFE-CO_2) are preferred for extracting lipid-based or membrane-bound agents. However, unsuitable solvent systems can result in protein precipitation, enzyme degradation, or the co-extraction of impurities that compromise the purity and functional activity of recovered bioactive compounds. Careful optimization of solvent polarity, pH, ionic strength, and extraction time is therefore vital to ensure compatibility with the target class of biomolecules and to minimize unwanted chemical alterations during processing (Sultana et al., 2024; Du et al., 2022; Vladić et al., 2022; Esquivel-Hernández et al., 2017).

3 Biochemical and bioactive composition of bacterial biomass and their derivatives

Bacteria and their derivatives contain a diverse set of structural biomolecules and metabolites that contribute directly to cosmetic efficacy. Their biochemical composition provides the molecular precursors for peptides, polysaccharides, organic acids, and lipids with moisturizing, antiaging, barrier-restoring, antioxidant, and antiinflammatory effects. These agents are also foundational to postbiotic agents such as lysates, ferment filtrates, cell wall fragments, and EPSs. Understanding the biochemical and bioactive profiles of bacterial biomass enables targeted strain selection and extraction methods for natural cosmetic and cosmeceutical formulations (Rotter et al., 2024; Rušanac et al., 2025; Khan et al., 2019; D'ambrosio et al., 2024; Lin et al., 2021; Sultana et al., 2024; Loo et al., 2025).

3.1 Biochemical composition of bacteria and their derivatives

The biochemical composition of bacterial biomass is typically dominated by proteins, EPSs, and lipids, with smaller fractions of nucleic acids, minerals, and vitamins. These categories are relevant to cosmetic and cosmeceutical applications because they serve as precursors or carriers of functional bioactives. For example, proteins yield bioactive peptides with antiaging activity, while polysaccharides contribute to hydration and film-forming effects, and lipids participate in barrier repair and emulsion stability. Bacterial composition varies by species, growth conditions, and extraction methods, but general ranges are well-established (Rotter et al., 2024; Rušanac et al., 2025; Khan et al., 2019; D'ambrosio et al., 2024; Lin et al., 2021; Sultana et al., 2024; Loo et al., 2025). Regarding the most common cosmetic-based bacteria of *Lactobacillus, Bifidobacterium, Streptococcus,* and *Bacillus* species, EPSs produced by LABs may account for even 5%–30% of the overall biomass and are particularly valuable for hydration and antipollution protection (Loo et al., 2025; Bang et al., 2017). In addition, lysates, ferment filtrates, and cell wall fragments retain many of these structural components, usually enriched in peptides, organic acids, and small metabolites depending on the extraction technique (Li and Luo, 2025; Cuevas-González et al., 2020; Martyniak et al., 2021; D'ambrosio et al., 2024).

Bacterial biomass and derivatives contain a wide spectrum of bioactives that directly influence skin physiology. These molecules mediate antioxidant, antiinflammatory, antimicrobial, antiaging, and moisturizing effects, making them highly relevant to natural cosmetic development. The type and concentration of bioactives depend on the bacterial strain, metabolic state, and bioprocessing method. The following classes represent the core bioactive groups identified in cosmetic-relevant bacteria, probiotics, and postbiotics (Rotter et al., 2024; Rušanac et al., 2025; Khan et al., 2019; D'ambrosio et al., 2024; Lin et al., 2021; Sultana et al., 2024; Loo et al., 2025). Table 16.2 represents the biochemical and bioactive composition of bacteria and their derivatives, while Fig. 16.2 summarizes the main bioactives from bacteria for natural cosmetics and cosmeceuticals.

TABLE 16.2 Biochemical composition of bacteria and their bioactive derivatives for natural cosmetic and cosmeceutical applications.

Bacteria-derived components	Examples of bacteria-derived components	Cosmetic relevance	References
Proteins and peptides	Structural or stress-response proteins and peptides (e.g., *S*-layer proteins and collagen-stimulating peptides)	Antiinflammatory, antioxidant, antiaging, antiwrinkle, collagen-promoting, and antimicrobial effects	(Loo et al., 2025; Bang et al., 2017; Aguirre-Garcia et al., 2025; Baracho and Lombardi, 2023)
Carbohydrates	EPSs, leucosin, and other cell wall polysaccharides	Moisturizing, antiaging, humectant, and film-forming properties	(Loo et al., 2025; Bang et al., 2017; Aguirre-Garcia et al., 2025; Baracho and Lombardi, 2023)
Lipids	Membrane phospholipids, glycolipids, and PUFAs/MUFAs	Barrier signaling, moisturizing, and skin-protective properties	(Loo et al., 2025; Bang et al., 2017; Aguirre-Garcia et al., 2025; Baracho and Lombardi, 2023)
Nucleic acids	DNA or RNA fragments	Signaling molecules or nutrient sources	(Bang et al., 2017; Schöpping et al., 2021)
Amino acids	Lysine, glutamic acid, glutamate, alanine, leucine, and tryptophan-derived metabolites	Natural moisturizing factors and cosmetic humectants	(Loo et al., 2025; Bang et al., 2017; Aguirre-Garcia et al., 2025; Camargo et al., 2023)
Fatty acids	Conjugated linoleic acid (CLA) and SCFAs (e.g., lactate, acetate, propionate, and butyrate)	Antiinflammatory, antioxidant, antiaging, immunomodulatory, and antimicrobial effects	(Loo et al., 2025; Aguirre-Garcia et al., 2025)
Vitamins	B-complex vitamins (e.g., B_2, B_3, B_6, B_7, B_9, and B_{12}) and vitamin K_2 (menaquinones)	Deep moisturizing, antiaging, immunomodulatory, antioxidant, and skin-health properties	(Loo et al., 2025; Aguirre-Garcia et al., 2025)

Bacteria-derived components	Examples of bacteria-derived components	Cosmetic relevance	References
Minerals	Calcium, magnesium, potassium, zinc, and iron	Enzymatic and antioxidant co-factors with deep moisturizing effects	(Bang et al., 2017; Schöpping et al., 2021)
Organic acids	Lactic, acetic, pyruvic, succinic, citric, 3-hydroxypropionic acid, and gamma-aminobutyric acid (GABA)	pH-regulating, mild-exfoliating, antipathogenic, and antimicrobial effects	(Loo et al., 2025; Bang et al., 2017; Aguirre-Garcia et al., 2025)
Bacteriocins	Nisin, lactacin, plantaricin, acidocin, and bifidocins	Antimicrobial, antiinflammatory, antioxidant, and antipathogen action	(Loo et al., 2025; Aguirre-Garcia et al., 2025)
Enzymes	Proteases, lipases, glycosidases, CAT, and SOD	Antioxidant and remodeling activities, mostly by being present in lysates	(Loo et al., 2025; Aguirre-Garcia et al., 2025)
Cell-wall fragments	Peptidoglycan fragments, lipoteichoic acids (LTAs), surface-layer proteins (SLPs), and teichoic acids	Important immune-modulating and postbiotic fractions	(Loo et al., 2025; Aguirre-Garcia et al., 2025; Maya-Martinez et al., 2019; Kohler et al., 2010)
Phenolic-like microbial metabolites and indole/alkaloid derivatives	Aromatic metabolites from amino acids, such as indole-3-lactic, acetic, and propionic acids, from LAB tryptophan and strain-dependent phenolic acids	Antimicrobial, antiinflammatory, antioxidant, immunomodulatory, and antiaging/antiwrinkle actions	(Loo et al., 2025; Aguirre-Garcia et al., 2025)
Carotenoid-like pigments (mainly found in pigmented bacteria)	For example, staphyloxanthin-like pigments in *Staphylococcus* spp. and several cyanobacteria	Antioxidant, skin appearance-enhancing, and colorant potential	(Koukouraki et al., 2020; Shiels et al., 2022; Favas et al., 2021; Mourelle et al., 2017; Pagels et al., 2021; Baracho and Lombardi, 2023; Shiels et al., 2021)

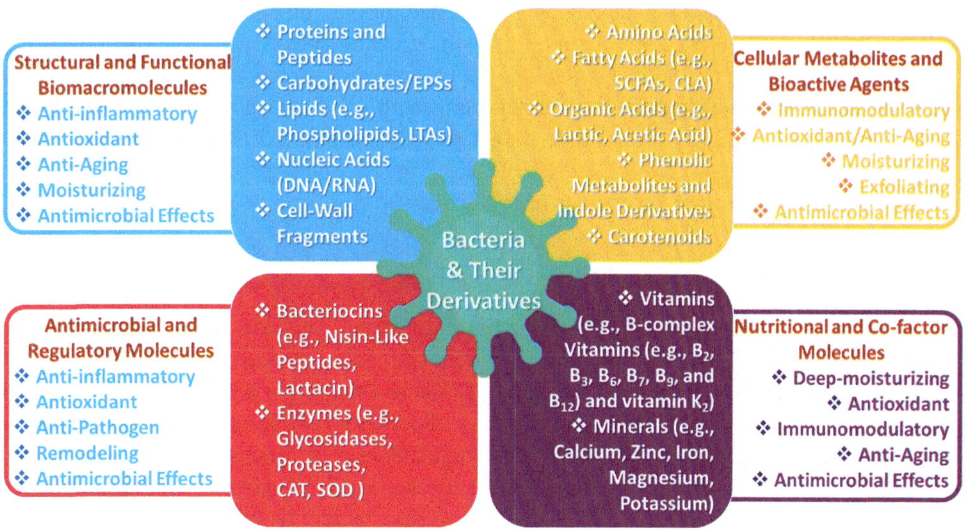

FIG. 16.2 Major classes of bacteria-derived bioactives relevant to cosmetics and cosmeceuticals.

4 Health-promoting properties of the bioactive constituents in bacteria and theirderivatives

Bacterial metabolic pathways, including those of LABs, peptides, EPSs, and SCFAs, offer several extracted components such as lysates, cell wall fragments, and other metabolites that exert multifunctional health-promoting effects on the skin. These compounds interact with key skin targets, including the stratum corneum, microbiome, keratinocytes, and immune

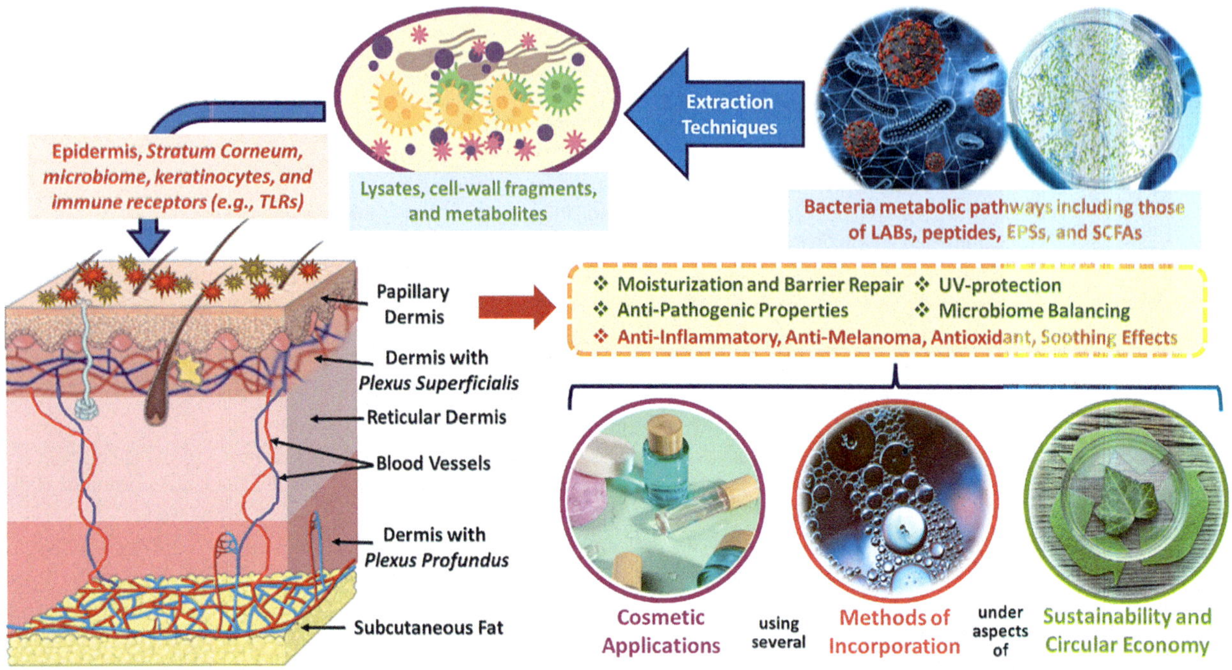

FIG. 16.3 Health-promoting effects of bacterial bioactives in cosmetics and cosmeceuticals. *(From Venetikidou, M., Lykartsi, E., Adamantidi, T., Prokopiou, V., Ofrydopoulou, A., Letsiou, S., Tsoupras, A., 2025. Proteolytic enzyme activities of bromelain, ficin, and papain from fruit by-products and potential applications in sustainable and functional cosmetics for skincare. Appl. Sci. 2076-3417. 15 (5), 2637. doi:10.3390/app15052637.)*

receptors [e.g., toll-like receptors (TLRs)], supporting homeostasis and improving skin condition. Their activities include moisturizing and barrier-repair functions, modulation of inflammatory pathways, ROS-scavenging, antimicrobial protection, UV-response support, and microbiome balancing. Overall, bacteria-derived components act through diverse biochemical mechanisms to enhance skin resilience and maintain physiological balance. Bioactive compounds from bacteria and their derivatives represent promising cosmetic agents that, with the correct incorporation techniques, could be integrated into novel cosmetic and cosmeceutical formulations under the principles of circular economy and sustainability (Li and Luo, 2025; Cuevas-González et al., 2020; Martyniak et al., 2021; Bulut et al., 2025; De Almeida et al., 2023; Puebla-Barragan and Reid, 2021; Shirkhan et al., 2024; Dou et al., 2023). Fig. 16.3 presents the health-promoting properties of the bioactive constituents in bacteria and their derivatives in cosmetics and cosmeceuticals.

4.1 Antioxidant activity of bacteria and their derivatives

Oxidative stress is a major factor contributing to skin aging, inflammation, and skin barrier impairment, primarily caused by ROS generated by environmental aggressors such as pollution, UV radiation, and chemical exposure. Bacteria and their several derivatives, including extracts, lysates, and metabolites, have emerged as a promising class of bioactive ingredients with inherent antioxidant properties. These derivatives can effectively neutralize ROS, regulating cellular antioxidant defense pathways, thereby reducing oxidative damage at the molecular level. Mechanistically, bacterial derivatives often contain enzymes such as superoxide dismutase (SOD) and catalase (CAT), small-molecule antioxidants, and bioactive peptides capable of scavenging free radicals or enhancing endogenous antioxidant systems. In addition, certain bacterial metabolites (e.g., SCFAs, EPSs, and phenolic-like microbial metabolites) contribute to redox homeostasis by modulating cellular signaling pathways such as the nuclear erythroid 2-related factor 2 (Nrf2), Kelch-like-associated protein 1 (Keap1), heme oxygenase-1 (HO-1), mitogen-activated protein kinases (MAPKs), nuclear factor kappa-light-chain-enhancer of activated B cells (NF-κB), and TLR-2 cascades, further supporting cytoprotective responses (Fu et al., 2024; Feng and Wang, 2020; Rinnerthaler et al., 2015; Jaffri, 2023; Fernandes et al., 2023; Pérez-Rivero and Pablo López-Gómez, 2023).

Dimarzio et al. (2008) evaluated the effects of a topical cream containing an ultrasonically treated *Streptococcus thermophilus* formulation on the ceramide levels of the stratum corneum and skin hydration in a group of 20 healthy elderly women (>60 years old, without skin disease). The experimental design involved a controlled, in vivo application, where each participant applied either a base cream or the same cream supplemented with the bacterial preparation to separate areas of the forearm. The treatment period lasted 2 weeks, with evaluations performed on stratum corneum sheets from the treated sites. Key parameters measured included ceramide content, transepidermal water loss (TEWL), and capacitance, which serve as indicators of skin barrier function and hydration status. The results demonstrated that the topical application of the cream containing *S. thermophilus* significantly elevated ceramide levels in the stratum corneum compared to the control treatment. This increase was attributed to the high neutral sphingomyelinase activity present in the bacterial preparation, which catalyzes the conversion of sphingomyelin to ceramides, thereby enhancing the lipid synthesis of the skin barrier. Moisturization values of the treated areas were also significantly higher than those of the control areas, indicating improved water retention and skin hydration. These findings collectively demonstrate that the topical probiotic preparation not only strengthened the skin barrier by increasing ceramide content, but also enhanced resistance to age-related dryness, leading to improved skin suppleness. This study provides one of the earliest mechanistic links between bacterial-derived enzymes and lipid remodeling in human skin, highlighting their relevance for antioxidant and barrier-protective cosmetics and cosmeceuticals (Dimarzio et al., 2008).

In a 2025 study (Augello et al., 2025), the antioxidant and antiaging properties of *S. thermophilus* lysate were evaluated using a hydrogen peroxide (H_2O_2)-induced aging model in human dermal fibroblasts, a widely accepted in vitro system that mimics oxidative stress-related skin aging. Exposure of skin fibroblasts to *S. thermophilus* lysate produced multiple protective effects against oxidative stress-induced aging. The lysate enhanced fibroblast proliferation and prevented cell aging, as evidenced by reduced β-galactosidase activity and decreased *p21* expression. Moreover, it promoted collagen I synthesis, indicating its potential to maintain or restore the structural integrity of the dermal matrix. Lysate-activated Nrf2-mediated signaling resulted in increased endogenous antioxidant defense, while simultaneously inhibiting NF-κB signaling, leading to a reduction in the levels of proinflammatory cytokines, including interleukins 1β and 6 (IL-1β and IL-6). Direct antioxidant assays revealed that the lysate possesses remarkable free radical scavenging capacity, iron chelation activity, and iron reduction power, all in a dose-dependent manner. These combined molecular effects suggest that *S. thermophilus* lysate acts as a multi-target antioxidant capable of protecting dermal cells from ROS-induced damage, promoting extracellular matrix (ECM) maintenance, and reducing inflammation, three vital mechanisms for antiaging skincare (Augello et al., 2025).

Levilactobacillus brevis BK3, derived from LABs isolated from Kimchi, a traditional Korean fermented food, revealed great antioxidant activity in 2,2-diphenyl-1-picryl-hydrazyl, 2,2′-azino-bis (3-ethylbenzothiazoline-6-sulfonic acid) assays, and total antioxidant capacity determination. Moreover, wrinkle improvement via the elastase and collagenase inhibitory activity, as well as intracellular activity assessment via human keratinocyte cells (HaCaT) and human fibroblasts (HFF-1), were also studied. The BK3 strain protected skin cells from oxidative stress induced by H_2O_2 and reduced intracellular ROS formation, while the expressions of SOD, CAT, and glutathione peroxidase (GPx) were upregulated. Meanwhile, matrix metalloproteinase-1 (MMP-1) and collagen type 1 alpha 1 (COL1A1), as major collagen synthesis and degradation contributors, were notably upregulated (Lee et al., 2024).

4.2 Antiinflammatory and antiskin disease activity of bacteria and their derivatives

Bacterial derivatives have been recognized for their antiinflammatory properties through interactions with skin cells such as keratinocytes, fibroblasts, and mast cells. These derivatives are able to selectively downregulate proinflammatory signaling cascades, such as NF-κB and MAPK, thereby reducing the secretion of cytokines such as IL-10, IL-6, and tumor necrosis factor alpha (TNF-α), while often enhancing the expression of antiinflammatory mediators like IL-10. Mechanistically, bacterial components such as LPSs, EPSs, and bioactive peptides are thought to regulate TLR signaling and other innate immune responses, promoting a balanced inflammatory response that protects tissue integrity without compromising host defense. Dose, strain, and molecular composition determine whether certain components (e.g., LPSs, EPSs, phenolic-like molecules) act as pro- or antiinflammatory mediators, rendering both formulation and characterization strategies critical (Rigauts et al., 2022; Thomas et al., 2016; Dinić et al., 2018; Lai and Gallo, 2008; Jenab et al., 2020).

Recently, *Lactobacillus rhamnosus* revealed in vitro and in vivo confirmed inhibitory activity against osteoclast differentiation by suppressing the TLR-2/NF-κB cascade. Using a macrophage colony-stimulating factor and receptor activator for NF-κB ligand, osteoclasts were induced. *L. rhamnosus* extracts (LREs) were obtained by ultrasonic crushing and centrifugation. All results were evaluated by western blotting. In addition, a mouse periodontitis model was established where LRE was injected into the gingival sulcus to evaluate the inhibitory effect of LRE on alveolar bone resorption (Fu et al., 2024). Fifty μg/mL of LRE was capable of inhibiting osteoclast differentiation without affecting apoptosis and proliferation mechanisms. This phenomenon was primarily attributed to the deactivation of the NF-κB/c-Fos/nuclear factor of activated T cells, cytoplasmic 1 (NFATc-1) via the TLR-2. In vivo study outcomes confirmed that a local LRE injection effectively suppressed osteoclast differentiation and alveolar bone resorption, providing an innovative strategy for the use of probiotics in the treatment of periodontitis (Fu et al., 2024).

Guéniche et al. (2010) investigated the impact of a *Bifidobacterium longum* (BL) lysate on skin inflammation and reactivity models, using an integrated in vitro, ex vivo, and in vivo design. Ex vivo treatment of human skin grafts with BL lysate significantly reduced markers of inflammation compared with the control, including vasodilatation, edema formation, mast-cell degranulation, and TNF-α release, indicating a direct antiinflammatory effect. Complementary in vitro tests using neuronal cell cultures showed that the lysate significantly inhibited capsaicin-induced release of calcitonin gene-related peptide, a neuropeptide involved in neurogenic inflammation and skin sensitivity, after 6 h of incubation. The clinical phase featured a 2-month randomized placebo-controlled trial with 66 women who applied a cream containing 10% BL lysate or a control cream twice daily to their face, hands, and feet for 2 months. Skin sensitivity (lactic acid prick test) and barrier recovery (TEWL after repeated tape stripping) were assessed at baseline, mid-point, and the end of the trial. The BL-lysate group showed a vast reduction in skin sensitivity and improved barrier resilience: participants required more tape strips to disrupt the barrier, indicating enhanced structural integrity and resistance to physical and chemical stress. Clinical and self-assessments reported lower dryness and discomfort and visible improvements in skin softness and hydration after 29 days. Overall, these results support the dual action of BL lysate as both an antiinflammatory and barrier-enhancing cosmetic active, with effects on both immune and neurogenic pathways for managing sensitive, irritated, or inflammation-prone skin (Guéniche et al., 2010).

Clinically, the multifaceted antiinflammatory action of bacterial strains is evident in topical bacterial or probiotic applications. A randomized controlled trial on patients with mild-to-moderate acne vulgaris compared a lotion derived from the cell-free supernatant of *Lactobacillus paracasei* MSMC 39-1 to 2.5% benzoyl peroxide. After 4 weeks, inflammatory lesion counts and erythema index were significantly decreased in both groups, while the probiotic-derived lotion was effective and had fewer side effects than benzoyl peroxide (Sathikulpakdee et al., 2022). Similarly, a pilot placebo-controlled in vivo study found that a daily topical application of *L. rhamnosus* and other lactobacilli, incorporated in a topical microcapsule formulation, could be a promising treatment for mild-to-moderate acne, as daily application of this formulation for 8 weeks reduced inflammatory lesions, with the beneficial effects persisting up to 4 weeks after discontinuation (Lebeer et al., 2022).

A 2020 randomized trial evaluated a topical cream containing live *Lactobacillus reuteri* DSM 17938 in adults with atopic dermatitis (AD). Participants applied either the probiotic-containing ointment or the control ointment twice daily for 8 weeks, while assessments at 4 and 8 weeks, included skin safety, tolerability, and clinical sensitivity (SCORAD). Both formulations were well-tolerated, whereas the probiotic ointment produced both statistically and clinically significant improvements in SCORAD and local SCORAD scores, indicating reduced inflammation and symptom severity of AD. These findings suggest that topically applied live probiotics can exert antiinflammatory, barrier-enhancing, and antimicrobial effects, making them valuable ingredients for cosmetic and therapeutic formulations targeting sensitive or inflamed skin (Butler et al., 2020).

4.3 Antiskin cancer activity of bacteria and their derivatives

Skin cancer, including melanoma and nonmelanoma types, poses a significant global health challenge due to its increasing incidence and metastatic risk. Traditional treatments, such as surgical excision, chemotherapy, and radiation therapy, often have substantial side effects and may not fully prevent recurrence. Therefore there is increasing interest in novel bioactive compounds that can enhance existing therapies by directly targeting cancer cells, modulating the tumor microenvironment, and strengthening host antitumor immunity. Bacteria and their derivatives have emerged as promising candidates for anticancer applications. Preclinical studies indicate that specific bacterial strains and their bioactive molecules can exert cytotoxic effects against melanoma cells, induce cell apoptosis, inhibit cell proliferation, and regulate angiogenesis and thrombosis, thereby impairing tumor growth and metastasis (Guo et al., 2024; Rahman et al., 2024).

Mechanistically, bacterial derivatives can stimulate immune-mediated anticancer responses, including the activation of cytotoxic T lymphocytes and antigen-presenting cells, and modulate inflammatory pathways that support tumor survival. In addition, some bacterial metabolites appear to sensitize tumor cells to conventional therapies (chemo- or radiotherapy) or promote immunogenic cell death, thereby potentiating combination approaches. While most evidence derives from in vitro and animal model studies, an increasing number of clinical investigations have explored bacterial derivatives as immunostimulants or adjunct topical interventions for skin cancers and precancerous lesions. These clinical data suggest that bacterial components may not only inhibit tumor growth but also improve skin barrier function and reduce inflammation linked to tumor progression. Taken together, the dual capacity to directly target cancer cells and modulate the cutaneous immune environment positions bacterial derivatives as versatile agents for both preventive and therapeutic strategies in skin oncology (Guo et al., 2024; Rahman et al., 2024; Liang et al., 2022; Torabi et al., 2025).

Nakatsuji et al. (2018) identified a novel anticancer mechanism whereby certain *S. epidermidis* strains produce 6-N-hydroxyaminopurine (6-HAP), a small molecule that inhibits DNA polymerase activity and selectively suppresses the proliferation of cancer cells. Using in vitro cancer cell assays, mouse melanoma models (B16F10), and metagenomic analyses, the study isolated and characterized 6-HAP and demonstrated its selective antiproliferative and cytotoxic action without harming primary keratinocytes. Mechanistic work revealed that some cancer cells possess mitochondrial enzymes, including mitochondrial amidoxime reducing component 1/2 (mARC1/2), that detoxify 6-HAP, explaining variable susceptibility across cell lines. In mice, systemic administration of 6-HAP significantly inhibited tumor growth with no observable systemic toxicity. Furthermore, topical colonization with 6-HAP-producing *S. epidermidis* reduced UV-induced tumor incidence compared with colonization by nonproducing strains. This work provides a compelling example of a symbiotic skin microbe producing a metabolite with direct chemopreventive and therapeutic potential (Nakatsuji et al., 2018).

An early clinical trial evaluated *Corynebacterium parvum* as an adjuvant to surgery in 260 patients with clinically detected stage I melanoma, randomized across 18 centers. Patients received either surgery alone or surgery plus *C. parvum* injections and were followed for at least 2 years. Multivariate analysis identified tumor thickness and anatomical site as prognostic variables. Overall 3-year disease-free survival (DFS) did not differ significantly between groups (81% in the *C. parvum* group versus 67% in the control group), but subgroup analysis suggested a benefit in patients with melanomas >3 mm in thickness (3-year DFS: 73% in the immunotherapy group vs. 33% in controls). Toxicity was minimal and transient. This trial illustrates the potential of bacterial immunotherapy to successfully augment anticancer and antitumor surveillance, particularly in higher-risk lesions, although confirmatory modern trials are lacking (Balch et al., 1982).

4.4 Moisturizing properties of bacteria and their derivatives

Maintaining adequate skin hydration is essential for preserving the skin barrier, elasticity, and overall cutaneous health. Disruption of barrier integrity or insufficient hydration can lead to dryness, irritation, premature aging, and heightened sensitivity to environmental stressors. In recent years, bacteria and their derivatives have emerged as promising bioactive ingredients for enhancing skin hydration. Certain bacterial strains, particularly LABs, such as *S. thermophilus* and *Lactobacillus* spp., produce enzymes, EPSs, and other metabolites that support the synthesis and maintenance of the skin's natural lipids, including ceramides and free fatty acids. These lipids are essential for the barrier function of the stratum corneum and the regulation of TEWL (Mazumder et al., 2024; Zheng et al., 2022).

Mechanistically, bacterial derivatives are able to stimulate endogenous ceramide production, strengthening the lipid matrix of the stratum corneum, while also regulating natural moisturizing factors, such as amino acids and peptides, which attract and retain water. In addition, they promote barrier restoration and increase skin resilience, especially in dry, sensitive, or aged skin. Several in vitro, ex vivo, and clinical studies have demonstrated that the topical application of bacterial lysates or probiotic-derived compounds increases skin hydration, improves barrier function, and mitigates dryness, supporting their use as functional ingredients in modern cosmetics and dermatocosmetics. Notably, research also highlights microbe-derived sphingolipid-modulating enzymes that directly enhance ceramide biosynthesis, further validating the role of bacterial metabolites in hydration-related cosmetic and cosmeceutical claims (Mazumder et al., 2024; Zheng et al., 2022).

The present clinical study evaluated the moisturizing effects of a cream formulation containing paraprobiotics like acidophilus paraprobiotics moisturizer (APM), which was prepared with thermally inactivated *Bifidobacterium lactis* and *Lactobacillus plantarum* (LP), and assessed its impact on the skin microbiome of healthy individuals. Fifty participants were randomized to either a treatment or control group. APM or a paraprobiotics-free moisturizer was applied to the right forearm. Skin hydration was evaluated by measuring TEWL and stratum corneum moisture (SCM) every hour for 4 h and again after 4 weeks of treatment. Moreover, epidermal samples were collected at baseline and after 4 weeks of treatment for microbiome analysis via next-generation sequencing. APM application significantly reduced TEWL and increased SCM relative to baseline and the control group, suggesting improved skin hydration. Microbiome analysis revealed changes in the relative abundance of *Cutibacterium*, *Corynebacterium*, and *Acinetobacter* following treatment. In addition, the proportions of Proteobacteria, Firmicutes, and Cyanobacteria decreased, while Planctomycetes, Chloroflexi, Verrucomicrobia, and Gemmatimonadetes increased. Importantly, APM suppressed *Corynebacterium tuberculostearicum*, a species associated with skin discomfort. These results suggest that moisturizers containing paraprobiotics can enhance skin hydration and promote a beneficial microbial community, providing preliminary evidence to inform future research, particularly given the current scarcity of studies focusing on bacteria-based skin hydration (Chaiyasut et al., 2022).

4.5 Anti-UV and photoprotective properties of bacteria and their derivatives

The skin is constantly exposed to UV radiation, which can cause DNA damage, oxidative stress, premature aging, and an increase in the risk of skin cancer. Recent research has highlighted the potential of certain bacteria and their derivatives to exert photoprotective effects, offering an emerging approach for reinforcing the skin's defense mechanisms. Probiotic and prebiotic bacteria, along with their metabolic products and by-products, have demonstrated the ability to produce UV-absorbing compounds, antioxidants, and enzymes that mitigate oxidative stress and DNA damage caused by UV exposure. For example, mycosporine-type amino acids, produced by certain bacterial species, function as natural sunscreens by absorbing UVA and UVB wavelengths and reducing free-radical formation. In addition, specific bacterial EPSs exhibit antiinflammatory properties that help reduce UV-induced erythema and maintain skin integrity (Souak et al., 2021; Guéniche et al., 2014; Lawrence et al., 2018).

Experimental studies indicate that the topical application of bacterial derivatives can enhance endogenous antioxidant defense systems, reduce ROS formation, and protect keratinocytes from UV-induced apoptosis. Some bacteria also modulate stress-response pathways, such as Nrf2 activation, further strengthening photoprotection. These findings support the idea that bacterial metabolites may serve as functional ingredients in sunscreens or daily skin care formulations (Souak et al., 2021; Guéniche et al., 2014; Lawrence et al., 2018). Although this field remains in its early stages, the photoprotective properties of bacteria and their derivatives represent a promising avenue for novel skincare. Further research, especially well-controlled clinical trials, is needed to validate efficacy, determine optimal formulation approaches, and assess long-term safety. The integration of microbial-derived photoprotective compounds may enable the development of next-generation sunscreens that not only prevent UV-induced damage but also support overall skin health through modulation of the cutaneous microbiome (Souak et al., 2021; Guéniche et al., 2014; Lawrence et al., 2018; Patra et al., 2020; Andersson et al., 2019).

Recently, Mondadori et al. (2025) assessed the photoprotective effects of five heat-treated probiotic strains (Skinbac) against UVA, UVB, and UVC radiation. Experiments were performed on HaCaT keratinocytes, normal human epidermal keratinocytes (NHEK), and a three-dimensional human skin model (Phenion Full-Thickness Skin Model). Protective effects were evaluated by monitoring cell viability and analyzing apoptosis-related gene expression (TP53), inflammation or immunosuppression (IL-6), and oxidative stress (HO-1) using quantitative real-time PCR. For UVC-irradiated NHEK cells, tight-junction proteins (claudin 1, claudin 4, and occludin) were quantified via ELISA to determine barrier integrity. All tested strains provided protection against UVA, UVB, and UVC damage. They maintained cell viability, reduced apoptosis and inflammatory responses, regulated oxidative-stress markers, and preserved tight-junction protein expression, indicating enhanced barrier protection. These results suggest that heat-treated probiotics may enhance the skin's defenses against UV-induced damage and could serve as innovative ingredients in probiotic-based skin care formulations (Mondadori et al., 2025).

Bouilly-Gauthier et al. (2010) investigated the effects of a dietary supplement (DS) combining *Lactobacillus johnsonii* La1 and nutritional doses of carotenoids on premature UV-induced skin damage in healthy adult women (Fitzpatrick skin types II–IV). Three clinical trials were conducted using different sources of UV radiation: nonextreme UVA-dominant UV radiation (UV-DL, CT1), extreme simulated solar radiation (UV-SSR, CT2), and natural sunlight (CT3). In CT1, early indicators of UV skin damage were evaluated histologically, including Langerhans cell density, type I dermal dendritic cells factor XIIIa^{+}, and dermal inflammatory cell levels. In CT2, minimal erythemal dose (MED) was measured clinically and colorimetrically, alongside changes in skin pigmentation. In CT3, dermatologists and participants assessed skin response under real-life sunlight exposure. After 10 weeks of supplementation, DS intake prevented Langerhans cell density decline and the increase in dermal dendritic cells normally induced by UV-DL, while also reducing inflammatory cell infiltration. MED increased by 20% (clinical) and 19% (instrumental), and colorimetric analysis revealed increased pigmentation (ΔE^*). Overall, the study showed that supplementation with La1 and carotenoids effectively reduced early UV-induced skin damage, suggesting long-term benefits in preventing photoaging (Bouilly-Gauthier et al., 2010).

4.6 Antiaging activity of bacteria and their derivatives

Skin aging is a multifactorial biological process influenced by intrinsic factors, such as genetics, cellular senescence, and hormonal alterations, and extrinsic factors, including oxidative stress, UV radiation, environmental pollution, and lifestyle habits. A key hallmark of cutaneous aging is the progressive degradation of structural ECM proteins, particularly collagen and elastin, leading to wrinkle formation, loss of elasticity, textural roughness, and impaired barrier function (Kim et al., 2024; Kanimozhi and Sukumar, 2025). Recently, bacteria and their derivatives have emerged as promising antiaging agents due to their ability to modulate skin physiology and promote collagen synthesis and ECM remodeling. Several bacterial species, including LABs, produce bioactive peptides, EPSs, and other metabolites capable of stimulating fibroblast activity, enhancing collagen and elastin synthesis, improving ECM organization, increasing skin firmness, and reducing the appearance of fine lines and wrinkles. These bioactives often exhibit complementary antioxidant, antiinflammatory, and reparative properties, further contributing to the attenuation of the skin-aging process. A growing body of in vitro studies and clinical trials has evaluated the effects of probiotic-, paraprobiotic-, and postbiotic-based interventions on skin parameters such as elasticity, hydration, wrinkle depth, dermal density, and overall skin appearance, providing promising evidence of their functional relevance in cosmetic and cosmeceutical formulations aimed at preventing or reducing skin aging (Kim et al., 2024; Kanimozhi and Sukumar, 2025; Liu and Sun, 2023).

In another study investigating photodamage-associated aging, tyndallized *Lactobacillus acidophilus* IDCC 3302 (ACT 3302) was evaluated against a UVB-induced photoaging model using HaCaT keratinocytes. Pretreatment with ACT 3302 notably reduced UVB-triggered upregulation of MMPs (MMP-1, 2, and 9), suppressed MAPK signaling activation, and lowered the expression of proinflammatory cytokines. ACT 3302 also helped preserve antioxidant enzyme activity, revealing a protective effect against oxidative stress and ECM degradation. These results highlight its potential as an antiphotoaging agent capable of mitigating UV-induced wrinkle formation (Im et al., 2019).

Clinically, Lee et al. (2015) conducted a randomized, double-blind, placebo-controlled clinical trial to evaluate the antiaging effects of LP HY7714 in 110 volunteers aged 41–59 years exhibiting dryness and visible wrinkles. Participants received either 1×10^{10} colony-forming units (CFU)/day of HY7714 or a placebo for 12 weeks. Skin hydration, wrinkle depth, radiance, and elasticity were measured every 4 weeks. The probiotic group exhibited significant increases in skin hydration on both the face and hands by week 12. TEWL decreased in both groups but showed a more pronounced reduction in the HY7714 group, particularly on the face and forearm. Wrinkle depth decreased significantly, skin radiance improved, and skin elasticity increased by 13.17% at week 4 and 21.73% at week 12. These findings provide clinical evidence supporting the use of HY7714 as a bioactive cosmetic ingredient capable of improving skin hydration, firmness, and visual signs of aging (Lee et al., 2015). Finally, in a broad human "skin health" 28-day study with a topical commensal probiotic integrating the Q24 *Micrococcus luteus* strain, BLIS Q24, 96 adults with self-reported normal or blemish-prone skin participated. Topical application of this probiotic serum led to reductions in blackheads, blemishes, oiliness, redness/rosacea, fine lines, wrinkles, and acne and improved overall skin quality (Jain et al., 2025).

4.7 Wound healing and antimicrobial activity of bacteria and their derivatives

Wound healing is a multistage biological process involving hemostasis, inflammation, proliferation, and tissue remodeling. Impaired wound healing is often associated with infection, chronic inflammation, or underlying medical conditions such as diabetes. Recently, bacteria and their derivatives, such as probiotics, prebiotics, postbiotics, symbiotics, paraprobiotics, and bacterial metabolites, have emerged as promising modulators of tissue repair and host defense. Bacterial derivatives exhibit broad-spectrum antimicrobial activity, including antibacterial, antifungal, and antiviral effects, which are essential for preventing infections that can delay wound closure. Their dual action, infection control combined with immunomodulatory and regenerative effects, offers a novel, multidimensional approach to clinical dermatology. Integrating these bioactive compounds into therapeutic strategies offers new opportunities for improving healing outcomes and reducing complications associated with delayed or impaired wound repair (Patra et al., 2020; Andersson et al., 2019; Mondadori et al., 2025).

A 2021 investigation (Golkar et al., 2021) evaluated the wound healing efficacy of metabiotics derived from *Lactobacillus fermentum*, *L. reuteri*, and *Bacillus subtilis* sp. natto, formulated into topical creams. Twenty-five Sprague Dawley rats were divided into five groups: three postbiotics-treated groups, a placebo cream group, and an untreated control. Wound healing was assessed by wound closure rate, hydroxyproline content, and histological analysis of the regenerated tissue. All postbiotic-based creams significantly accelerated wound closure compared to both the control and placebo groups. Hydroxyproline levels, an indicator of collagen synthesis, were markedly increased in treated animals, suggesting enhanced ECM formation. Histological analyses revealed improved epithelialization, collagen deposition, and angiogenesis. Among the formulations, the *B. subtilis* natto-derived metabiotics cream exhibited the strongest regenerating effects (Golkar et al., 2021).

Another study examined the therapeutic potential of LP on diabetic foot ulcer (DFU) wound healing and clarified its underlying mechanisms. Human umbilical vein endothelial cells were treated with advanced glycation end products to simulate diabetic stress. LP promoted cell viability and migration, reduced apoptosis, and decreased the secretion of proinflammatory cytokines IL-1β and IL-18. Mechanistically, LP inhibited activation of the NOD-like receptor family pyrin domain-containing 3 (NLRP3)/caspase-1/*p20*/Gasdermin D-N-terminal domain pyroptosis pathways, thereby suppressing inflammation-driven cell death (Wang et al., 2024a). In vivo, in streptozotocin-induced (STZ) diabetic rats, topical treatment accelerated wound closure and reduced NLRP3 and caspase-1 *p20* expression. Pearson correlation analysis confirmed an inverse relationship between LP levels and NLRP3, IL-1β, and IL-18 expression in DFU tissues. These findings reveal a previously unrecognized mechanism through which LP facilitates diabetic wound healing by targeting inflammasome-mediated pyroptosis, highlighting a promising therapeutic strategy for chronic diabetic wounds (Wang et al., 2024a).

A recent systematic review of oral or enteral probiotic therapy on skin or mucosal wound healing in humans included seven studies (348 individuals in total). Four of them reported positive effects on wound healing, while none reported serious adverse effects (Togo et al., 2022). In a triple-blind randomized trial, a topical-probiotic was found to be beneficial in episiotomy wound healing. Notably, oral supplementation with *Lactobacillus casei* accelerated the healing of episiotomy wounds compared with controls (Abdollahpour et al., 2023). Moreover, a study on infected chronic ischemic wounds treated with a multi-strain probiotic topical formulation reported eradication of pathogens and progress toward healing over ~3 weeks (Venosi et al., 2019). Recently, a first-in-human trial with a genetically modified probiotic, *L. reuteri* R2LC engineered to deliver a growth factor, showed that topical application (as "ILP100-Topical") was safe, well-tolerated, and linked to faster wound healing compared to the placebo, with several wounds healed by day 19 and reduced time to first recorded healing (Öhnstedt et al., 2023).

4.8 Other health-promoting benefits of bacteria and their derivatives

Beyond the skin-related benefits, including wound healing, antiaging, and photoprotective effects, bacteria and their derivatives also confer significant advantages to broader physiological systems. One of the most extensively studied areas is metabolic health, where specific bacterial strains and metabolites influence glucose homeostasis, insulin sensitivity, lipid metabolism, energy balance, and inflammation. Dysbiosis, or an imbalance of the gut microbiome, is strongly linked to intestinal barrier integrity, and modulating systemic metabolic pathways has been demonstrated for selected probiotics, postbiotics, and synbiotics (Roberfroid et al., 2010; Tenorio-Jiménez et al., 2020; Cani and Jordan, 2018; Lyu et al., 2024; Bernini et al., 2016) through multiple mechanisms. SCFAs, such as acetate, propionate, and butyrate, act as key signaling molecules that improve insulin sensitivity, regulate appetite, and reduce chronic inflammation. These metabolites are produced by SCFA-generating strains of *Lactobacillus* and *Bifidobacterium*. Certain bacterial metabolites also influence the expression of genes involved in lipogenesis and fatty acid β-oxidation, contributing to improved cholesterol and triglyceride profiles. Multiple clinical trials have shown that probiotic supplementation can lower fasting glucose, hemoglobin A1c HbA1c), and serum low-density lipoprotein (LDL) cholesterol, while increasing high-density lipoprotein (HDL) cholesterol and overall metabolic flexibility, supporting their role as adjunctive strategies for managing cardiometabolic and cardiovascular diseases (CVDs) (Roberfroid et al., 2010; Tenorio-Jiménez et al., 2020; Cani and Jordan, 2018; Lyu et al., 2024; Bernini et al., 2016).

Bernini et al. (2016) explored the effects of *B. lactis* HN019 in individuals with metabolic syndrome (MS). Fifty-one participants were randomly assigned to either a control or a probiotic group. For 45 days, the probiotic group consumed 80 mL/day of fermented milk containing 2.72×10^{10} CFU of *B. lactis* HN019. Significant reductions in body mass index, total cholesterol, LDL cholesterol, and the proinflammatory cytokines TNF-α and IL-6 were observed in the probiotic group, demonstrating improvements in metabolic, CVD, and inflammatory parameters (Bernini et al., 2016). Regarding cardiovascular health, bacteria and their derivatives are evidently able to modulate CVD risk factors such as blood pressure, lipid profile, inflammation, and endothelial function. Strains of *Lactobacillus* and *Bifidobacterium* reduced total cholesterol, LDL cholesterol, and triglycerides, while increasing HDL cholesterol. In addition, probiotics can downregulate circulating proinflammatory cytokines, mitigating endothelial dysfunction and atherosclerotic processes. Clinical trials indicate that daily probiotic consumption leads to modest but significant improvements in lipid profiles and inflammatory markers, suggesting their potential use alongside standard interventions for CVD risk reduction (Palathinkara et al., 2025; Jin et al., 2021; Xiao et al., 2003; Chen et al., 2014).

In a recent study, Noori et al. (2024) evaluated probiotic-fortified kefir containing *Lactobacillus helveticus* R0052 and BL R0175 in elderly individuals with high-CVD risk. Sixty-seven elderly participants were randomly assigned to two groups: a fortified kefir group, assigned to consume 240 mL of fortified kefir daily and a placebo group, that received regular kefir for 8 weeks. After 8 weeks, although classical lipid parameters (e.g., total cholesterol, HDL cholesterol, LDL cholesterol, triglycerides, non-HDL cholesterol, triglyceride/cholesterol index, or fasting blood glucose levels) did not differ significantly between the fortified kefir and placebo groups, improvements were observed in Castelli's Risk Index I and the atherogenic index. These results indicate a potentially favorable effect on CVD risk modulation, even in the absence of major changes in fasting lipid panels among elderly individuals (Noori et al., 2024).

Growing evidence supports a strong bidirectional communication system between the gut microbiota and the brain, known as the gut-brain axis. Probiotics capable of exerting psychological or neurological benefits are referred to as "psychobiotics." These microorganisms notably influence emotional and cognitive function through multiple mechanisms, including neurotransmitter regulation (e.g., serotonin, dopamine, gamma-aminobutyric acid) (Steenbergen et al., 2015; Gruenwald et al., 2002; Huang et al., 2016; Wallace and Milev, 2017). Clinical and preclinical studies have demonstrated that strains such as *L. rhamnosus*, *L. helveticus*, and BL can reduce anxiety-like behavior, improve mood, and enhance stress resilience. Probiotic supplementation has been correlated with lower cortisol levels, improved mood, and enhanced cognitive performance in specific populations. However, the effectiveness of psychobiotics appears to depend on baseline mental health status, strain specificity, and host factors such as nutrient status (e.g., vitamin D) (Steenbergen et al., 2015; Gruenwald et al., 2002; Huang et al., 2016; Wallace and Milev, 2017).

A clinical trial evaluating a probiotic formulation containing *L. helveticus* and *B. longum* in individuals with low mood was conducted. The study also examined whether factors such as irritable bowel syndrome symptoms, proinflammatory cytokine levels, brain-derived neurotrophic factor levels, and other blood biomarkers could affect treatment outcomes. Seventy-nine participants with moderate or higher self-reported mood scores, not being under psychotropic medication received in groups either the probiotic formulation or a matched placebo for 8 weeks (Romijn et al., 2017). No changes were observed in psychological outcomes (Cohen's d range = 0.07–0.16), inflammatory blood biomarkers, or neurotrophic factors. Specifically, 9 participants (23%) in the probiotic group and 10 participants (26%) in the placebo group demonstrated a >60% improvement on the Montgomery–Åsberg Depression Rating Scale, indicating no statistically significant treatment effects. The authors noted that baseline vitamin D levels moderated several results, whereas dry mouth and sleep disruption were reported more frequently in the placebo group. It was suggested that future research should focus on mild or antidepressant-naive populations with mild or acute symptoms or explore psychobiotics as adjunctive interventions rather than stand-alone treatments, while considering vitamin D levels as a potential moderator (Romijn et al., 2017).

5 Bacterial applications in natural cosmetic and cosmeceutical formulations

5.1 Skin care-based indicative applications of bacteria and their lysates

The incorporation of bacteria and their bioactive metabolites in skincare represents a shift toward biologically intelligent cosmetic design. Instead of acting merely as passive additives, selected bacterial strains and their derivatives actively interact with the skin ecosystem, supporting barrier integrity, regulating immune responses, and affecting microbiome composition. Commonly used probiotic or commensal strains include *L. rhamnosus*, known for its antiinflammatory and soothing effects, and *S. thermophilus*, which enhances hydration via the production of EPSs that reinforce the stratum corneum. Other strains, such as LP and *Bacillus coagulans,* contribute antioxidant activity and assist in regulating microbial balance. Through the production of antimicrobial peptides, SCFAs, EPSs, and antioxidant enzymes, these microorganisms help maintain epidermal homeostasis and strengthen the skin's natural defenses. Modern skincare is progressing toward more personalized and sustainable approaches that restore skin dysfunction, balancing, rather than sterilizing, the native microbiome (Jurášková et al., 2025; Jung et al., 2019; Majeed et al., 2020; Floch, 2014; Cicenia et al., 2014).

A study by Jung et al. (2019) investigated the effects of *L. rhamnosus* lysates on skin barrier function using in vitro and ex vivo models. Controlled lysis preserved key bioactives such as peptides, EPSs, and other skin-beneficial metabolites. This treatment significantly reduced TEWL, increased SCM, and improved lipid organization, while microscopic analyses confirmed strengthened structural integrity. The lysates were well-tolerated, with no cytotoxic effects, supporting their safety for topical use. These findings underscore the potential of probiotic-derived effluents to enhance barrier function, regeneration, hydration, and overall skin health by supporting endogenous repair mechanisms (Jung et al., 2019).

Another study evaluated a lysosomal bacterial cocktail composed of *Staphylococcus hominis* MBF12-19J, *Staphylococcus warneri* MBF02-19J, *M. luteus* MBF05-19J, and *B. subtilis* MBF10-19J. The optimized fermented lysate demonstrated strong inhibitory activity against *Propionibacterium acnes*, a key skin pathogen associated with acne, particularly when the strains were used at a specific ratio (*M. luteus* MBF05-19J: *B. subtilis* MBF10-19J: *S. warneri* MBF02-19J: *S. hominis* MBF12-19J: 1.5:1.5:0.5:0.5), supporting their broad synergistic activity. Mild antioxidant effects were observed, and no adverse skin reactions occurred in volunteer safety tests. The formulation remained stable after the incorporation of 12% sucrose as a lyoprotectant. This work illustrates how bacterial lysates can inhibit pathogenic microbes, provide antioxidant support, and maintain microbiome balance in topical formulations (Hawari et al., 2022).

Another research group investigated the skin symbiont *S. epidermidis* using in vitro keratinocyte co-cultures, transcriptomics, and in vivo mouse experiments. This co-culture increased keratinocyte proliferation and modulated cytokine secretion toward an immune-tolerant, antiinflammatory profile. Transcriptomic analysis revealed upregulation of genes involved in tight junctions, lipid metabolism, and antimicrobial defense. In vivo, topical application reduced TEWL, increased epidermal thickness, and improved overall barrier integrity. These results prove that native skin commensals such as *S.*

epidermidis actively support epidermal repair, immune balance, and long-term barrier resilience, providing a rationale for their use in microbiome-restoring skincare and corresponding cosmetics and dermatocosmetics (Zheng et al., 2022).

In the same context, the skin barrier is crucial for protecting against environmental stressors, preventing moisture loss, and regulating immune responses. In conditions such as AD, eczema, and sensitive skin disorders, this barrier becomes compromised, resulting in inflammation, dryness, and increased susceptibility to irritants and pathogens. Consequently, modern dermatological and cosmetic strategies focus not only on symptom relief but also on restoring barrier integrity. Increasing evidence shows that specific bacterial strains and their metabolites can directly enhance skin barrier structure, regulate immunity, and support microbiome balance (Betsi et al., 2008; Leung et al., 2004; Mukarram et al., 2025). Several bacterial strains, including *L. rhamnosus*, LP, *S. thermophilus,* and *S. epidermidis*, have demonstrated barrier-restoring and soothing effects by promoting ceramide production, enhancing epidermal renewal, modulating immune responses, and regulating the skin microbiome. These bioactivities complement moisturizers and emollients traditionally used for barrier repair, providing both immediate soothing and long-term resilience (Wu et al., 2017; Lombardi et al., 2022; Zheng et al., 2022).

A landmark clinical study by Myles et al. (2020) demonstrated the therapeutic potential of *Roseomonas mucosa* in pediatric AD. The research team conducted a clinical trial designed to assess its safety, tolerability, and efficacy in pediatric patients with moderate to severe eczema. Twenty children applied a topical spray containing live *R. mucosa* directly to the diseased skin areas twice weekly for 4 months. Seventeen out of 20 children (85%) showed a >50% reduction in eczema severity, with reduced itching, redness, dryness, and corticosteroid use. TEWL decreased, hydration increased, and metagenomic analyses confirmed enhanced microbial diversity and a significant reduction of *Staphylococcus aureus*. Lipidomic profiling revealed that *R. mucosa* produced sphingolipids that promote keratinocyte renewal and epidermal repair. The strain safely colonized the skin and persisted for up to 8 months posttreatment without adverse effects, establishing strong evidence for the safety and efficacy of live bacterial therapies in children (Myles et al., 2020).

A complementary study developed a living symbiotic hydrogel skin patch (Hy@Rm) that contained *R. mucosa.* The patch consisted of polyvinylpyrrolidone, polyvinyl alcohol, and sodium alginate, cross-linked via calcium ions and a freeze–thaw cycle to produce a porous, elastic structure. This patch created a stable microenvironment for bacterial survival, inhibited *S. aureus*, accelerated epidermal regeneration, and restored skin barrier function in an AD mouse model. Treated skin demonstrated improved hydration, reduced TEWL, normalized epidermal structure, collagen reorganization, and inflammatory cytokine suppression. The hydrogel was biocompatible, mechanistically protective, and enabled long-term bacterial viability, supporting the concept of next-generation bioactive, self-regenerating dressings (Liu et al., 2023).

5.2 Hair care-based applications of bacteria and their lysates

Recent advances in microbiome research have revealed that the scalp, like the skin, hosts a diverse microbial ecosystem vital for maintaining hair health. Dysbiosis of the scalp microbiome is linked to dryness, brittleness, dandruff, inflammation, and loss of shine. Leveraging beneficial bacteria and their bioactive metabolites in haircare formulations has, therefore, emerged as a promising strategy to rebalance the scalp environment, protect hair follicles, and enhance overall hair strength and appearance. Microbiome-friendly shampoos, conditioners, and leave-on scalp treatments enriched with live bacteria, bacterial lysates, or purified metabolites can deliver multiple benefits. Strains belonging to the *Lactobacillus* and *Bacillus* genera produce enzymes, peptides, and antioxidant metabolites that reinforce the hair shaft, improve moisture retention, and counteract oxidative stress on the scalp. These bioactives also help regulate microbial balance by suppressing pathogenic species linked to inflammation and follicular irritation. Consequently, the haircare industry is shifting toward novel products that move beyond cleansing and conditioning to restore scalp homeostasis, supporting structural resilience, shine, and hair vitality (Lousada et al., 2021; Paul et al., 2025; Woo et al., 2019; Nam et al., 2019, 2021).

Woo et al. (2019) evaluated the hair growth potential of LP hydrolysates (LPHs) using both in vitro and in vivo models. Human dermal papilla cells and MG-63 cells were treated with various LPHs to assess viability, cytotoxicity, and induction of the vascular endothelial growth factor (VEGF). Six groups of shaved male C57BL/6 mice were topically treated for 14 days with either hydrolysate (native or enzyme-treated), a control formulation (G1), LPHs (G2), LPHs treated with alcalase (G3), hydrolysates treated with bromelain (G4), hydrolysates treated with protamex (G5), and 5% minoxidil as a positive standard (G6). All LPH-treated groups (G2–G5) promoted significantly greater hair growth than minoxidil (G6), with substantial upregulation of VEGF and insulin-like growth factor 1, indicating enhanced angiogenesis and hair follicle activation. No cytotoxic effects were observed, confirming their safety. Histological analyses further showed accelerated follicular development and stronger hair formation. These results suggest that LPHs can safely modulate hair growth by activating proangiogenic and follicle-stimulating pathways (Woo et al., 2019).

Another study was conducted to examine the potential of *Leuconostoc holzapfelii*-derived extracellular vesicles (EVs), a bacterium isolated from human scalp hair, in promoting hair growth through their effects on hair follicle dermal papilla (HFDP) cells. The researchers aimed to investigate whether human scalp-derived *L. holzapfelii* extracellular vesicles (hs-LhEVs) could enhance cell proliferation, migration, and gene expression related to hair growth while reducing apoptosis, ultimately facilitating hair regeneration via the Wnt/β-catenin signaling pathway. EVs were isolated by ultracentrifugation and characterized in terms of size, morphology, and surface markers to ensure their purity and identity. HFDP cells were then treated with different concentrations of hs-LhEVs, up to 10^{10} particles, to evaluate their biological effects. Cell proliferation was measured using the CCK-8 assay, while cell migration was evaluated through wound healing assays. Flow cytometry was used to analyze cell cycle progression and apoptosis, with an emphasis on the ability of EVs to regulate cell division and prevent cell death.

A second study explored the hair-regenerative potential of EVs produced by *L. holzapfelii*, a bacterium naturally found on human scalp hair. Human HFDP cells were treated with increasing doses of hs-LhEVs to examine proliferation, migration, apoptosis, and gene activation. EV treatment significantly enhanced HFDP cell proliferation and migration in a dose-dependent manner while reducing apoptosis and cell cycle progression. Importantly, RT-PCR analysis revealed strong upregulation of the Wnt/β-catenin cascade genes [Wnt5a and Wnt10b ligands, β-catenin, and lymphoid enhancer-binding factor 1 (Lef1)], as well as hair-growth-correlated genes [versican, bone morphogenetic protein 2 (BMP-2), and BMP and activin membrane-bound inhibitor]. These findings demonstrate that hs-LhEVs promote hair follicle activation and regeneration by stimulating the Wnt/β-catenin axis, supporting their potential as microbiome-based hair growth enhancers (Yoon et al., 2022).

Kalenova et al. (2015) assessed the regenerative capacity of permafrost-derived *Bacillus* strains in a mouse burn model. BALB/c mice were treated topically with gels. The study included a cellulose gel as a control (G1), Solcoseryl gel (G2), a gel containing *Bacillus cereus* IP5832 (G3), and a gel containing *Bacillus* spp. MG8 at 2×10^6 CFU (G4). Over 13 days, the *Bacillus* spp. MG8 gel produced notable hair regrowth, outperforming both the control and *B. cereus* treatments. The accelerated hair regeneration suggests that specific *Bacillus* strains enhance wound repair while simultaneously activating hair follicles. These results highlight the potential of extremophile-derived *Bacillus* species as dual-action agents for skin and hair regeneration (Kalenova et al., 2015).

5.3 Examples from commercial products using bacteria and their lysates

A growing number of cosmetic formulations now incorporate bacterial strains, lysates, and postbiotic compounds, reflecting both their multifunctional properties and the growing recognition of the skin microbiome as a critical determinant of skin health. Commercial products commonly include *Lactobacillus* or *Bifidobacterium* lysates in creams, serums, shampoos, and lotions, where they provide soothing, antiinflammatory, and barrier-strengthening effects. Scalp-care applications frequently feature *Vitreoscilla filiformis* or *S. thermophilus* derivatives to support scalp microbial balance, reduce irritation, and enhance hair and scalp resilience. More advanced haircare formulations now integrate bacterial fermentation supernatants and postbiotic metabolites, which deliver antioxidant, immunomodulatory, and microbiome-regulating benefits while being produced via controlled biotechnological processes that ensure stability, reproducibility, and safety (Guéniche et al., 2010; Rušanac et al., 2025; Valpaços et al., 2023). Table 16.3 summarizes representative examples of commercial cosmetic products utilizing bacteria-derived ingredients, highlighting their intended functions and associated properties.

5.4 Safety and regulatory considerations for bacterial use in cosmetic applications

The incorporation of bacteria-derived compounds into cosmetic formulations offers potential benefits, including enhanced skin barrier function, antiinflammatory effects, and microbiome regulation, but their use is tightly governed by safety and regulatory requirements to ensure consumer protection. Within the European Union, bacterial ingredients in cosmetics fall under Regulation (EC) No. 1223/2009, which provides a harmonized legal framework across all member states. This regulation states that any cosmetics on the EU market must be safe under normal or reasonably foreseeable conditions of use. A designated responsible person within the EU must ensure product compliance, safety, quality, and correct labeling before market entry (EUR-Lex—02009R1223-20250901—EN—EUR-Lex n.d.; European Commission—Have your say. Eur Comm—Have Your Say, n.d.).

Prior to marketing, each cosmetic product undergoes a Cosmetic Product Safety Report (CPSR) performed by a qualified safety assessor, following the structure defined in Annex I of Regulation (EC) No. 1223/2009. For bacterial lysates, ferments, and other derivatives, the CPSR must specifically address the possible presence of endotoxins, residual metabolites, immunogenic fragments, and potential proinflammatory components, alongside toxicological profiles, dermal exposure

TABLE 16.3 Commercial and research-backed cosmetic agents or products derived from natural bioactives obtained from bacteria and their derivatives.

Cosmetic product	Cosmetic use	Bacteria strain	Beneficial impact	References
Clinique—Redness Solutions Soothing Cleanser with Microbiome Technology	Cleansing cream	*Lactobacillus* probiotic ferment	Nondrying face cleansing and irritation-reducing cosmeceutical formula	(Clinique (Paris), n.d.b.)
Clinique—Redness Solutions Daily Relief Cream with Microbiome Technology	Moisturizing cream	*Lactobacillus* probiotic ferment	Nourishing, soothing skin and comforting red spots	(Clinique (Paris), n.d.a.)
Antipodes—Culture Probiotic Night Recovery Water Cream	Night cream	*Lactobacillus* ferment	Moisturizing, calming stressed skin, and boosting skin health and firmness	(Antipodes Culture Probiotic Night Recovery Water Cream. Org Brands, n.d.)
Kilig—Probiotics Face Cream	Face cream	*Lactobacillus* ferment lysate	Sebum secretion reduction, pores, pimples, and blackhead reduction	(Organic Brands, n.d.)
Glowsophy—Cica Panthenol Soothing Moisturizer	Moisturizing cream	*Lactobacillus* ferment lysate, *Bifida* ferment lysate, *Streptococcus,* and *Thermophilus* ferment	Supporting the skin microbiome, enhancing the skin barrier, soothing, and hydrating the skin	(*Glowsophy Cica Panthenol Soothing Moisturiser (Ingredients Explained), n.d.*)
Masil—Probiotics Perfect Volume Shampoo	Shampoo	*Lactobacillus* ferment	Soothing and cleaning the scalp and hair, enhancing curls' elasticity and firmness	(*Masil 5 Probiotics Perfect Volume Shampoo (150 ml), n.d.*)
Skinesa—Defensin Probiotic Spray	Topical spray	*Roseomonas mucosa* Rsm 2015	Soothing itchy, rashy skin, retaining skin moisture, and enhancing skin barrier function	(SkinSAFE, n.d.)
Alimentum Labs—Derma Serum Skin-Restoring Serum	Serum	*Bacillus licheniformis, Bifidobacterium infantis, Lacticaseibacillus paracasei,* and *Ligilactobacillus salivarius*	Promoting a balanced skin microbiome, enhancing smooth, and glowing skin	(Alimentum Labs, n.d.)
Propaira—Microbiome Soft Shampoo 100 mL	Shampoo	*Saccharide* isomerate and*Lactococcus* ferment lysate	Repairing the scalp microbiome and skin barrier	(Microbiome Soft Shampoo. Propaira—Clin Ski, n.d.)
Propaira—Biotic Cream for Eczema	Cream	*Saccharide* isomerate and*Lactococcus* ferment lysate	Treating eczema-associated inflammation and irritation	(Microbiome Soft Shampoo. Propaira—Clin Ski, n.d.)
Revuele—ProBio Skin Balance Probiotic Cream Cleanser	Face cream cleanser	Probiotic *Lactobacillus* ferment lysate	Gentle cleansing for sensitive skin supports barrier function, microbiome balance, and prevents dryness	(Rev Beauty Care, n.d.)
The Pure Lotus—Youth Biotics Probiotic Concentrate Cream	Antiaging and moisturizing face cream	Probiotic *Lactobacillus* ferment, *Bifida* ferment lysate, *Lactococcus* ferment lysate, and *Streptococcus thermophilus* ferment	Intended for hydration, improved texture, antiaging, brightness, and microbiome-friendly skincare	(Lulula, n.d.)

estimates, and ingredient interactions. Validated stability, microbiological purity, and margin-of-safety calculations are mandatory components of the assessment (EUR-Lex—02009R1223-20250901—EN—EUR-Lex, n.d.; Registrar Corp, 2025; EU & GB Cosmetics Regulations Compliance, n.d.).

Regulation (EC) No. 1223/2009 also states that all cosmetic products must comply with strict microbiological quality criteria, remaining free from key pathogens such as *Candida albicans, Pseudomonas aeruginosa*, and *S. aureus*. Products incorporating bacterial derivatives must demonstrate resistance to contamination through validated preservation efficacy tests (challenge testing) and stability studies. Products intended for sensitive applications, such as infants or mucosal areas, are subject to stricter microbial limits (EUR-Lex—02009R1223-20250901—EN—EUR-Lex n.d.; Bonnet et al., 2020). The Product Information File must document ingredient origin, bacterial strain integrity, fermentation or extraction methods, proof of inactivation, and confirmation that no viable microorganisms are present in the final product cosmetic formulation (EU Cosmetics Regulation Comprehensive Guide. Biorius, n.d.; Biorius, 2021).

The Scientific Committee on Consumer Safety (SCCS) provides guidance for ingredient risk assessment, and its 2023 Notes of Guidance (12th revision) outline modern toxicological approaches, including in vitro, in silico, and next-generation risk assessment, replacing animal testing. For microbial-derived ingredients, SCCS requires detailed genotoxicity, skin sensitization, irritation, and systemic exposure data, as well as extensive documentation of the manufacturing process to ensure the absence of harmful contaminants or active pathogens (SCCS Notes of guidance for the testing of cosmetic ingredients and their safety evaluation—12th revision—Public Health, n.d.). In addition, according to the EU's safety-by-design principles, bacterial lysates and postbiotics are considered safe only when their purity, biological activity, structural integrity, and batch-to-batch consistency are fully verified. Compliance with good manufacturing practices (GMPs), typically ISO 22716:2007, is obligatory to ensure microbial quality and minimize contamination risk (Good manufacturing practice | European Medicines Agency (EMA), 2017; ISO, n.d.).

In the United States, cosmetics are regulated under the Federal Food, Drug, and Cosmetic Act. Unlike the EU, the FDA does not require premarket approval for cosmetics (except for color additives). Cosmetics must not be adulterated or misbranded, and the FDA retains authority to take action against unsafe products (FDA Regulation of Cosmetics and Personal Care Products Under the Modernization of Cosmetics Regulation Act of 2022 (MoCRA), n.d.; Commissioner O of the Microbiological Safety and Cosmetics, 2024). The FDA does not explicitly regulate or prohibit the use of live bacteria in cosmetics, but it also does not recognize probiotics as established cosmetic ingredients. Products containing live microorganisms raise concerns regarding viability, stability, interaction with preservatives, and microbiome effects, and claims suggesting therapeutic action may reclassify the product as a drug, triggering stringent regulatory requirements (Puebla-Barragan and Reid, 2021). FDA policy states that cosmetics do not need to be sterile but must meet acceptable microbial limits, such as <500 CFU/g for eye-area products and <1000 CFU/g for other cosmetics, while containing no pathogens (Program HF, 2025). Bacterial lysates, postbiotics, and fermentation-derived ingredients pose fewer regulatory challenges, but manufacturers must demonstrate the absence of viable microorganisms, validated microbial inactivation steps, and compliance with analytical methods like Bacteriological Analytical Manual methods, as well as standard preservative efficacy testing (Registrar Corp, 2025; EU & GB Cosmetics Regulations Compliance, n.d.).

Overall, the regulatory landscape reflects the innovation and complexity of microbiome-based cosmetics. EU legislation is grounded in premarket safety verification, while the United States relies more on manufacturer responsibility and postmarket surveillance. Although neither jurisdiction has explicit provisions addressing live bacteria, probiotics, or microbiome-modulating cosmetics, both frameworks prioritize microbiological purity, transparent labeling, GMP compliance, and the protection of consumer health. As research advances and bacterial derivatives become increasingly integrated into cosmeceutical science, regulatory systems continue to evolve to ensure that innovation proceeds without compromising safety.

6 Incorporation and encapsulation delivery systems of bacteria for several applications

The use of beneficial bacteria has expanded across fields such as nutrition, medicine, and cosmetics due to their diverse health-promoting properties. However, a major challenge in using these microorganisms lies in maintaining their viability, stability, and functional activity during processing, storage, and delivery to the target site. Environmental stressors like pH fluctuations, temperature changes, oxygen exposure, and enzymatic degradation can notably reduce bacterial survival. To overcome these limitations, researchers developed delivery systems that incorporate and encapsulate bacteria to stabilize or protect them, ensuring that they maintain their therapeutic potential and reach the intended site of action efficiently (Gupta et al., 2019; Pérez-Rivero and Pablo López-Gómez, 2023; Razavi et al., 2021; Agriopoulou et al., 2023).

Microencapsulation is a well-established technique in which bacteria are enclosed within natural or polymeric matrices to form protective microcapsules. Common encapsulating materials include agar, alginate, gelatin, and other biopolymers that create a physical barrier, shielding bacteria from harsh environmental conditions such as extreme pH levels, oxygen exposure, or temperature changes. This protection enhanced bacterial survival during storage, processing, and administration, while enabling controlled/targeted release at specific sites like the gastrointestinal tract or skin (Misra et al., 2021; Martín et al., 2015). Beyond simple protection, microencapsulation allows the co-encapsulation of multiple probiotic strains or bioactive compounds (e.g., prebiotics, antioxidants), enhancing synergistic interactions and broadening therapeutic efficacy. Due to its scalability and versatility, microencapsulation is widely used across functional foods, nutraceuticals, DSs, and cosmetic or cosmeceutical formulations (Misra et al., 2021; Martín et al., 2015; Vivek et al., 2023).

Nanoencapsulation represents a next-generation approach, utilizing nanoscale carriers to entrap bacteria or their derivatives (e.g., postbiotics, metabolites). The reduced particle size offers a high surface area, enhanced permeability, and improved interaction with biological tissues, enabling greater precision and more controlled release profiles than conventional microcapsules. It improves stability, bioavailability, and functional performance by protecting microorganisms from environmental stressors and enhancing their uptake by target tissues. It is especially valuable for applications requiring high precision and targeted delivery, including advanced pharmaceuticals, specialized nutraceuticals, and microbiome-modulating cosmetics (Arratia-Quijada et al., 2024; Shafique et al., 2023; Gutiérrez-Álzate et al., 2024). Using biodegradable and biocompatible nanomaterials reduced toxicity and improves safety for clinical or commercial applications. Overall, micro- and nanoencapsulation function as complementary delivery systems: microencapsulation provides robust protection, while nanoencapsulation offers enhanced targeting, controlled kinetics, and improved bioavailability (Arratia-Quijada et al., 2024; Shafique et al., 2023; Gutiérrez-Álzate et al., 2024).

Spray-drying and freeze-drying are widely used to convert live bacteria into stable, dry powders. Unlike encapsulation strategies, which focus on matrix-based protection and targeted delivery, these techniques primarily improve long-term stability, handling, storage, and transport of bacterial preparations (Luft and Mazutti, 2025). Spray-drying involves atomizing a bacterial suspension into a chamber with controlled hot airflow, producing fine-dried particles. The rapid evaporation of water leads to efficient drying but can stress bacterial cells. Therefore protective agents, such as sugars, proteins, or polysaccharides, are often added to preserve cell integrity and viability. Spray-drying is highly scalable and cost-efficient, making it ideal for the industrial production of probiotic powders for functional foods, beverages, DSs, and nutraceuticals (Huang et al., 2017; Xu et al., 2024). In contrast, freeze-drying removes water by sublimation at low temperature and pressure, imposing minimal thermal stress and preserving structural integrity, metabolic activity, and viability. It is especially suitable for sensitive or high-value bacterial strains used in pharmaceuticals and advanced functional foods. Cryoprotectants, such as trehalose or skim milk, are commonly used to enhance bacterial survival during freezing and drying (Wang et al., 2025; Ge et al., 2024). Both methods ensure extended shelf life, precise dosing, and easy incorporation into various products. While encapsulation ensures targeted delivery, drying techniques provide a complementary strategy for producing stable, functional bacterial agents.

Lipid-based systems, including liposomes, solid lipid nanoparticles, and other nano-vesicles, represent another advanced strategy for delivering beneficial bacteria or their bioactive derivatives. Unlike polymer-based micro- and nanoencapsulation or drying techniques that prepare bacteria in dehydrated form, lipid-based carriers use a biocompatible lipid bilayer that mimics natural cellular membranes. This structure provides excellent protection against oxygen, moisture, pH shifts, and enzymatic degradation, while enabling controlled and targeted release to tissues such as the gastrointestinal tract or skin. Modifying the lipid composition or particle size allows precise tuning of release kinetics, penetration depth, and bioavailability (Teleanu et al., 2025; Godase et al., 2024). Lipid-based carriers can also deliver multiple strains or co-formulated compounds (e.g., vitamins, antioxidants, prebiotics), enhancing the functional performance of bacterial products. These systems are increasingly used in functional foods, nutraceuticals, pharmaceuticals, and cosmetics, where they provide a versatile platform for integrating live or inactivated bacteria into complex formulations. Lipid-based systems complement encapsulation and drying technologies by offering enhanced protection, superior bioavailability, and improved therapeutic performance, forming a novel toolkit for stabilizing and delivering probiotics, postbiotics, and other beneficial bacterial derivatives (Sekurova et al., 2019; Teleanu et al., 2025; Godase et al., 2024; Wang et al., 2024b; Sun et al., 2023).

7 Limitations, challenges, and future perspectives

Bioactive compounds derived from bacteria have demonstrated strong potential for cosmetic applications due to their beneficial moisturizing, antioxidant, antiaging, anti-UV, antimicrobial, and regenerative properties. Despite these advantages, integrating such bioactives into cosmetic formulations presents several critical challenges related to safety, stability, efficacy, and consumer acceptance. Safety and allergenicity remain central concerns. Although many bacterial derivatives, particularly postbiotics and paraprobiotics, are nonviable and generally considered safe, certain residual cell wall fragments, metabolites, or processing impurities may still trigger skin irritation or allergic reactions, particularly in individuals with sensitive skin barriers or compromised skin. Inadequate processing of live probiotics can also pose a minimal but relevant risk of contamination with pathogenic microbes. Consequently, regulatory frameworks mandate rigorous safety testing, accurate microbial counts, contaminant screening, and transparent labeling, increasing both the complexity and cost of product development (Lundov et al., 2009; Smith and Alexander, 2005).

Another major barrier is the inherent instability of bacterial bioactives. Peptides, EPSs, lysates, and metabolites are highly sensitive to temperature, pH, light, and oxygen. Exposure to these stressors during manufacturing, storage, or daily application can cause degradation and loss of efficacy. In addition, interactions with common cosmetic agents, such as surfactants, emulsifiers, or preservatives, may de-stabilize or inactivate bacterial-derived molecules, complicating formulation design. Batch variability also represents a substantial limitation, as both the composition and potency of bacterial metabolites can differ based on strain specificity, culture media, fermentation duration, and extraction conditions, making standardization difficult (Lundov et al., 2009).

Consumer perception remains another significant challenge. Despite microbiome-focused skincare gaining popularity, some consumers remain reluctant to use products containing bacteria or their derivatives. Clear labeling, scientific communication, and consumer education are essential to explain the safety, nonviable nature, and scientifically validated benefits of bacterial ingredients. Overcoming this barrier is crucial for market acceptance (Habeebuddin et al., 2022; Kiprono et al., 2024). Formulation and delivery issues further complicate the incorporation of bacterial bioactives. Many of these agents require specialized protection systems, such as microencapsulation, nanoencapsulation, lipid-based carriers, spray or freeze-drying, to maintain stability, control release, and enhance skin penetration. These technologies substantially improve performance but also increase manufacturing complexity, production costs, and regulatory requirements (Puebla-Barragan and Reid, 2021; Saravanan et al., 2025; Jackson et al., 2019).

Sustainability-driven formulations introduce several constraints. The valorization of bacterial by-products aligns with circular economy principles, but extracting and purifying active compounds from fermentation residue biomass requires optimized, energy-intensive processes to preserve bioactivity and ensure safety, thereby limiting large-scale implementation (Gupta et al., 2019; Jackson et al., 2019). Even though bacterial derivatives hold substantial promise as innovative, multifunctional, and sustainable cosmetic agents, their practical use is constrained by safety concerns, instability, consumer perception, batch-to-batch variability, and formulation complexity. Future advancements in strain engineering, encapsulation methods, standardized fermentation protocols, and transparent consumer communication will be essential for enabling their safe and effective integration into next-generation microbiome-friendly skincare solutions.

8 Conclusions

Bioactive compounds derived from bacteria demonstrate multifunctional properties highly relevant to cosmetic science. Their moisturizing, antiaging, antioxidant, and anti-UV activities contribute to skin hydration, barrier restoration, elasticity, and dermal homeostasis, providing strong scientific justification for their integration into natural and microbiome-friendly products. These compounds can be extracted and integrated into cosmetics using conventional and advanced methods. Modern technologies, including micro- and nanoencapsulation, spray-drying, freeze-drying, and lipid-based delivery systems, offer superior stability, controlled release, and bioactivity preservation, while also supporting sustainability goals by valorizing bacterial biomass and fermentation by-products, minimizing waste, and promoting eco-conscious product development.

Despite encouraging findings from in vitro, in vivo, and preliminary clinical studies, current research focuses on oral probiotic benefits, with comparatively fewer systematic investigations into their topical cosmetic applications. To fully exploit the potential of bacterial derivatives in skincare, further work is needed to clarify their cutaneous mechanisms of action, optimize formulation strategies, ensure long-term safety, and validate their efficacy in real-world conditions. Overall, bacterial extracts and metabolites combine potent bioactivity with formulation feasibility and sustainability, positioning them as attractive candidates for next-generation natural cosmetics. Bridging current research gaps and prioritizing dermatological validation will be essential for establishing these ingredients as safe, effective, and environmentally responsible components of future cosmetic and cosmeceutical products.

Acknowledgments

The authors would like to thank the School of Chemistry in the Faculty of Sciences at Democritus University of Thrace for their continuous support.

Conflicts of interest

The authors declare no conflicts of interest.

Author contributions

A.T. was involved in conceptualization, methodology, validation, supervision, and project administration. A.T., A.V., T.A., and A.B. were involved in investigation and visualization. A.T., A.V., and T.A. were involved in writing—review and editing. All authors contributed to software and writing—original draft preparation and have read and agreed to the published version of the manuscript.

Funding

This research received no external funding.

References

Good manufacturing practice | European Medicines Agency (EMA), 2017. https://www.ema.europa.eu/en/human-regulatory-overview/research-development/compliance-research-development/good-manufacturing-practice. (Accessed 10 December 2025).

Commissioner O of the Microbiological Safety and Cosmetics, 2024. FDA.

Abdel-Nasser, A., Hathout, A.S., Badr, A.N., Barakat, O.S., Fathy, H.M., 2023. Extraction and characterization of bioactive secondary metabolites from lactic acid bacteria and evaluating their antifungal and antiaflatoxigenic activity. Biotechnol. Rep. 2215017X. 38. Available from: http://www.journals.elsevier.com/biotechnology-reports/. doi:10.1016/j.btre.2023.e00799.

Abdollahpour, D., Homayouni-Rad, A., Nourizadeh, R., Hakimi, S., Mehrabi, E., 2023. The effect of probiotic supplementation on episiotomy wound healing among primiparous women: a triple-blind randomized clinical trial. BMC Complement. Med. Ther. 2662-7671. 23 (1). doi:10.1186/s12906-023-03980-3.

Adebajo, S.O., Akintokun, P.O., Ojo, A.E., Akintokun, A.K., Badmos, O.A., 2020. Recovery of biosurfactant using different extraction solvent by rhizospheric bacteria isolated from rice-husk and poultry waste biochar amended soil. Egypt. J. Basic Appl. Sci. 2314808X. 7 (1), 252–266. Available from: https://www.tandfonline.com/toc/teba20/current. doi:10.1080/2314808X.2020.1797377.

Agriopoulou, S., Tarapoulouzi, M., Varzakas, T., Jafari, S.M., 2023. Application of encapsulation strategies for probiotics: from individual loading to co-encapsulation. Microorganisms. 2076-2607. 11 (12), 2896. doi:10.3390/microorganisms11122896.

Aguirre-Garcia, Y.L., Cerda-Alvarez, N.C., Santiago-Santiago, R.M., Chantre-López, A.R., Rangel-Ortega, S.D.C., Rodríguez-Herrera, R., 2025. The metabolites produced by lactic acid bacteria and their role in the microbiota–gut–brain axis. Fermentation. 23115637. 11 (7). Available from: www.mdpi.com/journal/fermentation. doi:10.3390/fermentation11070378.

Alimentum Labs, n.d. Derma Serum Skin Restoring Serum, 1 fl oz Ingredients and Reviews. SkinSAFE. https://www.skinsafeproducts.com/alimentum-labs-derma-serum-skin-restoring-serum-1-fl-oz. (Accessed 10 December 2025).

Allahkarami, S., Akhavan Sepahi, A., Hosseini, H., Razavi, M.R., 2021. Isolation and identification of carotenoid-producing *Rhodotorula* sp. from Pinaceae forest ecosystems and optimization of in vitro carotenoid production. Biotechnol. Rep. 2215017X. 32, e00687. doi:10.1016/j.btre.2021.e00687.

Andersson, T., Ertürk Bergdahl, G., Saleh, K., Magnúsdóttir, H., Stødkilde, K., Andersen, C.B.F., Lundqvist, K., Jensen, A., Brüggemann, H., Lood, R., 2019. Common skin bacteria protect their host from oxidative stress through secreted antioxidant RoxP. Sci. Rep. 20452322. 9 (1). Available from: www.nature.com/srep/index.html. doi:10.1038/s41598-019-40471-3.

Antipodes Culture Probiotic Night Recovery Water Cream. Org Brands, n.d. https://www.organicbrands.gr/el/product/7728/antipodes-culture-probiotic-night-recovery-water-cream?sz=16. (Accessed 10 December 2025).

Arratia-Quijada, J., Nuño, K., Ruíz-Santoyo, V., Andrade-Espinoza, B.A., 2024. Nano-encapsulation of probiotics: need and critical considerations to design new non-dairy probiotic products. J. Funct. Foods. 17564646. 116, 106192. doi:10.1016/j.jff.2024.106192.

Atallah, C., Abiad, A.E., Abiad, M.E., Nakad, M., Assaf, J.C., 2025. Bioengineered skin microbiome: the next frontier in personalized cosmetics. Cosmetics. 2079-9284. 12 (5), 205. doi:10.3390/cosmetics12050205.

Augello, F.R., Lombardi, F., Ciafarone, A., Altamura, S., Marazzato, M., Artone, S., Cinque, B., Palumbo, P., 2025. *Streptococcus thermophilus* CNCM I-5570 lysate counteracts the aging process in human dermal fibroblast cells by neutralizing harmful free radicals and impacting antioxidant and anti-inflammatory pathways, thus restoring their physiological functions. Biomed. Pharmacother. 07533322. 185, 117975. doi:10.1016/j.biopha.2025.117975.

Bajpai, V.K., Majumder, R., Rather, I.A., Kim, K., 2016. Extraction, isolation and purification of exopolysaccharide from lactic acid bacteria using ethanol precipitation method. Bangladesh J. Pharmacol. 1991-0088. 11 (3), 573. doi:10.3329/bjp.v11i3.27170.

Balch, C.M., Smalley, R.V., Bartolucci, A.A., Burns, D., Presant, C.A., Durant, J.R., 1982. A randomized prospective clinical trial of adjuvant *C. parvum* immunotherapy in 260 patients with clinically localized melanoma (Stage I): prognostic factors analysis and preliminary results of immunotherayp. Cancer. 10970142. 49 (6), 1079–1084. doi:10.1002/1097-0142(19820315)49:6<1079::AID-CNCR2820490604>3.0.CO;2-X.

Bang, J., Li, L., Seong, H., Kwon, Y.W., Jeong, E.J., Lee, D.Y., Han, N.S., 2017. Macromolecular and elemental composition analyses of leuconostoc mesenteroides ATCC 8293 cultured in a chemostat. J. Microbiol. Biotechnol. 17388872. 27 (5), 939–942. Available from: http://www.jmb.or.kr/journal/download.php?Filedir=./submission/Journal/027/&num=8470. doi:10.4014/jmb.1612.12038.

Baracho, D.H., Lombardi, A.T., 2023. Study of the growth and biochemical composition of 20 species of cyanobacteria cultured in cylindrical photobioreactors. Microb. Cell Fact. 14752859. 22 (1). Available from: https://microbialcellfactories.biomedcentral.com/. doi:10.1186/s12934-023-02035-z.

Bedair, H.M., Samir, T.M., Mansour, F.R., 2024. Antibacterial and antifungal activities of natural deep eutectic solvents. Appl. Microbiol. Biotechnol. 14320614. 108 (1). Available from: https://www.springer.com/journal/253. doi:10.1007/s00253-024-13044-2.

Bernini, L.J., Simão, A.N.C., Alfieri, D.F., Lozovoy, M.A.B., Mari, N.L., de Souza, C.H.B., Dichi, I., Costa, G.N., 2016. Beneficial effects of *Bifidobacterium lactis* on lipid profile and cytokines in patients with metabolic syndrome: a randomized trial. Effects of probiotics on metabolic syndrome. Nutrition. 18731244. 32 (6), 716–719. Available from: www.elsevier.com/locate/nut. doi:10.1016/j.nut.2015.11.001.

Betsi, G.I., Papadavid, E., Falagas, M.E., 2008. Probiotics for the treatment or prevention of atopic dermatitis. Am. J. Clin. Dermatol. 1175-0561. 9 (2), 93–103. doi:10.2165/00128071-200809020-00002.

Biorius, 2021. What Is a PIF (Product Information File) ? https://biorius.com/cosmetic-news/what-is-a-pif-product-information-file/. (Accessed 10 December 2025).

Bonnet, M., Lagier, J.C., Raoult, D., Khelaifia, S., 2020. Bacterial culture through selective and non-selective conditions: the evolution of culture media in clinical microbiology. New Microbes New Infect. 20522975. 34, 100622. doi:10.1016/j.nmni.2019.100622.

Bouilly-Gauthier, D., Jeannes, C., Maubert, Y., Duteil, L., Queille-Roussel, C., Piccardi, N., Montastier, C., Manissier, P., Piérard, G., Ortonne, J.-P., 2010. Clinical evidence of benefits of a dietary supplement containing probiotic and carotenoids on ultraviolet-induced skin damage. Br. J. Dermatol. 00070963. 163 (3), 536–543. doi:10.1111/j.1365-2133.2010.09888.x.

Bulut, S.D., Döndaş, H.A., Celebioglu, H.U., Sansano, J.M., Döndaş, N.Y., 2025. Recent insights about probiotics related pharmabiotics in pharmacology: prevention and management of diseases. Probiotics Antimicrob. Proteins. 18671314. 17 (4), 2262–2292. Available from: https://www.springer.com/journal/12602. doi:10.1007/s12602-025-10613-3.

Butler, É., Lundqvist, C., Axelsson, J., 2020. *Lactobacillus reuteri* DSM 17938 as a novel topical cosmetic ingredient: a proof of concept clinical study in adults with atopic dermatitis. Microorganisms. 2076-2607. 8 (7), 1026. doi:10.3390/microorganisms8071026.

Camargo, A.R.O., van Mastrigt, O., Bongers, R.S., Ben-Amor, K., Knol, J., Abee, T., Smid, E.J., Rantsiou, K., 2023. Quantitative physiology and proteome adaptations of *Bifidobacterium breve* NRBB57 at near-zero growth rates. Microbiol. Spectr. 2165-0497. 11 (3). doi:10.1128/spectrum.02568-22.

Cani, P.D., Jordan, B.F., 2018. Gut microbiota-mediated inflammation in obesity: a link with gastrointestinal cancer. Nat. Rev. Gastroenterol. Hepatol. 17595053. 15 (11), 671–682. Available from: http://www.nature.com/nrgastro/index.html. doi:10.1038/s41575-018-0025-6.

Carullo, D., Pataro, G., Donsì, F., Ferrari, G., 2020. Pulsed electric fields-assisted extraction of valuable compounds from *Arthrospira platensis*: effect of pulse polarity and mild heating. Front. Bioeng. Biotechnol. 2296-4185. 8. doi:10.3389/fbioe.2020.551272.

Chaiyasut, C., Sivamaruthi, B.S., Tansrisook, C., Peerajan, S., Chaiyasut, K., Bharathi, M., 2022. Influence of paraprobiotics-containing moisturizer on skin hydration and microbiome: a preliminary study. Appl. Sci. 2076-3417. 12 (23), 12483. doi:10.3390/app122312483.

Chen, Y., Liu, W., Xue, J., Yang, J., Chen, X., Shao, Y., Kwok, L.-Y., Bilige, M., Mang, L., Zhang, H., 2014. Angiotensin-converting enzyme inhibitory activity of *Lactobacillus helveticus* strains from traditional fermented dairy foods and antihypertensive effect of fermented milk of strain H9. J. Dairy Sci. 00220302. 97 (11), 6680–6692. doi:10.3168/jds.2014-7962.

Cicenia, A., Scirocco, A., Carabotti, M., Pallotta, L., Marignani, M., Severi, C., 2014. Postbiotic activities of *Lactobacilli*-derived factors. J. Clin. Gastroenterol. 0192-0790. 48 (Suppl. 1), S18. doi:10.1097/mcg.0000000000000231.

Clinique (Paris), n.d.a. Redness Solutions Daily Relief Cream With Microbiome Technology. Available from: https://www.clinique.gr/product/12517/6007/redness-solutions-daily-relief-cream-with-microbiome-technology. (Accessed 10 December 2025).

Clinique (Paris), n.d.b. Redness Solutions Soothing Cleanser. Available from: https://www.clinique.gr/product/12517/5800/redness-solutions-soothing-cleanser. (Accessed 10 December 2025).

Cuevas-González, P.F., Liceaga, A.M., Aguilar-Toalá, J.E., 2020. Postbiotics and paraprobiotics: from concepts to applications. Food Res. Int. 09639969. 136, 109502. doi:10.1016/j.foodres.2020.109502.

D'ambrosio, S., Dabous, A., Sadiq, S., Casillo, A., Schiraldi, C., Cassese, E., Bedini, E., Corsaro, M.M., Cimini, D., 2024. Bifidobacterium animalis subsp. lactis HN019 live probiotics and postbiotics: production strategies and bioactivity evaluation for potential therapeutic properties. Front. Bioeng. Biotechnol. 2296-4185. 12. doi:10.3389/fbioe.2024.1379574.

da Silva, J.D., Silva, F.A.M., Rodrigues, C.F., 2025. Microbial contamination in cosmetic products. Cosmetics. 20799284. 12 (5). Available from: www.mdpi.com/journal/cosmetics. doi:10.3390/cosmetics12050198.

De Almeida, C.V., Antiga, E., Lulli, M., 2023. Oral and topical probiotics and postbiotics in skincare and dermatological therapy: a concise review. Microorganisms. 2076-2607. 11 (6), 1420. doi:10.3390/microorganisms11061420.

Dimarzio, L., Cinque, B., Cupelli, F., De Simone, C., Cifone, M.G., Giuliani, M., 2008. Increase of skin-ceramide levels in aged subjects following a short-term topical application of bacterial Sphingomyelinase from *Streptococcus thermophilus*. Int. J. Immunopathol. Pharmacol. 0394-6320. 21 (1), 137–143. doi:10.1177/039463200802100115.

Dinić, M., Pecikoza, U., Djokić, J., Stepanović-Petrović, R., Milenković, M., Stevanović, M., Filipović, N., Begović, J., Golić, N., Lukić, J., 2018. Exopolysaccharide produced by probiotic strain *Lactobacillus paraplantarum* BGCG11 reduces inflammatory hyperalgesia in rats. Front. Pharmacol. 1663-9812. 9. doi:10.3389/fphar.2018.00001.

Dou, J., Feng, N., Guo, F., Chen, Z., Liang, J., Wang, T., Guo, X., Zhenshang, X., 2023. Applications of probiotic constituents in cosmetics. Molecules. 1420-3049. 28 (19), 6765. doi:10.3390/molecules28196765.

Du, M., Hou, Z., Liu, L., Xuan, Y., Chen, X., Fan, L., Zhuoxi, L., Benjin, X., 2022. Progress, applications, challenges and prospects of protein purification technology. Front. Bioeng. Biotechnol. 2296-4185. 10. doi:10.3389/fbioe.2022.1028691.

Esquivel-Hernández, D.A., Rodríguez-Rodríguez, J., Cuéllar-Bermúdez, S.P., García-Pérez, J.S., Mancera-Andrade, E.I., Núñez-Echevarría, J.E., Ontiveros-Valencia, A., Rostro-Alanis, M., García-García, R.M., Torres, J.A., Chen, W.N., Parra-Saldívar, R., 2017. Effect of supercritical carbon dioxide extraction parameters on the biological activities and metabolites present in extracts from *Arthrospira platensis*. Mar. Drugs. 16603397. 15 (6). Available from: http://www.mdpi.com/1660-3397/15/6/174/pdf. doi:10.3390/md15060174.

EU & GB Cosmetics Regulations Compliance, n.d. H2 Compliance. https://h2compliance.com/services/chemical-compliance/cosmetics/. (Accessed 10 December 2025).

EU Cosmetics Regulation Comprehensive Guide. Biorius, n.d. https://biorius.com/cosmetic-regulations/eu-cosmetics-regulation/. (Accessed 10 December 2025).

Favas, R., Morone, J., Martins, R., Vasconcelos, V., Lopes, G., 2021. Cyanobacteria and microalgae bioactive compounds in skin-ageing: potential to restore extracellular matrix filling and overcome hyperpigmentation. J. Enzyme Inhib. Med. Chem. 1475-6366. 36 (1), 1829–1838. doi:10.1080/14756366.2021.1960830.

Feng, T., Wang, J., 2020. Oxidative stress tolerance and antioxidant capacity of lactic acid bacteria as probiotic: a systematic review. Gut Microbes. 1949-0976. 12 (1), 1801944. doi:10.1080/19490976.2020.1801944.

Fernandes, A., Rodrigues, P.M., Pintado, M., Tavaria, F.K., 2023. A systematic review of natural products for skin applications: targeting inflammation, wound healing, and photo-aging. Phytomedicine. 09447113. 115, 154824. doi:10.1016/j.phymed.2023.154824.

Floch, M.H., 2014. Probiotics and Prebiotics. Gastroenterol. Hepatol. 10, 680–681.

Fournière, M., Latire, T., Souak, D., Feuilloley, M.G.J., Bedoux, G., 2020. *Staphylococcus epidermidis* and *Cutibacterium acnes*: two major sentinels of skin microbiota and the influence of cosmetics. Microorganisms. 2076-2607. 8 (11), 1752. doi:10.3390/microorganisms8111752.

Fu, J., Jia, L., Lili, W., Jiang, Y., Zhao, R., Juan, D., Guo, L., Zhang, C., Junji, X., Liu, Y., 2024. *Lactobacillus rhamnosus* inhibits osteoclast differentiation by suppressing the TLR2/NF-κB pathway. Oral Dis. 1354-523X. 30 (4), 2373–2386. doi:10.1111/odi.14712.

Ganesan, N.G., Rangarajan, V., 2021. A kinetics study on surfactin production from *Bacillus subtilis* MTCC 2415 for application in green cosmetics. Biocatal. Agric. Biotechnol. 18788181. 33, 102001. doi:10.1016/j.bcab.2021.102001.

Gao, T., Yixuan, L., Wang, X., Tao, R., Ren, F., 2023. *Bifidobacterium longum* 68S mediated gut-skin axis homeostasis improved skin barrier damage in aging mice. Phytomedicine. 09447113. 120, 155051. doi:10.1016/j.phymed.2023.155051.

Ge, S., Han, J., Sun, Q., Zhou, Q., Zhongdu, Y., Ping, L., Qing, G., 2024. Research progress on improving the freeze-drying resistance of probiotics: a review. Trends Food Sci. Technol. 09242244. 147, 104425. doi:10.1016/j.tifs.2024.104425.

Godase, S.S., Kulkarni, N.S., Dhole, S.N., 2024. A comprehensive review on novel lipid-based nano drug delivery. Adv. Pharm. Bull. 22517308. 14 (1), 34–47. Available from: https://apb.tbzmed.ac.ir/Article/apb-37690. doi:10.34172/apb.2024.012.

Golkar, N., Ashoori, Y., Heidari, R., Omidifar, N., Abootalebi, S.N., Mohkam, M., Gholami, A., 2021. A novel effective formulation of bioactive compounds for wound healing: preparation, in vivo characterization, and comparison of various postbiotics cold creams in a rat model. Evid. Based Complement. Alternat. Med. 17414288. 2021. Available from: http://www.hindawi.com/journals/ecam/contents.html. doi:10.1155/2021/8577116.

Gruenwald, J., Graubaum, H.J., Harde, A., 2002. Effect of a probiotic multivitamin compound on stress and exhaustion. Adv. Ther. 0741238X. 19 (3), 141–150. Available from: http://www.springer.com/springer+healthcare/journal/12325. doi:10.1007/BF02850270.

Guéniche, A., Bastien, P., Ovigne, J.M., Kermici, M., Courchay, G., Chevalier, V., Breton, L., Castiel-Higounenc, I., 2010. *Bifidobacterium longum* lysate, a new ingredient for reactive skin. Exp. Dermatol. 16000625. 19 (8), e1. doi:10.1111/j.1600-0625.2009.00932.x.

Guéniche, A., David, P., Philippe, B., Stephanie, B., Elif, B., Isabelle, C.-H., 2014. Probiotics for photoprotection. Dermato-Endocrinol. 1938-1980. 1 (5), 275–279. doi:10.4161/derm.1.5.9849.

Guo, C., Liu, J., Zhang, Y., 2024. Current advances in bacteria-based cancer immunotherapy. Eur. J. Immunol. 0014-2980. 54 (2). doi:10.1002/eji.202350778.

Gupta, P.L., Rajput, M., Oza, T., Trivedi, U., Sanghvi, G., 2019. Eminence of microbial products in cosmetic industry. Nat. Prod. Bioprospect. 21922209. 9 (4), 267–278. Available from: https://link.springer.com/journal/13659. doi:10.1007/s13659-019-0215-0.

Gutiérrez-Álzate, K., Beltrán-Cotta, L.A., Dos Santos Rekowsky, B.S., Cavalheiro, C.P., da Costa, M.P., 2024. Micro- and nanoencapsulation of probiotics: exploring their impact on animal-origin foods. ACS Food Sci. Technol. 26921944. 4 (12), 2799–2812. Available from: https://pubs.acs.org/page/afsthl/about.html. doi:10.1021/acsfoodscitech.4c00776.

Habeebuddin, M., Karnati, R.K., Shiroorkar, P.N., Nagaraja, S., Asdaq, S.M.B., Anwer, M.K., Fattepur, S., 2022. Topical probiotics: more than a skin deep. Pharmaceutics. 1999-4923. 14 (3), 557. doi:10.3390/pharmaceutics14030557.

Hawari, F.L., Almadea, T., Hananingsih, K., Baikuni, A., Malik, A., Arifianti, A.E., Ramadon, D., Tjampakasari, C.R., 2022. Development of bacterial cocktail of strains *Staphylococcus hominis*, *Staphylococcus warneri*, *Bacillus subtilis*, and *Micrococcus luteus* as active ingredients for Skin Care Formula. Indones. J. Pharm. 2338–9486. doi:10.22146/ijp.4174.

Huang, R., Wang, K., Jianan, H., 2016. Effect of probiotics on depression: a systematic review and meta-analysis of randomized controlled trials. Nutrients. 2072-6643. 8 (8), 483. doi:10.3390/nu8080483.

Huang, S., Vignolles, M.L., Chen, X.D., Loir, Y.L., Jan, G., Schuck, P., Jeantet, R., 2017. Spray drying of probiotics and other food-grade bacteria: a review. Trends Food Sci. Technol. 09242244. 63, 1–17. Available from: http://www.elsevier.com/wps/find/journaldescription.cws_home/601278/description#description. doi:10.1016/j.tifs.2017.02.007.

Im, A.R., Lee, B., Kang, D.J., Chae, S., 2019. Protective effects of tyndallized *Lactobacillus acidophilus* IDCC 3302 against UVB-induced photodamage to epidermal keratinocytes cells. Int. J. Mol. Med. 1791244X. 43 (6), 2499–2506. Available from: https://www.spandidos-publications.com/ijmm. doi:10.3892/ijmm.2019.4161.

ISO, n.d. ISO 22716:2007. https://www.iso.org/standard/36437.html. (Accessed 10 December 2025).

Jackson, S.A., Schoeni, J.L., Vegge, C., Pane, M., Stahl, B., Bradley, M., Goldman, V.S., Burguière, P., Atwater, J.B., Sanders, M.E., 2019. Improving end-user trust in the quality of commercial probiotic products. Front. Microbiol. 1664302X. 10. Available from: https://www.frontiersin.org/journals/microbiology#. doi:10.3389/fmicb.2019.00739.

Jaffri, J.M., 2023. Reactive oxygen species and antioxidant system in selected skin disorders. Malays. J. Med. Sci. 1394195X. 30 (1), 7–20. doi:10.21315/mjms2023.30.1.2.

Jain, R., Voss, A.L., Rosario, J.D., Hale, J.D.F., 2025. Efficacy of a topical live probiotic in improving skin health. Int. J. Cosmet. Sci. 0142-5463. 47 (3), 488–496. doi:10.1111/ics.13043.

Jenab, A., Roghanian, R., Emtiazi, G., 2020. Bacterial natural compounds with anti-inflammatory and immunomodulatory properties (Mini review). Drug Des. Dev. Ther. 11778881. 14, 3787–3801. Available from: https://www.dovepress.com/getfile.php?fileID=61577. doi:10.2147/DDDT.S261283.

Jha, A.K., Sit, N., 2022. Extraction of bioactive compounds from plant materials using combination of various novel methods: a review. Trends Food Sci. Technol. 09242244. 119, 579–591. Available from: http://www.elsevier.com/wps/find/journaldescription.cws_home/601278/description#description. doi:10.1016/j.tifs.2021.11.019.

Jin, L., Shi, X., Yang, J., Zhao, Y., Xue, L., Xu, L., Cai, J., 2021. Gut microbes in cardiovascular diseases and their potential therapeutic applications. Protein Cell. 1674-800X. 12 (5), 346–359. doi:10.1007/s13238-020-00785-9.

Jung, Y.O., Jeong, H., Cho, Y., Lee, E.O., Jang, H.W., Kim, J., Nam, K.T., Lim, K.M., 2019. Lysates of a probiotic, *Lactobacillus rhamnosus*, can improve skin barrier function in a reconstructed human epidermis model. Int. J. Mol. Sci. 14220067. 20 (17). Available from: https://www.mdpi.com/1422-0067/20/17/4289/pdf. doi:10.3390/ijms20174289.

Jurášková, D., Pires, V.C., Ribeiro, S.C., Ferreira, S.S., Bernardo, F., Evtyugin, D., Coimbra, M.A., Silva, C.C.G., 2025. Exopolysaccharide (EPS)-producing *Streptococcus thermophilus*: functional and probiotic potential. Foods. 23048158. 14 (17). Available from: www.mdpi.com/journal/foods. doi:10.3390/foods14173013.

Kahraman Ilıkkan, Ö., 2025. Lactobacillomics as a new notion in lactic acid bacteria research through omics integration. World J. Microbiol. Biotechnol. 0959-3993. 41 (2). doi:10.1007/s11274-025-04285-y.

Kalenova, L.F., Novikova, M.A., Subbotin, A.M., 2015. Effects of permafrost microorganisms on skin wound reparation. Bull. Exp. Biol. Med. 15738221. 158 (4), 478–482. Available from: www.wkap.nl/journalhome.htm/0007-4888. doi:10.1007/s10517-015-2789-9.

Kanimozhi, N.V., Sukumar, M., 2025. Aging through the lens of the gut microbiome: challenges and therapeutic opportunities. Arch. Gerontol. Geriatr. Plus. 29503078. 2 (2), 100142. doi:10.1016/j.aggp.2025.100142.

Khan, M.K., Chemat, F., Sattar, S., Muhammad, I., 2019. Extraction of bioactive molecules: conventional versus novel methods. In: Suleria, H.A.R., Barrow, C., Eds.. Bioactive Compounds from Plant Origin—Extraction, Applications, and Potential Health Benefits. Taylor and Francis Group, pp. 332. doi:10.1201/9780429029288.

Kim, J., Hwang, S.J., Lee, G.S., Lee, J.R., An, H.I., Im, H.S., Kim, M., Lee, S.S., Lee, H.J., Kim, C.S., 2024. Collagenase and tyrosinase inhibitory compounds from fish gut bacteria *Ruegeria atlantica* and *Pseudoalteromonas neustonica*. ACS Omega. 24701343. 9 (32), 34259–34267. Available from: https://www.pubs.acs.org/journal/acsodf. doi:10.1021/acsomega.3c09585.

Kiprono, S., Wambani, J., Rono, J., Langat, V., Shi, Z., Raballah, E., Yang, G., 2024. Microencapsulation of probiotics and their applications: a review of the literature. ES Food Agrofor. 26877309. 17. Available from: https://www.espublisher.com/journals/articledetails/1106/. doi:10.30919/esfaf1106.

Kohler, T., Xia, G., Kulauzovic, E., Peschel, A., 2010. Teichoic acids, lipoteichoic acids and related cell wall glycopolymers of gram-positive bacteria. In: Holst, O., Brennan, P.J., von Itzstein, M. (Eds.), Microbial Glycobiology. Academic Press, pp. 75–91. Available from: https://www.sciencedirect.com/science/book/9780123745460. doi:10.1016/B978-0-12-374546-0.00005-5.

Koukouraki, P., Tsoupras, A., Sotiroudis, G., Demopoulos, C.A., Sotiroudis, T.G., 2020. Antithrombotic properties of Spirulina extracts against platelet-activating factor and thrombin. Food Biosci. 22124292. 37, 100686. doi:10.1016/j.fbio.2020.100686.

Lai, Y., Gallo, R.L., 2008. Toll-like receptors in skin infections and inflammatory diseases. Infect. Disord. Drug Targets. 18715265. 8 (3), 144–155. Available from: http://www.ingentaconnect.com/content/ben/iddt/2008/00000008/00000003/art00003. doi:10.2174/187152608785587 [illegible]

Lawrence, K.P., Long, P.F., Young, A.R., 2018. Mycosporine-like amino acids for skin photoprotection. Curr. Med. Chem. 1875533X. 25 (40), 5512–5527. Available from: http://www.eurekaselect.com/152756/article. doi:10.2174/0929867324666170529124237.

Lebeer, S., Oerlemans, E.F.M., Claes, I., Henkens, T., Delanghe, L., Wuyts, S., Spacova, I., van den Broek, M.F.L., Tuyaerts, I., Wittouck, S., De Boeck, I., Allonsius, C.N., Kiekens, F., Lambert, J., 2022. Selective targeting of skin pathobionts and inflammation with topically applied lactobacilli. Cell Rep. Med. 26663791. 3 (2), 100521. doi:10.1016/j.xcrm.2022.100521.

Lee, D.E., Huh, C.S., Ra, J., Choi, I.D., Jeong, J.W., Kim, S.H., Ryu, J.H., Seo, Y.K., Koh, J.S., Lee, J.H., Sim, J.H., Ahn, Y.T., 2015. Clinical evidence of effects of *Lactobacillus plantarum* HY7714 on skin aging: a randomized, double blind, placebo-controlled study. J. Microbiol. Biotechnol. 17388872. 25 (12), 2160–2168. Available from: http://www.jmb.or.kr/journal/download.php?Filedir=./submission/Journal/025/&num=7338. doi:10.4014/jmb.1509.09021.

Lee, Y.S., Lee, S.J., Jang, W.J., Lee, E.W., 2024. Protective effects of the postbiotic *Levilactobacillus brevis* BK3 against H_2O_2 induced oxidative damage in skin cells. J. Microbiol. Biotechnol. 17388872. 34 (7), 1401–1409. Available from: https://www.jmb.or.kr/journal/view.html?uid=6457&vmd=Full. doi:10.4014/jmb.2403.03010.

Leung, D.Y.M., Boguniewicz, M., Howell, M.D., Nomura, I., Hamid, Q.A., 2004. New insights into atopic dermatitis. J. Clin. Invest. 00219738. 113 (5), 651–657. Available from: http://www.jci.org. doi:10.1172/JCI21060.

Li, Z., Luo, X., 2025. Probiotics, prebiotics, synbiotics, postbiotics, and paraprobiotics—new perspectives on functional foods and nutraceuticals. Foods. 2304-8158. 14 (15), 2613. doi:10.3390/foods14152613.

Liang, L., Qihang, S., Ma, Y., Zhao, S., Zhang, H., Gao, X., 2024. Research progress on the polysaccharide extraction and antibacterial activity. Ann. Microbiol. 1869-2044. 74 (1). doi:10.1186/s13213-024-01762-x.

Liang, S., Wang, C., Shao, Y., Wang, Y., Xing, D., Geng, Z., 2022. Recent advances in bacteria-mediated cancer therapy. Front. Bioeng. Biotechnol. 2296-4185. 10. doi:10.3389/fbioe.2022.1026248.

Lin, H., Zhang, J., Shiyang, L., Zheng, B., Jiamiao, H., 2021. Polysaccharides isolated from *Laminaria japonica* attenuates gestational diabetes mellitus by regulating the gut microbiota in mice. Food Front. 2643-8429. 2 (2), 208–217. doi:10.1002/fft2.79.

Liu, R., Sun, B., 2023. Lactic acid bacteria and aging: unraveling the interplay for healthy longevity. Aging Dis. 2152-5250. doi:10.14336/ad.2023.0926.

Liu, X., Qin, Y., Dong, L., Han, Z., Liu, T., Tang, Y., Yun, Y., Jingjie, Y., Tao, J., Zeng, X., Feng, J., Zhang, X.-Z., 2023. Living symbiotic bacteria-involved skin dressing to combat indigenous pathogens for microbiome-based biotherapy toward atopic dermatitis. Bioact. Mater. 2452199X. 21, 253–266. doi:10.1016/j.bioactmat.2022.08.019.

Lolou, V., Panayiotidis, M.I., 2019. Functional role of probiotics and prebiotics on skin health and disease. Fermentation. 2311-5637. 5 (2), 41. doi:10.3390/fermentation5020041.

Lombardi, F., Augello, F.R., Artone, S., Bahiti, B., Sheldon, J.M., Giuliani, M., Cifone, M.G., Palumbo, P., Cinque, B., 2022. Efficacy of probiotic *Streptococcus thermophilus* in counteracting TGF-β1-induced fibrotic response in normal human dermal fibroblasts. J. Inflamm. (U.K.). 14769255. 19 (1). Available from: https://journal-inflammation.biomedcentral.com/. doi:10.1186/s12950-022-00324-9.

Loo, J.S., Oslan, S.N.H., Mokshin, N.A.S., Othman, R., Amin, Z., Dejtisakdi, W., Prihanto, A.A., Tan, J.S., 2025. Comprehensive review of strategies for lactic acid bacteria production and metabolite enhancement in probiotic cultures: multifunctional applications in functional foods. Fermentation. 23115637. 11 (5). Available from: www.mdpi.com/journal/fermentation. doi:10.3390/fermentation11050241.

Lopes, G., Clarinha, D., Vasconcelos, V., 2020. Carotenoids from cyanobacteria: a biotechnological approach for the topical treatment of psoriasis. Microorganisms. 2076-2607. 8 (2), 302. doi:10.3390/microorganisms8020302.

Lousada, M.B., Lachnit, T., Edelkamp, J., Rouillé, T., Ajdic, D., Uchida, Y., Di Nardo, A., Bosch, T.C.G., Paus, R., 2021. Exploring the human hair follicle microbiome. Br. J. Dermatol. 0007-0963. 184 (5), 802–815. doi:10.1111/bjd.19461.

Luft, L., Mazutti, M.A., 2025. Freeze and spray drying technologies to produce solid microbial formulations for sustainable agriculture. Processes. 2227-9717. 13 (7), 2188. doi:10.3390/pr13072188.

Lulula, n.d. The Pure Lotus Youth Biotics Αντιρυτιδική Κρέμα Προσώπου με. https://www.lulula.gr/vendors/the-pure-lotus/the-pure-lotus-probiotic-concentrate-cream-50ml.htm. (Accessed 10 December 2025).

Lundov, M.D., Moesby, L., Zachariae, C., Johansen, J.D., 2009. Contamination versus preservation of cosmetics: a review on legislation, usage, infections, and contact allergy. Contact Dermat. 16000536. 60 (2), 70–78. doi:10.1111/j.1600-0536.2008.01501.x.

Lytras, F., Psakis, G., Gatt, R., Cebrián, G., Raso, J., Valdramidis, V., 2024. Exploring the efficacy of pulsed electric fields (PEF) in microbial inactivation during food processing: a deep dive into the microbial cellular and molecular mechanisms. Innov. Food Sci. Emerg. Technol. 14668564. 95, 103732. doi:10.1016/j.ifset.2024.103732.

Lyu, Q., Chen, R.A., Chuang, H.L., Zou, H.B., Liu, L., Sung, L.K., Liu, P.Y., Wu, H.Y., Chang, H.Y., Cheng, W.J., Wu, W.K., Wu, M.S., Hsu, C.C., 2024. Bifidobacterium alleviate metabolic disorders via converting methionine to 5'-methylthioadenosine. Gut Microbes. 19490984. 16 (1). Available from: http://www.tandfonline.com/toc/kgmi20/current. doi:10.1080/19490976.2023.2300847.

Mahmoud, Y.A.-G., Elkaliny, N.E., Elshikh, F.M., Ashraf, Y., Metwally, K., Yahya, G., Sherif, S., 2025. Cold plasma as a revolutionary antimicrobial modality: a multifaceted weapon against antibiotic resistance. Antibiotics. 2079-6382. 14 (9), 930. doi:10.3390/antibiotics14090930.

Majeed, M., Majeed, S., Nagabhushanam, K., Lawrence, L., Arumugam, S., Mundkur, L., 2020. Skin protective activity of lactosporin-the extracellular metabolite from *Bacillus coagulans* MTCC 5856. Cosmetics. 2079-9284. 7 (4), 76. doi:10.3390/cosmetics7040076.

Martín, M.J., Lara-Villoslada, F., Ruiz, M.A., Morales, M.E., 2015. Microencapsulation of bacteria: a review of different technologies and their impact on the probiotic effects. Innov. Food Sci. Emerg. Technol. 14668564. 27, 15–25. Available from: http://www.elsevier.com/locate/ifset. doi:10.1016/j.ifset.2014.09.010.

Martyniak, A., Medyńska-Przęczek, A., Wędrychowicz, A., Skoczeń, S., Tomasik, P.J., 2021. Prebiotics, probiotics, synbiotics, paraprobiotics and postbiotic compounds in IBD. Biomolecules. 2218-273X. 11 (12), 1903. doi:10.3390/biom11121903.

Maya-Martinez, R., Andrew, J., Alexander, N., Otten, C.F., Ayala, I., Vollmer, D., Gray, J., Bougault, C.M., Burt, A., Laguri, C., Fonvielle, M., Arthur, M., Strynadka, N.C.J., Vollmer, W., Simorre, J.-P., 2019. Recognition of peptidoglycan fragments by the transpeptidase PBP4 from *Staphylococcus aureus*. Front. Microbiol. 1664-302X. 9. doi:10.3389/fmicb.2018.03223.

Mazumder, M.A.R., Jubayer, M.F., Kayshar, M.S., Peter, D., Ranganathan, T.V., 2024. Bacteria as a source of bioactive cosmeceuticals. In: Kathuria, D., Sharma, A., Verma, M., Nayik, G.A. (Eds.), Bioprospecting of Natural Sources for Cosmeceuticals. Royal Society of Chemistry, Bangladesh, pp. 198–222. Available from: https://books.rsc.org/books/edited-volume/2186/Bioprospecting-of-Natural-Sources-for. doi:10.1039/9781837672288-00198.

McFarland, L.V., 2015. From yaks to yogurt: the history, development, and current use of probiotics. Clin. Infect. Dis. 1058-4838. 60 (suppl 2), S85. doi:10.1093/cid/civ054.

Meena, L., Malini, B., Byresh, T.S., Sunil, C.K., Ashish Rawson, N.V., 2024. Ultrasound as a pre-treatment in millet-based probiotic beverage: it's effect on fermentation kinetics and beverage quality. Food Chem. Adv. 2772753X. 4, 100631. doi:10.1016/j.focha.2024.100631.

Misra, S., Pandey, P., Mishra, H.N., 2021. Novel approaches for co-encapsulation of probiotic bacteria with bioactive compounds, their health benefits and functional food product development: a review. Trends Food Sci. Technol. 09242244. 109, 340–351. Available from: http://www.elsevier.com/wps/find/journaldescription.cws_home/601278/description#description. doi:10.1016/j.tifs.2021.01.039.

Mondadori, G., Amoruso, A., Visciglia, A., Deusebio, G., Pinto, D., Pane, M., Rinaldi, F., 2025. Heat-treated probiotics' role in counteraction of skin UVs-induced damage in vitro. Cosmetics. 2079-9284. 12 (3), 121. doi:10.3390/cosmetics12030121.

Mourelle, M.L., Gómez, C.P., Legido, J.L., 2017. The potential use of marine microalgae and cyanobacteria in cosmetics and thalassotherapy. Cosmetics. 20799284. 4 (4). Available from: https://www.mdpi.com/2079-9284/4/4/46/pdf. doi:10.3390/cosmetics4040046.

Mukarram, M., Rizzo, D., Omari, S., Grand, Z., Jackson, S., Jaing, J., Vinagolu-Baur, J., Jimoh, L., 2025. The impact of topical probiotic *Lactobacillus plantarum* on skin barrier repair in atopic dermatitis. ARC J. Dermatol. 24560022. 8 (3), 19–36. doi:10.20431/2456-0022.0803003.

Mussagy, C.U., Paz, A.V.C., Cornejo, P., Santander, C., González, F., Voloua, R.G., Besoain, X., Larach, A., Salinas, A., Godoy, K., Sangaré, D., 2025. CFD insights into microwave-assisted deep eutectic solvent for the recovery of astaxanthin from bacteria *Paracoccus carotinifaciens*: from extraction to agricultural applications. Sep. Purif. Technol. 13835866. 360, 131212. doi:10.1016/j.seppur.2024.131212.

Myles, I.A., Castillo, C.R., Barbian, K.D., Kanakabandi, K., Virtaneva, K., Fitzmeyer, E., Paneru, M., Otaizo-Carrasquero, F., Myers, T.G., Markowitz, T.E., Moore, I.N., Liu, X., Ferrer, M., Sakamachi, Y., Garantziotis, S., Swamydas, M., Lionakis, M.S., Anderson, E.D., Earland, N.J., Ganesan, S., Sun, A.A., Bergerson, J.R.E., Silverman, R.A., Petersen, M., Martens, C.A., Datta, S.K., 2020. Therapeutic responses to *Roseomonas mucosa* in atopic dermatitis may involve lipid-mediated TNF-related epithelial repair. Sci. Transl. Med. 19466242. 12 (560). Available from: https://stm.sciencemag.org/lookup/doi/10.1126/scitranslmed.aaz8631. doi:10.1126/SCITRANSLMED.AAZ8631.

EUR-Lex - 02009R1223-20250901 - EN - EUR-Lex, n.d. https://eur-lex.europa.eu/eli/reg/2009/1223/2025-09-01. (Accessed 10 December 2025).

European Commission - Have your say, n.d. Eur Comm—Have Your Say. https://ec.europa.eu/info/law/better-regulation/have-your-say/initiatives/13197-EU-chemicals-strategy-for-sustainability-Cosmetic-Products-Regulation-revision-/public-consultation_en. (Accessed 10 December 2025).

FDA Regulation of Cosmetics and Personal Care Products Under the Modernization of Cosmetics Regulation Act of 2022 (MoCRA), n.d. https://www.congress.gov/crs-product/R47826. (Accessed 10 December 2025).

Glowsophy Cica Panthenol Soothing Moisturiser (Ingredients Explained), n.d. https://skinsort.com/products/glowsophy/cica-panthenol-soothing-moisturiser. (Accessed 10 December 2025).

Masil 5 Probiotics Perfect Volume Shampoo (150 ml), n.d. https://www.zizel.gr/masil-5-probiotics-perfect-volume-shampoo-150ml. (Accessed 10 December 2025).

Microbiome Soft Shampoo. Propaira - Clin Ski, n.d. https://propaira.com/products/hair-scalp/microbiome-soft-shampoo. (Accessed 10 December 2025).

SCCS Notes of Guidance for the Testing of Cosmetic Ingredients and Their Safety Evaluation—12th Revision, n.d. Public Health. https://health.ec.europa.eu/publications/sccs-notes-guidance-testing-cosmetic-ingredients-and-their-safety-evaluation-12th-revision_en. (Accessed 10 December 2025).

Nakatsuji, T., Chen, T.H., Butcher, A.M., Trzoss, L.L., Nam, S.J., Shirakawa, K.T., Zhou, W., Oh, J., Otto, M., Fenical, W., Gallo, R.L., 2018. A commensal strain of *Staphylococcus epidermidis* protects against skin neoplasia. Sci. Adv. 23752548. 4 (2). Available from: http://advances.sciencemag.org/content/4/2/eaao4502/tab-pdf. doi:10.1126/sciadv.aao4502.

Nam, G.H., Jo, K.J., Park, Y.S., Kawk, H.W., Yoo, J.G., Jang, J.D., Kang, S.M., Kim, S.Y., Kim, Y.M., 2019. The peptide AC 2 isolated from Bacillus-treated *Trapa japonica* fruit extract rescues DHT (dihydrotestosterone)-treated human dermal papilla cells and mediates mTORC1 signaling for autophagy and apoptosis suppression. Sci. Rep. 20452322. 9 (1). Available from: www.nature.com/srep/index.html. doi:10.1038/s41598-019-53347-3.

Nam, W., Kim, H., Bae, C., Kim, J., Nam, B., Kim, J., Park, S., Lee, J., Sim, J., 2021. *Lactobacillus paracasei* HY7015 promotes hair growth in a telogenic mouse model. J. Med. Food. 1096-620X. 24 (7), 741–748. doi:10.1089/jmf.2020.4860.

Noori, M., Shateri, Z., Babajafari, S., Eskandari, M.H., Parastouei, K., Ghasemi, M., Afshari, H., Samadi, M., 2024. The effect of probiotic-fortified kefir on cardiovascular risk factors in elderly population: a double-blind, randomized, placebo-controlled clinical trial. BMC Nutr. 20550928. 10 (1). Available from: https://bmcnutr.biomedcentral.com/. doi:10.1186/s40795-024-00875-5.

Öhnstedt, E., Vågesjö, E., Fasth, A., Tomenius, H.L., Dahg, P., Jönsson, S., Tyagi, N., Åström, M., Myktybekova, Z., Ringstad, L., Jorvid, M., Frank, P., Hedén, P., Roos, S., Phillipson, M., 2023. Engineered bacteria to accelerate wound healing: an adaptive, randomised, double-blind, placebo-controlled, first-in-human phase 1 trial. eClinicalMedicine. 25895370. 60, 102014. doi:10.1016/j.eclinm.2023.102014.

Organic Brands, n.d. Kilig Probiotics Face Cream | Κρέμα Προσώπου με Προβιοτικά για Λιπαρές & Μεικτές Επιδερμίδες. https://www.organicbrands.gr/el/product/8028/kilig-probiotics-face-cream?sz=3. (Accessed 10 December 2025).

Pagels, F., Pereira, R.N., Vicente, A.A., Guedes, A.C., 2021. Extraction of pigments from microalgae and cyanobacteria—a review on current methodologies. Appl. Sci. 2076-3417. 11 (11), 5187. doi:10.3390/app11115187.

Palathinkara, M., Aljadah, M., Thorgerson, A., Dawson, A.Z., Widlansky, M.E., 2025. Association of probiotic supplementation and cardiovascular risk profiles of patients with coronary artery disease—a cross-sectional analysis of the NHANES database between 1999–2019. Front. Nutr. 2296861X. 12. Available from: https://www.journal.frontiersin.org/journal/nutrition. doi:10.3389/fnut.2025.1495633.

Papadopoulou, S.N.A., Adamantidi, T., Kranas, D., Cholidis, P., Anastasiadou, C., Tsoupras, A., 2025. A comprehensive review on the valorization of bioactives from marine animal by-products for health-promoting, biofunctional cosmetics. Mar. Drugs. 1660-3397. 23 (8), 299. doi:10.3390/md23080299.

Patra, V., Gallais Sérézal, I., Wolf, P., 2020. Potential of skin microbiome, pro- and/or pre-biotics to affect local cutaneous responses to UV exposure. Nutrients. 2072-6643. 12 (6), 1795. doi:10.3390/nu12061795.

Paul, J.K., Azmal, M., Omar Faruk Talukder, A.N.M.S.N.B.H., Meem, M., Ghosh, A., 2025. Unlocking the secrets of the hair microbiome: from scalp health to therapeutic advances. Microbe. 29501946. 7, 100353. doi:10.1016/j.microb.2025.100353.

Pérez-Rivero, C., Pablo López-Gómez, J., 2023. Unlocking the potential of fermentation in cosmetics: a review. Fermentation. 2311-5637. 9 (5), 463. doi:10.3390/fermentation9050463.

Płaza, G.A., Łukasik, K., Wypych, J., Nałecz-Jawecki, G., Berry, C., Brigmon, R.L., 2008. Biodegradation of crude oil and distillation products by biosurfactant-producing bacteria. Pol. J. Environ. Stud. 12301485. 17 (1), 87–94.

Program HF, 2025. BAM Chapter 23: methods for Cosmetics. FDA.

Puebla-Barragan, S., Reid, G., 2021. Probiotics in cosmetic and personal care products: trends and challenges. Molecules. 1420-3049. 26 (5), 1249. doi:10.3390/molecules26051249.

Rahman, M.M., Grice, I.D., Ulett, G.C., Wei, M.Q., 2024. Advances in bacterial lysate immunotherapy for infectious diseases and cancer. J. Immunol. Res. 23147156. 2024. Available from: http://www.hindawi.com/journals/jir/. doi:10.1155/2024/4312908.

Rakhuba, D., Novik, G., Dey, E.S., 2009. Application of supercritical carbon dioxide (scCO2) for the extraction of glycolipids from *Lactobacillus plantarum* B-01. J. Supercrit. Fluids. 08968446. 49 (1), 45–51. doi:10.1016/j.supflu.2008.11.016.

Razavi, S., Janfaza, S., Tasnim, N., Gibson, D.L., Hoorfar, M., 2021. Microencapsulating polymers for probiotics delivery systems: preparation, characterization, and applications. Food Hydrocoll. 0268005X. 120, 106882. doi:10.1016/j.foodhyd.2021.106882.

Registrar Corp, 2025. Cosmetic Product Safety Reports (CPSR) For EU & UK. https://www.registrarcorp.com/services/cosmetic-product-safety-report-cpsr/. (Accessed 10 December 2025).

Rev Beauty Care, n.d. Probio Skin Balance Probiotic Cream Cleanser, 150 Ml. https://www.revuele.com.gr/product/probio-skin-balance-probiotic-cream-cleanser-150-ml/. (Accessed 10 December 2025).

Rigauts, C., Aizawa, J., Taylor, S.L., Rogers, G.B., Govaerts, M., Cos, P., Ostyn, L., Sims, S., Vandeplassche, E., Sze, M., Dondelinger, Y., Vereecke, L., Van Acker, H., Simpson, J.L., Burr, L., Willems, A., Tunney, M.M., Cigana, C., Bragonzi, A., Coenye, T., Crabbé, A., 2022. *Rothia mucilaginosa* is an anti-inflammatory bacterium in the respiratory tract of patients with chronic lung disease. Eur. Respir. J. 13993003. 59 (5). Available from: https://erj.ersjournals.com/content/59/5/2101293. doi:10.1183/13993003.01293-2021.

Rinnerthaler, M., Bischof, J., Streubel, M.K., Trost, A., Richter, K., 2015. Oxidative stress in aging human skin. Biomolecules. 2218273X. 5 (2), 545–589. Available from: http://www.mdpi.com/2218-273X/5/2/545/pdf. doi:10.3390/biom5020545.

Roberfroid, M., Gibson, G.R., Hoyles, L., McCartney, A.L., Rastall, R., Rowland, I., Wolvers, D., Watzl, B., Szajewska, H., Stahl, B., Guarner, F., Respondek, F., Whelan, K., Coxam, V., Davicco, M.J., Léotoing, L., Wittrant, Y., Delzenne, N.M., Cani, P.D., Neyrinck, A.M., Meheust, A., 2010. Prebiotic effects: metabolic and health benefits. Br. J. Nutr. 14752662. 104 (2), S1. doi:10.1017/S0007114510003363.

Roca, C., Alves, V.D., Freitas, F., Reis, M.A.M., 2015. Exopolysaccharides enriched in rare sugars: bacterial sources, production, and applications. Front. Microbiol. 1664302X. 6. Available from: http://journal.frontiersin.org/article/10.3389/fmicb.2015.00288/full. doi:10.3389/fmicb.2015.00288.

Romijn, A.R., Rucklidge, J.J., Kuijer, R.G., Frampton, C., 2017. A double-blind, randomized, placebo-controlled trial of *Lactobacillus helveticus* and *Bifidobacterium longum* for the symptoms of depression. Aust. N. Z. J. Psychiatry. 14401614. 51 (8), 810–821. Available from: http://anp.sagepub.com/content/by/year. doi:10.1177/0004867416686694.

Rotter, A., Varamogianni-Mamatsi, D., Pobirk, A.Z., Matjaž, M.G., Cueto, M., Díaz-Marrero, A.R., Jónsdóttir, R., Sveinsdóttir, K., Catalá, T.S., Romano, G., Guler, B.A., Atak, E., Zrimec, M.B., Bosch, D., Deniz, I., Gaudêncio, S.P., Grigalionyte-Bembič, E., Klun, K., Zidar, L., Rius, A.C., Baebler, Š., Lukić Bilela, L., Rinkevich, B., Mandalakis, M., 2024. Marine cosmetics and the blue bioeconomy: from sourcing to success stories. iScience. 25890042. 27 (12), 111339. doi:10.1016/j.isci.2024.111339.

Rozas, M., de Ruijter, A.H., Fabrega, M.J., Zorgani, A., Guell, M., Paetzold, B., Brillet, F., 2021. From dysbiosis to healthy skin: major contributions of *Cutibacterium acnes* to skin homeostasis. Microorganisms. 2076-2607. 9 (3), 628. doi:10.3390/microorganisms9030628.

Rušanac, A., Škibola, Z., Matijašić, M., Čipčić Paljetak, H., Perić, M., 2025. Microbiome-based products: therapeutic potential for inflammatory skin diseases. Int. J. Mol. Sci. 1422-0067. 26 (14), 6745. doi:10.3390/ijms26146745.

Saravanan, C., Gopinath, N.K., Ganesan, R., Thirumurugan, D., 2025. Challenges and limitations in using bacterial metabolites as immunomodulators. Front. Cell. Infect. Microbiol. 22352988. 15. Available from: http://www.frontiersin.org/Cellular_and_Infection_Microbiology/archive. doi:10.3389/fcimb.2025.1535394.

Sathikulpakdee, S., Kanokrungsee, S., Vitheejongjaroen, P., Kamanamool, N., Udompataikul, M., Taweechotipatr, M., 2022. Efficacy of probiotic-derived lotion from *Lactobacillus paracasei* MSMC 39-1 in mild to moderate acne vulgaris, randomized controlled trial. J. Cosmet. Dermatol. 1473-2130. 21 (10), 5092–5097. doi:10.1111/jocd.14971.

Schöpping, M., Gaspar, P., Neves, A.R., Franzén, C.J., Zeidan, A.A., 2021. Identifying the essential nutritional requirements of the probiotic bacteria *Bifidobacterium animalis* and *Bifidobacterium longum* through genome-scale modeling. Npj Syst. Biol. Appl. 20567189. 7 (1). Available from: www.nature.com/npjsba/. doi:10.1038/s41540-021-00207-4.

Sekurova, O.N., Schneider, O., Zotchev, S.B., 2019. Novel bioactive natural products from bacteria via bioprospecting, genome mining and metabolic engineering. Microb. Biotechnol. 17517915. 12 (5), 828–844. Available from: http://onlinelibrary.wiley.com/journal/10.1111/(ISSN)1751-7915. doi:10.1111/1751-7915.13398.

Shafique, B., Ranjha, M.M.A.N., Murtaza, M.A., Walayat, N., Nawaz, A., Khalid, W., Mahmood, S., Nadeem, M., Manzoor, M.F., Ameer, K., Aadil, R.M., Ibrahim, S.A., 2023. Recent trends and applications of nanoencapsulated bacteriocins against microbes in food quality and safety. Microorganisms. 20762607. 11 (1). Available from: www.mdpi.com/journal/microorganisms. doi:10.3390/microorganisms11010085.

Shiels, K., Tsoupras, A., Lordan, R., Nasopoulou, C., Zabetakis, I., Murray, P., Saha, S.K., 2021. Bioactive lipids of marine microalga *Chlorococcum* sp. SABC 012504 with anti-inflammatory and anti-thrombotic activities. Mar. Drugs. 1660-3397. 19 (1), 28. doi:10.3390/md19010028.

Shiels, K., Tsoupras, A., Lordan, R., Zabetakis, I., Murray, P., Saha, S.K., 2022. Anti-inflammatory and antithrombotic properties of polar lipid extracts, rich in unsaturated fatty acids, from the Irish marine cyanobacterium *Spirulina subsalsa*. J. Funct. Foods. 17564646. 94, 105124. doi:10.1016/j.jff.2022.105124.

Shirkhan, F., Safaei, F., Mirdamadi, S., Zandi, M., 2024. The role of probiotics in skin care: advances, challenges, and future needs. Probiotics Antimicrob. Proteins. 1867-1306. 16 (6), 2132–2149. doi:10.1007/s12602-024-10319-y.

Silva, T.P., Alves, L., Salgado, F., Roseiro, J.C., Łukasik, R.M., Paixão, S.M., 2024. Ionic liquids toward enhanced carotenoid extraction from bacterial biomass. Molecules. 1420-3049. 29 (17), 4132. doi:10.3390/molecules29174132.

SkinSAFE, n.d. Skinesa Defensin Probiotic Spray Ingredients and Reviews. https://www.skinsafeproducts.com/skinesa-defensin-probiotic-spray. (Accessed 10 December 2025).

Smith, C.N., Alexander, B.R., 2005. The relative cytotoxicity of personal care preservative systems in Balb/C 3T3 clone A31 embryonic mouse cells and the effect of selected preservative systems upon the toxicity of a standard rinse-off formulation. Toxicol. Vitro. 08872333. 19 (7), 963–969. doi:10.1016/j.tiv.2005.06.014.

Souak, D., Barreau, M., Courtois, A., André, V., Duclairoir Poc, C., Feuilloley, M.G.J., Gault, M., 2021. Challenging cosmetic innovation: the skin microbiota and probiotics protect the skin from UV-induced damage. Microorganisms. 2076-2607. 9 (5), 936. doi:10.3390/microorganisms9050936.

Steenbergen, L., Sellaro, R., van Hemert, S., Bosch, J.A., Colzato, L.S., 2015. A randomized controlled trial to test the effect of multispecies probiotics on cognitive reactivity to sad mood. Brain Behav. Immun. 10902139. 48, 258–264. Available from: http://www.elsevier.com/inca/publications/store/6/2/2/8/0/0/index.htt. doi:10.1016/j.bbi.2015.04.003.

Strahl, H., Errington, J., 2017. Bacterial membranes: structure, domains, and function. Annu. Rev. Microbiol. 0066-4227. 71 (1), 519–538. doi:10.1146/annurev-micro-102215-095630.

Sultana, S., Sultana, R., Al-Mansur, M.A., Akbor, M.A., Bhuiyan, N.A., Ahmed, S., Yasmin, S., Jamal, A.H.M.S.I.M., 2024. An industrially potent rhamnolipid-like biosurfactant produced from a novel oil-degrading bacterium, *Bacillus velezensis* S2. RSC Adv. 20462069. 14 (34), 24516–24533. Available from: http://pubs.rsc.org/en/journals/journal/ra. doi:10.1039/d4ra02572e.

Sun, Q., Yin, S., Yingxu, H., Cao, Y., Jiang, C., 2023. Biomaterials and encapsulation techniques for probiotics: current status and future prospects in biomedical applications. Nanomaterials. 2079-4991. 13 (15), 2185. doi:10.3390/nano13152185.

Sun, S., Yu, Y., Jo, Y., Han, J.H., Xue, Y., Cho, M., Bae, S.J., Ryu, D., Park, W., Ha, K.T., Zhuang, S., 2025. Impact of extraction techniques on phytochemical composition and bioactivity of natural product mixtures. Front. Pharmacol. 16639812. 16. Available from: http://www.frontiersin.org/Pharmacology. doi:10.3389/fphar.2025.1615338.

Teleanu, R.I., Moldoveanu, E.T., Niculescu, A.G., Predescu, E., Roza, E., Tincu, I.F., Grumezescu, A.M., Teleanu, D.M., 2025. Liposomal and lipid-based drug delivery systems: bridging gut microbiota and pediatric disorder treatments. Pharmaceutics. 19994923. 17 (6). Available from: http://www.mdpi.com/journal/pharmaceutics. doi:10.3390/pharmaceutics17060707.

Tenorio-Jiménez, C., José Martínez-Ramírez, M., Gil, Á., Gómez-Llorente, C., 2020. Effects of probiotics on metabolic syndrome: a systematic review of randomized clinical trials. Nutrients. 2072-6643. 12 (1), 124. doi:10.3390/nu12010124.

Thomas, C.M., Saulnier, D.M.A., Spinler, J.K., Hemarajata, P., Gao, C., Jones, S.E., Grimm, A., Balderas, M.A., Burstein, M.D., Morra, C., Roeth, D., Kalkum, M., Versalovic, J., 2016. FolC2-mediated folate metabolism contributes to suppression of inflammation by probiotic *Lactobacillus reuteri*. MicrobiologyOpen. 20458827. 5 (5), 802–818. Available from: http://onlinelibrary.wiley.com/journal/10.1002/(ISSN)2045-8827. doi:10.1002/mbo3.371.

Togo, C., Zidorio, A.P., Gonçalves, V., Botelho, P., de Carvalho, K., Dutra, E., 2022. Does probiotic consumption enhance wound healing? A systematic review. Nutrients. 2072-6643. 14 (1), 111. doi:10.3390/nu14010111.

Torabi, S., Nahidi, Y., Ghasemi, S.Z., Reihani, A., Samadi, A., Ramezanghorbani, N., Nazari, E., Davoudi, S., 2025. Evaluation of skin cancer prevention properties of probiotics. Genes Nutr. 18653499. 20 (1). Available from: https://genesandnutrition.biomedcentral.com. doi:10.1186/s12263-025-00770-z.

Utami, L.A., Putri, D.H., 2020. The effect of ethanol solvent concentration on antimicrobial activities the extract of Andalas endophytic bacteria (*Morus macroura* Miq.) fermentation product. Eksakta. 2549-7464. 21 (1), 1–6. doi:10.24036/eksakta/vol21-iss1/210.

Valpaços, C., Leclerc-Mercier, S., Lopes, L., Svoboda, D., Miranda, D., Correia, P., Junior, J., Fernandes, E., Francois-Newton, V., Mandary, M.B., Gueniche, A., Tan, J., Kerob, D., 2023. Benefits of the dermocosmetic mineral 89 probiotic fractions adjunct to topical retinoids for anti-aging benefits. Clin. Cosmet. Investig. Dermatol.. 11787015. 16, 375–385. Available from: https://www.dovepress.com/getfile.php?fileID=87390. doi:10.2147/CCID.S396952.

Venosi, S., Ceccarelli, G., de Angelis, M., Laghi, L., Bianchi, L., Martinelli, O., Maruca, D., Cavallari, E.N., Toscanella, F., Vassalini, P., Trinchieri, V., Oliva, A., d'Ettorre, G., 2019. Infected chronic ischemic wound topically treated with a multi-strain probiotic formulation: a novel tailored treatment strategy. J. Transl. Med. 1479-5876. 17 (1). doi:10.1186/s12967-019-2111-0.

Vivek, K., Mishra, S., Pradhan, R.C., Nagarajan, M., Kumar, P.K., Singh, S.S., Manvi, D., Gowda, N.N., 2023. A comprehensive review on microencapsulation of probiotics: technology, carriers and current trends. Appl. Food Res. 27725022. 3 (1). Available from: https://www.journals.elsevier.com/applied-food-research. doi:10.1016/j.afres.2022.100248.

Vladić, J., Jerković, I., Radman, S., Jazić, J.M., Ferreira, A., Maletić, S., Gouveia, L., 2022. Supercritical CO_2 extract from microalga *Tetradesmus obliquus*: the effect of high-pressure pre-treatment. Molecules. 1420-3049. 27 (12), 3883. doi:10.3390/molecules27123883.

Wallace, C.J.K., Milev, R., 2017. The effects of probiotics on depressive symptoms in humans: a systematic review. Ann. Gen. Psychiatry. 1744859X. 16 (1). Available from: http://www.annals-general-psychiatry.com. doi:10.1186/s12991-017-0138-2.

Wang, J., Peng, W., Dhital, S., Aibing, Y., Chen, X.D., 2025. Impact of freezing and freeze drying on *Lactobacillus rhamnosus* GG survival: mechanisms of cell damage and the role of pre-freezing conditions and cryoprotectants. Foods. 2304-8158. 14 (10), 1817. doi:10.3390/foods14101817.

Wang, X., Li, X., Liu, J., Tao, Y., Wang, T., Li, L., 2024a. *Lactobacillus plantarum* promotes wound healing by inhibiting the NLRP3 inflammasome and pyroptosis activation in diabetic foot wounds. J. Inflamm. Res. 11787031. 17, 1707–1720. Available from: https://www.dovepress.com/getfile.php?fileID=97636. doi:10.2147/JIR.S449565.

Wang, X., Mengxi, Y., Jianming, Y., Liu, T., Jian, L., Zheng, X., Wang, Y., Song, W., Luo, Y., Yue, T., 2024b. Research advances on encapsulation of probiotics with nanomaterials and their repair mechanisms on intestinal barriers. Food Sci. Hum. Wellness. 2097-0765. 13 (6), 3095–3109. doi:10.26599/fshw.2022.9250246.

Wong, F., Amir, A., 2019. Mechanics and dynamics of bacterial cell lysis. Biophys. J. 00063495. 116 (12), 2378–2389. doi:10.1016/j.bpj.2019.04.040.

Woo, Y.M., Kim, O.J., Jo, E.S., Jo, M.Y., Ahn, M.Y., Lee, Y.H., Li, C.R., Lee, S.H., Choi, J.S., Ha, J.M., Kim, A., 2019. The effect of *Lactobacillus plantarum* hydrolysates promoting VEGF production on vascular growth and hair growth of C57BL/6 mice. J. Anal. Sci. Technol. 20933371. 10 (1). Available from: https://www.jast-journal.springeropen.com/. doi:10.1186/s40543-019-0178-0.

Wu, Y.J., Wu, W.F., Hung, C.W., Ku, M.S., Liao, P.F., Sun, H.L., Lu, K.H., Sheu, J.N., Lue, K.H., 2017. Evaluation of efficacy and safety of *Lactobacillus rhamnosus* in children aged 4–48 months with atopic dermatitis: an 8-week, double-blind, randomized, placebo-controlled study. J. Microbiol. Immunol. Infect.. 19959133. 50 (5), 684–692. Available from: http://www.elsevier.com/wps/find/journaldescription.cws_home/722895/description#description. doi:10.1016/j.jmii.2015.10.003.

Xiao, J.Z., Kondo, S., Takahashi, N., Miyaji, K., Oshida, K., Hiramatsu, A., Iwatsuki, K., Kokubo, S., Hosono, A., 2003. Effects of milk products fermented by *Bifidobacterium longum* on blood lipids in rats and healthy adult male volunteers. J. Dairy Sci. 00220302. 86 (7), 2452–2461. doi:10.3168/jds.s0022-0302(03)73839-9.

Xie, Y., Peng, Q., Yuyu, J., Xie, A., Yang, L., Shuzhen, M., Zhu, L., Tengxia, H., Xiao, Y., Zhao, J., Zhang, Q., 2021. Isolation and identification of antibacterial bioactive compounds from *Bacillus megaterium* L2. Front. Microbiol. 1664-302X. 12. doi:10.3389/fmicb.2021.645484.

Xu, Y., Dong, M., Xiao, H., Quek, S.Y., Ogawa, Y., Guangyuan, M., Zhang, C., 2024. Advances in spray-dried probiotic microcapsules for targeted delivery: a review. Crit. Rev. Food Sci. Nutr. 1040-8398. 64 (30), 11222–11238. doi:10.1080/10408398.2023.2235424.

Yadav, M.K., Song, J.H., Vasquez, R., Lee, J.S., Kim, I.H., Kang, D.K., 2024. Methods for detection, extraction, purification, and characterization of exopolysaccharides of lactic acid bacteria—a systematic review. Foods. 23048158. 13 (22). Available from: www.mdpi.com/journal/foods. doi:10.3390/foods13223687.

Yoon, Y.C., Ahn, B.H., Min, J.W., Lee, K.R., Park, S.H., Kang, H.C., 2022. Stimulatory effects of extracellular vesicles derived from *Leuconostoc holzapfelii* that exists in human scalp on hair growth in human follicle dermal papilla cells. Curr. Issues Mol. Biol. 14673045. 44 (2), 845–866. Available from: https://www.mdpi.com/1467-3045/44/2/58/pdf. doi:10.3390/cimb44020058.

Yuan, J., Donglin, M., Yang, Y., Zhao, Y., Ren, H., Liu, X., Tan, M., Kuntai, L., 2025. A review and prospects: multi-omics and artificial intelligence-based approaches to understanding the effects of lactic acid bacteria and yeast interactions on fermented foods. Innov. Food Sci. Emerg. Technol. 14668564. 99, 103874. doi:10.1016/j.ifset.2024.103874.

Zhang, Y., Liu, P., Hao, F., Wang, D., Zhao, D., Zhang, J., Wang, C., Meng, L., 2022. Effects of *Lactobacillus kefiri* fermentation supernatant on skin aging caused by oxidative stress. J. Funct. Foods. 17564646. 96, 105222. doi:10.1016/j.jff.2022.105222.

Zheng, Y., Hunt, R.L., Villaruz, A.E., Fisher, E.L., Liu, R., Liu, Q., Cheung, G.Y.C., Li, M., Otto, M., 2022. Commensal *Staphylococcus epidermidis* contributes to skin barrier homeostasis by generating protective ceramides. Cell Host Microbe. 19346069. 30 (3), 301. Available from: http://www.elsevier.com. doi:10.1016/j.chom.2022.01.004.

Zhou, J., Wang, M., Saraiva, J.A., Martins, A.P., Pinto, C.A., Prieto, M.A., Simal-Gandara, J., Cao, H., Xiao, J., Barba, F.J., 2022. Extraction of lipids from microalgae using classical and innovative approaches. Food Chem. 18737072. 384. Available from: www.elsevier.com/locate/foodchem. doi:10.1016/j.foodchem.2022.132236.

Zhou, X., Du, H.H., Ni, L., Ran, J., Hu, J., Yu, J., Zhao, X., 2021. Nicotinamide mononucleotide combined with *Lactobacillus fermentum* TKSN041 reduces the photoaging damage in murine skin by activating AMPK signaling pathway. Front. Pharmacol. 16639812. 12. Available from: http://www.frontiersin.org/Pharmacology. doi:10.3389/fphar.2021.643089.

Chapter 17

Fungi

Mehak Kaur[a,b], Kusum Kumari[a], Sunil Kumar Deshmukh[c], and Mayurika Goel[a]

[a]*Sustainable Agriculture Program, The Energy and Resources Institute, TERI-Gual Pahari, Gurugram, Haryana, India*

[b]*Department of Botany, University of Delhi, Delhi, India*

[c]*Research and Development, Greenvention Biotech Pvt. Ltd., Pune, Maharashtra, India*

1 Introduction

Nowadays, the majority of cosmetic products used in various forms consist of around 15–20 synthetic, petroleum-based, nonbiodegradable, and toxic chemicals (Oliver and Selinger, 2022). These include heavy metals, toxic elements, phthalates, parabens, and other chemicals identified as allergens, skin sensitizers, irritants, and acutely toxic substances (Panico et al., 2019). Benzophenones, a class of compounds used as ultraviolet (UV) filters in sunscreens, have been found to be procarcinogenic, hormone disruptors, and allergens. Furthermore, high absorption, long-term detection, and destruction of human tissues and environment have been linked to the compound owing to its lipophilic properties (Kerdivel et al., 2013). The harmful effects of preservatives such as parabens on keratinocytes, fibroblasts, and collagen expression and triclosan on the liver, hormones, muscles, and immunity have been reported since past decade (Dhillon et al., 2015; Lee et al., 2019; Dinwiddie et al., 2014; Matwiejczuk et al., 2020). The trace presence of heavy metals such as lead, aluminum, chromium, cadmium, zinc, titanium, and manganese in lip products has always been a major concern (Goyal and Jerold, 2023). This unknown exposure to hazardous chemicals calls for an urgent need of transition to nature-derived cosmetics. Besides the toxicity concerns, sustainability considerations such as environmental impact, cost-effectiveness, and long-term health benefits advocate for a shift from conventional to biobased cosmetics. The rapid depletion of nonrenewable resources and stringent environmental regulations have further increased the demand for high-performance, safe, sustainable, and natural products derived from plants and microorganisms in recent years (Goyal and Jerold, 2023).

Biocosmetics are made entirely of natural ingredients sourced from plants, animals, microbes, enzymes, insects, and organically grown crops and are used for topical and oral applications (Vandamme, 2001). These biobased personal care products offer advantages such as waste reduction, recyclability, low energy consumption, and safety (Secchi et al., 2016). They can be produced, sourced, and distributed more cost-effectively compared to their chemical counterparts, thanks to modern biorefinery technologies and biobased processes such as fermentation. The integration of pharmacy-like therapeutic properties with cosmetics results in cosmeceuticals, a marketing gimmick term that lacks a legal definition. Today's conscious consumers seek multifunctional cosmetic products, such as lipsticks that not only provide vibrant color but also repair chapped lips. Cosmeceuticals are classified according to the target conditions they address, such as skin lightening, sun protection, scar reduction, antioxidants, and antiaging effects. Naturally occurring secondary metabolites known as bioactives have been reported to either naturally possess such properties or can be biotechnologically manipulated to manifest cosmeceutical properties. When it comes to sources of bioactives, plants, microorganisms, and insects are the major market players. Bioactive isolation from plants for cosmetics is cumbersome, energy and cost-intensive, while yielding lower outputs. Insect bioactives, such as carmine, raise ethical concerns for some geopolitical communities. Microorganisms such as bacteria, fungi, and algae have recently emerged as sustainable, vegan, and natural solutions to these issues. Among them, fungi are well-known for their diverse bioactives and adaptable nature, making them a robust source for biobased cosmetic ingredients. For example, anthraquinones from *Monascus* are known to impart yellow to maroon shades while exhibiting in-built antioxidant, antimicrobial, and antiinflammatory properties (Kaur et al., 2023; Kalra et al., 2020). Mixed-culture (*Aspergillus oryzae* and *Rhizopus oryzae*) fermented rice bran, on the contrary, has been reported to possess cosmeceutical

Biofunctional Cosmetics for Health. https://doi.org/10.1016/B978-0-443-27500-5.00029-0

properties such as antipigmentation and antiaging effects (Abd Razak et al., 2017). This chapter, thus, unifies the cosmeceutical applications of fungi in incorporating new-generation safe ingredients into cosmetic products. Innovation results from the integration of basic, applied, and industrial research, leading to new fungal products and inevitable growth. Over the past two decades, fungal biotechnology has notably progressed from academic research to industrial applications, particularly in the pharmaceutical and cosmetic sectors. The natural compounds derived from fungal biotechnology are produced through sustainable methods and have demonstrated the ability to reduce harmful substances, benefiting humans, animals, plants, and the environment. In regard to these recent innovations, the regulatory framework and global market outlook are also discussed in further sections.

2 The cosmetic properties of fungi

Cuticle is the major skin barrier present in humans, containing keratinocytes along with protein-rich and lipid-rich cells. When it gets damaged, dryness, dullness, and invasion by external microbes and irritants occur, triggering inflammatory reactions, aging, cuticle damage, and other such symptoms. Therefore to establish healthy external beauty, internal skin repair is crucial (Ding et al., 2022). Fungal bioactives can be harnessed as sustainable and natural cosmetic ingredients with multifunctional properties, as shown in Fig. 17.1. These bioactives impart climate adaptability to fungi, enabling them to survive in distinct environmental conditions such as extreme hot springs, cold glaciers, and salty marine habitats (Agrawal et al., 2018). Some of the compounds derived from fungi for cosmetic applications include lactic acid, proteins, ceramides, antioxidants, and chitin–glucans, which enhance the esthetic appeal and impart cosmeceutical benefits to the skin (Table 17.1).

2.1 Skin repairing and wound healing

Conventional wound dressings can cause irritation while having poor wound compatibility and inefficiency in chronic wound treatment, highlighting the need for biocompatible alternatives that accelerate healing naturally (Jones et al., 2020). Natural protection of skin fibrocytes with antimicrobial properties is essential to address skin problems, and thus exploration of natural resources for multifunctional bioactives is needed. Utilizing antioxidants can protect and repair skin cells, boost their vitality and connectivity, enhance immune capacity, and reduce free radical damage. Bioactive indole derivatives isolated from the marine fungus *Hyrtios* sp. have shown antioxidant capacity similar to that of Trolox, a commercial antioxidant. An aromatic polyketone compound isolated from the sponge-derived fungus *Aspergillus versicolor*

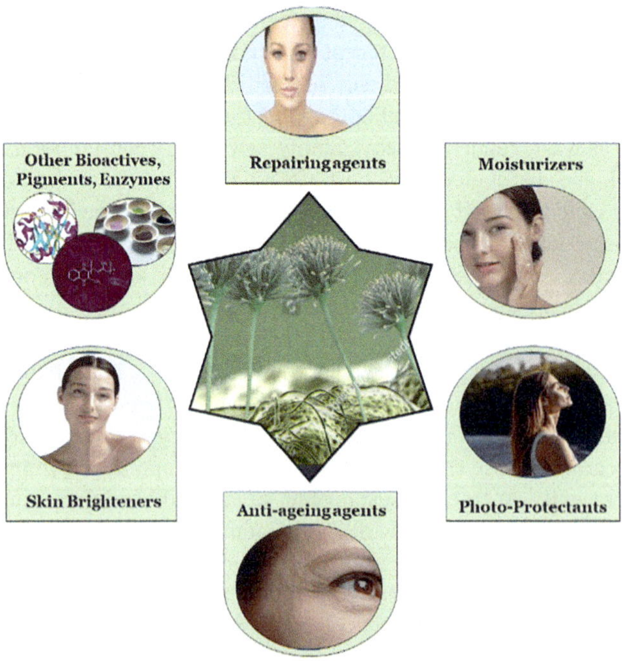

FIG. 17.1 Different types of cosmetic bioactives from fungi. The figure gives an idea about various applications of bioactives from fungi, viz., skin brightener, moisturizer, photoprotection, etc.

TABLE 17.1 Multifunctional properties of fungal bioactives.

Functional ingredient	Source	Cosmetic effect	Reference
Azelaic acid	*Malassezia furfur*	Hyperpigmentation, acne breakouts, skin inflammation and infections	(Ashbee and Bignell, 2010)
Chitin	Fungal cell wall	Antimicrobial, antiinflammatory, antioxidant, antiaging, firming, regenerative, and moisturizing effects, reinstating skin elasticity and stimulating collagen synthesis	(Sułkowska-Ziaja et al., 2023)
Coumarins	*Aspergillus, Fomitopsis officinalis, Penicillium, Talaromyces flavus, Xylaria* sp., *Trichosporon asahii*	Fixative in deodorants and perfumes, and antioxidant activity	(Costa et al., 2016)
Crude extract	Lichenised fungi *Bryoria capillaris*	UV protection, antioxidant capacity, and tyrosinase inhibitory activity	(Toksoz et al., 2023)
Lactic acid	*Rhizopus* genera	Moisturizing, antiaging, UV protection, skin-peeling, and exfoliating agent for lightening	(Gupta et al., 2019)
Lasiodiplodan	*Lasiodiplodia theobromae*	Antiaging and wound healing	(Cunha et al., 2019)
Mannosylerythritol lipids	*Candida*	Moisturizing, antioxidant, protective, and healing effects with repairing damaged hair	(Morita et al., 2015)
Mycelium culture medium	*Ceriporia lacerata*	Antiwrinkling, antiinflammatory, and wound healing activities	(Kim et al., 2021)
Pigments	*Monascus, Neurospora, Penicillium, Aspergillus, Alternaria, Talaromyces, Phaffia*	Color, antioxidant, antiinflammatory, UV protection, antimicrobial, anticancer, and wound healing	(Kalra et al., 2020)
Sophorolipids	*Candida bombicola*	Treatment of acne, dandruff, and body odors	(Dhevagi et al., 2021)

showed good antioxidant activity in experiments (Ding et al., 2022). ACCB (*Aspergillus chevalieri* TM2-S6 cultivation broth extract), a culture filtrate of *A.. chevalieri* TC2-S6 isolated from a marine sponge, contained two bioactives, tetrahydroauroglaucin and flavoglaucin, capable of protecting human fibrocytes under oxidative stress conditions (Ding et al., 2022). While these ideas offer methods for skin repair, the effective combination of these functional molecules to create novel skin repair products still requires experimental validation (Mishra et al., 2022). Application of powdered mycelium from *Aspergillus niger*, *Penicillium notatum*, and *Phycomyces mucor* on wounded rats increased the tensile strength of the skin, showing that it can withstand a higher amount of stress than untreated wounds (Prudden et al., 1970). Treated *Mucor mucedo*, *A. oryzae*, and *Phycomyces blakesleeanus* mycelia demonstrated increased cell proliferation in fibrocytes at low concentrations. Chitosan, known for enhancing skin healing, reducing scars, and its antiinflammatory, antioxidant, and antimicrobial properties, is a popular constituent in wound treatment technologies commercially derived from fungi of the family *Mucoraceae* (Jones et al., 2020).

2.2 Skin whitening

In reality, the societal promotion of fairness as a beauty standard leads to self-doubt and low confidence, which skin-whitening companies exploit to sell their products effectively. Melanin is the pigment responsible for determining skin color, and its production is controlled by tyrosinase, a target enzyme for skin-brightening cosmetics. Some of the compounds derived from fungi boasting skin-whitening qualities are kojic acid, azelaic acid, ellagic acid, and 3,4-dihydroxybenzaldehyde (Sułkowska-Ziaja et al., 2023). *A. niger* acts upon plant tannins to produce the compounds ellagic and gallic acid with antioxidant properties recommended for use in skin-whitening products such as Shu Uemura White Recovery EX + Brightening Oil (Hyde et al., 2010). Kojic acid, a compound known for increasing skin brightness and its antimicrobial properties, is produced by several *Aspergillus* and *Penicillium* species. It is also a mainstream by-product of fungal-fermented rice. The practice of making cosmeceutical kojic acid from fungal-fermented rice at home has been reported since ages, especially in Japan. Derivatives of kojic acid, such as kojic acid dimethyl ether and kojic acid monomethyl ether, as well as phomaligol A, identified from marine *Alternaria* sp., exhibit tyrosinase inhibitory activity (Corinaldesi et al., 2017). Screening of wild fungal isolates for melanolytic activity resulted in the identification of *Sporotrichum pruinosum*, the most promising fungus that decolorized synthetic melanin (Hyde et al., 2010). Similarly, azelaic acid, produced by the marine fungus *Malassezia* sp., is an inhibitor of tyrosinase. A competitive inhibitor of tyrosinase, similar to the structure of homothallin II, was isolated from the *Trichoderma viridae* strain H1-7 from marine sediments, which inhibited the enzyme by binding to its copper active site. The marine fungus *Botrytis* sp. was found to produce an α-pyrone derivative (6-[(E)-hept-1-enyl]-α-pyrone) characterized by antityrosinase activity (Agrawal et al., 2018). A cyclopentenone compound, myrothenone A, found in *Myrothecium* sp. strain MFA58 showed tyrosinase inhibitor activity that was greater than that of kojic acid. Two new sesquiterpene compounds, 1β, 5α, 6α, 14-tetraacetoxy-9α-benzoyloxy-7βH-eudesman-2β, 11-diol and 4α, 5α-diacetoxy-9α-benzoyloxy-7βH-eudesman-1β, 2β, 11, 14-tetraol, isolated from the marine fungus *Pestalotiopsis* sp. strain Z233, also exhibited tyrosinase inhibitory activity. Cydromicin, a secondary metabolite produced by *Tolypocladium* sp. strain SCSIO 40433, isolated from Arctic glacial sediments, also showed tyrosinase inhibitor activity (Ding et al., 2022).

2.3 Antiwrinkling/antiaging

In aging, the final pathway of all mechanisms involves the disruption of the network of collagen and elastin, which, along with dehydration, leads to fine wrinkles (Wu et al., 2016). Another primary factor causing skin aging in humans is the oxidative change in the body (Agrawal et al., 2018). Reactive oxygen species (ROS) are highly reactive radicals that aggressively seek to pair their unpaired electrons by attacking nearby chemical compounds. Antioxidants inhibit the oxidation reaction of free radicals by exchanging one of their own electrons with the free radical molecules to stabilize them (Kaur et al., 2024). Neutralizing these free or peroxide radicals with antioxidants is essential for protecting cells from oxidative stress. Using antioxidants is an effective approach for antiaging supplements, with marine fungi such as *Penicillium* and *Acremonium* being excellent sources of antioxidant compounds. Gallic acid isolated from *A. niger*, *Fusarium solani,* and *T. viridae* exhibited free radical scavenging activities (Gupta et al., 2019). Numerous antioxidant compounds, including tocopherols, phenolic compounds, ergosterol, benzoic acids, sesquiterpenes, gentisyl alcohol, gallic acid, lectins, and polysaccharides, have been identified in the *Penicillium* genus of fungi that can be utilized as cosmetic ingredients (Kaur et al., 2024). *Epicoccum* sp., derived from a macroalga, produced a compound with high α, α-diphenyl-picrylhydrazyl radical scavenging activity. Likewise, *Aspergillus wentii* EN-48 isolated from brown alga produced metabolites with antioxidant activities (Agrawal et al., 2018).

2.4 Moisturizing

Moisturizing products formulated with humectants or occlusive ingredients help retain water in the stratum corneum and suppress trans-epidermal water loss. Higher-molecular-weight polysaccharides form net-like structures that prevent water loss, offering better moisturizing retention properties (Yao and Baojun, 2022). Commercial moisturizers help in decelerating the loss of skin humidity and minimizing fine wrinkles (Wu et al., 2016). Chitosan, with its superior water-binding capacity compared to methyl cellulose, is ideal as a skin moisturizer and delivery system in antiaging cosmeceutical products. Zygomycetes are considered a good source of chitosan and chitin as they are the major constituents of the cell walls. Examples include *A. niger*, *R. oryzae*, and *Trichoderma reesei* (Huq et al., 2022). Trehalose, with its sulfate forms, is used as a moisture retention agent in some cosmetic creams and lotions, while its fatty acid esters act as surface-active agents (Ohtake and Wang, 2011). Trehalose has been found in several fungi such as *Aspergillus*, *Cryptococcus*, *Penicillium,* and others because of its role in stress adaption and has shown excellent antioxidant and high water-retaining properties. This makes it useful in moisturizer creams in cosmetic products (Ribeiro et al., 2024). In a study, it was found that *Mortierella* fungus produced cis-11-eicosenoic acid, which can be used in cosmetic creams for moisturizing benefits (Kikukawa et al., 2015). Glycosphingolipids, a constituent of lipid rafts found in filamentous fungi such as *Aspergillus,* act as a barrier function in the skin to retain moisture, which makes this compound a potent moisturizing ingredient (Jiang et al., 2021). Hyaluronic acid, which is a main component in moisturizing creams, can be extracted from fungi such as *Cryptococcus neoformans*, *Saccharomyces cerevisiae*, and *Pichia pastoris* (Shikina et al., 2022).

2.5 Photoprotective

Overexposure to UV rays can lead to mutagenic effects and damage to the epidermal layers of human skin. It also induces the formation of ROS, contributing to the loss of skin elasticity, skin cancer, or skin photoaging (Ding et al., 2022). Sunscreens help in reducing the damage caused by UV rays. Three novel benzodiazepine alkaloids, circumdatin I, C, and

G, isolated from the marine fungus *Exophiala,* showed good anti-UV activity and were more efficient than oxybenzone, which is currently used in sunscreen (Zhang et al., 2008). The same characteristics have been shown by the two compounds golmaenone and neoechinulin A, isolated from the marine fungus *Aspergillus* sp. (Ding et al., 2022). Marine organisms are known as sources of photoprotective compounds, including mycosporines, mycosporine-like amino acids (MAAs), and several other UV filters, such as carotenoids and scytonemin. Examples of mycosporine-producing marine fungi are *Trimmatostroma salinum*, *Phaeotheca triangularis*, *Cryptococcus liquefaciens*, *Aureobasidium pullulans*, and *Hortaea werneckii,* which absorb UV in the range of 310–320 nm. Three unidentified UV-absorbable compounds recognized as MAAs have been found in fungi inhabiting glaciers and high-salt waters. Other than the potential use of fungi in prevention, some fungal metabolites also help in treating the damaged parts of the skin, such as schizophyllan, a *Schizophyllum commune*-derived compound containing β-1,6-branched-β-1,3-glucan that decreases the irritation and inflammation caused by UV damage (Hyde et al., 2010). Glucomannans (GM) from fungal cell walls have significant photoprotective effects. GM has been shown to suppress ultraviolet-B (UVB)-induced decreases in keratinocyte viability, reduce caspase activation, and inhibit proinflammatory gene expression. It also decreases UV-induced skin erythema and phospholipase A2 activity, providing overall protection to human keratinocytes (Ruszova et al., 2008).

2.6 Pigments

Beautiful colors provide sensory enjoyment and are found in several cosmetics. Natural pigments, such as microbial pigments, are widely used in cosmetics such as sunscreen, makeup, skin lightening, and antiaging products due to their safety, efficacy, and stability (Gupta et al., 2019). Fungi are considered great sources of novel, stable, and safe biological pigments with therapeutic properties. Filamentous fungi, such as *Neurospora*, *Penicillium,* and *Monascus,* are primarily known for the production of pigmented compounds, including polyketides, terpenoids, polyphenols, anthocyanins, anthraquinones, and carotenoids (Kalra et al., 2020). Fungal pigments are found to have several pharmacological activities, such as prevention against photo-oxidation, UV protection, antioxidant, antiinflammatory, antimicrobial, wound healing, and protection against environmental stresses (Kalra et al., 2020). A pigment from a marine *Aspergillus nidulans* was found to be similar to 5,6-dihydroxyindole-2-carboxylic acid, the precursor of melanin, which can reduce ROS generation after UV irradiation and has the potential for use in sunscreen formulations (Ding et al., 2022). Melanin, with photoprotection and antioxidant effects, has been extracted from many fungal species, such as *C. neoformans*, *Colletotrichum lagenarium*, *Exophiala*, *Paracoccidioides brasiliensis*, *Magnaporthe grisea*, *Sporothrix schenckii*, and *Aspergillus fumigatus*. Alterporriols from *Alternaria*, Arpink Red from *Penicillium*, rubrocristin, and catenarin from *Aspergillus* are identified red pigments from fungal sources with cosmeceutical properties (Kalra et al., 2020). The red color extracts produced by *Talaromyces* and *Monascus* were found to have roles in the cosmetic sector as antioxidant, antimicrobial, anticancer, and antiinflammatory agents (Kaur et al., 2023; Mishra et al., 2021). *Monascus*-fermented rice, termed red koji rice, has been used since ancient times in cosmetics due to its cosmeceutical properties (Kaur et al., 2023). Carotenoids, which are responsible for most of the red, orange, and yellow colors in nature, are being used in cosmetics due to their stability in emulsions, solubility, and antioxidant properties. Astaxanthin, produced by fungi such as *Rhodotorula*, *Phaffia,* and *Xanthophyllomyces,* has wide applications in skin protection and as an antioxidant (Dhevagi et al., 2021). Astaxanthin has been added as an active ingredient in some cosmetics, such as Geisha Astaxanthin Refining Serum, Kose Becky Firming Essence, and Home Facial Pro Astaxanthin (Ding et al., 2022).

2.7 Enzymes

Enzymes derived from fungi are predominantly used in the food industry to enhance the flavor of foods, but they also play an important role in the cosmetic industry. Melanocytic enzymes extracted from fungi such as *S. pruinosum*, *Acrostaphylus* sp., *Galactomyces geotrichum*, and *Phanerochaete chrysosporium* demonstrated effective degradation of skin melanin, opening up possibilities for the skin-lightening industry (Mohorčič et al., 2007). An enzyme produced by *S. pruinosum* helps in degrading melanin rather than inhibiting its synthesis, as other skin-lightening products are mechanized to do (Mohorčič et al., 2007). There is potential for manganese peroxidase (MnP) purified from *Geotrichum* sp. to be used as a skin-lightening agent in the cosmetic industry (Kim and Jung-Mo Ahn, 2016). Lignin peroxidase, found to play an important role in the degradation of eumelanin, leads to the amplification of processes associated with skin lightening (Gupta, 2023). Lipase isolated from *Rhizomucor miehei* is used as a biocatalyst in the production of personal care products such as skin creams and bath oils (Kumar et al., 2023). Excessive oil secretion may affect the microbial environment of the face, leading to acne. Therefore it is particularly important to clean the face. Lipase can catalyze the hydrolysis of insoluble triglycerides into glycerol diesters and glycerol monomers, producing cleansing facial oil. These enzymes are, thus, employed in various formulations, including products for nasal washes, cosmetic facades, and hair care, due to their superior ability to digest lipids (Gupta, 2023).

2.8 Miscellaneous

Globally, >80% of people suffer from acne at some point in their lives. Over 80% of individuals who had clindamycin-resistant *Propionibacterium acnes* also had clindamycin-resistant *Staphylococcus epidermidis*. Therefore there is a need to discover new bioactive molecules against both *P. acnes* and *S. epidermidis*. The two unusual pyridones, trichodin A and trichodin B, extracted from the mycelia and culture broth of the marine fungus *Trichoderma* sp. strain MF106 showed antibiotic activity against *S. epidermidis*, with IC_{50} values of 24 μM and 4 μM, respectively (Agrawal et al., 2018). Biosurfactant extracted from the yeast *Scheffersomyces shehatae* has demonstrated effectiveness in makeup removal, comparable to the cleansing activity of a 1% sodium dodecyl sulfate solution and micellar water used for removing cosmetic products (Cedrola et al., 2024). Due to chitosan's bioadhesive properties, film formation ability, curl retention, and stiffness, it is used as an ingredient in various hair care products, including shampoos, hair gels, hair colorants, hair sprays, permanent wave agents, styling lotions, and hair tonics (Corinaldesi et al., 2017). In the cosmetic industry, formic acid works best as a fragrance ingredient. Fungal genera such as *Aspergillus*, *Penicillium*, *Rhizopus,* and *Trichoderma* are known to produce cosmetic organic acids such as formic acid, lactic acid, and citric acid (Gaur et al., 2024).

3 Current innovations in fungal cosmetics

3.1 Fungal fermentation for bioactives

Biotechnological processes impact the cosmetic industry by producing safe and effective fermented ingredients that are emerging as a new generation of active compounds (Gomes et al., 2020). In fermentation, microbes or enzymes act upon raw materials, enabling large-scale production of exopolysaccharides, enzymes, secondary metabolites, and other cosmetic ingredients. Kojic acid, hyaluronic acid, chitosan, resveratrol, sclerotium gum, superoxide dismutase, and photolyase are among the major cosmetic ingredients produced with the help of fungal fermentation (Abrashev et al., 2016; Peng et al., 2021). Several organic acids, such as citric acid, lactic acid, and glycolic acid, generated through fungal fermentation processes, are highly versatile and utilized as key ingredients in the cosmetic industry (Vandenberghe et al., 2017). Recently, anisic acid derivatives have been produced via fermentation using *Rhizopycnis vagum* isolated from the tissues of *Nicotiana tabacum* (Wang et al., 2018). Hemisqualane, synthesized through the fermentation of sugarcane by *Yarrowia lipolytica*, serves as a sustainable alternative to toxic cyclomethicone, a liquid silicone employed as a stabilizer in cosmetic products with issues of bioaccumulation (McPhee et al., 2014). Various types of exopolysaccharides are also produced by fungal fermentation; for example, schizophyllan, a bioactive polymer and humectant, is produced by *S. commune* (Selvasekaran et al., 2021). A cost-effective route has been developed by utilizing bagasse for the co-production of the biopolymer together with cellulolytic enzymes (Arunrattanamook et al., 2022). Sclerotium gum, an emulsifier, stabilizer, and thickener, is produced by *Sclerotium rolfsii* and commercialized under the Amigel and Actigum trade names. Pullulan, a fibrous polymer used for its photoprotective, binding, and film-forming properties, is produced via batch fermentation of *A. pullulans* (Pérez-Rivero and López-Gómez, 2023). Other polysaccharides, such as chitin and chitosan, with UV-protective, moisturizing, and film-forming properties, have been produced by *Mucor rouxii* and *R. oryzae* from whey medium and molasses (Aranaz et al., 2018). KitoZyme, Mycoved, and Chibio are companies that produce these multifunctional polysaccharides through fungal fermentation processes.

3.2 Endophytic fungi for bioactives

The extraction of bioactive compounds from plant sources is a cumbersome process, which necessitates the massive destruction of plants, causing disruption in ecosystems. This major constraint limits the large-scale production of natural active ingredients through plants. As a potential solution, endophytic fungi are being explored for the production of bioactive compounds in a free fermentative medium. Endophytic fungi exist in a symbiotic relationship with plant tissues, providing secondary defense metabolites to the plants. Endophytic fungi, namely, *Alternaria* sp. *MG1*, *Arcopilus aureus,* and *A. niger*, have been identified to synthesize resveratrol, a type of stilbene known for its antioxidant and antiaging properties (Dwibedi and Saxena, 2019; Liu et al., 2016; Shi et al., 2012). Biotechnological tools such as epigenetic modification, growth optimization with natural supplements, precursor feeding, chemical elicitors, and co-culturing have been employed to augment extracellular resveratrol production by the endophytic fungus *A. aureus* (Dwibedi and Saxena, 2019). This resulted in a cost-effective fermentation process for the production of resveratrol, addressing the increasing global demand for this compound. *Alternaria*, an endophytic fungus isolated from black grape, has been identified as the most potent and stable isolate for producing novel structural analogues of resveratrol with antitumor activity (Shi et al., 2012; Wang et al., 2014). Another endophytic fungal isolate from the same plant, *A. niger* C2J6 has also synthesized resveratrol in fermentation (Liu et al., 2016). One study has reported sucrose as the carbon source responsible for high-concentration resveratrol production from an endophytic *Aspergillus* strain (Roat and Saraf, 2016). Exploration of endophytic fungi for large-scale production of bioactive ingredients constitutes a relatively underexplored research domain, which requires attention from the cosmetic researchers' community.

3.3 Enzyme immobilization

Fungal enzymes play a major role in skin exfoliation, rejuvenation, and betterment. However, there are still some major barriers to their commercial application. Under harsh conditions, such as strong acidity or high temperature, free enzyme denaturation can occur, reducing their activity and substrate affinity (Franssen et al., 2013). To address these challenges, immobilization technologies have been employed to enhance enzymatic catalytic properties and stability. Immobilization optimizes enzyme–substrate interactions while minimizing nonspecific binding (Homaei et al., 2013). Immobilized enzymes offer prolonged operational stability, easy recovery, reusability, improved efficiency, and reduced process costs (Hassan et al., 2019; Datta et al., 2013). A variety of materials, including glass, natural and synthetic polymers, alginate, and activated carbon, serve as conventional supports for enzyme immobilization. Lactobionic acid (LBA) has recently gained attention as a valuable natural support for enzyme immobilization in the cosmetics industry. It can be produced by *Penicillium chrysogenum* through lactose conversion or enzymatically by catalase from *A. niger*. LBA is utilized in skincare products due to its moisturizing, cross-linking, antiaging, antioxidant, keratinizing, and solubilizing attributes (Alonso et al., 2013). The integration of fungal enzymes with immobilization signifies the advancing evolution of enzymatic technology aimed at enhancing the efficiency of biocatalysts for cosmetic active ingredients.

3.4 Nanotechnology

Nanotechnology (nanoparticles, NPs) has been extensively utilized in cosmetics and dermatological products, including soaps, antiwrinkle creams, perfumes, toothpastes, lipsticks, moisturizers, sunscreens, hair care products, skin cleansers, and nail care items (Lohani et al., 2014). Recently, significant attention has been directed toward the development of eco-friendly technologies employing biological agents such as bacteria, fungi, and plants for the synthesis of metal nanoparticles, including gold, silver, and platinum (Rai et al., 2008). Frequent use of phenoxyethanol and parabens as preservatives in cosmetics has been linked to skin irritation and enhanced sensitivity to UV radiation (Handa et al., 2006; Ishiwatari et al., 2007). Therefore researchers have long sought safer alternatives to these chemicals. Silver nanoparticles (Ag-NPs) are now widely employed as preservatives in cosmetic products such as deodorants, face packs, and antiaging creams due to their antimicrobial properties (Gajbhiye and Sakharwade, 2016). Endophytic fungal genera *Penicillium* have been employed to generate *Penicillium* Ag-NPs (PAg-NPs) with potent antimicrobial activity against *Bacillus subtilis, Escherichia coli, Pseudomonas aeruginosa, Staphylococcus aureus, Vibrio cholerae, A. niger, A. pullulans, Penicillium citrinum*, and many strains of *Candida* spp. at concentrations as low as 1 part per million (ppm) (Govindappa et al., 2016; Kim et al., 2008; Kokura et al., 2010). Furthermore, antiinflammatory, antioxidant, and wound healing properties with increased membrane stabilization have also been reported from PAg-NPs (Joel and Bhimba, 2012; Pretsch et al., 2014; Ruma et al., 2013). Phytochemicals, such as tannins, terpenoids, and saponins, isolated from *Penicillium*, can function as reducing and capping agents in the conversion of silver particles into nanoparticles (Govindappa et al., 2016). These agents are crucial to prevent the agglomeration of NPs and to provide stability to the final product (Rai et al., 2008). Titanium dioxide nanoparticles generated from *Aspergillus flavus* exhibited good antimicrobial properties and have found applications in sunscreens, whitening creams, and skin milks (DuPont, 2013; Rajakumar et al., 2012; Rai et al., 2008). In addition to enhancing bioactivities and product stability, nanoparticles can positively impact the appearance of cosmetic products by ensuring a homogeneous look and improving sensory qualities. They help maintain uniformity and prevent sedimentation, thereby supporting the product's esthetic and functional integrity for over a year (Kokura et al., 2010).

4 Regulatory framework for cosmetic ingredients

Due to its innovation, rapid development, and complexity, the cosmetic industry requires stringent regulation to ensure product safety and quality, thereby preventing negative health impacts on consumers. To regulate and continuously monitor them, major markets have established distinct regulatory frameworks, which influence the industry by limiting international trade, innovation, and market growth (Ferreira et al., 2022). International organizations have been established to overcome these regulatory barriers, such as the International Cooperation on Cosmetics Regulation (ICCR), which includes regulatory authorities from Brazil, Canada, Chinese Taipei, the European Union (EU), Japan, South Korea, and the United States. They meet annually to discuss cosmetic safety and regulation topics, such as alternatives to animal testing, nanotechnology, and microbiological limits. The Organization for Economic Co-operation and Development and the International Organization for Standardization also play crucial roles in the mutual acceptance of testing methods and the development of international cosmetic standards (Ferreira et al., 2022).

Regional regulatory frameworks for cosmetics vary significantly, including differing legal definitions of "cosmetic product." These definitions depend on the product's functions, the body parts to which it is applied, its mode of application, associated claims, and consumer perspectives in different regions. In the EU, the European Commission (EC) is responsible for controlling cosmetics through EC Regulation 1223/2009, and in the United States, the Food and Drug Administration (FDA) regulates cosmetics through the Federal Food, Drug, and Cosmetic Act, 1998 (Ferreira et al., 2022). In India, the Central Drugs Standard Control Organization has formed the Drugs and Cosmetics Act in 1940, which regulates the licensing and release of cosmetics, while the Bureau of Indian Standards regulates the ingredients that can be used in cosmetics (Table 17.2). In the EU, a cosmetic product is defined by its site of application and intended functions, and each product is classified into a single category (Couteau and Coiffard, 2010). In contrast, the United States allows a product to belong to both cosmetic and drug categories if it has dual intended uses (FDA, 2018). India takes a broader approach, classifying any product containing a cosmetic ingredient as a cosmetic (Ministry of Health and Family Welfare, Government of India, 2016). This variation between categories and regulations is a universal concern, necessitating further efforts to improve dialog and cooperation among countries.

When it comes to natural cosmetic ingredients, safety and toxicology assessment is still in a nascent form compared to synthetic counterparts. The evasion of the generic misconception that considers natural to be safe should be addressed through scientific validation (Silvério et al., 2023). Natural products, whether single compounds, purified fractions, or crude extracts, are complex and challenging to quantify, which complicates their safety assessments (Shipkowski et al., 2018). Regulatory authorities require safety and toxicological evaluations for new biological or natural extracts to ensure consumer health. New microbial ingredients are also subjected to similar regulations as novel natural ingredients not listed by entities such as the EU and India. The EU and Indian regulations have mandated positive lists for permissible ingredients

TABLE 17.2 Variation in cosmetic regulations across the world.

	European Union	United States	India
Regulation/Act	EC Regulation 1223/2009	Federal Food, Drug, and Cosmetic Act, 1998	The Drugs and Cosmetics Act, 1940, and the Bureau of Indian Standards
"Cosmetic" definition	"Any substance or mixture intended to be placed in contact with the external parts of the human body (epidermis, hair system, nails, lips, and external genital organs) or with the teeth and the mucous membranes of the oral cavity, with a view exclusively or mainly to cleaning them, perfuming them, changing their appearance, protecting them, keeping them in good condition, or correcting body odors"	"Articles intended to be rubbed, poured, sprinkled, or sprayed on, introduced into, or otherwise applied to the human body for cleansing, beautifying, promoting attractiveness, or altering the appearance"	"Any article intended to be rubbed, poured, sprinkled, or sprayed on, or introduced into, or otherwise applied to the human body or any part thereof for cleansing, beautifying, promoting attractiveness, or altering the appearance, and includes any article intended for use as a component of a cosmetic"
Regulation on ingredients	Bans >1400 chemicals, has positive and negative lists for permitted and restricted ingredients	Bans <20 ingredients with only a negative list of prohibited chemicals	Prohibits >1600 chemicals, has a list for prohibited, restricted, and allowed ingredients
New ingredient regulation[a]	A Product Information File (PIF) should be prepared and presented for approval by the concerned authority. Safety assessment through specified tests should be conducted, and the ingredient must be added to the positive list first before being released in the market	No particular certification or permission is required before releasing a new ingredient in the market; however, the manufacturer should maintain a record for product safety and adverse effects for the Cosmetic Ingredient Review (CIR) committee	Has a new section of *new cosmetic*, "a cosmetic which contains a novel ingredient that has not been used anywhere in the world or is not recognized for use in cosmetics in any national or international literature." The product should be assessed for safety through an accredited lab, and a manufacturing license is required from the Central Licensing Authority

[a]*New ingredient is roughly defined as an ingredient that is not available in the cosmetic ingredients list of the country and is not registered in the International Nomenclature of Cosmetic Ingredients (INCI) database.*

and negative lists for prohibited or restricted compounds in cosmetics. These ingredients have undergone rigorous safety testing, and cosmetic product safety reports have been submitted prior to their introduction in the market. For assessing the safety of a novel ingredient, the toxicological profile of the ingredient is formulated, which provides insights into the safe concentrations of the ingredient that can achieve the maximum desired efficacy (Manful et al., 2024). Furthermore, a risk assessment approach is also followed, which comprises the identification and characterization of a hazard, assessment of exposure, and characterization of the risk associated with it. A safety dossier must be submitted for approval, and once passed by the national regulating authorities, the new ingredient is included in the permissible list. Recent innovative materials, such as nanomaterials, can only be used once they are added to the positive lists, and to date, only five nanomaterials have been granted permission to be applied in cosmetics as UV filters and colorant (Manful et al., 2024).

The FDA maintains limited lists for controlling cosmetic ingredients compared to the comprehensive frameworks of the EU and India. Its approach involves listing a small number of prohibited and restricted ingredients, with color additives (excluding coal-tar hair dyes) requiring specific approval (Ferreira et al., 2022). The FDA also relies on assessments from the Cosmetic Ingredient Review, an industry-supported panel of scientific and medical experts evaluating the safety of various cosmetic ingredients (FDA, 2023). Countries such as Canada, Japan, China, Ethiopia, India, Cambodia, and Vietnam are similarly updating regulations or implementing bans on chemical ingredients to address public safety concerns, often issuing warnings on cosmetic labels to raise awareness (Goyal and Jerold, 2023). For green cosmetics, international standards such as Cosmetics Organic Standards (COSMOS) and private certification bodies such as Natrue, Vegan, Veganok, EU Ecolabel, Cosmebio, Soil Association, and Ecocert Greenlife have been assessing market products for their environmental and sustainable impact (Bozza et al., 2022). Fungal enzymes and fermentation products have received approval for use in cosmetics within the EU, although their bioactive components are currently undergoing assessment. Further evaluation and certification are necessary to ensure their safety and efficacy in cosmetic applications before market release, ensuring consumer safety and preventing a negative outlook on microbial products.

5 Fungus among us: Market outlook on current and future fungal cosmetics market

Modern consumers are becoming more informed and are prioritizing the inherent safety and sustainability of their daily products. In regard to this, there is a shift from traditional cosmetics focused on quick fixes and reactive measures to biocosmetics emphasizing long-term effectiveness, prevention, and a soothing user experience. Globally marketable and available biocosmetics are attracting their customer base with organic certifications such as Ecocert, COSMOS, and Natrue. The biocosmetics market developed through this setup presents vast opportunities for sustainability-based start-ups specializing in the development and alteration of ingredients and products catering to individual skin characteristics and environmental factors. These initiatives are gradually replacing fossil-based ingredients with natural, clean, vegan, sustainable, and high-efficacy alternatives. The influence of social media and beauty influencers with millions of virtual followers on the promotion of an organic and sustainable lifestyle is also pushing the market toward socially responsible practices. This evolving market demands accountability from companies regarding product design, ingredient safety and efficacy, recyclable packaging, and waste generation. Several cosmetic brands, such as Wedo, NatHabits, Alima Pure, Axiology, Aether Beauty, and RMS Beauty, are adopting zero-waste policies and emphasizing cruelty-free, vegan, and non-genetically modified organism (GMO) fermentable ingredients along with recyclable glass, fiber, biopolymer, and paper-based packaging to differentiate themselves from existing brands (Anagnosti et al., 2021). Increased government support and product approvals for biocosmetics are also creating a favorable environment for major cosmetic industry players such as The Estée Lauder Company (United States), L'Oréal (France), Nature's Gate (United States), Aubrey Organics (United States), and FANCL Corp. (Japan). The global biobased cosmetics market was valued at USD 4.95 billion in 2022 and is expected to register a CAGR of 6% during the forecast period of 2023–2032 (ER, 2023).

Biotechnological advancements enable sustainable production of natural ingredients with precise and targeted delivery formulations. For solubilizing bioactives both extracellularly and intracellularly, natural deep eutectic solvents are being optimized to provide eco-friendly and highly efficient solutions (Osowska and Ruzik, 2019; Jeliński et al., 2019). New-generation natural ingredients such as microbial bioactives, fermentation products, and nanomaterials are establishing their market with the concept of *beauty inside out*, where the product has efficacy as a cosmetic product while ensuring zero or positive effects on the environment. Fungal bioactives are isolated from fungi residing across diverse habitat conditions, tested for safety and efficacy, go through rigorous regulatory checkpoints, and then released to the market for commercial purposes (Fig. 17.2). Fungi-derived bioactives that are currently being employed in the cosmetics market include emollients, polysaccharides, and organic acids. Apart from these, several other fungi-based innovative products have been able to make it to the cosmetics market, such as Trehalose100, a soil fungus-based moisturizer by NagaseViita (Japan); fungal pigments-based lipsticks and eye shadows by Alchemical Mycology (England); and Time Revolution Night Repair

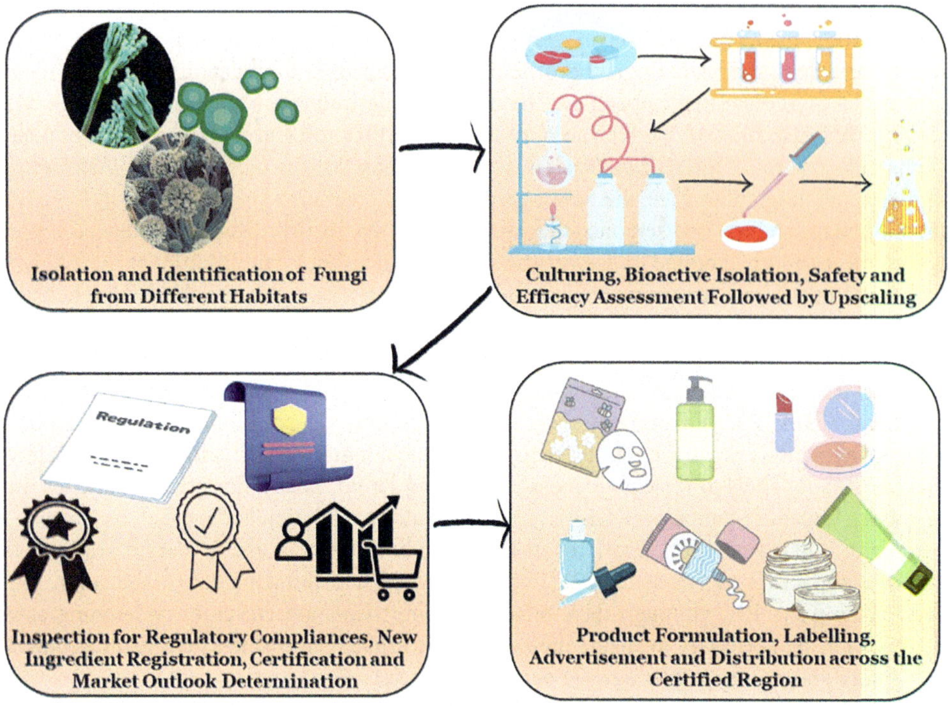

FIG. 17.2 Brief overview of the steps required to isolate, register, and market fungi-based cosmetic ingredients and products. The figure gives an idea about the isolation of fungi, cultivation, isolation of bioactive metabolites, upscaling, regulatory compliance, and, finally, marketing.

Ampoule by Missha (United States) (ER, 2023). An emerging market trend contributing to revenue growth is the increased consumer adoption of fermented ingredients and extracts in skincare products. While niche brands have previously offered cosmetics with fermented components, major industry players are now progressively adapting to meet evolving consumer expectations. Fermented extract of *Monascus* has been used in sunscreen (Relief Sun by Beauty of Joseon), toner (No.3 Super Glowing Essence Toner, No.3 Radiance Glowing Jumbo Essence Pad by Numbuzin), sheet mask (Deep Power Ringer Mask by Elizavecca), facial treatments (Secret Essence Fundamental Treatment by Su:m37), moisturizer (Rice Niacinamide Cream by Glamfox and Water-full Time Leap Water Gel Cream by Su:m37), and essence (Losec Summa Elixir 8 Miracle Power Essence by Su:m37). Furthermore, the fermented extract of turmeric and rice bran by *Monascus* is used as a power ingredient due to its high skin conditioning and protecting properties (Skinsort, 2024).

Even with the innovation and rapid growth in the biocosmetic industry, several challenges persist, particularly concerning microbe-based products. Issues include the slow efficacy of natural microbe-derived ingredients, high costs associated with pure or concentrated bioactive ingredients, limited shelf life, and nonvibrant color options with a restricted shade range. Concerns about brand reputation arise from the complex global supply chain of raw materials. There is also a lack of unified international standards for green cosmetic producers and risk assessment methods. Historical reports of adverse effects from plant extracts and some nondegradable natural substances highlight the necessity for rigorous safety analysis and adherence to green chemistry principles (Franca and Ueno, 2020). Moreover, many natural ingredients face difficulties in penetrating skin barriers, resulting in poor bioavailability, low solubility, and uncontrolled release (Dini and Laneri, 2021). Therefore further exploration of novel encapsulation methods for these natural bioactive substances is essential, as they are able to deliver immediate and tangible results.

6 Conclusion

The unknown exposure to hazardous chemicals in cosmetics necessitates an urgent transition to biobased alternatives. Beyond toxicity concerns, sustainability factors such as environmental degradation, carbon-intensive stress, and chemical pollution are also pushing the shift from conventional to biobased cosmetics. Among the natural sources, fungal bioactives have emerged as multifunctional, safe, sustainable, and innovative solutions for the biocosmetics market. Fungi offer unique advantages, such as high yield and rapid growth rates, which make them particularly suited for large-scale production. The feasibility of fungal systems for cosmetic ingredient production is particularly advantageous due to recent biotechnological advancements. Conventional biotechnology harnesses the capabilities of microorganisms through fermentation processes, whereas modern biotechnology involves the manipulation of genetic material and its integration into appropriate host systems to achieve specific applications. This dual approach enhances the versatility and efficiency of fungal bioactives in cosmetics. The existing regulatory framework and market forecast also favor fungal bioactives, provided they pass all safety and efficacy checkpoints established by different regulatory authorities across the world. The rapid depletion of nonrenewable resources and stringent environmental regulations have further increased the demand for high-performance, safe, sustainable, and natural cosmetic products derived from fungi in recent years. As the cosmetics industry continues to evolve, fungal bioactives are set to play a pivotal role in meeting the growing demand for eco-friendly and effective cosmetic solutions.

References

Abrashev, R., Feller, G., Kostadinova, N., Krumova, E., Alexieva, Z., Gerginova, M., Spasova, B., Miteva-Staleva, J., Vassilev, S., Angelova, M., 2016. Production, purification, and characterization of a novel cold-active superoxide dismutase from the Antarctic strain Aspergillus glaucus 363. Fungal Biol. 18786146. 120 (5), 679–689. doi:10.1016/j.funbio.2016.03.002.

Agrawal, S., Adholeya, A., Barrow, C.J., Deshmukh, S.K., 2018. Marine fungi: an untapped bioresource for future cosmeceuticals. Phytochem. Lett. 18767486. 23, 15–20. Available from: http://www.elsevier.com. doi:10.1016/j.phytol.2017.11.003.

Alonso, S., Rendueles, M., Díaz, M., 2013. Bio-production of lactobionic acid: current status, applications and future prospects. Biotechnol. Adv. 31 (8). doi:10.1016/j.biotechadv.2013.04.010.

Anagnosti, L., Varvaresou, A., Pavlou, P., Protopapa, E., Carayanni, V., 2021. Worldwide actions against plastic pollution from microbeads and microplastics in cosmetics focusing on European policies. Has the issue been handled effectively? Mar. Pollut. Bull. 0025326X. 162, 111883. doi:10.1016/j.marpolbul.2020.111883.

Aranaz, I., Acosta, N., Civera, C., Elorza, B., Mingo, J., Castro, C., Gandía, M.D.L.L., Caballero, A.H., 2018. Cosmetics and cosmeceutical applications of chitin, chitosan and their derivatives. Polymers 20734360. 10 (2). Available from: http://www.mdpi.com/2073-4360/10/2/213/pdf. doi:10.3390/polym10020213.

Arunrattanamook, N., Sornlake, W., Champreda, V., 2022. Co-production of schizophyllan and cellulolytic enzymes from bagasse by *Schizophyllum commune*. Biosci. Biotechnol. Biochem. 86 (8). doi:10.1093/bbb/zbac091.

Ashbee, R., Bignell, E., 2010. Pathogenic Yeasts. Springer-Verlag Berlin and Heidelberg GmbH & Co. K, pp. 365.

Bozza, A., Campi, C., Garelli, S., Ugazio, E., Battaglia, L., 2022. Current regulatory and market frameworks in green cosmetics: the role of certification. Sustain. Chem. Pharm. 23525541. 30, 100851. doi:10.1016/j.scp.2022.100851.

Cedrola, C.C., Barbosa, F.G., Marcelino, P.R.F., da Silvada Silva, N.P., Tavares, G.D., Barradas, T.N., da Silvada Silva, S.S., Vilela, F.M.P., 2024. Unlocking the beauty benefits: exploring biosurfactants from Scheffersomyces shehatae for cosmetics. J. Surfactants Deterg. 15589293. 27 (5), 801–811. Available from: http://link.springer.com/journal/11743. doi:10.1002/jsde.12739.

Corinaldesi, C., Barone, G., Marcellini, F., Dell'Anno, A., Danovaro, R., 2017. Marine microbial-derived molecules and their potential use in cosmeceutical and cosmetic products. Mar. Drugs. 1660-3397. 15 (4), 118. doi:10.3390/md15040118.

Costa, T.M., Tavares, L.B.B., de Oliveira, D., 2016. Fungi as a source of natural coumarins production. Appl. Microbiol. Biotechnol. 100 (15). doi:10.1007/s00253-016-7660-z.

Couteau, C., Coiffard, L., 2010. Regulation no 1223/2009 on cosmetic products. Nouvelles Dermatologiques 29 (5 PART 1), 217–221.

Cunha, M.A., Santos, V.A., Calegari, G.C., Sánchez Luna, W.N., Marin, S.L., Dekker, R.F., Barbosa-Dekker, A.M., 2019. Structure and Biological Properties of Lasiodiplodan: An Uncommon Fungal Exopolysaccharide of the (1 → 6)-β-D-Glucan Type. Springer Science and Business Media LLC, pp. 409–432. doi:10.1007/978-3-030-12919-4_10.

Datta, S., Christena, L.R., Rajaram, Y.R.S., 2013. Enzyme immobilization: an overview on techniques and support materials. 3 Biotech 3 (1). doi:10.1007/s13205-012-0071-7.

Dhevagi, P., Ramya, A., Priyatharshini, S., Thanuja, K.G., Ambreetha, S., Nivetha, A., 2021. Industrially Important Fungal Enzymes: Productions and Applications. Springer Science and Business Media LLC, pp. 263–309. doi:10.1007/978-3-030-68260-6_11.

Dhillon, G.S., Kaur, S., Pulicharla, R., Brar, S.K., Cledón, M., Verma, M., Surampalli, R.Y., 2015. Triclosan: current status, occurrence, environmental risks and bioaccumulation potential. Int. J. Environ. Res. Public Health 16604601. 12 (5), 5657–5684. Available from: http://www.mdpi.com/1660-4601/12/5/5657/pdf. doi:10.3390/ijerph120505657.

Ding, J., Wu, B., Chen, L., 2022. Application of marine microbial natural products in cosmetics. Front. Microbiol. 13. doi:10.3389/fmicb.2022.892505.

Dini, I., Laneri, S., 2021. The new challenge of green cosmetics: natural food ingredients for cosmetic formulations. Molecules. 1420-3049. 26 (13), 3921. doi:10.3390/molecules26133921.

Dinwiddie, M.T., Terry, P.D., Chen, J., 2014. Recent evidence regarding triclosan and cancer risk. Int. J. Environ. Res. Public Health 11 (2). doi:10.3390/ijerph110202209.

DuPont, 2013. Titanium oxide (Titania, TiO_2) nanoparticles – properties, applications. AZoNano. 06 March 2026. https://www.azonano.com/article.aspx?ArticleID=3357.

Dwibedi, V., Saxena, S., 2019. Diversity and phylogeny of resveratrol-producing culturable endophytic fungi from Vitis species in India. 3 Biotech. 2190-572X. 9 (5). doi:10.1007/s13205-019-1712-x.

ER, 2023. Bio Based Cosmetics Market, By Product Type (Emollients, Conditioning Polymers, Surfactants, and Others), By Source (Plants, Biopolymers, Microbes, and Others), By Application, By Distribution Channel, and By Region Forecast to 2032.

FDA, 2018. Federal Food, Drug, and Cosmetic Act (FD&C Act). https://www.fda.gov/regulatory-information/laws-enforced-fda/federal-food-drug-and-cosmetic-act-fdc-act.

FDA, 2023. Understanding How the FDA Regulates Food Additives and GRAS Ingredients. Sood and Drugs Authority, https://www.fda.gov/food/food-additives-and-gras-ingredients-information-consumers/understanding-how-fda-regulates-food-additives-and-gras-ingredients.

Ferreira, M., Matos, A., Couras, A., Marto, J., Ribeiro, H., 2022. Overview of cosmetic regulatory frameworks around the world. Cosmetics. 2079-9284. 9 (4), 72. doi:10.3390/cosmetics9040072.

Franca, C.C.V., Ueno, H.M., 2020. Green cosmetics: perspectives and challenges in the context of green chemistry. Desenvolv. Meio Ambiente 21769109. 53, 133–150. Available from: https://revistas.ufpr.br/made/article/view/62322/40588. doi:10.5380/dma.v53i0.62322.

Franssen, M.C.R., Steunenberg, P., Scott, E.L., Zuilhof, H., Sanders, J.P.M., 2013. Immobilised enzymes in biorenewables production. Chem. Soc. Rev. 14604744. 42 (15), 6491–6533. doi:10.1039/c3cs00004d.

Gajbhiye, S., Sakharwade, S., 2016. Silver nanoparticles in cosmetics. J. Cosmet. Dermatol. Sci. Appl.. 2161-4105. 06 (01), 48–53. doi:10.4236/jcdsa.2016.61007.

Gaur, S., Kaur, M., Kalra, R., Rene, E.R., Goel, M., 2024. Application of microbial resources in biorefineries: current trend and future prospects. Heliyon. 24058440. 10 (8), e28615. doi:10.1016/j.heliyon.2024.e28615.

Gomes, C., Silva, A.C., Marques, A.C., Lobo, J.S., Amaral, M.H., 2020. Biotechnology applied to cosmetics and aesthetic medicines. Cosmetics 20799284. 7 (2). Available from: https://res.mdpi.com/d_attachment/cosmetics/cosmetics-07-00033/article_deploy/cosmetics-07-00033.pdf. doi:10.3390/COSMETICS7020033.

Govindappa, M., Farheen, H., Chandrappa, C.P., Channabasava, R.V.R., Raghavendra, V.B., 2016. Mycosynthesis of silver nanoparticles using extract of endophytic fungi, *Penicillium* species of *Glycosmis mauritiana*, and its antioxidant, antimicrobial, anti-inflammatory and tyrokinase inhibitory activity. Adv. Nat. Sci. Nanosci. Nanotechnol. 20436262. 7 (3). Available from: http://iopscience.iop.org/article/10.1088/2043-6262/7/3/035014/pdf. doi:10.1088/2043-6262/7/3/035014.

Goyal, N., Jerold, F., 2023. Biocosmetics: technological advances and future outlook. Environ. Sci. Pollut. Res. 1614-7499. 30 (10), 25148–25169. doi:10.1007/s11356-021-17567-3.

Gupta, C., 2023. Role of Microbial Oxidative Enzymes in the Cosmetic Industry Microbial Oxidative Enzymes: Biotechnological Applications. De Gruyter, India, pp. 201–219. Available from: https://www.degruyter.com/document/doi/10.1515/9783111062235/html. doi:10.1515/9783111062235-010.

Gupta, P.L., Rajput, M., Oza, T., Trivedi, U., Sanghvi, G., 2019. Eminence of microbial products in cosmetic industry. Nat. Prod. Bioprospect. 21922209. 9 (4), 267–278. Available from: https://link.springer.com/journal/13659. doi:10.1007/s13659-019-0215-0.

Handa, O., Kokura, S., Adachi, S., Takagi, T., Naito, Y., Tanigawa, T., Yoshida, N., Yoshikawa, T., 2006. Methylparaben potentiates UV-induced damage of skin keratinocytes. Toxicology. 0300483X. 227 (1-2), 62–72. doi:10.1016/j.tox.2006.07.018.

Hassan, M.E., Yang, Q., Xiao, Z., Liu, L., Wang, N., Cui, X., Yang, L., 2019. Impact of immobilization technology in industrial and pharmaceutical applications. 3 Biotech 21905738. 9 (12). Available from: http://www.springerlink.com/content/2190-572x/. doi:10.1007/s13205-019-1969-0.

Homaei, A.A., Sariri, R., Vianello, F., Stevanato, R., 2013. Enzyme immobilization: an update. J. Chem. Biol. 18646166. 6 (4), 185–205. Available from: http://www.springer.com/chemistry/physical/journal/12154?cm_mmc=AD-_-enews-_-PSE1674-_-0&. doi:10.1007/s12154-013-0102-9.

Huq, T., Khan, A., Brown, D., Dhayagude, N., Zhibin, H., Yonghao, N., 2022. Sources, production and commercial applications of fungal chitosan: a review. J. Bioresour. Bioprod. 23699698. 7 (2), 85–98. doi:10.1016/j.jobab.2022.01.002.

Hyde, K.D., Bahkali, A.H., Moslem, M.A., 2010. Fungi - An unusual source for cosmetics. Fungal Divers. 43. doi:10.1007/s13225-010-0043-3.

Ishiwatari, S., Suzuki, T., Hitomi, T., Yoshino, T., Matsukuma, S., Tsuji, T., 2007. Effects of methyl paraben on skin keratinocytes. J. Appl. Toxicol. 0260-437X. 27 (1), 1–9. doi:10.1002/jat.1176.

Jeliński, T., Przybyłek, M., Cysewski, P., 2019. Natural deep eutectic solvents as agents for improving solubility, stability and delivery of curcumin. Pharm. Res. 36 (8). doi:10.1007/s11095-019-2643-2.

Jiang, C., Jinxin, G., Bin, H., Zeng, B., 2021. Glycosphingolipids in filamentous fungi: biological roles and potential applications in cosmetics and health foods. Front. Microbiol.. 1664-302X. 12. doi:10.3389/fmicb.2021.690211.

Joel, E.L., Bhimba, B.V., 2012. Fungi from mangrove plants: their antimicrobial and anticancer potentials. Int. J. Pharm. Pharm. Sci. 09751491. 4 (3), 139–142. Available from: http://www.ijppsjournal.com/Vol4Suppl3/3500.pdf.

Jones, M., Kujundzic, M., John, S., Bismarck, A., 2020. Crab vs. mushroom: a review of crustacean and fungal chitin in wound treatment. Mar. Drugs. 1660-3397. 18 (1), 64. doi:10.3390/md18010064.

Kalra, R., Conlan, X.A., Goel, M., 2020. Fungi as a potential source of pigments: harnessing filamentous fungi. Front. Chem. 8. doi:10.3389/fchem.2020.00369.

Kaur, M., Goel, M., Mishra, R.C., Lahane, V., Yadav, A.K., Barrow, C.J., 2023. Characterization of the red biochromes produced by the endophytic fungus *Monascus purpureus* CPEF02 with antimicrobial and antioxidant activities. Fermentation 23115637. 9 (4). Available from: https://www.mdpi.com/journal/fermentation. doi:10.3390/fermentation9040328.

Kaur, M., Peshwani, H., Goel, M., 2024. Penicillium: a treasure trove for antimycobacterial and antioxidant metabolites. In: Fungi Bioactive Metabolites: Integration of Pharmaceutical Applications. doi:10.1007/978-981-99-5696-8_9.

Kerdivel, G., Guevel, R.L., Habauzit, D., Brion, F., Ait-Aissa, S., Pakdel, F., Shioda, T., 2013. Estrogenic potency of benzophenone UV filters in breast cancer cells: proliferative and transcriptional activity substantiated by docking analysis. PLoS ONE. 1932-6203. 8 (4), e60567. doi:10.1371/journal.pone.0060567.

Kikukawa, H., Sakuradani, E., Nishibaba, Y., Okuda, T., Ando, A., Shima, J., Shimizu, S., Ogawa, J., 2015. Production of cis −11-eicosenoic acid by *Mortierella* fungi. J. Appl. Microbiol. 13645072. 118 (3), 641–647. doi:10.1111/jam.12725.

Kim, J.-W., Jung-Mo Ahn, O.-J.K., 2016. β-Glucan contents and anti-wrinkling effects of brown rice *Phellinus linteus* mycelium extracts fermented with *Lactobacillus plantarum*. Asian J. Beauty Cosmetol. 2466-2046. 14 (2), 127–137. doi:10.20402/ajbc.2016.0020.

Kim, J.H., An, C., Hwang, S.D., Kim, Y.S., 2021. Ceriporia lacerata mycelium culture medium as a novel anti-aging microbial material for cosmeceutical application. Cosmetics 20799284. 8 (4). Available from: https://www.mdpi.com/2079-9284/8/4/93/pdf. doi:10.3390/cosmetics8040101.

Kim, K.J., Sung, W.S., Moon, S.K., Choi, J.S., Kim, J.G., Lee, D.G., 2008. Antifungal effect of silver nanoparticles on dermatophytes. J. Microbiol. Biotechnol. 17388872. 18 (8), 1482–1484. Available from: http://www.jmb.or.kr/home/journal/include/downloadPdf.asp?articleuid={5555EA63-71F7-4E06-B904-C172A3AD3BF6}.

Kokura, S., Handa, O., Takagi, T., Ishikawa, T., Naito, Y., Yoshikawa, T., 2010. Silver nanoparticles as a safe preservative for use in cosmetics. Nanomed. Nanotechnol. Biol. Med.. 15499634. 6 (4), 570–574. doi:10.1016/j.nano.2009.12.002.

Kumar, A., Verma, V., Dubey, V.K., Srivastava, A., Garg, S.K., Singh, V.P., Arora, P.K., 2023. Industrial applications of fungal lipases: a review. Front. Microbiol. 1664302X. 14. Available from: https://www.frontiersin.org/journals/microbiology#. doi:10.3389/fmicb.2023.1142536.

Lee, J.D., Lee, J.Y., Kwack, S.J., Shin, C.Y., Jang, H.J., Kim, H.Y., Kim, M.K., Seo, D.W., Lee, B.M., Kim, K.B., 2019. Risk assessment of triclosan, a cosmetic preservative. Toxicol. Res. 22342753. 35 (2), 137–154. Available from: http://www.toxicolres.org/journal/download_pdf.php?doi=10.5487/TR.2019.35.2.137. doi:10.5487/TR.2019.35.2.137.

Liu, Y., Nan, L., Liu, J., Yan, H., Zhang, D., Han, X., 2016. Isolation and identification of resveratrol-producing endophytes from wine grape Cabernet Sauvignon. SpringerPlus. 2193-1801. 5 (1). doi:10.1186/s40064-016-2571-0.

Lohani, A., Verma, A., Joshi, H., Yadav, N., Karki, N., 2014. Nanotechnology-based cosmeceuticals. ISRN Dermatol. 2090-4606. 2014, 1–14. doi:10.1155/2014/843687.

Manful, M.E., Ahmed, L., Barry-Ryan, C., 2024. Cosmetic formulations from natural sources: safety considerations and legislative frameworks in the European Union. Cosmetics 11 (3), 72. doi:10.3390/cosmetics11030072.

Matwiejczuk, N., Galicka, A., Brzóska, M.M., 2020. Review of the safety of application of cosmetic products containing parabens. J. Appl. Toxicol. 40 (1). doi:10.1002/jat.3917.

McPhee, D., Pin, A., Kizer, L., Perelman, L., 2014. Squalane from sugarcane. Cosmet. Toiletries Mag. 129 (6), 1–6.

Ministry of Health and Family Welfare, Government of India, 2016. The Drugs and Cosmetics Act and Rules. The Gazaette of India, 1940. (As amended up to the 31st December, 2016).

Mishra, R.C., Barrow, C.J., Kalra, R., Dwivedi, N., Deshmukh, S.K., Goel, M., 2022. Phylogenetic diversity and antioxidant activity of selected fungi from ethno-medicinal plants and soil. Mycol. Prog. 18618952. 21 (2). Available from: http://link.springer.com/journal/11557. doi:10.1007/s11557-022-01776-2.

Mishra, R.C., Kalra, R., Dilawari, R., Deshmukh, S.K., Barrow, C.J., Goel, M., 2021. Characterization of an endophytic strain *Talaromyces assiutensis* CPEF04 with evaluation of production medium for extracellular red pigments having antimicrobial and anticancer properties. Front. Microbiol. 1664302X. 12. Available from: https://www.frontiersin.org/journals/microbiology#. doi:10.3389/fmicb.2021.665702.

Mohorčič, M., Friedrich, J., Renimel, I., André, P., Mandin, D., Chaumont, J.P., 2007. Production of melanin bleaching enzyme of fungal origin and its application in cosmetics. Biotechnol. Bioprocess Eng. 12268372. 12 (3), 200–206. doi:10.1007/BF02931093.

Morita, T., Fukuoka, T., Imura, T., Kitamoto, D., 2015. Mannosylerythritol Lipids: production and Applications. J. Oleo Sci. 1345-8957. 64 (2), 133–141. doi:10.5650/jos.ess14185.

Ohtake, S., Wang, Y.J., 2011. Trehalose: current use and future applications. J. Pharm. Sci. 15206017. 100 (6), 2020–2053. Available from: https://www.interscience.wiley.com/jpages/0022-3549. doi:10.1002/jps.22458.

Oliver, J., Selinger, B., 2022. The Chemistry of Cosmetics - Curious. Australian Academy of Science. http://www.nova.org.au/people-medicine/chemistry-cosmetics, https://curious.science.org.au/people-medicine/chemistry-cosmetics.

Osowska, N., Ruzik, L., 2019. New potentials in the extraction of trace metals using natural deep eutectic solvents (NADES). Food Anal. Methods. 1936-9751. 12 (4), 926–935. doi:10.1007/s12161-018-01426-y.

Panico, A., Serio, F., Bagordo, F., Grassi, T., Idolo, A., De Giorgi, M., Guido, M., Congedo, M., De Donno, A., 2019. Skin safety and health prevention: an overview of chemicals in cosmetic products. J. Prev. Med. Hyg. 24214248. 60 (1), E50. Available from: http://www.jpmh.org/index.php/jpmh/article/view/1080/pdf. doi:10.15167/2421-4248/jpmh2019.60.1.1080.

Peng, H., Guo, C., Tong, S., Ying, S., Feng, M., 2021. Two white collar proteins protect fungal cells from solar UV damage by their interactions with two photolyases in Metarhizium robertsii. Environ. Microbiol. 1462-2912. 23 (9), 4925–4938. doi:10.1111/1462-2920.15398.

Pérez-Rivero, C., López-Gómez, J.P., 2023. Unlocking the potential of fermentation in cosmetics: a review. Fermentation 23115637. 9 (5). Available from: https://www.mdpi.com/journal/fermentation. doi:10.3390/fermentation9050463.

Pretsch, A., Nagl, M., Schwendinger, K., Kreiseder, B., Wiederstein, M., Pretsch, D., Genov, M., Hollaus, R., Zinssmeister, D., Debbab, A., Hundsberger, H., Eger, A., Proksch, P., Wiesner, C., Proost, P., 2014. Antimicrobial and anti-inflammatory activities of endophytic fungi *Talaromyces wortmannii* extracts against acne-inducing bacteria. PLoS ONE. 1932-6203. 9 (6), e97929. doi:10.1371/journal.pone.0097929.

Prudden, J.F., Migel, P., Hanson, P., Friedrich, L., Balassa, L., 1970. The discovery of a potent pure chemical wound-healing accelerator. Am. J. Surg. 00029610. 119 (5), 560–564. doi:10.1016/0002-9610(70)90175-3.

Rai, M., Yadav, A., Gade, A., 2008. Mycofabrication, mechanistic aspect and multifunctionality of metal nanoparticles - WHERE are we ? And where should we go? Crit. Rev. Biotechnol. 28, 245–262.

Rajakumar, G., Rahuman, A.A., Roopan, S.M., Khanna, V.G., Elango, G., Kamaraj, C., Zahir, A.A., Velayutham, K., 2012. Fungus-mediated biosynthesis and characterization of TiO_2 nanoparticles and their activity against pathogenic bacteria. Spectrochim. Acta A Mol. Biomol. Spectrosc. 13861425. 91, 23–29. doi:10.1016/j.saa.2012.01.011.

Razak, D.L.A., Rashid, N.Y.A., Jamaluddin, A., Sharifudin, S.A., Kahar, A.A., Long, K., 2017. Cosmeceutical potentials and bioactive compounds of rice bran fermented with single and mix culture of Aspergillus oryzae and Rhizopus oryzae. J. Saudi Soc. Agric. Sci. 1658077X. 16 (2), 127–134. Available from: https://www.journals.elsevier.com/journal-of-the-saudi-society-of-agricultural-sciences/. doi:10.1016/j.jssas.2015.04.001.

Ribeiro, G.D., de Holanda Paranhos, L., Eleutherio, E.C.A., 2024. Trehalose promotes biological fitness of fungi. Fungal Biol. doi:10.1016/j.funbio.2024.03.004.

Roat, C., Saraf, M., 2016. Synergistic effect of xylose and sucrose enhances accumulation of stilbenes in endophytic fungus: *Aspergillus stellatus*. Int. J. Curr. Microbiol. Appl. Sci. 23197692. 5 (7), 571–575. doi:10.20546/ijcmas.2016.507.063.

Ruma, K., Sunil, K., Prakash, H.S., 2013. Antioxidant, anti-inflammatory, antimicrobial and cytotoxic properties of fungal endophytes from Garcinia species. Int. J. Pharm. Pharm. Sci. 5 (SUPPL 3), 889–897.

Ruszova, E., Pavek, S., Hajkova, V., Jandova, S., Velebny, V., Papezikova, I., Kubala, L., 2008. Photoprotective effects of glucomannan isolated from *Candida utilis*. Carbohydr. Res. 00086215. 343 (3), 501–511. doi:10.1016/j.carres.2007.11.010.

Secchi, M., Castellani, V., Collina, E., Mirabella, N., Sala, S., 2016. Assessing eco-innovations in green chemistry: life Cycle Assessment (LCA) of a cosmetic product with a bio-based ingredient. J. Clean. Prod. 09596526. 129, 269–281. doi:10.1016/j.jclepro.2016.04.073.

Selvasekaran, P., Mahalakshmi, F.R., Angalene, L.A., Chandini, T.S., Chidambaram, R., 2021. Fungal Exopolysaccharides: Production and Biotechnological Industrial Applications in Food and Allied Sectors. Springer Science and Business Media LLC, pp. 311–357. doi:10.1007/978-3-030-68260-6_12.

Shi, J., Zeng, Q., Liu, Y., Pan, Z., 2012. *Alternaria* sp. MG1, a resveratrol-producing fungus: isolation, identification, and optimal cultivation conditions for resveratrol production. Appl. Microbiol. Biotechnol. 0175-7598. 95 (2), 369–379. doi:10.1007/s00253-012-4045-9.

Shikina, E.V., Kovalevsky, R.A., Shirkovskaya, A.I., Toukach, P.V., 2022. Prospective bacterial and fungal sources of hyaluronic acid: a review. Comput. Struct. Biotechnol. J. 20010370. 20, 6214–6236. Available from: https://www.csbj.org. doi:10.1016/j.csbj.2022.11.013.

Shipkowski, K.A., Betz, J.M., Birnbaum, L.S., Bucher, J.R., Coates, P.M., Hopp, D.C., MacKay, D., Oketch-Rabah, H., Walker, N.J., Welch, C., Rider, C.V., 2018. Naturally complex: perspectives and challenges associated with Botanical Dietary Supplement Safety assessment. Food Chem. Toxicol. 18736351. 118, 963–971. Available from: https://www.elsevier.com/locate/foodchemtox. doi:10.1016/j.fct.2018.04.007.

Silvério, L.A.L., Coco, J.C., Macedo, L.M.D., Santos, É.M.D., Sueiro, A.C., Ataide, J.A., Tavares, G.D., Paiva-Santos, A.C., Mazzola, P.G., 2023. Natural product-based excipients for topical green formulations. Sustain. Chem. Pharm. 23525541. 33. Available from: http://www.journals.elsevier.com/sustainable-chemistry-and-pharmacy. doi:10.1016/j.scp.2023.101111.

Skinsort, 2024. Best products with monascus rice ferment. Skinsort. https://skinsort.com/products/products-with-monascus-rice-ferment.

Sułkowska-Ziaja, K., Trepa, M., Olechowska-Jarząb, A., Nowak, P., Ziaja, M., Kała, K., Muszyńska, B., 2023. Natural compounds of fungal origin with antimicrobial activity—potential cosmetic applications. Pharmaceuticals. 1424-8247. 16 (9), 1200. doi:10.3390/ph16091200.

Toksoz, O., Hur, J.S., Sesal, N.C., 2023. Endolichenic fungi extracts: a promising alternative for ultraviolet protection in cosmetics? J. Cosmet. Sci. 74 (4), 216–230.

Vandamme, E., 2001. Biocosmetics produced via microbial and enzymatic synthesis. Agro Food Ind. Hi-Tech 12 (1), 11–18.

Vandenberghe, L.P.S., Karp, S.G., de Oliveira, P.Z., de Carvalho, J.C., Rodrigues, C., Soccol, C.R., 2017. Solid-State Fermentation for the Production of Organic Acids Current Developments in Biotechnology and Bioengineering: Current Advances in Solid-State Fermentation. Elsevier, Brazil, pp. 415–434. Available from: https://www.sciencedirect.com/book/9780444639905/current-developments-in-biotechnology-and-bioengineering#:~:text=Description-,Current%20Developments%20in%20Biotechnology%20and%20Bioengineering%3A%20Current%20Advances%20in%20Solid,genetic%20engineering%2C%20metabolic%20engineering%20and. doi:10.1016/B978-0-444-63990-5.00018-9.

Wang, A., Li, P., Zhang, X., Han, P., Lai, D., Zhou, L., 2018. Two new anisic acid derivatives from endophytic fungus Rhizopycnis vagum Nitaf22 and their antibacterial activity. Molecules 14203049. 23 (3). Available from: http://www.mdpi.com/1420-3049/23/3/591/pdf. doi:10.3390/molecules23030591.

Wang, J., Cox, D.G., Ding, W., Huang, G., Lin, Y., Li, C., 2014. Three new resveratrol derivatives from the mangrove endophytic fungus *Alternaria* sp.. Mar. Drugs. 16603397. 12 (5), 2840–2850. Available from: http://www.mdpi.com/1660-3397/12/5/2840/pdf. doi:10.3390/md12052840.

Wu, Y., Choi, M.H., Li, J., Yang, H., Shin, H.J., 2016. Mushroom cosmetics: the present and future. Cosmetics 20799284. 3 (3). Available from: https://www.mdpi.com/2079-9284/3/3/22/pdf. doi:10.3390/cosmetics3030022.

Yao, Y., Baojun, X., 2022. Skin health promoting effects of natural polysaccharides and their potential application in the cosmetic industry. Polysaccharides. 2673-4176. 3 (4), 818–830. doi:10.3390/polysaccharides3040048.

Zhang, D., Yang, X., Kang, J.S., Choi, H.D., Son, B.W., 2008. Circumdatin I, a new ultraviolet-A protecting benzodiazepine alkaloid from a marine isolate of the fungus *Exophiala*. J. Antibiot. 00218820. 61 (1), 40–42. doi:10.1038/ja.2008.108.

Chapter 18

Protozoans

Nikolaos Toulis[a], Apostolos Beloukas[a], and Sophia Letsiou[a,b]
[a]*Department of Biomedical Sciences, School of Health and Care Sciences, University of West Attica, Athens, Greece*
[b]*Department of Food Science and Technology, Faculty of Food Sciences, University of West Attica, Athens, Greece*

1 Introduction: The rise of biofunctional cosmetics

Biofunctional cosmetics are a growing field that combines esthetic benefits with functional and therapeutic effects on the skin. This particular field has emerged to highlight the healing properties of products that create beauty, ranging from simpler structural organisms to the most complex ones. Biofunctional materials refer to substances formulated to engage with biological systems in a precise and advantageous manner. These materials are systematically developed to provide not merely structural or mechanical reinforcement but also to elicit biological functions, including the facilitation of cellular proliferation, tissue repair, antimicrobial responses, or biochemical communication (Williams, 2009). The intricate nature of biological systems necessitates effective molecular design for functional materials to address biomedical challenges. Biofunctional materials present extensive opportunities to tackle these issues (Zhou et al., 2017). These products often incorporate active ingredients derived from various biological sources, including plants, microorganisms, and marine life. In recent years, natural product-based cosmeceuticals have attracted significant attention from both researchers and the public due to perceptions of their safety compared with chemical compounds in skin-care products. The demand for biofunctional cosmeceuticals has surged, attributed to their distinctive chemical and biological properties absent in common ingredients used in cosmetic products (Alves et al., 2020). Among the lesser-explored yet highly promising sources of biofunctional compounds are protozoans, a diverse group of unicellular eukaryotic organisms. Despite being a significant food-borne public health problem across the world (Li et al., 2020) and one of the major causes of new cases associated with parasitic diseases in novel geographical areas by travelers and immigrants from **tropical and subtropical** regions (Norman et al., 2020), protozoans possess unique biochemical and antimicrobial properties that make them suitable for applications in skincare and cosmetics. This scholarly document investigates and elucidates the remarkable potential of protozoans in the realm of biofunctional cosmetics, while simultaneously emphasizing the significance of their diverse bioactive compounds, the intricate mechanisms of action, and the benefits that they confer upon cosmetic formulations. Furthermore, it examines the safety of protozoan-derived products in skin applications and, last but not least, suggests methods for the promotion of protozoan biomaterials synthesis utilizing biotechnological advancements.

2 Protozoans: Biology and relevance to biotechnology

Protozoans are single-celled eukaryotic chemoheterotrophic organisms, with many variations of this type of cell structure. Found in various environments, including freshwater, marine, and soil ecosystems, they exhibit a wide range of metabolic pathways and produce bioactive molecules, such as polysaccharides, lipids, peptides, and enzymes. These compounds have shown potential in various fields, including medicine, biotechnology, and cosmetics. The term "trophozoite" refers to the vegetative, active, and metabolically active growing form of a protozoan, i.e., the phase of its life cycle during which it grows, feeds on bacteria and small nutrient particles, and multiplies. Of the 20,000 protozoan species in nature, only a few are responsible for human infections. However, even these few pathogenic protozoans have significant public health and economic impacts. Malaria is the fourth leading cause of death in children in Africa.

The term "protozoan," derived from the Greek terms for "first" and "animal," pertains to a mode of nutrition that resembles that found in animals. Nonetheless, protozoa exhibit distinct characteristics that set them apart from animals; some possess the ability to perform photosynthesis, while numerous species exhibit complex life cycles that facilitate their transmission from one host organism to another. Recent genetic analyses have resulted in the reclassification of protozoa within the same kingdom as algae.

Biofunctional Cosmetics for Health. https://doi.org/10.1016/B978-0-443-27500-5.00006-X

2.1 Taxonomic overview

Protozoa have historically been classified as "first animals," yet molecular evidence has redefined their taxonomy, grouping them alongside algae and other protists. Protozoa primarily engage in asexual reproduction (monogonically) through mechanisms such as dichotomy, budding, or schizogony. Schizogony represents a form of multiple fission. In certain protozoan species, instances of sexual (bisexual) reproduction have been documented (Tortora et al., 2016).

Major groups relevant to biotechnology and cosmetics include:

1. **Ciliates** (e.g., *Tetrahymena* species)
2. **Ameboids** (e.g., *Acanthamoeba* species)
3. **Excavata, without mitochondria** (e.g., Giardia and Trichomonas species)
4. **Flagellates** (e.g., *Euglena* species)
5. **Apicomplexans** (e.g., *Toxoplasma* species, though primarily studied for medical applications)
6. Members of the taxonomic group Ciliates, or Ciliophora, possess cilia, which resemble whip-like structures, albeit of a reduced length. These cilia are systematically organized in parallel formations upon the surface of the ciliate and exhibit coordinated movement, facilitating the locomotion of the cell within its surroundings and the transport of nutritional particles toward its oral apparatus.

The ciliate *Tetrahymena thermophila* serves as a quintessential model organism that synergizes the capabilities of both forward and reverse genetics with an array of advantageous biochemical and cellular biological characteristics. *Tetrahymena* inhabits freshwater environments across a broad spectrum of ecological conditions. In its natural habitat, *Tetrahymena* predominantly consumes bacteria; however, laboratory strains are typically maintained as axenic cultures in nutrient-rich media (originating from tissue extracts) or in chemically defined media. Its populations exhibit rapid growth, with cellular division occurring every 2–3 h under optimal conditions. Each individual cell is relatively large, measuring between 30 and 50 μm in length, rendering them particularly suitable for investigations utilizing light and electron microscopy techniques. *T. thermophila* represents a ciliate model organism whose examination has contributed to significant discoveries and profound insights into both conserved and divergent biological mechanisms. Furthermore, it exhibits significant evolutionary divergence from the frequently investigated organisms within the opisthokont lineage, thereby facilitating the exploration of both distinctive and universally conserved biological phenomena (Ruehle et al., 2016).

Amebae represent a class of protozoa characterized by their mobility *via* pseudopodia, which are cytoplasmic extensions that facilitate morphological alteration and enable directed movement toward nutritional sources. These pseudopods extend outward from the ameba's body, with the remaining cellular structure following suit. Their nutritional acquisition occurs through the process of phagocytosis, wherein they encapsulate microorganisms or organic substrates, subsequently metabolizing these entities to extract essential nutrients. Depending on the taxonomic classification, some species exhibit a free-living lifestyle, exemplified by *Acanthamoeba* spp., while others are parasitic, such as *Entamoeba histolytica*, which is known to induce significant pathogenicity in human hosts. In response to adverse environmental stimuli, they can enter a dormant state by forming resilient cysts, which serve to safeguard their viability until the reestablishment of optimal conditions for their active morphological state (Tortora et al., 2016).

Acanthamoeba, which proliferates in aquatic environments, including domestic tap water, has the potential to invade the cornea, leading to severe visual impairment or blindness. The application of *Acanthamoeba* in the investigation of cellular differentiation mechanisms, motility, phagocytosis, bacterial pathogenesis, and evolutionary dynamics renders it a compelling model organism. There exists a considerable emphasis on *Acanthamoeba* as a "Trojan horse" for various other microbial entities, encompassing viral, bacterial, protist, and yeast pathogens. *Acanthamoeba* undergoes two distinct stages in its life cycle: an active trophozoite stage characterized by vegetative growth and a dormant cyst stage exhibiting minimal metabolic activity. Moreover, it serves as a causative agent for cutaneous lesions and sinus infections, vision-threatening keratitis, and a rare yet lethal form of encephalitis referred to as granulomatous amebic encephalitis (Siddiqui and Khan, 2012).

Single-celled eukaryotic protozoa, characterized by a digestive groove along their cytoskeleton, are categorized within the clade Excavata, which encompasses protozoa that create "excavating-like" cavities. The majority of these organisms are classified as atractomorphs and possess flagella. This supergroup comprises two phyla that are devoid of mitochondria (Diplomonads and Parabasalids), along with the Euglenozoa, which possess them.

Within the Diplomonads, protozoa exhibiting a dual-nucleus structure and multiple flagella are identified. Although they lack conventional mitochondria, they possess mitosomes, which are incapable of synthesizing ATP. A notable example of such a parasite is *Giardia intestinalis*, commonly referred to as *Giardia lamblia* or *Giardia duodenalis*. This parasite inhabits the small intestine of humans and various other mammals. It is excreted in an encysted form within feces and can persist in the environment for extended periods before being ingested by a subsequent host. The diagnosis of giardiasis, the infection induced by *G. intestinalis*, relies upon the detection of cysts present in fecal matter.

Conversely, within the Parabasalids class, the protozoa are classified as anaerobes and possess a parabasal body, a structure intricately associated with flagella. Instead of typical mitochondria, they contain hydrogenosomes that facilitate the production of hydrogen. An illustrative example of this class is *Trichomonas vaginalis*. Similar to other flagellates, *T. vaginalis* features a corrugated membrane that comprises a membrane enclosed by a flagellum. *T. vaginalis* lacks an encysted developmental stage, necessitating rapid transmission from one host to another prior to complete desiccation. This organism is located within the vaginal cavity of females and the urinary tract of males. Transmission typically occurs through sexual intercourse; however, it may also be spread through the use of towels, toilets, or other sanitary artifacts (Tortora et al., 2016).

Flagellates represent a distinct group of protozoa distinguished by the presence of one or multiple elongated, whip-like structures known as flagella, which serve the dual purpose of locomotion and occasionally food acquisition. These microorganisms inhabit a diverse array of ecological niches, encompassing freshwater and marine ecosystems, as well as acting as pathogens in both animal and human hosts. Flagellates may exist as free-living entities, exemplified by *Euglena*, which engages in photosynthetic activity, or as parasitic forms, such as *G. lamblia*, the etiological agent of giardiasis, and *Trypanosoma*, responsible for causing sleeping sickness. Reproductive processes among flagellates predominantly occur asexually *via* binary fission, and their remarkable adaptability to varied habitats renders them a compelling focus of investigation within the fields of microbiology and parasitology. Their structural attributes and motility capabilities enable them to fulfill significant ecological functions, including nutrient cycling and the facilitation of disease spread.

Euglenozoa constitutes a specific subgroup of flagellates, encompassing two categories of flagellate organisms, which are classified together owing to shared ribosomal RNA sequences, the presence of disc-shaped mitochondria, and the absence of sexual reproductive processes. These organisms are primarily photoautotrophic, characterized by a semirigid cellular membrane known as the pellicle, and exhibit propulsion *via* a flagellum that extends from their anterior margin. The majority of euglenoids possess a red photoreceptive organelle situated at their anterior extremity. This organelle, rich in carotenoids, functions to perceive light and orient the organism accordingly with the assistance of the flagellum. Certain Euglenozoa exhibit potential chemoheterotrophic capabilities, wherein, in the absence of illumination, they assimilate organic substances from their surroundings through structures known as cytostomes. Euglenozoa are frequently examined in conjunction with algae due to their photosynthetic characteristics (Tortora et al., 2016).

Euglena, in particular, represents a species of Euglenozoa that exhibits both autotrophic and heterotrophic traits. Species within this genus are extensively distributed across various ecosystems, predominantly inhabiting freshwater environments. The majority of these organisms are aerobic and utilize either photosynthesis or diverse organic compounds as interchangeable substrates for carbon and energy. The most extensively researched species is the readily cultivable *Euglena gracilis*, which, despite possessing a comparatively rigid surface structure, can be subjected to subfractionation to isolate nuclei, mitochondria, chloroplasts, flagella, and pellicles. The resulting subfractions exhibit several distinctive attributes: the nuclear envelope remains intact during mitotic division, chromosomes are consistently condensed throughout all stages of the cell cycle, the mitochondrial respiratory chain comprises two terminal oxidases, and chloroplasts possess three membranes, indicative of their endosymbiotic evolutionary lineage. Various species of *Euglena*, along with certain molecular constituents, demonstrate potential applications in environmental bioremediation and exhibit promising biomedical utility (Buetow, 2011).

The Apicomplexans (Sporozoa), in their fully developed state, are obligate endocytic parasites. They are distinguished by the presence of a specialized complex of organelles located at the apex of the cysts, which is the origin of the taxonomic designation (Apicomplexans, derived from the Latin terms "apical" and "complex"). The organelles comprising the apical complex harbor enzymes that facilitate the invasion of host tissues. In addition, Apicomplexans exhibit intricate life cycles, which encompass transmission among various host organisms.

Toxoplasma gondii represents another endocytic parasite classified within the Apicomplexans. The primary host for this parasite is the domestic feline. The trophozoites, referred to as tachyzoites, undergo both asexual and sexual reproduction within the infected feline host, ultimately leading to the formation of oocysts. These oocysts, each containing eight sporozoites, are expelled in the feces. Upon ingestion of the oocysts by humans or other animals, the sporozoites emerge from the oocyst as trophozoites and proliferate within the tissues of the newly infected host. *T. gondii* poses a significant risk to pregnant individuals due to its potential to cause congenital infection. Laboratory diagnosis is achieved through the identification of *T. gondii* in histological specimens. In addition, serum antibodies can be detected utilizing ELISA and indirect immunofluorescence techniques (Tortora et al., 2016).

3 Protozoan bioactive compounds with cosmetic potential

As eukaryotic organisms, protozoa exhibit a quintessential structural framework wherein numerous elements and organelles emblematic of mammalian cells are identifiable. Nevertheless, even among conventional organelles, these organisms demonstrate significant structural variability. Furthermore, certain structures in protozoa, including mitochondria, peroxisomes, and the Golgi complex, are notably absent. Conversely, innovative organelles such as hydrogenosomes, mitosomes, apicoplasts, kinetoplasts, glycosomes (which are specialized peroxisomes), rhoptries, micronemes, and dense granules serve as distinguishing characteristics of specific protozoan species. In addition, a variety of atypical cytoskeletal structures, some composed of yet unidentified proteins, are observed within these eukaryotic microorganisms that have the ability to interact with other eukaryotic cells. Thus protozoans produce a variety of bioactive compounds that can be harnessed for cosmetic applications (Souza, 2008).

3.1 Polysaccharides

Polysaccharides are ubiquitous across all living organisms; they demonstrate a wide array of biochemical configurations and fulfill critical functions in microorganisms, animals, and plants to provide defense mechanisms against pathogens, environmental perturbations, and climate variability. Microbial exopolysaccharides (EPSs) are integral to cellular adhesion and stress tolerance, and their utilization presents significant advantages in comparison with synthetic polysaccharides. The structural and physicochemical diversity of EPSs enables their application across various domains, including food science, medical therapeutics, agriculture, polymer industries, and cosmetics (Kumari et al., 2025).

3.1.1 Exopolysaccharides

Microbial EPSs represent a class of extracellular carbohydrate polymers that engender the formation of protective capsules or slimy coatings surrounding cellular structures (Kaur and Dey, 2023). Numerous microorganisms, alongside protozoans, are known for their capability to synthesize EPSs, which serve as a mechanism for enhancing their adaptability to environmental conditions and enduring extreme growth circumstances through the formation of protective biofilms on various surfaces. Biofilms are composed of a consortium of interconnected microbial cells affixed to a solid substrate, encapsulated within a viscous extracellular matrix that includes EPSs, proteins, DNA, and glycolipids. Microorganisms that are adept at biofilm formation exhibit heightened resistance to nutrient scarcity, fluctuations in temperature, alterations in pH, reactive oxygen species (ROS), disinfectants, and antibiotics in comparison with solitary microbial cells. The prominence of EPSs as the principal constituent of biofilms underscores the capacity of these molecules to insulate epidermal cells, thereby maintaining their hydration and obstructing the infiltration of environmental contaminants into the skin (Kumari et al., 2025).

3.1.2 Promastigote secretory gel

The promastigote stage of *Leishmania* is enveloped in a thick glycocalyx, which is predominantly constituted of a singular molecule identified as lipophosphoglycan (LPG). LPG is characterized by a repetitive polymer consisting of disaccharide phosphate units, which are affixed to the surface of the organism *via* a glycophosphatidylinositol (GPI) anchor. In numerous respects, LPG appears to exhibit functional and structural similarities to the lipopolysaccharides found in various prokaryotic entities. The prevalence of LPG on the surface of the parasite, which serves as the primary interface with the host organism, implies a pivotal function for this glycoconjugate within its infectious lifecycle. To date, LPG has been associated with the adhesion and release of the parasite within the midgut of the sand fly, the binding and internalization by macrophages, the evasion of oxidative stress, and, ultimately, facilitating the parasite's establishment of successful infections (Beverley and Turco, 1998). *Leishmania* parasites are conveyed to vertebrate hosts by female phlebotomine sand flies during their blood-feeding process, wherein they penetrate the upper capillaries of the dermis utilizing their barbed mouthparts. Within the midgut of the sand fly, proteophosphoglycans (PPGs) secreted by *Leishmania* establish a biological occlusion referred to as the PSG, which obstructs the gut and promotes the regurgitation of infectious parasites. The main substances of the PSG are filamentous PPGs and LPGs, but it also contains newly synthesized glucans, which give the gel a slimy texture and rich quantities of phosphate polysaccharides that bind ions and water (Giraud et al., 2018).

The relationship between the lesion induced by the sand fly bite and PSG remained largely unexplored for an extensive period. Recently, researchers employed nanoinjection techniques to administer a sand fly-ejected quantity of PSG into the dermal tissue of BALB/c mice, resulting in the differential expression of 7907 transcripts. These transcripts exhibited a transient upregulation during the initial 6 h postwound and were notably enriched in pathways pertinent to inflammation, cellular proliferation, fibrotic processes, epithelial cell differentiation, and wound remodeling. It has been demonstrated that PSG markedly expedited wound healing both *in vitro* and in murine models; this effect was correlated with an early upregulation of transcripts associated with inflammation [interleukin (IL)-1β, IL-6, IL-10, TNF-α] and the recruitment of inflammatory cells (CCL2, CCL3, CCL4, CXCL2), which was subsequently followed, after a period of 6 days, by an enhanced expression of transcripts related to epithelial cell proliferation, fibroplasia, and fibrosis [fibroblast growth factor receptor 2 (FGFR2), epidermal growth factor (EGF), epidermal growth factor receptor (EGFR), insulin-like growth factor 1 (IGF1)] (Giraud et al., 2018).

3.1.3 Mannose

Protein glycosylation in the trypanosomatid *Crithidia fasciculata* transpires through the transfer of an oligosaccharide characterized by the composition of Man7GlcNAc2 from dolichol-P-P to polypeptide chains. The molecular architecture of the oligosaccharide has been thoroughly elucidated. Subsequent to this discovery, analogous observations have been documented in other trypanosomatids, including *Trypanosoma cruzi* and *Leishmania mexicana*, as well as in certain mutant strains of the yeast *Saccharomyces cerevisiae*. The modification of protein-conjugated oligosaccharides of the *N*-glycosidic variety in lower eukaryotic organisms has exhibited distinctive characteristics that are not present in higher eukaryotes, such as the accumulation of a mannose-rich polysaccharide component on a portion of the oligosaccharide transferred from dolichol-P-P along with methyl groups (Mendelzon and Parodi, 1986). High-mannose-type oligosaccharides have been demonstrated to play pivotal roles in the quality control of proteins. A plethora of intracellular proteins, including lectins, chaperones, and glycan-processing enzymes, are implicated in this quality control mechanism. These encompass calnexin/calreticulin, uridine diphosphate (UDP)-glucose glycoprotein glucosyltransferase, cargo receptors (for instance, VIP36 and ERGIC-53), mannosidase-like proteins (such as ER-degradation-enhancing-alpha-mannosidase-protein-1, EDEM and Htm1p), and ubiquitin ligase (Fbs). It is posited that these molecules are capable of recognizing high-mannose-type glycans with subtly varying structural attributes, although the precise specificities remain to be elucidated. The process of protein quality control is paramount for the maintenance of cellular functionality, ensuring that only properly folded proteins are synthesized. The accumulation of misfolded proteins has been implicated in the etiology of various diseases. The mechanism of protein folding is facilitated by an array of chaperones, which are localized in diverse cellular compartments, including the cytosol, the endoplasmic reticulum (ER), and the mitochondria. Recent scholarly attention has been directed toward elucidating the roles of glycoprotein glycan chains in the realm of protein quality control. Glycosylation represents the most critical category of protein modification. The interactions among various classes of carbohydrate-recognizing proteins (lectins, chaperones, glycosidases, glycosyltransferases) with glycan chains carry significant importance, particularly concerning their roles in the quality control of proteins (Ito et al., 2005). Cells of the epidermis, which are subject to direct exposure to solar UV radiation, may potentially undergo genetic mutations, leading to substantial repercussions on the resultant protein products. These cell protein deformations can be prevented with the use of high-mannose-type oligosaccharides as a quality regulation mechanism.

3.1.4 β-Glucans

For an extended period, scholarly investigations have concentrated on β-glucans, which are polysaccharides extensively found within the cell walls of various microorganisms, including bacteria, algae, fungi, yeasts, and protozoa, due to their significant physicochemical properties that encompass thickening, stabilizing, emulsification, and gelation. Notably, the structural attributes of β-glucans, including the configuration of linear β-(1→3)- or β-(1→6)-chain cores, their molecular weight, length, and the quantity and degree of branching side chains, exert a profound influence on their solubility and conformational states in aqueous environments (e.g., single helix, triple helix, random coil conformation). Such structural characteristics endow β-glucans with various biological properties, including anticancer, antioxidative, and antiinflammatory effects. In immune cells, these biological mechanisms are facilitated through interactions with specific receptors for β-glucans, such as CR3 and/or Dectin-1. Although the Dectin-1 receptor is predominantly expressed in immune cells, it is also present on the surface of cutaneous cells, including fibroblasts and keratinocytes. Consequently, β-glucans are utilized within the cosmetic industry for their antioxidant and moisturizing properties, as well as serving as a texturizing agent in cosmetic formulations (Ozanne et al., 2020). (1,3)-β-Glucans and analogous glucans hold significant value both as storage polysaccharides (such as laminarins and paramylon) and as structural polysaccharides within the cell wall (including callose, cellulose, chitin, etc.) in protozoans, particularly within the protozoan group Euglenophyta (Euglenophyceae), as well as among the chromistans. The characteristics of these polysaccharides exhibit a degree of correlation with taxonomic classification; however, notable variability exists both between and occasionally within classes across each taxonomic division. Moreover, the composition and intricate structures of these polysaccharides are influenced by the organism's growth and developmental stages. The euglenid storage polysaccharides (paramylon) are characterized as (1,3)- or (1,3;1,6)-β-glucans; conversely, (1,3)-β-glucans and related glucans play a pivotal role as structural components of the cell wall in numerous protozoans and chromistans, encompassing callose ((1,3)-β-glucan), cellulose ((1,4)-β-glucan), chitin ((1,4)-β-N-acetylglucosamine), and (1,3:1,4)-β-glucans (Myklestad and Granum, 2009). Both structural glucans (cellulose and chitin) possess the potential and capacity to be utilized in cosmetic formulations.

One of the most prevalent organic polymers recognized by humanity is **cellulose**, a biopolymer that serves as a fundamental component of the cell walls in plant organisms. Derivatives of cellulose present numerous advantages, including recyclability, reproducibility, biocompatibility, biodegradability, economic efficiency, and the availability of diverse forms. Although cellulose can be extracted from sources such as wood, cotton, and various other plant fibers, wood pulp is predominantly utilized for the processing of cellulose. As elucidated by its molecular composition, cellulose is a carbohydrate polymer constituted of repetitive β-D-glucopyranose units, featuring three hydroxyl groups per anhydroglucose unit, which endows the cellulose molecule with significant functionality. Given its derivation from natural substrates, cellulose and its derivatives confer multiple benefits compared to their inorganic or synthetic alternatives. Specifically, they are characterized by their renewable nature, a broad spectrum of cellulose forms dependent on their source, elevated functionality attributable to extensive surface coverage of hydroxyl groups, biodegradability, cost-effectiveness, and easy accessibility (Dhar, 2010). Since 1980, cellulose has been employed in wound management, including the treatment of burns, due to its ability to maintain a moist environment, provide an effective physical barrier against pathogens, foster optimal conditions for tissue regeneration, and serve as a recommended temporary covering for skin wounds. This biocompatibility is attributed to its similarity with constituents of the extracellular matrix, such as collagen. Research has already explored the application of cellulose in meniscal cartilage implants, bone tissue implants, and primarily as a delivery mechanism for pharmaceuticals and other bioactive compounds (Bianchet et al., 2020).

Natural polymers such as **chitin** and its derivative chitosan have emerged as highly promising candidates for the formulation of skin care products due to a multitude of advantageous characteristics, including their antimicrobial and antioxidant activities, regenerative and cell-penetrating capabilities, as well as their nontoxic and nonimmunogenic nature. Chitin, recognized as the most prevalent natural amino polysaccharide, is extensively acknowledged for its composition of 2-acetamido-2-deoxy-β-D-glucose linked by a β (1→4) bond and is projected to be synthesized annually in quantities comparable to cellulose. Its significance has surged not solely due to its status as a largely untapped resource but also as a novel functional material with considerable potential across diverse domains, with recent advancements in chitin chemistry being particularly remarkable. Within the cosmetic sector, chitosan is employed for various applications, including the development of drug delivery systems, functioning as a chelating agent to enhance the stability of formulations, and serving as a therapeutic agent that promotes healing, stimulates tissue regeneration, and inhibits the process of fibrosis. Moreover, it has been evidenced that chitosan macromolecules, alongside their antiaging, antiinflammatory, and antioxidant attributes, possess the capability to absorb ultraviolet (UV) radiation. Research indicates that chitosan oligosaccharides significantly mitigate skin aging in hairless murine models subjected to UV exposure over a period of 10 weeks. The solubility of chitosan in diluted acidic solutions, coupled with its excellent film- and fiber-forming properties, facilitates the processing of chitosan and the preparation of chitosan-based materials of diverse structural and geometrical configurations. It is well documented that chitosan exhibits high solubility in a majority of acidic environments. Nonetheless, only a select variety of acids are applicable in the field of cosmetology, such as lactic acid, succinic acid, salicylic acid, and glycolic acid. Alpha hydroxy acids, including lactic, succinic, and glycolic acids, are known to stimulate the biosynthesis of collagen and elastin fibers, which are crucial for maintaining skin elasticity and resilience, enhance deep hydration of the skin, and exert antiaging effects. Beta hydroxy acids (BHAs), such as salicylic acid, are recognized for their ability to reduce pore size while exhibiting both antibacterial and antiinflammatory properties (Kodolova-Chukhontseva et al., 2023; Ravi Kumar, 2000).

3.2 Lipids and sterols

Lipids serve as a significant reservoir of stored energy, function as vital precursors in the organism's metabolic pathways, and comprise essential constituents of cellular membranes and other biological entities. In the realm of cosmetic formulations, lipids and their derivatives constitute a primary component. Various classes of lipids function effectively as moisturizing, emollient, and softening agents, serve as surfactants and emulsifiers, confer consistency to products, act as carriers for color and fragrance, function as preservatives to uphold product integrity, and may be integrated into the molecular delivery system. Historically, chemicals have been extensively utilized; however, contemporary market trends and consumer preferences are increasingly directed toward natural products (Hernandez, 2012; De Luca et al., 2021).

3.2.1 Phosphatidylserine

Parasitic protozoa are enveloped by membrane structures that exhibit a distinct lipid and protein composition in comparison with the membranes of the host organism. The membranes of the parasite are critically important not only from a structural perspective but also for other specific processes, such as the invasion of host cells, the acquisition of nutrients, and the evasion of the host's immune response (Vial et al., 2003). In protozoa belonging to the genus *Leishmania*, there exists a pivotal juncture within the host–parasite interaction, which encompasses the adhesion of the parasite to the intestinal epithelium, followed by a subsequent detachment and translocation to the proboscis of the insect vector. In mammalian hosts, this interaction entails adherence to and subsequent invasion of host macrophages, initially facilitated by metacyclic promastigotes and later by amastigotes. Both metacyclic promastigotes and amastigotes employ receptor-mediated phagocytosis as a mechanism for the invasion of mammalian cells. The phospholipid phosphatidylserine (PS) has been proposed as a significant ligand for the parasite in this particular process (Dos Santos et al., 2013). PS is a structural phospholipid typically situated on the inner surface of the plasma membrane. During apoptosis, cells undergo a loss of membrane asymmetry, resulting in the exposure of PS on the outer leaflet of the plasma membrane. The identification of PS on the surface of apoptotic cells prompts phagocytic cells to engulf these dying cells. In mammals, there exists a redundancy of receptors involved in the clearance of apoptotic cells. The majority of these receptors utilize PS as their ligand; however, the only receptor that can specifically and directly recognize PS is the recently characterized PS receptor (PSR). The interaction between PS and PSR stimulates macropinocytic activity in macrophages, thereby facilitating the endocytic pathway necessary for the removal of apoptotic cells. In addition, the recognition of PS by this receptor induces the production of transforming growth factor-beta 1 (TGF-β1) by phagocytic cells. This cytokine serves to inhibit the inflammatory response through both autocrine and paracrine mechanisms. Research has demonstrated that the amastigote forms of *Leishmania* (L.) *amazonensis* present PS on their surface and exploit this ligand to invade host macrophages. The recognition of PS is associated with increased secretion of TGF-β1 and the production of IL-10 mRNA. The pretreatment of amastigotes with annexin V, which binds to PS in the presence of elevated calcium concentrations, resulted in a reduction of amastigote infectivity by at least 50% and a significant decrease in TGF-β1 production by infected macrophages. Therefore PS signaling in amastigote forms functions similarly to that of apoptotic cells through a mechanism termed "apoptotic mimicry" (Wanderley et al., 2005). Leveraging the phagocytosis-inducing characteristics of PS extracts derived from *Leishmania* could potentially be employed within the cosmetic sector as exfoliants, promoting skin-cell regeneration, or may even have utility in the treatment of scar tissue. In fact, it is well-documented that PS promotes the differentiation of keratinocytes. Precisely, treatment with PS morphologically transitioned normal human keratinocytes (NHK) from a proliferative state to a differentiating state, thereby indicating that PS facilitates epidermal differentiation in NHK. In addition, it has been observed that topical administration of PS resulted in a significant reduction in transepidermal water loss that was induced by tape-stripping in hairless murine models. Furthermore, the concentration of ceramides (CERs) within the epidermis was markedly elevated in the PS-treated cohort in comparison with the vehicle-treated group *in vivo*. Specifically, the levels of nonhydroxyl CER exhibited a 1.4-fold increase, and glucosylceramide (GlcCer) demonstrated a 1.6-fold increase in the dermal tissue of hairless mice following topical treatment with PS (Chung et al., 2006).

3.2.2 Sterols

Sterols are integral to the biological functions of eukaryotic cells. They are crucial for the structural integrity and operational efficacy of cellular membranes and also serve as precursors in the biosynthesis of a variety of biomolecules, including steroid hormones. Trypanosomatids and fungi exhibit a critical dependence on ergosterol and other 24-alkyl sterols, which are lacking in mammalian cells, for their viability and proliferation. The biosynthesis of sterols, such as cholesterol and ergosterol, necessitates a minimum of 20 metabolic reactions that involve various specific enzymes (de Macedo-silva et al., 2015). In a manner analogous to fungi, trypanosomatid pathogens, including *Trypanosoma brucei*, *T. cruzi*, and several species of *Leishmania*, synthesize C24-alkylated, ergostane-derived sterols (Xu et al., 2014). Specifically, *Leishmania* and *Trypanosoma* parasites generate ergosterol-related sterols through a biosynthetic pathway akin to that utilized in pathogenic fungi, and their proliferation is sensitive to inhibitors of sterol biosynthesis (Roberts et al., 2003). The distinctiveness of ergosterol biosynthesis and homeostasis in *T. brucei* is primarily attributed to the enzymatic formation of a 24β-methyl group in the sterol side chain structure, a process catalyzed by sterol C24-methyl transferase (TbSMT), as well as to the quantity of the final product, ergosterol, that is employed for supporting growth. *T. brucei* encounters a range of environments throughout its life cycle, with the various developmental stages exhibiting markedly different sterol profiles. Despite possessing a complete ergosterol biosynthesis pathway in the procyclic forms, the bloodstream forms (BSFs) are typically regarded as deficient in ergosterol biosynthesis and are considered auxotrophic for sterols. At this juncture, the cells fulfill their sterol requirements through the dietary intake of cholesterol *via* lipoproteins present in the full-growth medium derived from the blood meal (Haubrich et al., 2015). In addition, ergosterol constitutes the predominant sterol identified in untreated *C. fasciculata*; however, substantial quantities of ergost-7-en-3-ol, ergosta-7,24(28)-dien-3β-ol, ergosta-5,72,224(28)-tetraen-3-ol, cholesta-8,24-dien-3β-ol, and, notably, an uncommon occurrence of 14α-methyl-cholesta-8,24-dien-3-ol were also detected (Rahman and Pascal, 1990).

Ergocalciferol (vitamin D2) represents the synthetic variant of vitamin D, and it is posited to exhibit a biological activity analogous to that of cholecalciferol. Adequate consumption of vitamin D is imperative for the prevention of rickets in pediatric populations and osteomalacia in adult individuals. Vitamin D3 is predominantly located in animal-derived products such as fish liver oils (exhibiting elevated concentrations), fish, eggs, butter, margarine (demonstrating moderate concentrations), as well as cheese and milk (providing sufficient concentrations). Consequently, strict vegetarians, who abstain from the consumption of dairy products, are predisposed to disorders associated with vitamin D deficiency. Vitamin D2 is the variant that has been predominantly utilized in dietary and pharmaceutical supplementation. In the natural environment, wild mushrooms contain measurable quantities of vitamin D2. Despite the low levels of vitamin D2 in mushrooms, prior investigations have identified them as a substantial source of ergosterol. Mushrooms are regarded as a delicacy, widely embraced by both vegetarians and nonvegetarians alike. Thus they may serve as a viable means to augment vitamin D2 levels in the diets of populations susceptible to symptoms of vitamin D deficiency, provided that their ergosterol content can be effectively converted into vitamin D (Jasinghe and Perera, 2005). Vitamin D2 is synthesized from its precursor ergosterol under the influence of UV light, a process that is also commercially executed to enhance vitamin D2 contents in mushrooms classified as "Novel Food," as mentioned (Sommer et al., 2023). In examining the impact of UV irradiation on the transformation of ergosterol to vitamin D2 in consumable mushrooms, it was observed that the conversion rate was maximized under ultraviolet radiation B (UVB; wavelength 290–315 nm) in comparison with ultraviolet radiation C (wavelength 190–290 nm). The influence of ultraviolet radiation A (wavelength 315–400 nm) on the conversion of ergosterol in mushrooms to vitamin D2 remains unclear (Jasinghe and Perera, 2005).

Vitamin D exists in two distinct isomeric forms, namely, ergocalciferol (vitamin D_2) and cholecalciferol (vitamin D_3). Exposure to solar radiation facilitates the synthesis of vitamin D exclusively in the form of D_3, whereas dietary sources are capable of providing both isomeric forms, which are widely considered by numerous experts to be functionally equivalent and interchangeable. Nonetheless, various arguments have been posited to contest this assumption, including the observation that the two forms exhibit differential effectiveness in elevating serum concentrations of 25-hydroxyvitamin D, characterized by the reduced binding affinity of vitamin D_2 metabolites to vitamin D binding protein in the plasma, alongside the identification of a nonphysiological metabolic pathway and a comparatively shorter shelf life associated with vitamin D_2. Yet, it remains the case that the predominant formulations of vitamin D available for medical prescription are predominantly in the form of vitamin D_2 rather than vitamin D_3. Multivitamins, conversely, may incorporate either vitamin D_2 or vitamin D_3 (Mostafa and Hegazy, 2015).

Skin aging constitutes a multifaceted phenomenon that is modulated by the total exposure to both intrinsic and extrinsic determinants throughout the human lifespan (termed the skin exposome), which is accountable for the progressive morphological and functional modifications observed in senescent skin. The principal internal determinants influencing chronological (physiological) skin aging encompass a decline in hormonal levels and alterations in gene expression with the progression of age. Moreover, the regenerative capabilities of the skin diminish with age due to the excessive senescence of keratinocytes, fibroblasts, and melanocytes over time, thereby contributing to the aging process of the skin. Senescent skin is typified by the presence of fine wrinkles and atrophy, accompanied by a decrease in elasticity. This chronological aging process impacts all regions of the skin; however, it manifests phenotypic variations across distinct anatomical areas and exhibits significant variability among diverse populations. The single-nucleotide polymorphisms within the MC1R gene (which serves as the principal regulator of melanin pigmentation) are notably correlated with the perceived age of the face, thereby establishing a novel molecular foundation for youthful appearances. The maintenance of adequate vitamin D_3 levels is critical for the overarching prevention of premature aging, thereby fostering a salutary skin aging process. Vitamin D_3 metabolites, encompassing both its classical form (1,25(OH)2D_3) and novel derivatives initiated by CYP11A1, exert a plethora of beneficial protective effects on the skin, which can significantly influence the mechanisms underlying premature aging, potentially leading to a postponement or mitigation of both chronological skin aging and photoaging. Skin-resident cells, including keratinocytes, fibroblasts, and sebocytes, possess the capacity to locally activate vitamin D_3 and manifest a variety of biological effects, such as photoprotection and immunosuppression, akin to those induced by UV radiation (Bocheva et al., 2021).

Photodamage pertains to the deleterious effects on the skin resulting from exposure to UV radiation. The consequences of UV-light exposure can vary with dosage, potentially resulting in DNA damage, eliciting inflammatory responses, inducing skin cell apoptosis (programmed cell death), accelerating skin aging, and increasing the risk of skin cancer. Various investigations, predominantly *in vitro* studies and murine models wherein 1,25-dihydroxyvitamin D_3 was applied topically to the dermis prior to or immediately following UV irradiation, have demonstrated that vitamin D possesses photoprotective properties. Documented outcomes on dermal cells encompass diminished DNA damage, lowered rates of apoptosis, enhanced cell viability, and reduced erythema. Furthermore, it has been hypothesized that the nongenomic mechanisms of vitamin D are integral to its photoprotective capabilities; such effects are associated with cellular signaling pathways that facilitate the opening of calcium channels. Given the aforementioned considerations, ergosterol extracts derived from protozoans possess the potential for incorporation into sunscreen formulations, facilitating the conversion to vitamin D_2 *via* exposure to solar UV radiation. In this manner, dermal cells will benefit through cellular protection against the sun's UV rays by absorbing them and subsequently transforming them into vitamin D_2, alongside the beneficial properties of vitamin D itself in dermatological applications (Fig. 18.1).

It is worth mentioning to acknowledge that 1,25-dihydroxyvitamin D3 exerts regulatory effects on the expression of cathelicidin, an antimicrobial protein that seemingly facilitates the mediation of innate immunity within the dermal layers

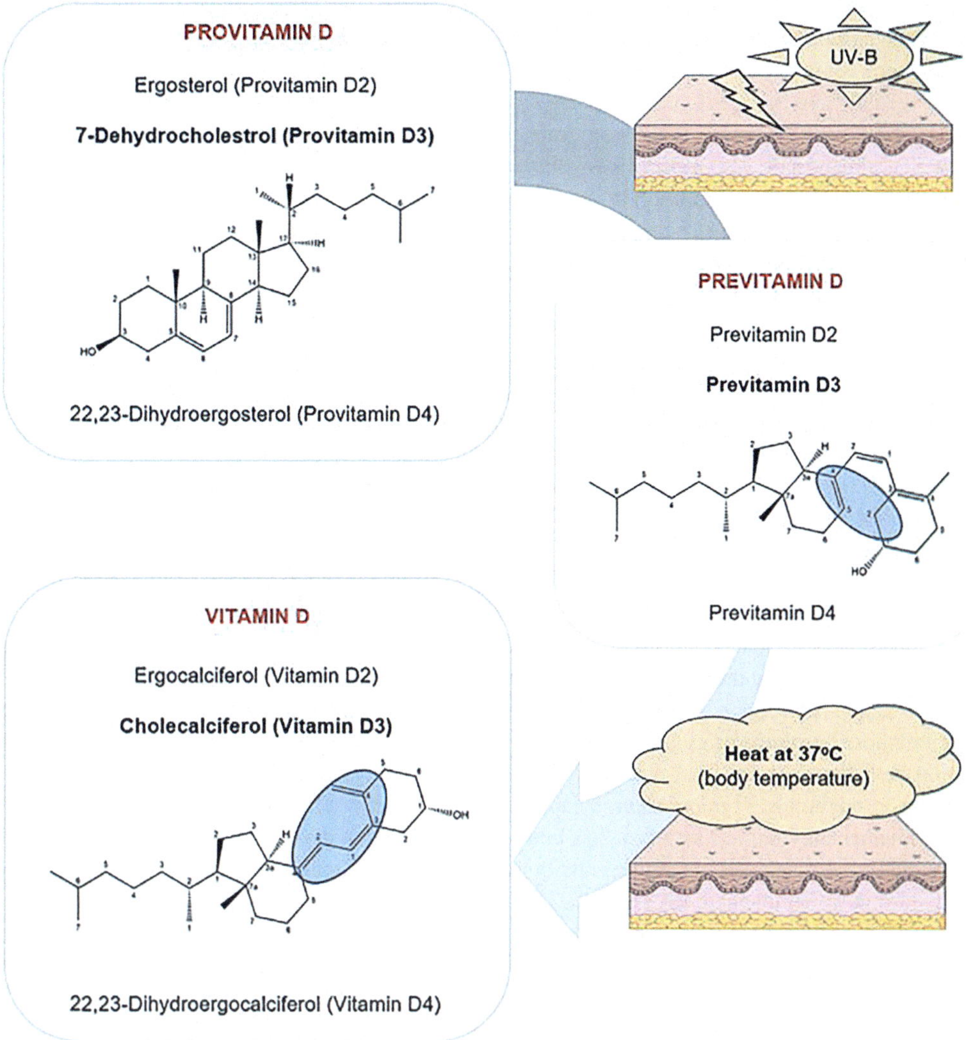

FIG. 18.1 The biosynthetic pathway of vitamin D upon exposure to UVB radiation. The provitamins D ergosterol, 7-dehydrocholesterol, and 22,23-dihydroergosterol undergo respective transformations into previtamins D2, D3, and D4, which are further subjected to thermal conversion, yielding ergocalciferol (vitamin D2), cholecalciferol (vitamin D3), and 22,23-dihydroergocalciferol (vitamin D4). *(From Janoušek, J., Pilařová, V., Macáková, K., Nomura, A., Veiga-Matos, J., Silva, D.D.d., Remião, F., Saso, L., Malá-Ládová, K., Malý, J., Nováková, L., Mladěnka, P., 2022. Vitamin D: sources, physiological role, biokinetics, deficiency, therapeutic use, toxicity, and overview of analytical methods for detection of vitamin D and its metabolites. Crit. Rev. Clin. Lab. Sci. 59 (8), 517–554. doi:10.1080/10408363.2022.2070595.)*

by enhancing the processes of wound healing and tissue regeneration. A study has shown that the expression of cathelicidin is significantly elevated during the initial phases of conventional wound healing. Additional research has indicated that cathelicidin plays a pivotal role in modulating inflammatory responses within the skin, stimulates angiogenesis, and promotes reepithelialization, an essential process for the restoration of the epidermal barrier, thereby reinstating a functional barrier that safeguards the underlying cellular structures from environmental adversities. The biologically active form of vitamin D, along with its analogs, has been demonstrated to induce the upregulation of cathelicidin expression in cultured keratinocyte models (Mostafa and Hegazy, 2015).

3.2.3 Sphingolipids

Sphingolipids (SLs) represent a significant category of lipids that are prevalent within the membranes of eukaryotic cells, notably the plasma membrane, in addition to being found in certain prokaryotic organisms and viruses. Since their initial identification, SLs have been a topic of considerable debate within the scientific community. Initially regarded solely as structural components, extensive research over the past several decades has elucidated their critical roles in a multitude of cellular functions, which encompass, but are not limited to, the establishment of structural domains, polarized intracellular trafficking, signal transduction, cellular proliferation, differentiation, and apoptosis.

Structurally, SLs are characterized by a sphingoid base backbone, such as sphingosine (SPH), which can undergo *N*-acylation to produce CER. To this CER, a diverse array of head groups—ranging from charged and neutral to phosphorylated and/or glycosylated—can be conjugated to generate complex SLs, such as sphingomyelin (SM), which serves as the principal complex SL in mammals, and inositol phosphorylceramide, found in fungi, plants, and various protozoa. These molecular entities exhibit both polar and nonpolar domains, imparting an amphipathic nature that facilitates their aggregation into membranous structures, while simultaneously preserving the capacity for interfacial interactions with a variety of partners, exemplified by the participation of glycosphingolipids (GSLs) in cellular recognition complexes, cellular adhesion, and the modulation of cellular growth.

The distinctive structural characteristics inherent to SLs influence their biophysical properties, thereby differentiating them from their glycerolipid counterparts, for instance, SM in contrast to phosphatidylcholine (PC). Such interfacial disparities confer upon complex SLs, like SM, a remarkable capacity to form both intra- and intermolecular hydrogen bonds, a property that is finely regulated by the presence of trans double bonds. This capability is evidenced by the propensity of SLs to cluster, diverging from the conventional behavior exhibited by typical "fluid" membrane lipids. Furthermore, the elongated saturated alkyl chains of SLs enable them to be densely associated with sterols, a process stabilized by hydrogen bonding, leading to the formation of laterally compact hydrophobic micro-domains commonly referred to as lipid rafts. These structures have been posited to play pivotal roles in a broad range of processes, including the polarized trafficking of lipid-modified proteins and the stabilization of various biological structures, such as lamellar bodies, as well as the assembly and activation of signal transduction complexes (Mina and Denny, 2018). These lipid rafts are hypothesized to be instrumental in a wide variety of processes, encompassing the polarized trafficking of lipid-modified proteins and the orchestration of signal transduction complex assembly and activation. In the case of the apicomplexan *Plasmodium* species, lipid rafts enriched in SLs have been implicated in the interaction between the parasite and the host erythrocyte, facilitated by the trafficking of glycosylphosphatidylinositol (GPI)-anchored proteins originating from both the host and the parasite. Moreover, studies employing tritiated serine incorporation have demonstrated that both *Plasmodium falciparum* and *T. gondii* possess the capability to synthesize SLs de novo. Similar to mammals, *P. falciparum* is capable of synthesizing the complex phosphosphingolipid SM, and an ortholog of the mammalian enzyme, SM synthase, has been identified within genomic databases (Pratt et al., 2013).

SLs may also act as bioactive signaling entities attributable to their distinct biophysical characteristics; for instance, the low pK a (7–8) of sphingosine phosphate (SP) enables it to exist in a partially uncharged state at physiological pH, thereby preserving its capacity to traverse cellular membranes. Similarly, CER, which is a neutral molecule, possesses the capability to spontaneously translocate across membranes. Numerous investigations have substantiated the presence of such signaling functionalities; for instance, SPH demonstrates multifaceted effects on protein kinases, CER orchestrates various cellular stress responses, including apoptosis regulation, and sphingosine-1-phosphate plays pivotal roles in cellular survival, migration, and inflammation (Mina and Denny, 2018).

3.2.4 Ceramides

CERs are also thought to be critical molecules in the maintenance and formation of the epidermal permeability barrier and important components in water retention within the skin. GlcCer, a common GSL found in many parasites and humans, is a glycosylated form of CER that does not exhibit cytostatic activity (Cummings, 2023; Štefanić et al., 2010). GlcCer is subject to hydrolysis by β-glucocerebrosidase within keratinocytes, yielding CER, which is subsequently sequestered in the stratum corneum. Concentrations of GlcCer exhibit a marked elevation during the process of epidermal differentiation, after which GlcCer undergoes enzymatic hydrolysis into CERs, thereby modulating the functionality of the permeability barrier. The concentration of CER within the epidermis is maintained through a delicate equilibrium governed by the activities of β-glucocerebrosidase, sphingomyelinase, and ceramidase. A deficiency or attenuation of β-glucocerebrosidase within the epidermal layer can lead to alterations in the distribution of CER and GlcCer, which, in turn, results in a compromised epidermal permeability barrier. Diminished levels of GlcCer and CER in murine models predisposed to atherosclerosis have been associated with skin inflammation, as well as alterations in hair pigmentation and loss. Previous investigations have established that all molecular species of CERs present in the stratum corneum are ultimately derived from GlcCer. Furthermore, GlcCer serves the dual purpose of mitigating dehydration in the stratum corneum while concurrently facilitating the restoration of the skin's barrier function. Consequently, GlcCers are integral to the enhancement of the epidermal permeability barrier function (Jiang et al., 2021).

Overall, SLs in the skin, akin to their presence in other mammalian cells, are pervasive constituents of cellular membranes and are implicated in numerous crucial biological processes, including growth regulation, cellular differentiation, and apoptosis. The modulation of these biological functions by SLs appears to be predominantly contingent upon the specific sphingoid bases present. SLs play a regulatory role in the receptors for platelet-derived growth factor and EGF. In addition, they partake in the co-evolution of transmembrane domains (TMDs) and the establishment of specialized microdomains enriched in GSLs (Popa, 2018).

3.3 Peptides and proteins

The advantageous implications of incorporating protein-rich compounds in the formulations of diverse topical applications are acknowledged by numerous scholars. Proteins have been swiftly regarded as valuable components for establishing an optimal environment conducive to the maintenance of healthy skin and hair due to their capacity to retain moisture within the stratum corneum and its appendages. Subsequent scientific studies were undertaken to explore the binding characteristics of proteins and peptides to the integument and hair, and their prospective function as hair conditioning agents was posited in the ensuing years, particularly at the onset of the 1960s. Proteins were deemed beneficial in bestowing luster, softness, and manageability owing to their substantivity. Furthermore, the majority of protein derivatives employed for cosmetic applications are derived from simple proteins (both fibrous and globular), while conjugated proteins (including proteoglycans and nucleoprotein derivatives) are utilized with significantly less frequency. Proteins sourced from both animal (mammalian and aquatic) and plant (angiosperm) origins may be utilized in the formulation of cosmetic ingredients; proteins extracted from lower organisms (e.g., algae and fungi) have only recently been considered for such applications (Secchi, 2008).

3.3.1 Amebapores

Apicomplexans exhibit substantial evolutionary divergence from extensively examined model eukaryotic cellular systems and, as obligate parasites, have demonstrated remarkable ingenuity in the formation and specialization of cellular structures and compartments. Upon the process of invasion, they engender and typically persist within a "parasitophorous vacuole" adorned with proteins secreted by the parasite. In addition, proteins secreted by the parasite target and modify preexisting compartments within the host, including the nucleus, mitochondrion, ER, cytoskeletal elements, and plasma membrane. In executing these modifications, they frequently disrupt the host's regulatory mechanisms governing defense and metabolic processes, induce reorganization of the host organelle positioning and associations, alter the mechanical characteristics of the host cell, and modify the interactions of infected cells with other host cells and tissues (Barylyuk et al., 2020).

Amebae implement mechanisms that may signify recognition, internalization, and subsequent destruction of foreign material at a profoundly primordial level, which may bear resemblance to those observed in phagocytic cells of advanced multicellular organisms. Ameboid organisms constitute a significant component of the protozoan domain and exhibit considerable phylogenetic diversity. *E. histolytica* is responsible for the global incidence of human amebiasis and is distinguished by its tissue-destructive capabilities and its extraordinary ability to eliminate host cells. These amebae have attracted the interest of immunologists due to their cytolytic responses, which resemble, in terms of contact-dependence and rapidity, the cytotoxic reactions exhibited by lymphocytes, and because they effectively eliminate immune effector cells such as neutrophils, lymphocytes, and macrophages. Notably, a nonpathogenic counterpart, *Entamoeba dispar*, exists. Within their natural habitat, namely, the human colon, both ameba species utilize bacteria as a primary nutritional resource. The virtually anaerobic conditions prevalent in the lower intestine negate the potential for amebae, akin to other phagocytes, to deploy antimicrobial agents such as oxygen-derived metabolites and nitric oxide. Consequently, *E. histolytica* appears to depend on an oxygen-independent mechanism (e.g., antibacterial peptides) to mitigate intracellular microbial proliferation within their digestive vacuoles.

A defining characteristic of numerous effector cells within innate immune systems is the presence of granules, which serve as storage for antimicrobial and cytolytic peptides that can be discharged for both intracellular and extracellular functionalities. Similarly, *E. histolytica*, despite being a representative of primitive eukaryotic cells, is laden with cytoplasmic granular vesicles believed to be integral to cellular digestion and the secretion of cytotoxic substances. It is plausible to assert that the molecular arsenal contained within the cytoplasmic granules of the ameba plays a crucial role in both the elimination of engulfed bacteria within phagosomes and the destruction of host cells when an appropriate stimulus, such as cell-cell contact, incites granular exocytosis into the localized environment of the contact zone. The cytoplasmic granular vesicles present in amebae harbor a specific family of peptides, referred to as amebapores, due to their ability to form pores in both artificial and natural membranes. Within the cytoplasmic granules of amebae, three distinct isoforms—amebapores A, B, and C—are identified; these peptides are uniformly composed of 77 amino acid residues and exhibit cytolytic properties against mammalian nucleated cells, while also demonstrating significant antibacterial efficacy, predominantly against Gram-positive bacteria. The proficient lysis of wall-less bacteria, or cytoplasts, from both Gram-positive and Gram-negative strains indicates that the bacterial cytoplasmic membrane represents the primary target for these peptides. The outer membrane of intact Gram-negative bacteria likely presents a state of heightened resistance to amebapores, attributable either to its unique biochemical composition or to its relatively low membrane potential. Furthermore, amebapores exhibit cytolytic activity against human nucleated cells, thus rendering them significant in the extracellular elimination of host cells (Leippe, 1999; Andrä et al., 2003).

Moreover, antimicrobial peptides (AMPs) are ubiquitous in the natural world and play a pivotal role in the internal defense mechanisms of all plant and animal species. To date, over 750 distinct AMPs have been identified, typically comprising 10–40 amino acid residues. In contrast to classical AMPs, NK-lysin and granulysin are remarkable in that they can be classified as small proteins rather than mere peptides; with sizes of 78 and 74 amino acid residues, respectively, they possess a distinct globular three-dimensional conformation. Notably, the archetype of this innovative class of defensive agents is found in amebae: the pore-forming proteins of *E. histolytica*, designated as amebapores. From an evolutionary perspective, successful molecules—those that are optimally adapted for their designated functions—are conserved across a diverse array of species. Nevertheless, it is striking that both the highly specialized, intricate immune system of mammals and a primitive phagocytic organism such as an ameba employ analogous molecules to achieve a comparable antimicrobial function (Bruhn et al., 2003).

Contemporary cosmetic formulations aspire to possess the capability to obstruct ion channels, deliver antioxidative and anti-inflammatory properties, diminish melanin synthesis through tyrosinase inhibition, stimulate cellular proliferation and renewal, among numerous other functions. Current scientific literature suggests that AMPs are proficient in facilitating such effects (Mazurkiewicz-Pisarek et al., 2023). Specifically, AMPs hold a critical position in the maintenance of skin barrier integrity and overall function, being synthesized in substantial quantities within the skin in reaction to a diverse array of stimuli, including particular cytokines, bacterial constituents, and inflammatory processes, contingent upon the specific peptide involved. These peptides exhibit the capacity to eradicate or impede the proliferation of a variety of microorganisms. This characteristic may also serve as a significant attribute for innovative cosmetic products, given the rising recognition of the significance of a balanced skin microflora. For example, in individuals suffering from atopic dermatitis (AD), a dysregulated skin microbiome is observable in both lesional and nonlesional areas, despite a similar overall baseline AMP production when comparing AD patients with healthy individuals. This finding underscores the critical nature of a balanced microflora, which constitutes an essential component of the skin's innate immune system, due to the fact that the microflora itself secretes AMPs. In light of the increasing consumer preference for biological products within the pharmaceutical and cosmetic sectors, as opposed to synthetic treatment options, interest in AMPs is progressively rising. Peptides are already integral to the cosmetic industry, exhibiting a myriad of applications attributable to their involvement in numerous biological processes (Alencar-Silva et al., 2018).

3.3.2 Calmodulin

Upon the stimulation of cells, Ca^{2+} serves as a conduit for a multitude of distinct signals, both directly and indirectly, that are associated with a diverse array of cellular activities, including exocytosis and endocytosis. This phenomenon is also applicable to ciliates; however, the investigation of Ca^{2+} signaling has been conducted with specificity only in Paramecium. In summary, the process of trichocyst exocytosis necessitates the mobilization of Ca^{2+} from alveolar sacs, with cortical Ca^{2+} reserves being closely monitored and augmented by an influx of Ca^{2+}. In general, the Ca^{2+} signal is conveyed through its interaction with various proteins, such as low-capacity/high-affinity Ca^{2+}-binding proteins characterized by specific Ca^{2+}-binding motifs. Among these, several proteins featuring EF-hand motifs are theoretically present, as exemplified by calmodulin—specifically, 13 genes encoding potential calmodulin isoforms have been identified in Paramecium—or proteins containing C2-domains, akin to the well-characterized Ca^{2+}-sensor, synaptotagmin. Calmodulin is recognized as essential for the formation of a functional site for trichocyst exocytosis. In mammalian cellular systems, calmodulin interacts with synaptobrevin, thereby influencing the configuration of soluble N-ethylmaleimide sensitive factor, vesicle fusing ATPase (NSF) attachment protein receptors. Through its engagement with the auxiliary protein Munc13, calmodulin additionally facilitates the priming process for neurotransmission. Nonetheless, due to its Ca^{2+}-binding characteristics and kinetic properties, calmodulin is generally regarded as unsuitable for functioning as a Ca^{2+} sensor during rapid exocytotic responses. Furthermore, calmodulin acts as a Ca^{2+} sensor for various types of endocytosis within nerve terminals, suggesting that it may fulfill a similar role in ciliates. In conclusion, calmodulin may represent a multifunctional element of dense core vesicle docking and exocytosis sites in ciliates as well (Plattner, 2010).

It has been established that calmodulin, which serves as the predominant cytosolic calcium-binding protein, exhibits the highest levels in maturing keratinocytes and sebaceous gland cells within normal skin. Specifically, its presence is significantly elevated in the epidermal regions adjacent to wound margins and in areas undergoing reepithelialization during periods characterized by maximal local calcium concentrations (Lansdown et al., 1999). A separate investigation elucidated the function of calmodulin-like skin protein (CLSP) in attenuating the elevation of senescence-associated β-galactosidase, which is provoked by hydrogen peroxide or UV irradiation in keratinocytes. CLSP was initially characterized as a homolog of calmodulin whose precise role remains to be elucidated; it is predominantly expressed in skin keratinocytes and associated epithelial cells. Several observations concerning the operational role of CLSP in cutaneous tissues have been documented. The expression of CLSP is stimulated by the differentiation of keratinocytes, and it is instrumental in facilitating keratinocyte differentiation, in conjunction with its binding partner 14-3-3σ. The murine ortholog of CLSP, designated

Scarf, may be integral to the reestablishment of the epidermal Ca^{2+} gradient during the processes of wound healing and the formation of the epidermal barrier. The expression of CLSP is notably heightened in conditions such as AD and psoriasis. In this mentioned investigation, utilizing primary keratinocytes subjected to hydrogen peroxide (H_2O_2) treatment or UV irradiation as models of keratinocyte senescence, researchers sought to ascertain the influence of CLSP on senescence within skin keratinocytes. The findings revealed that CLSP expression was significantly upregulated in keratinocytes exposed to H_2O_2 or UV. In summary, it was demonstrated that secreted CLSP mitigates senescence in keratinocytes. While the physiological implications of this discovery warrant further exploration, it may pioneer novel research directions for comprehending skin senescence (Takahara et al., 2019).

3.3.3 ATP-binding cassette proteins

The ATP-binding cassette (ABC) superfamily constitutes one of the most extensive families of proteins, with representatives distributed across all biological kingdoms. Members of this superfamily participate in a diverse array of transport mechanisms, facilitating the movement of substrates that range from diminutive ions to comparatively large polypeptides and polysaccharides, as well as engaging in various cellular processes, including DNA repair, translation, and the regulation of gene expression. The ABC transporter superfamily represents one of the most substantial protein families observed in both prokaryotic and eukaryotic organisms. While prokaryotes employ ABC transporters for both the import and export of substances, eukaryotic organisms are posited to utilize these transporters predominantly for export purposes (Sauvage et al., 2009). These proteins exhibit a highly conserved ATPase domain, denoted as the ABC, characterized by an amino acid sequence that encompasses three principal conserved motifs: the characteristic A and B motifs, as delineated by Walker et al. (1982), which are commonly identified in ATPases, alongside a distinctive sequence referred to as the "ABC signature," situated immediately upstream of the Walker B site. The ABC signature sequence is unique to ABC transporters and serves to differentiate them from other ATP-binding proteins. Predominantly, eukaryotic ABC proteins function as transporters that are structured with four domains within a singular polypeptide chain: two hydrophobic TMDs that facilitate substrate translocation pathways, and two cytoplasmic domains housing the nucleotide-binding domains (NBDs) that are integral for ATP binding and hydrolysis (Fig. 18.2). These "full-size" transporters, designated as (TMD-NBD)2, are primarily localized within the plasma membrane. A significant number of ABC transporters, referred

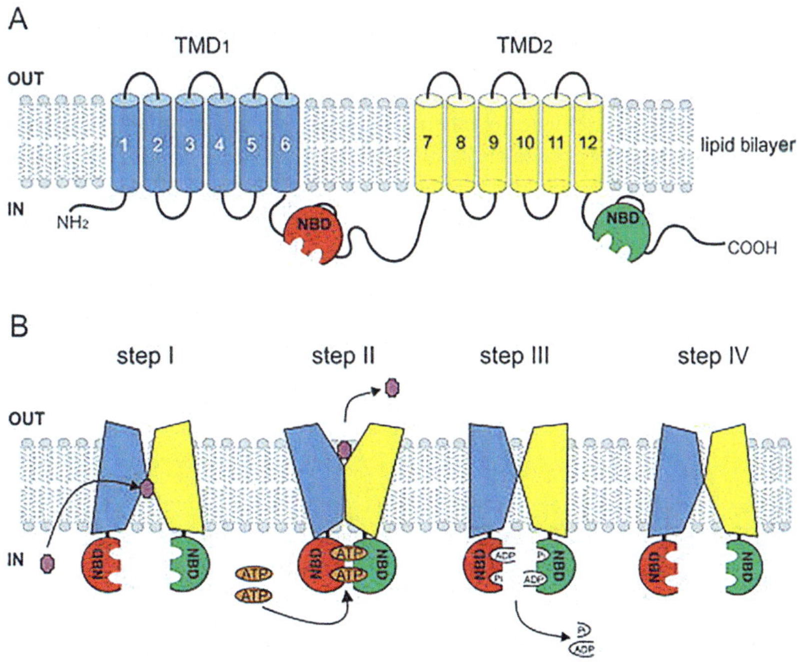

FIG. 18.2 The structural configuration of ABC full transporters and the ATP-switch model elucidating the transport cycle of an ABC transporter (exporter-type). (A) A prototypical structure of an ABC full transporter comprises two transmembrane domains (TMDs), TMD1 (colored blue) and TMD2 (colored yellow), each comprising six transmembrane (TM) segments, in addition to two nucleotide-binding domains (NBDs), NBD1 (colored red) and NBD2 (colored green). In the context of "long" multidrug resistance proteins (MRPs), an additional TMD (designated TMD0) is incorporated at the N-terminus. (B) The ATP-switch mechanism. The initiation of the transport cycle is triggered by the binding of a substrate (indicated by a purple cross) to a high-affinity binding pocket formed by the TMDs (illustrated as a blue-and-yellow pentagon). *(From Dermauw, W., Van Leeuwen, T., 2014. The ABC gene family in arthropods: comparative genomics and role in insecticide transport and resistance. Insect Biochem. Mol. Biol. 45 (1), 89–110. doi:10.1016/j.ibmb.2013.11.001.)*

to as "half-size" transporters, consist of a solitary ATPase domain fused to a single TMD, with the positioning at either the N- or C-terminal end determining the structural configuration of the protein (TMD-NBD or NBD-TMD). The homo- or heterodimerization of "half-size" transporters is essential for their functional activity. The principal physiological roles of ABC transporters in eukaryotes encompass the translocation of a broad spectrum of endogenous metabolites (including sugars, amino acids, ions, phospholipids, proteins, etc.) and cytotoxic compounds across both extra- and intracellular membranes. Recently, an exhaustive examination of the genomes of *Leishmania major* and *Leishmania infantum* for ABC sequences facilitated the identification of the complete ABC protein superfamily within *Leishmania*. Among the 42 ABC open reading frames (ORFs) identified, which account for 0.5% of the total gene complement in *L. major*, 32 were ascertained to encode ABC transporters, while 10 encoded ABC proteins devoid of any TMD. Notably, a comparative analysis revealed that the identical ABC data set was observed in both *L. major* and *L. infantum*, and that multiple homologous ORFs were retrieved from the genomes of *T. brucei* and *T. cruzi*. Within the ABCD, ABCE, and ABCF families, all *Trypanosoma* genes were found to be paired with an orthologous counterpart in the *Leishmania* genome (Sauvage et al., 2009).

Despite the sophisticated differentiation processes executed by the skin, keratinocytes, fibroblasts, and a lesser population of other cell types present within the dermal layer (including melanocytes, neural cells, and immune cells) are equipped to engage in the metabolism of xenobiotics that are introduced either from the exterior environment or *via* the circulatory system. ABC transporters are expressed within skin cells to safeguard against deleterious xenobiotics. Furthermore, these transmembrane proteins fulfill several additional roles that contribute to the maintenance of skin homeostasis. In addition, the exposure of skin cells to UV radiation frequently results in augmented activity of ABC transporters, as evidenced by observations related to multidrug resistance proteins, transport-associated proteins, cystic fibrosis transmembrane conductance regulator, and breast cancer resistance protein. Conversely, a distinct impact of oxidative stress has been noted concerning mitochondrial sulfonylurea receptors. Nevertheless, the scarcity of empirical data in the existing literature underscores the limited scope of experimental investigations addressing the function of ABC transporters in both the physiology and pathophysiology of skin cells and the integumentary system in its entirety.

It has been documented that the distribution of ABC transporters within the skin exhibits varying intensities between the epidermis and the dermis. For instance, MRP1 demonstrates a pronounced expression within comprehensive skin specimens and the dermis, while exhibiting a diminished expression in the epidermis. This differential expression facilitates the absorption of compounds from the epidermal layer and their subsequent secretion into the deeper strata of the skin. Moreover, by regulating the efflux of steroid hormones from normal human epidermal keratinocytes, ABC transporters contribute to the maintenance of appropriate hormonal equilibrium within the skin. The expression of ABC transporters in human skin biopsies has been found to correlate with sweat metabolites, thereby indicating their involvement in sweat secretion and, consequently, an indirect influence on thermoregulation in the body. By extricating contact allergens and exogenous substances, such as pathogen fragments, from the intracellular milieu, ABC transporters assume a significant role in the migration of Langerhans cells and aid in the preservation of a robust immune response within the skin. ABC transporters also facilitate the translocation of lipid metabolites across cellular organelles to regulate lipid homeostasis and avert the onset of disease. Research has indicated that a dysfunction in ABCA12, which is integral to the translocation of GlcCers into lamellar granules, results in a disruption of the skin's barrier functions and is even implicated in the etiology of the rare skin disorder known as harlequin ichthyosis. In light of the aforementioned considerations, ABCs have the potential to act as a balancing product that will regulate the skin's hormonal composition and fortify cellular integrity (Gęgotek and Skrzydlewska, 2023).

3.4 Enzymes

As all biological mechanisms fundamentally rely on enzymatic activity, these biocatalysts are integral to dermal care. Within the integumentary system, enzymes facilitate the dissociation of intricate inactive molecules, subsequently converting them into simpler and frequently more bioactive forms. For instance, proteases catalyze the cleavage or hydrolysis of proteins, glycosidases enhance the epidermis by increasing CER levels, and tyrosinase promotes melanin biosynthesis. In both the skin and the stratum corneum, enzymatic processes modulate keratinization, maintain intercorneocyte adhesion, stimulate tanning and autophotoprotection, influence the metabolism of sebaceous glands and adipocytes, exhibit depigmenting effects on age spots, bolster the skin's innate defense systems, and safeguard collagen and elastin fibers. Consequently, enzymes unequivocally represent promising natural active agents for targeted personal care formulations categorized as "functional cosmetics," "cosmeceuticals," or "therapeutic products" (Ansorge-Schumacher and Thum, 2013).

3.4.1 Proteases

Proteolytic enzymes appear to assume critical responsibilities within the life cycles of all protozoan parasites of medical significance, which encompass the pathogens responsible for malaria, trypanosomiasis, leishmaniasis, amebiasis, toxoplasmosis, giardiasis, cryptosporidiosis, and trichomoniasis. Protozoans utilize proteases derived from all four principal classes of proteolytic enzymes for a variety of functions, including the invasion of host cells and tissues, the degradation of immune response mediators, and the hydrolysis of host proteins for nutritional acquisition. The biochemical and molecular elucidation of protozoan proteases is yielding instruments to enhance the comprehension of the roles of these enzymes (Rosenthal, 1999).

Proteases facilitate the hydrolysis of peptide bonds, consequently dismantling protein substrates. Proteases that mediate the cleavage of an internal peptide bond within a protein are frequently designated as proteinases or, less commonly, endoproteases. Conversely, proteases that catalyze the cleavage of one or two amino acids from either the extreme amino terminus or carboxy terminus of a protein or peptide are classified as exopeptidases or, more specifically, as aminopeptidases and carboxypeptidases, contingent upon the terminal end of the substrate molecule from which the amino acids are liberated. These distinctions in substrate specificity among proteases are critical, as they often provide insights into the functional roles of the proteases (McKerrow et al., 1993). The majority of proteases exhibit the ability to hydrolyze only specific peptide bonds. In certain instances, highly selective enzymes hydrolyze solely a particular bond within a specific protein. Conversely, some proteases cleave multiple peptide bonds that conform to certain sequence or structural criteria. An assessment of the substrate specificity of a protease can be instrumental in elucidating the biological function of the enzyme. The hydrolysis of the authentic substrate of a protease or that of synthetic peptide substrates can be evaluated. Nevertheless, interpretations derived from such investigations should be approached with caution, as *in vitro* assessments of substrate cleavage may not accurately predict the specificity of the protease within its authentic biological milieu. Most proteases are categorized into one of four predominant classes. Serine proteases represent the largest family of proteolytic enzymes. They derive their name from the amino acid serine, whose hydroxyl group is integral to the binding and catalysis of the substrate at the active site. In cysteine or thiol proteases, the thiol group of the amino acid cysteine fulfills a comparable function. Metalloproteases incorporate a metal ion within the active site that is pivotal for substrate binding, while aspartyl proteases employ two aspartic acid side chains in the catalytic process. Serine and cysteine proteases depend on the nucleophilic properties of the serine, threonine, and cysteine side chains, respectively, to directly target the peptide bond, thus establishing a transient, covalent enzyme-substrate intermediate. Aspartic and metalloproteases utilize a water molecule for nucleophilic attack and do not generate a covalent intermediate. Subclassifying a protease into one of these distinct categories, such as determining whether it functions as a protease or an exopeptidase, holds significant importance as this classification yields insights into the enzyme's functional role *in vivo*. Proteases are most effectively categorized into one of these four classifications through the implementation of inhibitor studies. Specific inhibitors corresponding to each of the four protease classifications are readily accessible. Proteases are typically synthesized in the form of proenzymes, which subsequently undergo processing to yield mature, enzymatically active forms. The processing of proenzymes may arise from autohydrolysis or the catalytic action of other proteases. Numerous proteases associated with protozoan parasites have been identified and meticulously characterized. These encompass representatives from all four primary classes of proteases. In certain instances, the genes encoding pivotal proteases have been successfully isolated and sequenced, with molecular studies contributing to the elucidation of protease functionalities (Rosenthal, 1999; McKerrow et al., 1993; Klemba and Goldberg, 2002).

In these organisms, proteases perform "housekeeping" functions that are prevalent among many eukaryotic species, as well as roles that are highly specific to the life cycles of the parasites. An illustrative example of the protease diversity existing within a single organism can be observed in the proteases that operate during the erythrocytic cycle of the malaria parasite *P. falciparum*. Various mechanistic classes of proteases have evolved to address the peptide bond hydrolysis demands of the cell (Klemba and Goldberg, 2002).

While proteases are recognized for their capacity to degrade proteins, including those present in the skin, their judicious and strategic incorporation into cosmetic and therapeutic formulations can yield beneficial outcomes, such as enhanced exfoliation, ameliorated skin texture, and improved absorption of bioactive compounds (Mousavi Ghahfarrokhi et al., 2023).

The role of these proteases is pertinent to cellular turnover, facilitating the removal of desquamated cells from the epidermis and reinstating similar cellular populations, while exerting keratinolytic activity (Naveed et al., 2021).

Despite the historical utilization of proteolytic enzymes in skincare formulations, it remains uncertain whether their actions merely induce superficial exfoliation or possess the potential for long-term alterations in epidermal and dermal properties. Significant advancements have been achieved in elucidating the function of stratum corneum-localized proteases in the process of epidermal cell shedding through desmosomal degradation. With advancing age, these proteolytic activities tend to diminish, which may contribute to compromised barrier integrity and suboptimal esthetic characteristics (Smith et al., 2007).

3.4.2 Lipase

Lipases constitute an enzyme family that, under physiological conditions, catalyze the hydrolysis of carboxylic ester bonds within hydrophobic substrates such as triglycerides. In nonaqueous environments, their functional capabilities can be redirected toward alcoholysis, esterification, interesterification, and the transfer of acyl groups from esters to alternative nucleophiles, such as amines or thiols, involving both long- and short-chain carboxylic acids. Notably, they are distinguished by their exceptional compatibility with fatty, nonaqueous media and emulsions, which is essential for cosmetic formulation; extensive substrate acceptance, including a variety of nonnatural compounds; high chemo- and stereoselectivity; functionality without the necessity for costly cofactors; and comparatively robust process stability (Ansorge-Schumacher and Thum, 2013).

Phospholipases (PLs) and lyso-phospholipases (LysoPLAs) constitute a complex ensemble of enzymes that catalyze the cleavage of phospholipids and lyso-phospholipids. PLs are categorized as A1, A2, B, C, or D, while LysoPLAs are classified as LysoPLA1 and LysoPLA2, contingent upon the hydrolysis site. These enzymes cleave phospholipids within cell membranes and intracellular compartments, yielding an array of products such as lysophospholipids (LPL), free fatty acids (FFA), diacylglycerols (DG), choline phosphate, phosphoinositides, and phosphatidic acid, among others. Phospholipase A1 (PLA1) specifically hydrolyzes acyl groups from phospholipids at the sn-1 position, resulting in the production of FFA and LPL. PLA1 activities have been identified across various cell types and tissues from a diverse spectrum of organisms through the measurement of the hydrolysis of PC to lysophosphatidylcholine. However, despite their apparent ubiquity and diversity, a limited number of PLA1s have thus far been cloned and characterized. Accumulating evidence suggests that certain PLA1s possess the capability to generate bioactive lipids, a function traditionally attributed to PLA classes A2, C, and D, although the biological implications of this specific PLA warrant comprehensive investigation (Belaunzarán et al., 2011). Numerous LysoPLAs exhibit PLA1 activity in addition to their authentic LysoPLA activity. All of these lipases serve a multitude of biological functions, including the production of bioactive lipids that function as second messengers and modulators of the immune response. Some PLs are implicated in the recycling of membrane phospholipids, while others exert cytolytic effects. Notably, PLs are potent toxins found in the venom of bees and snakes, inducing blood and necrotic damage. In several pathogens, including *Pseudomonas*, *Rickettsia*, *Candida*, *Amoeba*, *Giardia*, *Toxoplasma*, and others, PLs are integral to the infection process and have been acknowledged as genuine virulence and pathogenic factors (Monic et al., 2022). Lipases have been recognized for their significance in the developmental life cycle, virulence, and transmission of a variety of parasitic organisms. Potential functions encompass the procurement of host-derived resources essential for energy metabolism, as well as serving as fundamental precursors for the biosynthesis of intricate parasite lipids that are crucial for membrane reorganization and structural integrity (Shakarian et al., 2010).

According to the existing literature and genomic analyses, kinetoplastids exhibit a variety of proteins with presumed PLA1 enzymatic activity, among which several have been subjected to experimental investigation. In the case of *T. cruzi*, a parasite characterized by an overwhelmingly intracellular existence, the sole identified PLA1 enzyme is a membrane-associated and secreted protein that modifies the lipid composition of the host through the generation of second messengers and the subsequent activation of protein kinase *C. Leishmania* spp. also harbor a PLA1 enzyme that may contribute to pathogenicity. It has been established that the pathogens *T. brucei* and *Trypanosoma congolense* exhibit greater PLA1 activity compared to the nonpathogenic *Trypanosoma lewisi*. Furthermore, in the mammalian forms of *T. brucei* (BSF), the PLA1 activity is markedly elevated in comparison with its insect forms. Lastly, significant PLA1 activity has been quantified specifically in tissue fluids derived from rabbits infected with *T. brucei*, and this activity demonstrates a positive correlation with the fluctuations of parasitemia. However, no PLA2 enzymes have been documented in *T. brucei* to date, nor have LysoPLAs. Collectively, these observations imply that PLA1 may play a pivotal role in the interactions between host and pathogen (Monic et al., 2022).

The significance of PLAs and LysoPLs in relation to virulence in pathogenic organisms, along with their capacity to modulate the host immune response, renders them particularly noteworthy within the framework of host-parasite interactions. Certain characterized PLAs in pathogenic protozoa appear to be integral to the survival of the parasite within its host and the initiation of an infection. Advances in genomic sequencing and the accessibility of numerous genomic resources have elucidated that the majority of protozoan parasites are likely to possess multiple PLA genes (Hervé et al., 2023).

In the realm of cosmetics, lipases are presently regarded as the most pivotal enzymes for biotechnological applications. Within the cosmetics manufacturing sector, these enzymes can serve both as active constituents in cosmetic formulations and as biocatalysts for the synthesis of specific cosmetic compounds. Active lipases are predominantly utilized in cosmetic products aimed at surface cleansing, anticellulite interventions, or overall body slimming, where they play a crucial role in the gentle loosening and removal of impurities and/or minute flakes of desquamated corneous tissue (i.e., exfoliation) and/or assist in the degradation of adipose deposits, frequently in conjunction with additional enzymes such as proteases. Additional applications have been documented for nasal cleansing, cosmetics, beauty masks, and hair care formulations. In an alternative application, lipases are incorporated into cosmetic formulations to facilitate controlled *in situ* release of an active ingredient (e.g., hydroxy acids) from an inactive precursor (e.g., hydroxy acid ester), a modality that has garnered particular attention in the domain of functional perfumery for the gradual and uniform development of fragrance over time (Ansorge-Schumacher and Thum, 2013; Ramos et al., 2025).

In addition, lipases have been extensively employed in the cosmetics and fragrance sectors for the production of various surfactants and aroma compounds. A range of surfactants derived from monoacylglycerols and DG is synthesized through lipase-mediated transesterification and resolution of racemic intermediates. Furthermore, esters of wax, cinnamic acid, ellagic acid, and ferulic acid are generated *via* lipase-catalyzed esterification, which can be utilized as flavor/fragrance agents and as additives in cosmetic products and sunscreens (Sarmah et al., 2018).

3.4.3 Superoxide dismutase

Aerobic organisms synthesize deleterious derivatives of oxygen through the reduction of molecular oxygen during the processes of aerobic metabolism. The predominant free radical species produced include the superoxide anion (O_2-), hydrogen peroxide (H_2O_2), and their subsequent breakdown or metabolic derivatives. Consequently, these organisms have developed intricate defense mechanisms to neutralize the toxic by-products of oxygen reduction. Superoxide dismutase (SOD) facilitates the dismutation of O_2- into H_2O_2 and O_2. The conversion of H_2O_2 to H_2O and O_2 is mediated by catalase, peroxidase, and glutathione peroxidase, the latter of which utilizes glutathione as the reducing agent. Two principal variants of SOD execute the dismutation of O_2- across diverse organisms and within various organelles and cellular compartments. These SODs are distinguished by the presence of metal ions (either Mn/Fe or Cu and Zn) at the enzyme's active site, along with their susceptibility to inhibition by cyanide, azide, and H_2O_2. Bacterial species possess either Mn/Fe- or Cu.Zn-SOD, whereas virtually all eukaryotic organisms encompass both forms of SOD. In the majority of eukaryotes, the activity of Mn-SOD is confined to the mitochondria and chloroplasts; this enzyme exhibits insensitivity to cyanide and H_2O_2. The enzyme Fe-SOD has been identified in plants and various free-living and parasitic protozoa; although it is inhibited by H_2O_2, it remains unaffected by cyanide.

In higher eukaryotes, cytosolic sources of O_2- are predominantly managed by Cu.Zn-SOD. Recently, this enzyme has also been identified within the periplasm of several bacterial species. This specific variant of SOD is inhibited by both cyanide and H_2O_2. All SOD variants are subject to inhibition by azide.

Numerous parasitic protozoa, including *E. histolytica*, *Giardia*, *Trichomonads*, *Trypanosoma*, *Leishmania*, and *Plasmodium*, have been demonstrated to exhibit anaerobic metabolic requirements. Nevertheless, metabolically, they have been characterized as microaerobic or microaerophilic. In certain instances, these organisms have been observed to produce H_2O_2 as a metabolic by-product and display heightened sensitivity to exogenous H_2O_2. Furthermore, these parasites, particularly the intracellular species, are inherently subjected to the deleterious oxygen metabolites produced by the effector immune cells of the host. However, numerous studies have indicated that many of these parasites lack, or exhibit significant deficiencies in, the enzymatic systems essential for the detoxification of H_2O_2 (e.g., catalase, glutathione peroxidase). Instead, they have evolved alternative detoxification mechanisms, which have been extensively characterized in particular prokaryotic organisms (Mehlotra, 1996).

An augmented generation of O_2-, or diminished levels of SOD, has been associated with a broad spectrum of pathological conditions, including cataract formation and senescence, inflammatory tissue necrosis, tumor proliferation, drug-induced liver necrosis (notably including acetaminophen-induced damage), asthma, and neurodegenerative diseases (such as amyotrophic lateral sclerosis (Lou Gehrig's disease), to enumerate a few instances.

Interestingly, in the model organisms *Caenorhabditis elegans* and *Drosophila melanogaster*, elevated production of SOD resulting from genetic mutations or transgenic expression correlates with substantial increases in both oxidant tolerance and lifespan. Therapeutic administration of SOD has demonstrated efficacy in mitigating tissue damage subsequent to injury induced by ischemia and irradiation, wherein oxidants are implicated as critical mediators of pathological processes (James, 1994).

These protective effects observed in experimental models underscore the relevance of SOD in human biology as well. When human skin is exposed to oxygen, it precipitates skin aging and damage. SOD acts as a potent scavenger of oxygen-free radicals, exhibiting pronounced sunscreen properties and protective effects against radiation. Concurrently, SOD functions as an antiinflammatory enzyme with well-documented antiinflammatory capabilities. Researchers have conducted extensive studies on the potential toxicity of SOD, demonstrating that it possesses no toxic side effects and is deemed very safe for cosmetic use. A specific study indicated that the migration of Langerhans cells to lymph nodes was compromised in EC-SOD transgenic mice. EC-SOD was shown to downregulate contact hypersensitivity by attenuating the inflammatory response, implying that EC-SOD may serve as a therapeutic agent for inflammatory dermatological conditions. In addition, one researcher utilized iodine-labeled SOD and applied it to the dermis of mice, with results indicating effective penetration and absorption into the skin.

Furthermore, a prior investigation revealed that pretreatment with SOD and a cell-penetrating peptide (TAT-SOD), administered to male subjects 1 h prior to exposure to UVB, resulted in an average increase of $36.6 \pm 18.4\%$ in the minimum erythema dose compared to control groups. In addition, TAT-SOD pretreatment diminished apoptotic sunburn cell formation by $47.6 \pm 8.6\%$ across all subjects. This substantiates that local application of SOD in conjunction with the cell-penetrating peptide (HIV-TAT) could significantly mitigate skin damage induced by UVB (Zheng et al., 2023).

In addition, the phenomenon of skin aging, alongside various other alterations, is typified by a reduction in collagen type I, collagen type III, and additional matrix constituents, as well as disrupted fibroblast–matrix interactions and compromised fibroblast interactions with organ parenchyma, predominantly with organ-specific epithelial cells and musculature. In human senescent dermal tissue, fibroblasts manifest growth arrest, morphological and functional transformations, and elevated concentrations of ROS, which have been documented both *in vitro* and *in vivo*. This is accompanied by an adaptive upregulation of SOD2 at the mRNA and protein levels, thereby offering empirical support for a shared response phenotype characteristic of cellular senescence (Treiber et al., 2012).

In summary, SOD is capable of efficiently scavenging oxygen free radicals, mitigating the effects of skin aging, enhancing the softness and smoothness of the skin, and facilitating moderate collagen cross-linking, while also stabilizing both collagen and elastin, ultimately contributing to the skin's elasticity. Furthermore, SOD acts in the capacity of an external coating agent for the prevention and treatment of certain dermatological conditions, effectively alleviating skin redness and swelling induced by irritation, and assisting in photoprotection.

3.4.4 Peroxiredoxins

Giardia is recognized for its absence of the conventional enzymatic systems associated with peroxide detoxification, including catalase and glutathione peroxidase, and for an extended duration, no H_2O_2-metabolizing enzymes had been definitively identified or elucidated within the parasite. Conversely, it is extensively acknowledged that H_2O_2 exerts toxic effects on *Giardia* trophozoites, precipitating a range of alterations, encompassing the inactivation of O_2 consumption, depletion of the cellular thiol pool, disruption of membrane potential and cellular motility, proteolytic degradation of the FDP, and the initiation of a distinct form of programmed cell death.

A plausible resolution to this apparent contradiction emerged upon the realization that the genome of *G. intestinalis* encodes two peroxiredoxins (Prxs), which are classified within the Prx1 subfamily: Prx1a and Prx1b. Ubiquitously present across all domains of life, from prokaryotes to mammals, Prxs are pervasive cysteine-dependent peroxidases capable of reducing H_2O_2 to H_2O. In addition to their role in H_2O_2 metabolism, these enzymes are also involved in the repair of oxidative damage, attributable to their capacity to reduce alkyl hydroperoxides, as well as in the detoxification of peroxynitrite ($ONOO^-$), a deleterious species generated through the interaction of NO with $O_2^{\cdot-}$.

To evaluate their functional characteristics, the Giardia protein Prx1a and a truncated variant of Prx1b (designated as ΔPrx1b) were expressed in *E. coli*, subsequently purified, and functionally examined. Notably, these proteins, exhibiting comparable efficacy, demonstrated the ability to metabolize H_2O_2, ONOO–, and two alkyl-hydroperoxide model compounds, namely, cumyl- and tert-butyl-hydroperoxide. These results substantiate the hypothesis that Giardia Prxs are instrumental not only in the management of oxidative stress but also in the repair of molecules suffering from oxidative damage (Mastronicola et al., 2016).

Concurrently, each of the *Plasmodium* species examined in this discourse possesses a set of five peroxiredoxins (Prxs): specifically, two belonging to the Prx1 subfamily (Prx1a and Prx1m), one PrxQ, one Prx5, and one Prx6. The enzymes Prx1a and Prx1m exhibit closer clustering with their homologs in other species than they do with each other, suggesting that the Prx1a and Prx1m lineages had already diverged from a common ancestor of the Plasmodia. The Plasmodia species that infect nonhuman mammals share this same Prx complement and will be incorporated into the discussion where pertinent. Investigations employing GFP fusion proteins have demonstrated that *P. falciparum* Prx1a and Prx6 are localized to the cytosol, while PfPrxQ is found exclusively in the nucleus, Prx1m is associated with the mitochondrion, and Prx5 is situated in the apicoplast, as illustrated in Fig. 18.3. In addition, Prx5 has been identified in *Toxoplasma* and *Naegleria fowleri* (Gretes et al., 2012; Guo et al., 2025).

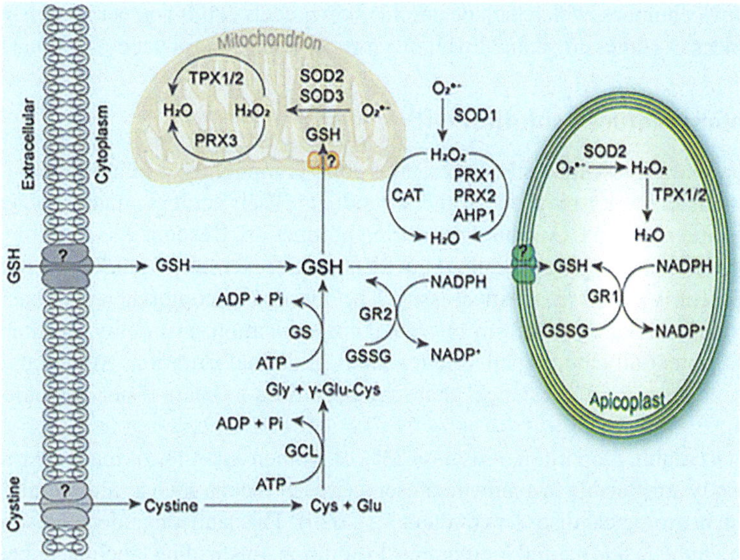

FIG. 18.3 The metabolic pathways for peroxide and glutathione within *Toxoplasma gondii* are distinctly compartmentalized across the cytoplasm, mitochondrion, and apicoplast. The zoonotic pathogen *T. gondii* exhibits an exceptionally resilient redox metabolism, demonstrating the ability to endure following the deletion of multiple peroxidases or essential enzymes required for the regeneration or de novo synthesis of glutathione (GSH). *(From Guo, Q., Pan, J., Guo, X., Zhao, M., Du, H., Wang, M., Deponte, M., Zhong, X., Xiao, L., Feng, Y., Xia, N., 2025. Toxoplasma survives the loss of key enzymes of peroxide and glutathione metabolism. FASEB J. 39 (5). doi:10.1096/fj.202402341r.)*

Recent empirical findings substantiate that Prx5 functions to safeguard epidermal keratinocytes from UVB-induced damage, including mitochondrial dysfunction and apoptosis, not solely through the direct removal of mitochondrial and cytosolic H_2O_2 but also by enhancing the catalytic efficacy of mitochondrial Prx3 and cytosolic Prx1 and Prx2 indirectly. It is plausible that fortifying Prx5 defenses could contribute to the prevention of UVB-induced dermal damage and could be utilized as a component in sunscreen formulations (Kim et al., 2023).

4 Safety and regulatory considerations

The cosmetic sector is experiencing a substantial transformation as consumer inclinations increasingly favor sustainability, the utilization of natural constituents, and ethical manufacturing processes. Microbial and biobased cosmetics present a viable solution to this emerging demand, employing natural raw materials alongside biotechnological advancements to supplant synthetic compounds. Nonetheless, this evolution also engenders intricate safety and ethical dilemmas that necessitate careful consideration to safeguard consumer welfare, uphold environmental standards, and promote equitable socioeconomic practices.

4.1 The promise and risk of microbial ingredients

Microbial biotechnology has markedly transformed a variety of industries—including healthcare, agriculture, pharmaceuticals, and cosmetics—by facilitating the creation of sustainable materials such as bioethanol, biogas, biosurfactants, and biopolymers. These microbially derived products frequently originate from organic waste, thereby contributing to the objectives of a circular economy by mitigating waste and generating renewable resources (Kumar et al., 2025). Within the realm of cosmetics, microbial products provide biodegradable and low-toxicity alternatives to synthetic ingredients. For instance, biosurfactants, including sophorolipids, rhamnolipids, and mannosylerythritol lipids, are emerging as efficacious and safer replacements for traditional surfactants, owing to their compatibility with skin and their minimal ecological footprint (Adu et al., 2020).

Despite these merits, apprehensions regarding the long-term safety and efficacy of microbial products remain prevalent. The employment of engineered microbial systems and biotechnological methodologies introduces uncertainties concerning toxicity, allergenicity, and unintended environmental repercussions (Ahmed, 2023). Although biosurfactant toxicity is generally low, it is dose-dependent, necessitating comprehensive *in vitro* investigations—often utilizing advanced 3D skin models—to accurately forecast their safety under actual conditions. The ethical obligation to minimize animal testing has catalyzed the advancement of such *in vitro* techniques, which include porcine skin models exhibiting permeability akin to that of human skin, representing significant strides in addressing animal welfare considerations in product evaluation (Adu et al., 2020).

4.2 Biobased cosmetics: Nature's solution with caveats

Biobased cosmetics, composed of essential oils, herbs, microbial compounds, and antibiotics, are regarded as safer and more environmentally sustainable alternatives to synthetic products. Their ecological advantages encompass low resource intensity, biodegradability, and reduced CO_2 emissions during production. Responsible sourcing, waste minimization, pollution mitigation, and sustainable packaging are integral to their environmentally friendly assertions (Paramita et al., 2024).

Nevertheless, safety concerns persist as a critical issue. The absence of comprehensive long-term safety data, coupled with inadequate regulatory oversight, can result in microbial contamination, instability, or interaction complications with other cosmetic ingredients, potentially inciting allergic reactions or dermal irritation. Numerous microbial extracts contain inherent toxins, allergens, or phototoxic substances that may pose risks to users if not meticulously processed and monitored (Bozza et al., 2022).

Research indicates that a notable proportion of users—23% of women and 14% of men—experience adverse reactions to cosmetics annually, frequently attributable to synthetic preservatives or metals such as aluminum, which have also been controversially associated with neurological disorders (Adu et al., 2020). This statistic underscores the imperative for enhanced safety assessments of both synthetic and natural ingredients. In addition, misleading labeling, subpar preservation techniques, and the lack of standardized testing for "natural" assertions heighten the potential for consumer risk (Paramita et al., 2024).

4.3 Regulatory and certification frameworks: Progress and gaps

The evolution of regulatory mechanisms pertaining to biobased cosmetics has been notably gradual. Until the recent past, there existed an absence of globally standardized benchmarks to delineate what qualifies as a "natural" or "organic" cosmetic. This deficiency enabled cosmetic manufacturers to assert unverified claims such as "green," "eco," or "bio," thereby misleading consumers who may conflate these terminologies with safety and environmental benefits (Bozza et al., 2022). Certification entities such as Ecocert, Cosmos, ICEA, and Natrue have contributed to the establishment of some degree of order by providing verification of ingredients and assessments of sustainability. ISO 16128, formulated by the International Organization for Standardization, supplies guidelines for defining and quantifying the natural and organic content present in cosmetic ingredients. Nevertheless, it remains a nonbinding standard and is devoid of specific safety protocols.

In addition, prevailing certifications frequently neglect significant health and environmental hazards, including allergenic compounds or the aquatic toxicity associated with certain bioderived substances. Numerous "natural" materials lack the capacity for easy biodegradation, leading to their potential accumulation in ecosystems and posing risks to aquatic organisms. There exists an acute necessity for ecotoxicological investigations and more stringent environmental impact evaluations of these substances prior to their approval (Bozza et al., 2022).

Within the European Union, a catalog of prohibited substances in cosmetics encompasses natural compounds known to present risks, and safety evaluations are mandated to incorporate assessments of both local and systemic effects. However, such stringent oversight is not uniformly enforced, particularly in emerging markets. Consequently, products exhibiting variable safety and quality may enter the global marketplace without adequate scrutiny.

4.4 Ethical imperatives in microbial and natural product development

The ethical considerations associated with the development of microbial and biobased cosmetics are extensive and profoundly impactful. These encompass apprehensions regarding biosafety, bioterrorism, public confidence, and equitable access to technological advancements. For example, the misuse of microbial technologies could result in the introduction of pathogens or genetically modified organisms into the environment or supply chain. Thus the implementation of robust containment protocols, adherence to ethical research practices, and the promotion of public transparency are of paramount importance (Ahmed, 2023).

Equity and access also represent critical dimensions of this discourse. Communities that contribute to the biodiversity or traditional knowledge underlying many natural ingredients frequently do not reap the benefits derived from their commercialization. This situation raises pertinent issues related to intellectual property rights, biopiracy, and benefit-sharing, necessitating legal and ethical rectification through frameworks such as the Nagoya Protocol and fair-trade agreements.

Moreover, the economic and social ramifications of supplanting conventional cosmetics with biobased alternatives warrant thorough consideration. While natural cosmetics may offer enhanced safety and sustainability, they are often accompanied by higher costs, thereby restricting accessibility for consumers with lower incomes.

Consequently, ethical product development must engage with issues of affordability, inclusive innovation, and the democratization of sustainable beauty. To foster public trust and ensure equitable practices, ethical governance should encompass:

- Transparency in ingredient sourcing and safety data.
- Inclusive standards that reflect both scientific rigor and societal values.
- Engagement with stakeholders from diverse regions and economic contexts.
- Certification systems that transcend marketing strategies to enforce genuine accountability.

5 Future perspectives

Prospects for the utilization of protozoans in biofunctional cosmetics are exceedingly auspicious, propelled by advancements in biotechnology and an increasing demand for natural, sustainable constituents. Protozoans, with their distinctive metabolic capabilities and bioactive compounds, possess potential for innovative dermatological applications such as anti-aging, hydration, UV protection, and antimicrobial functionalities. Novel research is commencing to elucidate the molecular mechanisms underlying these advantages, thereby facilitating the development of targeted formulations. As omics technologies and synthetic biology advance, it may become practicable to engineer protozoans or extract their metabolites with greater efficiency and safety. Regulatory transparency and consumer enlightenment will also assume pivotal roles in enhancing their acceptance and assimilation into mainstream cosmetic products. In addition to their biochemical adaptability, protozoans present a predominantly unexploited repository of novel compounds, such as enzymes, lipids, and polysaccharides, that can be utilized for a spectrum of cosmetic functionalities. Species such as *E. gracilis* have already demonstrated promise in synthesizing β-glucans and antioxidants, which contribute to dermal regeneration and protection. Future innovations may encompass the cultivation of specific protozoan strains under regulated conditions to maximize the yield of desired bioactive molecules. Furthermore, advancements in nanotechnology could facilitate the encapsulation and administration of protozoan-derived substances, augmenting their stability, penetration, and efficacy in topical applications.

The incorporation of protozoan-based ingredients also harmonizes effectively with the inclination toward eco-conscious and cruelty-free beauty products. Unlike certain conventional animal-derived components, protozoans can be cultivated sustainably with minimal ecological impact. Collaborations among cosmetic chemists, microbiologists, and bioengineers will likely expedite the identification of new protozoan species and metabolic pathways advantageous to skin health. As consumer consciousness expands and scientific validation progresses, protozoans may emerge as a fundamental element in the forthcoming generation of biofunctional and personalized cosmetic solutions.

Last but not least, the use of protozoans in the cosmetic industry will contribute to the minimization of chemical pollution. Adopting a "zero waste" policy is crucial for preventing cosmetic waste from contaminating humans *via* environmental pollution. The integration of zero waste and zero CO_2 emission protocols in the cosmetic industry's sourcing, production, and packaging stages is essential for fostering "Green Growth." Recycling industrial waste should be mandated to facilitate a circular economy. The significant environmental impact of conventional cosmetics containing microbeads, microplastics, and triclosan necessitates urgent attention. These diminutive particles are unremovable from oceans, integrate into natural cycles, and infiltrate the food chain. Volatile organic compounds in fragrances contribute to smog and air pollution. UV filters such as avobenzone, octocrylene, and oxybenzone in sunscreens contaminate systemic circulation, the environment, and agricultural productivity. Ultrafine crystalline silica nanoparticles in cosmetics can induce genetic alterations and severe mutations. Evidence suggests that nanoparticles can traverse the blood–brain barrier through inhalation and affect brain function. Synthetic antioxidants butylated hydroxyanisole (BHA) and butylated hydroxytoluene (BHT), used as cosmetic preservatives, disrupt aquatic species and lead to genetic changes (Goyal and Jerold, 2023).

6 Conclusions

The investigation into the use of protozoans in biofunctional cosmetics reveals their remarkable and largely unexplored potential. Protozoans offer a rich reservoir of bioactive compounds, including polysaccharides, lipids, peptides, and enzymes, capable of imparting significant functional and therapeutic benefits to cosmetic formulations. Specific examples, such as the wound healing properties of PSG, the protein quality control facilitated by high-mannose-type oligosaccharides, and the moisturizing and photoprotective effects of β-glucans and ergosterol-derived vitamin D2, underscore their diverse applications. Furthermore, PS shows promise for skin cell regeneration and scar tissue treatment. The increasing consumer demand for natural and sustainable ingredients aligns well with the cultivation of protozoans, which can be achieved with minimal ecological impact. Advancements in biotechnology and synthetic biology hold promise for optimizing the extraction and engineering of these beneficial molecules. However, comprehensive safety assessments, transparent labeling, and robust regulatory frameworks are crucial to ensure consumer confidence and address potential ethical considerations related to biosafety and equitable access. Continued interdisciplinary collaboration between cosmetic chemists, microbiologists, and bioengineers will be vital in unlocking the full potential of protozoans, leading to innovative and sustainable dermatological solutions.

References

Adu, S.A., Naughton, P.J., Marchant, R., Banat, I.M., 2020. Microbial biosurfactants in cosmetic and personal skincare pharmaceutical formulations. Pharmaceutics. 19994923. 12 (11), 1–21. Available from: https://www.mdpi.com/1999-4923/12/11/1099/pdf. doi:10.3390/pharmaceutics12111099.

Ahmed, I.A., 2023. Ethical Issues of Microbial Products for Industrialization. Springer Science and Business Media LLC, pp. 393–411. doi:10.1007/978-981-99-1737-2_20.

Alencar-Silva, T., Braga, M.C., Santana, G.O.S., Saldanha-Araujo, F., Pogue, R., Dias, S.C., Franco, O.L., Carvalho, J.L., 2018. Breaking the frontiers of cosmetology with antimicrobial peptides. Biotechnol. Adv. 07349750. 36 (8), 2019–2031. Available from: www.elsevier.com/inca/publications/store/5/2/5/4/5/5/index.htt. doi:10.1016/j.biotechadv.2018.08.005.

Alves, A., Sousa, E., Kijjoa, A., Pinto, M., 2020. Marine-derived compounds with potential use as cosmeceuticals and nutricosmetics. Molecules. 1420-3049. 25 (11), 2536. doi:10.3390/molecules25112536.

Andrä, J., Herbst, R., Leippe, M., 2003. Amoebapores, archaic effector peptides of protozoan origin, are discharged into phagosomes and kill bacteria by permeabilizing their membranes. Dev. Comp. Immunol. 0145305X. 27 (4), 291–304. doi:10.1016/s0145-305x(02)00106-4.

Ansorge-Schumacher, M.B., Thum, O., 2013. Immobilised lipases in the cosmetics industry. Chem. Soc. Rev. 0306-0012. 42 (15), 6475. doi:10.1039/c3cs35484a.

Barylyuk, K., Koreny, L., Huiling, K., Butterworth, S., Crook, O.M., Lassadi, I., Gupta, V., Tromer, E., Mourier, T., Stevens, T.J., Breckels, L.M., Pain, A., Lilley, K.S., Waller, R.F., 2020. A comprehensive subcellular atlas of the toxoplasma proteome via hyper LOPIT provides spatial context for protein functions. Cell Host Microbe. 19313128. 28 (5), 752. doi:10.1016/j.chom.2020.09.011.

Belaunzarán, M.L., Lammel, E.M., De Isola, E.L.D., 2011. Phospholipases A in trypanosomatids. Enzyme Res. 20900414. 2011 (1). doi:10.4061/2011/392082.

Beverley, S.M., Turco, S.J., 1998. Lipophosphoglycan (LPG) and the identification of virulence genes in the protozoan parasite Leishmania. Trends Microbiol. 0966842X. 6 (1), 35–40. doi:10.1016/S0966-842X(97)01180-3.

Bianchet, R.T., Cubas, A.L.V., Machado, M.M., Moecke, E.H.S., 2020. Applicability of bacterial cellulose in cosmetics—bibliometric review. Biotechnol. Rep. 2215017X. 27. Available from: http://www.journals.elsevier.com/biotechnology-reports/. doi:10.1016/j.btre.2020.e00502.

Bocheva, G., Slominski, R.M., Slominski, A.T., 2021. The impact of vitamin D on skin aging. Int. J. Mol. Sci. 1422-0067. 22 (16), 9097. doi:10.3390/ijms22169097.

Bozza, A., Campi, C., Garelli, S., Ugazio, E., Battaglia, L., 2022. Current regulatory and market frameworks in green cosmetics: the role of certification. Sustain. Chem. Pharm. 23525541. 30, 100851. doi:10.1016/j.scp.2022.100851.

Bruhn, H., Riekens, B., Berninghausen, O., Leippe, M., 2003. Amoebapores and NK-lysin, members of a class of structurally distinct antimicrobial and cytolytic peptides from protozoa and mammals: a comparative functional analysis. Biochem. J. 0264-6021. 375 (3), 737–744. doi:10.1042/bj20030250.

Buetow, D.E., 2011. Euglena Encyclopedia of Life Sciences. Wiley. doi:10.1002/9780470015902.a0001964.pub3.

Chung, S.-Y., Nam, S.-J., Choi, W.-K., Seo, M.-Y., Kim, J.-W., Park, C.-S., et al., 2006. Phosphatidylserine enhances skin barrier function through keratinocyte differentiation. J. Soc. Cosmet. Sci. Korea 32 (1), 17–22.

Cummings, R.D., 2023. Glycosphingolipids in human parasites. FEBS Open Bio. 22115463. 13 (9), 1625–1635. Available from: http://www.elsevier.com/wps/find/journaldescription.cws_home/726807/description#description. doi:10.1002/2211-5463.13662.

De Luca, M., Pappalardo, I., Limongi, A.R., Viviano, E., Radice, R.P., Todisco, S., Martelli, G., Infantino, V., Vassallo, A., 2021. Lipids from microalgae for cosmetic applications. Cosmetics. 20799284. 8 (2). Available from: www.mdpi.com/journal/cosmetics. doi:10.3390/cosmetics8020052.

de Macedo-silva, S., Souza, W., Rodrigues, J., 2015. Sterol biosynthesis pathway as an alternative for the anti-protozoan parasite chemotherapy. Curr. Med. Chem. 09298673. 22 (18), 2186–2198. doi:10.2174/0929867322666150319120337.

Dhar, N., 2010. Novel Cellulose Nanoparticles for Potential Cosmetic and Pharmaceutical Applications (Ph.D. thesis). University of Waterloo.

Dos Santos, M.G., Muxel, S.M., Zampieri, R.A., Pomorski, T.G., Floeter-Winter, L.M., 2013. Transbilayer dynamics of phospholipids in the plasma membrane of the Leishmania genus. PLoS One. 19326203. 8 (1). Available from: http://www.plosone.org/article/fetchObjectAttachment.action?uri=info%3Adoi%2F10.1371%2Fjournal.pone.0055604&representation=PD. doi:10.1371/journal.pone.0055604Brazil.

Gęgotek, A., Skrzydlewska, E., 2023. The role of ABC transporters in skin cells exposed to UV radiation. Int. J. Mol. Sci. 1422-0067. 24 (1), 115. doi:10.3390/ijms24010115.

Giraud, E., Lestinova, T., Derrick, T., Martin, O., Dillon, R.J., Volf, P., Müller, I., Bates, P.A., Rogers, M.E., Beverley, S.M., 2018. Leishmania proteophosphoglycans regurgitated from infected sand flies accelerate dermal wound repair and exacerbate leishmaniasis via insulin-like growth factor 1-dependent signalling. PLoS Pathog. 1553-7374. 14 (1), e1006794. doi:10.1371/journal.ppat.1006794.

Goyal, N., Jerold, F., 2023. Biocosmetics: technological advances and future outlook. Environ. Sci. Pollut. Res. 1614-7499. 30 (10), 25148–25169. doi:10.1007/s11356-021-17567-3.

Gretes, M.C., Poole, L.B., Karplus, P.A., 2012. Peroxiredoxins in parasites. Antioxid. Redox Signal. 15577716. 17 (4), 608–633. doi:10.1089/ars.2011.4404.

Guo, Q., Pan, J., Guo, X., Zhao, M., Huiyu, D., Wang, M., Deponte, M., Zhong, X., Xiao, L., Feng, Y., Xia, N., 2025. Toxoplasma survives the loss of key enzymes of peroxide and glutathione metabolism. FASEB J. 0892-6638. 39 (5). doi:10.1096/fj.202402341r.

Haubrich, B.A., Singha, U.K., Miller, M.B., Nes, C.R., Anyatonwu, H., Lecordier, L., Patkar, P., Leaver, D.J., Villalta, F., Vanhollebeke, B., Chaudhuri, M., Nes, W.D., 2015. Discovery of an ergosterol-signaling factor that regulates trypanosoma brucei growth. J. Lipid Res. 15397262. 56 (2), 331–341. Available from: http://www.jlr.org/. doi:10.1194/jlr.M054643.

Hernandez, E., 2012. Lipids, pharmaceutical and cosmetic use. Kirk-Othmer Encycl. Chem. Technol. 29, 1–19. doi:10.1002/0471238961.lipihern.a01.

Hervé, P., Monic, S., Bringaud, F., Rivière, L., 2023. Phospholipases A and lysophospholipases in protozoan parasites. Microb. Cell. 23112638. 10 (10), 204–216. doi:10.15698/mic2023.10.805.

Ito, Y., Hagihara, S., Matsuo, I., Totani, K., 2005. Structural approaches to the study of oligosaccharides in glycoprotein quality control. Curr. Opin. Struct. Biol. 0959440X. 15 (5), 481–489. doi:10.1016/j.sbi.2005.08.012.

James, E.R., 1994. Superoxide dismutase. Parasitol. Today. 01694758. 10 (12), 481–484. doi:10.1016/0169-4758(94)90161-9.

Jasinghe, V.J., Perera, C.O., 2005. Distribution of ergosterol in different tissues of mushrooms and its effect on the conversion of ergosterol to vitamin D2 by UV irradiation. Food Chem. 03088146. 92 (3), 541–546. Available from: www.elsevier.com/locate/foodchem. doi:10.1016/j.foodchem.2004.08.022.

Jiang, C., Jinxin, G., Bin, H., Zeng, B., 2021. Glycosphingolipids in filamentous fungi: biological roles and potential applications in cosmetics and health foods. Front. Microbiol. 1664-302X. 12. doi:10.3389/fmicb.2021.690211.

Kaur, N., Dey, P., 2023. Bacterial exopolysaccharides as emerging bioactive macromolecules: from fundamentals to applications. Res. Microbiol. 09232508. 174 (4), 104024. doi:10.1016/j.resmic.2022.104024.

Kim, S.R., Park, J.W., Lee, B.H., Lim, K.M., Chang, T.S., 2023. Peroxiredoxin V protects against UVB-induced damage of keratinocytes. Antioxidants. 20763921. 12 (7). Available from: www.mdpi.com/journal/antioxidants. doi:10.3390/antiox12071435.

Klemba, M., Goldberg, D.E., 2002. Biological roles of proteases in parasitic protozoa. Annu. Rev. Biochem. 00664154. 71, 275–305. doi:10.1146/annurev.biochem.71.090501.145453.

Kodolova-Chukhontseva, V.V., Rozova, E.Y., Dresvyanina, E.N., Nashchekina, Y.A., Dobrovol'skaya, I.P., Vlasova, E.N., Bystrov, S.G., Popova, E.N., Maslennikova, T.P., Yudin, V.E., Morganti, P., 2023. New composite materials based on chitosan films reinforced with chitin nanofibrils for cosmetic application. Cosmetics. 20799284. 10 (2). Available from: www.mdpi.com/journal/cosmetics. doi:10.3390/cosmetics10020051.

Kumar, D., Kumar, R., Sakshi, A.K., 2025. Ethical Implications and Regulatory Frameworks for Microbial Products and Processes: Microbial Contributions to a Circular Economy. Springer Science and Business Media LLC, pp. 401–418. doi:10.1007/978-981-96-4824-5_17.

Kumari, J., Kumawat, R., Prasanna, R., Jothieswari, D., Debnath, R., Ikbal, A.M.A., Palit, P., Rawat, R., Gopikrishna, K., Tiwari, O.N., 2025. Microbial exopolysaccharides: classification, biosynthetic pathway, industrial extraction and commercial production to unveil its bioprospection: a comprehensive review. Int. J. Biol. Macromol. 01418130. 297, 139917. doi:10.1016/j.ijbiomac.2025.139917.

Lansdown, A.B.G., Sampson, B., Rowe, A., 1999. Sequential changes in trace metal, metallothionein and calmodulin concentrations in healing skin wounds. J. Anat. 00218782. 195 (3), 375–386. Available from: http://onlinelibrary.wiley.com/journal/10.1111/(ISSN)1469-7580. doi:10.1046/j.1469-7580.1999.19530375.x.

Leippe, M., 1999. Antimicrobial and cytolytic polypeptides of amoeboid protozoa—effector molecules of primitive phagocytes. Dev. Comp. Immunol. 0145305X. 23 (4-5), 267–279. doi:10.1016/s0145-305x(99)00010-5.

Li, J., Wang, Z., Karim, M.R., Zhang, L., 2020. Detection of human intestinal protozoan parasites in vegetables and fruits: a review. Parasit. Vectors. 17563305. 13 (1). Available from: http://www.parasitesandvectors.com/. doi:10.1186/s13071-020-04255-3.

Mastronicola, D., Falabella, M., Forte, E., Testa, F., Sarti, P., Giuffrè, A., 2016. Antioxidant defence systems in the protozoan pathogen *Giardia intestinalis*. Mol. Biochem. Parasitol. 01666851. 206 (1-2), 56–66. doi:10.1016/j.molbiopara.2015.12.002.

Mazurkiewicz-Pisarek, A., Baran, J., Ciach, T., 2023. Antimicrobial peptides: challenging journey to the pharmaceutical, biomedical, and cosmeceutical use. Int. J. Mol. Sci. 1422-0067. 24 (10), 9031. doi:10.3390/ijms24109031.

McKerrow, J.H., Sun, E., Rosenthal, P.J., Bouvier, J., 1993. The proteases and pathogenicity of parasitic protozoa. Annu. Rev. Microbiol. 00664227. 47, 821–853. Available from: http://www.annualreviews.org/journal/micro. doi:10.1146/annurev.mi.47.100193.004133.

Mehlotra, R.K., 1996. Antioxidant defense mechanisms in parasitic protozoa. Crit. Rev. Microbiol. 1040841X. 22 (4), 295–314. doi:10.3109/10408419609105484.

Mendelzon, D.H., Parodi, A.J., 1986. N-linked high mannose-type oligosaccharides in the protozoa *Crithidia fasciculata* and *Crithidia harmosa* contain galactofuranose residues. J. Biol. Chem. 00219258. 261 (5), 2129–2133. doi:10.1016/s0021-9258(17)35907-0.

Mina, J.G.M., Denny, P.W., 2018. Everybody needs sphingolipids, right! Mining for new drug targets in protozoan sphingolipid biosynthesis. Parasitology. 14698161. 145 (2), 134–147. Available from: http://journals.cambridge.org/action/displayJournal?jid=PAR. doi:10.1017/S0031182017001081.

Monic, S.G., Lamy, A., Thonnus, M., Bizarra-Rebelo, T., Bringaud, F., Smith, T.K., Figueiredo, L.M., Rivière, L., 2022. A novel lipase with dual localisation in *Trypanosoma brucei*. Sci. Rep. 20452322. 12 (1). Available from: www.nature.com/srep/index.html. doi:10.1038/s41598-022-08546-w.

Mostafa, W.Z., Hegazy, R.A., 2015. Vitamin D and the skin: focus on a complex relationship: a review. J. Adv. Res. 20901232. 6 (6), 793–804. doi:10.1016/j.jare.2014.01.011.

Mousavi Ghahfarrokhi, S.S., Mahdigholi, F.S., Amin, M., 2023. Collateral beauty in the damages: an overview of cosmetics and therapeutic applications of microbial proteases. Arch. Microbiol. 1432072X. 205 (12). Available from: https://www.springer.com/journal/203. doi:10.1007/s00203-023-03713-7.

Myklestad, S.M., Granum, E., 2009. Biology of (1,3)-β-glucans and related glucans in protozoans and chromistans. In: Chemistry, Biochemistry, and Biology of 1-3 Beta Glucans and Related Polysaccharides. Academic Press, pp. 353–385. Available from: https://www.sciencedirect.com/science/book/9780123739711. doi:10.1016/B978-0-12-373971-1.00010-8.

Naveed, M., Nadeem, F., Mehmood, T., Bilal, M., Anwar, Z., Amjad, F., 2021. Protease—a versatile and ecofriendly biocatalyst with multi-industrial applications: an updated review. Catal. Lett. 1011-372X. 151 (2), 307–323. doi:10.1007/s10562-020-03316-7.

Norman, F.F., Comeche, B., Chamorro, S., Pérez-Molina, J.A., López-Vélez, R., 2020. Update on the major imported protozoan infections in travelers and migrants. Future Microbiol. 17460921. 15 (3), 213–225. Available from: http://www.futuremedicine.com/loi/fmb. doi:10.2217/fmb-2019-0212.

Ozanne, H., Toumi, H., Roubinet, B., Landemarre, L., Lespessailles, E., Daniellou, R., Cesaro, A., 2020. Laminarin effects, a β-(1,3)-glucan, on skin cell inflammation and oxidation. Cosmetics. 2079-9284. 7 (3), 66. doi:10.3390/cosmetics7030066.

Paramita, S., Kusuma, I.W., Sulistioadi, Y.B., Kiswanto,, 2024. Environmental and Safety Aspects of Bio-based Cosmetics in Indonesia Biomass-based Cosmetics: Research Trends and Future Outlook. Springer Nature, Indonesia, pp. 545–568. Available from https://link.springer.com/book/10.1007/978-981-97-1908-2. doi:10.1007/978-981-97-1908-2_22.

Plattner, H., 2010. Membrane Trafficking in Protozoa, Vol. 280, pp. 79–184. Elsevier BV. doi:10.1016/s1937-6448(10)80003-6.

Popa, I., 2018. The concept of sphingolipid rheostat in skin: a driving force for new active ingredients in cosmetic applications. OCL. 2272-6977. 25 (5), D507. doi:10.1051/ocl/2018043.

Pratt, S., Wansadhipathi-Kannangara, N.K., Bruce, C.R., Mina, J.G., Shams-Eldin, H., Casas, J., Hanada, K., Schwarz, R.T., Sonda, S., Denny, P.W., 2013. Sphingolipid synthesis and scavenging in the intracellular apicomplexan parasite, *Toxoplasma gondii*. Mol. Biochem. Parasitol. 18729428. 187 (1), 43–51. doi:10.1016/j.molbiopara.2012.11.007.

Rahman, M.D., Pascal, R.A., 1990. Inhibitors of ergosterol biosynthesis and growth of the trypanosomatid protozoan *Crithidia fasciculata*. J. Biol. Chem. 00219258. 265 (9), 4989–4996. doi:10.1016/s0021-9258(19)34073-6.

Ramos, G.R., Ostrosky, E.A., Lopes, P.S., Filho, N.A., Kakuda, L.L., da Silva Pinto, J.N., de Lima Viana, E., Morais, N.S., Rios, N.S., Gomes, A.P.B., Xavier, F.H., de Sousa, F.C., de Assis, C.F., 2025. Developing a cosmetic formulation containing lipase produced by the fungus *Aspergillus terreus*. PLoS One. 19326203. 20 (5). Available from: https://journals.plos.org/plosone/article?id=10.1371/journal.pone.0322106. doi:10.1371/journal.pone.0322106.

Ravi Kumar, M.N.V., 2000. A review of chitin and chitosan applications. React. Funct. Polym. 13815148. 46 (1), 1–27. doi:10.1016/S1381-5148(00)00038-9.

Roberts, C.W., McLeod, R., Rice, D.W., Ginger, M., Chance, M.L., Goad, L.J., 2003. Fatty acid and sterol metabolism: potential antimicrobial targets in apicomplexan and trypanosomatid parasitic protozoa. Mol. Biochem. Parasitol. 01666851. 126 (2), 129–142. doi:10.1016/s0166-6851(02)00280-3.

Rosenthal, P.J., 1999. Proteases of protozoan parasites. Adv. Parasitol. 0065308X. 43, 105–159. Available from: https://www.sciencedirect.com/bookseries/advances-in-parasitology. doi:10.1016/s0065-308x(08)60242-0.

Ruehle, M.D., Orias, E., Pearson, C.G., 2016. Tetrahymena as a unicellular model eukaryote: genetic and genomic tools. Genetics. 19432631. 203 (2), 649–665. Available from: http://www.genetics.org/content/genetics/203/2/649.full.pdf. doi:10.1534/genetics.114.169748.

Sarmah, N., Revathi, D., Sheelu, G., Rani, K.Y., Sridhar, S., Mehtab, V., Sumana, C., 2018. Recent advances on sources and industrial applications of lipases. Biotechnol. Prog. 8756-7938. 34 (1), 5–28. doi:10.1002/btpr.2581.

Sauvage, V., Aubert, D., Escotte-Binet, S., Villena, I., 2009. The role of ATP-binding cassette (ABC) proteins in protozoan parasites. Mol. Biochem. Parasitol. 01666851. 167 (2), 81–94. doi:10.1016/j.molbiopara.2009.05.005.

Secchi, G., 2008. Role of protein in cosmetics. Clin. Dermatol. 0738081X. 26 (4), 321–325. doi:10.1016/j.clindermatol.2008.04.004.

Shakarian, A.M., McGugan, G.C., Joshi, M.B., Stromberg, M., Bowers, L., Ganim, C., Barowski, J., Dwyer, D.M., 2010. Identification, characterization, and expression of a unique secretory lipase from the human pathogen *Leishmania donovani*. Mol. Cell. Biochem. 15734919. 341 (1-2), 17–31. doi:10.1007/s11010-010-0433-6.

Siddiqui, R., Khan, N.A., 2012. Biology and pathogenesis of Acanthamoeba. Parasit. Vectors. 17563305. 5 (1). doi:10.1186/1756-3305-5-6.

Smith, W.P., Bishop, M., Gillis, G., Maibach, H., 2007. Topical proteolytic enzymes affect epidermal and dermal properties. Int. J. Cosmet. Sci. 0142-5463. 29 (1), 15–21. doi:10.1111/j.1467-2494.2007.00354.x.

Sommer, K., Hillinger, M., Eigenmann, A., Vetter, W., 2023. Characterization of various isomeric photoproducts of ergosterol and vitamin D2 generated by UV irradiation. Eur. Food Res. Technol. 1438-2377. 249 (3), 713–726. doi:10.1007/s00217-022-04167-9.

Souza, W., 2008. An introduction to the structural organization of parasitic protozoa. Curr. Pharm. Des. 13816128. 14 (9), 822–838. doi:10.2174/138161208784041123.

Štefanić, S., Spycher, C., Morf, L., Fabriàs, G., Casas, J., Schraner, E., Wild, P., Hehl, A.B., Sonda, S., 2010. Glucosylceramide synthesis inhibition affects cell cycle progression, membrane trafficking, and stage differentiation in *Giardia lamblia*. J. Lipid Res. 00222275. 51 (9), 2527–2545. doi:10.1194/jlr.m003392.

Takahara, Y., Miyachi, N., Nawa, M., Matsuoka, M., 2019. Calmodulin-like skin protein suppresses the increase in senescence-associated β-galactosidase induced by hydrogen peroxide or ultraviolet irradiation in keratinocytes. Cell Biol. Int. 1065-6995. 43 (7), 835–843. doi:10.1002/cbin.11159.

Tortora, G.J., Funke, B.R., Case, C.L., 2016. Microbiology: An Introduction. Pearson.

Treiber, N., Maity, P., Singh, K., Ferchiu, F., Wlaschek, M., Scharffetter-Kochanek, K., 2012. The role of manganese superoxide dismutase in skin aging. Derm. -Endocrinol. 1938-1980. 4 (3), 232–235. doi:10.4161/derm.21819.

Vial, H.J., Eldin, P., Tielens, A.G.M., Van Hellemond, J.J., 2003. Phospholipids in parasitic protozoa. Mol. Biochem. Parasitol. 126 (2), 143–154. doi:10.1016/S0166-6851(02)00281-5.

Walker, J.E., Saraste, M., Runswick, M.J., Gay, N.J., 1982. Distantly related sequences in the alpha- and beta-subunits of ATP synthase, myosin, kinases and other ATP-requiring enzymes and a common nucleotide binding fold. EMBO J. 02614189. 1 (8), 945–951. doi:10.1002/j.1460-2075.1982.tb01276.x.

Wanderley, J.L.M., Benjamin, A., Real, F., Bonomo, A., Moreira, M.E.C., Barcinski, M.A., 2005. Apoptotic mimicry: an altruistic behavior in host/Leishmania interplay. Braz. J. Med. Biol. Res. 0100-879X. 38 (6), 807–812. doi:10.1590/S0100-879X2005000600001.

Williams, D.F., 2009. On the nature of biomaterials. Biomaterials. 01429612. 30 (30), 5897–5909. doi:10.1016/j.biomaterials.2009.07.027.

Xu, W., Hsu, F.-F., Baykal, E., Huang, J., Zhang, K., Horn, D., 2014. Sterol biosynthesis is required for heat resistance but not extracellular survival in Leishmania. PLoS Pathog. 1553-7374. 10 (10), e1004427. doi:10.1371/journal.ppat.1004427.

Zheng, M., Liu, Y., Zhang, G., Yang, Z., Weiwei, X., Chen, Q., 2023. The applications and mechanisms of superoxide dismutase in medicine, food, and cosmetics. Antioxidants. 2076-3921. 12 (9), 1675. doi:10.3390/antiox12091675.

Zhou, J., Jie, L., Xuewen, D., Bing, X., 2017. Supramolecular biofunctional materials. Biomaterials. 01429612. 129, 1–27. doi:10.1016/j.biomaterials.2017.03.014.

Chapter 19

Marine microorganisms

Katie Shiels, Margarida Matias, Jessica Walshe, Patrick Murray, and Sushanta Kumar Saha
Centre for Applied Bioscience Research, Technological University of the Shannon, Limerick, Ireland

1 Introduction

1.1 Overview of marine microalgae

Microalgae can be considered microscopic plants with either eukaryotic or prokaryotic types of cellular structures. They represent a very large group of phototrophic and heterotrophic organisms contributing to vast diversity in terms of their morphology, and are distributed ubiquitously throughout all habitats, including freshwater and marine environments. Marine microalgae, which also comprise both eukaryotic lineages and prokaryotic cyanobacteria, are among the most diverse groups of organisms in aquatic ecosystems (Hopes and Mock, 2015). These photoautotrophs form the base of marine food webs and biogeochemical cycles while accounting for about half of the global primary production with the generation of oxygen that sustains life on the planet Earth (Falkowski et al., 1998). They have been part of the Earth's environment for about 3.4 billion years, thanks to their exceptional metabolic diversity, which enabled them to adapt to a wide range of environmental conditions, such as variable salinity, nutrient limitation, ultraviolet radiation, desiccation, and temperature fluctuations (Carvalho et al., 2011).

Microalgae include taxa within the Chlorophyceae, Eustigmatophyceae, Bacillariophyceae, and Cyanobacteria (also known as blue–green algae), as well as a limited number of species within the Rhodophyceae. The evolutionary path of microalgae translates into biochemical heterogeneity. Microalgae produce an array of pigments such as chlorophylls (e.g., chlorophyll *a*, *b*, *c*, and *d*), carotenoids (e.g., β-carotene, astaxanthin, fucoxanthin, etc.), and phycobilipigments [allophycocyanin, phycocyanin (PC), and phycoerythrin] with distinct absorption spectra. Microalgae also biosynthesize polyunsaturated fatty acids (PUFAs) with unusual unsaturation patterns, sterols, vitamins, and complex polysaccharides (Levasseur et al., 2020). Many of these molecules are connected to stress defense mechanisms that confer survival advantages, for example, the accumulation of carotenoids under high light or nutrient deprivation, and the synthesis of mycosporine-like amino acids (MAAs) as natural sunscreens against UV damage, as well as their role in osmoregulation (Ngoennet et al., 2018). There appears to be an even greater metabolic potential, with genomic surveys uncovering new biosynthetic pathways and cryptic species whose metabolites are yet to be explored (Guiry, 2012; Leliaert et al., 2012). Recent molecular studies with environmental DNA continue to expand the known diversity of marine phytoplankton, indicating that numerous microalgal taxa with potential industrial applications remain undescribed and/or uncharacterized (De Vargas et al., 2015).

Microalgae are attractive candidates for biotechnological exploitation because of their rapid growth rate, small cell size, and relatively low nutrient requirements, as well as their ability to utilize solar or artificial light, which makes cultivation in sustainable, controlled systems feasible. They can be grown using seawater or even wastewater as their growth medium, reducing the need for freshwater or arable land (Pulz and Gross, 2004). In addition, microalgae can utilize concentrated carbon dioxide (CO_2) streams from industrial emissions, offering potential for greenhouse gas (GHG) mitigation while producing valuable biomass (Chisti, 2007; Wang et al., 2008). These properties make marine microalgae attractive organisms for the production of compounds with applications in various sectors like cosmetics, food, pharmaceuticals, and nutraceuticals (Gamal and Shreadah, 2024; Yarkent et al., 2020).

Biofunctional Cosmetics for Health. https://doi.org/10.1016/B978-0-443-27500-5.00007-1

1.2 Importance in cosmetics

Antiaging remains a major focus within the cosmetics sector, reflecting sustained global consumer demand. Oxidative stress is a central driver of skin aging and is a key contributor to the degradation of skin elasticity and the formation of premature wrinkles. Antioxidant compounds in cosmetic formulations can provide a preventative approach by targeting free radicals. Carotenoids such as astaxanthin from *Haematococcus pluvialis* and β-carotene from *Dunaliella salina* are among the most potent natural antioxidants reported, with well-documented bioactivity (Ambati et al., 2014; Higuera-Ciapara et al., 2006). MAAs produced by marine cyanobacteria and marine red microalgae absorb ultraviolet radiation in the 310–360 nm range, functioning as natural sunscreens that can reduce UV-induced DNA damage and erythema (skin inflammation), and therefore have been proposed as safer alternatives to synthetic UV filters, which are increasingly scrutinized for environmental toxicity (Al Qoh et al., 2025; Ngoennet et al., 2018). It was reported that the exopolysaccharides from *Chlorella vulgaris* and *Porphyridium cruentum* can provide hydration and film-forming properties, improving skin moisture retention and barrier protection (Wang et al., 2017; Raposo et al., 2013).

Microalgae are a recognized source of PUFAs, including eicosapentaenoic acid (EPA) and docosahexaenoic acid (DHA), which contribute to skin barrier integrity, elasticity, and antiinflammatory responses (Spolaore et al., 2006). Marine diatoms, including species of *Amphora*, have been reported as promising producers of marine-derived EPA, highlighting their relevance for cosmetic and nutraceutical applications (Nieri et al., 2023). Fucoxanthin, a carotenoid xanthophyll produced by brown algae and diatoms such as *Phaeodactylum tricornutum* and *Amphora* spp., has demonstrated inhibitory effects on melanogenesis, supporting its potential use in skin-brightening and antihyperpigmentation applications (Hogan et al., 2021; Peng et al., 2011). In addition to lipids and pigments, microalgae produce bioactive polysaccharides that exhibit moisturizing, antioxidant, and reported antihyaluronidase activity, contributing to improved skin hydration and reduced extracellular matrix degradation (Rosic, 2025). Moreover, microalgal extracts contain phenolic compounds, vitamins, and sterols that contribute to additional antioxidant and antiinflammatory effects, enhancing their potential as multifunctional cosmetic ingredients (Vo et al., 2012). Collectively, microalgae offer a diverse portfolio of bioactive compounds suitable for a wide range of cosmetic formulations, with particular emphasis on antiaging, skin-brightening, and moisturizing applications (Fig. 19.1).

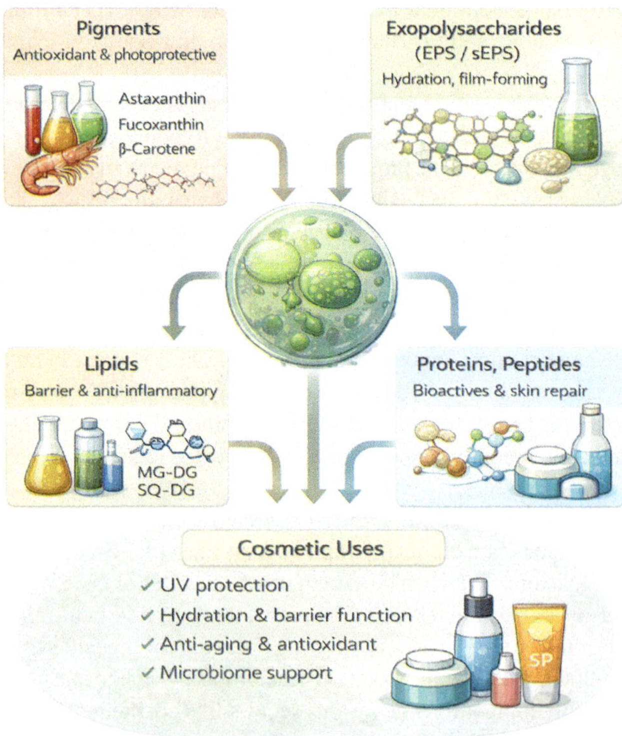

FIG. 19.1 Major classes of bioactive compounds derived from marine microalgae and their relevance for cosmetic applications. Marine microalgae produce a diverse range of metabolites, including pigments, exopolysaccharides, lipids, and proteins/peptides, each contributing distinct functional properties such as antioxidant and photoprotective activity, hydration and barrier support, antiinflammatory effects, and skin repair. Collectively, these compound classes underpin the multifunctional use of microalgal extracts in skincare, suncare, and cosmetic formulations.

The sustainability of production further enhances their appeal. Terrestrial plants have been used for centuries in cosmetics, but the cultivation of marine microalgae requires neither fertile land nor freshwater, a substantial distinction compared with terrestrial plant-based ingredients (Ubando et al., 2022). This ecological advantage aligns with consumer demand for natural, safe, and environmentally responsible products, which has fueled the rising incorporation of microalgal extracts into antiaging creams, sunscreens, moisturizers, and other personal care formulations (Kinawy et al., 2024). Scientometric analyses confirm a steady increase in both research publications and patents on microalgae-derived cosmetics over the last two decades, reflecting both scientific enthusiasm and growing industrial adoption (Chinjoo and Golzary, 2025; Dillon et al., 2012; Goncalves et al., 2024; Kinawy et al., 2024; Yaiser, 2016).

This chapter reviews marine microalgae as a source of cosmetic actives, integrating biological function, production technologies, and emerging commercial translation, while critically distinguishing between experimental evidence and market adoption.

2 Historical background

The industrial use of microalgae is a recent endeavor in human history; however, historical evidence indicates that their biomass was valued for nourishment and healing purposes long before their biochemical properties were understood. The Aztecs harvested *Arthrospira* from Lake Texcoco and prepared it as nutrient-rich cakes known as *tecuitlatl*. In East Asia, *Nostoc* species were used in China, Mongolia, and Japan, sometimes as food and sometimes in preparations with medicinal and restorative purposes (Gamal and Shreadah, 2024).

Microalgae remain strongly associated with health, with commercially available dietary supplements predominantly based on *Spirulina* and *Chlorella*. The discovery of the exceptional nutritional properties of *Spirulina* and *Chlorella* in the mid-20th century stimulated renewed interest in their exploitation, leading to investment in large-scale cultivation projects. *Chlorella*, in particular, was promoted in postwar Japan as a high-protein supplement, while *Spirulina* gained recognition from international bodies such as the United Nations and the World Health Organization as a potential solution for malnutrition (Belay, 2007).

During the same period, the biochemical characterization of microalgal pigments, PUFAs, and polysaccharides advanced significantly, and their potential applications expanded beyond food and nutrition into pharmaceuticals and cosmeceuticals. The late 20th century also saw the first commercial production of carotenoids such as β-carotene from the halotolerant marine microalga *D. salina* and the highly potent antioxidant astaxanthin from *H. pluvialis*, both of which are now widely incorporated into formulations for antiaging and photoprotective cosmetic products (Ambati et al., 2014). In addition to these established pigments, marine microalgae have emerged as promising sources of lutein, a xanthophyll carotenoid with notable cosmetic relevance. Lutein has been shown to exhibit antioxidant and blue-light-filtering properties, helping to protect skin cells from photooxidative stress, lipid peroxidation, and premature aging caused by ultraviolet and high-energy visible-light exposure. Furthermore, lutein has been associated with improved skin hydration, elasticity, and barrier function, supporting its use in skin-protective and antiaging formulations. Several marine and freshwater microalgal species have demonstrated potential for sustainable lutein production, highlighting microalgae as viable alternative sources for high-value cosmetic ingredients (Saha et al., 2020).

By the beginning of the 21st century, the groundwork had been laid for the systematic exploration of microalgae as a sustainable source of cosmetic actives. Advances in cultivation, extraction, and molecular biology during the last two decades built upon this historical trajectory and gave rise to the modern developments discussed in the following sections.

3 Modern advancements within an integrated perspective

Currently, microalgal compounds can be produced at an industrial rate, mainly due to major developments in cultivation systems. Traditional open raceway ponds remain useful for low-cost biomass production but are constrained by contamination risks and variable yields. In contrast, closed photobioreactors (PBRs) allow greater control over light, gas exchange, and sterility, leading to higher purity and consistency in metabolites destined for cosmetic formulations (Gamal and Shreadah, 2024; Levasseur et al., 2020). The trade-off is that PBRs require greater capital investment and energy input, which continues to be a barrier to low-cost scalability. Research in reactor geometry, light management, and hybrid designs that integrate open and closed systems has aimed to address this limitation, with promising but not yet definitive results (Deprá et al., 2025).

Likewise, there have been advances in the extraction and purification of microalgal bioactives. The preservation of bioactivity during recovery is critical for cosmetic applications, since key compounds such as the biofunctional pigments and proteins are difficult to stabilize once they are extracted from the cellular milieu. Supercritical carbon dioxide (SC-CO_2)

extraction has become a preferred green-extraction method for carotenoids, while microwave-assisted, ultrasound-assisted, and pressurized liquid extraction methods have enabled higher yields of thermolabile bioactive compounds (Ilhami et al., 2025). All these methods are based on green chemistry principles and are in line with the environmental expectations of the cosmetics market. Nevertheless, they demand significant investment in equipment and process optimization, which can slow adoption by small and medium enterprises.

Synthetic biology has also created further opportunities by allowing targeted improvement of metabolite yields. The application of CRISPR and related genome-editing systems has enabled precise modifications of metabolic pathways, increasing the accumulation of carotenoids, PUFAs, and other bioactives with potential cosmetic applications (Nymark et al., 2016). Yet, many microalgae are resistant to genetic transformation, and gene editing can lead to unpredictable or unstable outcomes. Regulatory uncertainty regarding genetically modified organisms in cosmetics adds another layer of difficulty. For these reasons, nontransgenic conventional approaches, including adaptive laboratory evolution (ALE), continue to play an important role alongside synthetic biology.

Another defining aspect of modern microalgal biotechnology has been the integration of artificial intelligence (AI) and digital tools into process control. Machine learning algorithms have been used to predict growth kinetics, optimize nutrient supply, and determine harvest times in both open and closed cultivation systems (Imamoglu, 2024). Digital twin models of PBRs allow researchers to simulate cultivation under different environmental conditions, reducing costs and accelerating the design of efficient bioprocesses.

In the context of environmental innovation, circular economy concepts have also reshaped the way microalgae are developed for cosmetics. Microalgal biorefineries, in which lipids, pigments, polysaccharides, and proteins are extracted in a cascading sequence from a single biomass source, represent a key development in this context (Occhipinti et al., 2024). This approach distributes production costs and minimizes waste, improving sustainability and economic feasibility. The valorization of residual biomass as animal feed, fertilizer, or bioenergy further enhances the environmental credentials of microalgal production systems. Life-cycle assessments (LCAs) consistently show that integrated models outperform standalone production, especially when coupled with wastewater treatment or industrial CO_2 capture (Arashiro et al., 2022; Ubando et al., 2022).

Formulation science has also matured over the last two decades, providing new opportunities for the use of microalgal metabolites. Since many are unstable, their encapsulation in biocompatible carriers or lipid nanoparticles is increasingly used to protect active molecules and ensure controlled release in creams, serums, and sunscreen products (Wang et al., 2017). These strategies improve stability and efficacy while ensuring compliance with cosmetic safety standards. Successful microalgae-based cosmetics require an integrated approach, starting with appropriate strain selection and green extraction, and extending to stabilization of active ingredients during formulation development.

Despite these modern advances, significant challenges persist. Biomass productivity in large-scale systems remains lower than what would be required for low-cost, widespread market penetration, with downstream processing contributing heavily to total costs. Variability in metabolite profiles across batches also persists, which complicates standardization. Global market expansion is hindered by differences in regulatory frameworks between regions, which slow global adoption. Consumer perceptions of genetically modified microalgae and skepticism toward new bioactives also influence market delivery. Addressing these barriers will require further improvements in the entire conceptual design and production of microalgae-based cosmetics (Fig. 19.2), as well as an adaptation to different consumer demands as the market itself changes. However, there is already a wide array of commercially available biocompounds, as well as emerging bioactives from microalgae, which are discussed in the following.

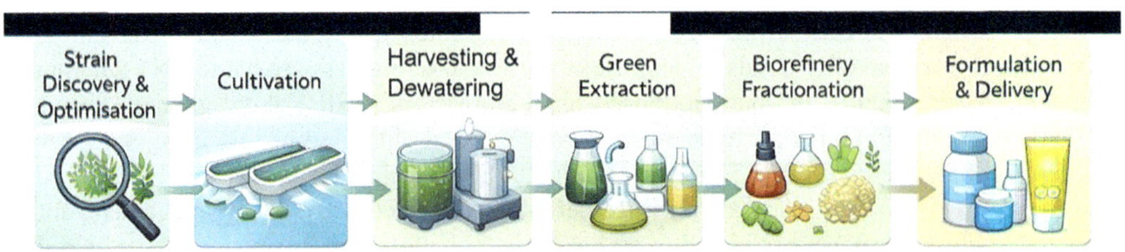

FIG. 19.2 Integrated pipeline for producing marine microalgal cosmetic actives. The process begins with strain selection and optimization, followed by controlled cultivation (open ponds or photobioreactors). Biomass is harvested and extracted using green methods (e.g., supercritical CO_2, pressurized liquid extraction), with downstream biorefinery steps to fractionate pigments, lipids, polysaccharides, peptides, and other bioactives. Extracts are then stabilized/encapsulated and formulated into topical products such as serums, creams, and sunscreens, reflecting a circular supply chain that maximizes resource use and sustainability.

4 Bioactive compounds from marine microalgae

Marine microalgae, together with their cyanobacterial relatives, have evolved under intense environmental pressures: high solar radiation, variable salinity, and nutrient competition (Rojas-Villalta et al., 2024; Bhardwaj et al., 2025). To thrive, microalgae synthesize a remarkable repertoire of secondary metabolites, many of which fortuitously align with the needs of human skincare and haircare. Over the past decade, these molecules have increasingly been scrutinized not only for their ecological roles but also for their potential as biofunctional ingredients in cosmetics (Perera et al., 2023; Shiels et al., 2021; Oliveira and Bragotto, 2022).

4.1 Pigments

Among the most recurrent industrial microalgal compounds are carotenoids, pigments that serve a dual purpose as colorants and potent antioxidants. Astaxanthin, primarily accumulated in the microalga *H. pluvialis*, has repeatedly been shown to quench singlet oxygen and neutralize reactive oxygen species (ROS) with high efficacy relative to many terrestrial antioxidants (Nishida et al., 2023; Catanzaro et al., 2020). Clinical studies suggest that oral supplementation in the range of 4–6 mg per day may be associated with improvements in skin elasticity, moisture, and wrinkle appearance in photoaged skin (Bjørklund et al., 2022; Ng et al., 2021). Beyond direct antioxidant effects, astaxanthin modulates matrix metalloproteinases and inflammatory pathways, thereby protecting dermal collagen (Siahaan et al., 2022). Importantly, circular bioeconomy studies demonstrate that even the by-products of *H. pluvialis* cultivation, once treated as waste, can be valorized into useful cosmetic ingredients (Ashokkumar et al., 2021; Mussagy et al., 2025; Villaró et al., 2021).

Equally compelling is fucoxanthin, the golden-brown pigment of diatoms such as *P. tricornutum* and *Amphora* spp. Fucoxanthin not only shields microalgal cells from excess light but has also been reported to exhibit antiphotoaging activity when applied in dermal contexts. Recent systematic reviews describe reductions in oxidative stress, inhibition of UV-induced mitochondrial membrane potential expression, and enhancements in skin moisture and elasticity (Mohibbullah et al., 2022; Mumu et al., 2022). Clinical investigations of a fucoxanthin-containing cream (0.03% concentrate) reported reductions in wrinkle appearance and improvements in hydration and elasticity (Khaw et al., 2022). Advances in cultivation have been particularly striking: by manipulating light quality and intensity, biotechnologists have achieved significant boosts in fucoxanthin yields, a crucial step toward a reliable commercial supply (Khaw et al., 2022).

β-Carotene, meanwhile, is a classic example of a stress-induced pigment that accumulates in the marine microalga *D. salina*. Comparative analyses indicate that while β-carotene exerts antioxidant and photoprotective effects, its potency is often eclipsed by that of astaxanthin (Hyrslova et al., 2022; Bhardwaj et al., 2025). Still, as a natural precursor of vitamin A, β-carotene continues to offer relevance in skin health formulations (Wang et al., 2022).

Cyanobacteria contribute an additional layer of interest through their phycobilipigments. These water-soluble pigments, such as PC, not only serve as striking blue colorants but also possess antiinflammatory and radical scavenging properties (Fernandes et al., 2023; Soliman et al., 2024). Recent Irish research has identified phycobilipigments in marine microalgae, underscoring their potential for application in novel skincare products (Shiels et al., 2025).

4.2 Polysaccharides

While pigments are primarily valued for their antioxidant properties, the maintenance of the skin barrier relies heavily on hydration, for which polysaccharides are particularly beneficial. Microalgal sulfated exopolysaccharides (sEPS) not only serve ecological functions but also possess remarkable bioactivity tied to their chemical structure and molecular weight. These sEPS are high-molecular-weight, anionic heteropolymers composed of monosaccharides such as glucose, xylose, galactose, and uronic acids, along with other substituents like methyl groups and proteins (Feng et al., 2023; Raposo et al., 2013).

Many microalgae secrete sEPS, which form hydrating biofilms around their cells. When transferred into cosmetics, these sEPS create invisible films on human skin, helping to retain moisture while contributing antioxidant and soothing effects (Magnabosco et al., 2025).

Going beyond moisture, sEPS from microalgae exhibit both antioxidant and anticoagulant properties, which are closely linked to their degree of sulfation and sugar composition. This dual bioactivity suggests that microalgal sEPS may exhibit functional similarities to glycosaminoglycans such as heparin, but with potentially lower toxicity and a more tunable structure (Mousavian et al., 2022). Microalgal sEPS are also being explored for immunomodulatory effects, particularly due to their capacity to influence complement activation pathways. Structural activity studies on marine algal polysaccharides have shown that not just sulfate content, but also molecular weight, branching, and monosaccharide ratios (e.g., galactose to fucose) determine their anticomplement efficacy (Feng et al., 2023).

In recent work, exopolysaccharides produced by an EMS-induced mutant of *P. cruentum* were reported to improve skin moisturization and elasticity, upregulate barrier-related genes, and accelerate wound closure in fibroblast scratch assays (Han et al., 2024). In parallel, polysaccharide fractions from newly isolated microalgae strains collected in Greek coastal lagoons demonstrated antioxidant, wound-healing, and moisture-retention activity in vitro (Vasilakis et al., 2025). Structural analyses also revealed that specific features of microalgal EPS influence collagen production and antiaging activity, underscoring their relevance as biofunctional cosmetic actives (Toucheteau et al., 2023).

Together, these findings highlight that EPS, once overlooked, represent valuable and sustainable ingredients for skincare. Their integration into cosmetic formulations aligns with consumer demand for green, circular approaches to beauty and wellness (Magnabosco et al., 2025).

Alguronic Acid, a proprietary algal polysaccharide formulation commercialized for cosmeceutical use, is representative of a broader class of microalgal exopolysaccharides whose physicochemical properties and biological activities make them attractive as hydrating, film-forming, and bioactive cosmetic ingredients. Although independent, peer-reviewed clinical data specific to alguronic acid are limited in the literature, the mechanistic rationale for its use is supported by studies of microalgal exopolysaccharides more generally (Laroche, 2022). Commercial intellectual property filings also describe isolated microalgal polysaccharide compositions and their formulation into topical products, documenting both methods of extraction and targeted cosmeceutical endpoints, which corroborate the translational pathway from algal biomass to finished skincare actives (Coragliotti et al., 2015).

4.3 Lipids: Essential fatty acids for skin barrier function

Among the most versatile metabolites of marine microalgae are their lipids, which consist of neutral triglycerides, glycolipids, and phospholipids. Of particular relevance to dermatology are PUFAs such as EPA (20:5n-3) and DHA (22:6n-3). These fatty acids are essential structural components of membranes and signaling molecules in microalgae, and in human skin, these fatty acids serve parallel roles: reinforcing the stratum corneum barrier, maintaining hydration, and modulating inflammatory responses.

Experimental studies began to reveal the molecular basis of these effects. For example, lipid extracts from the marine microalga *Nannochloropsis oceanica* were found to alter phospholipid and sphingolipid profiles in keratinocytes exposed to UVB radiation, increasing ceramide levels, key for barrier function and resilience, while reducing lipid species associated with inflammation (Łuczaj et al., 2023). Reviews of microalgal lipid fractions also reported suppression of proinflammatory cytokines such as IL-6, TNF-α, and IL-1β in vitro (Chwil et al., 2024; Conde et al., 2022). Taken together, findings from cellular and biochemical models support the potential of microalgae-derived lipids to contribute to barrier recovery and skin homeostasis.

Notably, these functional roles are mirrored in the reported bioactivity of microalgal lipid extracts. Recent reviews highlighted microalgal oils and polar lipids as sustainable emollients and sources of bioactive fatty acids for dermocosmetic formulations, with potential advantages over terrestrial oils in terms of both biocompatibility and ecological footprint (Papadopoulou et al., 2025; Martínez et al., 2025).

Shiels and colleagues examined an Irish green microalga, *Chlorococcum* sp. SABC 012504, and demonstrated that its PUFA-rich polar lipids, including glycolipids such as monogalactosyldiacylglycerols (MGDG) and sulfoquinovosyldiacylglycerols (SQDG), exhibited potent antiinflammatory and antithrombotic activity in human blood models (Shiels et al., 2021). Although the findings were discussed in a cardiovascular context, they reveal the antiinflammatory potential of microalgal polar lipids, a property that is relevant to soothing irritated skin as well.

A complementary study on the marine cyanobacterium *Spirulina subsalsa*, also isolated from Irish waters, reinforced this view. Polar-lipid fractions rich in ω-3 fatty acids were shown to significantly inhibit platelet-activating factor and thrombin-induced aggregation (Shiels et al., 2022). Again, the findings were discussed in relation to cardiovascular models; however, the demonstrated capacity of these extracts to suppress inflammatory cascades suggests their potential dermatological relevance. Formulations enriched with such microalgal lipids may simultaneously restore skin hydration and calm inflammation.

Together, these studies bridge ecological chemistry and skin physiology. The lipids that enable microalgae to thrive in dynamic marine environments also confer barrier-strengthening, antiinflammatory, and emollient effects on human skin. This convergence of function underscores why microalgal lipids are increasingly positioned as both nutritional and topical agents for maintaining cutaneous health and resilience.

4.4 Proteins, peptides, and amino acids

Like polysaccharides and lipids, microalgal proteins also harbor a wealth of bioactivity. Once hydrolyzed, they release peptides with notable effects on skin biology. Recent investigations have shown that microalgal hydrolysates can generate peptides capable of neutralizing oxidative stress and calming inflammatory pathways, while also inhibiting enzymes such as collagenase and elastase that erode the dermal matrix (Aurino et al., 2025; Mirzapour-Kouhdasht et al., 2024). These functions directly link microalgal proteins to antiaging and skin-protective applications.

Even more intriguing is the discovery of small amino acid derivatives with neuromodulatory effects. Extracts of the unicellular marine red microalga *Rhodosorus marinus* were found to contain γ-aminobutyric acid (GABA) and GABA-alanine, which were associated with reductions in inflammatory mediators in keratinocytes and reconstructed epidermis, hinting at their role in soothing neurogenic skin irritation (Scandolera et al., 2018). Likewise, a biodiscovery study of marine cyanobacteria isolated from Irish waters has confirmed their ability to synthesize GABA through glutamate decarboxylase activity, expanding the catalog of naturally occurring amino acids with cosmetic potential (Shiels et al., 2019).

Together, these findings suggest that proteins and amino acid derivatives from marine microalgae are more than structural reserves: they represent a biochemical toolkit that may help defend the skin against oxidative stress, inflammation, and environmental aggressors. From collagen-protecting peptides to GABA-mediated soothing effects, microalgae open promising new avenues for functional skincare formulations grounded in marine biotechnology.

4.5 Phenolics and polyphenols

Other promising metabolites of microalgae are the phenolic compounds, a diverse group that includes phenolic acids, flavonoids, and tannin-like molecules. These compounds act as frontline antioxidants, neutralizing ROS, while also tempering inflammatory pathways. Some phenolics have been reported to exhibit tyrosinase inhibition, a mechanism directly linked to pigmentation control and skin-brightening applications, highlighting their potential for future cosmetic research from microalgal sources (Mahrous et al., 2025).

A defining feature of microalgal phenolics is their metabolic plasticity. Their abundance in microalgae is not fixed but varies with abiotic factors like light intensity, salinity, and nutrient supply. This means that, unlike many plant phenolics locked into seasonal cycles, microalgal phenolics can be steered by cultivation design, allowing researchers and industry to optimize extracts for specific cosmetic functions (Cichoński and Chrzanowski, 2022). Advances in extraction and analytical workflows now enable more consistent recovery and standardization, bringing these compounds closer to formulation-ready status (Bermudez et al., 2024). Although still less explored than carotenoids, phenolics represent the next frontier for natural antioxidant and skin-brightening actives.

4.6 Mycosporine-like amino acids

MAAs serve complementary photoprotective and osmoregulatory roles. They are secondary metabolites biosynthesized by cyanobacteria, microalgae, and other organisms, and their cellular content is enhanced upon exposure to harmful UV radiation. These small, colorless molecules absorb UV radiation between 310 and 360 nm and dissipate the absorbed energy primarily as heat. MAAs are water-soluble, low-molecular-weight compounds (<400 Da). Other types of MAAs have recently been reported with molecular weights of 478, 508, 612, or 1050 Da, depending on the types and numbers of associated sugars. Their natural role is to protect microalgal cells from photodamage, yet this function aligns neatly with human needs for chemical-based sunscreen alternatives. Unlike many synthetic UV filters, MAAs are photostable, water-soluble, and biodegradable, qualities that make them attractive as "reef-safe" actives.

Scientific interest in MAAs has surged in recent years, with reviews highlighting not only their photoprotective capacity but also their antiinflammatory and antioxidant roles, expanding their potential beyond sun protection (Geraldes and Pinto, 2021; Görünmek et al., 2024; Rosic, 2019). Browne et al. (2023) documented strong UV-absorbing compounds in cyanobacteria collected from Irish coastal waters, suggesting that local strains may represent natural reservoirs of MAAs (Browne et al., 2023). These findings position Irish marine biodiversity within the broader global discussion on sustainable, eco-conscious sunscreen product development.

4.7 Vitamins and minerals

Microalgae can also be a source of micronutrients that support skin health in more subtle ways. They accumulate β-carotene (provitamin A), tocopherols (vitamin E), vitamin C, and a spectrum of B-complex vitamins, along with trace minerals such as selenium and zinc. Though rarely used as isolated cosmetic actives, these micronutrients work in synergy with pigments, polysaccharides, and lipids to broaden antioxidant defenses, strengthen the skin barrier, and promote repair processes (Del Mondo et al., 2020; Prates, 2025).

A recent review highlighted how these vitamins not only reinforce redox balance but also enhance the performance of whole algal extracts in antiaging and protective skincare formulations (Martínez et al., 2025). Advances in microalgal

TABLE 19.1 Major bioactive compounds from marine microalgae and their cosmetic relevance.

Compound class	Representative microalgal sources	Key bioactivity	Cosmetic relevance	Key references
Carotenoids (e.g., astaxanthin, fucoxanthin, β-carotene)	*Haematococcus pluvialis, Phaeodactylum tricornutum, Dunaliella salina*	Antioxidant activity; UV absorption; modulation of oxidative stress pathways	Antiaging, photoprotection, skin-brightening, color stabilization	(Ambati et al., 2014; Catanzaro et al., 2020; Hogan et al., 2021; Bhardwaj et al., 2025)
Mycosporine-like amino acids (MAAs)	Marine cyanobacteria; red microalgae (*Porphyridium, Rhodosorus*)	UV absorption (310–360 nm); antioxidant and antiinflammatory effects	Natural photoprotective actives; reef-considerate sunscreen formulations	(Geraldes and Pinto, 2021; Rosic, 2019; Browne et al., 2023)
Sulfated exopolysaccharides (sEPS)	*Porphyridium cruentum, Chlorella vulgaris*	Film-forming; hydration; antioxidant and immunomodulatory activity	Moisturizing, barrier reinforcement, skin conditioning	(Raposo et al., 2013; Feng et al., 2023; Han et al., 2024)
Lipids and polyunsaturated fatty acids (PUFAs)	*Nannochloropsis, Amphora, Chlorococcum, Spirulina subsalsa*	Barrier support; antiinflammatory effects; modulation of ceramide metabolism	Emollients; barrier repair; soothing formulations	(Spolaore et al., 2006; Shiels et al., 2021; Łuczaj et al., 2023)
Proteins and bioactive peptides	*Spirulina, Chlorella,* marine cyanobacteria	Antioxidant activity; enzyme inhibition (collagenase, elastase); antiinflammatory effects	Antiaging; skin-protective and soothing formulations	(Mirzapour-Kouhdasht et al., 2024; Aurino et al., 2025)
Phenolic compounds	Diverse marine microalgae (species-dependent)	Antioxidant activity; tyrosinase inhibition	Skin-brightening; antioxidant support	(Cichoński and Chrzanowski, 2022; Mahrous et al., 2025)
Vitamins and micronutrients (e.g., provitamin A, vitamin E, B-complex)	*Chlorella, Spirulina,* mixed microalgal biomass	Synergistic antioxidant and barrier-supporting effects	Supportive actives within whole-extract formulations	(Del Mondo et al., 2020; Arora and Philippidis, 2023)

biotechnology further indicate that vitamin-rich microalgal biomass can sustainably be cultivated and processed, creating a renewable source of micronutrients for cosmeceutical formulations (Arora and Philippidis, 2023). In this way, microalgae provide not just isolated molecules but an integrated biochemical toolkit for maintaining cutaneous resilience.

Taken together, the evidence underscores the remarkable biochemical breadth of marine microalgae and cyanobacteria (Table 19.1). From carotenoids that defend against oxidative and photoinduced stress, to polysaccharides that hydrate and reinforce the skin barrier, to lipids, peptides, phenolics, MAAs, vitamins, and minerals that offer antiinflammatory, soothing, and photoprotective benefits, these organisms provide a multilayered toolkit for skin health. What unites these diverse compounds is not only their ecological role in helping microalgae survive fluctuating and harsh environments, but also their growing translation into biofunctional ingredients for dermocosmetics. As research continues to refine cultivation methods, extraction technologies, and mechanistic understanding, microalgal metabolites are increasingly being explored as sustainable, multifunctional alternatives to synthetic additives in the cosmetics industry.

5 Applications in cosmetics

Marine microalgae are increasingly transitioning from natural marine environments, through laboratory development, into commercial cosmetic products. Their bioactive compounds are increasingly being formulated into skincare, suncare, and haircare products, driven both by science and consumer demand. What began as an ecological adaptation is now being translated into functional attributes relevant to skin hydration, protection, and cosmetic performance. Many cosmetic companies, including L'Oréal, Unilever, and La Prairie, have incorporated microalgae-derived ingredients into selected product lines, including antiwrinkle creams, hydrating serums, sunscreens, and facial masks.

5.1 Skincare

Microalgal extracts have emerged as a compelling class of cosmetic actives due to their chemically diverse and biologically responsive metabolite profiles. Pigments, polysaccharides, and lipids derived from these microorganisms are no longer restricted to controlled laboratory investigations but are now incorporated into advanced topical formulations aimed at mitigating oxidative stress and supporting epidermal barrier function. This transition from experimental systems to commercial skincare reflects both the maturation of microalgal biotechnology and a growing recognition of the relevance of algal metabolites for skincare applications. In a 2025 review, Martínez-Ruiz and colleagues describe how carotenoids, phenolics, and exopolysaccharides from microalgae are now standardized into topical applications that have been reported to improve skin hydration and provide protection against UV-induced damage (Martínez et al., 2025).

Clinical testing has begun to support these claims. In one study, lotions containing *Spirulina* and *Ulva* extracts measurably improved hydration and reduced wrinkle depth, suggesting that the antioxidant and antiinflammatory activities observed in vitro may translate to effects in human skin (Kim et al., 2018). In this context, microalgae are not used as sources of isolated compounds but rather as complex extracts, further highlighting the need for additional clinical and mechanistic studies.

5.2 Haircare

Hair, like skin, is vulnerable to oxidative stress, UV, and pollution. Here too, microalgae are beginning to play a role. A recent review of *Spirulina* in eco-cosmetics describes how proteins and pigments incorporated into shampoos and conditioners enhance fiber strength, improve hydration, and protect against oxidative fading (Ramos et al., 2025). Laboratory models suggest microalgal peptides can bind to keratin fibers, while phycobiliproteins act as natural colorants with added radical scavenging properties. For consumers, this translates into shampoos that cleanse while also helping to protect the hair shaft, reflecting a convergence of functional performance and haircare.

5.3 Sun protection

Among cosmetic applications, sun care represents an area where microalgal compounds may offer particularly significant potential. The discovery of MAAs and carotenoids, such as fucoxanthin and astaxanthin, has opened new avenues for the development of natural UV-filtering agents. These molecules absorb or dissipate harmful radiation while also counteracting the inflammation and oxidative stress triggered by sunlight. A 2025 article reviewed how MAA-rich extracts are already being tested in sunscreen prototypes, praised for their photostability and reef-safe credentials (Najafi et al., 2025).

This builds on a growing body of evidence. Reviews by Rosic (2019) and Görünmek et al. (2024) outlined not just UV absorption but broader antioxidant roles, suggesting these compounds may replace or complement synthetic filters in multifunctional sunscreens (Görünmek et al., 2024; Rosic, 2019). These developments suggest a potential shift toward bioderived sunscreen actives sourced from marine microalgae, offering an alternative to petrochemical-based filters.

The progression from ecological chemistry to cosmetic efficacy is supported by diverse studies. Proteomic surveys are beginning to explore how algal peptides may modulate skin aging pathways, reduce oxidative stress, and influence repair-related signaling (Rosic, 2025). In parallel, human trials, like those with *Spirulina* extracts by Kim et al. (2018), showed tangible improvements in hydration and wrinkle reduction. Together, these findings provide a conceptual bridge, suggesting that mechanisms conferring stress tolerance in microalgae may also be relevant to protecting human skin.

5.4 Commercial products

Evidence that microalgae have transitioned from experimental research into mainstream cosmetic use can be observed in the increasing number of commercial products incorporating microalgae-derived ingredients. Ingredient labeling increasingly reflects the incorporation of microalgae-derived compounds into creams, serums, sunscreens, and body care products across a wide range of market segments.

Prestige skincare brands were among the earliest commercial adopters of microalgal ingredients. Elemis Pro-Collagen Marine Cream includes *P. cruentum* extract, a red microalga rich in sEPS that are associated with film-forming and hydration-supporting properties (SpecialChem, 2021). ISDIN incorporates *P. cruentum* extracts in its Fusion Water Magic SPF 50, where the ingredient is positioned to support moisture retention and provide antioxidant complementarity to conventional UV filters.

Antioxidant-rich green microalgae have also entered the cosmetic market. *H. pluvialis* extracts, prized as the natural source of astaxanthin, appear in antioxidant serums and creams across multiple brands, capitalizing on published evidence that astaxanthin exhibits strong antioxidant activity relative to many terrestrial antioxidants (Ambati et al., 2014; Catanzaro et al., 2020), alongside widespread documentation of its inclusion in commercial formulations (Incidecoder, n.d.a).

Extracts of the marine microalga *D. salina*, a recognized source of β-carotene, feature in moisturizers marketed for radiance and skin tone correction (Incidecoder, n.d.b). Extracts of *Nannochloropsis oculata* have been incorporated into "instant lifting" serums, where polysaccharide- and protein-rich fractions are marketed to create temporary skin-tightening effects at the surface (Incidecoder, n.d.c).

Luxury antiaging product lines frequently incorporate microalgae within proprietary ingredient complexes. Shiseido's Benefiance Wrinkle Smoothing Cream highlights a proprietary KOMBU-Bounce Complex derived from brown, red, and green algae and lists *Chlorella* extract among its active components (Shiseido, 2024). The inclusion of *Chlorella*, rich in proteins and antioxidants, reflects how microalgae are now positioned not only as supporting ingredients but also as signature actives in global prestige franchises.

Niche cosmetic brands have also leveraged microalgae to differentiate formulations within a competitive market. MARA Beauty's Sea Vitamin C Serum blends *Chlorella* with vitamin C, marketing the extract as a stabilizing, soothing partner to ascorbic acid (MARA, n.d.). Indie innovators such as Nuworld Botanicals offer a Whipped Blue *Spirulina* Body Cream, leveraging the antioxidant-rich pigment PC for both its radical scavenging properties and its striking natural color (Incidecoder, n.d.d). Mass-market retailers, including Sephora, also list *Chlorella* extract in selected products, indicating broader acceptance of microalgal ingredients beyond niche positioning (Sephora Collection, n.d.).

The cyanobacterium *Spirulina* deserves special mention. Beyond supplements, it has found a foothold in topical products: Viva's Face Tonic *Spirulina* and multiple indie creams list *Spirulina platensis* extracts as a skin-conditioning and antioxidant active (SpecialChem, n.d.). These uses are consistent with clinical findings reporting improvements in skin hydration and barrier-related parameters following the application of Spirulina extracts, making it one of the few microalgal ingredients with both experimental evidence and shelf presence.

Even sun care is beginning to embrace microalgae. While still emerging, products incorporating algal actives, such as astaxanthin, fucoxanthin, or MAA-rich extracts, are marketed as environmentally considerate alternatives or adjuncts to conventional SPF formulations. Industry reports have highlighted pilot launches of "microalgae sunscreens," a space likely to expand as regulatory and consumer pressure mounts against traditional UV filters (Najafi et al., 2025).

Together, these examples illustrate that microalgae are now deeply integrated into commercial cosmetics, no longer relegated to theoretical white papers or patent filings (Table 19.2). Microalgal actives, whether derived from *Porphyridium*, *Haematococcus*, *Nannochloropsis*, *Chlorella*, *Spirulina*, or *Phaeodactylum*, serve as a bridge between marine biochemistry, clinical validation, and consumer-facing products. For instance, Comfort Zone's *Skin Regimen LX Microalgae Essence* utilizes an extract of *Euglena gracilis*, a unicellular microalga associated with the support of cellular energy metabolism and improved skin hydration, thereby reinforcing the ingredient's positioning as both a bioactive and hydrating component in formulations targeting stressed skin (Comfort Zone, n.d.). In a different yet complementary innovation, the Algalip lipstick project by Eleonora Rombolà demonstrates how microalgae biomass and pigment production can be leveraged in color cosmetics: the formulation replaces conventional oil, wax, and pigment components with algae-derived oils and

TABLE 19.2 Examples of commercial cosmetic products incorporating microalgae-derived ingredients.

Brand/product	Microalgal source	Ingredient function (as positioned)	Product category	Source
Elemis—Pro-Collagen Marine Cream	*Porphyridium cruentum*	Hydration support; film-forming polysaccharides	Antiaging skincare	SpecialChem, 2021
ISDIN—Fusion Water Magic SPF 50	*Porphyridium cruentum*	Moisture support; antioxidant complement to UV filters	Sun care	ISDIN product information
Shiseido—Benefiance Wrinkle Smoothing Cream	*Chlorella* spp.	Antioxidant and skin-conditioning component within a proprietary complex	Antiaging skincare	Shiseido, 2024
MARA Beauty—Sea Vitamin C Serum	*Chlorella* extracts	Soothing and stabilizing partner to ascorbic acid	Facial serum	MARA, n.d.
NuWorld Botanicals—Whipped Blue Spirulina Body Cream	*Spirulina platensis*	Antioxidant activity; natural pigmentation	Body care	Incidecoder, n.d.d
Sephora Collection—Bronzing Drops	*Chlorella* extracts	Skin-conditioning and formulation support	Color cosmetics	Sephora Collection, n.d.
Viva—Face Tonic Spirulina	*Spirulina platensis*	Skin-conditioning; antioxidant support	Facial toner	SpecialChem, n.d.
Comfort Zone—Skin Regimen LX Microalgae Essence	*Euglena gracilis*	Support for cellular energy metabolism; hydration	Essence/ serum	Comfort Zone, n.d.

pigments, and even fabricates the packaging from compostable, algae-based 3D-printing filament, thereby aligning sustainable design with circular microalgal bioprocessing (Rombolà, 2020).

Note: Examples are illustrative and based on ingredient listings and manufacturer disclosures; inclusion does not imply clinical efficacy.

6 Sustainable sourcing of marine microalgae for cosmetic actives

Sourcing bioactive ingredients from marine microalgae offers a sustainability benefit that is difficult to match with terrestrial crops traditionally used in cosmetics (Prates, 2025). As photosynthetic microscopic plants capable of thriving in saline, brackish, or even nutrient-rich wastewaters, microalgae can be cultivated without competing for arable land or freshwater, decoupling ingredient production from agricultural supply chains that are increasingly constrained by climate and water stress (Yu et al., 2024). Their high aerial productivities under controlled growth conditions and tolerance of nonpotable water directly translate into lower land and freshwater footprints per unit of bioactive compounds, especially when cultivation is strategically sited on marginal land or co-located with existing industrial infrastructure (Udayan et al., 2022).

A second pillar of sustainability is achieved by integrating microalgae cultivation with environmental remediation, where PBRs or optimized pond reactors are coupled to wastewater treatment systems. Such systems enable the simultaneous removal of nitrogen and phosphorus while generating biomass that can further be valorized, transforming a treatment obligation into a productive resource stream (Ferreira et al., 2019). LCAs and comparative analyses show that these configurations reduce eutrophication potential and overall environmental burden when nutrient removal is aligned with co-product recovery within a biorefinery model (Arashiro et al., 2022; Ubando et al., 2022). Within this context, sEPS produced by species such as *Porphyridium* have gained interest as hydrating and film-forming cosmetic actives, and their recovery directly from spent culture media or lightly clarified supernatants enables the valorization of an otherwise discarded process stream (Feng et al., 2023; Levasseur et al., 2020).

This integrated approach therefore strengthens both the environmental and economic performance of microalgal production chains by improving mass and energy balances while generating high-value biomolecules. Carbon management provides a third and often under-appreciated sustainability feature. Microalgal cultivation directly utilizes inorganic carbon, and sparging with concentrated CO_2, potentially sourced from fermentation off-gas or industrial flue gas, can boost productivity while providing a pathway for point-source CO_2 utilization (Singh et al., 2025). When LCAs allocate appropriate credits for avoided emissions and when downstream products displace petrochemical-derived materials, overall GHG balances can be markedly improved (Blanco et al., 2022). Critically, sustainable sourcing is not only about where and how microalgae are grown but also about how bioactives are recovered. Downstream processing, harvesting, dewatering, and drying of microalgal biomass remain the dominant energy "hotspot" in most LCAs, irrespective of their end use (Bradley et al., 2023).

For cosmetic supply chains, process design plays a crucial role in maintaining the ecological advantages of microalgal cultivation. Achieving higher steady-state cell densities reduces volumetric handling, while prioritizing low-energy primary concentration methods, such as gravity thickening, flotation, or membrane-based approaches, minimizes the need for full thermal drying, which can compromise compound quality. Harvesting and primary concentration strategies, such as sedimentation, flotation, and membrane separation, have been widely studied as energy-efficient ways to concentrate microalgal biomass prior to downstream processing, reducing the energy and cost bottlenecks associated with commercial-scale cultivation (Vandamme, 2017). Two-step thickening and dewatering schemes further optimize process economics by increasing biomass concentration before drying (Ahmed et al., 2022). Alternative dewatering methods like electroflotation also demonstrate how innovative process design reduces energy demands while preserving valuable cellular compounds (Jeevanandam et al., 2020).

Moreover, the adoption of green, solvent-lean extraction methods applied to wet or near-wet biomass, including SC-CO_2 extraction for carotenoids and other bioactives, as well as pressurized liquid and ultrasound-assisted techniques for thermolabile components, helps to preserve compound integrity while reducing dependence on harmful organic solvents. SC-CO_2 is widely recognized as an environmentally favorable approach for recovering lipids, pigments, and other high-value metabolites from microalgae, while ultrasound- and pressurized liquid-based methods provide complementary, low-impact options for sensitive biomolecules. Collectively, these operational strategies are critical for ensuring that the sustainability and bioactivity advantages inherent to microalgal valorization are fully realized (Correa et al., 2022; Tzima et al., 2023; Morón-Ortiz et al., 2024).

Collectively, these approaches highlight the integration of cultivation and downstream processing as a systems-level challenge, emphasizing that environmental benefits are contingent on holistic process optimization. Strategic site selection, high-density cultivation, and green extraction methods collectively reduce the carbon, water, and land footprints of microalgal bioactives while enabling high-quality cosmetic ingredients (Mittal and Ranade, 2023). When aligned with

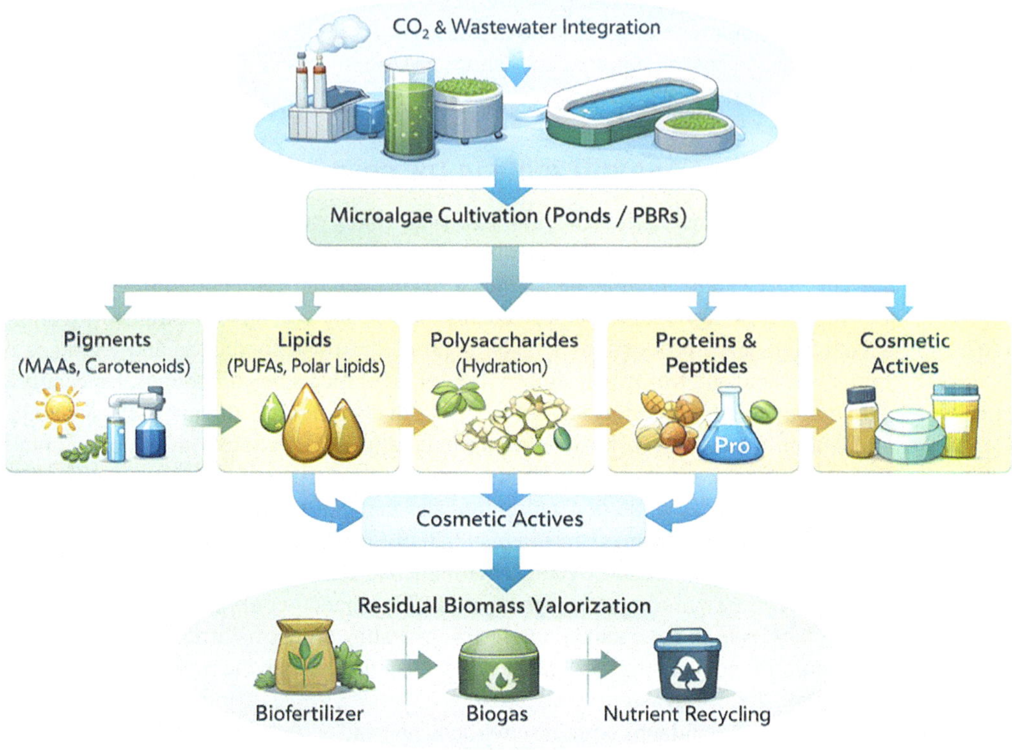

FIG. 19.3 Circular biorefinery model for sustainable production of marine microalgal cosmetic actives. This schematic illustrates how cultivation integrates with CO_2 utilization and wastewater treatment, how multiple product streams (pigments, polysaccharides, lipids, proteins, peptides, vitamins) are co-recovered through cascading fractionation, and how residual biomass is valorized into biofertilizer or bioenergy, closing material and energy loops for enhanced sustainability.

industrial-scale bioprocesses, microalgae represent a promising platform for sustainable production that meets both ecological and commercial criteria (Geng et al., 2025).

Sustainability also benefits from adopting a biorefinery concept across the product pipeline. Rather than extracting a single "target" molecule, cascading recovery of lipids (emollients; PUFA-rich polar lipids), pigments (astaxanthin, fucoxanthin), sEPS (hydration/barrier support), proteins/peptides (antioxidant, antiprotease), and vitamin-rich fractions distributes both energy inputs and environmental burdens across multiple value streams (Ranaprathap Katakojwala, 2021). Residual biomass can be directed to biofertilizers and/or anaerobic digestion (AD), and nutrient-rich digestates recycled to cultivation, further tightening elemental cycles. When paired with digital optimization (e.g., AI-assisted control of light and nutrients to time harvests at pigment or sEPS maxima), such integrated designs accelerate both environmental and economic performance (Budzianowski and Postawa, 2016; Ghatak, 2011).

Finally, the regulatory and market context for "green" cosmetics increasingly rewards transparent, auditable sourcing. Although certification schemes are not substitutes for LCA, the practices they encourage, including restricted auxiliary chemicals, solvent recovery, renewable energy sourcing, and improved traceability, tend to correlate with better environmental outcomes and smoother technology transfer from pilot to commercial scale (Kralisch et al., 2014).

In summary, marine microalgae provide a credible route to low-impact cosmetic actives because they (1) avoid pressure on fertile soils and freshwater, (2) can be integrated with wastewater cleaning and CO_2 utilization, and (3) lend themselves to biorefinery-based, green-chemistry extraction (Fig. 19.3). Realizing this potential requires disciplined attention to the known hotspots of dewatering and drying, and rigorous process integration that demonstrates measurable reductions in life-cycle impacts (Papadaki et al., 2024).

7 Future trends and innovations in cosmetic applications of marine microalgae

The next wave of microalgae-enabled cosmetics will be shaped by various converging forces, such as (1) discovery of new strains and chemistries; (2) precision bioprocessing for reliable, low-impact supply; (3) delivery technologies that unlock efficacy at the skin interface; (4) regulatory and market pull for verifiable "reef-safe" and biodegradable ingredients; and

(5) circular product design (Lucía Morocho-jácome et al., 2022). Together, these trends point toward ingredients that are not only natural but also engineered for performance, safety, and sustainability.

First, the discovery pipeline is accelerating beyond cultured model species. Environmental DNA surveys and improved culturing of extremotolerant taxa are expanding the accessible chemodiversity, including microalgae and cyanobacteria adapted to high light, salinity, and UV, precisely the pressures that select for photoprotective pigments, MAAs, and bioactive exopolysaccharides (Raj et al., 2021). Systematic screening has already revealed strong UV-absorbing MAAs in Irish coastal cyanobacteria, an example of regionally unique biodiversity feeding a global need for eco-conscious sun care. The near term is likely to see targeted bioprospecting of underexplored habitats (coastal lagoons, hypersaline pools, polar/brackish niches) coupled with rapid dereplication and metabolomics, with an emphasis on phenolics, MAAs, and sEPS (Browne et al., 2023; Rastogi et al., 2023).

Second, precision strain engineering and non-GMO route optimization will increasingly deliver "designed" ingredient profiles. While CRISPR/Cas systems have also been validated in marine microalgae for pathway edits that elevate carotenoids (astaxanthin, fucoxanthin), tailor fatty acid unsaturation, or modulate polysaccharide sulfation patterns relevant to hydration and barrier support (Banerjee et al., 2018). However, ALE and spectral/photonic control will remain attractive where GMO regulation or consumer perception is restrictive: for instance, manipulating light intensity/quality to push fucoxanthin and accessory pigment yields in *P. tricornutum* or other diatoms (Elshobary et al., 2025). A practical hybrid model is likely to use nontransgenic factors (light, nutrients) for market-facing production, while retaining engineered strains for closed systems and intermediate manufacture of high-value actives.

Third, digitalization will make cultivation and harvesting both smarter and greener. Machine learning-guided feeding, gas management, and harvest timing have already demonstrated gains in productivity and product consistency, and "digital twin" frameworks for PBRs are emerging as powerful tools for process development, monitoring, and optimization in microalgal cultivation systems. These tools will be applied not only to growth rate but to "quality by design" targets, such as maintaining specific MAAs or EPS molecular-weight distributions that correlate with UV absorption or film-forming performance, respectively. Expect AI-assisted control to couple with sustainability metrics so that setpoints optimize both yield and life-cycle impacts (Sheik et al., 2024; Syed et al., 2024).

Fourth, the manufacturing envelope will shift from single-molecule extraction to true microalgal biorefineries serving cosmetic industries. Cascading recovery of pigments, lipids, proteins/peptides, and sulfated EPS will distribute costs and environmental burdens while creating multifunctional ingredient systems (Sarker and Kaparaju, 2024). In this context, two concrete innovations are poised for growth: (1) wet or near-wet extraction (e.g., SC-CO_2 for carotenoids; pressurized liquid or ultrasound-assisted extraction for thermolabile polysaccharides and peptides) to minimize energy and solvent use while preserving bioactivity; and (2) valorization of side streams, such as EPS-rich culture media or lipid-extracted biomass recycled for biofertilizer use or biogas production through AD, tightening elemental cycles and improving LCA outcomes (Laroche, 2022; Seeger et al., 2025).

On the formulation front, delivery science will become as important as discovery science. Encapsulation of bioactive ingredients in lipid nanoparticles or biopolymeric carriers will be used not just for stability but for controlled localization in the stratum corneum, translating in vitro antioxidant or antiinflammatory effects into clinical gains (Rehman et al., 2024). Structure-function tuning is likely to focus on, for example, engineering EPS sulfation and molecular weight for film persistence and Transepidermal Water Loss reduction, or enriching polar lipids (MGDG/SQDG) that support ceramide metabolism and barrier repair. In proteins, bioactive peptide discovery from controlled hydrolysis will target collagenase/elastase inhibition and neurosoothing effects (GABA derivatives), with safety workflows addressing allergenicity and sensitization early in development (Ngoc et al., 2023).

Two cross-cutting themes will also frame future products. Microbiome-aware design will favor microalgal actives that modulate inflammation without disrupting commensals; polar lipids and gentle polysaccharides are candidates for "barrier-plus-microbiome" positioning grounded in cell and ex vivo skin models (Hong et al., 2025). Traceability and certification are likely to move from peripheral considerations to central procurement criteria: solvent recycling, renewable electricity, wastewater/CO_2 integration, and restricted auxiliaries map directly onto COSMOS/EcoCert expectations and LCA improvements, strengthening claims of low-impact, ethically sourced ingredients (Bozza et al., 2022).

8 Overall conclusion

Marine microalgae and their cyanobacterial relatives have transitioned from being ecological curiosities to bona fide platforms for high-value cosmetic actives. Biologically, they are prolific producers of photoprotective pigments (e.g., astaxanthin, fucoxanthin, β-carotene, and lutein), sulfated and neutral polysaccharides, PUFAs and polar lipids, peptides, phenolics, vitamins, GABA, and MAAs. These metabolites evolved to counter intense light, salinity, desiccation, and nutrient stress in the euphotic ocean (Prates, 2025). Many of these compounds align directly with dermatological needs: antioxidant and antiphotoaging defense, hydration and barrier reinforcement, modulation of inflammation, pigment control, and photoprotection. Early human data, though still limited, indicate potential translatability from in vitro and ex vivo models to clinical endpoints such as wrinkle reduction and improved hydration, while MAA-rich extracts and carotenoids are increasingly being explored within "reef-safe" and multifunctional suncare concepts (Zhou et al., 2021).

Industrial production of β-carotene from the marine microalga *D. salina* provided one of the first generations of microalgal actives with clear cosmetic relevance (Wang et al., 2022). Today, these ingredients anchor a growing product landscape alongside marine red microalga *Porphyridium's* exopolysaccharides and *Nannochloropsis* complexes in prestige and mass-market formulations, with evidence-led claims relating to hydration, antioxidant support, and short-term skin-tightening effects (Liu et al., 2025). Notably, regional bioprospecting adds scientific and commercial specificity: Irish marine biodiversity has yielded cyanobacterial MAAs with strong UV signatures and PUFA-rich polar lipids from *Chlorococcum* sp. and *S. subsalsa* that exhibit antiinflammatory bioactivity relevant to barrier recovery (Browne et al., 2023; Shiels et al., 2022, 2021).

With continued progress in microalgal cultivation technology, green extraction methods, analytics, encapsulation/delivery, clinical validation, and careful attention to the well-known sustainability hotspots, marine microalgal bioactives are poised not merely to supplement but to contribute to the evolution of future dermocosmetic portfolios (Chinjoo and Golzary, 2025). With coordinated work across academia, industry, and regulators, microalgal ingredients can progress from occasional target actives to interoperable, circular platforms that have the potential to influence the development of skincare, suncare, and haircare applications (Chinjoo and Golzary, 2025; Ubando et al., 2022; Bearth et al., 2024). More research with clinical evidence of microalgal bioactives, along with technological improvements (both cultivation and downstream processing), suggests that microalgae hold significant promise for driving sustainable, environmentally friendly innovation in the cosmetics industry.

References

Ahmed, A.S., et al., 2022. Microalgae to Biofuel: Cutting-edge Harvesting and Extraction Techniques. Energy Science & Engineering.

Al Qoh, S., Amine, J., Assobhei, O., Etahiri, S., 2025. Investigation of UV protection and anti-aging properties of mycosporine-like amino acids in the Moroccan red alga *Gracilaria gracilis* (Gracilariales, Rhodophyta). J. Appl. Phycol. 0921-8971. 37 (2), 1341–1356. doi:10.1007/s10811-024-03406-8.

Ambati, R.R., Moi, P.S., Ravi, S., Aswathanarayana, R.G., 2014. Astaxanthin: sources, extraction, stability, biological activities and its commercial applications - A review. Mar. Drugs 16603397. 12 (1), 128–152. Available from: http://www.mdpi.com/1660-3397/12/1/128/pdf. doi:10.3390/md12010128.

Arashiro, L.T., Josa, I., Ferrer, I., Van Hulle, S.W.H., Rousseau, D.P.L., Garfí, M., 2022. Life cycle assessment of microalgae systems for wastewater treatment and bioproducts recovery: natural pigments, biofertilizer and biogas. Sci. Total Environ. 18791026. 847. Available from: https://www.elsevier.com/locate/scitotenv. doi:10.1016/j.scitotenv.2022.157615.

Arora, N., Philippidis, G.P., 2023. The prospects of algae-derived vitamins and their precursors for sustainable cosmeceuticals. Processes. 2227-9717. 11 (2), 587. doi:10.3390/pr11020587.

Ashokkumar, V., Chen, W.-H., Kumar, G., Satjarak, A., Chanthapatchot, W., Ngamcharussrivichai, C., 2021. A biorefinery approach for high value-added bioproduct (astaxanthin) from alga Haematococcus sp. and residue pyrolysis for biochar synthesis and metallic iron production from hematite (Fe2O3). Fuel. 00162361. 304, 121150. doi:10.1016/j.fuel.2021.121150.

Aurino, E., Mora, L., Marzocchella, A., Kuchendorf, C.M., Ackermann, B., Hayes, M., 2025. Functional and bioactive benefits of selected microalgal hydrolysates assessed in silico and in vitro. Mar. Drugs 16603397. 23 (2). Available from: http://www.mdpi.com/journal/marinedrugs. doi:10.3390/md23020053.

Banerjee, A., Banerjee, C., Negi, S., Chang, J.S., Shukla, P., 2018. Improvements in algal lipid production: a systems biology and gene editing approach. Crit. Rev. Biotechnol. 15497801. 38 (3), 369–385. doi:10.1080/07388551.2017.1356803.

Bearth, A., Otten, C.D., Cohen, A.S., 2024. Consumers' perceptions and acceptance of genome editing in agriculture: insights from the United States of America and Switzerland. Food Res. Int. 178, 113982. doi:10.1016/j.foodres.2024.113982.

Belay, A., 2007. Spirulina (Arthrospira): production and quality assurance. In: Spirulina in Human Nutrition and Health, CRC Press.

Bermudez, G., Terenzi, C., Medri, F., Andrisano, V., Montanari, S., 2024. Extraction and analytical methods for the characterization of polyphenols in marine microalgae: a review. Mar. Drugs. 1660-3397. 22 (12), 538. doi:10.3390/md22120538.

Bhardwaj, R., Yadav, A., Swapnil, P., Meena, M., 2025. Characterization of microalgal β-carotene and astaxanthin: exploring their health-promoting properties under the effect of salinity and light intensity. Biotechnol. Biofuels Bioprod. 18. doi:10.1186/s13068-025-02612-x.

Bjørklund, G., Gasmi, A., Lenchyk, L., Shanaida, M., Zafar, S., Mujawdiya, P.K., Lysiuk, R., Antonyak, H., Noor, S., Akram, M., Smetanina, K., Piscopo, S., Upyr, T., Peana, M., 2022. The role of astaxanthin as a nutraceutical in health and age-related conditions. Molecules. 1420-3049. 27 (21), 7167. doi:10.3390/molecules27217167.

Blanco, J., Linares, M., López Granados, M., Agirre, I., Gandarias, I., Arias, P.L., Iglesias, J., Moreno, J., García, A., 2022. Integrated environmental and exergoeconomic analysis of biomass-derived maleic anhydride. Adv. Sustain. Syst. 23667486. 6 (9). Available from: https://www.advsustainsys.com. doi:10.1002/adsu.202200121.

Bozza, A., Campi, C., Garelli, S., Ugazio, E., Battaglia, L., 2022. Current regulatory and market frameworks in green cosmetics: the role of certification. Sustain. Chem. Pharm. 23525541. 30, 100851. doi:10.1016/j.scp.2022.100851.

Bradley, T., Rajaeifar, M.A., Kenny, A., Hainsworth, C., Del Pino, V., Del Valle Inclán, Y., Povoa, I., Mendonça, P., Brown, L., Smallbone, A., Roskilly, A.P., Joyce, S., Heidrich, O., 2023. Life cycle assessment of microalgae-derived biodiesel. Int. J. Life Cycle Assess. 16147502. 28 (5), 590–609. Available from: https://www.springer.com/journal/11367. doi:10.1007/s11367-023-02140-6.

Browne, N., Otero, P., Murray, P., Saha, S.K., 2023. Rapid screening for mycosporine-like amino acids (MAAs) of Irish marine cyanobacteria and their antioxidant potential. Sustainability. 2071-1050. 15 (4), 3792. doi:10.3390/su15043792.

Budzianowski, W.M., Postawa, K., 2016. Total Chain Integration of sustainable biorefinery systems. Appl. Energy 03062619. 184, 1432–1446. Available from: http://www.elsevier.com/inca/publications/store/4/0/5/8/9/1/index.htt. doi:10.1016/j.apenergy.2016.06.050.

Carvalho, A.P., Silva, S.O., Baptista, J.M., Malcata, F.X., 2011. Light requirements in microalgal photobioreactors: an overview of biophotonic aspects. Appl. Microbiol. Biotechnol. 01757598. 89 (5), 1275–1288. doi:10.1007/s00253-010-3047-8.

Catanzaro, E., Bishayee, A., Fimognari, C., 2020. On a beam of light: photoprotective activities of the marine carotenoids astaxanthin and fucoxanthin in suppression of inflammation and cancer. Mar. Drugs 18, 544. doi:10.3390/md18110544.

Chinjoo, N., Golzary, A., 2025. Microalgae: revolutionizing skin repair and enhancement. Biotechnol. Rep. 2215017X. 47, e00911. doi:10.1016/j.btre.2025.e00911.

Chisti, Y., 2007. Biodiesel from microalgae. Biotechnol. Adv. 07349750. 25 (3), 294–306. doi:10.1016/j.biotechadv.2007.02.001.

Chwil, M., Mihelič, R., Matraszek-Gawron, R., Terlecka, P., Skoczylas, M.M., Terlecki, K., 2024. Comprehensive review of the latest investigations of the health-enhancing effects of selected properties of Arthrospira and Spirulina microalgae on skin. Pharmaceuticals. 1424-8247. 17 (10), 1321. doi:10.3390/ph17101321.

Cichoński, J., Chrzanowski, G., 2022. Microalgae as a source of valuable phenolic compounds and carotenoids. Molecules. 1420-3049. 27 (24), 8852. doi:10.3390/molecules27248852.

Comfort Zone, n.d. Skin Regimen LX Microalgae Essence [WWW Document]. https://us.comfortzoneskin.com/products/skin-regimen-lx-microalgae-essence (Accessed 15 September 2025).

Conde, T., Lopes, D., Łuczaj, W., Neves, B., Pinto, B., Maurício, T., Domingues, P., Elżbieta Skrzydlewska, M.R.D., 2022. Algal lipids as modulators of skin disease: a critical review. Metabolites. 2218-1989. 12 (2), 96. doi:10.3390/metabo12020096.

Coragliotti, A., Franklin, S., Day, A.G., Decker, S.M., 2015. Microalgal polysaccharide compositions. US8927522B2.

Correa, T., Godoy, M.G., Bazylinski, D.A., Abreu, F., 2022. Continuous production of biogenic magnetite nanoparticles by the marine bacterium Magnetovibrio blakemorei strain MV-1T with a nitrous oxide injection strategy. Mar. Drugs 16603397. 20 (11). Available from: http://www.mdpi.com/journal/marinedrugs. doi:10.3390/md20110724.

De Vargas, C., Audic, S., Henry, N., Decelle, J., Mahé, F., Logares, R., Lara, E., Berney, Ć., Bescot, N.L., Probert, I., Carmichael, M., Poulain, J., Romac, S., Colin, S., Aury, J.M., Bittner, L., Chaffron, S., Dunthorn, M., Engelen, S., Flegontova, O., Guidi, L., Horák, A., Jaillon, O., Lima-Mendez, G., Lukeš, J., Malviya, S., Morard, R., Mulot, M., Scalco, E., Siano, R., Vincent, F., Zingone, A., Dimier, C., Picheral, M., Searson, S., Kandels-Lewis, S., Acinas, S.G., Bork, P., Bowler, C., Gorsky, G., Grimsley, N., Hingamp, P., Iudicone, D., Not, F., Ogata, H., Pesant, S., Raes, J., Sieracki, M.E., Speich, S., Stemmann, L., Sunagawa, S., Weissenbach, J., Wincker, P., Karsenti, E., Boss, E., Follows, M., Karp-Boss, L., Krzic, U., Reynaud, E.G., Sardet, C., Sullivan, M.B., Velayoudon, D., 2015. Eukaryotic plankton diversity in the sunlit ocean. Science 10959203. 348 (6237). Available from: http://www.sciencemag.org/content/348/6237/1261605.full.pdf. doi:10.1126/science.1261605.

Del Mondo, A., Smerilli, A., Sané, E., Sansone, C., Brunet, C., 2020. Challenging microalgal vitamins for human health. Microb. Cell Fact. 1475-2859. 19 (1). doi:10.1186/s12934-020-01459-1.

Deprá, M.C., Dias, R.R., Zepka, L.Q., Jacob-Lopes, E., 2025. Tackling old challenges in microalgal biotechnology: the role of photobioreactors to advance the technology readiness level. Processes 22279717. 13 (1). Available from: http://www.mdpi.com/journal/processes. doi:10.3390/pr13010051.

Dillon, H.F., Zaman, A., Day, A.G., Coragliotti, A., 2012. Microalgae-derived compositions for improving the health and appearance of skin. US8277849B2.

Elshobary, M.E., Abo-Shanab, W.A., Ende, S.S.W., Alquraishi, M., El-Shenody, R.A., 2025. Optimizing Phaeodactylum tricornutum cultivation: integrated strategies for enhancing biomass, lipid, and fucoxanthin production. Biotechnol. Biofuels Bioprod. 27313654. 18 (1). Available from: https://biotechnologyforbiofuels.biomedcentral.com/. doi:10.1186/s13068-024-02602-5.

Falkowski, P.G., Barber, R.T., Smetacek, V., 1998. Biogeochemical controls and feedbacks on ocean primary production. Science 281, 200–206. doi:10.1126/science.281.5374.200.

Feng, Y., Wassie, T., Gan, R., Xin, W., 2023. Structural characteristics and immunomodulatory effects of sulfated polysaccharides derived from marine algae. Crit. Rev. Food Sci. Nutr. 1040-8398. 63 (24), 7180–7196. doi:10.1080/10408398.2022.2043823.

Fernandes, R., Campos, J., Serra, M., Fidalgo, J., Almeida, H., Casas, A., Toubarro, D., Barros, A.I.R.N.A., 2023. Exploring the benefits of phycocyanin: from Spirulina cultivation to its widespread applications. Pharmaceuticals 14248247. 16 (4). Available from: https://www.mdpi.com/journal/pharmaceuticals. doi:10.3390/ph16040592.

Ferreira, A., Reis, A., Vidovic, S., Vladic, J., Gkelis, S., Melkonyan, L., Avetisova, G., Congestri, R., Acién, G., Muñoz, R., Collet, P., Gouveia, L., 2019. Combining microalgae-based wastewater treatment with biofuel and bio-based production in the frame of a biorefineryIn: Hallmann, A., Rampelotto, P.H. (Eds.), Grand Challenges in Algae Biotechnology, Springer International Publishing, Cham, pp. 319–369. doi:10.1007/978-3-030-25233-5_9.

Gamal, R., Shreadah, M.A., 2024. Marine microalgae and their industrial biotechnological applications: a review. J. Genet. Eng. Biotechnol. 1687157X. 22 (4), 100407. doi:10.1016/j.jgeb.2024.100407.

Geng, Y., Shaukat, A., Azhar, W., Raza, Q.U.A., Tahir, A., Abideen, M.Z.U., Zia, M.A.B., Bashir, M.A., Rehim, A., 2025. Microalgal biorefineries: a systematic review of technological trade-offs and innovation pathways. Biotechnol. Biofuels Bioprod. 27313654. 18 (1). Available from: https://biotechnologyforbiofuels.biomedcentral.com/. doi:10.1186/s13068-025-02694-7.

Geraldes, V., Pinto, E., 2021. Mycosporine-like amino acids (MAAs): biology, chemistry and identification features. Pharmaceuticals. 1424-8247. 14 (1), 63. doi:10.3390/ph14010063.

Ghatak, H.R., 2011. Biorefineries from the perspective of sustainability: feedstocks, products, and processes. Renew. Sustain. Energy Rev. 13640321. 15 (8), 4042–4052. doi:10.1016/j.rser.2011.07.034.

Goncalves, O., Probert, I., Pruvost, J., Massé, A., Decamp, A., Maugard, T., Arnaudin, I., Bridiau, N., Toucheteau, C., Le, C.D., Picton, L., Dulong, V., Rihouey, C., Gaignard, C., Laroche, C., Pierre, G., Delattre, C., Dubessay, P., Michaud, P., 2024. New depolymerized exopolysaccharides, derived from microalgae, their preparation process and their uses in cosmetics to delay the effects of skin aging. FR3120309B1.

Görünmek, M., Ballık, B., Çakmak, Z.E., Çakmak, T., 2024. Mycosporine-like amino acids in microalgae and cyanobacteria: biosynthesis, diversity, and applications in biotechnology. Algal Res. 22119264. 80, 103507. doi:10.1016/j.algal.2024.103507.

Guiry, M.D., 2012. How many species of algae are there? J. Phycol. 15298817. 48 (5), 1057–1063. doi:10.1111/j.1529-8817.2012.01222.x.

Han, S.I., Heo, Y.M., Jeon, M.S., Kyung, S., Kang, S., Kwon, S.J., Ryu, J.H., Kim, J.H., Ahn, J.W., 2024. The effect of exopolysaccharides from EMS-induced Porphyridium cruentum mutant on human epidermal and dermal layers. Front. Mar. Sci. 22967745. 11. Available from: https://www.frontiersin.org/journals/marine-science#. doi:10.3389/fmars.2024.1365311.

Higuera-Ciapara, I., Félix-Valenzuela, L., Goycoolea, F.M., 2006. Astaxanthin: a review of its chemistry and applications. Crit. Rev. Food Sci. Nutr. 46, 185–196. doi:10.1080/10408690590957188.

Hogan, P., Otero, P., Murray, P., Saha, S.K., 2021. Effect of biomass pre-treatment on supercritical CO_2 extraction of lipids from marine diatom *Amphora* sp. and its biomass evaluation as bioethanol feedstock. Heliyon. 24058440. 7 (1), e05995. doi:10.1016/j.heliyon.2021.e05995.

Hong, J.Y., Kwon, D., Park, K.Y., 2025. Microbiome-based interventions for skin aging and barrier function: a comprehensive review. Ann Dermatol 37, 259–268. doi:10.5021/ad.25.009.

Hopes, A., Mock, T., 2015. Evolution of Microalgae and Their Adaptations in Different Marine Ecosystems Encyclopedia of Life Sciences. Wiley, pp. 1–9. doi:10.1002/9780470015902.a0023744.

Hyrslova, I., Krausova, G., Mrvikova, I., Stankova, B., Branyik, T., Malinska, H., Huttl, M., Kana, A., Doskocil, I., 2022. Functional properties of *Dunaliella salina* and its positive effect on probiotics. Mar. Drugs. 1660-3397. 20 (12), 781. doi:10.3390/md20120781.

Ilhami, S., Rahman, S.N.S.A., Iqhrammullah, M., Hamid, Z., Chai, Y.H., Lam, M.K., 2025. Polyhydroxyalkanoates production from microalgae for sustainable bioplastics: a review. Biotechnol. Adv. 07349750. 79. Available from: https://www.sciencedirect.com/science/journal/07349750. doi:10.1016/j.biotechadv.2025.108529.

Imamoglu, E., 2024. Artificial intelligence and/or machine learning algorithms in microalgae bioprocesses. Bioengineering. 2306-5354. 11 (11), 1143. doi:10.3390/bioengineering11111143.

Incidecoder, n.d.a. Haematococcus pluvialis extract [WWW Document]. https://incidecoder.com/ingredients/haematococcus-pluvialis-extract (Accessed 15 September 2025).

Incidecoder, n.d.b. *Dunaliellasalina* extract [WWW Document]. https://incidecoder.com/ingredients/dunaliella-salina-extract (Accessed 15 September 2025).

Incidecoder, n.d.c. *Nannochloropsisoculata* extract [WWW Document]. https://incidecoder.com/ingredients/nannochloropsis-oculata-extract (Accessed 15 September 2025).

Incidecoder, n.d.d. Nuworld Botanicals Whipped Blue Spirulina Superfood Body Cream ingredients [WWW Document]. https://incidecoder.com/products/nuworld-botanicals-whipped-blue-spirulina-superfood-body-cream (Accessed 15 September 2025).

Jeevanandam, J., Harun, M.R., Lau, S.Y., Sewu, D.D., Danquah, M.K., 2020. Microalgal biomass generation via electroflotation: a cost-effective dewatering technology. Appl. Sci. (Switz.) 20763417. 10 (24), 1–24. Available from: https://www.mdpi.com/2076-3417/10/24/9053/pdf. doi:10.3390/app10249053.

Khaw, Y.S., Yusoff, F.M., Tan, H.T., Mazli, N.A.I.N., Nazarudin, M.F., Shaharuddin, N.A., Omar, A.R., Takahashi, K., 2022. Fucoxanthin production of microalgae under different culture factors: a systematic review. Mar. Drugs 16603397. 20 (10). Available from: http://www.mdpi.com/journal/marinedrugs. doi:10.3390/md20100592.

Kim, J.H., Lee, J.E., Kim, K.H., Kang, N.J., 2018. Beneficial effects of marine algae-derived carbohydrates for skin health. Mar. Drugs 16603397. 16 (11). Available from: https://www.mdpi.com/1660-3397/16/11/459/pdf. doi:10.3390/md16110459.

Kinawy, R.N., Fathy, W.A., Hammouda, O., Abdelhameed, M.S., Sayed, A.F., Shaban, A.M., 2024. Revealing the utilization of microalgae in cosmetics: insights from a comprehensive scientometric analysis over the last two decades. Int. Aquat. Res. 20086970. 16 (4), 375–397. Available from: https://intelaquares.tonekabon.iau.ir/article_710115_0037866ea16daf26bb2d265cba7c9dc6.pdf. doi:10.22034/iar.2024.2008952.1753.

Kralisch, D., Ott, D., Gericke, D., 2014. Rules and benefits of Life Cycle Assessment in green chemical process and synthesis design: a tutorial review. Green Chem. 17, 123–145. doi:10.1039/C4GC01153H.

Laroche, C., 2022. Exopolysaccharides from microalgae and cyanobacteria: diversity of strains, production strategies, and applications. Mar. Drugs. 1660-3397. 20 (5), 336. doi:10.3390/md20050336.

Leliaert, F., Smith, D.R., Moreau, H., Herron, M.D., Verbruggen, H., Delwiche, C.F., De Clerck, O., 2012. Phylogeny and molecular evolution of the green algae. Crit. Rev. Plant Sci. 15497836. 31 (1), 1–46. doi:10.1080/07352689.2011.615705.

Levasseur, W., Perré, P., Pozzobon, V., 2020. A review of high value-added molecules production by microalgae in light of the classification. Biotechnol. Adv. 41, 107545. doi:10.1016/j.biotechadv.2020.107545.

Liu, R., Xue, W., Ling, X., Li, L., He, Y., Guo, M., 2025. Porphyridium purpureum culture extract as an ecologically safe agent against PM2.5 - induced skin toxicity. Ecotoxicol. Environ. Saf. 10902414. 303. Available from: https://www.sciencedirect.com/science/journal/01476513. doi:10.1016/j.ecoenv.2025.119034.

Lucía Morocho-jácome, A., Dos Santos, B.B., de Carvalho, J.C.M., de Almeida, T.S., Rijo, P., Valéria Robles Velasco, M., Rosado, C., Rolim Baby, A., 2022. Microalgae as a sustainable, natural-oriented and vegan dermocosmetic bioactive ingredient: the case of neochloris oleoabundans. Cosmetics. 2079-9284. 9 (1), 9. doi:10.3390/cosmetics9010009.

Łuczaj, W., Gęgotek, A., Conde, T., Domingues, M.R., Domingues, P., Skrzydlewska, E., 2023. Lipidomic assessment of the impact of Nannochloropsis oceanica microalga lipid extract on human skin keratinocytes exposed to chronic UVB radiation. Sci. Rep. 20452322. 13 (1). Available from: https://www.nature.com/srep/. doi:10.1038/s41598-023-49827-2.

Magnabosco, C., Santaniello, G., Romano, G., 2025. Microalgae: a promising source of bioactive polysaccharides for biotechnological applications. Molecules 30, 2055. doi:10.3390/molecules30092055.

Mahrous, M.H., Abdel-dayem, S.I.A., Adel, I.M., El-Dessouki, A.M., El-Shiekh, R.A., 2025. Efficacy of natural products as tyrosinase inhibitors in hyperpigmentation therapy: anti-melanogenic or anti-browning effects. Chem. Biodivers. 16121880. 22 (8). Available from: http://onlinelibrary.wiley.com/journal/10.1002/(ISSN)1612-1880. doi:10.1002/cbdv.202403324.

MARA, n.d. Mini Sea Vitamin C Serum [WWW Document]. https://themarabeauty.com/products/sea-vitamin-c-serum (Accessed 15 September 2025).

Martínez, R.J.G., Rivas García, F., March Cerdá, J.C., Hernández-Ruíz, Á., González Castro, M.I., Valverde-Merino, M.-I., Huertas Camarasa, F.J., Lloris Meseguer, F., López-viota Gallardo, M., 2025. Bioactive substances and skin health: an integrative review from a pharmacy and nutrition perspective. Pharmaceuticals (Basel) 18, 373. doi:10.3390/ph18030373.

Mirzapour-Kouhdasht, A., Garcia-Vaquero, M., Huang, J.-Y., 2024. Algae-derived compounds: bioactivity, allergenicity and technologies enhancing their values. Bioresour. Technol. 406, 130963. doi:10.1016/j.biortech.2024.130963.

Mittal, R., Ranade, V., 2023. Bioactives from microalgae: a review on process intensification using hydrodynamic cavitation. J. Appl. Phycol. 0921-8971. 35 (3), 1129–1161. doi:10.1007/s10811-023-02945-w.

Mohibbullah, M., Haque, M.N., Sohag, A.A.M., Hossain, M.T., Zahan, M.S., Uddin, M.J., Hannan, M.A., Moon, I.S., Choi, J.S., 2022. A systematic review on marine algae-derived fucoxanthin: an update of pharmacological insights. Mar. Drugs 16603397. 20 (5). Available from: https://www.mdpi.com/1660-3397/20/5/279/pdf. doi:10.3390/md20050279.

Morón-Ortiz, Á., Mapelli-Brahm, P., Meléndez-Martínez, A.J., 2024. Sustainable green extraction of carotenoid pigments: innovative technologies and bio-based solvents. Antioxidants 13, 239. doi:10.3390/antiox13020239.

Mousavian, Z., Safavi, M., Azizmohseni, F., Hadizadeh, M., Mirdamadi, S., 2022. Characterization, antioxidant and anticoagulant properties of exopolysaccharide from marine microalgae. AMB Express. 2191-0855. 12 (1). doi:10.1186/s13568-022-01365-2.

Mumu, M., Das, A., Emran, T.B., Mitra, S., Islam, F., Roy, A., Karim, M.M., Das, R., Park, M.N., Chandran, D., Sharma, R., Khandaker, M.U., Idris, A.M., Kim, B., 2022. Fucoxanthin: a promising phytochemical on diverse pharmacological targets. Front. Pharmacol. 16639812. 13. Available from: http://www.frontiersin.org/Pharmacology. doi:10.3389/fphar.2022.929442.

Mussagy, C.U., Caicedo-Paz, A.V., Figueroa, D., Santander, C., González, F., Tropea, A., Mondello, L., Spadaro, D., Trocino, S., Piazza, R.D., Marques, R.F.C., Godoy, K., Cornejo, P., 2025. Maximizing Haematococcus biorefineries: ionic liquid-based astaxanthin recovery, biocosmetic formulation, solar cell applications, and biofertilizer valorization. Bioresour. Technol. 18732976. 426. Available from: https://www.sciencedirect.com/science/journal/09608524. doi:10.1016/j.biortech.2025.132347.

Najafi, A., Heidary, M., Martinez, R.M., Baby, A.R., Morowvat, M.H., 2025. Microalgae-based sunscreens as green and sustainable cosmetic products. Int. J. Cosmet. Sci. 14682494. 47 (2), 213–222. Available from: http://onlinelibrary.wiley.com/journal/10.1111/(ISSN)1468-2494. doi:10.1111/ics.13019.

Ng, Q.X., De Deyn, M.L.Z.Q., Loke, W., Foo, N.X., Chan, H.W., Yeo, W.S., 2021. Effects of astaxanthin supplementation on skin health: a systematic review of clinical studies. J. Diet. Suppl. 1939022X. 18 (2), 169–182. Available from: http://www.tandfonline.com/loi/ijds20. doi:10.1080/19390211.2020.1739187.

Ngoc, L.T.N., Moon, J.-Y., Lee, Y.-C., 2023. Insights into bioactive peptides in cosmetics. Cosmetics 10, 111. doi:10.3390/cosmetics10040111.

Ngoennet, S., Nishikawa, Y., Hibino, T., Waditee-Sirisattha, R., Kageyama, H., 2018. A method for the isolation and characterization of mycosporine-like amino acids from cyanobacteria. Methods Protoc. 2409-9279. 1 (4), 46. doi:10.3390/mps1040046.

Nieri, P., Carpi, S., Esposito, R., Costantini, M., Zupo, V., 2023. Bioactive molecules from marine diatoms and their value for the nutraceutical industry. Nutrients. 2072-6643. 15 (2), 464. doi:10.3390/nu15020464.

Nishida, Y., Berg, P., Shakersain, B., Hecht, K., Takikawa, A., Tao, R., Kakuta, Y., Uragami, C., Hashimoto, H., Misawa, N., Maoka, T., 2023. Astaxanthin: past, present, and future. Mar. Drugs. 1660-3397. 21 (10), 514. doi:10.3390/md21100514.

Nymark, M., Sharma, A.K., Sparstad, T., Bones, A.M., Winge, P., 2016. A CRISPR/Cas9 system adapted for gene editing in marine algae. Sci. Rep. 20452322. 6. Available from: https://www.nature.com/srep/index.html. doi:10.1038/srep24951.

Occhipinti, P.S., Russo, N., Foti, P., Zingale, I.M., Pino, A., Romeo, F.V., Randazzo, C.L., Caggia, C., 2024. Current challenges of microalgae applications: exploiting the potential of non-conventional microalgae species. J. Sci. Food Agric. 10970010. 104 (7), 3823–3833. Available from: http://onlinelibrary.wiley.com/journal/10.1002/(ISSN)1097-0010. doi:10.1002/jsfa.13136.

Oliveira, A.P.F.D., Bragotto, A.P.A., 2022. Microalgae-based products: food and public health. Future Foods 6, 100157. doi:10.1016/j.fufo.2022.100157.

Papadaki, S., Tricha, N., Panagiotopoulou, M., Krokida, M., 2024. Innovative bioactive products with medicinal value from microalgae and their overall process optimization through the implementation of life cycle analysis—an overview. Mar. Drugs. 1660-3397. 22 (4), 152. doi:10.3390/md22040152.

Papadopoulou, S.N.A., Adamantidi, T., Kranas, D., Cholidis, P., Anastasiadou, C., Tsoupras, A., 2025. A comprehensive review on the valorization of bioactives from marine animal by-products for health-promoting, biofunctional cosmetics. Mar. Drugs 16603397. 23 (8). Available from: http://www.mdpi.com/journal/marinedrugs. doi:10.3390/md23080299.

Peng, J., Yuan, J.P., Wu, C.F., Wang, J.H., 2011. Fucoxanthin, a marine carotenoid present in brown seaweeds and diatoms: metabolism and bioactivities relevant to human health. Mar. Drugs 16603397. 9 (10), 1806–1828. Available from: http://www.mdpi.com/1660-3397/9/10/1806/pdf. doi:10.3390/md9101806.

Perera, R.M.T.D., Herath, K.H.I.N.M., Sanjeewa, K.K.A., Jayawardena, T.U., 2023. Recent reports on bioactive compounds from marine cyanobacteria in relation to human health applications. Life 20751729. 13 (6). Available from: https://www.mdpi.com/journal/life/. doi:10.3390/life13061411.

Prates, J.A.M., 2025. Applications of bioactive compounds from marine microalgae in health, cosmetics, and functional foods. Appl. Sci. 2076-3417. 15 (11), 6144. doi:10.3390/app15116144.

Pulz, O., Gross, W., 2004. Valuable products from biotechnology of microalgae. Appl. Microbiol. Biotechnol. 0175-7598. 65 (6), 635–648. doi:10.1007/s00253-004-1647-x.

Raj, S., Kuniyil, A.M., Sreenikethanam, A., Gugulothu, P., Jeyakumar, R.B., Bajhaiya, A.K., 2021. Microalgae as a source of mycosporine-like amino acids (MAAs); advances and future prospects. Int. J. Environ. Res. Public Health 16604601. 18 (23). Available from: https://www.mdpi.com/1660-4601/18/23/12402/pdf. doi:10.3390/ijerph182312402.

Ramos, S.D.P., Bürck, M., Costa, S.F.F.D., Assis, M., Braga, A.R.C., 2025. Spirulina as a key ingredient in the evolution of eco-friendly cosmetics. BioTech 26736284. 14 (2). Available from: https://www.mdpi.com/journal/biotech. doi:10.3390/biotech14020041.

Ranaprathap Katakojwala, S.V.M., 2021. A critical view on the environmental sustainability of biorefinery systems. Curr. Opin. Green Sustain. Chem. 24522236. 27, 100392. doi:10.1016/j.cogsc.2020.100392.

Raposo, M.F.D.J., De Morais, R.M.S.C., Bernardo de Morais, A.M.M., 2013. Bioactivity and applications of sulphated polysaccharides from marine microalgae. Mar. Drugs 11, 233–252. doi:10.3390/md11010233.

Rastogi, R.P., Shree, A., Patel, H.M., Chaudhry, S., Madamwar, D., 2023. Characterization, UV-induction, antioxidant function and role in photo-protection of mycosporine-like amino acids (MAAs) in a unicellular cyanobacterium, *Euhalothece* sp.WR7. Algal Res. 22119264. 70. Available from: http://www.sciencedirect.com/science/journal/aip/22119264. doi:10.1016/j.algal.2023.103030.

Rehman, M., Tahir, N., Sohail, M.F., Qadri, M.U., Duarte, S.O.D., Brandão, P., Esteves, T., Javed, I., Fonte, P., 2024. Lipid-based nanoformulations for drug delivery: an ongoing perspective. Pharmaceutics 19994923. 16 (11). Available from: http://www.mdpi.com/journal/pharmaceutics. doi:10.3390/pharmaceutics16111376.

Rojas-Villalta, D., Rojas-Rodríguez, D., Villanueva-Ilama, M., Guillén-Watson, R., Murillo-Vega, F., Gómez-Espinoza, O., Núñez-Montero, K., 2024. Exploring extremotolerant and extremophilic microalgae: new frontiers in sustainable biotechnological applications. Biology. 2079-7737. 13 (9), 712. doi:10.3390/biology13090712.

Rombolà, E., 2020. Algalip, The Lipstick Made From Algae [WWW Document]. https://isola.design/Designer-Projects-algalip-the-lipstick-made-from-algae (Accessed 15 September 2025).

Rosic, N., 2019. Mycosporine-like amino acids: making the foundation for organic personalised sunscreens. Mar. Drugs. 1660-3397. 17 (11), 638. doi:10.3390/md17110638.

Rosic, N., 2025. Unveiling the anti-aging potential of marine natural bioproducts. Mar. Drugs. 1660-3397. 23 (4), 165. doi:10.3390/md23040165.

Saha, S.K., Ermis, H., Murray, P., 2020. Marine microalgae for potential lutein production. Appl. Sci. 10, 6457. doi:10.3390/app10186457.

Sarker, N.K., Kaparaju, P., 2024. Microalgal bioeconomy: a green economy approach towards achieving sustainable development goals. Sustainability. 2071-1050. 16 (24), 11218. doi:10.3390/su162411218.

Scandolera, A., Hubert, J., Humeau, A., Lambert, C., De Bizemont, A., Winkel, C., Kaouas, A., Renault, J.H., Nuzillard, J.M., Reynaud, R., 2018. GABA and GABA-alanine from the red microalgae rhodosorus marinus exhibit a significant neuro-soothing activity through inhibition of neuro-inflammation mediators and positive regulation of TRPV1-related skin sensitization. Mar. Drugs 16603397. 16 (3). Available from: http://www.mdpi.com/1660-3397/16/3/96/pdf. doi:10.3390/md16030096.

Seeger, J., Zäh, M., Wendisch, V.F., Brandenbusch, C., Henke, N.A., 2025. Supercritical carbon dioxide extraction of astaxanthin from Corynebacterium glutamicum. Bioresour. Bioprocess. 21974365. 12 (1). Available from: https://bioresourcesbioprocessing.springeropen.com. doi:10.1186/s40643-025-00882-9.

Sephora Collection, n.d. Melting Cleansing Balm with Algae Extract [WWW Document]. https://www.kohls.com/product/prd-5267853/sephora-collection-melting-cleansing-balm-with-algae-extract.jsp (Accessed 15 September 2025).

Sheik, A.G., Kumar, A., Ansari, F.A., Raj, V., Peleato, N.M., Patan, A.K., Kumari, S., Bux, F., 2024. Reinvigorating algal cultivation for biomass production with digital twin technology - a smart sustainable infrastructure. Algal Res. 22119264. 84. Available from: https://www.sciencedirect.com/science/journal/22119264. doi:10.1016/j.algal.2024.103779.

Shiels, K., Murray, P., Saha, S.K., 2019. Marine cyanobacteria as potential alternative source for GABA production. Bioresour. Technol. Rep. 8, 100342. doi:10.1016/J.BITEB.2019.100342.

Shiels, K., Saha, S.K., Murray, P., 2025. Bioactive compounds for cyanobacteria and microalgae for human health applications: RUN-EU Student Research Colloquium 2025.

Shiels, K., Tsoupras, A., Lordan, R., Nasopoulou, C., Zabetakis, I., Murray, P., Saha, S.K., 2021. Bioactive lipids of marine microalga *Chlorococcum* sp. SABC 012504 with anti-inflammatory and anti-thrombotic activities. Mar. Drugs 16603397. 19 (1). Available from: https://www.mdpi.com/1660-3397/19/1/28/pdf. doi:10.3390/MD19010028.

Shiels, K., Tsoupras, A., Lordan, R., Zabetakis, I., Murray, P., Saha, S.K., 2022. Anti-inflammatory and antithrombotic properties of polar lipid extracts, rich in unsaturated fatty acids, from the Irish marine cyanobacterium *Spirulina subsalsa*. J. Funct. Foods. 17564646. 94, 105124. doi:10.1016/j.jff.2022.105124.

Shiseido, 2024. Benefiance Wrinkle Smoothing Cream [WWW Document]. https://www.shiseido.com/us/en/benefiance-wrinkle-smoothing-cream-0730852149533.html (Accessed 15 September 2025).

Siahaan, E.A., Agusman, R.P., Shin, K.H., Kim, S.K., 2022. Potential cosmetic active ingredients derived from marine by-products. Mar. Drugs 16603397. 20 (12). Available from: http://www.mdpi.com/journal/marinedrugs. doi:10.3390/md20120734.

Singh, U., Naaz, F., Hawkins, T.R., Weinberg, E., Banerjee, S., Mroz, R., Ohri, N., Zhang, J., Lee, -Y.-Y., Chen, F., Hill, R., Yantao, L., 2025. Direct flue gas capture for algae cultivation and subsequent valorization: evaluating life cycle emissions and costs. Sustain. Energy Fuels. 2398-4902. 9 (16), 4392–4403. doi:10.1039/d5se00329f.

Soliman, T.N., El-Dein, A.N., Al-Diam, S.A., Allayeh, A., Awad, H., Flefil, N.S., 2024. Characterization of C-phycocyanin antioxidant, anti-inflammatory, anti-tumour, and anti-HCoV-229E activities and encapsulation for implementation in an innovative functional yogurt. Heliyon 24058440. 10 (11). Available from: https://www.sciencedirect.com/science/journal/24058440. doi:10.1016/j.heliyon.2024.e31642.

SpecialChem, 2021. *Porphyridiumcruentum* extract [WWW Document]. https://www.specialchem.com/cosmetics/inci-ingredients/porphyridium-cruentum-extract (Accessed 15 September 2025).

SpecialChem, n.d. *Spirulinaplatensis* extract [WWW Document]. https://www.specialchem.com/cosmetics/inci-ingredients/spirulina-platensis-extract (Accessed 15 September 2025).

Spolaore, P., Joannis-Cassan, C., Duran, E., Isambert, A., 2006. Commercial applications of microalgae. J. Biosci. Bioeng. 13891723. 101 (2), 87–96. doi:10.1263/jbb.101.87.

Syed, T., Krujatz, F., Ihadjadene, Y., Mühlstädt, G., Hamedi, H., Mädler, J., Urbas, L., 2024. A review on machine learning approaches for microalgae cultivation systems. Comput. Biol. Med. 00104825. 172, 108248. doi:10.1016/j.compbiomed.2024.108248.

Toucheteau, C., Deffains, V., Gaignard, C., Rihouey, C., Laroche, C., Pierre, G., Lépine, O., Probert, I., Cerf, D.L., Michaud, P., Arnaudin-Fruitier, I., Bridiau, N., 2023. Thierry Maugard, Role of some structural features in EPS from microalgae stimulating collagen production by human dermal fibroblasts. Bioengineered. 2165-5979. 14 (1). doi:10.1080/21655979.2023.2254027.

Tzima, S., Georgiopoulou, I., Louli, V., Magoulas, K., 2023. Recent advances in supercritical CO_2 extraction of pigments, lipids, and bioactive compounds from microalgae. Molecules. 1420-3049. 28 (3), 1410. doi:10.3390/molecules28031410.

Ubando, A.T., Anderson, E., Ng, S., Chen, W.H., Culaba, A.B., Kwon, E.E., 2022. Life cycle assessment of microalgal biorefinery: a state-of-the-art review. Bioresour. Technol. 18732976. 360. Available from: https://www.elsevier.com/locate/biortech. doi:10.1016/j.biortech.2022.127615.

Udayan, A., Sirohi, R., Sreekumar, N., Sang, B.I., Sim, S.J., 2022. Mass cultivation and harvesting of microalgal biomass: current trends and future perspectives. Bioresour. Technol. 18732976. 344. Available from: https://www.elsevier.com/locate/biortech. doi:10.1016/j.biortech.2021.126406.

Vandamme, D., 2017. Harvesting, thickening and dewatering processes for microalgae biomass production. In: Pires, J.C.M. (Ed.), Microalgae as a Source of Bioenergy: Products, Processes and Economics. Bentham Science Publishers, pp. 202–223.

Vasilakis, G., Marka, S., Ntzouvaras, A., Zografaki, M.E., Kyriakopoulou, E., Kalliampakou, K.I., Bekiaris, G., Korakidis, E., Papageorgiou, N., Christofi, S., Vassilaki, N., Moschopoulou, G., Tzovenis, I., Economou-Amilli, A., Papanikolaou, S., Flemetakis, E., 2025. Wound healing, antioxidant, and antiviral properties of bioactive polysaccharides of microalgae strains isolated from Greek coastal lagoons. Mar. Drugs 16603397. 23 (2). Available from: http://www.mdpi.com/journal/marinedrugs. doi:10.3390/md23020077.

Villaró, S., Ciardi, M., Morillas-España, A., Sánchez-Zurano, A., Acién-Fernández, G., Lafarga, T., 2021. Microalgae derived astaxanthin: research and consumer trends and industrial use as food. Foods. 2304-8158. 10 (10), 2303. doi:10.3390/foods10102303.

Vo, T.-S., Ngo, D.-H., Kim, S.-K., 2012. Marine algae as a potential pharmaceutical source for anti-allergic therapeutics. Process Biochem. 47, 386–394. doi:10.1016/j.procbio.2011.12.014.

Wang, B., Li, Y., Wu, N., Lan, C.Q., 2008. CO_2 bio-mitigation using microalgae. Appl. Microbiol. Biotechnol. 01757598. 79 (5), 707–718. doi:10.1007/s00253-008-1518-y.

Wang, H.M.D., Li, X.C., Lee, D.J., Chang, J.S., 2017. Potential biomedical applications of marine algae. Bioresour. Technol. 18732976. 244, 1407–1415. Available from: https://www.elsevier.com/locate/biortech. doi:10.1016/j.biortech.2017.05.198.

Wang, J., Xinge, H., Chen, J., Wang, T., Huang, X., Chen, G., 2022. The extraction of β-carotene from microalgae for testing their health benefits. Foods. 2304-8158. 11 (4), 502. doi:10.3390/foods11040502.

Yaiser, T., 2016. Cosmetic compositions comprising microalgal oil. EP2996672A1.

Yarkent, Ç., Gürlek, C., Oncel, S.S., 2020. Potential of microalgal compounds in trending natural cosmetics: a review. Sustain. Chem. Pharm. 17, 100304. doi:10.1016/j.scp.2020.100304.

Yu, B.S., Pyo, S., Lee, J., Han, K., 2024. Microalgae: a multifaceted catalyst for sustainable solutions in renewable energy, food security, and environmental management. Microb. Cell Fact. 14752859. 23 (1). Available from: https://microbialcellfactories.biomedcentral.com/. doi:10.1186/s12934-024-02588-7.

Zhou, X., Cao, Q., Orfila, C., Zhao, J., Zhang, L., 2021. Systematic review and meta-analysis on the effects of astaxanthin on human skin ageing. Nutrients. 2072-6643. 13 (9), 2917. doi:10.3390/nu13092917.

Section IV

Health benefits of bioactive ingredients from sustainable animal-based sources

Chapter 20

Mollusks

Alexandros Tsoupras[a], Theodora-Evelina Traga[a], and Chryssa Anastasiadou[b]
[a]*Hephaestus Laboratory, School of Chemistry, Faculty of Sciences, Democritus University of Thrace, Kavala University Campus, Kavala, Greece*
[b]*Fisheries Research Institute, Hellenic Agricultural Organization-DIMITRA (ELGO-DIMITRA), Kavala, Greece*

1 Introduction

It is now well established that the cosmetics industry is increasingly seeking novel natural bioactive compounds as alternatives to synthetic chemicals. As skin, hair, and nail care have become integral components of everyday routines, the demand for safe, sustainable, and biologically active ingredients continues to rise (Fonseca et al., 2023). For decades, cosmetic formulations have relied heavily on synthetic substances such as parabens, phthalates, and petrochemicals (Nowak et al., 2021). However, growing concerns regarding their potential adverse effects on human health and the environment have accelerated a shift toward natural and eco-friendly alternatives. This transition is largely driven by increased consumer awareness of issues such as endocrine disruption, microbial resistance, and bioaccumulation within ecosystems. In this context, marine-derived polysaccharides, peptides, and lipids have attracted significant attention due to their ability to effectively replace conventional synthetic ingredients. These compounds exhibit antioxidant and photoprotective properties and often demonstrate superior biocompatibility (Nurkolis, 2025). Consequently, the integration of marine bioactives offers a sustainable and innovative solution for next-generation cosmetic formulations without compromising product efficacy.

Covering approximately 70% of the Earth's surface and serving as the origin of life, the marine environment represents an immense reservoir of biodiversity, encompassing an estimated 500,000 species distributed across nearly 28 phyla. Despite this vast biological diversity, natural product research has traditionally focused on only a limited number of marine organism groups, primarily nine categories, including mollusks, sponges, algae, phytoplankton, microorganisms, coelenterates, and bryozoans (Wen-Yu et al., 2021). In recent years, the cosmetics industry has increasingly emphasized the valorization of marine by-products into high-value cosmeceutical ingredients, thereby supporting sustainable blue economy initiatives through circular resource utilization (Rotter et al., 2024). Initial efforts concentrated on primary compounds derived from fish and algae, such as marine collagen and alginates. Over time, this focus has evolved toward the incorporation of advanced bioactive molecules with specific functional properties. Furthermore, innovations in extraction methodologies, including enzyme-assisted extraction, have enabled the isolation of high-purity compounds with notable antioxidant and antiaging potential. This progression reflects a broader shift from the use of crude marine materials to functionally active biomolecules, highlighting marine organisms as a largely untapped yet highly valuable source for next-generation cosmetic innovation (Brunt and Burgess, 2018).

Within marine ecosystems, mollusks have gained increasing attention due to their high-quality nutrients and bioactives with promising health-related properties. Beyond their importance as a food source, mollusks exhibit substantial potential in biotechnology and cosmetic applications (Papadopoulou et al., 2025). Numerous by-products generated during seafood processing, which are often discarded, can be repurposed into high-value ingredients for skincare and personal care formulations (Ngandjui et al., 2024). For instance, shells from oysters, mussels, and clams are rich in calcium carbonate and can be utilized in toothpaste formulations, mineral-based cosmetics, or as natural exfoliating agents (Mititelu et al., 2021). Even more valuable are soft tissues, such as the mantle and viscera, which are abundant in bioactive peptides, amino acids, and enzymes known to promote skin regeneration and hydration. In addition, cephalopod ink, rich in melanin, possesses antioxidant and UV-protective properties, while chitin and its derivative chitosan exhibit antimicrobial activity and beneficial effects in dermatological applications (Guo et al., 2023; Kulka and Sionkowska, 2023).

Biofunctional Cosmetics for Health. https://doi.org/10.1016/B978-0-443-27500-5.00018-6

Collectively, these natural compounds of marine (mollusks) not only serve as effective substitutes for synthetic additives but also enhance sustainability through the circular utilization of marine resources, positioning mollusks as a practical and eco-friendly option for future cosmeceutical innovation.

2 Mollusks and their by-products as sustainable sources of valuable marine bioactives for functional cosmetics

2.1 Mollusks and their by-products

Mollusca ranks as the second-largest animal phylum globally, encompassing over 90,000 known species. These organisms play essential roles and provide critical services across both marine and land-based ecosystems (Apostolou et al., 2024). These organisms, commonly known as mollusks, include familiar species such as snails, clams, squids, and octopuses. They are also known for their soft, unsegmented bodies. These, in many cases, are protected by a calcareous shell, which is not present in all mollusks, such as octopuses. They are widespread across marine, freshwater, and even terrestrial ecosystems, but the majority inhabit oceanic environments such as seas and oceans. Mollusks exhibit a wide variety of feeding behaviors and ecological roles, ranging from herbivory and predation to filter feeding and scavenging (Ngandjui et al., 2024; Haszprunar and Wanninger, 2012). With an estimated 100,000–200,000 species globally, of which around 52,000 are marine, they represent roughly 7% of all known animal life. Their morphological diversity and ecological adaptability make them highly significant both biologically and economically (Ngandjui et al., 2024). Mollusks are categorized into several distinct classes according to their structural features and ecological roles. Typically, the phylum is divided into seven major groups, each with unique characteristics and environmental adaptations (Fig. 20.1).

The first three largest groups contain gastropods, bivalves, and cephalopods. There are also four categories in which mollusks are classified, and these are Polyplacophora, Scaphopoda, Monoplacophora, and Aplacophora. Some familiar mollusks from the first three groups are snails in gastropods, clams in bivalves, and squids in cephalopods (Haszprunar and Wanninger, 2012). The largest group, gastropods, encompasses about 100,000 species, including snails, limpets, and sea slugs. These animals vary significantly in size, from under a millimeter to up to one meter, and may have coiled or

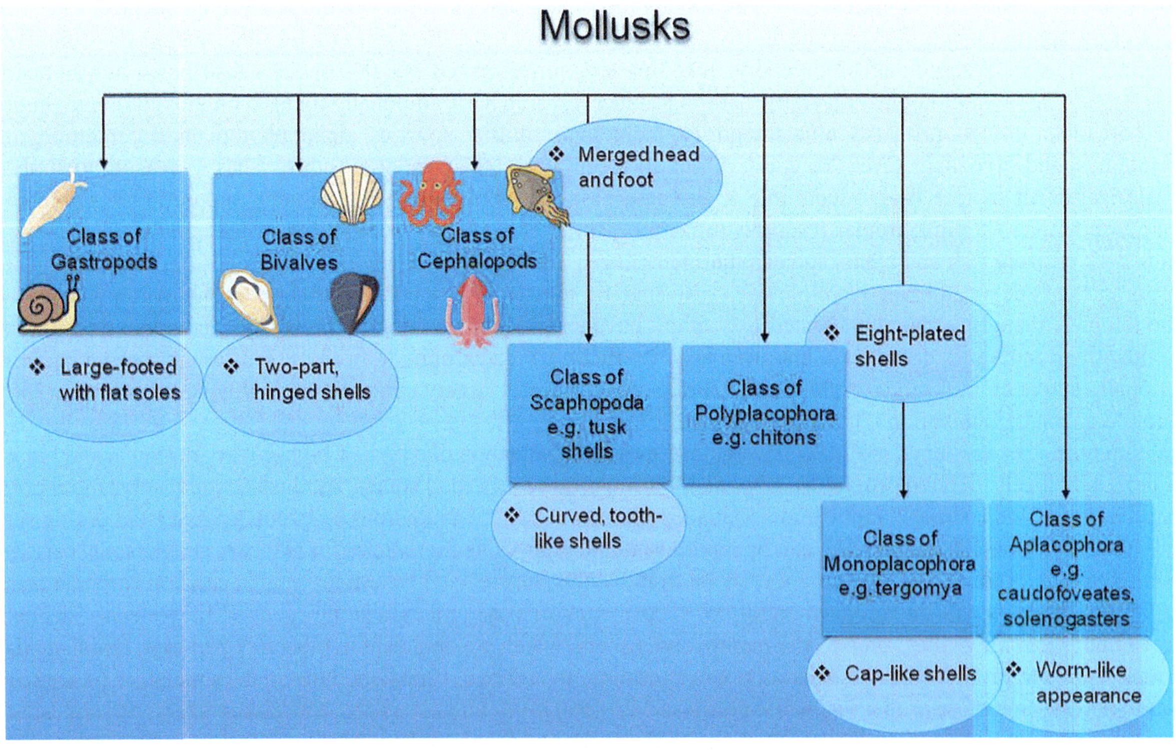

FIG. 20.1 Representative examples and classification of mollusks. *(From Papadopoulou, S.N.A., Adamantidi, T., Kranas, D., Cholidis, P., Anastasiadou, C., Tsoupras, A., 2025. A comprehensive review on the valorization of bioactives from marine animal by-products for health-promoting, biofunctional cosmetics. Mar. Drugs 16603397. 23 (8). Available from: https://www.mdpi.com/journal/marinedrugs. doi:10.3390/md23080299.)*

reduced shells. Gastropods are found in nearly every marine environment and display a range of feeding habits, including herbivory and carnivory (Apostolou et al., 2024; Haszprunar and Wanninger, 2012).

The second largest group is bivalves, consisting of mussels, clams, oysters, and scallops. There are almost 20,000 species, with their size ranging from 1 mm to over 150 cm. Opposed to gastropods, they have a two-part shell and are primarily filter feeders. They use specialized gills to extract food particles from the water. Bivalves are ecologically important for water filtration and as a food source for other animals (Ngandjui et al., 2024; Haszprunar and Wanninger, 2012). The third group of cephalopods includes 30,000 species, with 1000 being marine, and their reported size ranges from 3 cm to 7 cm (Haszprunar and Wanninger, 2012). This group has a special property, as animals within it seem to have advanced nervous systems and exhibit complex behaviors. They also have larger brains evolving with time (Haszprunar and Wanninger, 2012; Amodio et al., 2019). They are symmetrical with a prominent head and strong arms or tentacles equipped with suckers. In this class, there are squids, nautiluses, cuttlefish, and octopuses.

The class Polyplacophora, commonly referred to as chitons, represents a group within the Mollusca phylum that includes approximately 1,000 marine species. These marine organisms range in body length from 3 mm to 30 cm (Haszprunar and Wanninger, 2012). They are characterized by an oval-shaped body and a distinctive dorsal shell made up of eight overlapping plates or valves. Most chitons are herbivorous or detritivorous, using a specialized rasping structure called a radula to feed. They are typically found in intertidal zones (Ngandjui et al., 2024; Haszprunar and Wanninger, 2012).

In addition, the class Scaphopoda, or tusk shells, comprises 800 marine species. These mollusks possess elongated, tubular shells that resemble elephant tusks, ranging in size from 2 mm to 20 cm. They live buried in soft sediments, using a conical foot for digging and specialized tentacles called captacula to capture microscopic prey (Ngandjui et al., 2024; Haszprunar and Wanninger, 2012). The class Monoplacophora includes very few extant species, fewer than 30 known to science, such as Tergomya. These animals have a segmented body and a single cap-like dorsal shell. Once believed to be extinct, they were rediscovered in deep-sea environments at depths ranging from 200 to 7000 m. Although their feeding mechanisms are similar to chitons, they are distinct in structure due to their unique shell form (Ngandjui et al., 2024; Haszprunar and Wanninger, 2012). Lastly, the Aplacophora class consists of small, worm-like mollusks that either lack a shell entirely or have spicule-like structures in their skin. Typically ranging from 1 to 3 mm in length, these deep-sea species feed on invertebrates (Ngandjui et al., 2024; Haszprunar and Wanninger, 2012).

In general, molluskan shells, such as those of oysters, mussels, abalone, and nautilus, exhibit a highly specialized hierarchical structure composed of three primary layers (Song et al., 2019). These include an outer organic layer known as the periostracum, followed by two calcified layers: the prismatic (outer) and the nacreous (inner) layers (Saruwatari et al., 2009). The periostracum is a thin, flexible, leathery organic coating that serves as a protective barrier against environmental stress and shell degradation. Beneath this layer lies the prismatic layer, which is composed of elongated, columnar calcite crystals arranged perpendicular to the shell surface, providing mechanical strength and rigidity. The innermost nacreous layer, also referred to as mother-of-pearl, consists of aragonite crystals organized in a laminar, brick-wall-like architecture, a structure that confers exceptional fracture resistance and durability to the shell (Marie et al., 2012; Marin et al., 2012; Huang and Zhang, 2022; Marin et al., 2007).

Shell formation occurs through a tightly regulated biomineralization process mediated by the mantle epithelium, which secretes both organic and inorganic components (Huang and Zhang, 2022). These secretions include calcium carbonate minerals along with a complex organic matrix composed of proteins, peptides, glycoproteins, chitin, lipids, carbohydrates, acidic polysaccharides, and structural proteins (Marin et al., 2007). Collectively, these components form the shell matrix, which plays a critical role in controlling crystal nucleation, growth, and orientation. The unique combination of organic and inorganic materials results in a robust, multifunctional natural composite, making molluskan shells a valuable and versatile biomaterial for various industrial and biomedical applications.

Overall, mollusks are fundamental to marine ecosystems, playing vital roles in the food chain as both predators and prey. Many contribute to nutrient cycling and sediment stabilization. Beyond their ecological significance, certain mollusk species offer remarkable potential for industrial and cosmetic applications.

2.2 Mollusk-derived bioactive compounds with health-promoting properties

Mollusks are commonly classified as edible shellfish and have long been consumed as functional foods due to their recognized health benefits (Ngandjui et al., 2024; Wright et al., 2018). Marine mollusks have attracted considerable scientific interest because of their important role as valuable raw materials for the food industry and their wide range of benefits for human health, either through direct consumption or after processing into value-added products (Boulajfene, 2022), including functional foods (Ngandjui et al., 2024) and cosmetics (Papadopoulou et al., 2025). Owing to their high nutritional value, marine mollusks have served as dietary staples in many cultures for centuries (Ab Lah et al., 2017). They are rich sources of essential nutrients, including omega-3 (ω3) PUFA), including eicosapentaenoic acid (EPA; C20:5ω3) and docosahexaenoic acid (DHA; C22:6ω3), polar lipids, high-quality proteins, vitamins, and minerals (Larsen et al., 2011).

Among the seven molluskan classes, bivalves (such as mussels, oysters, clams, and scallops), cephalopods (including squid, cuttlefish, and octopus), and gastropods (such as whelks, sea snails, cockles, and abalone) are of greatest economic importance and are widely consumed as seafood, providing a balanced and valuable source of dietary protein (Chakraborty and Joy, 2020). These species also supply essential amino acids that are crucial for overall health, muscle development, and metabolic functions (Šimat et al., 2020). Consequently, mollusks represent a rich reservoir of chemical diversity and bioactive substances, supporting the development of nutritional supplements, functional food products, nutricosmetics, and cosmeceuticals. It is important to note that the composition of marine mollusks can vary significantly depending on factors such as species, habitat, diet, and harvesting practices (Boulajfene, 2022; Chakraborty and Joy, 2020; Khan and Liu, 2019).

A wide range of bioactive compounds derived from marine mollusks have demonstrated beneficial health effects and potential applications in food, cosmetics, and medical fields. These include proteins and peptides (such as collagen, gelatin, and albumins), polysaccharides (including carrageenan, agar-agar, fucans, fucoidans, chitin, chitosan, and their derivatives), lipids (mainly amphiphilic ones like phospholipids, but also more lipophilic ones like sterols and fatty acids), polyphenolic and carotenoid pigments (such as phlorotannins, β-carotene, chlorophylls, and lutein), enzymes (including gastric proteases, pepsins, gastricsins, chymosins, serine and cysteine proteases, lipases, and transglutaminase), as well as both fat- and water-soluble vitamins (Boulajfene, 2022; Šimat et al., 2020).

2.2.1 Amphiphilic and lipophilic lipid-based bioactives

Lipids are among the most important nutritional components of mollusks, performing essential biological roles as structural elements of cell membranes, signaling molecules, and energy storage compounds (Moruf et al., 2021; Zhukova, 2014). Molluskan lipids include fatty acids and their derivatives—such as tri-, di-, and monoacylglycerols, polar lipids (phospholipids and glycolipids)—as well as sterol-containing molecules, including cholesterol (Parrish, 2013; Tran et al., 2019). Most marine mollusks, particularly fatty species such as squid and octopus, are rich sources of ω3 PUFA, including EPA and DHA (Ahmad et al., 2019). These PUFA are associated with cardiovascular health, neurodevelopment, and antiinflammatory effects. They are widely used in the nutraceutical industry in products such as fish oil capsules and are also incorporated into livestock feed and infant formulas (Suleria et al., 2015). In bivalves like *Perna canaliculus*, the presence of PUFA contributes to antiinflammatory and antiarthritic effects (Mutalipassi et al., 2021). Despite their benefits, the overall PUFA content in mollusks is typically lower than that of other lipid classes, such as phospholipids and sterols.

Thus the amphiphilic marine polar lipids, and especially marine phospholipids, are the predominant lipid class in mollusks, likely due to their central role as structural components of biological membranes (Fokina et al., 2017). Analyses of nudibranch species such as *Chromodoris tinctoria*, *Chromodoris michaeli*, *Chromodoris geometrica*, *Chromodoris* sp., *Glossodoris cincta*, *Glossodoris atromarginata*, *Risbecia tryoni*, and *Platydoris* sp. revealed that phospholipids accounted for 73.8%–81.7% of total lipids (Zhukova, 2014). Similarly, in *Chromodoris* sp. and *Phyllidia coelestis*, phospholipids represented 85.7% and 54.9% of total lipids, respectively (Zhukova, 2007). In bivalves such as *Anadara broughtonii*, phosphatidylcholine (PC) and phosphatidylethanolamine (PE) were the principal phospholipids, comprising 45.0%–54.0% of total phospholipid content. Comparable proportions were observed in *Mytilus* species (*Mytilus edulis* and *Mytilus galloprovincialis*), with PC ranging from 36.8% to 43.1% and PE from 25.3% to 38.5% (Tabakaeva and Tabakaev, 2016).

More importantly, the bioactive marine polar lipids from mollusks, including phospholipids and glycolipids, are rich in beneficial PUFA like EPA and DHA, which contribute to significant antiinflammatory effects, modulating pathways involved in chronic conditions and supporting cardiovascular health. The structures and amphiphilic nature of these marine polar lipids help them integrate into cell membranes, providing antioxidant and antiinflammatory effects by inhibiting proinflammatory mediators and pathways, offering potential for nutraceuticals and functional products (functional foods/cosmetics), especially those with low omega-6/omega-3 ratios (Fig. 20.2) (Papadopoulou et al., 2025; Tsoupras et al., 2022).

More specifically, mollusks' bioactive polar lipids are, on the one hand, a good source of the essential ω3 PUFA, EPA, and DHA, known for their antiinflammatory properties, while, on the other hand, these polar lipids also contribute to health through antiinflammatory activity, acting as inhibitors of proinflammatory mediators that influence cellular immune processes like platelet-activating factor (PAF; 1-O-alkyl-2-acetyl-sn-glyceryl-3-phosphorylcholine), which modulates inflammation at the cellular level (Papadopoulou et al., 2025; Tsoupras et al., 2022). Such marine polar lipids can also reduce the production of inflammatory molecules such as nitric oxide (NO), TNF-α, IL-1β, and PGE2 by suppressing enzymes like COX-2 and 5-LOX, and they can modulate inflammatory pathways and interfere with key signaling transcription factors like NF-κB (Papadopoulou et al., 2025; Tsoupras et al., 2022).

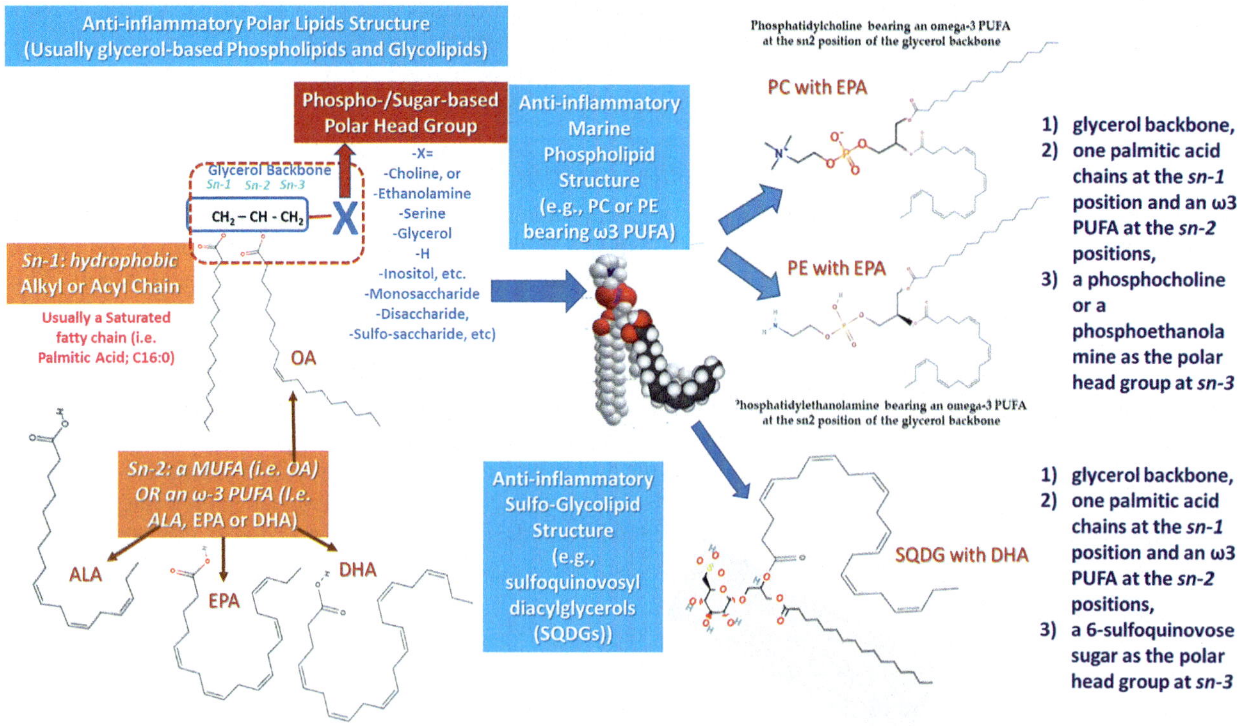

FIG. 20.2 Representative 2D and 3D structures of mollusk-derived PL bioactives, with antiinflammatory and antithrombotic health-promoting properties. Abbreviations: *ALA*, alpha-linolenic acid (C18:3ω3); *DHA*, docosahexaenoic acid (C22:6ω3); *EPA*, eicosapentaenoic acid (C20:5ω3); *PC*, phosphatidylcholines; *PE*, phosphatidylethanolamines; *PL*, polar lipids (either phospholipids or glycolipids); *SQDQ*, a specific class of sulfo-glycolipids containing 6-sulfoquinovose as the sulfo-sugar polar head group and two fatty acids esterified in the glycerol backbone. *(Some structures were obtained from the open access free platform Molview.Org (Accessed 30 November 2025).)*

Common mollusks, like the common octopus and squid, are indeed rich in such polar lipids, as well as mussels, such as the New Zealand Green-Lipped Mussel (*P. canaliculus*). In addition, species like *Bursatella leachii*, *Dicathais orbita*, and *Crassostrea madrasensis* also yield compounds with antiinflammatory or analgesic properties. Polar lipids from mollusks are being explored as ingredients for functional foods and supplements to combat chronic inflammation for cardiovascular health, based on their antiinflammatory and antithrombotic properties that support heart health. They are also being studied for their potential against neurodegenerative diseases, as they show promise in attenuating inflammation and oxidative stress relevant to such conditions (Papadopoulou et al., 2025; Ngandjui et al., 2024).

Marine sterols are another important but more lipophilic lipid class in mollusks, found in nudibranchs (*Chromodoris* spp., *Glossodoris* spp., *R. tryoni*, *Platydoris* sp.) (Zhukova, 2014). Sterols such as fucosterol and saringasterol possess antiinflammatory and antioxidant properties and have been investigated for multiple health benefits, including anticancer, antiobesity, antidiabetic, antiaging, and neuroprotective effects (Rahman et al., 2021). Sterols accounted for 13.5%–16.1% of total lipids in nudibranchs and approximately 13% in *Chromodoris* sp. and *P. coelestis* (Zhukova, 2014, 2007). Other more lipophilic lipids are mainly storage ones, including triacylglycerols and monoalkyl diacylglycerols, which usually represent minor fractions, ranging from 2.6% to 3.4% of total lipids (Zhukova, 2014).

2.2.2 *Polyphenolic and carotenoid pigments*

Marine polyphenolic compounds are present in several natural sources, including mollusks. Shellfish, such as clams and oysters, contain marine polyphenols and other micronutrients with biological activity (Pereira and Cotas, 2023). Among these, carotenoids such as astaxanthin and zeaxanthin are the most prevalent and are recognized for their potent antioxidant and antiinflammatory properties (Nag et al., 2022). These compounds are primarily acquired through the diet, as mollusks consume algae and other marine organisms rich in polyphenols and carotenoids (Quitério et al., 2021). Additional marine polyphenols, including catechins and procyanidins—also found in terrestrial sources such as tea, fruits, vegetables, and brown seaweeds—have been identified in shellfish and are associated with a wide range of health benefits, particularly antioxidant and antiinflammatory effects (Pereira and Cotas, 2023; Di Salvo et al., 2023).

2.2.3 Terpenes and other bioactive metabolites in mollusks

Mollusks represent one of the most chemically diverse groups among marine invertebrates and are particularly rich in terpenoid compounds. Terpenoids, also referred to as isoprenoids, constitute the largest class of natural products and exhibit remarkable structural diversity, enabling interactions with a wide range of biological targets. These compounds are commonly multicyclic, oxygenated molecules and are known for their broad spectrum of biological activities (Avila, 2020).

Marine and estuarine mollusks synthesize a diverse array of terpenoid metabolites, including chamigrene-, amphilectane-, and cembrane-type derivatives. Many of these compounds possess uncommon functional groups, such as isothiocyanates, dichloroimines, isonitriles, isocyanates, and halogen substitutions, which contribute to their unique bioactivity. Terpene biosynthesis in mollusks may occur de novo via the mevalonate pathway, leading to the formation of complex terpenes, including sesterterpenes. In nudibranch gastropods (Opisthobranchia), these small bioactive molecules play essential ecological roles, particularly in chemical communication, reproductive processes, and defense mechanisms against predators (Mudianta et al., 2014; Benkendorff, 2010).

2.2.4 Polysaccharides

Marine mollusks, particularly shellfish species, are valuable sources of structurally diverse polysaccharides with important applications in the food and biomedical industries. These include carrageenan, agar-agar, fucans, fucoidans, chitin, chitosan, and their derivatives (Senadheera et al., 2023). Polysaccharides obtained from molluskan shells, especially chitin and chitosan, are widely used as gelling agents, edible coatings, clarifying agents, and acidity regulators. In addition to their technological functions, these compounds exhibit antitumor, bactericidal, and fungicidal activities, while also enhancing dietary fiber intake and reducing lipid absorption (Suleria et al., 2015; Abdelmalek et al., 2017). Chitin and chitosan isolated from various molluskan species, such as chitons, the eggs of *Rapana venosa*, and the cephalopod *Sepia prashadi*, have demonstrated antioxidant, antimicrobial, antiviral, and antihypertensive properties (Mutalipassi et al., 2021). Moreover, bivalves such as *P. canaliculus* contain GAG-based compounds (Biolane and GlycOmega-PLUS) with documented antiinflammatory and antiarthritic effects (Mutalipassi et al., 2021).

2.2.5 Proteins and peptides

Marine mollusks are an abundant source of high-quality proteins, providing essential amino acids and a wide range of bioactive peptides, including collagen, gelatin, and albumins, which exhibit antioxidant, antihypertensive, and anticoagulant activities (Patra, 2021). These protein-derived compounds contribute to cardiovascular health, tissue regeneration, immune function, and muscle development (Li et al., 2007). Albumins isolated from mollusks have demonstrated both antioxidant and anticoagulant properties and are widely used in the food industry as whipping, stabilizing, and suspending agents (Suleria et al., 2015). Gelatin extracted from the tunics of giant squid (*Dosidicus gigas*) has shown notable antioxidant activity following enzymatic hydrolysis with proteases such as trypsin, chymotrypsin, and pepsin. Similarly, protein hydrolysates and peptides derived from bivalves, including *Sepia officinalis*, have exhibited significant antioxidant potential (Mutalipassi et al., 2021).

2.2.6 Marine enzymes

Mollusks are also a source of biologically active enzymes, particularly serine and cysteine proteases, which have found applications in food processing, including meat tenderization, prevention of undesirable color changes, herring curing, and squid fermentation (Suleria et al., 2015). The discovery and characterization of novel molluskan enzymes remain an active area of research. For example, the enzyme fucoidanase has been isolated and purified from the digestive glands of the marine mollusk *Lambis* sp. (Silchenko et al., 2014). In addition, the Antarctic mollusk *Nacella concinna* has been reported to produce proteolytic (keratinolytic) and glycolytic enzymes, such as α-L-rhamnosidases (Berezkina et al., 2020). Enzymatically active bacterial isolates obtained from gastropod species (*Conus ebraeus* L. 1758 and *Morula aspera*) and the bivalve *Hiatula chinensis* have also demonstrated strong enzymatic potential, further expanding the scope of mollusk-associated biocatalysts (Setyati et al., 2023).

2.2.7 Minerals and vitamins

Most molluskan species, including oysters and mussels, are rich in essential minerals such as calcium, iron, zinc, selenium, copper, manganese, phosphorus, and iodine, as well as water-soluble vitamins, including B-complex vitamins (B_{12}, B_6, and riboflavin), vitamin D, and vitamin A (Wright et al., 2018). These minerals play critical roles in bone health, immune function, antioxidant defense, and thyroid regulation, while vitamins are essential for energy metabolism, immune support, vision, and overall physiological health. As a result, molluskan-derived minerals and vitamins are widely utilized in the food, nutraceutical, pharmaceutical, and cosmetics industries (Papadopoulou et al., 2025; Suleria et al., 2015; Mutalipassi et al., 2021).

2.3 Cephalopods: Protein-rich tissues, bioactive mucus, and functional ink

Cephalopods, including octopus, squid, and cuttlefish, are a rich source of bioactive compounds with significant biotechnological, pharmaceutical, nutraceutical, and cosmeceutical potential (Paz et al., 2024; Pérez-Polo et al., 2023; Hamdi et al., 2024). Their skin mucus, ink, and various processing by-products contain a wide range of biologically active molecules, making them valuable marine resources. The skin mucus, which represents the primary interface between the organism and its environment, functions as a crucial defensive barrier and is particularly rich in bioactive substances exhibiting antioxidant, antimicrobial, antihypertensive, antiparasitic, and immunomodulatory activities (Pérez-Polo et al., 2023).

Cephalopod tissues are notably rich in proteins and peptides, including high levels of collagen and mucins (Pérez-Polo et al., 2023). Mucins, the main structural components of mucus, play essential roles in maintaining hydration, lubrication, and homeostasis while preventing desiccation and microbial invasion (Fernández-Boo et al., 2020). In both cephalopods and humans, mucins form a protective barrier over epithelial surfaces, supporting immune defense and wound healing (Pérez-Polo et al., 2023). Other proteins and peptides identified in cephalopod mucus include hemocyanins, histones, titin, leucine, and various muscle-related proteins such as myosin, paramyosin, and tropomyosin, some of which may arise from muscle tissue during sampling (Pérez-Polo et al., 2023). Hemocyanins exhibit notable antiviral and antitumor activities through immune stimulation, while histones derived from cephalopods have demonstrated antimicrobial activity against bacteria, fungi, viruses, and parasites. Titin contributes to muscle elasticity and repair, and leucine is a key amino acid involved in protein synthesis, tissue regeneration, and metabolic regulation (Pérez-Polo et al., 2023). Although respiration in cephalopods primarily occurs through the gills, the presence of hemocyanin in skin mucus may also suggest a supplementary role in gas exchange (Pérez-Polo et al., 2023; Madan and Wells, 1996). Importantly, noninvasive collection and analysis of skin mucus represent a sustainable approach for the valorization of seafood by-products, particularly in species such as *Octopus vulgaris*, which holds considerable biological and economic value (Pérez-Polo et al., 2023).

A distinctive and highly valuable feature of cephalopods is their ability to produce ink, a dark secretion primarily composed of melanin granules suspended in a colorless medium (Hamdi et al., 2024). Ink, produced mainly by squids and octopuses, serves as a chemical defense mechanism against predators but has also emerged as a multifunctional bioactive material with diverse therapeutic properties. Cephalopod ink contains melanin, tyrosinase, catecholamines, free amino acids, and trace metals (Derby, 2014; Ghattavi et al., 2022; Mikheil et al., 2017; Lucero et al., 1994; Russo et al., 2003; Palumbo, 2003; Kicklighter et al., 2005; Villanueva et al., 2004; Derby et al., 2007; Abdel-Malek, Moustafa and Salem, 2024). Melanin is a complex biopolymer derived from amino acids and occurs in two main forms: eumelanin and pheomelanin. Eumelanin, derived from 5,6-dihydroxyindole and 5,6-dihydroxyindole-2-carboxylic acid, exhibits a dark brown coloration, whereas pheomelanin, synthesized in the presence of cysteine from benzothiazine and benzothiazole units, displays orange-red hues (Ghattavi et al., 2022; Mikheil et al., 2017). Tyrosinase, a key enzyme in melanin biosynthesis, is abundantly present in cephalopod ink (Derby, 2014).

Cephalopod ink also contains low nanomolar to micromolar concentrations of catecholamines, such as dihydroxyphenylalanine (DOPA) and dopamine, along with high levels of free amino acids, including taurine, glutamate, lysine, leucine, and arginine. These compounds contribute to the ink's chemical defense through phagomimetic and deterrent properties (Lucero et al., 1994; Russo et al., 2003; Palumbo, 2003; Kicklighter et al., 2005; Villanueva et al., 2004; Derby et al., 2007). In addition, trace metals, such as copper, lead, and cadmium, have been detected and may act as cofactors in enzymatic processes involved in melanin synthesis (Derby et al., 2007; Abdel-Malek, Moustafa and Salem, 2024).

Functionally, cephalopod ink exhibits strong antioxidant activity, including free radical scavenging capacity and the reduction of molybdenum (VI) to molybdenum (V), effects largely attributed to its melanin content (Hamdi et al., 2024). It has demonstrated potent antibacterial activity against both Gram-positive bacteria (e.g., *Bacillus subtilis*, *Streptococcus faecalis*) and Gram-negative bacteria (e.g., *Escherichia coli*, *Pseudomonas aeruginosa*), as well as antifungal effects against *Aspergillus flavus* and *Candida albicans* (Hamdi et al., 2024). Anticancer activity has also been reported against several human cancer cell lines, including breast and liver cancers. Squid ink, particularly from *Loligo duvauceli*, exhibits antioxidant, antibacterial, and antiretroviral properties, and the antimicrobial protein Lolduvin-s has been isolated from Indian squid ink. Moreover, polysaccharides extracted from squid ink have shown strong inhibitory effects against oxidative stress by scavenging DPPH and hydroxyl radicals (Hamdi et al., 2024). Ink from cuttlefish species such as *Sepia aculeata*, *Sepia pharaonis*, and *Sepia kobiensis* has demonstrated significant antifungal and antitumor activities.

Beyond mucus and ink, cephalopod by-products are also rich in bioactive lipids. The common octopus (*O. vulgaris*) and various squid species contain high levels of ω3 PUFA, particularly EPA and DHA, which are associated with cardiovascular, neurological, antiinflammatory, and immune health benefits (Paz et al., 2024). Bioactive marine polar lipids from cephalopods exhibit strong antiinflammatory properties. Owing to their amphiphilic structure, these lipids readily integrate into cell membranes, where they modulate inflammatory pathways by inhibiting proinflammatory mediators such as PAF and reducing the production of inflammatory molecules, including NO, TNF-α, IL-1β, and PGE_2 through suppression of COX-2, 5-LOX, and NF-κB signaling (Papadopoulou et al., 2025; Tsoupras et al., 2022). Collectively, these properties support cardiovascular health and highlight the potential of molluskan polar lipids for use in nutraceuticals, functional food, and cosmetic products, particularly those with favorable omega-6/omega-3 ratios (Papadopoulou et al., 2025; Tsoupras et al., 2022). Fatty acids extracted from *Cuttlefish viscera*, including monounsaturated and saturated fatty acids, further contribute to antimicrobial, antiinflammatory, and cardioprotective effects. In addition, tocopherols (α- and γ-tocopherol), identified in by-products from Patagonian squid (*Doryteuthis gahi*), act as lipophilic antioxidants and contribute to both biological protection and food lipid stability (Paz et al., 2024).

Overall, the diverse bioactive compounds present in cephalopod mucus, ink, tissues, and by-products highlight their considerable potential as sustainable marine resources for functional foods, pharmaceuticals, nutraceuticals, and next-generation cosmetic formulations.

2.4 Gastropods and bivalves: Minerals, metabolites, and bioactive compounds

Gastropods and bivalves represent important classes of mollusks that are rich in minerals, secondary metabolites, and bioactive compounds with significant nutritional, pharmaceutical, and cosmeceutical potential (Papadopoulou et al., 2025; Ngandjui et al., 2024). Marine gastropods are particularly abundant in essential minerals such as potassium, iron, zinc, selenium, sodium, and sulfur, often exhibiting higher iron and selenium levels compared to other molluskan groups (Ab Lah et al., 2017; Durazzo et al., 2022). Their metabolite profiles are characterized by substantial proportions of terpenes (≈55%) and sterols (≈3%), along with notable levels of alkaloids (5%–6%) and polypropionates (13%–32%), whereas nitrogen-containing compounds are comparatively less prevalent (Benkendorff, 2010). In contrast, bivalves typically contain higher sterol content (≈41%) and lower terpene levels (≈5%), a difference that may be linked to metabolic variations in reproductive pathways (Benkendorff, 2010).

Gastropods have emerged as valuable sources of biologically active compounds with diverse therapeutic properties. A well-studied example is *R. venosa*, a carnivorous marine gastropod distributed in the Black Sea and other marine environments. Extracts from its soft tissues are rich in GAGs, which exhibit strong antioxidant and antiproliferative activities. These GAGs demonstrate effective radical scavenging capacity in DPPH and FRAP assays and have been shown to selectively inhibit the proliferation of Hep-2 human carcinoma cells while displaying low cytotoxicity toward normal fibroblasts, highlighting their promise for anticancer applications (Gaspar-Pintiliescu et al., 2024). Structurally, these GAGs resemble those found in human cartilage and possess additional antiinflammatory properties, suggesting potential benefits for joint health as well as nutraceutical and cosmetic applications.

Other gastropod species, such as the freshwater snail *Cipangopaludina lecythis*, also contain a diverse array of bioactive compounds in both their soft tissues and shells. Identified constituents include 6-gingerol, chitin, linoleic acid, eicosane, and octacosanol, which are associated with antioxidant, antiinflammatory, and regenerative activities (Ngangbam et al., 2024). The shell matrix is rich in chitin, a biodegradable and nontoxic polysaccharide with applications in cosmetic formulations, while additional compounds such as allantoin, also used in dermatological formulations, contribute skin-soothing and cell-regenerative properties. The presence of dihydrotachysterol, a vitamin D analog, further suggests potential roles in calcium metabolism and bone health (Ngangbam et al., 2024). Collectively, these findings highlight gastropods as a promising and underexplored source of marine bioactives.

Bivalves, including mussels, scallops, clams, and oysters, are affordable and nutritionally rich seafood resources, providing high-quality proteins, essential amino acids, minerals, and vitamins (Astorga España et al., 2007). They are particularly rich in zinc (226 ± 560 mg/kg) and copper (41 ± 110 mg/kg), with moderate levels of iron and selenium, and contain high concentrations of vitamins D and E (notably tocotrienols) (Durazzo et al., 2022; Khanna et al., 2010; Sen et al., 2007). Bivalves also accumulate carotenoids such as astaxanthin, canthaxanthin, mytiloxanthin, zeaxanthin, and their esters, which contribute to antioxidant and antiinflammatory activities (Maoka, 2011).

Numerous bioactive compounds isolated from bivalves have demonstrated anticoagulant, antibacterial, antiinflammatory, wound healing, and anticancer properties (Gaspar-Pintiliescu et al., 2024; Adler et al., 2024; Hafez et al., 2022). GAGs extracted from mussels such as *Anodonta anodonta* and *P. canaliculus* exhibit anticoagulant activity, while chondroitin sulfate-rich GAGs from *P. canaliculus* promote neurite outgrowth. In addition, heparan sulfate isolated from *Nodipecten nodosus* has been shown to inhibit arterial thrombosis without adverse effects, indicating pharmaceutical relevance (Gaspar-Pintiliescu et al., 2024). Bioactive lipids and amino acids from *M. galloprovincialis* have demonstrated wound healing properties by enhancing dermal and epidermal regeneration (Gaspar-Pintiliescu et al., 2024).

The valorization of blue mussels (*Mytilus* spp.), particularly from the Baltic Sea, offers significant opportunities for sustainable nutraceutical and functional food development (Adler et al., 2024). Mussels are excellent sources of complete proteins containing all essential amino acids, including glutamic acid, leucine, and lysine. Enzymatic hydrolysis of mussel proteins facilitates the release of bioactive peptides and amino acids with antihypertensive, antioxidant, and antimicrobial activities (Adler et al., 2024). In addition, mussels contain ω3 PUFA, notably EPA and DHA, which are associated with antiinflammatory and cardioprotective effects. Nevertheless, the primary fatty acids found are palmitic, myristic, and oleic acids. Other important components include glycogen, a key energy reserve that can act as a prebiotic when structurally preserved during extraction, supporting gut microbiota and overall intestinal health (Adler et al., 2024).

Clams and oysters further expand the bioactive potential of bivalves. Aqueous extracts from the giant clam *Tridacna squamosa* have shown strong antibacterial activity against *Salmonella enterica*, attributed to high levels of marine phenolic compounds such as gallic acid, chlorogenic acid, methyl gallate, and flavonoids, while maintaining low cytotoxicity, making them suitable for food-related applications (Hafez et al., 2022). Oysters, in particular, are well recognized for their exceptionally high zinc content, especially in soft tissues (Jianpeng et al., 2019). Their shells consist predominantly of calcium carbonate (≈95%), accompanied by a minor fraction of organic matrix proteins that form the skeletal framework (Upadhyay and Thiyagarajan, 2016). Calcinated oyster shell powder has attracted attention for its antibacterial and biocidal properties and favorable biocompatibility.

Beyond mineral components, oyster shells and tissues contain a wide range of organic compounds, including polysaccharides (mainly chitin), soluble and insoluble proteins (glycoproteins, collagen, gelatin, and albumins), lipids, free amino acids, short peptides, and pigments (Marin et al., 2012; Addadi et al., 2006). Bioactive peptides derived from oyster tissues and mantle exhibit strong antioxidant and immunomodulatory effects, while antimicrobial peptides present in oyster hemocytes, gills, and mantle are under active investigation as promising candidates for marine-derived therapeutic agents (Ulagesan et al., 2022). Overall, gastropods and bivalves represent highly valuable and sustainable marine resources, offering diverse bioactive compounds with broad applications in the food, nutraceutical, pharmaceutical, and cosmetic industries.

3 Mollusk-derived bioactive compounds in functional cosmetics applications

Marine mollusks, such as octopuses, squids, and snails, have significantly vital by-products, some of which include mollusk skin, shell structure, skin mucus, and the nacre layer. Their strong bioactivity has led to various applications in several industries. The cosmetics sector, utilizing bioactive compounds derived from marine by-products such as mollusks, has developed significantly in recent years. These bioactive compounds contain collagen, chitin, peptides, minerals, and omega-3 fatty acids. These substances contribute to various skin benefits, including antiaging effects, antioxidant activity, UV protection, and skin regeneration, making them ideal for use in products like creams, serums, and sunscreens (Hou et al., 2023; Lulu et al., 2022; Valeria et al., 2024; Zhang et al., 2023). Table 20.1 summarizes examples of bioactives present in mollusks for cosmetic applications, while Table 20.2 summarizes commercial cosmetic and cosmeceutical products that incorporate bioactives from marine mollusk by-products as active ingredients.

3.1 Mussel by-products in cosmetic ingredients

The beauty industry faces a significant challenge in removing microplastics, which harm the ecosystem, from products (Lulu et al., 2022). What is helpful is mussel adhesive proteins (MAPs). These proteins behave naturally as a strong glue in mussels, allowing them to stick firmly to various surfaces. MAPs are biodegradable and safe for living organisms. Their adhesive capability comes from two key compounds: L-DOPA and lysine. L-DOPA facilitates adhesion through metal coordination and hydrogen bonds, while lysine contributes via electrostatic interaction. By mimicking this natural process, a C–L–D (chitosan–graft-L-lysine-L–DOPA), a biodegradable material, has been developed. With its ability to create strong

TABLE 20.1 A summary of the bioactives present in mollusks with biological activities and cosmetic functions.

Category	Bioactive compound/ type	Mollusk source/ by-product	Key biological/ cosmetic function	References
Proteins and peptides	Collagen	Squid skin, cephalopod tissues, bivalves	Skin regeneration, fibroblast proliferation, antiaging	(Papadopoulou et al., 2025; Suleria et al., 2015; Mutalipassi et al., 2021; Patra, 2021; Li et al., 2007; Hou et al., 2023)
	Gelatin	Tunics of giant squid (*Dosidicus gigas*)	Antioxidant, wound healing, cosmetic formulations	(Papadopoulou et al., 2025; Mutalipassi et al., 2021)
	Albumins	Bivalves, mollusk soft tissues	Antioxidant, anticoagulant, stabilizing agent	(Papadopoulou et al., 2025; Suleria et al., 2015)
	Bioactive peptides	Bivalves, mollusk hydrolysates	Antioxidant, antihypertensive, immunomodulatory	(Papadopoulou et al., 2025; Mutalipassi et al., 2021)
Lipids	ω3 PUFA (EPA, DHA)	Squid, octopus, mussels, bivalves	Antiinflammatory, cardiovascular, skin barrier function	(Papadopoulou et al., 2025; Ahmad et al., 2019; Suleria et al., 2015; Mutalipassi et al., 2021; Fokina et al., 2017; Zhukova, 2007; Tabakaeva and Tabakaev, 2016; Rahman et al., 2021)
	Polar lipids (phospholipids, glycolipids)	Nudibranchs, cephalopods (i.e., squid, octopus), mussels	Antiinflammatory, antioxidant, skin, and cardiovascular health	(Papadopoulou et al., 2025; Zhukova, 2014; Fokina et al., 2017; Zhukova, 2007; Tabakaeva and Tabakaev, 2016)
	Sterols (fucosterol, saringasterol)	Nudibranchs, *Chromodoris* spp.	Antiinflammatory, antioxidant, antiaging, neuroprotective	(Zhukova, 2014; Zhukova, 2007; Rahman et al., 2021; Ngandjui et al., 2024)
	Triacylglycerols, monoalkyl diacylglycerols	Nudibranchs, other mollusks	Energy storage, minor cosmetic/nutraceutical roles	(Papadopoulou et al., 2025; Zhukova, 2014)
Polysaccharides	Chitin, chitosan	Chitons, cephalopod shells, mollusk shells	Antimicrobial, gelling, skin repair, antiaging	(Papadopoulou et al., 2025; Suleria et al., 2015; Mutalipassi et al., 2021; Senadheera et al., 2023)
	Glycosaminoglycans (GAGs)	*Perna canaliculus*, *Rapana venosa*	Antiinflammatory, anticoagulant, skin regeneration	(Papadopoulou et al., 2025; Gaspar-Pintiliescu et al., 2024; Mutalipassi et al., 2021)
	Carrageenan, agar-agar, fucoidans	Bivalves, mollusks	Gelling, antioxidant, antimicrobial, skin benefits	(Papadopoulou et al., 2025; Senadheera et al., 2023; Abdelmalek et al., 2017)
Minerals and vitamins	Calcium, iron, zinc, selenium, copper, manganese, phosphorus, iodine	Shells and soft tissues of bivalves and gastropods	Bone health, skin health, antioxidants, enzymatic cofactor	(Papadopoulou et al., 2025; Wright et al., 2018; Suleria et al., 2015; Mutalipassi et al., 2021)
	Vitamins A, B-complex, D	Bivalves, mollusk tissues	Skin health, immune function, antioxidant	(Papadopoulou et al., 2025; Wright et al., 2018; Suleria et al., 2015; Mutalipassi et al., 2021)
Pigments	Polyphenols (gallic acid, chlorogenic acid, methyl gallate, catechins, procyanidins, flavonoids)	Sepia, clams, oysters, giant clam	Antioxidant, antiinflammatory, antibacterial	(Papadopoulou et al., 2025; Hafez et al., 2022; Pereira and Cotas, 2023; Nag et al., 2022; Quitério et al., 2021; Di Salvo et al., 2023; Abdel-Malek, Moustafa and Salem, 2024)
	Carotenoids (astaxanthin, canthaxanthin, zeaxanthin, mytiloxanthin, β-carotene, lutein)	Bivalves, mussels, nudibranchs	Antioxidant, antiinflammatory, skin protection	(Papadopoulou et al., 2025; Nag et al., 2022; Quitério et al., 2021; Maoka, 2011)

Category	Bioactive compound/ type	Mollusk source/ by-product	Key biological/ cosmetic function	References
	Melanin	Cephalopod ink	Antioxidant, UV protection, photoprotection	(Papadopoulou et al., 2025; Hamdi et al., 2024; Derby, 2014; Ghattavi et al., 2022; Russo et al., 2003; Palumbo, 2003; Derby et al., 2007; Abdel-Malek, Moustafa and Salem, 2024)
	Tyrosinase	Cephalopod ink	Melanin synthesis, pigmentation	(Papadopoulou et al., 2025; Derby, 2014; Ghattavi et al., 2022; Russo et al., 2003; Palumbo, 2003; Derby et al., 2007; Abdel-Malek, Moustafa and Salem, 2024)
Terpenes and secondary metabolites	Terpenoids (chamigrene, amphilectane, cembrane type)	Nudibranchs, marine gastropods	Antiinflammatory, antioxidant, defense, cosmeceutical potential	(Papadopoulou et al., 2025; Avila, 2020; Mudianta et al., 2014; Benkendorff, 2010)
	Alkaloids, Polypropionates	Gastropods, bivalves	Antioxidant, antiinflammatory, antimicrobial	(Papadopoulou et al., 2025; Benkendorff, 2010; Maoka, 2011)
Enzymes	Serine and cysteine proteases	*Nacella concinna*, gastropods, bivalves	Food processing, cosmetic applications, protein modification	(Papadopoulou et al., 2025; Suleria et al., 2015; Silchenko et al., 2014; Berezkina et al., 2020; Setyati et al., 2023)
	Fucoidanase, α-L-rhamnosidases	Lambis sp., *Nacella concinna*	Polysaccharide modification, bioactive compound production	(Papadopoulou et al., 2025; Ngandjui et al., 2024)
Special mollusk-derived components	Mucus (rich in mucins, hemocyanins, histones, and peptides)	Cephalopods (octopus, squid)	Antioxidant, antimicrobial, skin regeneration, wound healing	(Papadopoulou et al., 2025; Pérez-Polo et al., 2023; Hamdi et al., 2024; Fernández-Boo et al., 2020; Madan and Wells, 1996)
	Nacre/Mother-of-pearl	Pearl oysters (*Pteria martensii*)	Collagen formation, fibroblast proliferation, antiaging, hair follicle regeneration	(Papadopoulou et al., 2025; Siahaan et al., 2022; Boulajfene, 2022)
	Mussel adhesive proteins (MAPs: L-DOPA and lysine)	Mussels	Biodegradable adhesives, microplastic-free cosmetic formulations	(Lulu et al., 2022)
	Snail mucus (with allantoin, hyaluronic acid)	*Helix aspersa* Muller	Skin regeneration, antioxidants, antiinflammatory properties, wound healing, and UV protection	(Valeria et al., 2024)
	Squid skin collagen	*Stenoteuthis oualaniensis*	Fibroblast proliferation, antiaging, skin regeneration	(Hou et al., 2023)

adhesion between surfaces, it can be used in cosmetic applications, especially in fragrance maintenance for hair, cotton fabric, and skin. Through this use, the elimination of microplastics becomes possible, offering a sustainable and innovative approach for the personal care industry (Lulu et al., 2022). Another biomimetic material, polydopamines (PDAs), inspired by the adhesion processes of mussels, has been used in sunscreen to protect the skin. PDAs, along with ZnO, have the ability to remain on the surface of the skin, protecting it from UV radiation and acting as an antiaging skin factor (Zhang et al., 2023).

The complex biochemical composition of the total lipid extract in mussel meat gives it valuable therapeutic properties. The high content of unsaturated fatty acids, along with fat-soluble vitamins, makes the extract a valuable ingredient for cosmetic preparations with emollient, nourishing, antioxidant, and regenerative properties (Burdge and Wootton, 2002; Ameur et al., 2012). In addition, it has been found experimentally that the extract also has antiinflammatory action

TABLE 20.2 Representative examples of commercial cosmetic products utilizing bioactive ingredients from Mollusks and their by-products.

Patent name or cosmetic formulation	Marine bioactives derived from fish sources (formulation content)	Cosmetic-associated benefits and commercial use	References
Crodarom Black Pearl (Croda Beauty, Yorkshire, UK)	Aragonite and conchiolin from Tahitian black pearls from the black-lip oyster (*Pinctada margaritifera*)	• Revitalizing, moisturizing, and nourishing propertiesProtecting skin against environmental damageSuitable for decorative cosmetics, radiance creams, or gloss shampoos	(Badilli and Inal, 2025)
Creanatural SEPIA MELANIN (The Innovation Company, France)	Creanatural Sepia Melanin derived from squid ink	• Photoprotective and antioxidant propertiesEffective UV filter for skin, sun, and hair-care cosmetics	(Rotter et al., 2024)
Akoshine (Akott Evolution, Milan, Italy)	Oyster shell pearl powder	• Moisturizing, sun-protective, antiaging, and smoothing productSoft and silky touch for creams, gels, lotions, massage formulations, body talc, tonics, powders, nail creams, and foundations	(Akott, n.d.)
Oligoceane pH (Croda Beauty, UK)	Oyster shell extract and sea salt extract	• Nourishing, moisturizing, conditioning, and skin-repairing agent in after-sun, body-, face-, neck-, skin-, and foot/leg-care products	(Croda, n.d.)
Huzhou Pearl Powder (Huzhou Shengtao Biotech, Huzhou, Zhejiang, China)	Amino acids and minerals from the jib clam of a natural Naidinae animal or the wrinkle clam of a bivalve mollusk	• Antiinflammatory, antiwrinkle, whitening, and skin-healing/smoothing properties-Eliminates black spots and can slow down senile wrinkles in the skin	(Huzhou Pearl Powder, n.d.)

(Flock et al., 2013; Stillwell and Wassall, 2003; Mititelu et al., 2020). Compared to the protein content, the lipid fraction is found in a much smaller proportion in the meat of mussels, up to 4% of the dry matter, but it must be remembered that it has a particular biological value. With the total lipid extract isolated and purified from mussel meat, containing mostly lipid vitamins and ω3 PUFA, a series of topical preparations for external use were developed: three emollient and nourishing cosmetic creams, an antiinflammatory ointment, and a healing ointment (Dermatocosmetic Preparations with Marine Lipids, n.d.). The control tests carried out on the prepared preparations showed a homogeneous appearance for all preparations, good stability, and a pH compatible with that of the skin. Rheological studies have also shown good consistency for all preparations. Cosmetic creams have a good stretching capacity and, in addition, when applied to the skin, are not sticky or oily, leaving behind a pleasant feeling of softness. Future investigations will highlight the optimal way to capitalize on this extract in various pharmaceutical forms.

3.2 Snail by-products in cosmetic ingredients

Snail by-products, such as snail mucus, have gained a lot of interest in the last few years for their use in cosmetic industry applications (Valeria et al., 2024). Snail mucus from *H. aspersa* Muller plays a significant role in cosmetics due to its ability to maintain healthy skin conditions. It has regenerative and protective effects. It is also recognized for its antioxidant and antimicrobial activity, as well as its wound repair capability. Snail mucus can repair signs of photoaging by stimulating the formation of collagen, elastin, and other dermal components. Its contribution to antioxidant compounds seems vital, as it counteracts damage from free radicals due to the presence of hyaluronic acid and various antioxidants. A key bioactive compound is allantoin, which is found in snail mucus. This compound has the ability to increase water content in the extracellular matrix and heal wounds (Valeria et al., 2024).

It has been found that the raw snail mucus application extract cannot be directly applied to the skin due to its lack of pharmacokinetics regarding its bioactive compounds. In addition, it tends to form a thick, insoluble film on cellular surfaces. For these reasons, a snail mucus extract coated with gold nanoparticles has been developed. This formulation allows for improved applications (Valeria et al., 2024). It can maintain significant antioxidant action, and the coated snail mucus exhibits high sun protection properties. This makes it a promising component for designing sunscreen formulations that could reduce conventional products. Antiinflammatory properties for skin protection have also been identified (Valeria et al., 2024).

3.3 Squid by-products in cosmetic ingredients

Bioactive compounds derived from mollusks, particularly collagen from marine sources, are gaining significant attention for future cosmetic use. Collagen is a major extracellular protein and is widely utilized in the food industry, medicine, and cosmetics industries due to its functional and biological properties (Hou et al., 2023). The Indian Ocean's iris squid (*Stenoteuthis oualaniensis*) is a promising source for type I collagen. This collagen, referred to as squid skin collagen, has been characterized for its effects on L-929 fibroblast cells, which are crucial for skin health and regeneration. It promotes the proliferation of L-929 fibroblast cells, and this is a vital benefit for cosmetic applications, as enhanced fibroblast proliferation can contribute to skin tissue regeneration and potentially offer antiaging effects by supporting skin vitality. Squid skin collagen and its derivatives could increase cell viability (Hou et al., 2023). They activate crucial intracellular signaling pathways, stimulating the PI3K/AKT and Ras/RAF/MAPK pathways. These are fundamental to cellular operations, such as metabolism, proliferation, and cell survival. By activating them, the collagen promotes cell growth and increases cell viability, while simultaneously inhibiting the expression of pro-apoptotic genes, thereby reducing programmed cell death. For these reasons, they play a key role in maintaining cell health and function, making it a significant compound for skin creams and other cosmetic applications (Hou et al., 2023).

3.4 Collagen uses in cosmetic applications

Collagen supplements play a significant role in dermatology and cosmetics by slowing the aging process and reducing the appearance of wrinkles. It has been found that both oral and topical forms of collagen are widely used in antiaging products. The mechanism by which collagen exerts its effects involves supplying essential components necessary for the production of both elastin and collagen within the skin. In addition, it interacts with fibroblast receptors in the dermis, thereby stimulating the generation of elastin and hyaluronic acid. Oral collagen, in the form of bioactive peptides, is absorbed quickly due to its lower molecular weight, facilitating its distribution across various body tissues. Collagen boosts the number of fibroblasts and the production of extracellular matrix proteins, which can improve skin health and help slow down skin aging (Al-Atif, 2022). While topical collagen can improve skin elasticity and texture, its complete infiltration into the skin may be limited due to its high molecular weight. However, it has been found that the topical application of collagen can promote antiwrinkling effects (Al-Atif, 2022).

3.5 Nacre use in cosmetic applications

Shell by-products from mollusks are valuable sources of health-promoting compounds. Among the most notable are conchiolins, which are insoluble proteins, and nacre, also known as mother of pearl. Nacre is the inner layer of bivalve shells; it is calcified and made up of aragonite crystals embedded in an organic matrix rich in proteins and polysaccharides. Increasingly, powdered nacre and pearl shell extracts are being explored for their cosmetic potential due to their unique biochemical properties (Siahaan et al., 2022).

Nacre obtained from pearl oysters (*Pteria martensii*) can promote wound healing, especially in deep burns, by stimulating collagen formation and encouraging fibroblast proliferation. In combination with hydrogels, nacre pearl powder has been shown to reduce inflammation and cell apoptosis in skin cells (Siahaan et al., 2022). There has been a lot of interest in the oral intake of nacre extract, as it has shown antiaging effects and benefits for skin health (Fokina et al., 2017). It can suppress skin aging and increase the skin's water content. In addition, nacre extract can counteract the reduction in the thickness of both the epidermal and dermal layers, which are characteristic signs of natural skin aging. Furthermore, it has helped to ameliorate the disrupted arrangement of collagen fibers in the dermis, a common age-related change (Yamamoto et al., 2024).

Nacre extract is not only effective for skin-related issues, but also beneficial for hair follicles. As the years pass, hair follicles tend to decrease; however, the administration of nacre extract helps them recover (Fokina et al., 2017). It has the potential to suppress the aging of the skin's dermal papilla cells and epithelial cells that form hair follicles, contributing to the prevention of age-related hair loss. The composition of nacre is primarily calcium carbonate and organic components, including proteins, polysaccharides, amino acids, vitamins, and peptides, which constitute a significant amount of bioactive compounds. Specific proteins, such as conchiolin, and sulfated polysaccharides have demonstrated biological activity (Yamamoto et al., 2024).

3.6 Melanin use in cosmetic applications

Melanin is a natural component that can be found in the ink of mollusks such as octopus, squid, and cuttlefish. As a nontoxic natural pigment, it serves as an effective natural colorant in cosmetics. Its antioxidant and anti-UV properties allow it to function as a photoprotective agent in cosmetics, thereby extending the antiaging period of such products. In addition, similar to vitamins C and E, melanin exerts an effect on the skin as an antiaging agent (Liberti et al., 2020).

Melanin plays a crucial role as a UV filter due to its significant impact on epidermal homeostasis, which is closely linked to melanocyte behavior. Melanin protects the skin from UV rays by absorbing them and releasing the absorbed energy as heat, effectively preventing direct UV radiation from reaching the DNA of the epidermal cells. In addition, melanin scavenges reactive oxygen species, which are generated in the skin during UV-induced oxidative stress. The amount of melanin present in the skin is determined by its phototype. However, in most cases, the natural melanin levels are insufficient to provide adequate UV protection during the summertime. For that reason, it is essential to use melanin in sunscreens as photoprotective molecules (Solano, 2020; Núñez-Pons et al., 2018).

Melanins, including allomelanin, neuromelanin, eumelanin, pheomelanin, and pyomelanin, found in cephalopod ink, marine bacteria, and fungi, have offered significant antiinflammatory and antioxidant cosmetic benefits (Shahidi and Saeid, 2025). Cephalopod ink has been incorporated into mascara, eyeshadow, and other cosmetic products. These displayed satisfactory outcomes in terms of the level of aspect, texture, color, and covering capacity of the formulated cosmetic products (Derby, 2014).

4 Conclusions, limitations, and future perspectives

Marine mollusks represent a highly diverse, sustainable, and largely underexploited source of bioactive compounds with significant potential for functional cosmetic and cosmeceutical applications. As highlighted in this review, mollusk-derived lipids, proteins, peptides, polysaccharides, pigments, enzymes, minerals, and vitamins exhibit a wide range of biological activities, including antioxidant, antiinflammatory, antimicrobial, photoprotective, wound healing, and antiaging effects. These properties, combined with their favorable biocompatibility, position molluskan bioactives as effective natural alternatives to synthetic cosmetic ingredients.

Importantly, the valorization of mollusk by-products—such as shells, skin mucus, ink, viscera, and processing residues—supports circular economy principles and aligns with current sustainability goals in the cosmetics industry. Advances in extraction technologies and biomimetic approaches have further enabled the development of high-value functional ingredients from mollusks, facilitating their incorporation into innovative skincare, haircare, and photoprotective formulations. Overall, marine mollusks emerge as a promising and eco-friendly resource capable of contributing to the next generation of natural, high-performance cosmetic products.

Despite the growing body of evidence supporting the cosmetic potential of mollusk-derived bioactives, several limitations remain. A significant portion of existing research is based on in vitro studies or preliminary bioactivity assays, while in vivo studies and well-designed clinical trials are still limited. Consequently, the long-term safety, efficacy, and skin bioavailability of many molluskan compounds in cosmetic formulations require further validation.

In addition, the chemical composition and bioactivity of mollusk-derived ingredients can vary considerably depending on species, habitat, seasonality, diet, and harvesting practices, which may affect reproducibility and standardization. Challenges also persist in scaling up extraction and purification processes while maintaining sustainability, cost-effectiveness, and compound stability. Regulatory hurdles, limited consumer awareness, and potential allergenicity issues may further restrict the rapid industrial adoption of mollusk-based cosmetic ingredients.

Future research should focus on advancing sustainable and green extraction technologies, including enzyme-assisted, supercritical fluid, and solvent-free methods, to improve yield, purity, and environmental compatibility. Greater emphasis on mechanistic studies, in vivo models, and clinical evaluations will be essential to substantiate the cosmetic efficacy and safety of mollusk-derived bioactives.

In addition, the development of standardized processing protocols and quality control frameworks will be crucial for ensuring consistency across raw materials and final products. Emerging strategies, such as nanotechnology, encapsulation systems, and biomimetic formulations, may enhance the stability, skin penetration, and targeted delivery of molluskan compounds.

From an industrial and environmental perspective, integrating mollusk by-product valorization into seafood-processing chains represents a promising pathway toward zero-waste biorefineries and sustainable blue economy models. With continued interdisciplinary collaboration among marine biologists, chemists, cosmetic scientists, and industry stakeholders, mollusks are poised to become a key marine resource for the development of safe, effective, and environmentally responsible functional cosmetic products.

Acknowledgments

The authors would like to thank the School of Chemistry, Faculty of Sciences at the Democritus University of Thrace, and the Fisheries Research Institute in Kavala, Greece, for their continuous support.

Conflicts of interest

The authors declare no conflicts of interest.

Funding

This research received no external funding.

Author contributions

A.T. was involved in conceptualization, methodology, validation, visualization, and supervision. T.E.T. and A.T. were involved in investigation and writing—original draft preparation. C.A. and A.T. were involved in writing—review and editing. All authors contributed to software and have read and agreed to the published version of the manuscript.

References

Ab Lah, R., Smith, J., Savins, D., Dowell, A., Bucher, D., Benkendorff, K., 2017. Investigation of nutritional properties of three species of marine turban snails for human consumption. Food Sci. Nutr. 2048-7177. 5 (1), 14–30. doi:10.1002/fsn3.360.

Abdel-Malek, A.R., Moustafa, A.Y., Salem, S.H., 2024. Antimicrobial and cytotoxic activities of flavonoid and phenolics extracted from *Sepia pharaonis* ink (Mollusca: Cephalopoda). BMC Biotechnol. 14726750. 24 (1). Available from: https://bmcbiotechnol.biomedcentral.com/. doi:10.1186/s12896-024-00880-3.

Abdelmalek, B.E., Sila, A., Haddar, A., Bougatef, A., Ayadi, M.A., 2017. β-Chitin and chitosan from squid gladius: biological activities of chitosan and its application as clarifying agent for apple juice. Int. J. Biol. Macromol. 18790003. 104, 953–962. Available from: https://www.elsevier.com/locate/ijbiomac. doi:10.1016/j.ijbiomac.2017.06.107.

Addadi, L., Joester, D., Nudelman, F., Weiner, S., 2006. Mollusk shell formation: a source of new concepts for understanding biomineralization processes. Chem. Eur. J. 0947-6539. 12 (4), 980–987. doi:10.1002/chem.200500980.

Adler, I., Kotta, J., Robal, M., Humayun, S., Vene, K., Tuvikene, R., 2024. Valorization of Baltic Sea farmed blue mussels: chemical profiling and prebiotic potential for nutraceutical and functional food development. Food Chem. X. 25901575. 23, 101736. doi:10.1016/j.fochx.2024.101736.

Ahmad, T.B., Rudd, D., Kotiw, M., Liu, L., Benkendorff, K., 2019. Correlation between fatty acid profile and anti-inflammatory activity in common Australian seafood by-products. Mar. Drugs 16603397. 17 (3). Available from: https://www.mdpi.com/1660-3397/17/3/155/pdf. doi:10.3390/md17030155.

Akott, n.d. Akoshine Oyster Shell Pearl Powder. Available online: https://cosmetics.specialchem.com/product/i-akott-akoshine-oyster-shell-pearl-powder (Accessed on 24 June 2025).

Al-Atif, H., 2022. Collagen supplements for aging and wrinkles: a paradigm shift in the field of dermatology and cosmetics. Dermatol. Pract. Concept. 2160-9381. 12 (1), e2022018. doi:10.5826/dpc.1201a18.

Ameur, A., Enroth, S., Johansson, Å., Zaboli, G., Igl, W., Johansson, A.C.V., Rivas, M.A., Daly, M.J., Schmitz, G., Hicks, A.A., Meitinger, T., Feuk, L., van Duijn, C., Oostra, B., Pramstaller, P.P., Rudan, I., Wright, A.F., Wilson, J.F., Campbell, H., Gyllensten, U., 2012. Genetic adaptation of fatty-acid metabolism: a human-specific haplotype increasing the biosynthesis of long-chain omega-3 and omega-6 fatty acids. Am. J. Hum. Genet. 00029297. 90 (5), 809–820. doi:10.1016/j.ajhg.2012.03.014.

Amodio, P., Boeckle, M., Schnell, A.K., Ostojíc, L., Fiorito, G., Clayton, N.S., 2019. Grow smart and die young: why did cephalopods evolve intelligence? Trends Ecol. Evol. 01695347. 34 (1), 45–56. doi:10.1016/j.tree.2018.10.010.

Apostolou, K., Radea, C., Meziti, A., Kormas, K.A., 2024. Bacterial diversity associated with terrestrial and aquatic snails. Microorganisms 13 (1), 8.

Astorga España, M.S., Rodríguez Rodríguez, E.M., Díaz Romero, C., 2007. Comparison of mineral and trace element concentrations in two molluscs from the Strait of Magellan (Chile). J. Food Compos. Anal. 08891575. 20 (3-4), 273–279. doi:10.1016/j.jfca.2006.06.007.

Avila, C., 2020. Terpenoids in marine heterobranch molluscs. Mar. Drugs. 1660-3397. 18 (3), 162. doi:10.3390/md18030162.

Badilli, U., Inal, O., 2025. Current approaches in cosmeceuticals: peptides, biotics and marine biopolymers. Polymers. 2073-4360. 17 (6), 798. doi:10.3390/polym17060798.

Benkendorff, K., 2010. Molluscan biological and chemical diversity: secondary metabolites and medicinal resources produced by marine molluscs. Biol. Rev. 1464-7931. 85 (4), 757–775. doi:10.1111/j.1469-185x.2010.00124.x.

Berezkina, A.Y., Avdiuk, K.V., Gudzenko, O.V., Kharkhota, M.A., Utevsky, A.Y., 2020. Bacterial enzymes associated with gastropod mollusc nacella concinna from the water area of the Argentine islands (West Antarctica). Probl. Cryobiol. Cryomed. 23076143. 30 (3), 295. Available from: http://cryo.org.ua/journal/index.php/probl-cryobiol-cryomed/article/view/1673/1776. doi:10.15407/CRYO30.03A.295.

Boulajfene, W., 2022. Nutritional and health benefits of marine mollusks. In: Kim, S.-K. (Ed.), Marine Biochemistry. Taylor & Francis, Abingdon, UK, pp. 435–453.

Brunt, E.G., Burgess, J.G., 2018. The promise of marine molecules as cosmetic active ingredients. Int. J. Cosmet. Sci. 0142-5463. 40 (1), 1–15. doi:10.1111/ics.12435.

Burdge, G.C., Wootton, S.A., 2002. Conversion of α-linolenic acid to eicosapentaenoic, docosapentaenoic and docosahexaenoic acids in young women. Br. J. Nutr. 00071145. 88 (4), 411–420. Available from: http://journals.cambridge.org/BJN. doi:10.1079/bjn2002689.

Chakraborty, K., Joy, M., 2020. High-value compounds from the molluscs of marine and estuarine ecosystems as prospective functional food ingredients: an overview. Food Res. Int. 09639969. 137, 109637. doi:10.1016/j.foodres.2020.109637.

Croda, n.d. Oligoceane PH. Available online: https://cosmetics.specialchem.com/product/i-croda-oligoceane-ph (Accessed on 24 June 2025).

Derby, C., 2014. Cephalopod ink: production, chemistry, functions and applications. Mar. Drugs. 1660-3397. 12 (5), 2700–2730. doi:10.3390/md12052700.

Derby, C.D., Kicklighter, C.E., Johnson, P.M., Zhang, X., 2007. Chemical composition of inks of diverse marine molluscs suggests convergent chemical defenses. J. Chem. Ecol. 15731561. 33 (5), 1105–1113. doi:10.1007/s10886-007-9279-0.

Dermatocosmetic Preparations with Marine Lipids, n.d. https://nutriterra.org/ro/dermatocosmetic-preparations-marine-lipids/ (Accessed on 3 January 2026).

Di Salvo, E., Gangemi, S., Genovese, C., Cicero, N., Casciaro, M., 2023. Polyphenols from Mediterranean plants: biological activities for skin photoprotection in atopic dermatitis, psoriasis, and chronic urticaria. Plants. 2223-7747. 12 (20), 3579. doi:10.3390/plants12203579.

Durazzo, A., Di Lena, G., Gabrielli, P., Santini, A., Lombardi-Boccia, G., Lucarini, M., 2022. Nutrients and bioactive compounds in seafood: quantitative literature research analysis. Fishes. 2410-3888. 7 (3), 132. doi:10.3390/fishes7030132.

Fernández-Boo, S., Gervais, O., Prado-Alvarez, M., Chollet, B., Claverol, S., Lecadet, C., Dubreuil, C., Arzul, I., 2020. Is pallial mucus involved in *Ostrea edulis* defenses against the parasite Bonamia ostreae? J. Invertebr. Pathol. 00222011. 169, 107259. doi:10.1016/j.jip.2019.107259.

Flock, M.R., Harris, W.S., Kris-Etherton, P.M., 2013. Long-chain omega-3 fatty acids: time to establish a dietary reference intake. Nutr. Rev. 17534887. 71 (10), 692–707. doi:10.1111/nure.12071.

Fokina, N.N., Ruokolainen, T.R., Nemova, N.N., 2017. Lipid Composition Modifications in the Blue Mussels (Mytilus Edulis L.) from the White Sea. IntechOpen. doi:10.5772/67811.

Fonseca, S., Amaral, M.N., Reis, C.P., Custódio, L., 2023. Marine natural products as innovative cosmetic ingredients. Mar. Drugs. 1660-3397. 21 (3), 170. doi:10.3390/md21030170.

Gaspar-Pintiliescu, A., Stefan, L.M., Mihai, E., Sanda, C., Manoiu, V.S., Berger, D., Craciunescu, O., Grigorov, B., 2024. Antioxidant and antiproliferative effect of a glycosaminoglycan extract from Rapana venosa marine snail. PLOS ONE. 1932-6203. 19 (2), e0297803. doi:10.1371/journal.pone.0297803.

Ghattavi, K., Homaei, A., Kamrani, E., Kim, S.-K., 2022. Melanin pigment derived from marine organisms and its industrial applications. Dyes Pigments. 01437208. 201, 110214. doi:10.1016/j.dyepig.2022.110214.

Guo, L., Li, W., Gu, Z., Wang, L., Guo, L., Ma, S., Li, C., Sun, J., Han, B., Chang, J., 2023. Recent advances and progress on melanin: from source to application. Int. J. Mol. Sci. 24 (5), 4360.

Hafez, M.S.M.A.E., et al., 2022. Antibacterial potential of *Tridacna* sp. and pearl oyster aqueous extracts on food spoilage *Salmonella enterica*. Egypt. J. Aquat. Biol. Fish. 2536-9814. 26 (6), 737–749. doi:10.21608/ejabf.2022.275509.

Hamdi, S.A.H., El-Shazly, M.A.M., Fol, M.F., Mossalem, H.S., Ghareeb, M.A., Ibrahim, A.M., Aloufi, A.S., El-Ghany, M.N.A., Korany, S.M., 2024. Octopus vulgaris ink chemical profiling and validation of its potential as antioxidant, antimicrobial, anti-cancer as well as anti-Schistosomal drug in vitro. Arq. Bras. Med. Vet. Zootec. 1678-4162. 76 (5). doi:10.1590/1678-4162-13217.

Haszprunar, G., Wanninger, A., 2012. Molluscs. Curr. Biol. 09609822. 22 (13), R510. doi:10.1016/j.cub.2012.05.039.

Hou, C., Lei, Y., Li, N., Wei, M., Wang, S., Rahman, S.U., Bao, C., Bao, B., Elango, J., Wenhui, W., 2023. Collagen from Iris squid grafted with polyethylene glycol and collagen peptides promote the proliferation of fibroblast through PI3K/AKT and Ras/RAF/MAPK signaling pathways. Int. J. Biol. Macromol. 01418130. 247, 125772. doi:10.1016/j.ijbiomac.2023.125772.

Huang, J., Zhang, R., 2022. The mineralization of molluscan shells: some unsolved problems and special considerations. Front. Mar. Sci. 2296-7745. 9. doi:10.3389/fmars.2022.874534.

Huzhou Pearl Powder, n.d. Huzhou Nanxun Shengtao Botanical. Available online: https://cosmetics.specialchem.com/product/i-huzhou-shengtao-biotech-huzhou-pearl-powder (Accessed on 24 June 2025).

Jianpeng, L., Gong, C., Wang, Z., Gao, R., Ren, J., Zhou, X., Wang, H., Xu, H., Xiao, F., Cao, Y., Zhao, Y., 2019. Oyster-derived zinc-binding peptide modified by plastein reaction via zinc chelation promotes the intestinal absorption of zinc. Mar. Drugs. 1660-3397. 17 (6), 341. doi:10.3390/md17060341.

Khan, B.M., Liu, Y., 2019. Marine mollusks: food with benefits. Compr. Rev. Food Sci. Food Saf. 15414337. 18 (2), 548–564. Available from: http://onlinelibrary.wiley.com/journal/10.1111/(ISSN)1541-4337. doi:10.1111/1541-4337.12429.

Khanna, S., Parinandi, N.L., Kotha, S.R., Roy, S., Rink, C., Bibus, D., Sen, C.K., 2010. Nanomolar vitamin e α-tocotrienol inhibits glutamate-induced activation of phospholipase A2 and causes neuroprotection. J. Neurochem. 14714159. 112 (5), 1249–1260. doi:10.1111/j.1471-4159.2009.06550.x.

Kicklighter, C.E., Shabani, S., Johnson, P.M., Derby, C.D., 2005. Sea hares use novel antipredatory chemical defenses. Curr. Biol. 09609822. 15 (6), 549–554. Available from: http://www.elsevier.com/journals/current-biology/0960-9822. doi:10.1016/j.cub.2005.01.057.

Kulka, K., Sionkowska, A., 2023. Chitosan based materials in cosmetic applications: a review. Molecules 28 (4), 1817.

Larsen, R., Eilertsen, K.E., Elvevoll, E.O., 2011. Health benefits of marine foods and ingredients. Biotechnol. Adv. 07349750. 29 (5), 508–518. doi:10.1016/j.biotechadv.2011.05.017.

Li, P., Yin, Y.L., Li, D., Kim, W.S., Wu, G., 2007. Amino acids and immune function. Br. J. Nutr. 14752662. 98 (2), 237–252. doi:10.1017/S000711450769936X.

Liberti, D., Alfieri, M.L., Monti, D.M., Panzella, L., Napolitano, A., 2020. A melanin-related phenolic polymer with potent photoprotective and antioxidant activities for dermo-cosmetic applications. Antioxidants. 2076-3921. 9 (4), 270. doi:10.3390/antiox9040270.

Lucero, M.T., Farrington, H., Gilly, W.F., 1994. Quantification of L-Dopa and dopamine in squid ink: implications for chemoreception. Biol. Bull. 0006-3185. 187 (1), 55–63. doi:10.2307/1542165.

Lulu, X., Liu, J., Ma, X.Y.D., Zibiao, L., Chaobin, H., Xuehong, L., 2022. Facile anchoring mussel adhesive mimic tentacles on biodegradable polymer cargo carriers via self-assembly for microplastic-free cosmetics. J. Colloid Interface Sci. 00219797. 612, 13–22. doi:10.1016/j.jcis.2021.12.141.

Madan, J.J., Wells, M.J., 1996. Cutaneous respiration in *Octopus vulgaris*. J. Exp. Biol. 0022-0949. 199 (11), 2477–2483. doi:10.1242/jeb.199.11.2477.

Maoka, T., 2011. Carotenoids in marine animals. Mar. Drugs. 1660-3397. 9 (2), 278–293. doi:10.3390/md9020278.

Marie, B., Joubert, C., Tayalé, A., Zanella-Cleón, I., Belliard, C., Piquemal, D., Cochennec-Laureau, N., Marin, F., Gueguen, Y., Montagnani, C., 2012. Different secretory repertoires control the biomineralization processes of prism and nacre deposition of the pearl oyster shell. Proc. Natl. Acad. Sci. U. S. A. 10916490. 109 (51), 20986–20991. Available from: http://www.pnas.org/content/109/51/20986.full.pdf+html. doi:10.1073/pnas.1210552109.

Marin, F., Luquet, G., Marie, B., Medakovic, D., 2007. Molluscan shell proteins: primary structure, origin, and evolution. Curr. Top. Dev. Biol. 80. doi:10.1016/S0070-2153(07)80006-8.

Marin, F., Roy, N.L., Marie, B., 2012. The formation and mineralization of mollusk shell. Front. Biosci. Scholar 19450524. 4 (3), 1099–1125. Available from: http://www.bioscience.org/fbs/getfile.php?FileName=/2012/v4s/af/321/321.pdf. doi:10.2741/s321.

Mikheil, D., Prabhakar, K., Jayanthy, A.-S., Setaluri, V., 2017. Coat color mutations, animals. In: Reference Module in Life Sciences, Elsevier, Amsterdam, The Netherlands, B9780128096338062324, ISBN 978-0-12-809633-8.

Mititelu, M., Nicolescu, T.O., Moroşan, E., Pop, A.L., Nicolescu, F., 2020. Study of hypolipemiant activity of some mussel extracts. Proceedings of 6 th International Conference on Interdisciplinary Management of Diabetes Mellitus and its Complications INTERDIAB (Bucharest, Romania, 5-7 March 2020), Filodiritto Editore – Proceedings, pp.338–343, 978-88-85813-79-3.

Mititelu, M., Stanciu, G., Drăgănescu, D., Ioniţă, A.C., Neacşu, S.M., Dinu, M., Stefan-van Staden, R.I., Moroşan, E., 2021. Mussel shells, a valuable calcium resource for the pharmaceutical industry. Mar. Drugs 20 (1), 25. https://www.mdpi.com/1660-3397/20/1/25.

Moruf, R.O., Ogunbambo, M.M., Taiwo, M.A., Afolayan, O.A., 2021. Marine bivalves as a dietary source of high-quality lipid: a review with special reference to natural n-3 long-chain polyunsaturated fatty acids. Bulletin of University of Agricultural Sciences and Veterinary Medicine Cluj-Napoca. Food Sci. Technol. 2344-5300. 78 (1), 11–18. doi:10.15835/buasvmcn-fst:2020.0064.

Mudianta, I.W., White, A.M., Suciati, K.P.L., Krishnaraj, R.R., Winters, A.E., Mollo, E., Cheney, K.L., Garson, M.J., 2014. Chemoecological studies on marine natural products: terpene chemistry from marine mollusks. Pure Appl. Chem. 13653075. 86 (6), 995–1002. http://www.degruyter.com/view/j/pac. doi:10.1515/pac-2013-1111.

Mutalipassi, M., Esposito, R., Ruocco, N., Viel, T., Costantini, M., Zupo, V., 2021. Bioactive compounds of nutraceutical value from fishery and aquaculture discards. Foods. 2304-8158. 10 (7), 1495. doi:10.3390/foods10071495.

Nag, M., Lahiri, D., Dey, A., Sarkar, T., Pati, S., Joshi, S., Bunawan, H., Mohammed, A., Edinur, H.A., Ghosh, S., Ray, R.R., 2022. Seafood discards: a potent source of enzymes and biomacromolecules with nutritional and nutraceutical significance. Front. Nutr. 2296861X. 9. Available from: https://journal.frontiersin.org/journal/nutrition. doi:10.3389/fnut.2022.879929.

Ngandjui, Y.A.T., Kereeditse, T.T., Kamika, I., Madikizela, L.M., Msagati, T.A.M., 2024. Nutraceutical and medicinal importance of marine molluscs. Mar. Drugs. 1660-3397. 22 (5), 201. doi:10.3390/md22050201.

Ngangbam, A.K., Nongmaithem, B.D., Dai, V.T., Lenin, L., Khundrakpam, L., Pinky, L., Irom, P., Sharma, H.S.S., 2024. Advancing the discovery of bioactive compounds, its extraction and identification from the underexplored mollusc, *Cipangopaludina lecythis* (W. H. Benson, 1836). Fish. Aquat. Sci. 2234-1757. 27 (9), 539–551. doi:10.47853/fas.2024.e51.

Nowak, K., Jabłońska, E., Ratajczak-Wrona, W., 2021. Controversy around parabens: alternative strategies for preservative use in cosmetics and personal care products. Environ. Res. 00139351. 198, 110488. doi:10.1016/j.envres.2020.110488.

Núñez-Pons, L., Avila, C., Romano, G., Verde, C., Giordano, D., 2018. UV-protective compounds in marine organisms from the Southern Ocean. Mar. Drugs. 1660-3397. 16 (9), 336. doi:10.3390/md16090336.

Nurkolis, F., 2025. Marine bioactives: pioneering sustainable solutions for advanced cosmetics and therapeutics. Pharmacol. Res. 10436618. 218, 107868. doi:10.1016/j.phrs.2025.107868.

Palumbo, A., 2003. Melanogenesis in the ink gland of *Sepia officinalis*. Pigment Cell Res. 08935785. 16 (5), 517–522. doi:10.1034/j.1600-0749.2003.00080.x.

Papadopoulou, S.N.A., Adamantidi, T., Kranas, D., Cholidis, P., Anastasiadou, C., Tsoupras, A., 2025. A comprehensive review on the valorization of bioactives from marine animal by-products for health-promoting, biofunctional cosmetics. Mar. Drugs 16603397. 23 (8). Available from: https://www.mdpi.com/journal/marinedrugs. doi:10.3390/md23080299.

Parrish, C.C., 2013. Lipids in marine ecosystems. ISRN Oceanogr 2013, 604045.

Patra, D.D., 2021. Marine-based nutraceuticals vis-à-vis therapeutic potential: a summary. Examines Mar. Biol. Oceanogr 4, 1–5.

Paz, D., Trigo, M., Martínez, S., Aubourg, S.P., 2024. Bioactive lipid-enriched concentrates from squid discards by one-step and two-step extractions with non-halogenated solvents. Int. J. Food Sci. Technol. 0950-5423. 59 (8), 5806–5817. doi:10.1111/ijfs.17336.

Pereira, L., Cotas, J., 2023. Therapeutic potential of polyphenols and other micronutrients of marine origin. Mar. Drugs. 1660-3397. 21 (6), 323. doi:10.3390/md21060323.

Pérez-Polo, S., Imran, M.A.S., Dios, S., Pérez, J., Barros, L., Carrera, M., 2023. Camino Gestal: identifying natural bioactive peptides from the common octopus (*Octopus vulgaris* Cuvier, 1797) skin mucus by-products using proteogenomic analysis. Int. J. Mol. Sci. 1422-0067. 24 (8), 7145. doi:10.3390/ijms24087145.

Quitério, E., Soares, C., Ferraz, R., Delerue-Matos, C., Grosso, C., 2021. Marine health-promoting compounds: recent trends for their characterization and human applications. Foods. 2304-8158. 10 (12), 3100. doi:10.3390/foods10123100.

Rahman, M.A., Dash, R., Sohag, A.A.M., Alam, M., Rhim, H., Ha, H., Moon, I.S., Uddin, M.J., Hannan, M.A., 2021. Prospects of marine sterols against pathobiology of Alzheimer's disease: pharmacological insights and technological advances. Mar. Drugs 16603397. 19 (3). Available from: https://www.mdpi.com/1660-3397/19/3/167/pdf. doi:10.3390/MD19030167.

Rotter, A., Varamogianni-Mamatsi, D., Pobirk, A.Z., Matjaž, M.G., Cueto, M., Díaz-Marrero, A.R., Jónsdóttir, R., Sveinsdóttir, K., Catalá, T.S., Romano, G., Guler, B.A., Atak, E., Zrimec, M.B., Bosch, D., Deniz, I., Gaudêncio, S.P., Grigalionyte-Bembič, E., Klun, K., Zidar, L., Rius, A.C., Baebler, Š., Lukić Bilela, L., Rinkevich, B., Mandalakis, M., 2024. Marine cosmetics and the blue bioeconomy: from sourcing to success stories. iScience. 25890042. 27 (12), 111339. doi:10.1016/j.isci.2024.111339.

Russo, G.L., De Nisco, E., Fiore, G., Di Donato, P., D'Ischia, M., Palumbo, A., 2003. Toxicity of melanin-free ink of *Sepia officinalis* to transformed cell lines: identification of the active factor as tyrosinase. Biochem. Biophys. Res. Commun. 0006291X. 308 (2), 293–299. Available from: http://www.sciencedirect.com/science/journal/0006291X. doi:10.1016/S0006-291X(03)01379-2.

Saruwatari, K., Matsui, T., Mukai, H., Nagasawa, H., Kogure, T., 2009. Nucleation and growth of aragonite crystals at the growth front of nacres in pearl oyster, *Pinctada fucata*. Biomaterials. 01429612. 30 (16), 3028–3034. doi:10.1016/j.biomaterials.2009.03.011.

Sen, C.K., Khanna, S., Roy, S., 2007. Tocotrienols in health and disease: the other half of the natural vitamin E family. Mol. Aspects Med. 00982997. 28 (5-6), 692–728. doi:10.1016/j.mam.2007.03.001.

Senadheera, T.R.L., Hossain, A., Shahidi, F., 2023. Marine bioactives and their application in the food industry: a review. Canada Appl. Sci. (Switz.) 20763417. 13 (21). Available from: https://www.mdpi.com/journal/applsci/. doi:10.3390/app132112088.

Setyati, W.A., Pringgenies, D., Soenardjo, N., Pramesti, R., 2023. Enzyme-producing symbiotic bacteria in gastropods and bivalves molluscs: candidates for bioindustry materials. Biodiversitas 20854722. 24 (1), 20–25. Available from: https://smujo.id/biodiv/article/view/12759/6379. doi:10.13057/biodiv/d240103.

Shahidi, F., Saeid, A., 2025. Bioactivity of marine-derived peptides and proteins: a review. Mar. Drugs. 1660-3397. 23 (4), 157. doi:10.3390/md23040157.

Siahaan, E.A., Agusman, R.P., Shin, K.-H., Kim, S.-K., 2022. Potential cosmetic active ingredients derived from marine by-products. Mar. Drugs. 1660-3397. 20 (12), 734. doi:10.3390/md20120734.

Silchenko, A.S., Kusaykin, M.I., Zakharenko, A.M., Menshova, R.V., Khanh, H.H.N., Dmitrenok, P.S., Isakov, V.V., Zvyagintseva, T.N., 2014. Endo-1,4-fucoidanase from Vietnamese marine mollusk *Lambis* sp. which producing sulphated fucooligosaccharides. J. Mol. Catal. B Enzym. 18733158. 102, 154–160. Available from: https://www.elsevier.com/locate/molcatb. doi:10.1016/j.molcatb.2014.02.007.

Šimat, V., Elabed, N., Kulawik, P., Ceylan, Z., Jamroz, E., Yazgan, H., Čagalj, M., Regenstein, J.M., Özogul, F., 2020. Recent advances in marine-based nutraceuticals and their health benefits. Mar. Drugs 16603397. 18 (12). Available from: https://www.mdpi.com/1660-3397/18/12/627. doi:10.3390/md18120627.

Solano, F., 2020. Photoprotection and skin pigmentation: melanin-related molecules and some other new agents obtained from natural sources. Molecules. 1420-3049. 25 (7), 1537. doi:10.3390/molecules25071537.

Song, X., Liu, Z., Wang, L., Song, L., 2019. Recent advances of shell matrix proteins and cellular orchestration in marine molluscan shell biomineralization. Front. Mar. Sci. 2296-7745. 6. doi:10.3389/fmars.2019.00041.

Stillwell, W., Wassall, S.R., 2003. Docosahexaenoic acid: membrane properties of a unique fatty acid. Chem. Phys. Lipids 00093084. 126 (1), 1–27. Available from: https://www.elsevier.com/locate/chemphyslip. doi:10.1016/S0009-3084(03)00101-4.

Suleria, H.A.R., Osborne, S., Masci, P., Gobe, G., 2015. Marine-based nutraceuticals: an innovative trend in the food and supplement industries. Mar. Drugs 16603397. 13 (10), 6336–6351. Available from: http://www.mdpi.com/1660-3397/13/10/6336/pdf. doi:10.3390/md13106336.

Tabakaeva, O.V., Tabakaev, A.V., 2016. Phospholipids from Soft Tissues of the Bivalve Mollusk Anadara broughtonii. Chem. Nat. Compd. 0009-3130. 52 (2), 299–300. doi:10.1007/s10600-016-1620-9.

Tran, Q.T., Le, T.T.T., Pham, M.Q., Do, T.L., Vu, M.H., Nguyen, D.C., Bach, L.G., Bui, L.M., Pham, Q.L., 2019. Fatty acid, lipid classes and phospholipid molecular species composition of the marine clam meretrix lyrata (Sowerby 1851) from Cua Lo Beach, Nghe An Province, Vietnam. Molecules 14203049. 24 (5). Available from: https://www.mdpi.com/1420-3049/24/5/895/pdf. doi:10.3390/molecules24050895.

Tsoupras, A., Brummell, C., Kealy, C., Vitkaitis, K., Redfern, S., Zabetakis, I., 2022. Cardio-protective properties and health benefits of fish lipid bioactives: the effects of thermal processing. Mar. Drugs. 1660-3397. 20 (3), 187. doi:10.3390/md20030187.

Ulagesan, S., Krishnan, S., Nam, T.-J., Choi, Y.-H., 2022. A review of bioactive compounds in oyster shell and tissues. Front. Bioeng. Biotechnol. 2296-4185. 10. doi:10.3389/fbioe.2022.913839.

Upadhyay, A., Thiyagarajan, V., 2016. Proteomic characterization of oyster shell organic matrix proteins (OMP). Bioinformation. 09738894. 12 (05), 266–278. doi:10.6026/97320630012266.

Valeria, C., Salvatore, P., Luca, V., Maria, G., Ludovica, M., Cristina, S., Lucia, M., Angela, C., Valeria, S., 2024. Innovative snail-mucus-extract (SME)-coated nanoparticles exhibit anti-inflammatory and anti-proliferative effects for potential skin cancer prevention and treatment. RSC Adv. 2046-2069. 14 (11), 7655–7663. doi:10.1039/d4ra00291a.

Villanueva, R., Riba, J., Ruíz-Capillas, C., González, A.V., Baeta, M., 2004. Amino acid composition of early stages of cephalopods and effect of amino acid dietary treatments on Octopus vulgaris paralarvae. Aquaculture 00448486. 242 (1-4), 455–478. Available from: http://www.journals.elsevier.com/aquaculture/. doi:10.1016/j.aquaculture.2004.04.006.

Wen-Yu, L., Hui-Jing, L., Qin-Ying, L., Yan-Chao, W., 2021. Application of marine natural products in drug research. Bioorg. Med. Chem. 09680896. 35, 116058. doi:10.1016/j.bmc.2021.116058.

Wright, A.C., Fan, Y., Baker, G.L., 2018. Nutritional value and food safety of bivalve molluscan shellfish. J. Shellfish Res. 07308000. 37 (4), 695–708. Available from: http://www.bioone.org/loi/shre. doi:10.2983/035.037.0403.

Yamamoto, H., Shimomura, N., Hasegawa, Y., 2024. Oral administration of nacre extract from pearl oyster shells has anti-aging effects on skin and muscle, and extends the lifespan in SAMP8 mice. Pharmaceuticals. 1424-8247. 17 (6), 713. doi:10.3390/ph17060713.

Zhang, Z., Wang, Y., Ting, L., Junjie, W., Huang, J., Jiang, J., Chen, M., Dong, W., 2023. Mussel-inspired anti-permeation hybrid sunscreen with reinforced UV-blocking and safety performance. Colloids Surf. A Physicochem. Eng. Asp. 09277757. 676, 132140. doi:10.1016/j.colsurfa.2023.132140.

Zhukova, N.V., 2007. Lipid classes and fatty acid composition of the tropical nudibranch mollusks *Chromodoris* sp. and *Phyllidia coelestis*. Lipids. 00244201. 42 (12), 1169–1175. doi:10.1007/s11745-007-3123-8.

Zhukova, N.V., 2014. Lipids and fatty acids of nudibranch mollusks: potential sources of bioactive compounds. Mar. Drugs 16603397. 12 (8), 4578–4592. Available from: http://www.mdpi.com/1660-3397/12/8/4578/pdf. doi:10.3390/md12084578.

Chapter 21

Crustaceans and shellfish

Alexandros Tsoupras[a], Evangelia Tsikopoulou[a], and Chryssa Anastasiadou[b]
[a]*Hephaestus Laboratory, School of Chemistry, Faculty of Sciences, Democritus University of Thrace, Kavala University Campus, Kavala, Greece*
[b]*Fisheries Research Institute, Hellenic Agricultural Organization-DIMITRA (ELGO-DIMITRA), Kavala, Greece*

1 Introduction

The growing emphasis on self-care in modern lifestyles has further fueled demand for novel cosmetic concepts and innovative ingredients (Rafatullah et al., 2024). Consumers increasingly seek products designed to enhance and maintain the appearance of skin, hair, and nails, driving the cosmetics industry toward natural and functional formulations (Fonseca et al., 2023). Although synthetic ingredients continue to be widely used, they often fail to fully meet consumer expectations, leading to a rising preference for natural alternatives perceived as safer, more sustainable, and environmentally friendly (Fonseca et al., 2023). Historically, natural products have been pivotal in the management of chronic inflammatory and skin-related disorders, as well as other lingering health issues. Thus they continue to be essential resources and form the foundation of modern drug discovery (Ghareeb et al., 2020; Lu et al., 2021; Oliver et al., 1994), with ongoing importance in modern medicine and cosmetics (Ghareeb et al., 2020).

A vast array of natural bioactives with an exceptional chemical diversity has traditionally been sourced from terrestrial plants and microorganisms; however, over the past three decades, marine organisms have emerged as significant contributors to novel marine natural products (MNPs) (Rafatullah et al., 2024). Covering approximately 70% of the Earth's surface and representing the origin of life, the oceans harbor immense biodiversity, encompassing nearly 500,000 species across about 28 phyla. Marine ecosystems are recognized as sources of structurally unique bioactive compounds rarely encountered in terrestrial organisms, largely due to the extreme environmental conditions in which many marine species thrive. Marine microorganisms, microalgae, fungi, sponges, and macroalgae—key components of aquatic food webs—produce a wide range of bioactives that can accumulate through trophic chains. Despite this richness, only a limited number of marine taxa have been extensively explored for natural product discovery.

Since the first biologically active MNP was reported by Bergmann in the late 1950s (Bergmann and Feeney, 1950), marine ecosystems have been increasingly acknowledged for their direct and indirect contributions to human health and well-being, extending beyond nutrition to include climate regulation, biogeochemical cycling, and cultural and recreational services. Compared to plant-derived ingredients, which may suffer from slow growth rates and seasonal or geographical variability in chemical composition, marine resources offer unparalleled biodiversity and chemical novelty. Advances in aquaculture technologies have further enabled the efficient and cost-effective cultivation of marine organisms—including crustaceans—as sustainable sources of bioactives for multiple applications, including functional cosmetics (Fonseca et al., 2023; Alves et al., 2020). In parallel, modern "omics" technologies, such as genomics, proteomics, and metabolomics, are increasingly employed to accelerate the discovery of marine-derived compounds and to elucidate their mechanisms of action in skin physiology, thereby supporting targeted ingredient development and robust safety and efficacy assessments (Brunt and Burgess, 2018).

In this context, marine-derived by-products—particularly those originating from crustaceans—represent a vast yet largely untapped reservoir of bioactive compounds with considerable potential for cosmetic applications. Commonly discarded as waste by fisheries (i.e., as fish by-catch), aquaculture, and seafood-processing industries, these materials are rich in diverse biofunctional constituents, including chitosan, collagen, peptides, amino acids, fatty acids, polar lipids (PLs), lipid-soluble vitamins, carotenoids, pigments, phenolic compounds, and minerals.

Biofunctional Cosmetics for Health. https://doi.org/10.1016/B978-0-443-27500-5.00021-6

Bioactive compounds from crustaceans and their by-products can be recovered using a variety of extraction techniques, with increasing emphasis on environmentally sustainable and "green" approaches. Once isolated, these compounds exhibit a broad spectrum of skin-beneficial properties, such as antioxidant, antiaging, antiinflammatory, antitumor, antiwrinkle, antihyperpigmentation, and wound healing activities (Papadopoulou et al., 2025). Materials traditionally regarded as biological waste therefore represent a valuable source of innovation in dermal science and cosmetic formulation. Consequently, the incorporation of crustacean- and fish-derived bioactives into cosmetic science has gained particular importance, especially in light of the rapid growth and innovation observed in this sector (Alves et al., 2020).

Several studies have already highlighted the potential of marine-derived bioactives in cosmetic applications. This chapter provides a comprehensive overview of bioactive compounds obtained from crustacean sources, with particular emphasis on cultured species and their by-products as sustainable resources of MNPs for functional cosmetic development. In addition, it discusses their cosmetic applications—especially in skincare—along with current limitations, challenges, and future perspectives for their industrial utilization.

2 Crustaceans and their by-products as sustainable sources of valuable marine bioactives for functional cosmetics

2.1 Crustaceans

Crustaceans are a diverse group of aquatic arthropods belonging to the subphylum *Crustacea* within the phylum *Arthropoda* (Eduardo Rebolledo Ranz, 2021). They are characterized by having a hard exoskeleton made of chitin, segmented bodies, and jointed appendages. Crustaceans include familiar animals such as crabs, lobsters, shrimp, crayfish, and barnacles. They inhabit a wide range of environments, primarily marine and freshwater ecosystems, and play crucial roles in aquatic food webs. The group is notably diverse, with an estimated 50,000 to 75,000 species described (Eduardo Rebolledo Ranz, 2021; Nugroho Susanto, 2021).

2.1.1 Habitat

Crustaceans inhabit a wide range of aquatic environments, occurring in both freshwater and marine ecosystems. Their distribution spans from the Arctic to the Antarctic and extends from high-altitude freshwater habitats, reaching elevations of up to 16,000 feet above sea level, including regions such as the Himalayas, to depths far below sea level (Hendrickx, 1996). Their bodies are segmented into the head, thorax, and abdomen, with various types of articulated appendages adapted for functions such as locomotion, feeding, and respiration. Large crustaceans breathe through gills, while smaller species depend on diffusion across their body surfaces for gas exchange. Most crustaceans are dioecious, with distinct male and female individuals, although reproductive strategies vary greatly among species. Ecologically, crustaceans play a vital role as a primary food source for humans and form a key trophic link in marine ecosystems, serving as prey for many predators, including whales, fish, and pinnipeds (Diarte-Plata and Escamilla-Montes, 2020).

2.1.2 Economy

As for their participation at the level of the economy, crustaceans hold substantial economic importance as a vital source of nutrition for humans and support global fisheries and aquaculture industries. Moreover, their by-products, such as chitosan, are utilized across various sectors, including pharmaceuticals, cosmetics, and the food industry, due to their bioactive properties. Concurrently, crustaceans serve as bioindicators of environmental health and are employed in ecological studies to monitor the quality of aquatic ecosystems (Nugroho Susanto, 2021). The primary taxonomic groups within Crustacea include several distinct subclasses. Branchiopoda comprises small, primarily freshwater species such as fairy shrimp, clam shrimp, tadpole shrimp, and water fleas. Remipedia consists of elongate, eyeless crustaceans typically found in anchialine cave systems. Cephalocarida, considered a primitive lineage, includes benthic crustaceans that also lack visual organs, such as horseshoe shrimps. Ostracoda encompasses minute, bivalved crustaceans—commonly referred to as seed shrimps—that inhabit both marine and freshwater environments. In addition, the groups Maxillopoda and Malacostraca represent more morphologically and ecologically diverse clades within the subphylum (, 2010).

2.1.3 Categories

Crustaceans are a large class of marine organisms that can be classified into several subclasses, each of which has unique characteristics, while they all share some common ones (Fig. 21.1). More specifically, the subclass Maxillopoda comprises several diverse groups of crustaceans, each with distinct morphological and ecological traits. Notably, Copepoda includes

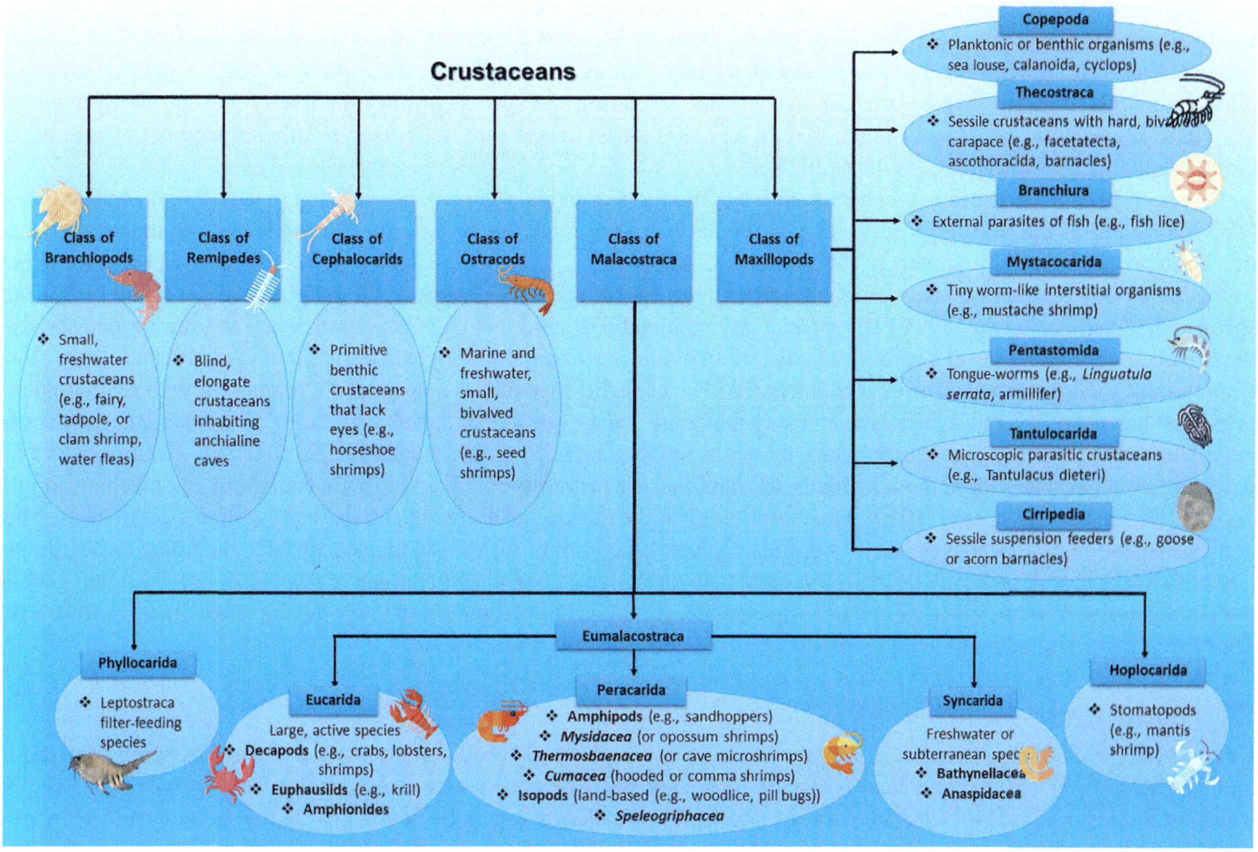

FIG. 21.1 Representative examples and classification of crustaceans. *(From Papadopoulou, S.N.A., Adamantidi, T., Kranas, D., Cholidis, P., Anastasiadou, C., Tsoupras, A., 2025. A comprehensive review on the valorization of bioactives from marine animal by-products for health-promoting, biofunctional cosmetics. Mar. Drugs 16603397. 23 (8). Available from: https://www.mdpi.com/journal/marinedrugs. doi:10.3390/md23080299.)*

predominantly planktonic or benthic organisms such as sea lice, calanoids, and cyclopoids. Thecostraca encompasses sessile crustaceans characterized by a hard, bivalved carapace, including groups such as Facetotecta, Ascothoracida, and barnacles. Branchiura consists of ectoparasites of fish, commonly known as fish lice. Mystacocarida includes minute, worm-like interstitial crustaceans exemplified by mustache shrimps. Pentastomida, or tongue worms, represent a parasitic lineage, with notable species such as *Linguatula serrata* and *Armillifer*. Tantulocarida comprises microscopic parasitic crustaceans such as *Tantulacus dieteri*, while Cirripedia includes sessile suspension feeders like goose and acorn barnacles. In contrast, the subclass Malacostraca is traditionally divided into three major groups: Phyllocarida, comprising filter-feeding leptostracan species; Hoplocarida, which includes the highly specialized stomatopods (e.g., mantis shrimp); and Eumalacostraca, the most diverse clade. Eumalacostracans can be further subdivided into these categories: Eucarida, consisting of large and motile taxa such as decapods (e.g., crabs, lobsters, shrimp), euphausiids (krill), and the rarely encountered amphionides; Syncarida, including primarily freshwater and subterranean forms such as Bathynellacea and Anaspidacea; and lastly, Peracarida, a highly diverse assemblage encompassing orders like Amphipoda (e.g., sandhoppers), Mysidacea (opossum shrimps), Thermosbaenacea (cave-dwelling microshrimps), Cumacea (comma or hooded shrimps), Tanaidacea (tanaids), Speleogriphacea, and Isopoda, the latter including terrestrial representatives such as woodlice and pill bugs (, 2010; Maasri and Thorp, 2024).

2.1.4 Anatomy

As for the anatomy of crustaceans, they are invertebrate organisms characterized by a bilaterally symmetrical, segmented body, an open circulatory system—in which hemolymph circulates freely within body cavities rather than through closed vessels—and a rigid exoskeleton known as the carapace. This external structure, composed primarily of chitin reinforced with calcium carbonate, provides mechanical protection against predators and minimizes water loss in terrestrial or semi-terrestrial species. These organisms possess multiple pairs of jointed appendages, typically more than four, which serve various functional roles, including locomotion, feeding, and sensory perception. The central nervous system consists of a ventral nerve cord and paired cerebral ganglia located anteriorly near the base of the antennae. Crustaceans commonly exhibit compound eyes mounted on mobile stalks, allowing for a wide field of vision. Internally, their digestive system comprises a linear alimentary canal equipped with a gastric mill for the mechanical processing of food, supported by paired digestive glands (hepatopancreas) involved in enzymatic digestion and nutrient absorption. Excretion is primarily achieved via a pair of specialized antennal (green) glands, and respiration occurs through gills, typically situated at the base of the thoracic appendages or antennae (Vittori, 2024).

The body plan of crustaceans is generally divided into three principal regions: the cephalon (head), thorax, and abdomen (also referred to as the *pleon*). In many taxa, particularly among more derived groups, the cephalon and thorax are fused into a single structural unit known as the cephalothorax, which is typically encased by a robust, unified carapace. Each of the three body regions may bear biramous, articulated appendages, a hallmark of the subphylum. Across all crustacean species, the head bears two pairs of antennae, a pair of mandibles, and two pairs of maxillae, at least during one stage of the life cycle. The presence of two distinct pairs of antennae is a key morphological feature that distinguishes crustaceans from insects, their terrestrial arthropod counterparts. The cephalic appendages consist of six primary structures: compound eyes, first antennae (which are biramous in many malacostracans), second antennae, mandibles, first maxillae, and second maxillae. Functionally, the antennae primarily serve sensory roles, such as chemoreception and mechanoreception for detecting food particles, while the mandibles and maxillae are primarily involved in food acquisition and mechanical processing (Bergmann and Feeney, 1950). The morphology of the thorax and abdomen, particularly with respect to the number and specialization of appendages, varies significantly across taxonomic groups. In malacostracans, including decapods and amphipods, the thorax generally bears five to eight pairs of thoracic appendages (termed *thoracopods* or *pereiopods*), while the abdomen typically includes six pairs of appendages, composed of pleopods and uropods, the latter often forming a tail fan structure used in locomotion and reproductive functions (Kenny et al., 2014).

2.1.5 Structure

Crustaceans have an open circulatory system, where hemolymph flows through body cavities instead of being confined to a closed network of vessels. The heart is usually located dorsally and plays a key role in circulating hemolymph. Oxygen transport in crustaceans involves different respiratory pigments depending on the taxonomic group: hemocyanin, a copper-based oxygen-binding protein, is common in Malacostraca, while hemoglobin is more frequently found in groups like copepods, ostracods, barnacles, and brachiopods. The digestive system features a linear alimentary canal, which includes a specialized grinding structure known as the gastric mill, functionally analogous to a gizzard. This organ facilitates mechanical digestion prior to enzymatic processing. Flanking the midgut are paired digestive glands (hepatopancreas), which are involved in enzyme secretion and nutrient absorption. Additional internal structures include excretory organs analogous to kidneys, such as the antennal (green) glands, and a relatively simple yet functionally compartmentalized nervous system. The central nervous system comprises a supraesophageal ganglion (brain) located near the base of the antennae, as well as a subesophageal ganglionic mass situated ventrally, beneath the alimentary canal (McMahon, 2001).

2.1.6 Molting

Crustaceans undergo periodic molting (ecdysis) throughout their development due to the rigidity and nonexpandable nature of their exoskeletons. This process, which can range in duration from several minutes to several hours, involves the formation of a new, pliable exoskeleton beneath the existing one, followed by the shedding of the old cuticle. During the molting phase, crustaceans experience increased vulnerability until the newly formed exoskeleton fully hardens and provides adequate protection. Notably, crustaceans can achieve an immediate increase in body size ranging between 40% and 80% postmolt. Reproduction in most crustacean species occurs sexually, with distinct male and female individuals facilitating genetic exchange (Diarte-Plata and Escamilla-Montes, 2020). Crustaceans are also categorized according to body size into two broad groups: the smaller Entomostraca and the larger Malacostraca. It is important to highlight that Entomostraca does not constitute a valid taxonomic clade due to the significant heterogeneity among its members. Conversely, Malacostraca is recognized as a well-defined taxonomic class distinguished by several morphological characteristics, including the presence of abdominal appendages, a functional gastric mill, an eight-segmented thorax, and an abdomen typically composed of six segments, although seven or eight segments may occasionally be present (Nugroho Susanto, 2021).

2.1.7 Mating system: Eggs

The majority of crustacean species exhibit sexual reproduction, characterized by distinct male and female individuals. Notably, recent research on *Tigriopus californicus* has demonstrated that male mate selection may be influenced by female diet, with a preference shown for females fed on algae rather than yeast-based diets. Although less common, hermaphroditism is observed in certain groups, including barnacles, remipedes, and Cephalocarida. Moreover, some species exhibit sequential hermaphroditism, undergoing sex reversal at different life stages. In addition, parthenogenesis—a form of asexual reproduction in which females produce viable offspring without fertilization—is widely documented in crustaceans. This reproductive strategy occurs in various taxa, including numerous branchiopods, select ostracods, certain isopods, and even among some more advanced crustaceans, such as the Marmorkrebs (marbled crayfish), a parthenogenetic species capable of clonal propagation (Cholidis et al., 2024).

In many crustacean species, fertilized eggs are directly released into the water column, allowing for external development. However, a significant number of taxa have evolved diverse reproductive strategies to retain and protect embryos until hatching. Among decapods, females commonly carry the eggs attached to the pleopods, facilitating aeration and protection. In contrast, peracarids, notostracans, anostracans, and numerous isopod species possess a brood pouch (marsupium), formed through modifications of the carapace and thoracic appendages, where embryonic development occurs. Branchiuran females, however, do not carry eggs in external ovisacs but instead attach them in linear arrangements to hard substrates such as rocks or aquatic vegetation. Most leptostracans and krill carry their eggs between the thoracic limbs, ensuring mechanical protection. Among copepods, reproductive strategies vary: some species enclose their eggs in specialized, thin-walled ovisacs, whereas others attach them in elongated, tangled strings for external incubation (Sachindra and Mahendrakar, 2005).

2.1.8 Well-established cosmeceutical applications

From a cosmeceutical standpoint, by-products derived from crustaceans, including their shells and exoskeletons, serve as significant reservoirs of chitin and its deacetylated derivative, chitosan. These biopolymers are extensively utilized in dermatological formulations due to their excellent biocompatibility, hydrating effects, wound healing capabilities, and inherent antimicrobial activity. Furthermore, certain crustacean species, such as krill and shrimp, are abundant sources of astaxanthin, a carotenoid pigment exhibiting potent antioxidant properties that contribute to the protection of skin against oxidative damage and ultraviolet (UV) radiation-induced harm (Saini and Keum, 2018; Treyvaud Amiguet et al., 2012).

2.2 Bioactive compounds and structural components of crustaceans

Compared with alternative biological sources (e.g., algae, yeast, bacteria, plants), marine by-products offer a cost-effective and sustainable source of astaxanthin, enabling value recovery from processing residues while simultaneously generating additional marketable co-products.

Crustaceans and their processing by-products represent an abundant and underexploited source of high-value bioactive compounds with significant potential for cosmetic, nutraceutical, and biomedical applications. While crustaceans are widely recognized for their nutritional value, their shells, heads, viscera, and exoskeletons—often discarded as industrial waste—are particularly rich in structurally and biologically active molecules. These by-products account for a substantial proportion of crustacean biomass and pose environmental and economic challenges due to disposal costs and rapid degradation. For example, even though processed shrimp represents a high-value commodity, shrimp-processing residues—primarily shells and heads—constitute approximately 45%–60% of total body mass, depending on species and processing methods (Jinxia et al., 2019; Sánchez-Camargo et al., 2011; Tsoupras et al., 2025). However, they are increasingly regarded as valuable secondary raw materials within circular economy frameworks.

Among the most important crustacean-derived bioactives are polysaccharides such as chitin, chitosan, and their derivatives, as well as glycosaminoglycans and hyaluronic acid (HA). These compounds exhibit excellent biocompatibility, biodegradability, and a wide range of biological activities, including antioxidant, antimicrobial, antiinflammatory, wound healing, moisturizing, and film-forming properties, making them particularly attractive for cosmetic and dermal applications (Nugroho Susanto, 2021). Crustacean by-products also contain high-quality proteins and peptides, minerals (e.g., calcium and magnesium), valuable and bioactive lipids, and pigments such as astaxanthin, a naturally occurring carotenoid pigment with potent antioxidant activities commonly found in shrimp and crab shells (Cahú et al., 2012). Compared with alternative biological sources (e.g., algae, yeast, bacteria, plants), crustaceans' by-products, and in general marine by-products, offer a cost-effective and sustainable source of astaxanthin, enabling value recovery from processing residues while simultaneously generating additional marketable co-products. Numerous studies have also demonstrated that shrimp by-products are valuable sources of high-added-value compounds apart from astaxanthin, such as omega-3 (ω3) polyunsaturated fatty acids (PUFAs) like eicosapentaenoic acid (EPA, 20:5ω3) and docosahexaenoic acid (DHA, 22:6ω3) (Tsoupras et al., 2025; Šimat et al., 2022), as well as PLs rich in these PUFA, phenolics, and several carotenoids with potent antioxidant and antiinflammatory capacities (Hossain and Shahidi, 2024). Shrimp residues also provide essential amino acids widely used in several applications (Yan and Chen, 2015) (Fig. 21.2).

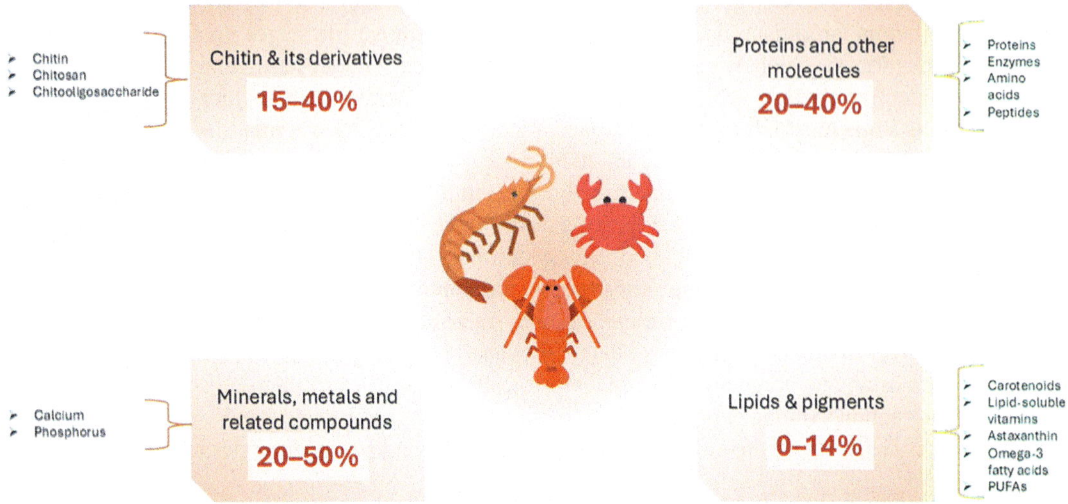

FIG. 21.2 Bioactive compounds derived from crustaceans. Representative crustaceans' bioactives. *(From Nugroho Susanto, G., 2021. Crustacea: the increasing economic importance of crustaceans to humans. In: Eduardo Rebolledo Ranz, R. (Ed.), Arthropods - are They Beneficial for Mankind? IntechOpen. ISBN: 978-1-78984-165-7.)*

Bioactive compounds from crustacean by-products can be recovered using diverse extraction and processing techniques, with increasing emphasis on environmentally friendly and "green" methodologies. These approaches not only improve extraction efficiency but also enhance sustainability by reducing solvent use and energy consumption. Once isolated, crustacean-derived bioactives have demonstrated significant efficacy in skincare formulations, contributing to antiaging, skin barrier reinforcement, UV protection, and improved hydration (Nugroho Susanto, 2021). Chitosan-based materials, in particular, are widely used as delivery systems and functional ingredients in creams, gels, masks, and wound dressings.

The valorization of crustacean by-products aligns closely with circular economy principles by transforming biological waste into high-value functional ingredients. This strategy reduces environmental burdens associated with waste disposal while enabling the development of innovative, sustainable cosmetic products. Continued advances in extraction technologies, formulation science, and mechanistic understanding of crustacean bioactives will further expand their industrial applicability and support the transition toward more sustainable and resource-efficient cosmetic and cosmeceutical industries.

2.2.1 Shell structure of crustaceans

Crustacean shells are complex biomaterials primarily composed of chitin (15%–40%), proteins (20%–40%), calcium carbonate (20%–50%), and lipids (0%–14%), along with notable concentrations of ω3 fatty acids, pigments, and various minor constituents. The exact composition is influenced by factors such as species and seasonal variation (Wenner and Kuris, 2020; Morin-Crini et al., 2019; Casadidio et al., 2019). These components exhibit a broad spectrum of potential applications. For instance, calcium carbonate is commonly employed as a fertilizer, filler, or white pigment, while shell-derived proteins can serve as animal feed or agricultural fertilizer (Jinjing et al., 2025). Chitin, in particular, offers remarkable versatility, with applications extending to water purification, biomaterials, functional foods, pharmaceuticals, and cosmetics (Hatchett, 1799). In greater detail, chitin and its derivatives, including chitin itself, chitosan, and chitooligosaccharides (COSs), constitute approximately 15%–40% of the total shell composition. Proteins and other nitrogen-containing compounds, such as enzymes, amino acids, and peptides, account for an additional 20%–40%. Furthermore, minerals, metals, and phosphorus collectively represent about 20%–50% of the shell's content. Lastly, lipids and pigments, including carotenoids, lipid-soluble vitamins, astaxanthin, ω3 fatty acids, and PUFAs, make up approximately 0%–14% of the shell mass (Ravi Kumar, 2000).

2.2.2 Chitin and its derivatives

Chitin and its derivatives include chitin, chitosan, and COS. Chitin ($C_8H_{13}O_5N$) is the second most abundant polysaccharide in nature, following cellulose. It consists of (1→4)-linked N-acetyl-D-glucosamine (NAG) monomers (Yanat and Schroën, 2023; Melton et al., 2019) and is structurally analogous to cellulose, with the key distinction being the incorporation of 2-acetamido-2-deoxy-β-D-glucose (NAG) units, joined via β(1→4) glycosidic bonds (Yanat and Schroën, 2023). Chitin typically appears as a white to pale yellow, highly hydrophobic biopolymer that is both tasteless and odorless (Younes and Rinaudo, 2015). Its crystalline structure is reinforced by extensive intramolecular hydrogen bonding, which contributes to its insolubility in water and most organic solvents (Cheung et al., 2015). Only a limited range of solvent systems, including fluorinated solvents (e.g., hexafluoropropanol, hexafluoroacetone), mixtures of chloroalcohols with mineral acids, and dimethylacetamide containing 5% lithium chloride, have proven effective in dissolving chitin (Klinger et al., 2019).

Chitosan is obtained through the deacetylation of chitin, typically via enzymatic or chemical hydrolysis processes (Aam et al., 2010). It is a linear heteropolymer composed of D-glucosamine (deacetylated units) and NAG (acetylated units), connected by $\beta(1\rightarrow4)$ glycosidic linkages (Klinger et al., 2019). In essence, the deacetylation process introduces a proton to the -NH_2 group of the repeating D-glucosamine units, thereby converting the neutral polysaccharide into a cationic polyelectrolyte under acidic conditions (Hamed et al., 2016). Chitosan is an acid-soluble, cationic biopolymer found in the exoskeletons of crustaceans, mollusks, arthropods, and insects (Cheung et al., 2015; Guan et al., 2020). Its physicochemical properties—and, by extension, its functional applications—are largely determined by its degree of acetylation (Cheung et al., 2015).

Hydrolysis of chitin or chitosan yields COSs. Various physical and chemical methods, including hydrothermal treatment, microwave irradiation, ultrasound, chemical hydrolysis, acid hydrolysis, and enzymatic degradation, have been employed to depolymerize these polymers and produce COS (Jinjing et al., 2025; Klinger et al., 2019). COSs are characterized by short chain length, low molecular weight, water solubility, and low viscosity. They exhibit a range of bioactive properties, including antibacterial, anticancer, cholesterol-lowering, and immunostimulatory effects (Hatchett, 1799; Díaz-Santana-Iturrios et al., 2022).

The term "chitin" derives from the Greek word "chiton," signifying "a coat of mail" (Melton et al., 2019). Chitin is a natural polysaccharide that serves as a key structural component in the exoskeletons of many arthropods, including crustaceans, insects, and some fungi. Chemically, it is a long-chain polymer of N-acetylglucosamine, a derivative of glucose. Chitin provides both strength and flexibility to the structures it forms, making it ideal for protective shells and cell walls. It is similar in function to cellulose in plants but differs in chemical structure. Chitin is biodegradable, biocompatible, and has applications in medicine, agriculture, and materials science. In crustaceans, chitin forms a scaffold that is often hardened by the deposition of calcium carbonate, creating a durable yet lightweight exoskeleton (Jia et al., 2014). Structurally, chitin is organized into highly ordered microfibrillar arrangements and constitutes a primary biopolymer in the exoskeletons of marine arthropods such as crustaceans and insects, as well as in fungal cell walls and cephalopod beaks (Yanat and Schroën, 2023; Díaz-Santana-Iturrios et al., 2022; Riaz Rajoka et al., 2020). The polysaccharide was first isolated by Hatchett in 1799 via mineral acid extraction from the shells of prawns, crayfish, and mollusks (Ahmad et al., 2020). The isolation procedure from crustacean shells involves rigorous sequential demineralization and deproteinization to obtain chitin. Despite its inherent insolubility due to extensive hydrogen bonding and crystalline structure, chitin derivatives, particularly chitosan, have been extensively investigated and utilized across biomedical, nutraceutical, agricultural, and cosmetic sectors owing to their favorable biocompatibility, biodegradability, low toxicity, recyclability, and multifunctional bioactivity. These derivatives demonstrate a broad spectrum of pharmacological and biological functionalities, encompassing antineoplastic (Díaz-Santana-Iturrios et al., 2022; Riaz Rajoka et al., 2020), antimicrobial (Kim, 2014; Jae-Young et al., 2006), antioxidative (Azuma et al., 2015; Tzeng et al., 2022), antihypertensive (Priyanka et al., 2022), antiinflammatory (Kalita et al., 2022), antidiabetic (Silva et al., 2021; Sajith et al., 2024), hypocholesterolemic (Tsoupras et al., 2025; Zhang et al., 2024), and anticoagulant effects (Ahmadkelayeh and Hawboldt, 2020).

2.2.3 Essential and bioactive amphiphilic and lipophilic lipid-based compounds and pigments

Lipids and pigments that constitute 0%–14% of the shell include amphiphilic carotenoids like astaxanthin, PLs, and phenolics, as well as lipid-soluble vitamins and the more lipophilic free fatty acids, such as ω3 PUFAs, triglycerides, terpenes, terpenoids, and several lipid esters, ethers, and sterols. For example, crustacean shells are a notable source of ω3 PUFAs, particularly EPA (C20:5ω3) and DHA (C22:6ω3), as well as lipid-soluble vitamins, including vitamins A, D, E, and K. Recent studies have also identified the presence of antiinflammatory bioactive PLs in certain crustacean species (Treyvaud Amiguet et al., 2012; Albalat et al., 2016). The lipid composition, however, is highly variable and influenced by multiple factors such as species, sex, climatic conditions, and environmental parameters (Balzano et al., 2017; Wang et al., 2019), as well as extraction processes. Lipid accumulation is most prominent in specific anatomical regions, including the hepatopancreas (liver and pancreas) in shrimp, the cephalothoracic region (head) in lobsters, and the gonads in crabs. According to Albalat et al. (2016), lobsters generally exhibit the highest total lipid content in comparison to shrimp and crabs. Furthermore, comparative analyses have shown that crabs possess significantly lower lipid concentrations in edible tissues relative to shrimp (Yabuzaki, 2017).

From four different extraction methods applied, Folch, two-step, Soxhlet, and enzyme-assisted aqueous extractions, the two latter methods showed higher lipid yields, carotenoid content, and improved oxidative stability compared with the other methods in lipids obtained from the hepatopancreas of Chinese mitten crab (*Eriocheir sinensis*) (Wang et al., 2019). Palmitic acid (C16:0), oleic acid (C18:1), and linoleic acid (C18:2) were the predominant fatty acids (FAs), primarily present as triglycerides. Untargeted metabolomic analysis of the enzyme-extracted lipids further identified carotenoids, PUFAs, sterols, amino acids, lipid β-oxidation products, ATP degradation metabolites, phosphatidylethanolamine, and astaxanthin. The Chinese mitten crab is a highly valued aquatic species in China, with the hepatopancreas serving as its main lipid storage organ and a key contributor to flavor. Comparative evaluation of extraction methods is essential for optimizing lipid recovery and quality from crab hepatopancreas. Given their high content of PUFAs and astaxanthin, crab hepatopancreas lipids show strong potential as functional ingredients and natural flavor enhancers in several applications.

Tsoupras et al. (2025) demonstrated that shrimp-derived extracts are rich in amphiphilic marine bioactive compounds, as they contain significant concentrations of marine phenolics, carotenoids, and PLs rich in unsaturated fatty acids (UFAs). These extracts exhibited robust antioxidant activity, primarily attributed to their phenolic and carotenoid content. More notably, they also displayed pronounced antiinflammatory and antithrombotic properties against specific mediators of inflammation, such as platelet-activating factor (PAF), and against platelet-related thrombosis induced by classic platelet agonists like ADP. LC–MS-based lipidomics and structure–activity relationship analyses revealed that the antiinflammatory and antithrombotic potency of these shrimp-derived extracts can mainly be attributed to the presence of UFA in the structures of shrimp-derived PLs, including the monounsaturated fatty acid (MUFA) oleic acid (C18:1n9), and particularly the ω3 PUFAs, EPA and DHA, which presented favorable antiinflammatory potential as evidenced by their strong anti-PAF potency, but also supported by their low n6/n3 PUFA ratio (Fig. 21.3). These amphiphilic bioactive PLs, particularly those rich in UFA have presented stronger anti-inflammatory effects than the free fatty acids against the PAF-pathway, but also through several dinstict intracellular mechanisms (Tsoupras et al., 2025). These findings underscore the potential of shrimp-derived amphiphilic bioactives as functional ingredients for the development of health-promoting, antiinflammatory, and antiaging cosmetic applications, including nutricosmetics and cosmeceuticals, aligned with the principles of sustainable resource utilization and circular bioeconomy (Papadopoulou et al., 2025).

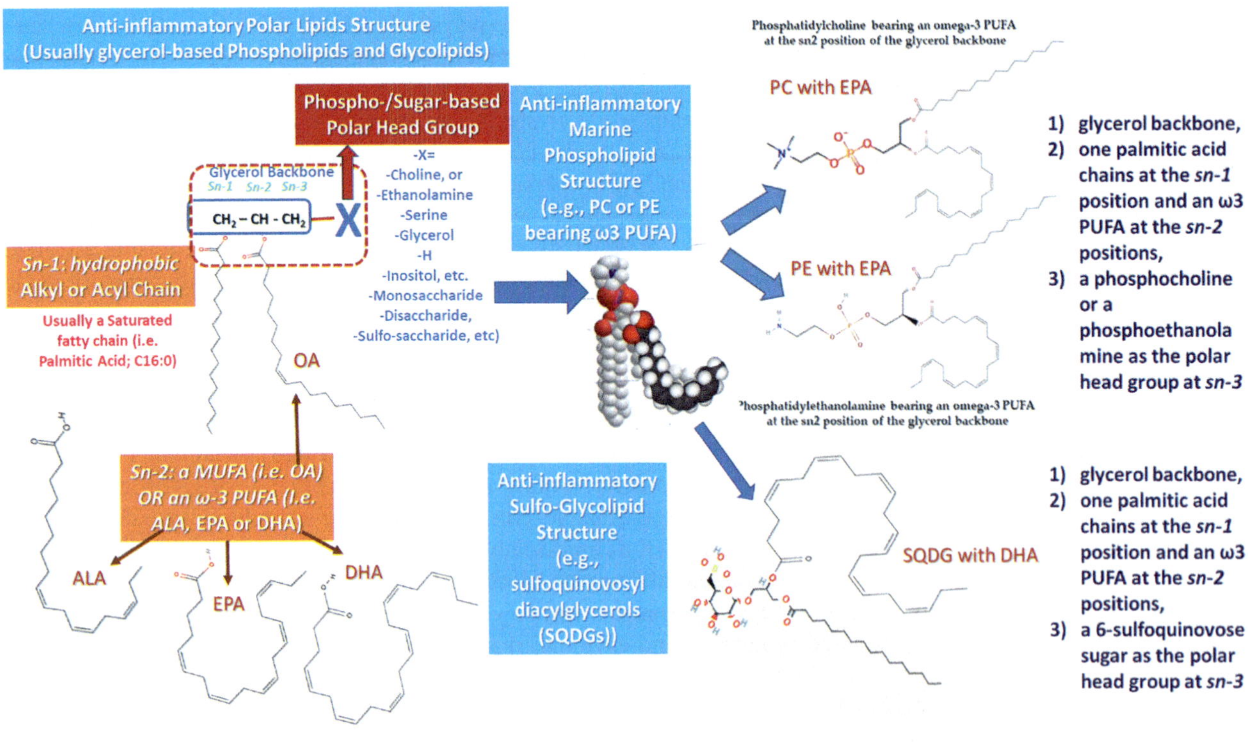

FIG. 21.3 Representative 2D and 3D structures of shrimp-derived PL bioactives, with antiinflammatory and antithrombotic health-promoting properties. *(Some structures were obtained from the free open-access platform Molview.Org.)*

The occurrence of carotenoids in marine organisms represents a significant biochemical feature due to their diverse functional roles and pronounced bioactivity. Carotenoids are lipophilic isoprenoid pigments, typically exhibiting red, orange, or yellow hues, and are biosynthesized by a broad spectrum of photosynthetic and nonphotosynthetic microorganisms, including bacteria and fungi. These compounds are renowned for their antioxidant capacity, which arises from their extended conjugated polyene chains that facilitate the effective neutralization of reactive oxygen species (ROS) and singlet oxygen (Morin-Crini et al., 2019; Klinger et al., 2019; Steven et al., 2022). Beyond their bioactivity, carotenoids are also primarily responsible for the pigmentation observed in various fruits (e.g., tomato, mango), vegetables (e.g., broccoli, spinach), and other plant-derived materials. According to recent data, >1200 naturally occurring carotenoids have been identified across 722 distinct biological sources (Fakhri et al., 2018). Structurally, over 95% of carotenoids are composed of repeating isoprene units (C_5) and are categorized based on their total carbon number into C_{40} (eight isoprenoid units), C_{45} (nine units), C_{50} (ten units), and C_{60} (twelve units). Among these, C_{40} carotenoids are the most ubiquitous, produced by organisms across all domains of life, bacteria, archaea, and eukaryotes. In contrast, the biosynthesis of C_{30} and C_{50} carotenoids is limited to bacteria and archaea, while only select bacterial taxa are capable of synthesizing C_{45} carotenoids.

In addition, several truncated derivatives, referred to as apocarotenoids, have been identified, which are typically produced through enzymatic or oxidative cleavage of canonical C_{40} carotenoid backbones. Notable examples include crocetin (C_{20}) and bixin (C_{25}), both of which exhibit biological relevance in various organisms. Furthermore, in specific contexts, vitamin A (retinol) is classified as an apocarotenoid, as it results from the symmetrical cleavage of β-carotene, yielding two retinal (C_{20}) molecules (Yang et al., 2021; Brotosudarmo et al., 2020). Structurally, carotenoids are broadly classified into two major categories: carotenes and xanthophylls.

Carotenes are composed exclusively of hydrocarbons and are typically characterized by linear or cyclic polyene chains, with prominent representatives, including β-carotene and lycopene. In contrast, xanthophylls are oxygenated derivatives of carotenes, containing one or more functional oxygen groups such as hydroxyl, keto, epoxy, or methoxy moieties. This structural differentiation imparts distinct physicochemical and biological properties to each group. Marine-derived xanthophylls of particular interest include astaxanthin, zeaxanthin, violaxanthin, cryptoxanthin, and capsanthin, which are known for their potent antioxidant activity and various health-promoting effects (Morin-Crini et al., 2019; Brotosudarmo et al., 2020).

Astaxanthin ($C_{40}H_{52}O_4$; 3,3′-dihydroxy-β,β-carotene-4,4′-dione) is a well-recognized, marine-derived carotenoid belonging to the xanthophyll subclass (Morin-Crini et al., 2019). It is a red-orange, lipophilic ketocarotenoid, structurally defined by the presence of both hydroxyl (–OH) and keto (C=O) functional groups at each terminal ring, which confer enhanced polarity and contribute to its potent antioxidant activity (Klinger et al., 2019; Wang et al., 2019; Fang et al., 2018; Ambati et al., 2014). The astaxanthin molecule contains two chiral centers at the C3 and C3′ positions, giving rise to multiple optical isomers and stereoisomeric configurations (Qiu et al., 2012; Saini et al., 2015). Astaxanthin exists in both geometric isomeric forms—namely, cis (Z) and trans (E)—and enantiomeric forms such as (3S,3′S) and (3R,3′R) (Higuera-Ciapara et al., 2006; Nishida et al., 2023). In biological matrices, astaxanthin is frequently found either esterified with fatty acids or noncovalently associated with proteins (as carotenoproteins), affecting its solubility, stability, and bioavailability.

Astaxanthin is an amphiphilic xanthophyll biosynthetically derived from β-carotene and zeaxanthin through the enzymatic action of β-carotene hydroxylase and β-carotene ketolase (Fig. 21.4) (Rahman, 1988; Camargo et al., 2021). It exhibits exceptionally potent antioxidant activity, reported to be approximately 10 times greater than that of zeaxanthin, lutein, β-carotene, and canthaxanthin, and up to 100 times more effective than α-tocopherol (Balzano et al., 2017). Astaxanthin occurs in both free (unesterified) and esterified forms (mono- and di-esterified), which significantly influence its chemical stability and biological functionality (Morin-Crini et al., 2019; Wang et al., 2019). The free form is inherently unstable and susceptible to oxidative degradation under exposure to light, elevated temperatures, oxygen, and extreme pH conditions. The hydroxyl groups of astaxanthin readily undergo esterification with various fatty acids, including linoleic, palmitic, oleic, and stearic acids, enhancing its lipophilicity and stabilizing its molecular structure. In addition, astaxanthin can form noncovalent complexes with proteins or lipoproteins—such as carotenoproteins and carotenolipoproteins—which are commonly observed in marine organisms like crustaceans. These complexes contribute to both the bioavailability and physiological activity of astaxanthin in biological systems (Klinger et al., 2019; Wang et al., 2019; Nagasawa, 2012).

2.2.4 *Protein and other molecules*

Protein hydrolysates represent approximately 40% of crustacean processing by-products and comprise a complex mixture of amino acids (e.g., arginine, glycine), peptides, oligopeptides, and nonprotein nitrogenous compounds such as nucleotides, all of which serve as valuable nutritional and functional components (Klinger et al., 2019; Balzano et al., 2017; Genodepa, 2015). These hydrolysates are typically generated through acid, alkaline, or enzymatic hydrolysis, processes that enhance the solubility, emulsifying capacity, and bioactive potential of the resulting products (Vittori, 2024; Genodepa, 2015). The

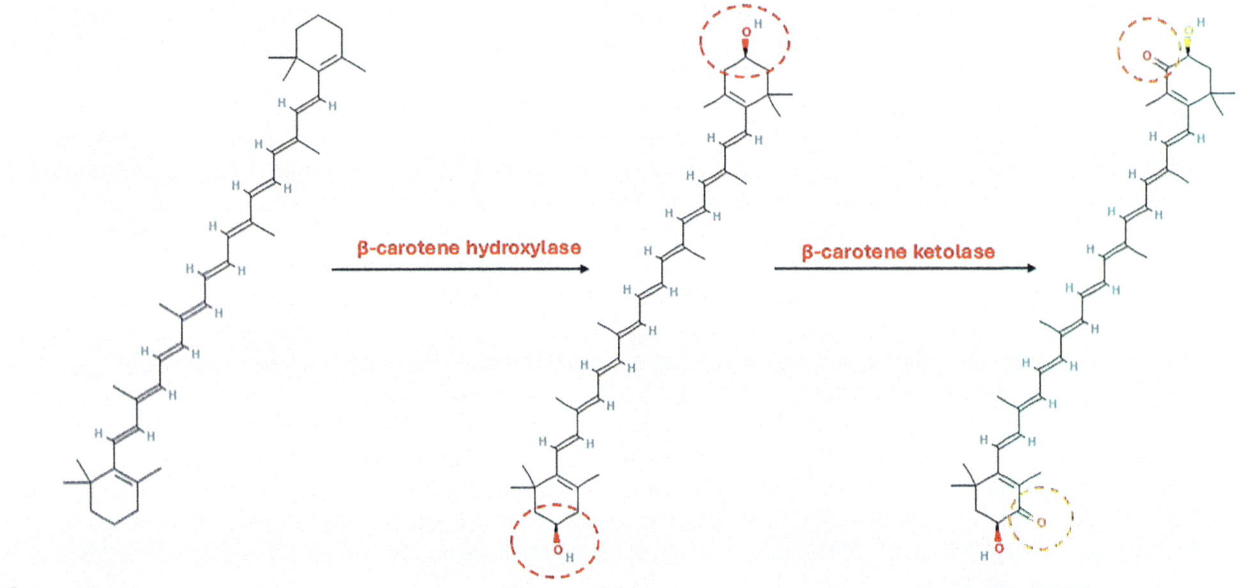

FIG. 21.4 Biochemical modification of main carotenoids into astaxanthin. Conversion of β-carotene and zeaxanthin into astaxanthin. *(From Nugroho Susanto, G., 2021. Crustacea: the increasing economic importance of crustaceans to humans. In: Eduardo Rebolledo Ranz, R. (Ed.), Arthropods - Are They Beneficial for Mankind? IntechOpen. ISBN: 978-1-78984-165-7.)*

protein content of crustacean by-products is influenced by multiple variables, including species, environmental conditions, seasonal variation, reproductive status, and the specific processing methods employed (Vittori, 2024). Furthermore, the size and molecular weight distribution of peptides within the hydrolysates can influence the availability of free amino acids and overall bioactivity (Klinger et al., 2019). Comparative studies have indicated that shrimp species generally exhibit higher protein content in their by-products relative to crabs (Vittori, 2024). Proteins in crustaceans serve a wide range of structural, enzymatic, hormonal, and immune functions. These proteins are critical to survival, as they support everything from exoskeleton formation and molting to digestion, reproduction, and defense against pathogens.

Structural proteins

In crustaceans, structural proteins play a crucial role in forming and maintaining the integrity of the exoskeleton. Cuticular proteins are embedded in the outer layers of the cuticle and bind with chitin to create a strong yet flexible matrix that provides mechanical strength and elasticity. During molting, new cuticular proteins are synthesized and cross-linked with chitin to build the new exoskeleton (Bouallegui, 2021). Sclerotin is a dark-colored, hardened protein formed through cross-linking reactions involving phenols and quinones (mediated by the enzyme phenoloxidase), contributing to the rigidity and pigmentation of the shell. Resilin is a highly elastic protein found in joints and movable appendages; it functions like a spring by storing and releasing mechanical energy to enable efficient movement, such as the rapid tail flicking seen in shrimp. Arthropodin is another protein that acts as a precursor to sclerotin and becomes involved in the hardening process of the exoskeleton. Together, these structural proteins are essential for the strength, flexibility, and overall functionality of the crustacean body (Kulkarni et al., 2021).

Enzymatic proteins

Crustaceans rely on a wide range of enzymatic proteins that are essential for digestion, molting, and immune responses. Most digestive enzymes are produced in the hepatopancreas, an organ responsible for nutrient absorption and metabolism. These include proteases, such as trypsin and chymotrypsin, which break down proteins; amylases, which digest carbohydrates; and lipases, which are responsible for lipid digestion. These enzymes enable crustaceans to process a diverse diet that may include detritus, algae, or animal prey. Another important enzyme is chitinase, which degrades chitin during molting and plays a role in remodeling the cuticle, as well as defending against fungal pathogens. In addition, phenoloxidase is a key component of the crustacean immune system, specifically within the prophenoloxidase-activating system. It contributes to both melanization the deposition of melanin around wounds or invading pathogens, and the sclerotization (hardening) of the newly formed exoskeleton after molting (Chang and Mykles, 2011).

Imunne-related proteins

Crustaceans rely heavily on innate immunity, and proteins play a central role in their defense mechanisms. One of the most important immune-related proteins is hemocyanin, a large copper-containing molecule that primarily functions as an oxygen carrier but also contributes to antimicrobial defense and shares structural similarities with phenoloxidase, an enzyme involved in immune responses (Andriamanalina et al., 2023). Another crucial group includes antimicrobial peptides such as penaeidins, crustins, and antilipopolysaccharide factors, which actively combat bacteria, fungi, and viruses by disrupting the integrity of their cell membranes. In addition, lectins and pattern recognition proteins detect pathogen-associated molecular patterns and initiate immune responses, such as phagocytosis or the activation of the prophenoloxidase cascade, ultimately leading to pathogen elimination. Together, these proteins form a robust first line of defense, allowing crustaceans to effectively respond to microbial threats in the absence of an adaptive immune system (Londono-Zuluaga et al., 2019).

Hormonal and regulatory proteins

Hormonal and regulatory proteins in crustaceans are essential for coordinating growth, development, reproduction, and metabolic functions. During the molting process, proteins such as ecdysone receptors and ultraspiracle act as transcription factors that regulate gene expression in response to ecdysteroids, controlling the synthesis of structural and enzymatic proteins necessary for the formation of a new exoskeleton. In females, vitellogenin is a key reproductive protein that serves as a precursor to yolk proteins, supporting oocyte development and successful reproduction. In addition, various neuropeptides, which are small protein-based signaling molecules, play crucial roles in regulating molting, reproduction, feeding behavior, and osmoregulation. Notable examples include the molt-inhibiting hormone, which prevents premature molting, and the crustacean hyperglycemic hormone, which regulates glucose levels and influences other physiological processes. Together, these proteins ensure the proper timing and coordination of critical life functions in crustaceans (Gbenebor et al., 2016).

Proteins in crustaceans play integral roles across virtually all physiological and developmental processes. Structural proteins, such as sclerotin and resilin, are fundamental to the formation, rigidity, and elasticity of the exoskeleton. Enzymatic proteins are essential for digestive functions and the regulation of the molting cycle, while immune-related proteins mediate defense mechanisms against microbial pathogens. In addition, hormonal proteins are critical regulators of growth, development, and reproductive processes. The molecular diversity and functional specialization of these proteins underscore the evolutionary adaptability and ecological success of crustaceans across a wide range of aquatic and terrestrial habitats.

2.2.5 Minerals and metals

Crustacean shells are a significant source of essential minerals, including phosphorus, magnesium, calcium, and nitrogen (Balzano et al., 2017). The concentration and composition of these minerals are influenced by factors such as species variability, extraction techniques, and demineralization protocols employed (Brunt and Burgess, 2018; Siahaan et al., 2022). Through the application of various acids under controlled conditions of temperature, duration, and acid concentration, a range of calcium salts can be synthesized. Among these, calcium carbonate is predominant, existing primarily in forms such as calcite, amorphous calcium carbonate, and tricalcium phosphate (hydroxyapatite) (Rotter et al., 2024).

3 Crustacean-derived marine bioactives in functional cosmetics applications

Marine-derived bioactives, including those derived from crustaceans and their by-products, are increasingly employed in cosmetic formulations due to their high content of biologically active compounds such as collagen, chitin, peptides, PUFA, and their organic derivatives, as well as inorganic compounds like valuable minerals. These bioactives exhibit a range of beneficial properties, including antiaging, moisturizing, antioxidant, UV-protective, and skin-regenerative effects, making them highly suitable for use in products such as creams, serums, facial masks, and sunscreens. Beyond enhancing the functional performance of cosmetics, their utilization also contributes to environmental sustainability by promoting the valorization of seafood processing waste (Ferreira et al., 2021; Zou et al., 2023; Kroeger et al., 1975). Representative examples of specific cosmetic products containing marine natural bioactives from crustaceans and/or their by-products are shown in Table 21.1.

3.1 Crustacean-derived polysaccharides in functional cosmetics applications

Polysaccharides are increasingly recognized as critical constituents in cosmetic formulations, owing to their multifunctional roles as moisturizers, emulsifiers, viscosity modifiers, and wound healing agents. Their utility is largely attributed to a wide range of bioactivities, including antimicrobial, antioxidant, antiaging, antiinflammatory, anticancer, antifungal,

TABLE 21.1 Representative examples of commercial cosmetic products utilizing bioactive ingredients from crustaceans and their by-products.

Patent name or cosmetic formulation	Marine bioactives (formulation content)	Cosmetic-associated benefits and commercial use	References
System4 R (Finland)	Chitosan from marine crustacean exoskeleton	• Hair smoothing, moisturizing, and perfume-free products • Leave-in chitosan spray • Lightweight consistency for both normal and oily hair	(Kroeger et al., 1975; Kroeger et al., 1975)
DHC Astaxanthin Power Cream (DHC, United States)	Astaxanthin is found in large amounts in the shells of crustaceans and in salmon	• Lightweight, fast-absorbing facial moisturizer that tones, hydrates, and brightens the skin for achieving a radiant-looking skin complexity	(Ifuku et al., 2009; Carrasqueira et al., 2025)
Marin Soothing Hydration Cream (Marin Skincare, ME, United States)	Marine lobster glycoproteins	• Skin-soothing and antiirritating agents that increase natural hyaluronic acid production and overall skin cell viability • Soothing hydration cream (lobster lotion) and lip treatment products	(Morganti et al., 2014; Wu et al., 2024)
Crodarom Black Pearl (Croda Beauty, Yorkshire, UK)	Aragonite and conchiolin from Tahitian black pearls from the black-lip oyster (*Pinctada margaritifera*)	• Revitalizing, moisturizing, and nourishing properties • Protecting skin against environmental damage • Suitable for decorative cosmetics, radiance creams, or gloss shampoos	(Morganti et al., 2016; Aranaz et al., 2018)

and matrix metalloproteinase (MMP) inhibitory properties. Among the various polysaccharides, chitin, chitosan, and their derivatives have attracted considerable interest for cosmetic applications (Terkula Iber et al., 2022; Marniemi and Parkki, 1975; Hesse, 1979). Crustaceans are known to contain substantial amounts of chitin and its derivatives. These compounds represent highly valuable constituents in the field of cosmetology. They have been proposed for incorporation into products intended for the skin, oral cavity, hair, and nails, addressing a broad spectrum of dermatological and esthetic concerns (Terkula Iber et al., 2022).

While chitin is a highly crystalline and structurally rigid polysaccharide with limited solubility, chitosan, its deacetylated derivative, exhibits solubility in acidic environments and the ability to form diverse structures such as films, fibers, scaffolds, and particles at various scales (micro-, nano-, and milli-sized). Moreover, specific oligosaccharides and chemically modified derivatives of chitin and chitosan display water solubility at physiological pH, often possessing enhanced or novel biological activities. In cosmetic formulations, these polysaccharides serve either as bioactive agents or as functional carriers for other therapeutic molecules, benefiting from their physicochemical versatility and biocompatibility (Kong et al., 2018).

Within the European Union (EU), cosmetic substances are regulated under the Cosmetic Products Regulation (EC No. 1223/2009). According to the CosIng database, chitin is listed in eight entries, primarily as an abrasive and bulking agent, whereas chitosan appears in 55 entries, predominantly noted for its film-forming and hair-fixing capabilities (Ito et al., 2015).

Chitosan and its derivatives are particularly promising for skincare applications due to their high molecular weight (HMW) and polycationic nature, which enhance adhesion to the skin's surface (Kroeger et al., 1975) (Table 21.2). Their demonstrated safety, nontoxicity, biodegradability, and biocompatibility further support their inclusion as active or auxiliary ingredients in a variety of cosmetic products, including moisturizers, lotions, creams, foundations, eye shadows, lipsticks, cleansing wipes, and bath preparations (Terkula Iber et al., 2022; Ifuku et al., 2009).

3.1.1 *Antiaging and moisturizing*

Chitosan can be used as an antiaging and moisturizing agent. Skin aging is a complex, multifactorial process that may be classified as either intrinsic—linked to genetic and chronological factors—or extrinsic, which is primarily driven by environmental exposures such as UV radiation, smoking, and air pollution. Key clinical manifestations of skin aging include dryness, loss of elasticity, increased roughness, and skin laxity. UV radiation, in particular, significantly contributes to wrinkle formation and hyperpigmentation, collectively leading to photoaging. Chitosan, especially in its HMW form, has emerged as a promising cosmetic ingredient due to its ability to form a transparent, breathable film on the skin surface. This film reduces transepidermal water loss, thereby enhancing skin hydration, elasticity, and smoothness, attributes critical to mitigating the visible signs of aging (Terkula Iber et al., 2022). In a study by Morganti et al. (2014), the application of chitin and chitosan nanofibril–hyaluronan delivery systems—formulated either as nanoemulsions or nonwoven

TABLE 21.2 Representative examples of marine polysaccharides from crustaceans with cosmetic-related functions and applications.

Crustaceans' sources	Bioactive peptides	Biological activity	Cosmetic-related functions	References
Shrimp shell	Chitosan oligosaccharide	Antiaging and antioxidant potential	• Antioxidant potential: increased superoxide dismutase (SOD), catalase (CAT), glutathione (GSH), and Glutathione Peroxidase (GSH-Px)Decreased malondialdehyde levels (MDA) and increased serum immunoglobulin G (IgG)Inhibited D-galactose upregulation of alanine aminotransferase (ALT), aspartate transaminase (AST), alkaline phosphatase (ALP), uric acid (UA), and creatinine levels	(Akamatsu et al., 1975; Morganti et al., 2014)
Crab (*Portunus sanguinolentus*)	Crab chitin nanofibrils	Anti-UV$_B$ and photoprotective potential	• Protected against UVB irradiationAntiinflammatory, antioxidant, and photoprotective benefits	(Silvestre et al., 2021; Nitulescu et al., 2023; Morganti et al., 2016; Afonso et al., 2019)

films—demonstrated significant antiaging effects. These systems not only increased collagen synthesis in dermal tissues but also inhibited collagenase activity, a major contributor to dermal matrix degradation. Notably, lutein encapsulated within chitosan–hyaluronan nanocarriers exhibited a complete release within 20 h, whereas chitin-based carriers demonstrated a more prolonged release profile. Further, in vitro assessments revealed that nanoemulsions comprising a liposomal complex of HA, phosphatidylcholine, and chitin enhanced collagen production, while a formulation enriched with a melatonin–vitamin E–β-glucan antioxidant complex achieved a remarkable ~ 90% inhibition of collagenase activity. Both topical and oral applications of these bioengineered complexes significantly promoted dermal repair and moisture balance in photoaged or acne-affected skin. In addition, in vivo studies involving chitin nanofibril and nanolignin composite masks indicated a downregulation of MMP-1 and upregulation of collagen type I, validating their antiaging and skin-rejuvenating potential in a clinical cohort of 30 women (Chen et al., 2017). Afonso et al. (2019) further reported that re-acetylated chitosan films offered a biocompatible and noncytotoxic matrix for the efficient delivery of antioxidants such as vitamin C, achieving rapid release (~52% within 15 min) while maintaining mechanical flexibility and functional stability. Similarly, Chaiwong et al. (2020) demonstrated that carboxymethyl chitosan (CMCH) derivatives with varying molecular weights significantly enhanced water solubility—by 96%, 90%, and 89% for low, moderate, and high MW-CMCH, respectively—compared to native chitosan. High MW-CMCH, tested using a Corneometer on porcine skin, exhibited superior moisturizing efficacy at a 0.5% concentration and also showed potential for use as a thickening agent and emulsion stabilizer in cosmetic emulsions. Moreover, Chen et al. (2017) developed montmorillonite-quaternized CMCH composites with synergistic UV-protective and hydrating properties, positioning them as promising multifunctional ingredients in advanced antiaging formulations.

3.1.2 UV protector

The use of chitosan as a UV-protective agent is also of significant importance. Chitin and chitosan exhibit excellent film-forming capabilities, resulting in the production of stable, water-resistant, and cytocompatible films that effectively absorb UV radiation at wavelengths below 400 nm. These characteristics make them highly promising candidates for incorporation into protective dermocosmetic formulations (Terkula Iber et al., 2022). UV radiation, specifically UVA (320–400 nm) and UVB (290–320 nm), constitutes the most biologically active portion of solar radiation and is associated with a spectrum of adverse dermatological effects. These include erythema, premature skin aging (photoaging), photosensitivity, phototoxicity, immunosuppression, and photocarcinogenesis (Silvestre et al., 2021; Nitulescu et al., 2023). Notably, squid pens have been identified as a sustainable and efficient source of chitosan, which can be further valorized for the development of scaffolds or UV-protective biomedical materials (Ntohogian et al., 2018). The inherent bioadhesive properties of both chitin and chitosan, demonstrated through their interactions with both positively charged polysaccharides and negatively charged keratin structures, further support their application in topical delivery systems (Morsy et al., 2017). Accordingly, sunscreens incorporating chitosan, in combination with other high-efficacy photoprotective agents, are employed to mitigate UV-induced skin damage during prolonged solar exposure (Tunku Mahmud et al., 2015; Guzmán et al., 2022).

Ntohogian et al. (2018) reported the utilization of chitosan nanoparticles as bioactive carriers and stabilizers for the encapsulation of natural and purified sunscreen agents, such as annatto and saffron, leading to the development of UV-protective nanoemulsion-based formulations. These emulsions demonstrated low cytotoxicity and remained stable over a 90-day storage period, while achieving sun protection factor (SPF) values ranging from 2.15 to 4.85. In a related study, Morsy et al. (2017) explored the formulation of a multifunctional hydroxyapatite–chitosan (HAP–chitosan) gel with antibacterial and UV-protective properties. Within this hybrid system, hydroxyapatite nanoparticles were homogeneously distributed throughout the chitosan matrix, resulting in a biofunctional film capable of attenuating the detrimental effects of UV exposure.

3.1.3 Skin-cleansing

Skin-cleansing cosmetic formulations are specifically designed to remove exogenous substances from the skin's surface, including environmental pollutants, microbial contaminants, and cosmetic residues. Due to their intrinsic cationic nature, chitosan and its derivatives serve as effective positively charged carriers in personal care formulations. Their electrostatic interaction with the anionic functional groups present on the skin's surface enables targeted delivery and controlled release of cleansing agents, enhancing formulation efficacy and skin adherence (Theerawattanawit et al., 2022; Rejinold et al., 2021). Tangkijngamvong et al. (2020) demonstrated the potential of chitosan-based nanoparticles as effective sebum-regulating systems. Specifically, chitosan particles and chitosan–proretinal nanoparticles significantly reduced sebum production, while the latter also mitigated erythema (skin redness), indicating antiinflammatory properties. Similarly, Theerawattanawit et al. (2022) reported that chitosan gels effectively decreased sebum levels without eliciting adverse dermatological responses. This effect is attributed to chitosan's ability to form complexes with sebum lipids, thereby facilitating their removal from the skin surface. Moreover, chitosan's film-forming capacity contributes to the formation of a transient barrier that inhibits subsequent sebum accumulation (Rejinold et al., 2021).

3.1.4 Antibacterial

Chitosan exhibits broad-spectrum antibacterial properties, primarily attributed to its polycationic nature. Its positively charged amino groups electrostatically interact with the negatively charged components of bacterial cell walls, leading to disruption of membrane integrity, cellular shrinkage, and eventual cell death. This widely accepted mechanism underpins the topical antibacterial efficacy of chitosan-based formulations. The magnitude of antibacterial activity is influenced by both the molecular weight and the charge density of chitosan chains, with higher molecular weight variants generally demonstrating enhanced bactericidal effects (Liu et al., 2022). Verma et al. (2021) reported that chitosan treatment resulted in a > 90% reduction in bacterial proliferation, underscoring its potent antimicrobial potential. Deng et al. (2022) developed a multifunctional, biobased hydrogel composed of quaternized chitosan and dialdehyde bacterial cellulose, which exhibited significant wound healing capacity and antibacterial activity. In a similar context, Liu et al. (2022) fabricated a hydrogel by cross-linking CMCH with polyvinyl alcohol using borax as a cross-linker. The hydrogel displayed excellent self-healing behavior and was further enhanced with the incorporation of highly stable silver nanoparticles (AgNPs), leading to pronounced antibacterial effects against *Escherichia coli* and *Staphylococcus aureus*. These multifunctional hydrogels hold considerable promise for applications in wound management and infection control.

3.1.5 Nail care

Nails are keratinized appendages of the skin, derived from the epidermal layer, and serve as protective and functional extensions of the integumentary system (Monti et al., 2022). Onychomycosis, a prevalent fungal infection of the nail apparatus, is pathologically distinct from other dermal mycoses. Effective treatment often requires the combination of topical broad-spectrum antifungal agents and systemic oral therapies. Predisposing factors include preexisting cutaneous fungal infections and nail trauma, both of which compromise the integrity of the nail barrier. Trauma may arise from mechanical insult or repeated chemical exposure, rendering the nail more susceptible to pathogenic invasion (Palmieri et al., 2014). Among topical treatments, nail lacquers offer superior efficacy compared to creams and solutions due to their enhanced film-forming properties and prolonged residence time at the site of infection (Ghannoum et al., 2015). Hydroxypropyl chitosan (HPCH), a semisynthetic chitosan derivative, has emerged as a promising excipient for nail drug delivery systems. HPCH forms a biocompatible, protective film on the nail plate, preserving keratin integrity, enhancing hydration, and improving overall nail condition. It has shown efficacy in reducing dystrophic symptoms in psoriatic nails and serves as a barrier against fungal reinfection (Csuka et al., 2023; Morganti et al., 2021). Repeated application of HPCH-based lacquers outperforms conventional treatments such as isopropyl alcohol and urea in preventing recurrent fungal infections. In addition, HPCH has been demonstrated to improve biomechanical properties—including hardness, tensile strength, and flexural strength—of keratinized tissues (e.g., hooves) in vitro. It also significantly reduced the extent of fungal colonization and structural degradation following dermatophyte invasion and abrasion (Akanno et al., 2020).

3.1.6 Hair care

Hair shafts, or piliferous ends, are primarily composed of keratin—a fibrous structural protein rich in amino acids such as cysteine and lysine—alongside melanin, which determines hair pigmentation (Terkula Iber et al., 2022). Hair is vulnerable to a variety of damaging factors, including thermal stress from high-temperature styling tools, chemical stress from coloring and bleaching agents, and environmental exposure to UV radiation and chlorinated water. These factors contribute to both structural and chemical degradation of the hair fiber, resulting in dryness, brittleness, and loss of luster (Fernández-Peña and Guzmán, 2020). Chitin and chitosan exhibit unique properties that render them particularly suitable for hair care applications. These include their ability to enhance hydration, promote the repair of damaged fibers, and improve hair sheen. Consequently, chitosan is widely used in numerous hair care products—including shampoos, rinses, waving agents, hair sprays, dyes, tonics, and styling formulations—where it serves to enhance rheological properties and improve ingredient adherence to the hair surface (Saini and Keum, 2018; Rejinold et al., 2021; Wang et al., 2020).

Conditioning, a fundamental step in hair care, typically employs cationic polymers like chitosan to restore manageability and texture to chemically or mechanically compromised hair. Damaged hair exhibits a denatured protein structure with exposed negatively charged groups, which cannot be repaired through biological pathways. Thus physicochemical approaches are employed, wherein cationic polymers form protective films over the damaged areas, mitigating breakage and restoring tactile qualities (Mohamed et al., 2025; Sionkowska et al., 2017). Chitosan and its derivatives electrostatically interact with the negatively charged keratin surface, creating a transparent, elastic coating that imparts strength, softness, and moisture retention to hair fibers (Martins et al., 2024). Mohamed et al. (2025) developed organic hair conditioners (OHCs) using chitosan conjugates—chitosan-(ethylthio-thiadiazole) and chitosan-(benzylthio-thiadiazole)—blended with natural fragrances. The formulations exhibited optimal pH values (4.2–4.7) to minimize dermal irritation. Select formulations (CH, E2, and B2) demonstrated superior performance in hydration, detangling, styling facilitation, antifrizz effects, antiinflammatory properties, and the formation of a protective hair barrier. Similarly, Sionkowska et al. (2017) evaluated ternary conditioning systems comprising chitosan, collagen, and HA. Their findings revealed that these biopolymers synergistically improved the mechanical integrity, water stability, and surface energy of hair conditioning films, enhancing the elasticity and resilience of hair fibers. Beyond chitosan-based systems, modern hair care has adopted peptide-based technologies such as Olaplex and K18, which employ bioactive peptides to penetrate the hair cortex, repairing disulfide bonds and damaged polypeptide chains. While these systems provide molecular-level repair, chitosan contributes surface-level reinforcement and conditioning, making the combination of both approaches a comprehensive strategy for hair restoration and maintenance (Ganguly et al., 2017).

3.1.7 Oral cavity-protective

The oral cavity comprises several key anatomical structures, including the teeth and gingiva—soft connective tissues that encase the teeth and line the alveolar processes—both of which are fundamental to maintaining oral health (Jormalainen, 1998). A wide range of dental pathologies, including dental caries, anodontia, bruxism, tooth wear, gingivitis, and periodontitis, can affect these tissues. Preventive and therapeutic strategies targeting conditions such as oral mucositis, plaque accumulation, microbial colonization, and periodontal disorders increasingly incorporate chitosan and its derivatives in various formulations, including gels, sprays, chewing gums, mouthwashes, dentifrices, and microspheres (Nguyen et al., 2017a; Samiraninezhad et al., 2023).

In oral healthcare, polymers—particularly chitosan—serve dual functional roles: as vehicles (e.g., in toothpaste, mouth rinses, dental varnishes, and chewing gums) and as carriers for active ingredients such as sodium fluoride (NaF), chlorhexidine, or phytochemicals. Chitosan exhibits a wide range of oral bioactivities, including pH buffering, antibacterial action, inhibition of biofilm formation, and antiabrasive effects, making it a valuable ingredient for maintaining oral hygiene and preventing dental disease (Saini and Keum, 2018).

Ganguly et al. (2017) developed periodontal gels incorporating natural polymers such as babul gum, karaya gum, and chitosan. Their findings indicated that the gels' surface pH varied depending on the polymer type and concentration. Importantly, when moxifloxacin hydrochloride was added, the gels demonstrated strong antimicrobial activity, indicating their potential utility in the treatment of periodontitis.

Nguyen et al. (2017) formulated fluoride-loaded nanoparticles using a tri-polymer system of chitosan, alginate, and pectin, with NaF serving as the active agent. Chitosan played a critical role in producing monodisperse, spherical nanoparticles with high stability. These nanoparticles enabled a sustained, low-concentration release of fluoride, with accelerated release under acidic conditions, an environment conducive to dental caries. This pH-responsive delivery system highlights chitosan's promise for improving fluoride bioavailability and caries prevention.

In another study, Samiraninezhad et al. (2023 synthesized hydrogels composed of chitosan, alginate, gelatin, and HA for targeted oral drug delivery. These natural polymer-based hydrogels demonstrated significant advantages over conventional formulations, offering controlled release kinetics, reduced systemic side effects, and enhanced therapeutic efficacy. Their application could be particularly beneficial in the management of oral lesions, mucosal conditions, and localized infections.

3.1.8 Other crustacean-derived oligosaccharides/polysaccharides in cosmetic applications

D-glucosamine and NAG monomers can be obtained from chitin isolated from crustaceans, while these chitin derivatives have also been used in the cosmetics industry in several applications, including hair, skin, and oral care products, considering the need to address the acceptability of this resource by vegan consumers (Rotter et al., 2024; Barthel and Markwardt, 1975; Bissett, 2006; Makar et al., 1975). D-glucosamine and NAG are found in the skin, serving as precursors for the biosynthesis of HA and acting as natural moisturizing factors. Furthermore, double-blind clinical trials have proven that oral NAG supplements are a promising treatment against wrinkles, while their topical application improves hyperpigmentation (Treyvaud Amiguet et al., 2012; Jinxia et al., 2019; Sánchez-Camargo et al., 2011; Makar et al., 1975). As a result, glucosamines are currently incorporated as ingredients in several creams and serums.195

3.2 Amphiphilic (phenolics, carotenoids, and PLs) and other lipid-based (fatty acids) marine bioactives for potential cosmetic applications

Crustaceans and their by-products also contain high-quality, valuable bioactive lipids, pigments like astaxanthin, and several other amphiphilic bioactives such as marine phenolics (Jinxia et al., 2019; Sánchez-Camargo et al., 2011; Treyvaud Amiguet et al., 2012; Cholidis et al., 2024; Ermolenko et al., 2023; Tsoupras et al., 2025; Ermolenko et al., 2023; Shuang et al., 2022). The majority of the studies have been conducted on shrimps, crabs, and their by-products, as they are an important component of aquaculture and the marine food industry and represent a rich source of bioactive compounds with documented health benefits (Cholidis et al., 2024; Sánchez-Camargo et al., 2011). Among these, shrimp-derived PLs play a key role in cell signaling, lipid metabolism, and cardiovascular protection, while also exhibiting antiinflammatory properties relevant to chronic inflammatory conditions (Sánchez-Camargo et al., 2011).

In parallel, astaxanthin—a major carotenoid found in shrimp—modulates inflammatory responses by regulating the expression of proinflammatory cytokines such as interleukin-1β (IL-1β), tumor necrosis factor-α (TNF-α), and interleukin-6 (IL-6). It further inhibits key inflammatory signaling pathways, including NF-κB and Jun-kinasaes (JNK), while interacting with the Nrf2 pathway (Sánchez-Camargo et al., 2011).

The antiinflammatory potential of shrimp lipids has been extensively demonstrated in zebrafish models, in which treatment with shrimp head lipid extracts resulted in a marked reduction in macrophage migration to injured tail regions (Sánchez-Camargo et al., 2011; Gómez-Guillén et al., 2018), compared to $CuSO_4$-treated controls, where inflammatory markers, including COX-2, TNF-α, and IL-1β, are usually induced and increased (Gómez-Guillén et al., 2018). Similar antiinflammatory effects were observed in tail-amputation models, where shrimp-derived phospholipids significantly decreased macrophage accumulation at higher concentrations, confirming their capacity to attenuate inflammatory responses in vivo (Bjørklund et al., 2022).

In vitro evidence further supports the antiinflammatory effects of shrimp-derived lipids. At the cellular level, shrimp lipid extracts from Litopenaeus vannamei cephalothorax—rich in oleic, palmitic, linoleic, stearic, arachidonic acids, EPA, and DHA—were evaluated using RAW 264.7 macrophages. These cells produce nitric oxide (NO) in response to inflammatory stress, and reduced NO levels indicate antiinflammatory activity. Encapsulated shrimp lipid extracts significantly reduced NO production (from 42.42 μM to 27.51 μM at 100 μg/mL), whereas nonencapsulated extracts showed negligible effects due to limited water solubility (Sangsuriyawong et al., 2019). Moreover, Tsoupras et al. (2025) demonstrated that shrimp-derived extracts are rich in amphiphilic marine bioactives, including phenolic compounds, carotenoids, and PLs rich in UFAs. These extracts exhibited strong antioxidant activity when assayed by the DPPH (2,2-diphenyl-1-picrylhydrazyl), ABTS (2,2′-azino-bis-3-ethylbenzothiazoline-6-sulfonic acid), and FRAP (Ferric Reducing Antioxidant Power) bioassays that evaluate entioxidant capacity by different mechanisms of action. The antioxidant activities pbserved in all these three assays were largely attributed to their phenolic and carotenoid content. These extracts also showed pronounced antiinflammatory and antithrombotic effects on human platelets. In particular, they inhibited key inflammatory mediators such as PAF and reduced platelet-related thrombosis induced by classical agonists like ADP. LC–MS-based lipidomic and structure–activity relationship analyses revealed that these bioactivities were primarily associated with UFA-rich PLs, notably those containing oleic acid (C18:1n9) and ω3 PUFAs (EPA and DHA). The high anti-PAF potency of these lipids, together with their favorable low n-6/n-3 PUFA ratio (Fig. 21.3), underscores their strong antiinflammatory potential. These findings highlighted that shrimp-derived amphiphilic PLs seem to be promising, sustainable functional ingredients for antiinflammatory and antiaging cosmetic applications, including nutricosmetics and cosmeceuticals, in line with circular bioeconomy principles (Vittori, 2024). Overall, shrimp lipids, phenolics, and carotenoids like astaxanthin demonstrate strong antiinflammatory potential, supporting their use in nutraceutical, pharmaceutical, and cosmetic applications.

Astaxanthin is a particularly potent antioxidant due to its unique molecular structure and amphiphilicity, which enables efficient scavenging of free radicals in both lipophilic and hydrophilic environments (Gómez-Guillén et al., 2018; e Silva et al., 2021). Using DPPH assays, astaxanthin-loaded liposomes exhibited high radical scavenging activity (up to 81.76%), with formulations containing 70% phosphatidylcholine showing superior stability and metal-chelating capacity during storage (Messina et al., 2019). Additional studies using multiple antioxidant assays (total antioxidant caqpacity, TAC, ferric reducing power, hydroxyl radical scavenging, DPPH, and oxygen radical absorbance capacity, ORAC) confirmed that shrimp oils with higher astaxanthin content displayed enhanced antioxidant activity, particularly following heat-assisted extraction, which improved astaxanthin recovery (Li et al., 2020).

At the cellular level, encapsulated shrimp lipid extracts demonstrated significantly higher antioxidant activity than nonencapsulated forms in RAW 264.7 cells, as measured by photochemiluminescence assays for lipid- and water-soluble antioxidant capacity (Lima et al., 2021). Astaxanthin extracted from shrimp by-products also protected human fibroblast (HS68) cells from oxidative damage, increasing cell viability from 59.1% to 83.6% at nontoxic concentrations (0.2 nM), with efficacy comparable to the synthetic antioxidant N-acetyl cysteine (Chintong et al., 2019). In vivo zebrafish models further confirmed the antioxidant capacity of shrimp head lipids, which reduced ROS overproduction and apoptosis induced by metronidazole exposure (Siahaan et al., 2022). Collectively, these findings highlight shrimp extracts as effective and sustainable antioxidants.

Given their antioxidant and antiinflammatory properties, shrimp-derived bioactives—particularly astaxanthin—are promising candidates for cosmetic applications as natural alternatives to synthetic ingredients (Nguyen et al., 2017b). Astaxanthin extracted from *L. vannamei* demonstrated strong singlet oxygen scavenging activity in human dermal fibroblasts, with an EC_{50} of 9.2 ± 0.5 μg/mL, indicating effective protection against ROS implicated in skin aging and inflammatory disorders. In addition, astaxanthin inhibited tyrosinase activity (IC_{50} = 12.2 ± 1.5 μg/mL), suggesting potential skin-whitening and pigmentation-regulating effects. Cytotoxicity studies in WS1 fibroblasts showed no adverse effects, with cell viability exceeding 90% and no morphological alterations after treatment, confirming its safety for topical use (Šimat et al., 2022).

Crustacean processing by-products constitute a significant natural source of astaxanthin, where it usually occurs either in free form or complexed with proteins (carotenoproteins) or chitin, with concentrations varying widely according to species and season (de Carvalho and Caramujo, 2017). Reported levels in crustacean shells range from 2.9 to 1203 μg/g dry weight, making astaxanthin the predominant carotenoid in these by-products (Jinxia et al., 2019; Villaró et al., 2021; Ahmadkelayeh et al., 2022). Although microalgae-derived astaxanthin is currently the main commercial source for cosmetic applications, crustacean waste represents a promising and underutilized alternative (Hamdi et al., 2024).

Astaxanthin can be recovered from crustacean carapaces using various extraction techniques, including conventional organic solvent extraction, oil-based extraction, and increasingly, green and sustainable methodologies. Ethanol extraction followed by chromatographic purification has been successfully applied to crayfish shells (Nunes et al., 2021), while fish oil has been used as an effective green solvent for astaxanthin recovery from shrimp by-products (Vicente et al., 2022). Enhanced yields have also been achieved through biological pretreatments, such as yeast fermentation prior to solvent extraction (Niu et al., 2018). Advanced technologies, including supercritical fluid extraction combined with microwave-assisted processes, as well as integrated biorefinery approaches targeting astaxanthin, proteins, and chitin, further highlight the potential for efficient and sustainable recovery from crustacean waste streams (Chintong et al., 2019; Chou et al., 2016).

Astaxanthin exhibits a broad spectrum of biological activities relevant to skin health, including antioxidant, photoprotective, antiaging, antiwrinkle, moisturizing, wound healing, antiinflammatory, and antipigmentation effects. In vitro studies have demonstrated its ability to enhance skin cell proliferation and collagen synthesis through modulation of VEGF expression, inhibition of MMPs, and upregulation of tissue inhibitors of metalloproteinases (TIMP-1; Hama et al., 2012).

Natural astaxanthin from shrimp shells has demonstrated potent antioxidant activities against DPPH and ABTS radicals, prevented the bleaching of β-carotene, and quenched singlet oxygen, while it also showed antityrosinase activities, as well as no toxicity (Prajaputra et al., 2024). More specifically, the astaxanthin extract could inhibit tyrosinase activity (IC50 12.2 ± 1.5 μg/mL) and had no toxic effects on human dermal fibroblast cells. These results suggested that shrimp astaxanthin would be a promising dietary supplement for skin health applications. Moreover, unlike conventional antioxidants, astaxanthin may exert its protective effects by regulating intracellular redox signaling rather than directly scavenging free radicals.

Both oral delivery and topical delivery of astaxanthin have shown beneficial effects on skin health. Topical application of astaxanthin-loaded liposomal systems has been shown to prevent UV-induced skin thickening, collagen degradation, and melanogenesis in in vivo models (Suresh et al., 2018). Astaxanthin liposomes also demonstrated superior photoprotective efficacy and lower cytotoxicity compared to liposomal formulations containing other carotenoids or tocopherols (Yan and Chen, 2015). Alternative delivery systems, such as nanoemulsions and biopolymer-based films, further enhance astaxanthin stability, skin penetration, and bioavailability. For example, astaxanthin nanoemulsions formulated with CMCH exhibited good skin permeability and cellular safety, while astaxanthin–collagen films derived from marine sources promoted accelerated wound healing and tissue regeneration in animal models (Liu et al., 2022; Lai-Cheong and McGrath, 2021).

Despite strong experimental evidence supporting the cosmeceutical potential of astaxanthin, studies specifically focused on astaxanthin derived from crustacean by-products remain limited. Given potential differences in composition, bioavailability, and biological response between animal- and microalgae-derived astaxanthin, further clinical and translational research is needed to fully validate the safety and efficacy of crustacean-derived astaxanthin in cosmetic applications.

In summary, crustacean-derived carotenoids like astaxanthin, phenolics, and lipid extracts rich in PLs bearing UFA exhibit strong antioxidant, antiinflammatory, and skin-protective properties, supporting their incorporation into cosmetic formulations aimed at combating oxidative stress, inflammation, and environmentally induced skin damage.

3.3 Protein hydrolysates for potential cosmetic applications

Among several marine invertebrate organisms, some crustaceans, like shrimps, contain considerable amounts of proteins of high nutritional value, including collagen (Yan and Chen, 2015). The processing of crustacean seafood, most commonly prawns, shrimp, crabs, and lobsters, results in a significant amount of waste, consisting of the carapace and the head of the crustacean. About 60%–80% of shrimp, 60%–70% of crab, 60%–85% of lobster, 65%–70% of crayfish, and 70%–75% of krill are discarded as waste during processing (Suresh et al., 2018; Hiransuchalert et al., 2021; Mechri et al., 2020). The by-product could be separated into its component chemicals: 15%–40% chitin, 20%–40% protein, and 20%–50% calcium carbonate (Yan and Chen, 2015; Nguyen et al., 2023). Collagen extraction from crustaceans, like shrimp and crab shells, faces challenges when using acid solutions, and the purification process is intricate due to the presence of noncollagenous proteins, rendering it less efficient. The reason for this limitation is that the structure of collagen from crustaceans is highly resistant to acid treatment. This resistance to acid extraction is due to the specific chemical composition and structure of crustacean collagen. Therefore enzymatic methods are often used to isolate collagen from crustaceans. These methods are better suited for breaking down the tough collagen fibers and preserving their integrity.

Enzymatic extraction, in particular, involves the use of specific enzymes that can break down collagen without damaging its properties. Hiransuchalert et al. (2021) and Piccirillo et al. (2014) have isolated the muscle of several mantis shrimp, such as *Miyakea nepa*, *Harpiosquilla harpax*, *Uropeltis woodmasoni*, and *Odontodactylus cultrifer*. The results showed that the primary collagen found in shrimp muscles resembles type I collagen found in vertebrate muscles. Although the collagen content percentage is relatively low, ranging from 0.015% to 0.4878%, some other crustaceans may display noteworthy collagen content variations along with differences in the types of collagen they produce. Moreover, such protein hydrolysates from these marine sources have also shown interesting bioactivities for cosmetic applications. For example, shrimp by-product protein hydrolysates (hyd) prepared using two bacterial-purified serine alkaline proteases showed potent antioxidant activities (DPPH, FRAP, and β-carotene protection) and inhibitory effects against angiotensin I-converting enzyme, tyrosinase (Tyr), and amylase (Amy) enzymes (Siahaan et al., 2022). Nevertheless, further studies, including more in vivo investigations on such protein hydrolysates coupled with a peptidomic analysis, molecular docking approaches, and prediction of peptide structures, are still required to evaluate the peptides responsible for the observed potential activities for cosmetic applications.

3.4 Marine substrates and minerals from crustaceans as cosmetic ingredients

Despite the extensive use of both synthetic and natural calcium phosphates (CaPs) in cosmetic products—including skincare, haircare, deodorants, and oral care—studies specifically investigating fish- and crustacean-derived CaPs as cosmetic ingredients remain limited. Recent evidence suggests that marine by-products may represent a promising alternative source. For example, calcium extracted from lobster shells has been shown to significantly promote bone and skin cell proliferation in vitro, indicating its potential as a functional cosmetic and cosmeceutical ingredient (Kodali et al., 2022).

Owing to its crystalline nanostructure and low photoreactivity, marine hydroxyapatite, a biocompatible CaP, may function as a physical UV filter that minimizes oxidative damage and skin irritation, making it suitable for broad-spectrum sunscreen formulations (Rotter et al., 2024). Marine-derived CaPs may exhibit distinct biological activities compared to those obtained from terrestrial sources due to differences in trace mineral composition. Consequently, further research is needed to establish robust scientific evidence supporting their cosmetic applications (Ferreira et al., 2021). Beyond UV protection, marine hydroxyapatite is being explored for skin and dental remineralization, wound healing delivery systems, and skin rejuvenation. Trace elements naturally associated with marine hydroxyapatite, such as zinc and magnesium, may enhance collagen synthesis, promote skin cell proliferation, and exert antiinflammatory effects. In addition, marine-derived magnesium and zinc are already incorporated into mineral sunscreens and antiacne formulations due to their antiinflammatory and sebum-regulating properties.

4 Conclusions, limitations, and future perspectives for crustacean-derived bioactives in cosmetic applications

Crustaceans and their processing by-products constitute a largely underexploited yet highly valuable source of structurally diverse and biologically potent compounds with significant potential for cosmetic and cosmeceutical applications. Bioactives derived from crustacean shells, exoskeletons, heads, and viscera—such as chitin and chitosan, proteins and peptides, lipid bioactives, pigments (notably astaxanthin), minerals, and CaPs—exhibit a broad range of skin-beneficial properties, including antioxidant, antiinflammatory, antiaging, antimicrobial, UV-protective, moisturizing, and wound healing effects. Their natural origin, biocompatibility, and multifunctionality make them attractive alternatives to synthetic cosmetic ingredients across skincare, haircare, oral care, and sun protection products. Importantly, the valorization of crustacean by-products aligns strongly with circular economy principles by transforming biological waste into high-value functional ingredients while reducing environmental burden.

Despite their promise, several challenges currently limit the large-scale adoption of crustacean-derived bioactives in cosmetic formulations. Variability in raw material composition due to species differences, seasonal availability, and environmental conditions complicates standardization and quality control. In addition, the availability of crustacean bioactives may be affected by climate change–driven alterations in marine ecosystems, including shifts in species distribution and changes in biochemical composition. These factors introduce uncertainty in supply chains and underscore the need for adaptive sourcing strategies that integrate environmental monitoring, controlled aquaculture, and systematic bioactive profiling.

Further limitations include insufficient in vivo and clinical evidence supporting the efficacy and long-term safety of many crustacean-derived ingredients, as well as challenges related to scalable extraction, cost efficiency, and regulatory approval. Ethical and environmental concerns, coupled with limited consumer awareness of marine by-product valorization, may also hinder market acceptance. Addressing these issues will require expanded clinical validation, harmonized regulatory frameworks, transparent sustainability assessments, and improved communication of environmental benefits.

Future research should focus on optimizing green and sustainable extraction technologies, advancing analytical characterization, and developing innovative encapsulation and delivery systems to enhance the stability, bioavailability, and performance of crustacean bioactives in cosmetic formulations. The integration of circular economy models, marine biorefineries, and biotechnological approaches—such as fermentation and enzyme-assisted processing—offers promising pathways to ensure a consistent supply while minimizing ecological impact. Cross-disciplinary collaboration among marine scientists, cosmetic chemists, toxicologists, and regulatory bodies will be essential to translate laboratory findings into commercially viable products.

In conclusion, as consumer demand increasingly shifts toward natural, sustainable, and multifunctional cosmetics, crustacean-derived bioactives provide a compelling foundation for next-generation cosmetic and cosmeceutical innovation. With continued scientific, technological, and regulatory advancements, these marine by-products have the potential to play a central role in the development of safe, effective, and environmentally responsible cosmetic products.

Acknowledgments

The authors would like to thank the School of Chemistry, Faculty of Sciences at the Democritus University of Thrace, and the Fisheries Research Institute in Kavala, Greece, for their continuous support.

Conflicts of interest

The authors declare no conflicts of interest.

Funding

This research received no external funding.

Author contributions

A.T. was involved in conceptualization, methodology, validation, visualization, and supervision. E.T. and A.T. were involved in investigation and writing—original draft preparation. C.A. and A.T. were involved in writing—review and editing. All authors contributed to software and have read and agreed to the published version of the manuscript.

References

Aam, B.B., Heggset, E.B., Norberg, A.L., Sørlie, M., Vårum, K.M., Eijsink, V.G.H., 2010. Production of chitooligosaccharides and their potential applications in medicine. Mar. Drugs 16603397. 8 (5), 1482–1517. Available from: http://www.mdpi.com/1660-3397/8/5/1482/pdf. doi:10.3390/md8051482.

Afonso, C.R., Hirano, R.S., Gaspar, A.L., Chagas, E.G.L., Carvalho, R.A., Silva, F.V., Leonardi, G.R., Lopes, P.S., Silva, C.F., Yoshida, C.M.P., 2019. Biodegradable antioxidant chitosan films useful as an anti-aging skin mask. Int. J. Biol. Macromol. 01418130. 132, 1262–1273. doi:10.1016/j.ijbiomac.2019.04.052.

Ahmad, S.I., Ahmad, R., Khan, M.S., Kant, R., Shahid, S., Gautam, L., Hasan, G.M., Hassan, M.I., 2020. Chitin and its derivatives: structural properties and biomedical applications. Int. J. Biol. Macromol. 18790003. 164, 526–539. Available from: https://www.elsevier.com/locate/ijbiomac. doi:10.1016/j.ijbiomac.2020.07.098.

Ahmadkelayeh, S., Cheema, S.K., Hawboldt, K., 2022. Extraction of astaxanthin from atlantic shrimp by-products using fish oil: process optimization and operational parameter effects. J. Clean. Prod. 09596526. 371, 133609. doi:10.1016/j.jclepro.2022.133609.

Ahmadkelayeh, S., Hawboldt, K., 2020. Extraction of lipids and astaxanthin from crustacean by-products: a review on supercritical CO2 extraction. Trends Food Sci. Technol. 09242244. 103, 94–108. doi:10.1016/j.tifs.2020.07.016.

Akamatsu, N., Nakajima, H., Ohno, M., Miura, Y., 1975. Increase in acetyl CoA synthetase activity after phenobarbital treatment. Biochem. Pharmacol. 00062952. 24 (18), 1725–1727. doi:10.1016/0006-2952(75)90013-1.

Akanno, A., Guzmán, E., Ortega, F., Rubio, R.G., 2020. Behavior of the water/vapor interface of chitosan solutions with an anionic surfactant: effect of polymer-surfactant interactions. Phys. Chem. Chem. Phys. 14639076. 22 (40), 23360–23373. Available from: http://pubs.rsc.org/en/journals/journal/cp. doi:10.1039/d0cp02470h.

Albalat, A., Collard, A., Brucem, C., Coates, C.J., Fox, C.J., 2016. Physiological condition, short-term survival, and predator avoidance behavior of discarded Norway lobsters (*Nephrops norvegicus*). J. Shellfish Res. 07308000. 35 (4), 1053–1065. Available from: http://www.bioone.org/loi/shre. doi:10.2983/035.035.0428.

Alves, A., Sousa, E., Kijjoa, A., Pinto, M., 2020. Marine-derived compounds with potential use as cosmeceuticals and nutricosmetics. Molecules. 1420-3049. 25 (11), 2536. doi:10.3390/molecules25112536.

Ambati, R., Phang, S.-M., Ravi, S., Aswathanarayana, R., 2014. Astaxanthin: sources, extraction, stability, biological activities and its commercial applications—a review. Mar. Drugs. 1660-3397. 12 (1), 128–152. doi:10.3390/md12010128.

Andriamanalina, T.M., Andrianandrasana, M.D., Ravonizafy, C., Andrianandrasana, E.R., 2023. Calcium salts from the demineralization of crab (*Scylla serrata*) wastes. Am. J. Innov. Sci. Eng. 2158-7205. 2 (1), 25–29. doi:10.54536/ajise.v2i1.1273.

Aranaz, I., Acosta, N., Civera, C., Elorza, B., Mingo, J., Castro, C., Gandía, M., Caballero, A.H., 2018. Cosmetics and cosmeceutical applications of chitin, chitosan and their derivatives. Polymers. 2073-4360. 10 (2), 213. doi:10.3390/polym10020213.

Azuma, K., Osaki, T., Minami, S., Okamoto, Y., 2015. Anticancer and anti-inflammatory properties of chitin and chitosan oligosaccharides. J. Funct. Biomater. 2079-4983. 6 (1), 33–49. doi:10.3390/jfb6010033.

Balzano, M., Pacetti, D., Lucci, P., Fiorini, D., Frega, N.G., 2017. Bioactive fatty acids in mantis shrimp, crab and caramote prawn: their content and distribution among the main lipid classes. J. Food Compos. Anal. 08891575. 59, 88–94. Available from: http://www.elsevier.com/inca/publications/store/6/2/2/8/7/8/index.htt. doi:10.1016/j.jfca.2017.01.013.

Barh, D., Azevedo, V. (Eds.), 2018 . Omics Technologies and Bio-Engineering: towards Improving Quality of Life. In: Emerging Fields, Animal and Medical Biotechnologies. Academic Press, London, United Kingdom; San Diego, CA, United States, pp. 1–625. ISBN: 978-0-12-804659-3.

Barthel, W., Markwardt, F., 1975. Aggregation of blood platelets by Adrenaline and its uptake. Biochem. Pharmacol. 00062952. 24 (20), 1903–1904. doi:10.1016/0006-2952(75)90415-3.

Bergmann, W., Feeney, R.J., 1950. The isolation of a new thymine pentoside from sponges. J. Am. Chem. Soc. 15205126. 72 (6), 2809–2810. doi:10.1021/ja01162a543.

Bissett, D.L., 2006. Glucosamine: an ingredient with skin and other benefits. J. Cosmet. Dermatol. 14732165. 5 (4), 309–315. doi:10.1111/j.1473-2165.2006.00277.x.

Bjørklund, G., Gasmi, A., Lenchyk, L., Shanaida, M., Zafar, S., Mujawdiya, P.K., Lysiuk, R., Antonyak, H., Noor, S., Akram, M., Smetanina, K., Piscopo, S., Upyr, T., Peana, M., 2022. The role of astaxanthin as a nutraceutical in health and age-related conditions. Molecules. 1420-3049. 27 (21), 7167. doi:10.3390/molecules27217167.

Bouallegui, Y., 2021. A comprehensive review on crustaceans' immune system with a focus on freshwater crayfish in relation to crayfish plague disease. Front. Immunol. 1664-3224. 12. doi:10.3389/fimmu.2021.667787.

Brotosudarmo, T.H.P., Limantara, L., Setiyono, E., Heriyanto, 2020. Structures of astaxanthin and their consequences for therapeutic application. Int. J. Food Sci. 23145765. 2020. Available from: http://www.hindawi.com/journals/ijfs/. doi:10.1155/2020/2156582.

Brunt, E.G., Burgess, J.G., 2018. The promise of marine molecules as cosmetic active ingredients. Int. J. Cosmet. Sci. 0142-5463. 40 (1), 1–15. doi:10.1111/ics.12435.

Cahú, T.B., Santos, S.D., Mendes, A., Córdula, C.R., Chavante, S.F., Carvalho, L.B., Nader, H.B., Bezerra, R.S., 2012. Recovery of protein, chitin, carotenoids, and glycosaminoglycans from Pacific white shrimp (*Litopenaeus vannamei*) processing waste. Process Biochem. 13595113. 47 (4), 570–577. doi:10.1016/j.procbio.2011.12.012.

Camargo, T.R., Mantoan, P., Ramos, P., Monserrat, J.M., Prentice, C., Fernandes, C.C., Zambuzzi, W.F., Valenti, W.C., 2021. Bioactivity of the protein hydrolysates obtained from the most abundant crustacean bycatch. Mar. Biotechnol. 14362236. 23 (6), 881–891. Available from: http://link.springer.com/journal/volumesAndIssues/10126. doi:10.1007/s10126-021-10072-1.

Carrasqueira, J., Bernardino, S., Bernardino, R., Afonso, C., 2025. Marine-derived polysaccharides and their potential health benefits in nutraceutical applications. Mar. Drugs. 1660-3397. 23 (2), 60. doi:10.3390/md23020060.

Casadidio, C., Peregrina, D.V., Gigliobianco, M.R., Deng, S., Censi, R., Di Martino, P., 2019. Chitin and chitosans: characteristics, eco-friendly processes, and applications in cosmetic science. Mar. Drugs 16603397. 17 (6). Available from: https://www.mdpi.com/1660-3397/17/6/369/pdf. doi:10.3390/md17060369.

Chaiwong, N., Leelapornpisid, P., Jantanasakulwong, K., Rachtanapun, P., Seesuriyachan, P., Sakdatorn, V., Leksawasdi, N., Phimolsiripol, Y., 2020. Antioxidant and moisturizing properties of carboxymethyl chitosan with different molecular weights. Polymers. 2073-4360. 12 (7), 1445. doi:10.3390/polym12071445.

Chang, E.S., Mykles, D.L., 2011. Regulation of crustacean molting: a review and our perspectives. Gen. Comp. Endocrinol. 10956840. 172 (3), 323–330. Available from: http://www.sciencedirect.com/science/journal/00166480. doi:10.1016/j.ygcen.2011.04.003.

Chen, K., Guo, B., Luo, J., 2017. Quaternized carboxymethyl chitosan/organic montmorillonite nanocomposite as a novel cosmetic ingredient against skin aging. Carbohydr. Polym. 01448617. 173, 100–106. doi:10.1016/j.carbpol.2017.05.088.

Cheung, R., Tzi, N., Wong, J., Chan, w., 2015. Chitosan: an update on potential biomedical and pharmaceutical applications. Mar. Drugs. 1660-3397. 13 (8), 5156–5186. doi:10.3390/md13085156.

Chintong, S., Phatvej, W., Rerk-Am, U., Waiprib, Y., Klaypradit, W., 2019. In vitro antioxidant, antityrosinase, and cytotoxic activities of astaxanthin from shrimp waste. Antioxidants. 2076-3921. 8 (5), 128. doi:10.3390/antiox8050128.

Cholidis, P., Kranas, D., Chira, A., Galouni, E.A., Adamantidi, T., Anastasiadou, C., Tsoupras, A., 2024. Shrimp lipid bioactives with anti-inflammatory, antithrombotic, and antioxidant health-promoting properties for cardio-protection. Mar. Drugs 16603397. 22 (12). Available from: http://www.mdpi.com/journal/marinedrugs. doi:10.3390/md22120554.

Chou, H.Y., Lee, C., Pan, J.L., Wen, Z.H., Huang, S.H., Lan, C.W.J., Liu, W.T., Hour, T.C., Hseu, Y.C., Hwang, B.H., Cheng, K.C., Wang, H.M.D., 2016. Enriched astaxanthin extract from haematococcus pluvialis augments growth factor secretions to increase cell proliferation and induces MMP1 degradation to enhance collagen production in human dermal fibroblasts. Int. J. Mol. Sci. 14220067. 17 (6). Available from: http://www.mdpi.com/1422-0067/17/6/955/pdf. doi:10.3390/ijms17060955.

Csuka, D.A., Csuka, E.A., Juhász, M.L.W., Sharma, A.N., Mesinkovska, N.A., 2023. A systematic review on the lipid composition of human hair. Int. J. Dermatol. 13654632. 62 (3), 404–415. Available from: http://onlinelibrary.wiley.com/journal/10.1111/(ISSN)1365-4632. doi:10.1111/ijd.16109.

de Carvalho, C.C.C.R., Caramujo, M.J., 2017. Carotenoids in aquatic ecosystems and aquaculture: a colorful business with implications for human health. Front. Mar. Sci. 22967745. 4. Available from: http://journal.frontiersin.org/article/10.3389/fmars.2017.00093/full. doi:10.3389/fmars.2017.00093.

Deng, L., Wang, B., Wenying, L., Han, Z., Chen, S., Wang, H., 2022. Bacterial cellulose reinforced chitosan-based hydrogel with highly efficient self-healing and enhanced antibacterial activity for wound healing. Int. J. Biol. Macromol. 01418130. 217, 77–87. doi:10.1016/j.ijbiomac.2022.07.017.

Diarte-Plata, G., Escamilla-Montes, R. (Eds.), 2020. Crustacea. IntechOpen, Erscheinungsort nicht ermittelbar, 978-1-78985-629-3.

Díaz-Santana-Iturrios, M., Zepeda-Benitez, V., Pacheco-Ovando, R., Cornejo, C.F., Cerda, J.M., Salinas-Zavala, C.A., Granados-Amores, J., 2022. Northeastern pacific octopus beak shape for species-level detection. Malacologia 00762997. 64 (2), 169–184. Available from: http://www.bioone.org/loi/mala. doi:10.4002/040.064.0202.

E Silva, D., Karla, D., Penha, R., Maristela, A., Angela, C., Thaís, P., de Sousa Jr., F., de Assis, C., 2021. Chemical characteristics and antioxidant activity of astaxanthin extracted from shrimp residues using soybean oil. J. Braz. Chem. Soc. 01035053. 32 (6). doi:10.21577/0103-5053.20210030.

Eduardo Rebolledo Ranz, R. (Ed.), 2021. Arthropods - are They Beneficial for Mankind? IntechOpen, 978-1-78984-165-7.

Ermolenko, E., Sikorskaya, T., Grigorchuk, V., 2023. Crabs *Eriocheir japonica* and *Paralithodes camtschaticus* are a rich source of lipid molecular species with high nutritional value. Foods. 2304-8158. 12 (18), 3359. doi:10.3390/foods12183359.

Fakhri, S., Abbaszadeh, F., Dargahi, L., Jorjani, M., 2018. Astaxanthin: a mechanistic review on its biological activities and health benefits. Pharmacol. Res. 10436618. 136, 1–20. doi:10.1016/j.phrs.2018.08.012.

Fang, S., Huang, B., Liu, J., 2018. The carotenoids of shrimps (Decapoda: Caridea and Dendrobranchiata) cultured in China. J. Crustac. Biol. 0278-0372. 38 (5), 523–530. doi:10.1093/jcbiol/ruy049.

Fernández-Peña, L., Guzmán, E., 2020. Physicochemical aspects of the performance of hair-conditioning formulations. Cosmetics. 2079-9284. 7 (2), 26. doi:10.3390/cosmetics7020026.

Ferreira, M.S., Resende, D.I.S.P., Lobo, J.M.S., Sousa, E., Almeida, I.F., 2021. Marine ingredients for sensitive skin: market overview. Mar. Drugs 16603397. 19 (8). Available from: https://www.mdpi.com/1660-3397/19/8/464/pdf. doi:10.3390/MD19080464.

Fonseca, S., Amaral, M.N., Reis, C.P., Custódio, L., 2023. Marine natural products as innovative cosmetic ingredients. Mar. Drugs 16603397. 21 (3). Available from: http://www.mdpi.com/journal/marinedrugs. doi:10.3390/md21030170.

Galliard, T., Phillips, D.R., Matthew, J.A., 1975. Enzymic reactions of fatty acid hydroperoxides in extracts of potato tuber II. Conversion of 9- and 13-hydroperoxy-octadecadienoic acids to monohydroxydienoic acid, epoxyhydroxy- and trihydroxymonoenoic acid derivatives. Biochim. Biophys. Acta Lipids Lipid Metab. 00052760. 409 (2), 157–171. doi:10.1016/0005-2760(75)90151-4.

Ganguly, A., Ian, C.K., Sheshala, R., Sahu, P.S., Al-Waeli, H., Meka, V.S., 2017. Application of diverse natural polymers in the design of oral gels for the treatment of periodontal diseases. J. Mater. Sci. Mater. Med. 15734838. 28 (3). Available from: https://www.wkap.nl/journalhome.htm/0957-4530. doi:10.1007/s10856-017-5852-4.

Gao, H., Nan, W., Wang, N., Jie, L., Sun, J., Peng, Q., 2022. Chitosan-based therapeutic systems and their potentials in treatment of oral diseases. Int. J. Biol. Macromol. 01418130. 222 (Pt B), 3178–3194. doi:10.1016/j.ijbiomac.2022.10.090.

Gbenebor, O.P., Adeosun, S.O., Lawal, G.I., Jun, S., 2016. Role of $CaCO_3$ in the physicochemical properties of crustacean-sourced structural polysaccharides. Mater. Chem. Phys. 02540584. 184, 203–209. doi:10.1016/j.matchemphys.2016.09.043.

Genodepa, J.G., 2015. Digestive Enzyme Dynamics during Early Life Stages of the Mud Crab, *Scylla serrata* and the Spiny Lobster, *Panulirus ornatus*, James Cook University.

Ghannoum, M.A., Long, L., Isham, N., Bulgheroni, A., Setaro, M., Caserini, M., Palmieri, R., Mailland, F., 2015. Ability of hydroxypropyl chitosan nail lacquer to protect against dermatophyte nail infection. Antimicrob. Agents Chemother. 0066-4804. 59 (4), 1844–1848. doi:10.1128/aac.04842-14.

Ghareeb, M.A., Tammam, M.A., El-Demerdash, A., Atanasov, A.G., 2020. Insights about clinically approved and Preclinically investigated marine natural products. Curr. Res. Biotechnol. 25902628. 2, 88–102. Available from: https://www.journals.elsevier.com/current-research-in-biotechnology/. doi:10.1016/j.crbiot.2020.09.001.

Gómez-Guillén, M.C., Montero, P., López-Caballero, M.E., Baccan, G.C., Gómez-Estaca, J., 2018. Bioactive and technological functionality of a lipid extract from shrimp (*L. vannamei*) cephalothorax. LWT. 00236438. 89, 704–711. doi:10.1016/j.lwt.2017.11.052.

Gromkowska-Kępka, K.J., Puścion-Jakubik, A., Markiewicz-Żukowska, R., Socha, K., 2021. The impact of ultraviolet radiation on skin photoaging — review of in vitro studies. J. Cosmet. Dermatol. 14732165. 20 (11), 3427–3431. Available from: http://onlinelibrary.wiley.com/journal/10.1111/(ISSN)1473-2165. doi:10.1111/jocd.14033.

Guan, F., Han, Y., Yan, K., Zhang, Y., Zhang, Z., Ningfeng, W., Tian, J., 2020. Highly efficient production of chitooligosaccharides by enzymes mined directly from the marine metagenome. Carbohydr. Polym. 01448617. 234, 115909. doi:10.1016/j.carbpol.2020.115909.

Guzmán, E., Ortega, F., Rubio, R.G., 2022. Chitosan: a promising multifunctional cosmetic ingredient for skin and hair care. Cosmetics. 2079-9284. 9 (5), 99. doi:10.3390/cosmetics9050099.

Hama, S., Takahashi, K., Inai, Y., Shiota, K., Sakamoto, R., Yamada, A., Tsuchiya, H., Kanamura, K., Yamashita, E., Kogure, K., 2012. Protective effects of topical application of a poorly soluble antioxidant astaxanthin liposomal formulation on ultraviolet-induced skin damage. J. Pharm. Sci. 00223549. 101 (8), 2909–2916. doi:10.1002/jps.23216.

Hamdi, S.A.H., Ghonaim, G.M., Sayed, R.R.E., Rodríguez-Couto, S., El-Ghany, M.N.A., 2024. Bioprocess of astaxanthin extraction from shrimp waste via the common microorganisms Saccharomyces cerevisiae and Lactobacillus acidophilus in comparison to the chemical method. Biomass Convers. Biorefin. 21906823. 14 (7), 8333–8339. Available from: https://www.springer.com/journal/13399. doi:10.1007/s13399-022-02984-2.

Hamed, I., Özogul, F., Regenstein, J.M., 2016. Industrial applications of crustacean by-products (chitin, chitosan, and chitooligosaccharides): a review. Trends Food Sci. Technol. 09242244. 48, 40–50. Available from: http://www.elsevier.com/wps/find/journaldescription.cws_home/601278/description#description. doi:10.1016/j.tifs.2015.11.007.

Hatchett, C., 1799. XVIII. Experiments and observations on shell and bone. Philos. Trans. R. Soc. Lond. 0261-0523. 89, 315–334. doi:10.1098/rstl.1799.0019.

Hendrickx, M.E., 1996. Habitats and biodiversity of decapod crustaceans in the SE Gulf of California, México. Rev. Biol. Trop. 44 (2), 603–617.

Hesse, G.W., 1979. Chronic zinc deficiency alters neuronal function of hippocampal mossy fibers. Science. 00368075. 205 (4410), 1005–1007. doi:10.1126/science.224456.

Higuera-Ciapara, I., Félix-Valenzuela, L., Goycoolea, F.M., 2006. Astaxanthin: a review of its chemistry and applications. Crit. Rev. Food Sci. Nutr. 1040-8398. 46 (2), 185–196. doi:10.1080/10408690590957188.

Hiransuchalert, R., Oonwiset, N., Imarom, Y., Chindudsadeegul, P., Laongmanee, P., Arnupapboon, S., 2021. Extraction and characterization of pepsin-soluble collagen from different mantis shrimp species. Fish. Aquat. Sci. 2234-1757. 24 (12), 406–414. doi:10.47853/fas.2021.e42.

Hossain, A., Shahidi, F., 2024. Upcycling shellfish waste: distribution of amino acids, minerals, and carotenoids in body parts of North Atlantic crab and shrimp. Foods. 2304-8158. 13 (17), 2700. doi:10.3390/foods13172700.

Ifuku, S., Nogi, M., Abe, K., Yoshioka, M., Morimoto, M., Saimoto, H., Yano, H., 2009. Preparation of chitin nanofibers with a uniform width as α-chitin from crab shells. Biomacromolecules. 1525-7797. 10 (6), 1584–1588. doi:10.1021/bm900163d.

Ito, I., Yoneda, T., Omura, Y., Osaki, T., Ifuku, S., Saimoto, H., Azuma, K., Imagawa, T., Tsuka, T., Murahata, Y., Ito, N., Okamoto, Y., Minami, S., 2015. Protective effect of chitin urocanate nanofibers against ultraviolet radiation. Mar. Drugs. 1660-3397. 13 (12), 7463–7475. doi:10.3390/md13127076.

Jae-Young, J., Park, P.-J., Kim, B., Kim, S.-K., 2006. Antihypertensive activity of chitin derivatives. Biopolymers. 0006-3525. 83 (3), 250–254. doi:10.1002/bip.20553.

Jia, M., Yang, L., Yang, X., Huang, Y., Hongjie, W., Huang, Y., Lin, J., Yanxiu, L., Hou, Z., Zhang, Q., 2014. Development of both methotrexate and mitomycin C loaded PEGylated chitosan nanoparticles for targeted drug codelivery and synergistic anticancer effect. ACS Appl. Mater. Interfaces. 1944-8244. 6 (14), 11413–11423. doi:10.1021/am501932s.

Jinjing, M., Chu, D., Rakhimovna, V.N., Wang, P., Zhu, S., Xie, H., Liu, Q., Yin, H., 2025. Efficient and green extraction of chitin from mantis shrimp shell using deep eutectic solvents at room temperature. Bioresour. Technol. 09608524. 435, 132888. doi:10.1016/j.biortech.2025.132888.

Jinxia, H., Weihang, L., Mei, L., Wang, Y., Ding, R., Wang, L., 2019. Extraction and purification of astaxanthin from shrimp shells and the effects of different treatments on its content. Rev. Bras. Farmacogn. 0102695X. 29 (1), 24–29. doi:10.1016/j.bjp.2018.11.004.

Jormalainen, V., 1998. Precopulatory mate guarding in crustaceans: male competitive strategy and intersexual conflict. Q. Rev. Biol. 0033-5770. 73 (3), 275–304. doi:10.1086/420306.

Kalita, P., Ahmed, A.B., Sen, S., Chakraborty, R., 2022. A comprehensive review on polysaccharides with hypolipidemic activity: occurrence, chemistry and molecular mechanism. Int. J. Biol. Macromol. 18790003. 206, 681–698. Available from: https://www.elsevier.com/locate/ijbiomac. doi:10.1016/j.ijbiomac.2022.02.189.

Kenny, N., Sin, Y., Shen, X., Zhe, Q., Wang, W., Chan, T., Tobe, S., Shimeld, S., Chu, K., Hui, J., 2014. Genomic sequence and experimental tractability of a new decapod shrimp model, *Neocaridina denticulata*. Mar. Drugs. 1660-3397. 12 (3), 1419–1437. doi:10.3390/md12031419.

Kim, S.-K., 2014. Marine Carbohydrates: Fundamentals and Application; Advances in Food and Nutrition Research. Elsevier Academic Press, London San Diego, CA, 978-0-12-800268-1.

Klinger, C., ółtowska-Aksamitowska, S.Z., Wysokowski, M., Tsurkan, M.V., Galli, R., Petrenko, I., Machałowski, T., Ereskovsky, A., Martinović, R., Muzychka, L., Smolii, O.B., Bechmann, N., Ivanenko, V., Schupp, P.J., Jesionowski, T., Giovine, M., Joseph, Y., Bornstein, S.R., Voronkina, A., Ehrlich, H., 2019. Express method for isolation of ready-to-use 3D chitin scaffolds from *Aplysina archeri* (aplysineidae: verongiida) demosponge. Mar. Drugs 16603397. 17 (2). Available from: https://www.mdpi.com/1660-3397/17/2/131/pdf. doi:10.3390/md17020131.

Kodali, D., Hembrick-Holloman, V., Gunturu, D.R., Samuel, T., Jeelani, S., Rangari, V.K., 2022. Influence of fish scale-based hydroxyapatite on forcespun polycaprolactone fiber scaffolds. ACS Omega 24701343. 7 (10), 8323–8335. Available from: https://pubs.acs.org/journal/acsodf. doi:10.1021/acsomega.1c05593.

Kong, S.Z., Li, J.C., Li, S.D., Liao, M.N., Li, C.P., Zheng, P.J., Guo, M.H., Tan, W.X., Zheng, Z.H., Hu, Z., 2018. Anti-aging effect of chitosan oligosaccharide on d-galactose-induced subacute aging in mice. Mar. Drugs 16603397. 16 (6). Available from: http://www.mdpi.com/1660-3397/16/6/181/pdf. doi:10.3390/md16060181.

Kroeger, H., Donner, I., Skiello, G., 1975. Influence of a new virostatic compound on the induction of enzymes in rat liver. Arzneim.-Forsch. 25 (9), 1426–1429.

Kulkarni, A., Krishnan, S., Anand, D., Uthaman, S.K., Otta, S.K., Karunasagar, I., Valappil, R.K., 2021. Immune responses and immunoprotection in crustaceans with special reference to shrimp. Rev. Aquac. 17535131. 13 (1), 431–459. Available from: http://onlinelibrary.wiley.com/journal/10.1111/(ISSN)1753-5131. doi:10.1111/raq.12482.

Kumar, M.N.V.R., 2000. A review of chitin and chitosan applications. React. Funct. Polym. 13815148. 46 (1), 1–27. doi:10.1016/S1381-5148(00)00038-9.

Lai-Cheong, J.E., McGrath, J.A., 2021. Structure and function of skin, hair and nails. Medicine (United Kingdom) 13654357. 49 (6), 337–342. Available from: http://www.elsevier.com/wps/find/journaldescription.cws_home/709606/description#description. doi:10.1016/j.mpmed.2021.03.001.

Li, X., Li, C., Zhu, Y., Shi, Y., Zhang, X., Zhang, S., Wang, L., Lin, H., Hou, H., Hsiao, C.D., Han, L., Liu, K., 2020. Lipid fingerprinting of different material sources by UPLC-Q-Exactive Orbitrap/MS approach and their zebrafish-based activities comparison. J. Agric. Food Chem. 15205118. 68 (7), 2007–2015. Available from: http://pubs.acs.org/journal/jafcau. doi:10.1021/acs.jafc.9b06132.

Lima, S.G.M., Freire, M.C.L.C., Oliveira, V.D.S., Solisio, C., Converti, A., de Lima, Á.A.N., 2021. Astaxanthin delivery systems for skin application: a review. Mar. Drugs 16603397. 19 (9). Available from: https://www.mdpi.com/1660-3397/19/9/511. doi:10.3390/MD19090511.

Liu, Y., Mao, J., Guo, Z., Yufang, H., Wang, S., 2022. Polyvinyl alcohol/carboxymethyl chitosan hydrogel loaded with silver nanoparticles exhibited antibacterial and self-healing properties. Int. J. Biol. Macromol. 01418130. 220, 211–222. doi:10.1016/j.ijbiomac.2022.08.061.

Londono-Zuluaga, C., Jameel, H., Gonzalez, R.W., Lucia, L., 2019. Crustacean shell-based biosorption water remediation platforms: status and perspectives. J. Environ. Manag. 10958630. 231, 757–762. Available from: https://www.sciencedirect.com/science/journal/03014797. doi:10.1016/j.jenvman.2018.10.096.

Lu, W.Y., Li, H.J., Li, Q.Y., Wu, Y.C., 2021. Application of marine natural products in drug research. Bioorg. Med. Chem. 14643391. 35. Available from: http://www.journals.elsevier.com/bioorganic-and-medicinal-chemistry/. doi:10.1016/j.bmc.2021.116058.

Maasri, A., Thorp, J.H., 2024. Identification and Ecology of Freshwater Arthropods in the Mediterranean Basin. Elsevier, Amsterdam, 978-0-12-821844-0.

Makar, A.B., McMartin, K.E., Palese, M., Tephly, T.R., 1975. Formate assay in body fluids: application in methanol poisoning. Biochem. Med. 00062944. 13 (2), 117–126. doi:10.1016/0006-2944(75)90147-7.

Marniemi, J., Parkki, M.G., 1975. Radiochemical assay of glutathione S-epoxide transferase and its enhancement by phenobarbital in rat liver in vivo. Biochem. Pharmacol. 00062952. 24 (17), 1569–1572. doi:10.1016/0006-2952(75)90080-5.

Marques, I., Botelho, G., Guiné, R., 2019. Comparative study on nutritional composition of fish available in Portugal. Nutr. Food Sci. 0034-6659. 49 (5), 925–941. doi:10.1108/nfs-11-2018-0311.

Martins, E., Castro, P., Ribeiro, A.B., Pereira, C.F., Casanova, F., Vilarinho, R., Moreira, J., Ramos, Ó.L., 2024. Bleached hair as standard template to insight the performance of commercial hair repair products. Cosmetics 20799284. 11 (5). Available from: https://www.mdpi.com/journal/cosmetics. doi:10.3390/cosmetics11050150.

McMahon, B.R., 2001. Control of cardiovascular function and its evolution in crustacea. Can. J. Exp. Biol. 00220949. 204 (5), 923–932. Available from: https://journals.biologists.com/jeb/. doi:10.1242/jeb.204.5.923.

Mechri, S., Sellem, I., Bouacem, K., Jabeur, F., Chamkha, M., Hacene, H., Bouanane-Darenfed, A., Jaouadi, B., 2020. Antioxidant and enzyme inhibitory activities of *Metapenaeus monoceros* by-product hydrolysates elaborated by purified alkaline proteases. Waste Biomass Valorization. 1877-2641. 11 (12), 6741–6755. doi:10.1007/s12649-020-00942-5.

Melton, L.D., Shahidi, F., Varelis, P. (Eds.), 2019. Encyclopedia of Food Chemistry. Elsevier, Amsterdam, Netherlands ; Oxford, United Kingdom ; Cambridge, MA, 978-0-12-814045-1.

Messina, C.M., Manuguerra, S., Renda, G., Santulli, A., 2019. Biotechnological applications for the sustainable use of marine by-products: in vitro antioxidant and pro-apoptotic effects of astaxanthin extracted with supercritical CO_2 from *Parapeneus longirostris*. Mar. Biotechnol. 14362236. 21 (4), 565–576. Available from: http://link.springer.com/journal/volumesAndIssues/10126. doi:10.1007/s10126-019-09904-y.

Mohamed, A.E., Elgammal, W.E., Ibrahim, A.G., Dawaba, H.M., Nossier, E.S., Dawaba, A.M., 2025. Thiadiazole chitosan conjugates as a novel cosmetic ingredient for rinse-off hair conditioners: design, formulation, characterization and in silico-molecular docking studies. BMC Chem. 2661801X. 19 (1). Available from: https://bmcchem.biomedcentral.com/. doi:10.1186/s13065-025-01404-6.

Monti, D., Tampucci, S., Paganini, V., Burgalassi, S., Chetoni, P., Galván, J., Celandroni, F., Ghelardi, E., 2022. Ciclopirox hydroxypropyl chitosan (CPX-HPCH) nail lacquer and breathable cosmetic nail polish: in vitro evaluation of drug transungual permeation following the combined application. Life. 2075-1729. 12 (6), 801. doi:10.3390/life12060801.

Morganti, P., Morganti, G., Coltelli, M.B., 2021. Smart and sustainable hair products based on chitin-derived compounds. Cosmetics 20799284. 8 (1). Available from: https://www.mdpi.com/2079-9284/8/1/20. doi:10.3390/cosmetics8010020.

Morganti, P., Palombo, M., Carezzi, F., Nunziata, M., Morganti, G., Cardillo, M., Chianese, A., 2016. Green nanotechnology serving the bioeconomy: natural beauty masks to save the environment. Cosmetics. 2079-9284. 3 (4), 41. doi:10.3390/cosmetics3040041.

Morganti, P., Palombo, M., Tishchenko, G., Yudin, V., Guarneri, F., Cardillo, M., Ciotto, P.D., Carezzi, F., Morganti, G., Fabrizi, G., 2014. Chitin-hyaluronan nanoparticles: a multifunctional carrier to deliver anti-aging active ingredients through the skin. Cosmetics. 2079-9284. 1 (3), 140–158. doi:10.3390/cosmetics1030140.

Morin-Crini, N., Lichtfouse, E., Torri, G., Crini, G., 2019. Applications of chitosan in food, pharmaceuticals, medicine, cosmetics, agriculture, textiles, pulp and paper, biotechnology, and environmental chemistry. Environ. Chem. Lett. 1610-3653. 17 (4), 1667–1692. doi:10.1007/s10311-019-00904-x.

Morsy, R., Ali, S.S., El-Shetehy, M., 2017. Development of hydroxyapatite-chitosan gel sunscreen combating clinical multidrug-resistant bacteria. J. Mol. Struct. 00222860. 1143, 251–258. Available from: https://www.elsevier.com/inca/publications/store/5/0/0/8/5/0/index.htt. doi:10.1016/j.molstruc.2017.04.090.

Nagasawa, H., 2012. The crustacean cuticle structure composition and mineralization. Front. Biosci. 1945-0494. E4 (2), 711–720. doi:10.2741/e412.

Nguyen, S., Escudero, C., Sediqi, N., Smistad, G., Hiorth, M., 2017a. Fluoride loaded polymeric nanoparticles for dental delivery. Eur. J. Pharm. Sci. 09280987. 104, 326–334. doi:10.1016/j.ejps.2017.04.004.

Nguyen, T.T., Barber, A.R., Corbin, K., Zhang, W., 2017b. Lobster processing by-products as valuable bioresource of marine functional ingredients, nutraceuticals, and pharmaceuticals. Bioresour. Bioprocess. 21974365. 4 (1). Available from: https://bioresourcesbioprocessing.springeropen.com. doi:10.1186/s40643-017-0157-5.

Nguyen, T.T., Hoang, T., Pham, T., Truong, V.K., Luo, X., Qin, J., Zhang, W., 2023. High solubility and bioavailability of lobster shell-derived calcium for significantly proliferating bone and skin cells in vitro. Mar. Drugs 16603397. 21 (6). Available from: http://www.mdpi.com/journal/marinedrugs. doi:10.3390/md21060358.

Nishida, Y., Berg, P., Shakersain, B., Hecht, K., Takikawa, A., Tao, R., Kakuta, Y., Uragami, C., Hashimoto, H., Misawa, N., Maoka, T., 2023. Astaxanthin: past, present, and future. Mar. Drugs. 1660-3397. 21 (10), 514. doi:10.3390/md21100514.

Nitulescu, G., Lupuliasa, D., Adam-Dima, I., Nitulescu, G.M., 2023. Ultraviolet filters for cosmetic applications. Cosmetics 20799284. 10 (4). Available from: https://www.mdpi.com/journal/cosmetics. doi:10.3390/cosmetics10040101.

Niu, T., Xuan, R., Jiang, L., Wei, W., Zhen, Z., Song, Y., Hong, L., Zheng, K., Zhang, J., Qingshan, X., Tan, Y., Yan, X., Chen, H., 2018. Astaxanthin induces the Nrf2/HO-1 antioxidant pathway in human umbilical vein endothelial cells by generating trace amounts of ROS. J. Agric. Food Chem. 0021-8561. 66 (6), 1551–1559. doi:10.1021/acs.jafc.7b05493.

Ntohogian, S., Gavriliadou, V., Christodoulou, E., Nanaki, S., Lykidou, S., Naidis, P., Mischopoulou, L., Barmpalexis, P., Nikolaidis, N., Bikiaris, D.N., 2018. Chitosan nanoparticles with encapsulated natural and UF-purified annatto and saffron for the preparation of UV protective cosmetic emulsions. Molecules. 1420-3049. 23 (9), 2107. doi:10.3390/molecules23092107.

Nugroho Susanto, G., 2021. Crustacea: the increasing economic importance of crustaceans to humans. In: Eduardo Rebolledo Ranz, R. (Ed.), Arthropods - Are They Beneficial for Mankind? IntechOpen. ISBN: 978-1-78984-166-4. doi:10.5772/intechopen.96255.

Nunes, A.N., Roda, A., Gouveia, L.F., Fernández, N., Bronze, M.R., Matias, A.A., 2021. Astaxanthin extraction from marine crustacean waste streams: an integrated approach between microwaves and supercritical fluids. ACS Sustain. Chem. Eng. 21680485. 9 (8), 3050–3059. Available from: http://pubs.acs.org/journal/ascecg. doi:10.1021/acssuschemeng.0c06534.

Oliver, J.M., Ross, E.L., Frank, E.K., 1994. The discovery of marine natural products with therapeutic potential. In: Gullo, V.P. (Ed.), Discovery of Novel Natural Products with Therapeutic Potential. Elsevier, pp. 109–174. ISBN: 978-0-7506-9003-4.

Palmieri, R., Cantoresi, F., Caserini, M., Bidoli, A., Maggio, F., Marino, R., Carnevale, C., Sorgi, P., 2014. Randomized controlled trial of a water-soluble nail lacquer based on hydroxypropyl-chitosan (HPCH), in the management of nail psoriasis. Clin. Cosmet. Investig. Dermatol.. 1178-7015. 7, 185. doi:10.2147/CCID.S61659.

Papadopoulou, S.N.A., Adamantidi, T., Kranas, D., Cholidis, P., Anastasiadou, C., Tsoupras, A., 2025. A comprehensive review on the valorization of bioactives from marine animal by-products for health-promoting biofunctional cosmetics. Mar. Drugs 16603397. 23 (8). Available from: https://www.mdpi.com/journal/marinedrugs. doi:10.3390/md23080299.

Piccirillo, C., Rocha, C., Tobaldi, D.M., Pullar, R.C., Labrincha, J.A., Ferreira, M.O., Castro, P.M.L., Pintado, M.M.E., 2014. A hydroxyapatite–Fe_2O_3 based material of natural origin as an active sunscreen filter. J. Mater. Chem. B. 2050-750X. 2 (36), 5999–6009. doi:10.1039/C4TB00984C.

Prajaputra, V., Isnaini, N., Maryam, S., Ernawati, E., Deliana, F., Haridhi, H.A., Fadli, N., Karina, S., Agustina, S., Nurfadillah, N., Arisa, I.I., Desiyana, L.S., Bakri, T.K., 2024. Exploring marine collagen: sustainable sourcing, extraction methods, and cosmetic applications. S. Afr. J. Chem. Eng. 10269185. 47, 197–211. Available from: https://www.journals.elsevier.com/south-african-journal-of-chemical-engineering/. doi:10.1016/j.sajce.2023.11.006.

Priyanka, D.N., Prashanth, K.V.H., Tharanathan, R.N., 2022. A review on potential anti-diabetic mechanisms of chitosan and its derivatives. Carbohydr. Polym. Technol. Appl. 26668939. 3, 100188. doi:10.1016/j.carpta.2022.100188.

Qiu, D., Yue-Chan, W., Zhu, W., Yin, H., Long-Tao, Y., 2012. Identification of geometrical isomers and comparison of different isomeric samples of astaxanthin. J. Food Sci. 0022-1147. 77 (9). doi:10.1111/j.1750-3841.2012.02842.x.

Rafatullah, M., Siddiqui, M.R., Khan, M.A., Kapoor, R.T. (Eds.), 2024. Multidisciplinary Applications of Marine Resources: A Step Towards Green and Sustainable Future. Springer Nature Singapore, Singapore, 978-981-97-5056-6.

Rahman, A. (Ed.), 1988. Studies in Natural Products Chemistry. Elsevier, Amsterdam ; New York, 978-0-444-42970-4.

Rajoka, M.S.R., Mehwish, H.M., Wu, Y., Zhao, L., Arfat, Y., Majeed, K., Anwaar, S., 2020. Chitin/chitosan derivatives and their interactions with microorganisms: a comprehensive review and future perspectives. Crit. Rev. Biotechnol. 15497801. 40 (3), 365–379. Available from: http://www.tandfonline.com/loi/ibty20. doi:10.1080/07388551.2020.1713719.

Rejinold, N.S., Choi, G., Choy, J.H., 2021. Chitosan hybrids for cosmeceutical applications in skin, hair and dental care: an update. Emerg. Mater. 2522574X. 4 (5), 1125–1142. Available from: https://springer.com/journal/42247. doi:10.1007/s42247-021-00280-9.

Rotter, A., Varamogianni-Mamatsi, D., Pobirk, A.Z., Matjaž, M.G., Cueto, M., Díaz-Marrero, A.R., Jónsdóttir, R., Sveinsdóttir, K., Catalá, T.S., Romano, G., Guler, B.A., Atak, E., Zrimec, M.B., Bosch, D., Deniz, I., Gaudêncio, S.P., Grigalionyte-Bembič, E., Klun, K., Zidar, L., Rius, A.C., Baebler, Š., Lukić Bilela, L., Rinkevich, B., Mandalakis, M., 2024. Marine cosmetics and the blue bioeconomy: from sourcing to success stories. iScience 25890042. 27 (12). Available from: https://www.sciencedirect.com/science/journal/25890042. doi:10.1016/j.isci.2024.111339.

Sachindra, N.M., Mahendrakar, N.S., 2005. Process optimization for extraction of carotenoids from shrimp waste with vegetable oils. Bioresour. Technol. 09608524. 96 (10), 1195–1200. doi:10.1016/j.biortech.2004.09.018.

Saini, R.K., Keum, Y.S., 2018. Carotenoid extraction methods: a review of recent developments. Food Chem. 18737072. 240, 90–103. Available from: https://www.elsevier.com/locate/foodchem. doi:10.1016/j.foodchem.2017.07.099.

Saini, R.K., Nile, S.H., Park, S.W., 2015. Carotenoids from fruits and vegetables: chemistry, analysis, occurrence, bioavailability and biological activities. Food Res. Int. 09639969. 76, 735–750. Available from: https://www.elsevier.com/inca/publications/store/4/2/2/9/7/0. doi:10.1016/j.foodres.2015.07.047.

Sajith, M.P., Pitchai, A., Ramasamy, P., 2024. Anticoagulant protective effects of sulfated chitosan derived from the internal bone of spineless cuttlefish (*Sepiella inermis*). Cureus. 2168-8184. 16 (7). doi:10.7759/cureus.64558.

Samiraninezhad, N., Asadi, K., Rezazadeh, H., Gholami, A., 2023. Using chitosan, hyaluronic acid, alginate, and gelatin-based smart biological hydrogels for drug delivery in oral mucosal lesions: a review. Int. J. Biol. Macromol. 01418130. 252, 126573. doi:10.1016/j.ijbiomac.2023.126573.

Sánchez-Camargo, A.P., Meireles, M.A.A., Lopes, B.L.F., Cabral, F.A., 2011. Proximate composition and extraction of carotenoids and lipids from Brazilian redspotted shrimp waste (Farfantepenaeus paulensis). J. Food Eng. 02608774. 102 (1), 87–93. doi:10.1016/j.jfoodeng.2010.08.008.

Sangsuriyawong, A., Limpawattana, M., Siriwan, D., Klaypradit, W., 2019. Properties and bioavailability assessment of shrimp astaxanthin loaded liposomes. Food Sci. Biotechnol. 1226-7708. 28 (2), 529–537. doi:10.1007/s10068-018-0495-x.

Shuang, L., Xie, S., Liang, Y., Long, X., Liangbin, H., Hongbo, L., Haizhen, M., 2022. Comprehensive lipidomic analysis of the lipids extracted from freshwater fish bones and crustacean shells. Food Sci. Nutr. 2048-7177. 10 (3), 723–730. doi:10.1002/fsn3.2698.

Siahaan, E.A., Agusman, R.P., Shin, K.H., Kim, S.K., 2022. Potential cosmetic active ingredients derived from marine by-products. Mar. Drugs 16603397. 20 (12). Available from: http://www.mdpi.com/journal/marinedrugs. doi:10.3390/md20120734.

Silva, I.M.V., Machado, F., Moreno, M.J., Nunes, C., Coimbra, M.A., Coreta-Gomes, F., 2021. Polysaccharide structures and their hypocholesterolemic potential. Molecules 14203049. 26 (15). Available from: https://www.mdpi.com/1420-3049/26/15/4559/pdf. doi:10.3390/molecules26154559.

Silvestre, J., Delattre, C., Michaud, P., de Baynast, H., 2021. Optimization of chitosan properties with the aim of a water resistant adhesive development. Polymers. 2073-4360. 13 (22), 4031. doi:10.3390/polym13224031.

Šimat, V., Rathod, N., Čagalj, M., Hamed, I., Mekinić, I.G., 2022. Astaxanthin from crustaceans and their byproducts: a bioactive metabolite candidate for therapeutic application. Mar. Drugs. 1660-3397. 20 (3), 206. doi:10.3390/md20030206.

Sionkowska, A., Kaczmarek, B., Michalska, M., Lewandowska, K., Grabska, S., 2017. Preparation and characterization of collagen/chitosan/hyaluronic acid thin films for application in hair care cosmetics. Pure Appl. Chem. 1365-3075. 89 (12), 1829–1839. doi:10.1515/pac-2017-0314.

Steven, R., Humaira, Z., Natanael, Y., Dwivany, F.M., Trinugroho, J.P., Dwijayanti, A., Kristianti, T., Tallei, T.E., Emran, T.B., Jeon, H., Alhumaydhi, F.A., Radjasa, O.K., Kim, B., 2022. Marine microbial-derived resource exploration: uncovering the hidden potential of marine carotenoids. Mar. Drugs 16603397. 20 (6). Available from: https://www.mdpi.com/1660-3397/20/6/352/pdf?version=1653559838. doi:10.3390/md20060352.

Suresh, P.V., Kudre, T.G., Johny, L.C., 2018. Sustainable valorization of seafood processing by-product/discard. In: Singhania, R.R., Agarwal, R.A., Kumar, R.P., Sukumaran, R.K. (Eds.), Waste to Wealth (Energy, Environment, and Sustainability). Springer Singapore, Singapore, pp. 111–139, 978-981-10-7430-1.

Tangkijngamvong, N., Phaiyarin, P., Wanichwecharungruang, S., Kumtornrut, C., 2020. The anti-sebum property of chitosan particles. J. Cosmet. Dermatol. 1473-2130. 19 (8), 2135–2140. doi:10.1111/jocd.13274.

Terkula Iber, B., Kasan, N.A., Torsabo, D., Omuwa, J.W., 2022. A review of various sources of chitin and chitosan in nature. J. Renew. Mater. 2164-6341. 10 (4), 1097–1123. doi:10.32604/jrm.2022.018142.

Theerawattanawit, C., Phaiyarin, P., Wanichwecharungruang, S., Noppakun, N., Asawanonda, P., Kumtornrut, C., 2022. The efficacy and safety of chitosan on facial skin sebum. Skin Pharmacol. Physiol. 1660-5527. 35 (1), 23–30. doi:10.1159/000517965.

Thorp, J.H., Covich, A.P. (Eds.), 2010 . Ecology and Classification of North American Freshwater Invertebrates, third ed. In: Aquatic Ecology Series. Academic Press, Amsterdam; Boston, pp. 1–1056. ISBN: 978-0-12-690647-9. doi:10.1016/B978-0-12-690647-9.X5000-5.

Treyvaud Amiguet, V., Kramp, K.L., Mao, J., McRae, C., Goulah, A., Kimpe, L.E., Blais, J.M., Arnason, J.T., 2012. Supercritical carbon dioxide extraction of polyunsaturated fatty acids from Northern shrimp (*Pandalus borealis* Krøyer) processing by-products. Food Chem. 18737072. 130 (4), 853–858. doi:10.1016/j.foodchem.2011.07.098.

Tsoupras, A., Cholidis, P., Kranas, D., Galouni, E.A., Ofrydopoulou, A., Efthymiopoulos, P., Shiels, K., Saha, S.K., Kyzas, G.Z., Anastasiadou, C., 2025. Anti-Inflammatory, antithrombotic, and antioxidant properties of amphiphilic lipid bioactives from shrimp. Pharmaceuticals 14248247. 18 (1). Available from: https://www.mdpi.com/journal/pharmaceuticals. doi:10.3390/ph18010025.

Tunku Mahmud, T.H.T., Abdul-Aziz, A., Muda, R., 2015. A review on the potential use of chitosan-based delivery system in mild facial cleansing formulation. Int. J. Polym. Mater. Polym. Biomater. 1563535X. 64 (8), 432–437. Available from: https://www.tandf.co.uk/journals/titles/00914037.asp. doi:10.1080/00914037.2014.958832.

Tzeng, H.P., Liu, S.H., Chiang, M.T., 2022. Antidiabetic properties of chitosan and its derivatives. Mar. Drugs 16603397. 20 (12). Available from: http://www.mdpi.com/journal/marinedrugs. doi:10.3390/md20120784.

Verma, M., Gahlot, N., Singh, S.S.J., Rose, N.M., 2021. UV protection and antibacterial treatment of cellulosic fibre (cotton) using chitosan and onion skin dye. Carbohydr. Polym. 01448617. 257. Available from: http://www.elsevier.com/wps/find/journaldescription.cws_home/405871/description#description. doi:10.1016/j.carbpol.2020.117612.

Vicente, F.A., Ventura, S.P.M., Passos, H., Dias, A.C.R.V., Acosta, M.A.T., Novak, U., Likozar, B., 2022. Crustacean waste biorefinery as a sustainable cost-effective business model. SSRN 15565068. Available from: https://www.ssrn.com/index.cfm/en/. doi:10.2139/ssrn.4004674.

Villaró, S., Ciardi, M., Morillas-España, A., Sánchez-Zurano, A., Acién-Fernández, G., Lafarga, T., 2021. Microalgae derived astaxanthin: research and consumer trends and industrial use as food. Foods. 2304-8158. 10 (10), 2303. doi:10.3390/foods10102303.

Vittori, M., 2024. Structural diversity of crustacean exoskeletons and its implications for biomimetics. Interface Focus. 2042-8901. 14 (2). doi:10.1098/rsfs.2023.0075.

Wang, F., Lin, W., Lv, S., Jiang, S., Lin, L., Lu, J., 2019. Comparison of lipids extracted by different methods from Chinese mitten crab (*Eriocheir sinensis*) hepatopancreas. J. Food Sci. 17503841. 84 (12), 3594–3600. Available from: http://onlinelibrary.wiley.com/journal/10.1111/(ISSN)1750-3841. doi:10.1111/1750-3841.14946.

Wang, W., Xue, C., Mao, X., 2020. Chitosan: structural modification, biological activity and application. Int. J. Biol. Macromol. 01418130. 164, 4532–4546. doi:10.1016/j.ijbiomac.2020.09.042.

Wenner, A., Kuris, A. (Eds.), 2020. Crustacean Egg Production, first ed., CRC Press, 978-1-003-07256-0.

Wu, Q., Cheng, N., Fang, D., Wang, H., Rahman, F.U., Hao, H., Zhang, Y., 2024. Recent advances on application of polysaccharides in cosmetics. J. Dermatol. Sci. Cosmet. Technol. 2950306X. 1 (1). Available from: https://www.keaipublishing.com/en/journals/journal-of-dermatologic-science-and-cosmetic-technology/. doi:10.1016/j.jdsct.2024.100004.

Yabuzaki, J., 2017. Carotenoids Database: structures, chemical fingerprints and distribution among organisms. Database. 1758-0463. 2017 (1). doi:10.1093/database/bax004.

Yan, N., Chen, X., 2015. Sustainability: don't waste seafood waste. Nature. 0028-0836. 524 (7564), 155–157. doi:10.1038/524155a.

Yanat, M., Schroën, K., 2023. Advances in chitin-based nanoparticle use in biodegradable polymers: a review. Carbohydr. Polym. 01448617. 312, 120789. doi:10.1016/j.carbpol.2023.120789.

Yang, J., Hua, S., Huang, Z., Zhengbiao, G., Cheng, L., Hong, Y., 2021. Comparison of bioaccessibility of astaxanthin encapsulated in starch-based double emulsion with different structures. Carbohydr. Polym. 01448617. 272, 118475. doi:10.1016/j.carbpol.2021.118475.

Younes, I., Rinaudo, M., 2015. Chitin and chitosan preparation from marine sources: structure, properties, and applications. Mar. Drugs. 1660-3397. 13 (3), 1133–1174. doi:10.3390/md13031133.

Zhang, Z., Ma, Z., Song, L., Farag, M.A., 2024. Maximizing crustaceans (shrimp, crab, and lobster) by-products value for optimum valorization practices: a comparative review of their active ingredients, extraction, bioprocesses and applications. J. Adv. Res. 20901232. 57, 59–76. Available from: https://www.sciencedirect.com/science/journal/20901232. doi:10.1016/j.jare.2023.11.002.

Zou, Y., Heyndrickx, M., Debode, J., Raes, K., de Pascale, D., Behan, P., Giltrap, M., O'Connor, C., Solstad, R.G., Lian, K., Altintzoglou, T., Dragøy, R., Scheers, N., Undeland, I., Robbens, J., 2023. Valorisation of crustacean and bivalve processing side streams for industrial fast time-to-market products: a review from the European Union regulation perspective. Front. Mar. Sci. 22967745. 10. Available from: https://www.frontiersin.org/journals/marine-science#. doi:10.3389/fmars.2023.1068151.

Chapter 22

Fish and fish biowastes

Alexandros Tsoupras[a], Eleni Kourmazou[a], and Chryssa Anastasiadou[b]

[a]Hephaestus Laboratory, School of Chemistry, Faculty of Sciences, Democritus University of Thrace, Kavala University Campus, Kavala, Greece

[b]Fisheries Research Institute, Hellenic Agricultural Organization-DIMITRA (ELGO-DIMITRA), Nea Peramos, Kavala, Greece

1 Introduction

Self-care has become an essential aspect of modern lifestyles, driving the beauty industry to pursue innovative concepts and novel ingredients for cosmetic and skincare formulations (Rafatullah et al., 2024). Consumers are increasingly interested in products designed to enhance and modify the appearance of skin, hair, and nails (Fonseca et al., 2023).

In recent decades, the cosmetics industry has turned toward natural products (NPs), including those derived from the largely unexplored and complex realm of marine resources, uncovering a vast array of valuable information from ocean environments (Alves et al., 2020). Although synthetic chemicals are still widely used in cosmetic formulations, many do not fully satisfy consumer expectations. Consequently, there is a growing demand for products containing natural ingredients, which are perceived as safer, more sustainable, and environmentally friendly alternatives (Fonseca et al., 2023)

Historically, NPs have played a crucial role in treating chronic inflammatory conditions, skin disorders, and other health-related ailments, and they continue to be fundamental to modern drug development (Ghareeb et al., 2020). NPs are distinguished by their remarkable chemical diversity, which fosters innovation in pharmaceutical research. While terrestrial plants and bacteria have traditionally been the primary sources of NPs, marine organisms—including invertebrates, plants, and microorganisms—have emerged over the past three decades as significant contributors to novel bioactive compounds known as marine natural products (MNPs) (Rafatullah et al., 2024)

Covering approximately 70% of the Earth's surface and representing the origin of life, the oceans constitute an immense reservoir of biodiversity, encompassing nearly 500,000 species across approximately 28 phyla. Despite this diversity, only a limited number of marine taxa have been extensively studied for NP isolation, including several fish species (Lu et al., 2021; Oliver et al., 1994; Ciavatta et al., 2020; Papikinou et al., 2024). Marine ecosystems are regarded as a rich source of structurally unique bioactive compounds rarely found in terrestrial organisms, mostly due to the extreme environments where the initial sources for such bioactives live, meaning the marine microorganisms, microalgae, fungi, sponges, and macroalgae, which are the main food sources for several fish or for other organisms that fish eat through the food chain of these ecosystems. These bioactives are commonly classified into terpenoids, sterols, polyethers, unsaturated fatty acids, alkaloids, glycosides, polysaccharides, peptides, and macrolides (Lu et al., 2021).

The first biologically active MNP was reported by Bergmann in the late 1950s (Bergmann and Feeney, 1950). Since then, marine ecosystems have been widely acknowledged for their direct and indirect contributions to human well-being. Beyond serving as sources of nutrients and raw materials, these ecosystems play essential roles in biogeochemical cycling, climate regulation, and atmospheric gas balance, as well as supporting recreational and cultural activities (Bergmann and Feeney, 1950).

Although plant-derived ingredients are widely used in cosmeceuticals, they present certain limitations, including slow growth rates and variability in chemical composition due to seasonal and geographical factors. In contrast, marine ecosystems offer unparalleled biodiversity and chemical diversity, providing access to unique biomolecules. With the support of modern aquaculture techniques, many marine organisms, and especially fish, can be cultivated efficiently and cost-effectively as sustainable sources of not only food but also marine bioactives for several applications, including functional cosmetics (Fonseca et al., 2023; Alves et al., 2020).

Furthermore, advanced technologies such as genomics, proteomics, and metabolomics—the "omics" sciences—are increasingly employed to accelerate the discovery of marine-derived compounds and to elucidate their mechanisms of

Biofunctional Cosmetics for Health. https://doi.org/10.1016/B978-0-443-27500-5.00022-8

action in human skin physiology. These approaches enable targeted ingredient development and enhance safety and efficacy screening (Barh and Azevedo, 2018; Brunt and Burgess, 2018).

Several studies have already addressed the potential and existing applications of marine-derived bioactives in the cosmetic industry. This chapter aims to provide a comprehensive overview of bioactive compounds from fish sources, with emphasis on cultured fish species and fish by-products as sustainable sources of marine bioactives for functional cosmetics. Moreover, potential cosmetic applications of these compounds, emphasizing their benefits in skincare formulations, as well as limitations and future perspectives, are also addressed in this chapter.

2 Fish and its by-products as sustainable sources of valuable marine bioactives for functional cosmetics

2.1 Composition, nutritional value, and valuable bioactive compounds from fish and its by-products

Fish are aquatic vertebrates that inhabit both open seas and oceans, as well as freshwater environments such as rivers, lakes, and marshes. The places where they live and survive, as well as their characteristics, are influenced by climatic, geographical, and anthropogenic factors (Manel et al., 2020).

The body of fish is usually hydrodynamic (elliptical or spindle-shaped), i.e., it is specially shaped to reduce hydrodynamic resistance when swimming and to optimize energy consumption. The body is functionally divided into the head, trunk, and tail. On the body are scales, a mucus layer, and fins that provide propulsion, direction, and stability. The morphology of the scales and the ratio of types (e.g., cellular/osteodermal) vary between species and are related to lifestyle and ecological niche (Traverso et al., 2024).

The head contains basic sensory organs, such as eyes, olfactory epithelia, openings, and the muscular structures of the mouth (for food collection). In most fish, the gills are the main organs of gas exchange; the thin, broad surface of the lamellae allows efficient diffusion of oxygen from the water into the blood and excretion of carbon dioxide (Park et al., 2014).

The lateral line is a specialized system consisting of neuromasts that allows the perception of hydrodynamic changes, currents, subtle vibrations, and movements of neighboring bodies. Neuromasts can be either superficial or embedded in channels. This mechanism enables them to swim in a directed manner, engage in collective behavior (schooling/congregation), and locate prey or predators even in limited visibility (Edgley et al., 2024). The fins (dorsal, caudal, pelvic, pectoral, anal) have specialized roles: propulsion (mainly caudal), flexible movement (pectoral/pelvic), and stabilization (dorsal/anal). The shape and mechanism of use of the fins depend on the swimming style (e.g., continuous rapid propulsion in pelagic species or bursts of acceleration in predators). The muscle mass of fish is mainly characterized by four main components: moisture, protein, lipids, and ash.

Primary analytical studies show that the chemical composition of fish includes mainly moisture, which accounts for the largest percentage (59.1–87.8%), proteins that vary widely (9%–24%), and lipids that also show great variation (0.8%–23%), while ash (inorganic salts) represents the smallest percentage (1%–1.5%) (Afreen and Ucak, 2020; Awuchi et al., 2022; Proximate composition of New Zealand Marine Finfish and Shellfish, n.d.). These values vary depending on the fish species, age, and physiological condition, as estimated by the Food and Agriculture Organization (based on 62 species) (Fig. 22.1). For example, fish living in cold, pelagic waters tend to have a different fatty composition (e.g., higher levels of polyunsaturated omega-3 fatty acids) than species living in warmer or freshwater environments, differences that have been measured in primary composition studies.

It is widely recognized that fish and marine organisms are rich sources of high-quality nutrients like proteins and healthy fats, but also of a plethora of diverse bioactive compounds. Fish flesh is also rich in proteins, several amino acids, polyunsaturated fatty acids (PUFAs), minerals, micronutrients, and dietary vitamins A, B3, B6, B12, D, and E (Marques et al., 2019; Suleria et al., 2015; Lall and Kaushik, 2021). Moreover, fish oil contains sterols, vitamins, minerals, polyphenols, and pigments, along with fatty acids, including PUFAs [e.g., docosahexaenoic acid (DHA), eicosapentaenoic acid (EPA), arachidonic acids (AAs)], monounsaturated fatty acids (MUFAs, e.g., gondoic, palmitoleic, and oleic acids), and saturated fatty acids (SFAs, e.g., stearic and palmitic acids) (Awuchi et al., 2022; Ucak and Nayik, 2022; Mata-Sotres et al., 2021; Caballero et al., 2003). Fresh, dried, fermented, and salted fish exhibit high lipid content, as well as a wide range of macromolecules, minerals, and amino acids (Chen and Hou, 2016; Zhuang and Sun, 2011). Calcium has been found in fish bones, crude enzymes were extracted from the viscera, and proteins were traced in both fish skin and head (Alves et al., 2017). Finally, fish also contain essential minerals such as potassium (K), phosphorus (P), sodium (Na), zinc (Zn), magnesium (Mg), calcium (Ca), iron (Fe), selenium (Se), and iodine (I) (Marques et al., 2019; Nerhus et al., 2018). Several of these nutrients and secondary metabolites from fish are highly bioactive compounds with antioxidant, antiaging, antiinflammatory, antimicrobial, and healing properties, among several other bioactives. Because of these attributes, fish-derived bioactives are increasingly used as raw materials in health-related and cosmetic industries.

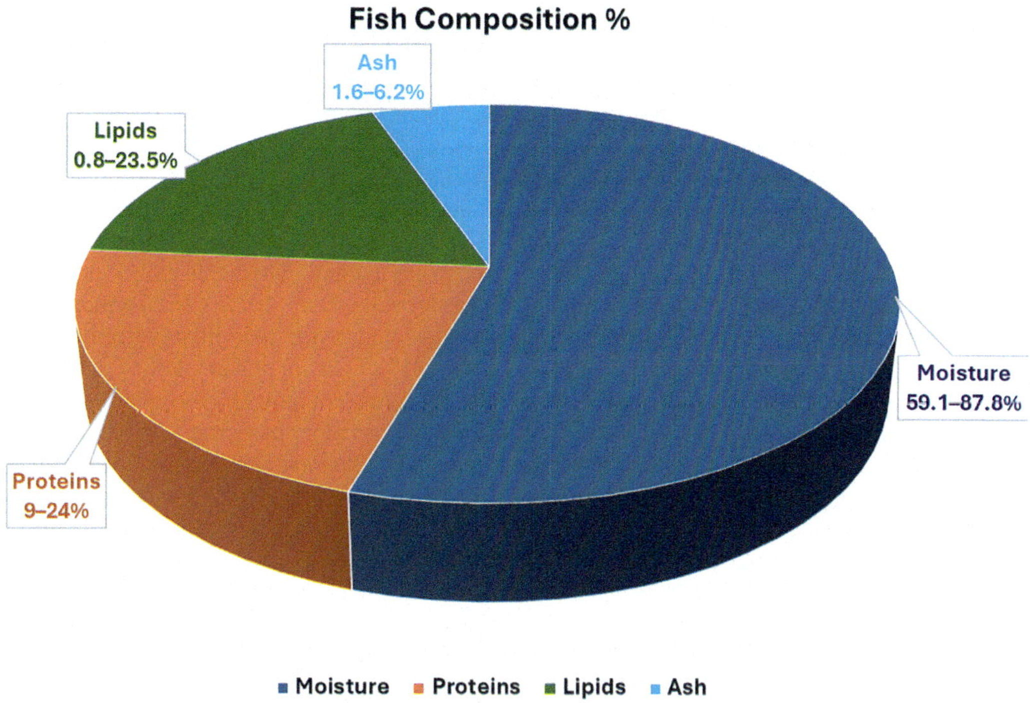

FIG. 22.1 Average (%) chemical composition of fish. *(From Papadopoulou, S.N.A., Adamantidi, T., Kranas, D., Cholidis, P., Anastasiadou, C., Tsoupras, A., 2025a. A comprehensive review on the valorization of bioactives from marine animal by-products for health-promoting, biofunctional cosmetics. Mar. Drugs. 16603397. 23 (8). Available from: https://www.mdpi.com/journal/marinedrugs. doi:10.3390/md23080299.)*

However, a significant issue in the fishing and marine processing industries involves bycatch (nontarget species caught unintentionally) and especially the fish by-products, such as fish skin, bones, scales, heads, and viscera. These are among the various components of the marine biomass that account for approximately 50%–70% of total fish weight and are typically discarded as biological waste during processing. Nevertheless, these components are regarded as secondary raw materials with high valorization potential, and thus the excessive accumulation of such fishery organic waste discards—comprising both fishery by-catch and processing by-products—presents both environmental and economic challenges and concerns (Caruso et al., 2020). For example, these discards are difficult to handle and must be managed as certified by-products due to their high content of polyunsaturated lipids and endogenous proteolytic enzymes, which accelerate degradation. Thus on the one hand, they are high in healthy fats, including marine polar lipids (PLs), ω3 PUFA, and lipid vitamins, as well as in valuable minerals; on the other hand, they also contain endogenous enzymes like proteases, which promote rapid spoilage, release of unpleasant odors, and microbiological degradation. Moreover, the cost of proper disposal places a financial burden on fisheries and fish processing industries. Thus proper storage under hygienic and temperature-controlled conditions is essential, adding to logistical and operational costs.

Given these concerns, the valorization and full utilization of fish by-products are gaining increasing attention as a sustainable and resource-efficient solution. This practice is aligned with the principles of the circular economy, which promotes sustainable development by minimizing waste, enhancing resource efficiency, and thus contributing to the long-term sustainability of the fishing sector (Teixeira et al., 2024; Suuronen and Gilman, 2020). Through proper utilization, companies can reduce waste management costs and environmental burdens, while simultaneously capitalizing on the valuable bioactive molecules within these by-products.

Bioactive compounds obtained from fish and their by-products can be used in various industries, including food, agriculture, cosmetics, nutraceuticals, and pharmaceuticals (Caruso et al., 2020). Thus various sectors such as the food and feed industries, agriculture, cosmetics, and pharmaceutical fields can benefit from these resources. Both fatty and lean fish species—including salmon, mackerel, sardines, herring, cod, and tuna—are viable sources. The bioactive compound profile depends heavily on factors such as fish species, anatomical part, lipid content, and even seasonal variations. For instance, fatty fish such as salmon, sardines, and herring are notably high in ω3 PUFA, like EPA and DHA, as well as in bioactive marine PLs, carotenoids, and lipid vitamins (Papadopoulou et al., 2025a; Tsoupras et al., 2019a; Redfern et al., 2021; Tsoupras et al., 2018, 2019a, 2022). Lean fish such as cod also contain considerable amounts of these lipid bioactives; however, they are mainly known for being especially rich in high-quality collagen and gelatin (Honrado et al., 2022; Vázquez et al., 2019).

By-products from fish processing contain a broad spectrum of bioactive substances. These include structural and functional proteins (collagen, gelatin, myosin, actin), essential fatty acids (EFAs) (notably EPA and DHA), fat-soluble vitamins such as A, D, and E, PL bioactives rich in ω3 PUFA, trace minerals like calcium, zinc, and selenium, and biologically active enzymes (e.g., proteases and lipases) (Papadopoulou et al., 2025a; Tsoupras et al., 2022). Furthermore, fish tissues also contain valuable pigments and carotenoids such as astaxanthin, which is especially concentrated in the skin of salmon (Papadopoulou et al., 2025a; Tsoupras et al., 2022; Adamantidi et al., 2025).

Many of these compounds are already used in commercial products (Papadopoulou et al., 2025a; Adamantidi et al., 2025) and cosmeceutical applications (Jimenez-Champi et al., 2024; Coppola et al., 2021; Kandyliari et al., 2020; Ghalamara et al., 2024). Fish-derived collagen and peptide derivatives from fish are integral ingredients in modern antiaging creams, hydrating gels, facial masks, and therapeutic wound dressings (Papadopoulou et al., 2025a). Furthermore, antioxidant-rich fish protein hydrolysates (FPH) and bioactive peptides are increasingly studied for their photoprotective, antiwrinkle, and antipigmentation potential (Rajabimashhadi et al., 2023; Alves et al., 2017). Fish oil, rich in marine lipid bioactives, including sterols, amphiphilic marine phenolics, and especially various fatty acids (not only PUFA, but also MUFAs and SFAs), is incorporated into skincare formulations for its regenerative and antiinflammatory properties and barrier-restoring effects. These fatty acids support skin health by enhancing hydration, reducing inflammation, and minimizing oxidative stress. Fish oil has also demonstrated photoprotective, antiwrinkling, and antimelanogenic effects (Papadopoulou et al., 2025a).

Each anatomical part of the fish offers different opportunities for the extraction and application of bioactive components. The fish head, which was once discarded as waste, is now recognized as a valuable source of oils (rich in EPA and DHA), proteins, peptides, and hyaluronic acid (HA). The backbone and spines are utilized for gelatin production and are also rich in minerals like calcium and phosphorus, as well as collagen. The swim bladder is a specialized organ that yields high-quality collagen and functional peptides. The skin and fins are known for their high concentrations of collagen and gelatin, making them ideal for cosmetic applications. Viscera contain oils, protamine (a bioactive peptide), and a range of digestive enzymes, which are of interest in pharmacology. Muscle tissue, aside from being a protein-rich food source, is also rich in ω3 PUFA, marine amphiphilic bioactives (i.e., marine PL bioactives, carotenoids, and phenolics), and bioactive peptides (Papadopoulou et al., 2025a). Fish are also nutritionally dense in essential minerals, including potassium, phosphorus, sodium, zinc, magnesium, calcium, iron, selenium, and iodine. The muscle flesh of fish is a complete protein source, offering essential amino acids and a suite of vitamins, notably A, B3 (niacin), B6, B12, D, and E, all of which contribute to human health (Papadopoulou et al., 2025a).

Not only fish, but their by-products such as fish heads, skins, bones, viscera, and fish by-catch are abundant in valuable bioactive compounds too, including polysaccharides (e.g., chitin, chitosan, and their derivatives, HA, GAGs, and fucoidans), fatty acids (e.g., SFAs, MUFAs, and mainly PUFAs like LA, DHA, EPA, ALA, or AA), lipid bioactives and PLs (e.g., lecithin, phospholipids, glycolipids, sphin-golipids, sulfolipids, or marinosomes), lipid vitamins (e.g., A, B, D, E, or K), water-soluble vitamins (especially B3, B6, and B12), amino acids [all 20 standard residues and mostly mycosporine-like amino acids (MAAs)], proteins (e.g., collagen, elastin, gelatin), bioactive peptides (small amino acid chains and collagen and gelatin hydrolysates), carotenoids and other pigments (e.g., astaxanthin, melanins like allomelanin, neuromelanin, eumelanin, pheomelanin, and pyomelanin, lutein, β-carotene, halocynthiaxanthin, and fucoxanthin), phenolic compounds (e.g., polyphenols, PBDEs, phlorotannins like diphlorethol, triphlo-roethol, trifuhalol, and tetrafuhalol, phloroglucinol, eckol, and eckstolonol), marine terpenoids and alkaloids, and several substrates and minerals (e.g., hydroxyapatite, CaPs, minerals like Ca, Mg, and Zn), among others (Table 22.1) (Papadopoulou et al., 2025a).

These compounds exhibit a broad spectrum of biological activities, such as antioxidant, antiinflammatory, antimicrobial, antiaging, moisturizing, and UV-protective properties, making them ideal for cosmetic use (Papadopoulou et al., 2025a). Their extraction not only supports the development of functional skincare products but also contributes to environmental sustainability by promoting the circular use of marine resources.

Table 22.2 summarizes the challenges and benefits in the valorization of fish by-products, while in Fig. 22.2, a schematic diagram is provided illustrating the valorization of different fish by-products, highlighting the valuable bioactive compounds that can be extracted from various parts of a fish, and in Fig. 22.3, a summary of the bioactives present in fish bycatch and by-products is structurally illustrated.

Thus several valuable bioactive compounds can be extracted from various parts of a fish and its by-products, while different anatomical sections, often considered waste from fish processing, can be utilized to obtain beneficial components for various applications (e.g., functional foods, nutraceuticals, cosmetics). The diagram in Fig. 22.1 segments a fish into several key anatomical parts (head, backbone and thorns, skin and fins, swim bladder, viscera, and muscle), listing for each part specific valuable compounds. Specifically, the head (green circle) is indicated as a source of oils (e.g., EPA, DHA), proteins, peptides, and HA, while from the backbone and thorns (blue circle), gelatin, minerals (e.g., Ca, P), and collagen can be extracted. Swim bladders (light blue circle) are a valuable source of collagen and other peptides. Skin and fins (yellow

TABLE 22.1 Valuable bioactive compounds derived from fish processing by-products.

Fish by-product	Percentage (%w/w)	Valuable compounds	References
Skin	3.5	Collagen, gelatin, antimicrobial compounds (e.g., cathelicidins, defensins), and ω3 PUFA	(Caruso et al., 2020; Atef and Ojagh, 2017; Ashraf et al., 2020)
Bones	10–15	Calcium phosphate (hydroxyapatite), collagen, gelatin, ω3 PUFA, lipids, and P	(Caruso et al., 2020; Coppola et al., 2021; Kandyliari et al., 2020; Suresh et al., 2018)
Scales	2	Collagen, chitin, chitosan, minerals (e.g., Zn, Ca), and glycoproteins	(Caruso et al., 2020; Molina-Ramírez et al., 2021)
Head	10–15	Protein hydrolysates, gelatin, and bioactive peptides, enzymes (e.g., pepsin, trypsin), and bioactive lipids	(Prihanto et al., 2019; Kuang and Mohtar, 2018; Wang (2021); Zhang et al., 2021; Tsoupras et al., 2019b)
Viscera	12–18	Fish oil (e.g., EPA, DHA), digestive enzymes (trypsin, lipase), probiotics, bile acids, and vitamin D	(Caruso et al., 2020; Wang, 2021; Wang et al., 2019)
Swim bladder	39.2	Type I and II collagen, gelatin, GAGs, and elastin	(Abdallah et al., 2020; Yushuang et al., 2022; Rocha et al., 2024)
Fins	~1%–2% (estimated[a])	CS, HA, and collagen	(Abdallah et al., 2020; Urbi et al., 2022)
Cartilage	-[b]	CS, GS, and protein-polysaccharide complexes	(Abdallah et al., 2020; Jerosch, 2011)
Liver	~5%–15% (estimated[c])	Vitamins A and D_3, ω3 PUFA, and antioxidant enzymes	(Ashraf et al., 2020; Abdallah et al., 2020; Mata-Sotres et al., 2021)

ω3 PUFA, omega 3 polyunsaturated fatty acids; *EPA*, eicosapentenoic acid; *DHA*, docosahexaenoic acid; *GAGs*, glycosaminoglycans, *CS*, chondroitin sulfate; *GS*, glucosamine sulfate; *HA*, hyaluronic acid.

[a]*Percentages are estimated based on species and processing method. Exact values for fins, cartilage, and liver are not widely standardized in the literature.*

[b]*Percentages are estimated based on species and processing method. Exact values for fins, cartilage, and liver are not widely standardized in the literature.*

[c]*Percentages are estimated based on species and processing method. Exact values for fins, cartilage, and liver are not widely standardized in the literature.*

TABLE 22.2 Challenges and opportunities of fishery bycatch and by-products.

Challenges	Benefits
• Negative environmental impact due to discards and waste accumulation	• Promote fishery sustainability and enable environmentally friendly waste management
• Loss of high-value bioactives through the discarding of heads, skins, viscera, bones, etc.	• Valorization of compounds like enzymes, lipids, and peptides for high-end uses
• Lack of standardized extraction protocols	• Advances in green and selective extraction methods (e.g., enzymatic hydrolysis, membrane filtration)
• High operating and processing costs for waste handling	• Resource-efficient use through biorefinery models and circular economy integration
• Short shelf life and high perishability due to lipids and enzymes	• Stabilization techniques improve raw material storage for long-term industrial use
• Regulatory restrictions for classifying and reusing by-products	• Growing acceptance and guidance under the EU Circular Economy Action Plan (CEAP) and the Food and Agriculture Organization (FAO) sustainability goals
• Consumer perception issues regarding waste-derived ingredients	• Increasing demand for natural, marine-origin, clean-label bioactives in cosmetics and supplements

From Papadopoulou, S.N.A., Adamantidi, T., Kranas, D., Cholidis, P., Anastasiadou, C., Tsoupras, A., 2025a. A comprehensive review on the valorization of bioactives from marine animal by-products for health-promoting, biofunctional cosmetics. Mar. Drugs. 16603397. 23 (8). Available from: https://www.mdpi.com/journal/marinedrugs. doi:10.3390/md23080299.

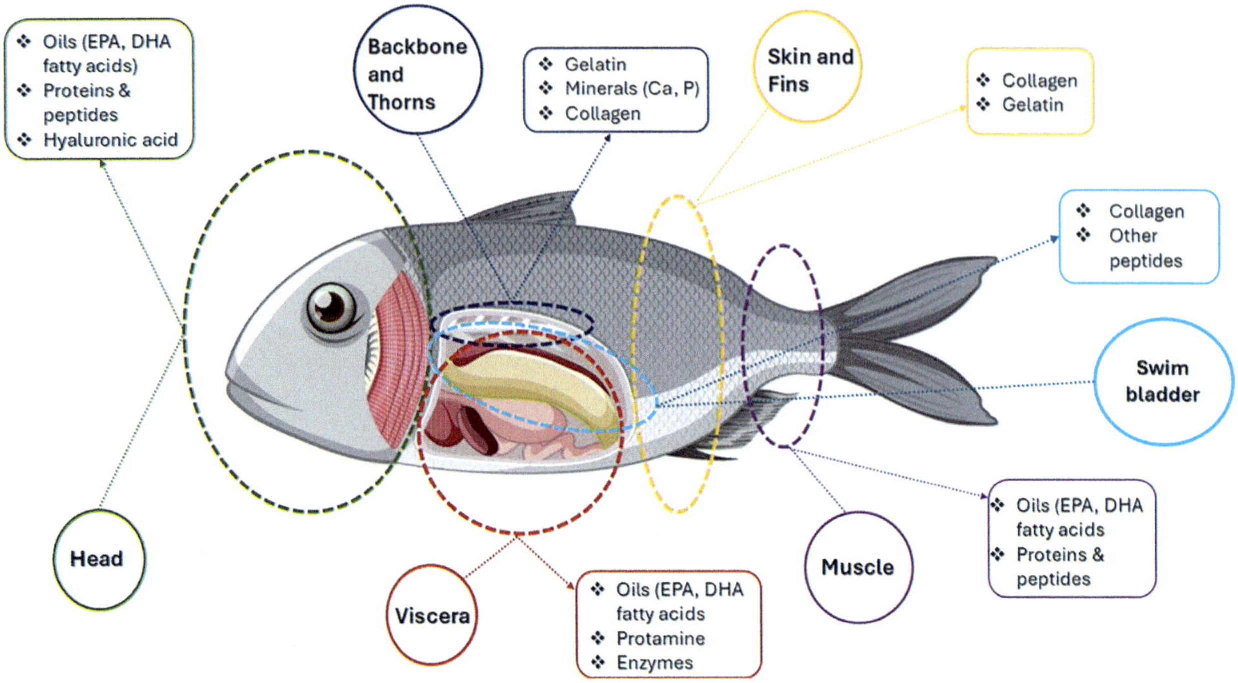

FIG. 22.2 A schematic diagram illustrating the valorization of different fish by-products, highlighting the valuable bioactive compounds that can be extracted from various parts of a fish. *(From Papadopoulou, S.N.A., Adamantidi, T., Kranas, D., Cholidis, P., Anastasiadou, C., Tsoupras, A., 2025a. A comprehensive review on the valorization of bioactives from marine animal by-products for health-promoting, biofunctional cosmetics. Mar. Drugs. 16603397. 23 (8). Available from: https://www.mdpi.com/journal/marinedrugs. doi:10.3390/md23080299.)*

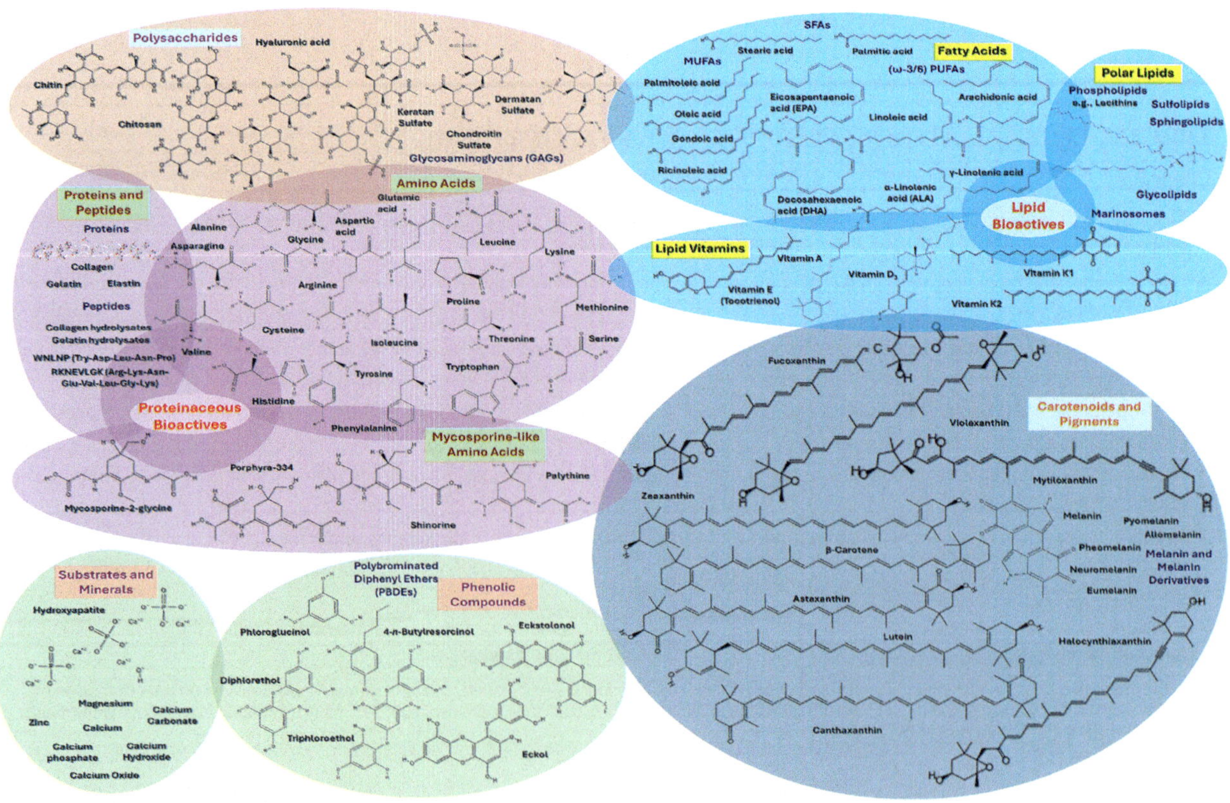

FIG. 22.3 An overview of bioactive compounds and their structures present in fish bycatch and by-products. *(From Papadopoulou, S.N.A., Adamantidi, T., Kranas, D., Cholidis, P., Anastasiadou, C., Tsoupras, A., 2025a. A comprehensive review on the valorization of bioactives from marine animal by-products for health-promoting, biofunctional cosmetics. Mar. Drugs. 16603397. 23 (8). Available from: https://www.mdpi.com/journal/marinedrugs. doi:10.3390/md23080299.)*

circle) are rich in collagen and gelatin, viscera are a significant source of oils like EPA and DHA, protamine, and enzymes, and the muscle may yield, for instance, EPA and/or DHA oils, proteins, and peptides. The visualization emphasized the concept of a "zero-waste" approach in the fishing industry, where by-products are not discarded but rather processed to recover high-value compounds (Awuchi et al., 2022; Atef and Ojagh, 2017; Sinha and Häder, 2020; Sousa et al., 2020), and it also provides characteristic examples of natural marine bioactives derived mainly from fish processing by-products.

In conclusion, marine organisms, and especially fish, provide a wide array of bioactive substances that offer numerous therapeutic and cosmetic benefits. These include antioxidant, antiinflammatory, antimicrobial, healing, neuroprotective, cardioprotective, hepatoprotective, and antiaging effects. The sustainable exploitation of these resources, especially through the valorization of by-products, represents a promising strategy for enhancing human health while reducing environmental impact. Moreover, continuous research and technological advancements in extraction, purification, and formulation methods will further unlock the potential of marine bioactives, paving the way for novel applications in the biomedical, cosmetic, nutraceutical, and food sectors. Embracing the full potential of marine biodiversity not only supports economic innovation but also aligns with global goals for environmental sustainability and public health (Ahmmed et al., 2021).

2.2 Fish protein-based bioactive compounds

Fish proteins—particularly those like immunoglobulins—exhibit protective effects against pathogenic microorganisms, including viruses and bacteria. They also play a role in preventing protein-energy malnutrition in vulnerable populations. Fish proteins are rich in essential (e.g., leucine, lysine) and nonessential (e.g., aspartic, glutamic) amino acids. Fish bioactive peptides (protein fragments), consisting of 2–20 amino acids, exist in fish proteins in an inactive form (Wang, 2021) and are released through in vivo proteolysis or in vitro enzymatic hydrolysis (Wang, 2021; Zamora-Sillero et al., 2018). Functional derivatives of fish proteins include FPH and hydrolyzed animal proteins (HAP). These are produced via enzymatic hydrolysis of muscle, which contains ~65%–75% of the total fish protein (Kim, 2013), skin, and waste (e.g., head, trimmings, fins, viscera, frames) (Sinha and Häder, 2020), by using proteases to break down complex proteins from these fish sources into protein hydrolysates that contain several peptides, among them some bioactive ones. For instance, protein-rich fish by-products such as backbone, skin, head, viscera, and blood can be used to formulate collagen, gelatin, and proteoglycans (Barba and Lorenzo, 2020). Several fish-derived bioactive peptides have been found to help regulate oxidative stress, modulate inflammation, and promote skin regeneration by stimulating fibroblasts and enhancing collagen production. At the same time, they inhibit metalloproteinases—enzymes that break down collagen—thereby slowing skin aging and improving tissue integrity.

Fish by-products, including skin, bones, and cartilage, represent abundant sources of collagen (Rajabimashhadi et al., 2023; Prajaputra et al., 2024; Martins et al., 2023). It is estimated that filleting residues may account for up to 75% of the total fish weight, with skin and bones comprising a substantial proportion of this collagen-rich biomass (Alfaro et al., 2015). Collagen is a fibrous structural protein that forms the extracellular matrix (ECM) in fish, providing mechanical support and maintaining the physiological integrity of tissues such as cartilage, skin, tendons, bones, and cranial structures. Accounting for approximately 25% of the total protein content in fish, collagen is the most abundant individual protein. Although multiple collagen types exist, type I collagen is the predominant form present in fish by-products and is primarily located in connective tissues, muscles, skin, bones, and corneas (Shahidi, 2010; Nurilmala et al., 2022; Subhan et al., 2021; Raman and Gopakumar, 2018). Collagen is characterized by a high content of glycine, proline, and hydroxyproline residues. Under acidic conditions, the native collagen structure can be denatured, leading to its conversion into soluble proteins such as gelatin (Alfaro et al., 2015).

Marine collagen, including fish-derived collagen for several applications, is primarily extracted from fish by-products, including scales, bones, and mainly skin. It has extensive use in skincare due to its moisturizing and antiaging properties. Upon hydrolysis, collagen breaks down into gelatin and bioactive peptides, which can penetrate the skin barrier and stimulate the production of endogenous collagen (Papadopoulou et al., 2025a). Marine collagen is highly valued due to its superior bioavailability and low allergenicity compared to land-animal-derived collagens. In addition, dietary supplementation with marine collagen peptides has shown promise in managing neurodegenerative disorders by offering neuroprotective effects and improving cognitive functions.

When collagen undergoes acid or alkaline pretreatment, followed by heating above its thermal transition temperature, the native triple-helical structure denatures, leading to the formation of gelatin (Sinha and Häder, 2020; Ashraf et al., 2020). Gelatin is a colorless, odorless, protein-based macromolecule and biodegradable biopolymer. Owing to its structural similarity to collagen, gelatin retains many of collagen's functional properties, making it particularly suitable for the production of edible and biodegradable films capable of extending the shelf life of food products (Barba and Lorenzo, 2020; Alfaro et al., 2015; Ashraf et al., 2020).

The functional properties of gelatin are strongly influenced by the fish species from which it is derived. Gelatin obtained from cold-water fish generally exhibits lower industrial value than that from temperate- or warm-water species. This is primarily attributed to the reduced thermal stability of collagen in cold-water fish, which results from lower levels of proline and hydroxyproline in their protein structures (Tkaczewska et al., 2018). Notably, gelatin derived from warm-water fish shares many physicochemical characteristics with porcine gelatin, highlighting its potential as a viable alternative to mammalian gelatin in pharmaceutical applications. In contrast, gelatin sourced from cold-water fish is particularly well-suited for applications such as vitamin microencapsulation and other pharmaceutical uses (Ashraf et al., 2020).

Although fish skin has traditionally been the primary raw material for gelatin extraction, recent studies have demonstrated that several other fish by-products are also valuable sources of gelatin. Examples include gelatin obtained from the skins of Pacific cod (*Gadus macrocephalus*) and seabass (*Lates calcarifer*), as well as from the scales of bighead carp (*Hypophthalmichthys nobilis*), the heads of mackerel (*Scomber scombrus*), and the bones of black tilapia (Caruso et al., 2020; Joy et al., 2024; Valcarcel et al., 2021; He et al., 2022).

Enzymes like proteases and lipases extracted from fish tissues are of significant commercial interest due to their high catalytic efficiency. In cosmetics, these enzymes are utilized in exfoliating formulations, where they aid in the removal of dead skin cells, promote epidermal regeneration, and enhance skin texture. Beyond cosmetics, fish-derived enzymes are also used in wound debridement products and in food processing as natural tenderizers or flavor enhancers. Recent studies have highlighted their use in biosensors, biodegradable packaging, and even biofuel production, making them multifaceted assets across various industries (Saranya et al., 2018).

In summary, fish proteins are rich in both essential (e.g., leucine, lysine) and nonessential (e.g., glutamic acid, aspartic acid) amino acids. These form the building blocks for structural compounds such as collagen, gelatin, and proteoglycans, all of which are beneficial for human health and are increasingly being utilized in cosmeceutical and pharmaceutical products (González-Serrano et al., 2022).

2.3 Fish amphiphilic and lipophilic lipid-based bioactives for functional cosmetics

2.3.1 *Fish-derived bioactive fatty acids*

Fatty acids consist of a chain of carbon atoms with a carboxyl group (COOH) at one end and a methyl group (CH_3) at the other. According to their degree of saturation—determined by chain length, number of double bonds, and hydrogen atom arrangement—they are classified as SFA (e.g., stearic and palmitic acids), MUFA (e.g., gondoic, oleic, and palmitoleic acids), and PUFA [e.g., the ω3 EPA, DHA, and α-linolenic acid (ALA), and the ω6 AA]. Among these, PUFA include EFAs (ω3 and ω6), which cannot be synthesized by the human body and therefore must be obtained from the diet, especially from marine sources, mainly fish sources (Awuchi et al., 2022; Ashraf et al., 2020; Kundam et al., 2018). The primary ω3 PUFA are EPA, DHA, and ALA, with ALA serving as the metabolic precursor for the endogenous synthesis of EPA and DHA (Ozogul et al., 2021).

Fish species are categorized by lipid content into very low-fat, low-fat, medium-fat, and high-fat groups. This classification affects the concentration and type of fatty acids and lipids they offer, influencing their nutritional and functional value. For example, high-fat species like mackerel and herring offer abundant ω3s, while low-fat species provide mainly lean protein and collagen (Zheng et al., 2025). PUFA composition is also strongly influenced by environmental and biological factors such as temperature, salinity, ecosystem characteristics, and diet (e.g., algae and plankton) (Ashraf et al., 2020; Catala, 2017). Fish lipid content is another important consideration, as fish are classified as very low-fat, low-fat, medium-fat, or high-fat species depending on whether they are wild or farmed (Catala, 2017). In addition, marine fish oils—particularly those derived from the liver, head, and viscera—are rich sources of PUFA (predominantly ω3 ones), as well as fat-soluble vitamins A, D, and E (Jimenez-Champi et al., 2024).

Ω3 PUFA, especially EPA and DHA, are essential for maintaining the structural and functional integrity of cellular membranes. They also modulate the production of inflammatory mediators and are known to enhance skin hydration, elasticity, and resilience by strengthening the skin's lipid barrier. Marine fish oils, particularly from species like salmon, sardines, herring, and mackerel, are rich in these fatty acids and in fat-soluble vitamins (A, D, and E). Ω3s also influence critical signaling pathways, including nuclear factor kappa B (NF-κB), Toll-like receptors, transforming growth factor-beta (TGF-β), and peroxisome proliferator-activated receptors, which are central to inflammation, immunity, and cell proliferation (Tsoupras et al., 2022).

2.3.2 *Fish-derived bioactive PLs*

PLs, such as phospholipids and glycolipids, are characterized by amphipathic structures and are essential for cell membrane architecture and function. Fish are excellent sources of ω3-PUFA-rich PLs, especially PL rich in EPA and DHA. These molecules enhance membrane fluidity, assist in the transport of fat-soluble vitamins, and participate in immune modulation and inflammation resolution. Omega-3 fatty acids are present in both free and esterified forms. Esterified omega-3s are bound to PL or triacylglycerides (TAG), while depending on the species, up to one-third of EPA and DHA in fish may be found in PL form. Clinical trials on the benefits of fish oils have shown that, instead of the classic, so-far-used neutral forms of ω3 PUFA esterified in TAG or ethyl esters, the PLs that are rich in ω3 PUFA seem to better contribute to cardiovascular, neuroprotective, and antiinflammatory benefits by maintaining membrane homeostasis, regulating gene expression, and balancing omega-6 to omega-3 fatty acid ratios (Tsoupras et al., 2022).

PL in general are composed of two fatty acids attached to a glycerol or sphingosine backbone and a phosphate or sugar polar head group (Fig. 22.4), which allows them to possess an amphiphilic nature and thus to form micelles and liposomes in watery environments essential for cellular and intracellular membrane integrity, but also for facilitating nutrient delivery and cell signaling. TAG, consisting of three fatty acids, serve as energy reservoirs and are less polar, highly hydrophobic/lipophilic molecules, whereas PLs are amphiphilic compounds (having both polar heads and nonpolar fatty acid groups). Thus although PLs are present in lower quantities in fish compared to TAG, especially those bearing ω3 PUFA or MUFA in their structures, they are considered more bioavailable and biologically active fish bioactives than the more lipophilic free fatty acids (FFAs), TAG, and ethyl esters (Tsoupras et al., 2022).

Marine PLs, and especially fish PL, are rich in ω3 fatty acids and are particularly abundant in oily fish like salmon, herring, sardines, and mackerel. Phosphatidylcholine (PC) is the predominant PL found in fish, typically enriched with omega-3s in the sn-2 position of its glycerol backbone. Other important PL include phosphatidylethanolamine (PE), phosphatidylserine, phosphatidylinositol, lyso-phosphatidylcholine (lyso-PC), sphingomyelin, and several marine glycolipids with simple (monogalactosyldiacylglycerols or digalactosyldiacylglycerols) or more complex sugar polar heads, like those in several sphingoglycolipids, ceramides, and gangliosides. All these bioactive fish-derived PLs are usually rich in EPA and DHA, and to a lesser extent, docosapentaenoic acid, oleic acid, and stearidonic acid (Tsoupras et al., 2022) (Fig. 22.4). Fish-derived glycolipids also possess functional roles in cellular recognition and signal transduction. Their bioactivities include antimicrobial, antimalarial, antiviral, anticancer, immunomodulatory, and neurogenic effects. Glycolipids with sulfated sugar moieties, often originating from marine microalgae and accumulating through the food web into fish, exhibit potent antiinflammatory and antithrombotic properties (Fig. 22.5).

Several PL molecules, and especially those bearing MUFA or ω3 PUFA in their structures, are highly bioactive molecules. It is suggested that fish PLs can transport ω3 PUFAs more efficiently, enhancing their antithrombotic and antiinflammatory

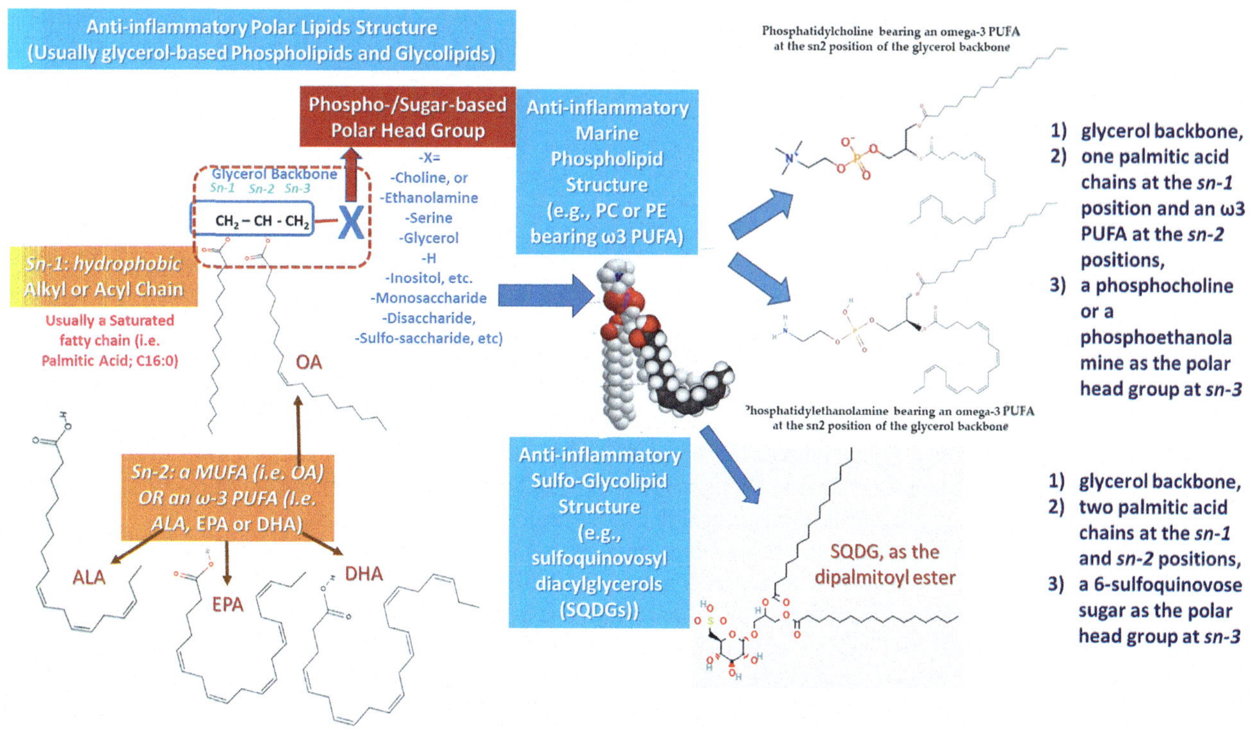

FIG. 22.4 Representative 2D and 3D structures of fish PL bioactives, with antiinflammatory and antithrombotic health-promoting properties. *PC*, phosphatidylcholines; *PE*, phosphatidylethanolamines; *PL*, polar lipids (either phospholipids or glycolipids); *SQDQ*, a specific class of sulfo-glycolipids containing 6-sulfoquinovose as the sulfo-sugar polar head group and 2 fatty acids esterified in the glycerol backbone. *(Source: Some structures are from the free open-access platform MolView.Org.)*

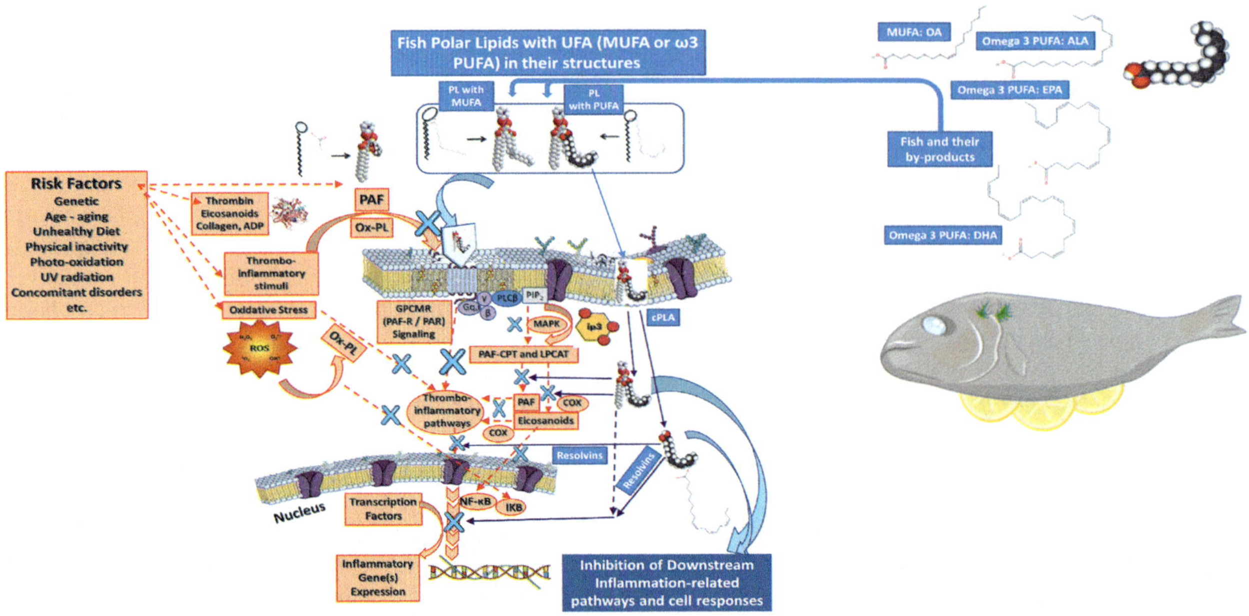

FIG. 22.5 Mechanisms of action of biofunctional polar lipids with UFA (MUFA or ω3 PUFA) in their structures, derived from fish and their by-products, against thrombo-inflammatory signaling and associated inflammatory cell responses and manifestations. Red colors: representative signaling of thrombo-inflammatory stimuli induced by the presence of several risk factors, such as those of PAF and thrombin, which, via the pathways shown, propagate the inflammatory cell responses. Blue colors: bioactive polar lipids (PLs) rich in UFA (MUFA or ω3 PUFA) from fish or their by-products can beneficially affect all these signaling pathways and transcription factors, thus further inhibiting the expression of thrombo-inflammatory genes and associated cell responses (the blue X represents an inhibitory effect on a pathway and/or an enzyme and/or a receptor and/or a transcription factor and/or the expression of thrombo-inflammatory genes by fish-derived bioactive polar lipids, as indicated by the blue arrows). *ADP*, adenosine diphosphate; *ALA*, alpha-linolenic acid; *COX*, cyclooxygenase; *cPLA2*, cytoplasmic phospholipase A2; *GPCMR*, G-protein-coupled membrane receptors; *IKB*, inhibitor of NF-kB; *IP3*, inositol trisphosphate; *MAPK*, mitogen-activated protein kinase; *MUFA*, monounsaturated fatty acids; *NF-kB*, nuclear factor kappa beta; *OA*, oleic acid; *Ox-PL*, oxidized phospholipids; *PAF*, platelet-activating factor; *PAF-CPT* and *LPCAT*, the basic biosynthetic enzymes of the two distinct pathways of PAF-synthesis, PAF-cholinephosphotransferase and lyso-phosphatidylcholine acetyltransferase 2, respectively; *PAF-R*, PAF-receptor; *PAR*, protease-activated receptors for thrombin; *PL*, polar lipids; *PLCβ*, phospholipase C beta; *PUFA*, poly-unsaturated fatty acids; *ROS*, reactive oxygen species; *UFA*, unsaturated fatty acid. *(From Papadopoulou, S.N.A., Adamantidi, T., Kranas, D., Cholidis, P., Anastasiadou, C., Tsoupras, A., 2025a. A comprehensive review on the valorization of bioactives from marine animal by-products for health-promoting, biofunctional cosmetics. Mar. Drugs. 16603397. 23 (8). Available from: https://www.mdpi.com/journal/marinedrugs. doi:10.3390/md23080299.)*

efficacy against specific signaling pathways and cascades of inflammation. For example, numerous studies have shown that PLs possess the ability to regulate the metabolism of platelet-activating factor (PAF), a potent inflammatory mediator involved in atherogenesis. In particular, an in vivo study in rabbits demonstrated that the administration of fish PLs led to a slowing of atherosclerosis progression through suppression of PAF biosynthesis and simultaneous enhancement of PAF catabolism (Nasopoulou et al., 2011), as overviewed by Tsoupras et al. (2022) (Fig. 22.5).

The antiinflammatory effect of PLs is also documented at the cellular level. In macrophage cultures, marine phospholipids inhibited lipopolysaccharide (LPS)-induced inflammatory responses through suppression of the mitogen-activated protein kinase (MAPK) and NF-κB signaling pathways (Papadopoulou et al., 2025a) (Fig. 22.4), while the preferential high incorporation of dietary fish PL in high-density lipoprotein cholesterol (HDL-C) increases HDL-C levels and also its antiinflammatory and antioxidant functionality (Velissaridou et al., 2024). These findings clearly indicate that their effects are not only limited to the regulation of PAF but extend to central mechanisms of inflammation.

Oily fish, including salmon and herring, are abundant sources of ω3 PUFAs and exhibit pronounced antiinflammatory and antithrombotic effects. They are characterized by a low ω6/ω3 PUFA ratio, which enhances the antiinflammatory and cardioprotective properties of fish PLs. A lower ω6/ω3 PUFA ratio is associated with improved protection against inflammation (Tsoupras et al., 2019a; Redfern et al., 2021; Tsoupras et al., 2018, 2019a). Moreover, apart from the direct effects that such PLs possess, they can also exhibit beneficial indirect effects through their fatty acid content. ω3 PUFA-rich PLs are transported via plasma lipoproteins to cellular membranes, where phospholipase A_2 (PLA_2) catalyzes the release of ω3 PUFAs from the sn-2 position of PLs. Even at lower concentrations, the EPA and DHA content of fish PLs is of great importance against inflammation, since when they are released by PLA_2 from cell membrane PLs, these ω3 PUFAs usually act as critical precursors for other bioactive lipid mediators and immune system regulators. More specifically, these liberated ω3 PUFAs subsequently act through eicosanoid pathways, involving cyclooxygenase (COX) enzymes, to resolve inflammation and regulate inflammatory cell responses (Fig. 22.5). These mediators are associated with cardiovascular protection, fetal brain and visual development, and neuroprotective actions against Alzheimer's disease and related neurodegenerative conditions (Tsoupras et al., 2022). Furthermore, it has been shown that the incorporation of ω3 PUFAs into platelet phospholipid membranes directly affects their function. In a classical study, it was found that this incorporation modifies the properties of the membranes and leads to a reduced adhesion capacity, contributing to an antithrombotic effect (Fig. 22.5).

Mackerel, another oily fish, contains comparable bioactive PL that exhibit strong antithrombotic and antiinflammatory activity through both platelet-activating factor (PAF) and thrombin pathways. Research indicates that these PL are more potent inhibitors of PAF and thrombin than neutral lipids, thereby conferring greater antiatherogenic potential (Nigam et al., 1996) Sardines, also classified as oily fish, are rich in such ω3 PUFA and demonstrate significant inhibitory activity against PAF. Raw sardines, in particular, possess PL with high ω3 PUFA levels and an exceptionally low ω6/ω3 PUFA ratio, which underpin their pronounced antiinflammatory and cardioprotective effects (Nasopoulou et al., 2013). Interestingly, not only oily fish, but also cod—a lean white fish—has been found to provide biofunctional lipids of nutritional importance. PLs derived from cod have shown strong antiplatelet activity against aggregation induced by PAF and thrombin, indicating that raw cod exhibits notable antiatherogenic and cardioprotective properties (Panayiotou et al., 2000).

Overall, fish PLs are not just structural components of membranes, but bioactive cell regulators with direct involvement in inflammatory and thrombotic mechanisms. Their incorporation into the diet may contribute substantially to the reduction of atherosclerosis and related cardiovascular diseases, paving the way for the development of not only new functional foods and nutraceuticals, but also nutricosmetic applications (Papadopoulou et al., 2025a). Moreover, the utilization of such highly bioactive fish PLs against skin inflammation and for cosmetic-related health-promoting applications is still in its infancy and needs further attention and research.

2.3.3 Fish-derived bioactive carotenoids and other pigments with similar structures

Pigments play a key role in producing the diverse coloration observed in fish and are therefore important indicators of quality. The most common carotenoids found in fish include lutein (green-yellow, predominantly in freshwater species), astaxanthin (yellow to red-pink, notably in salmon and present in both marine and freshwater species), canthaxanthin (orange-red), zeaxanthin (yellow-orange), β-carotene (orange), α- and β-doradexanthins (yellow), and tunaxanthin, which is commonly found in yellow-colored fish species such as *Scombrina, Caragana, Percina*, and *Seriola quinqueradiata* (Ashraf et al., 2020b). Some carotenoids are specific to certain fish species, and their generally low concentrations are influenced by dietary intake and the physiological status of the fish (PDF, Use of natural carotenoids for pigmentation in fishes, 2025).

Fish carotenoids have been widely used in cosmetic applications, initially for their pigmentation capacities, but lately, more and more for their potential bioactivities and health benefits. For example, astaxanthin, a red-orange carotenoid prevalent in salmon, shrimp, and other marine organisms, has drawn scientific interest due to its potent antioxidant capacity. It effectively neutralizes reactive oxygen species (ROS), particularly those generated by ultraviolet (UV) radiation, thus protecting skin cells from oxidative damage and delaying photoaging. Astaxanthin also exhibits strong antiinflammatory activity, further enhancing its utility in skincare formulations aimed at antiaging and sun protection (Xie et al., 2017).

Not only astaxanthin, but several such bioactive carotenoids and pigments of similar structures possess strong antioxidant properties that enable them to neutralize ROS and protect skin cells from oxidative damage caused by environmental stressors such as UV radiation and pollution. In addition, carotenoids can enhance skin tone and radiance, making them attractive components of plant-based and eco-conscious cosmetic formulations (Adamantidi et al., 2025).

Vitamin A, either derived from fish directly and/or through the metabolism of fish carotenoids, as well as vitamin A derivatives, including retinol and retinoic acid, plays a critical role in regulating epidermal cell turnover, stimulating collagen synthesis, and addressing common skin concerns such as fine lines, wrinkles, and hyperpigmentation. Although their use has historically been associated with irritation and photosensitivity, recent advances in encapsulation technologies and controlled-release delivery systems have significantly mitigated these drawbacks. Vitaminoids, particularly retinoids, are also essential for maintaining skin hydration, supporting barrier integrity, and promoting repair mechanisms, and they are compatible with a wide range of skincare formulations (Adamantidi et al., 2025).

Recent developments in cosmetic science have focused on enhancing the stability, bioavailability, and targeted delivery of these active compounds through detailed investigation of their molecular structure, biochemical behavior, and skin-related functions. Studies examining bioactive compounds such as vitamin A, vitaminoids, and carotenoids derived from several sources, including marine sources like fish and its by-products, have demonstrated their effectiveness in skin regeneration, wound healing, management of hyperpigmentation and acne, as well as in improving hydration, elasticity, and barrier repair. Notably, emerging technologies such as nanoemulsions and microencapsulation have further increased their efficacy and synergistic potential in skincare applications while reducing the risk of adverse effects (Adamantidi et al., 2025).

2.3.4 Fish-derived bioactive marine phenolics

Phenolic compounds are present in substantial amounts in marine organisms and encompass a diverse group of substances, including bromophenolic compounds, simple phenolic acids (such as hydroxycinnamic and hydroxybenzoic acids), flavonoids, and phlorotannins (Mateos et al., 2020). Among these classes, flavonoids are the most extensively studied and include compounds such as quercetin, rutin, and catechins, which are primarily found in algae and subsequently in fish through the food chain (Rathod et al., 2023).

For example, numerous cyanobacteria and macroalgae have been identified as rich sources of bromophenolic compounds, which can be transferred through the marine food web from macroalgae to invertebrate grazers and subsequently to fish. The characterization of these compounds is particularly important, as some bromophenols may exhibit toxic properties (Bidleman et al., 2019). Bromophenols—including hydroxylated and methoxylated bromodiphenyl ethers—are thought to originate largely from natural sources and from the biotransformation of both natural and anthropogenic compounds, given the limited evidence of their industrial use (Malmvärn et al., 2005). Natural marine bromophenols are mainly detected in red algae but are subsequently accumulated in several marine organisms too, including fish through dietary transfer. Notably, higher concentrations of hydroxylated and methoxylated polybrominated diphenyl ethers (PBDEs) have been reported in finfish than in shellfish, as reported by Malmvärn et al. (2005). According to data compiled by Koch and Sures (2018), tribromophenol concentrations in fish range from 3.7 to 230 ng/g wet weight (w/w).

It is well-established that phenolic compounds exhibit strong antioxidant, antiinflammatory, and anticancer activities, highlighting their potential relevance in nutrition, pharmaceuticals, and cosmeceutical applications.

2.4 Fish-derived vitamins, vitaminoids, and minerals

Apart from the aforementioned amphiphilic and lipophilic lipid-based fish-derived bioactive compounds, fish are also rich sources of lipid vitamins A, D_3, and E, as well as water-soluble B-complex vitamins, primarily obtained through the consumption of fish and/or fish oils (Awuchi et al., 2022; Kundam et al., 2018; Balami et al., 2019).

In addition, marine species contain notably high levels of essential and trace mineral elements. Compared with terrestrial foods, seafood provides greater amounts of several vital minerals, particularly in fish muscle tissue, including sodium (Na), potassium (K), calcium (Ca), magnesium (Mg), phosphorus (P), sulfur (S), iron (Fe), manganese (Mn), zinc (Zn), copper (Cu), selenium (Se), fluorine (F), and iodine (I) (Kundam et al., 2018; Jiang et al., 2014; Mogobe et al., 2015). Moreover, fish bones have been shown to be especially rich in calcium and phosphorus, as well as HA (Jimenez-Champi et al., 2024).

2.5 Fish-derived bioactive polysaccharides

Specific fish species are also rich sources of several bioactive polysaccharides, especially complex polysaccharide biopolymers like chitosan and glycosaminoglycans (GAGs) (i.e., chondroitin, glucosamine, and HA). The ECM and synovial fluid are largely composed of GAGs, including chondroitin sulfate (CS), glucosamine sulfate, and HA. GAGs are anionic heteropolysaccharides consisting of repeating disaccharide units of amino sugars and uronic acids linked by glycosidic bonds. They play essential roles in cellular signaling, tissue hydration, and the maintenance of structural integrity (Castrogiovanni et al., 2016). Among them, CS is a particularly important GAG that can be efficiently extracted from marine sources, especially blue shark (*Prionace glauca*) cartilage, which represents a rich and sustainable source of CS. Marine-derived CS typically has a lower molecular weight than terrestrial-derived CS, resulting in improved bioavailability and absorption. Research has shown that CS obtained from blue shark cartilage exhibits antiinflammatory and chondroprotective properties due to its amino acid composition, supporting joint health and cartilage regeneration. In addition, it has applications in cosmeceutical formulations, particularly for skin hydration and antiaging purposes (Golovach et al., 2023; López-Álvarez et al., 2020; Agustin et al., 2025).

GAGs are generally classified into sulfated and nonsulfated forms. Sulfated GAGs include CS, dermatan sulfate (DS), keratan sulfate, and heparin/heparan sulfate (HS), whereas HA is the only nonsulfated GAG (Paththuwe Arachchi et al.,

2025). CS is widely distributed within the ECM of connective tissues such as the brain, skin, tendons, and cartilage (Medeiros et al., 2021). Notably, CS can be extracted from various fish tissues, including the head, skin, eyes, cartilage, and fins (Urbi et al., 2022; Abdallah et al., 2020b). Glucosamine, a crystalline compound commonly found in connective tissues and cartilage—particularly as a structural component of chitin—serves as a key precursor in GAG biosynthesis (Ashraf et al., 2020; Jerosch, 2011). Lastly, HA, a major ECM constituent, is present in high concentrations in synovial fluid, skin, and the vitreous body of the eye (Abdallah et al., 2020; Elhiss et al., 2024).

Chitosan is another biopolymer derived from the deacetylation of chitin, which is abundant in the exoskeletons of crustaceans and certain fish. It has been shown to possess antimicrobial and moisturizing properties. In cosmetics, chitosan serves as a film-forming agent and stabilizer, commonly found in products such as facial masks, shampoos, conditioners, and moisturizers. It supports skin hydration by forming a semipermeable film that reduces transepidermal water loss (TEWL). In addition, chitosan-based materials are being explored for drug delivery, wound healing applications, and tissue engineering scaffolds, owing to their biocompatibility and biodegradability (Kumari et al., 2017).

3 Fish-derived bioactive compounds in functional cosmetics applications

In recent years, there has been a notable and steadily increasing trend toward the use of fish and fish by-products, including fish skin, heads, bones, scales, internal organs, shells, and tissues, which are increasingly being incorporated into cosmetic formulations due to their high content of bioactive compounds, such as polysaccharides, collagen, gelatin, peptides, minerals, fish oil, and several lipid bioactives, including ω3 PUFA, PLs, lipid vitamins, and carotenoid pigments. This trend is also driven by the recently developed modern green technologies for isolating these compounds from raw fish-derived sources. These bioactives provide antiaging, moisturizing, antioxidant, UV-protective, and skin-repairing effects, making them particularly attractive and valuable ingredients for applications in the field of cosmetology, including creams, serums, masks, and sunscreens. Their use not only enhances the functional performance of cosmetic products but also promotes sustainability by valorizing seafood processing waste (Brunt and Burgess, 2018; Ferreira et al., 2021; Rotter et al., 2024; Siahaan et al., 2022). Table 22.3 summarizes examples of commercial cosmetic and cosmeceutical products that incorporate marine by-products as active ingredients.

3.1 Fish-derived polysaccharides in functional cosmetics applications

Several polysaccharides can be retrieved from several marine sources, including fish, but mainly from its by-products (i.e., skin, scales, bones, heads, etc.). Marine polysaccharides play a vital role in cosmetics, serving as moisturizers, emulsifiers, thickening agents, and wound healing agents due to their broad spectrum of bioactivities. These include antimicrobial, antioxidant, antiaging, matrix metalloproteinase (MMP)—inhibitory, anticancer, antiinflammatory, antifungal, and other therapeutic properties. Among them, chitin, chitosan, and their derivatives have garnered special attention for cosmetic use (Carrasqueira et al., 2025; Casadidio et al., 2019; Wu et al., 2024). These compounds have been proposed for use in formulations targeting the skin, oral cavity, nails, and hair, allowing the treatment of various related conditions (Casadidio et al., 2019).

3.1.1 Chitin and chitosan in functional cosmetics applications

Chitin is a rigid polysaccharide with low solubility, making it challenging to work with. In contrast, chitosan is soluble in acidic solutions and can form films, scaffolds, fibers, and micro-, nano-, and milli-particles. At physiological pH, certain oligosaccharides and derivatives of chitin and chitosan are water-soluble, exhibiting enhanced or novel properties. In cosmetics, chitin, chitosan, and their derivatives act either as active ingredi-ents due to their bioactivities or as carriers for other bioactive agents owing to their tech-nological adaptability (Aranaz et al., 2018).

In the European Union (EU), cosmetic ingredients are regulated under the Cosmetic Product Regulation (2009) (https://health.ec.europa.eu/system/files/2016-11/cosmetic_1223_2009_regulation_en_0.pdf, accessed 6 June 2025). The CosIng database lists eight entries under "chitin," mostly cited as abrasive and bulking agents. The search term "chitosan" yields 55 entries, where chitosan is primarily characterized as a film-forming and hair-fixing agent (CosIng—Cosmetics—GROWTH—European Commission, n.d.).

Chitosan and its derivatives are excellent candidates for skincare formulations due to their high molecular weight (HMW) and cationic nature, which promote skin adhesion (Rotter et al., 2024). Their safety, nontoxicity, biocompatibility, and biodegradability make them suitable as excipients or active ingredients in cosmetics (Casadidio et al., 2019). They are used in various cosmetic products, including lotions, skin moisturizers, creams, foundations, eye shadows, lip-sticks, cleansing wipes, and bath products (Hesse, 1979). Chitosan has been utilized for several functional cosmetics applications.

TABLE 22.3 Examples of commercial cosmetic products utilizing bioactive ingredients from fish and its by-products.

Patent name or cosmetic formulation	Marine bioactives derived from fish sources (formulation content)	Cosmetic-associated benefits and commercial use	References
Marine Hydrolyzed Collagen IMW (Ashland Global Holdings, Wilmington, DE, United States)	Marine collagen oligopeptides, upcycled from fish skin	• Biofunctional cosmetic ingredient for scalp and hair purposes • Collagen boosting and glow-enhancing results • Use in skin-care, hair-care, makeup, and bath products	(Badilli and Inal, 2025)
Affinisphere (BASF, Ludwigshafen, Germany)	Marine atelocollagen microspheres from shark fins	• Oily skin improvement • Perfect for impure and oily skin during summer and humid climates • Mattifying cream and serum products	(Badilli and Inal, 2025)
Marine Filling Spheres (BASF, Ludwigshafen, Germany)	Dehydrated microspheres of marine collagen and GAGs from shark fins	• Moisturization and antiwrinkle properties • Skin soothing and surface-smoothing results • Use in antiaging, facial skin health, and lip-care products	(Badilli and Inal, 2025)
COLLASURGE (Croda Beauty, Yorkshire, UK)	Marine collagen amino acids from fish species	• Moisturizing, hydrating, nourishing, repairing, soothing, cooling, and softening properties for creams, gels, skin- and hair-care products	(Badilli and Inal, 2025)
Ichtyocollagen (Sederma by Croda Beauty, Snaith, UK)	pH-soluble marine collagen from fish skin extract	• Moisturizing, hydrating, nourishing, repairing, and film-forming properties • Used in creams and gels	(Badilli and Inal, 2025)
Finn Canada (Canada)	FINN's salmon skin collagen (Salmonollagen)	• Improves skin condition, treating wrinkles, spots, dryness, dulness, and acne • Used in cleansing foams, scrub cleansing foams, gels, creams, extracts, toning, and milk lotions	(Siahaan et al., 2022)
Pure Marine Collagen (Kenney and Ross Limited, Port Saxon, Nova Scotia, Canada)	Hydrolyzed collagen from the skin of deep-sea wild fish	• Promotes healthy skin, nails, and hair outcomes • Improves skin hydration, elasticity, and firmness • Used as a protein additive in cosmetics, nutraceuticals, or food products	(Siahaan et al., 2022)
Collagen HM Sol, Elastin TM, Glycosann Sol, and Protein M+ (220 Rue du Petit Port, France)	Hydrolyzed marine collagen, elastin, chondroitin sulfate, and cartilage extract from fish by-products	• Moisturizing, cell firmness, regeneration, and elasticity benefits for antiaging and antiwrinkle purposes	(Sotelo et al., 2021)
ThalaCol (Thai Union Ingredients (Global), Bangkok, Thailand)	Contains 100% pure, hydrolyzed marine collagen peptides from wild tuna skin	• Provides more radiant and youthful skin, offering effective incorporation into topical skincare cosmetics like moisturizer sticks	(Premium High-Purity Marine Collagen Peptides | Thala, n.d.)
Nutricoll Natural Marine Collagen Powder (Chitinor, Seagarden, Norway)	Natural fish collagen peptide derived from wild cod	• Antiaging, antiwrinkle, moisturizing, and hair protection bioactive, free from artificial additives and preservatives • Used in face masks, creams, serums, lotions, hair balms, shampoos, and conditioners	(Nutricoll Natural Marine Collagen Powder—Chitinor, n.d.)
Cropure Orange Roughy (Croda Beauty, UK)	Orange roughy oil (*Hoplostethus atlanticus*)	• Good-spreading, nongreasy, emollient, softening, and moisturizing agent in creams, lotions, sun-care, color, and bath cosmetics	(Cropure Orange Roughy—Croda, n.d.)
Zellulin ZelluGEN 10% Solution (Avant, Old Street, London)	Hydrolyzed fish-derived minnow muscle cell lysate biopeptides	• Regenerating, revitalizing, skin-smoothing agent used in leave-on body care and cosmetic products • Antiaging agent that promotes elastic skin, collagen production, and skin hydration benefits	(Zellulin® ZelluGEN 10% Solution—Avant, n.d.)
Earthen InstantPeel Exfoliant (Earthen SkinCare, Pleasantville, New York)	Shrimp extract, fish oil, and hydrolyzed collagen from fish	• Gentle exfoliation and moisturization properties • Exfoliant aimed to improve skin texture (smooth, soft, and luminous looking)	(InstantPeelTM Exfoliant, n.d.)

Patent name or cosmetic formulation	Marine bioactives derived from fish sources (formulation content)	Cosmetic-associated benefits and commercial use	References
DHC Astaxanthin Power Cream (DHC, United States)	Astaxanthin is found in large amounts in salmon	• Lightweight, fast-absorbing facial moisturizer that tones, hydrates, and brightens the skin for achieving a radiant-looking skin complexion	(Astaxanthin Collagen All-in-One Gel, n.d.)

From Papadopoulou, S.N.A., Adamantidi, T., Kranas, D., Cholidis, P., Anastasiadou, C., Tsoupras, A., 2025a. A comprehensive review on the valorization of bioactives from marine animal by-products for health-promoting, biofunctional cosmetics. Mar. Drugs. 16603397. 23 (8). Available from: https://www.mdpi.com/journal/marinedrugs. doi:10.3390/md23080299.

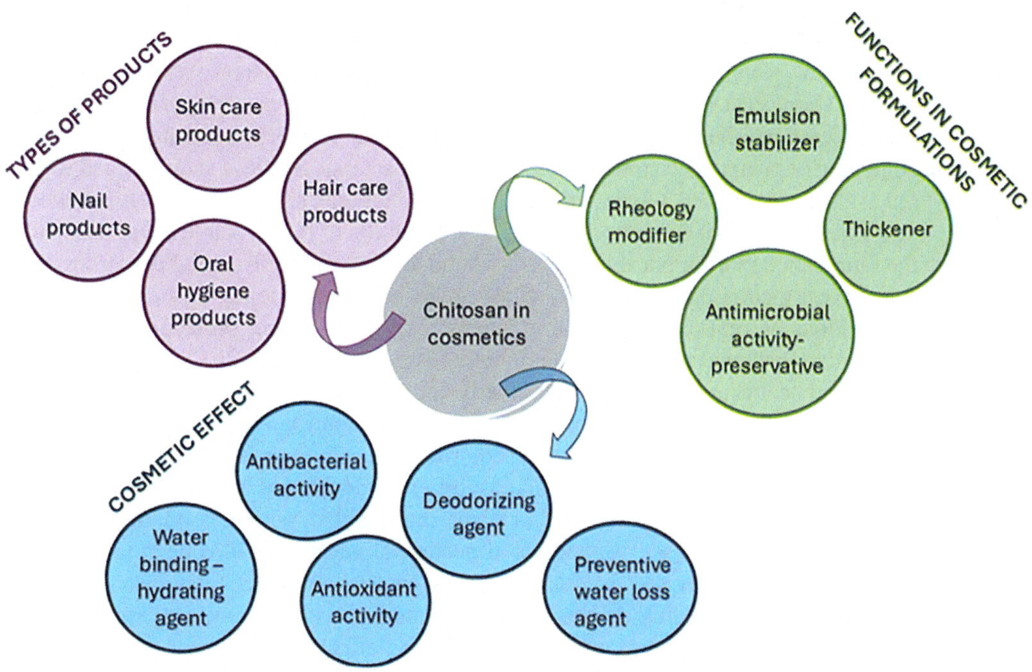

FIG. 22.6 A summary of chitosan applications in cosmetics. *(From Papadopoulou, S.N.A., Adamantidi, T., Kranas, D., Cholidis, P., Anastasiadou, C., Tsoupras, A., 2025a. A comprehensive review on the valorization of bioactives from marine animal by-products for health-promoting, biofunctional cosmetics. Mar. Drugs. 16603397. 23 (8). Available from: https://www.mdpi.com/journal/marinedrugs. doi:10.3390/md23080299.)*

For example, it has been widely used as an antiaging and moisturizing agent, as a UV-radiation-protective agent, as a skin-cleansing agent, as a nail-care agent, and as a hair-care agent, as well as an antibacterial agent and an oral-cavity-protective agent, among other uses (Papadopoulou et al., 2025a). A summary of well-documented chitosan applications in cosmetics is depicted in Fig. 22.6.

For example, chitosan—particularly in its high-molecular-weight (HMW) form—forms a transparent film on the skin that reduces TEWL and enhances skin elasticity and smoothness, making it an effective moisturizing agent in cosmetic formulations (Casadidio et al., 2019). In addition, Morganti et al. (2014) demonstrated that chitin- and chitosan-based nanofibril–hyaluronan carriers, formulated as nanoemulsions or nonwoven films, promoted collagen synthesis while inhibiting collagenase activity. Nanoemulsions containing a liposomal complex of HA, phosphatidylcholine, and chitin increased collagen production, whereas formulations enriched with an antioxidant complex of melatonin, vitamin E, and β-glucan (MEB) exhibited strong collagenase inhibition of approximately 90%. Further in vitro studies showed that both oral and topical administration of chitin nanofibril-hyaluronan MEB formulations enhanced skin repair in acne-affected and photo-irradiated areas while restoring dermal moisture balance.

Afonso et al. (2019) reported that re-acetylated chitosan films enabled a more efficient release of antioxidants with anti-aging potential, such as vitamin C, while maintaining flexibility and noncytotoxicity, achieving a rapid release of approximately 52% of active compounds within 15 min. These findings suggest that chitosan-based films are promising materials for antiaging facial masks. Moreover, Chaiwong et al. (2020) showed that carboxymethyl chitosan (CMCH) with varying molecular weights significantly improved water solubility and skin hydration.

Chen et al. (2017) developed montmorillonite-quaternized CMCH composites that enhanced UV protection and moisture retention, highlighting their potential as effective antiaging cosmetic ingredients. Chitin and chitosan form stable, water-resistant, cytocompatible films that absorb UV below 400 nm, making them a perfect candidate for protective cream formulations as well (Casadidio et al., 2019). Therefore to prevent negative skin reactions caused by prolonged sun exposure, sun-screens incorporating chitosan and other highly protective ingredients are utilized (Nitulescu et al., 2023; Ntohogian et al., 2018). For instance, according to Ntohogian et al. (2018), chitosan nanoparticles have been utilized as active carriers and stabilizers for encapsulating natural and purified annatto and saffron (sunscreen agents) to formulate UV-protective sunscreen emulsions. Morsy et al. (2017) developed a multifunctional hydroxyapatite-chitosan (HAP-chitosan) gel as a hybrid antibacterial sunscreen system that can also reduce the negative effects of exposure to UV radiation.

In general, positively charged chitosan interacts with the negatively charged bacterial cell walls, leading to membrane destabilization and subsequent cell shrinkage. This interaction represents a widely accepted mechanism underlying the topical antibacterial activity of chitosan. The extent of bacterial inactivation depends on both the molecular weight and charge density of the chitosan polymer chains. Notably, antibacterial efficacy has been shown to increase with higher chitosan molecular weight (Rejinold et al., 2021). Verma et al. (2021) further confirmed the antimicrobial potential of chitosan, reporting a reduction of >90% in bacterial proliferation following chitosan treatment. Deng et al. (2022) found that a multifunctional, biobased hydrogel formulation composed of quaternized chitosan and dialdehyde bacterial cellulose showed good wound healing and antibacterial activity. Liu et al. (2022) studied a hydrogel formulation from borax cross-linked polyvinyl alcohol (PVA) and CMCH that demonstrated excellent self-healing properties, while the addition of highly stable silver nanoparticles (AgNPs) to the hydrogel made the formulation more applicable for both wound healing and antibacterial properties.

Chitosan and its derivatives, incorporated into gels, sprays, chewing gums, mouth-washes, dentifrices, and microspheres, have found applications as oral-cavity-protective agents too, by providing protection against conditions like oral mucositis, plaque formation, bacterial growth, and periodontal issues (Gao et al., 2022a; Zúñiga-López et al., 2024; Ramadhany et al., 2018). In oral healthcare, polymers, particularly chitosan, can function either as a vehicle or as a carrier. Examples of the former include their use in toothpaste, mouth rinse, chewing gum, and dental varnishes, while they can also act as a carrier for sodium fluoride (NaF), herbal extracts, and chlorhexidine. Chitosan's activities in the oral cavity include buffering mouth pH, antimicrobial action, inhibiting biofilm adsorption, and acting as an antiabrasive agent (Aranaz et al., 2018). Chitosan has been used in periodontal gels with excellent antimicrobial activities (Ganguly et al., 2017), while fluoride-loaded nanoparticles based on chitosan, alginate, and pectin polymers have also been used for dental delivery (Nguyen et al., 2017). Finally, hydrogels derived from natural polymers such as chitosan, alginate, gelatin, and HA have demonstrated considerable potential as oral drug delivery systems compared with conventional approaches. These hydrogels enable sustained release of therapeutic agents, reduce systemic side effects, and enhance treatment efficacy, making them suitable for the management of oral lesions.

Hydroxypropyl chitosan (HPCH) is an effective nail-care agent that delivers active ingredients while forming a protective, hydrating film that preserves keratin and improves nail structure (Monti et al., 2022; Cantoresi et al., 2014). It helps reduce dystrophic symptoms, lowers the risk of recurrent fungal infections, and enhances mechanical properties such as hardness and strength, while also protecting nails from fungal penetration and physical damage (Ghannoum et al., 2015).

Finally, chitin and chitosan can also improve hair hydration, repair damaged strands, and enhance shine, making them widely used in shampoos, conditioners, hair sprays, and styling products (Aranaz et al., 2018; Guzmán et al., 2022; Smart and Sustainable Hair Products Based on Chitin-Derived Compounds, n.d.; Sionkowska et al., 2017; Liu et al., 2025; Mohamed et al., 2025). As cationic polymers, chitosan and its derivatives bind to negatively charged keratin on damaged hair, forming a protective, elastic film that strengthens and softens hair (Akanno et al., 2020; Fernández-Peña and Guzmán, 2020; Wang et al., 2020). Studies show that chitosan-based formulations, especially when combined with collagen, HA, or thiadiazole conjugates, improve moisture retention, elasticity, and hair manageability (Sionkowska et al., 2017; Mohamed et al., 2025). Complementary peptide-based treatments, such as Olaplex and K18, repair hair at the molecular level, providing a combined surface- and cortex-level restoration for healthier hair (Martins et al., 2024).

3.1.2 HA, GAGs, carrageenan, and fucoidans as cosmetic ingredients

Apart from chitin and chitosan, several other marine polysaccharides derived from fish, including HA and GAGs, have also emerged as promising cosmetic ingredients due to their diverse structural features and multifaceted bioactivities. For example, HA, which is usually isolated from by-products of the fishing industry, such as fish skin and scales, has been increasingly used in moisturizing and antiaging formulations (Papadopoulou et al., 2025a).

HA from fish sources, such as bluefin tuna by-products, exhibits strong moisturizing and antiinflammatory properties, making it a promising ingredient for cosmetic and cosmeceutical applications (Elhiss et al., 2024). Fish-derived GAGs, including CS and glucosamine from shark cartilage, contribute to skin hydration, tissue architecture, and ECM regulation. Clinical-grade fish cartilage hydrolysates, rich in CS and collagen peptides, have been shown in ex vivo and randomized trials to enhance fibroblast activity, stimulate endogenous hyaluronan and elastin synthesis, suppress MMPs, and improve skin hydration, elasticity, and barrier function, thereby reducing signs of photoaging (Abdallah et al., 2020; Kim, 2023; Vázquez et al., 2013; Yuan et al., 2024; Wauquier et al., 2022).

In addition, fucose-rich polysaccharides and sulfated compounds present in fish mucus provide antioxidant, antiinflammatory, and collagen-supporting effects. These fish-derived molecules can enhance moisture retention, promote skin repair, and reduce UV-induced aging, making them valuable for serums and antiaging creams (Mourão et al., 2018; Wang et al., 2023; Kang et al., 2024).

3.2 Proteins, protein hydrolysates, peptides, and amino acids in functional cosmetics applications

3.2.1 Collagen

Collagen is one of the most studied and widely used biopolymers in cosmetics because it acts as a natural moisturizer and hydrating ingredient, while also helping to preserve the elasticity and structural integrity of the skin. Collagen is the primary structural protein in connective tissues and usually forms a triple-helix structure that provides strength and elasticity. It also regulates cellular activity, making it valuable in regenerative medicine and wound healing. While traditionally sourced from bovine and porcine by-products, these sources carry risks of disease transmission and face cultural or religious restrictions. As a result, marine collagen is emerging as a safe and effective alternative for biomedical and cosmetic applications (Manel et al., 2020). Thus recently, there has been intense interest in research on collagen of marine origin, especially on the use of fish-derived sustainable collagen from fish by-products like fish skin in cosmetics, because of its beneficial bioactive properties for skin regeneration and healing, as well as due to its superior absorption capabilities (Venkatesan et al., 2017).

Marine collagen, particularly type I collagen derived from fish such as salmon, cod, tilapia, and gray mullet, is a highly effective and versatile ingredient for both cosmetic and wound healing applications (Papadopoulou et al., 2025a). Its lower molecular weight allows faster absorption than mammalian collagen, providing deep hydration, forming a protective barrier, and improving skin elasticity, firmness, and moisture retention. In cosmetics, creams and serums containing fish collagen enhance skin hydration, elasticity, and firmness; reduce wrinkles and pore size; counteract photoaging; and alleviate acne, with hydrolyzed collagen preferred for better solubility, dermal penetration, and water-binding ability (Venkatesan et al., 2017; Sionkowska et al., 2020; Sugibayashi et al., 2019; Allard et al., 2003; Xhauflaire-Uhoda et al., 2008; Al-Atif, 2022; Wang et al., 2018; Li et al., 2022; Salvatore et al., 2020; Klimaszewska et al., 2019; Jimbo et al., 2016; Hou et al., 2012; Shibuya et al., 2014; Rahman et al., 2024; Elbialy et al., 2020; Shalaby et al., 2020). Fish collagen also exhibits antiaging effects by supporting fibroblast proliferation, promoting collagen and elastin repair, regulating the type I/III collagen ratio, and potentiating vitamin C derivatives. In wound healing, it stimulates keratinocyte proliferation, fibroblast differentiation, angiogenesis, ECM synthesis, and collagen deposition, while reducing inflammation and metalloproteinase activity. Compared with mammalian sources, fish collagen offers a more diverse and stable protein composition, lower risk of zoonotic disease transmission, mild odor, good mechanical strength, and compatibility with halal requirements. Derived from fish by-products, it represents a sustainable and valuable resource that aligns with circular economy and waste reduction strategies (Azarian and Sutapun, 2022; Mititelu et al., 2022; Ngandjui et al., 2024).

3.2.2 Gelatin

Gelatin derived from marine fish by-products, such as cod, salmon, and tilapia, is a partially hydrolyzed form of collagen that exhibits strong antioxidant, antiinflammatory, and photoprotective properties. In cosmetics, fish gelatin and its hydrolysates are widely used as thickening and stabilizing agents in creams, lotions, shampoos, hair sprays, sunscreens, and bath products (Papadopoulou et al., 2025a). They protect the skin from UV-induced damage by preserving lipids, supporting collagen synthesis, reducing oxidative stress, and modulating the TGF-β/Smad and NF-κB pathways (Barba and Lorenzo, 2020; Venkatesan et al., 2017; Al-Nimry et al., 2021; Chen and Hou, 2016). Marine gelatin peptides, including sequences like Leu–Ser–Gly–Tyr–Gly–Pro, limit lipid peroxidation, enhance collagen deposition (indicated by increased hydroxyproline), and maintain skin architecture, thereby preventing photoaging and improving skin hydration and firmness (Zhuang and Sun, 2011; Sun et al., 2013; Chen et al., 2016). These properties make marine gelatin and its derivatives valuable, multifunctional ingredients for antiaging, photoprotective, and regenerative cosmetic formulations (Awuchi et al., 2022; Proximate composition of New Zealand Marine Finfish and Shellfish, n.d.).

3.2.3 Other proteins: Enzymes

In addition to collagen, other bioactive molecules in fish, such as enzymes and peptides, are also believed to have significant antiaging properties. For example, it has been reported that an enzyme isolated from salmon eggs has a remarkable rejuvenating effect on skin tissue. Of particular interest is the serine endoprotease (known as Zonase), which, in its normal function, participates in the breakdown of the egg shell during hatching without affecting the embryo. The enzyme Zonase from salmon eggs has attracted research interest in the cosmetics sector for its antiaging properties, as it has exhibited moisturizing and antiaging effects comparable to, or even superior to, those of certain conventional cosmetic ingredients, while mimicking the skin's endogenous molecules responsible for maintaining moisture (Brunt and Burgess, 2018). Thus in cosmetic applications, this enzyme has been shown to effectively remove dead keratinocytes through enzymatic exfoliation, while promoting the proliferation of new cells in the skin.

Topical application of salmon (*Salmo salar*) egg extracts has been associated with a reduction in wrinkles, a reduction in erythema, an improvement in pigmentation uniformity, and an enhancement of skin hydration, without causing side effects. This extract contains a variety of bioactive components, such as unsaturated fatty acids, proteins, nucleic acids (DNA, RNA), vitamins, and trace elements. It is estimated that unsaturated fatty acids, such as oleic and linoleic acids (LAs), contributed to improving transdermal absorption, allowing active compounds to penetrate deeper into the dermis. The most pronounced effect recorded was a reduction in wrinkles. This result appears to be due to the synergistic action of vitamin A, amino acids, and minerals such as zinc and copper, which support the maintenance of skin elasticity and the stability of the ECM, thereby limiting sagging and the formation of new wrinkles.

3.2.4 Amino acids, their combinations in small peptides, and several bioactive peptides in functional cosmetics

Marine-derived amino acids are essential for maintaining skin structure and function, as they serve as building blocks for proteins like collagen, elastin, and keratin (Wu, 2020; Cadar et al., 2024; Al Hajj et al., 2024). Key amino acids from marine sources—such as glycine, proline, hydroxyproline, lysine, arginine, histidine, and taurine—support collagen stability, wound healing, skin hydration, barrier repair, and microcirculation (Al Hajj et al., 2024; Murakami et al., 2012). Deficiencies in these amino acids can impair protein synthesis, leading to wrinkles, sagging, dryness, and delayed wound healing. Furthermore, epidermal keratinocytes require amino acids to synthesize certain antimicrobial peptides (e.g., cathelicidins and defensins), which combat pathogens and maintain a balanced skin microbiome (Cadar et al., 2024; Solano, 2020). Marine amino acids are safe, nontoxic, and sustainable, derived from natural sources that do not trigger allergic reactions, possessing antioxidant effects and promoting collagen production, making them valuable cosmeceutical ingredients (Solano, 2020). Key amino acids—such as histidine, lysine, arginine, glycine, proline, and leucine (abundant in collagen)—contribute to wound healing, skin firmness, and wrinkle reduction. In practice, each of the 20 standard amino acids, derived from various marine sources, contributes to the creation and maintenance of smooth, healthy, and youthful-looking skin while also regulating the aging process.

Commercially, several amino acid-based skincare products are currently available. Characteristic examples include the MAAs, which are abundant in marine organisms, including fish, algae, and invertebrates, function as natural UV-absorbing compounds, and thus protect against UVA and UVB radiation without generating free radicals. In addition, they exhibit antioxidant and antiphotoaging properties, improve skin elasticity, and reduce fine lines, sunburn, and, therefore, photoaging (Prajaputra et al., 2024; Rasal and Khajure, 2024). They scavenge ROS such as hydroxyl radicals, singlet oxygen, and superoxide anions, thereby protecting the skin from oxidative stress induced by UV exposure or environmental stimuli. MAAs can enhance endogenous antioxidant defenses by upregulating enzymes such as superoxide dismutase (SOD) and catalase (CAT), supporting skin photoprotection. Together, marine amino acids and MAAs provide hydration, antiaging, UV protection, and skin repair benefits, making them highly valuable ingredients in cosmetic and cosmeceutical formulations (Cadar et al., 2024; Al Hajj et al., 2024; Murakami et al., 2012; Solano, 2020; Rasal and Khajure, 2024; Beaumont and Blachier, 2020; Yoshimura et al., 2023; Rosic, 2019; Oda et al., 2017; Eckes et al., 2015; Brotherton and Balskus, 2015; Urrea-Victoria et al., 2025; Chavda et al., 2023; Wada et al., 2015; Lawrence et al., 2018; Gacesa et al., 2018; Kageyama et al., 2019; Waditee-Sirisattha and Kageyama, 2021).

Moreover, for skin care, important ones from the classic amino acids also include the cationic histidine, lysine, and arginine, as well as the neutral glycine, proline, and leucine, the latter being particularly abundant in collagen. Beyond their role in protein synthesis, these amino acids contribute to essential skin functions. They act complementarily, meaning no single amino acid is inherently the most important (Lee et al., 2023). Studies have shown that lysine, combined with arginine, can accelerate wound healing, enhance biocompatibility and hydrophilicity, and help prevent infections, while the combination of leucine, glycine, and proline improves skin firmness and reduces wrinkles (Park et al., 2017).

Several other combinations have also been studied, along with the incorporation of a fatty chain to increase amphiphilicity, such as a palmitoyl chain, which has a wide range of cosmetic and skin-protective effects (Papadopoulou et al., 2025a). Some combinations promote wound healing and enhance collagen synthesis by stimulating fibroblasts and upregulating type I collagen, DS, HS, and ECM gene expression, thereby increasing skin firmness and elasticity. They improve skin hydration by upregulating aquaporin-3 and strengthen the skin barrier, while their antioxidant activity protects DNA, scavenges superoxide radicals, inhibits lipid peroxidation, and activates Nrf2-dependent enzymes to prevent UV-induced damage (Solano, 2020; Bojarska, 2020; Lei et al., 2025; Husein El Hadmed and Castillo, 2016; Liu et al., 2024; Henseler, 2023; Waszkielewicz and Mirosław, 2024; Peptides in Cosmetics: From Pharmaceutical Breakthroughs to Skincare Innovations, n.d.; Pintea et al., 2025; Xie et al., 2018; Deng et al., 2020; Tałałaj et al., 2019; Mota et al., 2025; Resende et al., 2021; Usage of Synthetic Peptides in Cosmetics for Sensitive Skin, n.d.). Some such small amino acid combinations also provide antiinflammatory benefits, reduce wrinkle depth and volume, smooth skin texture, and soften wrinkles (Solano, 2020; ; Lei et al., 2025; Husein El Hadmed and Castillo, 2016; Liu et al., 2024; Henseler, 2023; Waszkielewicz and Mirosław, 2024; Peptides in Cosmetics: From Pharmaceutical Breakthroughs to Skincare Innovations, n.d.; Pintea et al., 2025; Xie et al., 2018; Deng et al., 2020; Tałałaj et al., 2019; Mota et al., 2025; Resende et al., 2021; Usage of Synthetic Peptides in Cosmetics for Sensitive Skin, n.d.). In addition, they exhibit whitening potential through tyrosinase inhibition, modulate antiaging molecular pathways, and increase tissue inhibitors of MMP1 and MMP2 while downregulating MMP9 (Solano, 2020; ; Husein El Hadmed and Castillo, 2016; Liu et al., 2024). Their neurocosmetic properties include blocking calcium channels and inhibiting acetylcholine release, functioning in a nontoxic manner similar to enkephalins (; Husein El Hadmed and Castillo, 2016). Mixed with palmitic acid or elaidic acid, they further reduce wrinkle depth, improve texture, and enhance overall skin appearance (Solano, 2020; ; Lei et al., 2025; Husein El Hadmed and Castillo, 2016; Waszkielewicz and Mirosław, 2024; Peptides in Cosmetics: From Pharmaceutical Breakthroughs to Skincare Innovations, n.d.; Tałałaj et al., 2019). Clinical studies have demonstrated that creams containing such small combinations can achieve up to a 27% reduction in periorbital wrinkle depth, highlighting their potent antiaging, moisturizing, antioxidant, antiinflammatory, and photoprotective properties (; Husein El Hadmed and Castillo, 2016; Henseler, 2023).

Apart from such small peptide formulations derived from simple amino acid combinations, several other marine-derived bioactive peptides, particularly those derived from fish and other seafood by-products and hydrolysates, are also valuable functional ingredients in skincare and cosmeceuticals due to their wide range of antioxidant, antimicrobial, antiphotoaging, antiwrinkle, and skin-protective properties (Papadopoulou et al., 2025a), as well as immunomodulatory, antihypertensive, and anticancer effects (Xia et al., 2021a; Kang et al., 2019; Peng et al., 2022; Hu et al., 2012; Fernando et al., 2023). Such marine-derived bioactive peptides, typically 3–20 amino acids long, are released from marine proteins via enzymatic hydrolysis using proteases like trypsin, pepsin, chymotrypsin, alcalase, and papain (Marine Bioactive Peptides: Anti-Photoaging Mechanisms and Potential Skin Protective Effects, n.d.). Several of these marine peptides have been found to protect the skin against UV-induced damage by inhibiting ROS, regulating MMPs, promoting collagen synthesis, and modulating pathways such as TGF-β/Smad and MAPK (Siahaan et al., 2022; Chen et al., 2016; Xia et al., 2021; Yang et al., 2023; Lu et al., 2017; Lønne et al., 2013; Zhang et al., 2011; Chotphruethipong et al., 2021; Chen et al., 2019; Maia Campos et al., 2021; Fu et al., 2022; Gao et al., 2022a). Notable examples include cod skin gelatin hydrolysates, tilapia gelatin peptides, and marine collagen peptides from *Pollachius virens*, *Hippoglossus hippoglossus*, and *Pleuronectes platessa* (Venkatesan et al., 2017; Cadar et al., 2024; Lu et al., 2017; Yang et al., 2023).

The use of peptides derived from fish by-products is particularly attractive for cosmetics, as it combines high bioactivity with sustainability. These peptides contribute to antiaging, photoprotection, skin hydration, wrinkle reduction, and overall skin health, supporting the development of innovative skincare and antiaging formulations (Marques et al., 2019). Specific examples of fish-derived marine bioactive peptides in functional cosmetics applications are shown in Table 22.4.

3.3 Amphiphilic and lipophilic marine bioactive compounds of lipid nature in functional cosmetics applications

Apart from the more polar sugar-based marine polysaccharides and amino acid-based marine-derived compounds (proteins, enzymes, protein hydrolysates and simple amino acids), a vast array of several other bioactive compounds exist in fish sources, which, due to their less polar nature, are usually classified as either amphiphilic or lipophilic substances, usually of lipid nature. Within these marine bioactives, classic lipid molecules are usually included, such as FFAs, triglycerides, esters, long-chain hydrocarbon-based compounds, along with not-so-lipophilic but more amphiphilic compounds like lipid vitamins, carotenoids, and other pigments of similar structures and PLs, while some more polar substances like marine phenolics are also included in this broad category of marine amphiphilic bioactives. Depending on their structures and the

TABLE 22.4 Examples of fish-derived peptides in cosmetic-related functions and applications.

Fish species	Bioactive peptides	Biological activity	Cosmetic-related functions	References
Tilapia	Skin-collagen peptides	Oral mucosal ulcers	• 75% marine collagen peptides promoted the proliferation and migration of L929 cells • Enhanced ulcer healing • Suppressed inflammation • Upregulated expression of the vascular endothelial growth factor (VEGF) and fibroblast growth factors (FGF)	(Gao et al., 2022b)
Tuna (*Thunnus obesus*)	Collagen peptide from skin (TSCP) and bone (TBCP)	UVB protection, photoaging, and radical scavenging/antioxidant effects	• *Reduced skin photoaging via MAPK and TGF-β signaling pathways* • Inhibited phosphorylated (p)-*p38* activation, enhanced TGF-β1, and decreased p-ERK, p-Janus kinase inhibitor (JNK), and MMP-1 • ROS scavenging antioxidant action • Improved cell viability, suppressed mRNA, and protein expression • Inhibited skin water loss (TEWL)	(Fu et al., 2022)
Black pomfret (*Parastromateus niger*)	Peptides	Antiaging potential	• Improved skin aging due to the free radical scavenging and antiaging activity of the peptides	(Xia et al., 2021)
Hydrolyzed fish cartilage	Collagen peptides	Antiaging potential	• Reduced wrinkles and increased dermis echogenicity • Enhanced collagen morphology and decreased elastosis • Improved morphological skin characteristics and thickness	(Maia Campos et al., 2021)
Giant croaker (*Nibea japonica*)	Swim bladder collagen peptides: acid- and pepsin-solubilized collagen (ASC and PSC)	Wound healing and antioxidant potential	• ASC and PSC displayed antioxidant and radical scavenging properties • Collagen sponge peptides accelerated wound healing (scratch closure rate) • Decreased IL-1β, IL-6, and tumor necrosis factor α (TNF-α) levels (antiinflammatory benefits)	(Chen et al., 2019)
Sea bass (*Late calcarifer*)	Hydrolyzed collagen from the defatted Asian sea bass (Asbs-HC)	Antioxidant, skin nourishment, and wound healing potential	• Pro-Hyp and Pro-Hyp-Gly were the peptides present in the sea bass • Asbs-HC (1000 μg/mL) showed the best cell proliferation and migration • Accelerated the wound healing process by increasing fibroblast mobility at the site of the injury	(Chotphruethipong et al., 2021)
Crimson snapper	Crimson snapper scale peptides (CSSPs)	Antioxidant and antiaging potential	• Enhanced the antioxidant enzyme activity and upregulated the expression of antioxidant genes • Prolonged the mean lifespan of the skin	(Yang et al., 2023)
Salmon and codfish skin	Collagen peptides	Antiaging and skin-related health potential	• Revealed good moisture absorption • Prevented skin dehydration • Presented nontoxic and nonirritating outcomes	(Siahaan et al., 2022)
Chum salmon skin	Marine collagen peptides (MCPs)	Wound healing and antiangiogenesis potential	• Accelerated tissue regeneration at the wound site (wound healing) • Improved angiogenesis • Formed thicker and more organized collagen deposition	(Zhang et al., 2011)
Salmon skin	Gelatin and hydrolysates	Antiaging, anti-UV, and antiphotoaging potential	• Improved UV-irradiation-induced pathological alterations in skin texture and morphology • Decreased hydroxyproline content in photoaging skin • Increased SOD, CAT, glutathione (GSH), and its peroxidase (GSH-P_X) (antioxidant potential) • Participated in collagen synthesis	(Chen et al., 2016)
Atlantic salmon egg extract (*Salmo salar*)	Serine endoproteases, oleic, and linoleic acid	Antiwrinkle, antiaging, and skin-health-promoting	• Improved wrinkles, pigmentation, redness, brightness, and hydration • Neither skin irritation nor sensitization was observed	(Lønne et al., 2013)

From Papadopoulou, S.N.A., Adamantidi, T., Kranas, D., Cholidis, P., Anastasiadou, C., Tsoupras, A., 2025a. A comprehensive review on the valorization of bioactives from marine animal by-products for health-promoting, biofunctional cosmetics. Mar. Drugs. 16603397. 23 (8). Available from: https://www.mdpi.com/journal/marinedrugs. doi:10.3390/md23080299.

substrates they are incorporated into, each one of the molecules belonging to any of these categories and subcategories exhibits varied biological activities, some of which are of great interest to the cosmetics sector (Papadopoulou et al., 2025a).

3.3.1 Fatty acids

Marine ω3 PUFA, particularly DHA and EPA, are potent immunomodulatory and antiinflammatory agents, with multiple mechanisms of action (Parolini, 2024). Structurally, they feature a double bond between carbons 3 and 4, with DHA being especially abundant in fresh lean and oily fish (Calder, 2015). Their biological effects are exerted through three main pathways: serving as substrates for specialized proresolving mediators, incorporation into cell membrane PLs, and acting as agonists for cellular receptors (Tsoupras et al., 2022). Antiinflammatory activity primarily arises from their integration into cell membranes, which reduces AA content, thereby inhibiting AA metabolism, COX gene expression, and decreasing the production of AA-derived eicosanoids such as prostaglandins, thromboxanes, and leukotrienes. Upon inflammatory stimulation, phospholipase A2 hydrolyzes sn-2 glycerol phospholipids, releasing free AA, EPA, or DHA, which then enter enzymatic pathways involving COX, lipoxygenase, and cytochrome P450 (CYP450) to produce mediators that regulate inflammation (Parolini, 2020). Overall, their main mechanism is related to competition with AA and the inhibition of inflammatory eicosanoid synthesis, while at the same time, they have a decisive influence on the production and function of cytokines, which are involved in the tissue healing process.

Nevertheless, all the PUFAs found in fish oil, both the ω3 ones (DHA and EPA) and the ω6 ones (LA and ALA), have been documented to have protective and therapeutic effects on the skin (Papadopoulou et al., 2025a). According to available research data, the PUFAs in fish oil help improve the skin barrier and water balance, limit the effects of photoaging, accelerate wound healing, inhibit hyperpigmentation, and reduce the likelihood of developing or progressing skin cancer lesions. The most recent skin-related applications of fatty acids derived from fish oil include their use in the treatment of photoaging, melanogenesis, dermatitis, cancer, and wound healing. The administration of PUFAs has demonstrated efficacy in alleviating symptoms associated with these dermatological conditions. Certain fatty acids are licensed for preventive or therapeutic use in clinical trials. In addition, some formulations containing fish oil have been approved to treat a variety of skin conditions in both animal- and cell-based research (Yang et al., 2020; Huang et al., 2018).

Thus marine fatty acids have been successfully incorporated into creams, emulsions, cosmetic masks, lipsticks, bath products, and nail polishes due to their antiinflammatory potential (Papadopoulou et al., 2025a). Topical studies demonstrate the efficacy of marine ω3 PUFA in skincare: for example, sardine extract (rich in DHA and EPA) combined with ketoprofen significantly enhanced skin penetration and inhibited UVB-induced erythema by 60.5%, outperforming mackerel extracts or individual treatments (Huang et al., 2018). In addition, FFAs from cod liver oil enhance drug permeation through the skin and oral mucosa with minimal toxicity. These properties underscore the value of marine ω3 PUFAs as safe, effective, and multifunctional ingredients in cosmeceutical and dermatological applications (Loftsson et al., 2016).

In addition, omega-3 fatty acids, mainly EPA and DHA, thanks to their antiinflammatory actions, appear to have therapeutic potential in acne, especially in cases of deficiency of these fatty acids (Guertler et al., 2024). At the same time, it has been observed that fish lipid extracts, rich in EPA and DHA, significantly suppress the production of MMP-1 in human skin fibroblasts. MMP-1 is an enzyme that plays a key role in collagen breakdown, a process that leads to reduced elasticity and premature photoaging. Therefore these findings indicate that fish oils and fish lipid extracts can be innovative bioactive ingredients for antiaging cosmetic products, as well as for skin care products designed to limit damage from UV radiation (Lee et al., 2022).

In particular, with regard to photoaging, beyond sunscreens, novel photoprotective agents are sought, with fatty acids, particularly ω3 PUFA like ALA, EPA, and DHA, showing promise, as they can reduce proinflammatory eicosanoid production by competing with AA metabolism (Huang et al., 2018; Calder, 2012), and inhibit UV-induced keratinocyte responses through COX-2, NF-κB, and MAPK/ERK pathways, thereby protecting the skin from UV damage (Pilkington et al., 2011; Desai et al., 2018). Moreover, both ω6 and ω3 PUFA can affect fibroblast activation and proliferation, and affect the synthesis of collagen and ECM components either directly or indirectly (Reilly and Lozano, 2021). DHA and EPA predominantly appear to reduce the expression of proinflammatory markers such as IL-8, regulate enzyme activity (e.g., COX-2, MMP-1), and enhance the production and activation of antioxidant protective mediators and transcription factors such as Nrf2 and heme oxygenase 1 (HO-1), exerting beneficial effects both topically and via dietary intake, thus contributing significantly to photoprotection and antiaging skin care.

These actions have been documented both in topical application and through dietary intake. In women from a cross-sectional study, photoaging incidences were inversely associated with higher EPA intake and vegetable oil-derived ALA, suggesting that ω3 PUFA supplementation can provide a positive nutricosmetic impact on skin aging; yet, further epidemiological studies are needed (Latreille et al., 2013). Topical application of ω3 PUFA is also believed to improve aged skin, implying its efficacy toward enriching fatty acids or sterols with therapeutic benefits and limiting harmful ones (Wang and Wu, 2019). For example, an antiaging ω3 PUFA-enriched gel cream reduced the secretion of proinflammatory, photoaging agents, induced beneficial ECM remodeling, increased skin hydration and elasticity, reduced crow's feet wrinkle area and volume, lowered fine-line wrinkle volume, decreased subepidermal low-echogenic band, and also reduced the red spot area and count, thus enhancing the antiaging effects and strengthening the beneficial dermocosmetic properties of such functional cosmetics (Cohen et al., 2023).

With regard to hyperpigmentation, DHA has also been shown to reduce melanogenesis and thus hyperpigmentation by promoting tyrosinase degradation, while the ω3 PUFA ALA and the ω6 PUFA LA inhibit tyrosinase activity, limit melanin production, and enhance skin brightness, with liposomal forms of LA showing improved stability and whitening efficacy in skin whitening applications (Huang et al., 2018).

Fish oil ω3 PUFAs, such as DHA and EPA, demonstrate protective effects against several skin inflammation-related disorders, including skin malignancies, including melanoma and nonmelanoma skin carcinoma, by preventing cutaneous carcinogenesis during both the initiation and promotion phases. Fatty acids modulate melanoma biology differently; palmitic acid increases melanin, while DHA suppresses tumor proliferation. Thus SFAs and PUFAs exert opposing effects on melanin content and actin polymerization, influencing melanosome trafficking. DHA also interacts with RACK1 to inhibit melanoma cell proliferation via protein kinase C (PKC) signaling suppression (Huang et al., 2018). The anticancer effect of ω3 PUFAs is ascribed to their ability to downregulate proinflammatory eicosanoid synthesis from COX-2 (Huang et al., 2018).

Experimental studies show that DHA and EPA inhibit the growth of premalignant keratinocytes (HaCaT cells), and combinations with anticancer drugs or topical agents enhance therapeutic outcomes (Nikolakopoulou et al., 2013). For instance, co-administration of fish oil with imiquimod in mouse models reduced tumor growth and increased antiinflammatory IL-10 levels. Similarly, quercetin fatty acid esters (e.g., quercetin–ALA or quercetin–LA) improve apoptosis, mechanical properties, and ERK pathway modulation in A375 melanoma cells, decreasing cell viability and phosphorylated ERK expression while enhancing cell–cell adhesion (Aghamohammadi et al., 2022). Overall, ω3 PUFA provides antiinflammatory, antimelanogenic, and anticancer effects, supporting both skin photoprotection and potential adjunctive therapy in skin carcinogenesis.

Marine PUFA, particularly ω3 PUFA like EPA and DHA, support skin hydration, barrier integrity, and wound healing. The ω6 PUFA, LA, contributes to ceramide synthesis, strengthening the stratum corneum lipid matrix and preventing water loss. Fish oil fatty acids enhance collagen structure, promote fibroblast activation, stimulate angiogenesis, and accelerate tissue regeneration via receptors like GPR120 and molecular mediators such as TGF-β and involucrin. They modulate inflammatory pathways, reducing excessive cytokine activity while maintaining necessary repair signals, thus providing both therapeutic and cosmeceutical benefits in dermatitis, psoriasis, acne, and general skin aging (Brunt and Burgess, 2018)

For example, marine-derived fatty acids, particularly ω3 PUFAs, have demonstrated significant therapeutic benefits in dermatitis as well, by reducing inflammation, enhancing skin hydration, and improving barrier function. Clinical studies showed that topical ω3 PUFA creams decreased the increased TEWL in irritant contact dermatitis (Ivic et al., 2024), while γ-linolenic acid-enriched fabrics reduced erythema and pruritus in atopic dermatitis (Yang et al., 2020). Microneedling with ω3 PUFA-containing formulations enhanced skin redness, brightness, texture, and overall hydration (Nip et al., 2025). Novel ointments combining cod liver oil with natural excipients also improved the quality of life in patients with recessive dystrophic epidermolysis bullosa by promoting blister healing and reducing pain (Ahmad and Akhtar, 2023).

Marine fatty acids have proven beneficial in other inflammatory skin disorders too, such as psoriasis and acne vulgaris. ω3 PUFA supplementation complemented the therapeutic actions of topical tretinoin-oleic acid vesicles by reducing psoriasis severity, nail involvement, scalp lesions, pruritus, erythema, and scaling (Márquez-Balbás et al., 2011; Zhao et al., 2023). Higher fish consumption also correlates with reduced severity of acne vulgaris, a chronic inflammation of pilosebaceous follicles (Das et al., 2024; Di Landro et al., 2012).

3.3.2 *Classic amphiphilic compounds of lipid nature (PLs and lipid-soluble vitamins)*

Marine-derived PLs and lipid-soluble vitamins are increasingly valued in cosmetic science for their combined roles in skin hydration, barrier reinforcement, antiinflammatory action, and antiaging protection (Papadopoulou et al., 2025a). Sourced from marine organisms, including fish and their by-products, PLs—including phospholipids, glycolipids, sphingolipids, and sulfolipids—are particularly bioactive against inflammation-related complications and disorders, either on their own by inhibiting specific thrombo-inflammatory mediators or/and due to their high EPA and DHA content and their indirect antiinflammatory potential when released from these PLs intracellularly (Tsoupras et al., 2022).

PLs are valuable ingredients in dermatological science thanks to their characteristic amphiphilic nature (hydrophobic and hydrophilic regions). This dual behavior makes them ideal emollients, contributing significantly to maintaining skin hydration and restoring the functionality of the skin barrier (Ahmad and Ahsan, 2020). Marine PLs, especially those derived from fish, offer a vast array of combined benefits: they improve skin moisture and elasticity, strengthen the barrier, and have a mild cleansing action. These lipids integrate into the stratum corneum lipid matrix, reducing TEWL, enhancing elasticity, repairing barrier function, and providing antiinflammatory, photoprotective, and hydrating effects (Danby et al., 2022; Lopes et al., 2021; Caffrey et al., 2023), while also acting as emulsifiers, emollients, and delivery systems through liposomes and nanocarriers (Rotter et al., 2024; Lopes et al., 2021; Caffrey et al., 2023; Haq et al., 2021). Therefore their incorporation into cosmetic formulations is not limited to bioactivity, but also contributes to the luxurious feel and high quality of the products.

At a functional level, phospholipids have specialized roles: phosphatidylcholine creates a protective membrane on the skin's surface, limiting transdermal water loss and enhancing the moisture of the stratum corneum, while phosphatidyl ethanolamine is associated with cell membrane renewal processes, contributing to tissue elasticity and structural stability. At the same time, PLs with antiinflammatory properties protect membranes from oxidative damage and regulate inflammatory mechanisms, such as NF-κB activation, giving them significant antiaging and cytoprotective value.

The use of marine phospholipids is already evident in advanced cosmetic products, initially as emulsifiers in natural cosmetics, but recently either in the form of highly active serums or in moisturizing and antiaging creams. Research data show that fishery by-products, such as skin, scales, bones, and fish oil, are rich sources of bioactive lipid components suitable for cosmetic use. Their application leads to formulas with powerful moisturizing, regenerative, and antiaging properties, which improve skin elasticity and protect it from damage caused by UV radiation (Haq et al., 2021; Lens, 2025; Alfutaimani et al., 2024; van Hoogevest and Fahr, 2019). Furthermore, lecithin extracted from rainbow trout, fish, eggs, and other marine organisms has displayed notable emulsifying, moisturizing, and skin-penetrating benefits, better delivery, and long-term stability in cosmetics (Topuz et al., 2021; Thy et al., 2025). Fish-derived phospholipids, such as phosphatidylcholine and PE, further support moisture retention, membrane renewal, and tissue elasticity, while regulating inflammatory pathways like NF-κB.

In addition, certain marine lipids are incorporated into specialized dermatological formulas to treat conditions such as acne and improve the overall appearance and texture of the skin (Nimisha, 2024). Marine sources supply lipid-soluble vitamins A, D, and E, which contribute to collagen stimulation, normalization of keratinocyte turnover, antioxidant and UV-protective defense, regulation of hyperproliferative skin conditions, and improved microcirculation (Adamantidi et al., 2025; Rotter et al., 2024; Huang et al., 2018; Zasada and Budzisz, 2019; Akbaş et al., 2023; Holick, 2007; Papadopoulou et al., 2025a; Formisano et al., 2023; Yang and McClements, 2013). Together, marine PLs and such vitamins—often delivered via advanced systems such as liposomes, nanoemulsions, and solid lipid nanoparticles—enable the development of high-performance, sustainable cosmetic and cosmeceutical formulations with moisturizing, regenerative, antiaging, and protective benefits (Rotter et al., 2024; Haq et al., 2021; Papadopoulou et al., 2025b).

3.3.3 Other amphiphilic marine compounds of lipid (carotenoids and pigments of similar structure) and nonlipid nature (phenolics)

While algae dominate the marine pigment sector, several nonalgal marine organisms, including fish, produce or accumulate pigments with notable cosmetic and cosmeceutical potential. For example, astaxanthin, zeaxanthin, lutein B, tunaxanthin, halocynthiaxanthin, fucoxanthin, and β-carotene from the Japanese mackerel (*Scomber japonicus/Pneumatophorus japonicus*), rainbow trout (*Oncorhynchus mykiss*), and salmon have shown vast antioxidant, anti-UV, and radical scavenging potential for integration into cosmetics and cosmeceuticals (Brunt and Burgess, 2018). Fish by-product carotenoids are extensively used as preservatives in cosmetics, together with other antioxidants, as well as in creams and lotions offering sun protection (Ashraf et al., 2020; Vílchez et al., 2011). Astaxanthin is a well-known marine pigment extracted from algae but also from fish sources like salmon, especially from its by-products, and has been widely applied in cosmetics and cosmeceuticals (Galasso et al., 2017).

Marine carotenoids exhibit strong photoprotective and antioxidant activities, protecting epidermal keratinocytes from UV-induced inflammation and oxidative damage while effectively inhibiting lipid peroxidation (Papadopoulou et al., 2025a). Experimental studies have shown that carotenoids isolated from marine organisms possess antioxidant capacities up to 40–600 times greater than α-tocopherol, with compounds such as astaxanthin, fucoxanthin, zeaxanthin, lutein, and β-carotene demonstrating exceptional in vivo ROS-scavenging ability; notably, astaxanthin is up to 94 times more potent than α-tocopherol in neutralizing hypochlorous acid.

Despite this strong bioactivity, their broader cosmetic application remains limited due to insufficient systematic in vivo topical studies, even as market demand for natural carotenoids continues to rise. Fish species such as mackerel, trout, and amberjack represent rich, sustainable sources of carotenoids with antioxidant, anti-UV, and radical scavenging potential, often utilized as preservatives or active ingredients in sun-protective cosmetics (Ashraf et al., 2020; Vílchez et al., 2011).

Among them, astaxanthin stands out as the most important marine carotenoid, as it has gained widespread acceptance mainly as an antioxidant in skincare formulations (Galasso et al., 2017), while also offering antiaging, moisturizing, antiwrinkle, photoprotective, antiinflammatory, wound healing, and antitumor effects (Veeruraj et al., 2019; Bose et al., 2023; Ikarashi et al., 2020; Imokawa, 2019; Eren et al., 2019). Mechanistically, astaxanthin activates the Nrf2/HO-1 antioxidant pathway (Niu et al., 2018), improves epidermal barrier function, reduces TEWL (Ito et al., 2018; Komatsu et al., 2017), enhances aquaporin-3-mediated hydration (Ikarashi et al., 2020), inhibits tyrosinase, and suppresses inflammatory signaling pathways, including NF-κB, COX-2, iNOS, and STAT3 (Komatsu et al., 2017; Fang et al., 2017; Meephansan et al., 2017; Ito et al., 2018; Dutta et al., 2023; Davinelli et al., 2018; Patruno et al., 2021; Park et al., 2018; Park et al., 2019). Clinical and preclinical studies consistently demonstrate its ability to reduce UV-induced erythema, wrinkles, inflammation, dermatitis severity, and oxidative stress, while promoting wound healing and skin elasticity, firmly establishing marine carotenoids—and astaxanthin in particular—as highly promising bioactives for advanced cosmetic and cosmeceutical formulations. However, its low solubility and stability necessitate advanced delivery systems (Šimat et al., 2022), such as nanoemulsions, liposomes, nanoparticles, cyclodextrin complexes, and hydrogels, which enhance skin penetration, stability, and bioavailability [474-480].

Another class of marine-derived colorants and pigments are the marine phenolics, which, even though they are more polar nonlipid molecules compared to all the previously mentioned compounds of lipid nature, are still classified as the more polar amphiphilic bioactives. Marine organisms contain abundant phenolic compounds, including bromophenols, simple phenolic acids, flavonoids, and phlorotannins, many of which are transferred through the marine food chain from algae to invertebrates and fish (Mateos et al., 2020; Rathod et al., 2023). Flavonoids such as quercetin, rutin, and catechins—commonly found in algae and fish (Rathod et al., 2023)—are among the most extensively studied, while all types of marine phenolics have exhibited strong antioxidant, antiinflammatory, and anticancer properties (Pereira and Cotas, 2023). Bromophenolic compounds, primarily originating from red algae and subsequently accumulating in fish and shellfish, show variable concentrations across marine species and require careful characterization because some may exhibit toxicity (Bidleman et al., 2019; Malmvärn et al., 2005; Koch and Sures, 2018). Phlorotannins and related phenolics from marine algae and fish have demonstrated significant antioxidant, UV-protective, radical scavenging, tyrosinase inhibitory, and antimelanogenic effects in both in vitro and in vivo studies, highlighting their potential for skin protection and hyperpigmentation management (Brunt and Burgess, 2018). However, due to their sensitivity to environmental and processing conditions, encapsulation technologies are increasingly applied to marine phenolics to enhance stability, bioavailability, controlled release, and sensory acceptability in cosmetic and cosmeceutical applications (Franco et al., 2023).

3.3.4 Other lipophilic compounds (squalene)

Squalene ($C_{30}H_{50}$) is a polyunsaturated hydrocarbon belonging to the triterpenes and consisting of six isoprene units. It is found in high concentrations in certain fish oils, with shark liver oil being the main source, although it is also found in vegetable oils but in smaller quantities. In human sebum, it accounts for approximately 13% of its lipid composition, making it a key component. Squalane, the saturated derivative of squalene, is also found in these sources. Scientific interest in squalene increased significantly when its presence in shark liver oil, which has been used for decades in traditional medicine, was studied.

A series of studies has highlighted multiple bioactivities of both squalene and squalane, most notably their anticancer, antioxidant, detoxifying, moisturizing, and emollient properties, which have been observed in both in vitro experiments and animal models. The two molecules are now considered particularly promising for applications in pharmaceuticals and functional foods.

As a powerful monophotonic oxygen receptor, squalene has been proposed as a molecule with high cosmetic value, especially after the recognition of its widespread presence in human sebum, hair lipids, and other surface lipid layers. At the same time, it is classified among compounds with chemoprotective actions, as well as properties that enhance the body's resistance to toxic stress.

An important action of squalene is the protection of the skin from lipid peroxidation caused either by UV radiation or other sources of oxidative stress. Its ability to neutralize singlet oxygen at an extremely high rate explains its strong antioxidant properties. In addition, squalene has been shown to effectively protect human breast epithelial cells from DNA damage resulting from oxidative stress.

In recent years, research data have shown that squalene has a protective effect against carcinogens. In fact, when administered in combination with anticancer drugs, it can inhibit or prevent tumor growth in various experimental models.

In dermatology and cosmetology, squalene is preferred because of its powerful emollient properties. It easily penetrates the deeper layers of the skin, enhancing elasticity and softness without leaving oily residues. In addition, it helps increase hydration by creating a protective film on the skin's surface and retaining moisture in the stratum corneum.

Research efforts have examined the use of squalene in combination with other lipids, such as triglycerides, cholesterol, ceramides, and fatty acids, to create mixtures with properties similar to those of protective casein varnish, which is used as a barrier for moisturizing skin with insufficient defenses. The results showed that formulations containing squalene could improve skin barrier function to a degree comparable to that of the varnish.

Another study investigated the application of an aqueous gel containing squalene in dialysis patients with mild uremic pruritus. After 2 weeks of treatment, a clear improvement in dryness and a reduction in itching were observed. However, 2 weeks after discontinuing treatment, itching reappeared, and 40% of patients experienced dryness again, highlighting the beneficial but temporary effect of the treatment (Kim and Karadeniz, 2012).

3.4 Fish-derived substrates and minerals as cosmetic ingredients

Although synthetic and naturally sourced calcium phosphates (CaPs) are widely used in cosmetic products such as skincare, haircare, deodorants, and oral care, research specifically focusing on fish-derived CaPs remains limited. Recent studies suggest that marine by-products are promising alternative sources of functional cosmetic minerals (Carella et al., 2021). For example, hydroxyapatite derived from cod bones demonstrated excellent biocompatibility and strong UV absorption across a wide UVA/UVB range without generating free radicals, likely due to its crystalline nanostructure and low photoreactivity, making it suitable as a broad-spectrum sunscreen ingredient (Piccirillo et al., 2014). Further work using hydroxyapatite obtained from Fringescale sardine bones showed that hydrogels formulated with unmodified hydroxyapatite and trace-element-doped variants achieved SPF values of 20 (hydroxyapatite), 40 (hydroxyapatite-Mn), and 50 (hydroxyapatite-Fe), underscoring the role of mineral doping in enhancing photoprotective performance (Siahaan et al., 2022).

Because marine-derived CaPs possess distinct trace mineral compositions compared with terrestrial sources, they may offer additional benefits, such as promoting collagen synthesis, skin cell proliferation, antiinflammatory activity, wound healing, skin rejuvenation, and skin and tooth remineralization (Kodali et al., 2022). In parallel, marine minerals such as magnesium and zinc are already incorporated into sunscreens and antiacne products for their antiinflammatory and sebum-regulating effects (Ferreira et al., 2021; Rotter et al., 2024).

Beyond CaPs, pearls, and nacre from bivalves have attracted cosmetic interest due to their antioxidant, skin-brightening, ECM-stimulating, regenerative, hydrating, and wound healing properties, attributed in part to bioactive proteins such as conchiolin (Siahaan et al., 2022; Loh et al., 2021). Collectively, these findings support the growing potential of fish- and shellfish-derived mineral by-products as sustainable, multifunctional ingredients for advanced cosmetic and cosmeceutical formulations, while also highlighting the need for further targeted research.

4 Conclusions, limitations, and future perspectives

Marine ecosystems, and especially sustainable fish sources, including cultured fish, fish bycatch, and fish by-products, represent a largely untapped reservoir of structurally unique and biologically potent compounds with significant potential in cosmetic science. These natural, biocompatible, and sustainable bioactives exhibit a wide range of cosmetic benefits, including antiinflammatory, antioxidant, antiaging, skin-whitening, antimicrobial, UV-protective, and moisturizing effects, making them attractive alternatives to synthetic ingredients in skincare, haircare, nail care, oral care, and sun protection products. The extreme marine environment—characterized by high salinity, pressure, and UV exposure—drives the biosynthesis of highly resilient and effective molecules, while the valorization of marine by-products such as fish skin, scales, bones, and heads supports circular economy and sustainability principles.

Nevertheless, climate change is reshaping the distribution of marine organisms, driving the poleward migration of macroalgae, mollusks, and fish, and altering the availability and composition of valuable marine bioactives such as PUFAs, pigments, peptides, and polysaccharides. While warming oceans may expand access to certain bioactives in temperate and polar regions, they may also diminish cold-water species that produce unique compounds, creating uncertainty in supply. To address these shifts, future sourcing strategies must integrate environmental monitoring, adaptive harvesting, cultivation, and bioactive profiling to ensure sustainability, quality control, and resource security.

Moreover, despite strong interest in marine-derived cosmetic ingredients, their large-scale adoption is limited by insufficient clinical validation, variability in raw materials, challenges in standardization, scalability, cost, and regulatory uncertainty, particularly for fish-, mollusk-, and crustacean-derived compounds. Ethical and environmental concerns, along with limited consumer awareness, further constrain market acceptance. Future progress will depend on expanded in vivo and clinical studies, regulatory harmonization, and transparent sustainability frameworks.

Although substantial progress has been made in identifying and characterizing fish-derived compounds, further optimization of extraction methods, clinical validation of efficacy, and regulatory harmonization are needed. Advances in green extraction technologies, analytical characterization, encapsulation, and delivery systems are expected to significantly enhance the stability, efficacy, and bioavailability of marine bioactives. Emphasis on circular economy models, marine biorefineries, and biotechnology approaches such as fermentation and synthetic biology can reduce waste and ecological pressure while ensuring a consistent supply. Overall, the next phase of marine cosmetic research will focus on sustainable innovation, mechanistic understanding, advanced delivery systems, regulatory clarity, and cross-sector collaboration to fully realize the potential of marine-derived ingredients in safe, effective, and environmentally responsible skincare products.

By utilizing all the above, and as consumer demand increasingly favors natural, eco-friendly, and multifunctional cosmetics, fish-derived bioactives offer a promising and innovative foundation for the development of next-generation cosmetic and cosmeceutical products.

Acknowledgments

The authors would like to thank the School of Chemistry, Faculty of Sciences at the Democritus University of Thrace, and the Fisheries Research Institute in Kavala, Greece, for their continuous support.

Conflicts of interest

The authors declare no conflicts of interest.

Author contributions

A.T. was involved in conceptualization, methodology, validation, visualization, and supervision. E.K. and A.T. were involved in investigation and writing—original draft preparation. C.A. and A.T. were involved in writing—review and editing. All authors contributed to software and have read and agreed to the published version of the manuscript.

Funding

This research received no external funding.

References

(PDF) Use of natural carotenoids for pigmentation in fishes, 2025. ResearchGate.

Abdallah, M.M., Fernández, N., Matias, A.A., Bronze, M.D.R., 2020. Hyaluronic acid and chondroitin sulfate from marine and terrestrial sources: extraction and purification methods. Carbohydr. Polym. 01448617. 243. Available from: http://www.elsevier.com/wps/find/journaldescription.cws_home/405871/description#description. doi:10.1016/j.carbpol.2020.116441.

Adamantidi, T., Lafara, M.-P., Venetikidou, M., Likartsi, E., Toganidou, I., Tsoupras, A., 2025. Utilization and bio-efficacy of carotenoids, vitamin A and its vitaminoids in nutricosmetics, cosmeceuticals, and cosmetics' applications with skin-health promoting properties. Appl. Sci. 2076-3417. 15 (3), 1657. doi:10.3390/app15031657.

Afonso, C.R., Hirano, R.S., Gaspar, A.L., Chagas, E.G.L., Carvalho, R.A., Silva, F.V., Leonardi, G.R., Lopes, P.S., Silva, C.F., Yoshida, C.M.P., 2019. Biodegradable antioxidant chitosan films useful as an anti-aging skin mask. Int. J. Biol. Macromol. 01418130. 132, 1262–1273. doi:10.1016/j.ijbiomac.2019.04.052.

Afreen, M., Ucak, I., 2020. Fish processing wastes used as feed ingredient for animal feed and aquaculture feed. J. Surv. Fish. Sci. 23687487. 6 (2), 55–64. doi:10.18331/sfs2020.6.2.7.

Aghamohammadi, M., Zolghadr, L., Nezhad, N.S., Yazdi, H.A., Esfahani, A.J., Gheibi, N., 2022. Investigating the effects of quercetin fatty acid esters on apoptosis, mechanical properties, and expression of ERK in melanoma cell line (A375). Life Sci. 18790631. 310. Available from: www.elsevier.com/locate/lifescie. doi:10.1016/j.lfs.2022.121007.

Agustin, T., Nursyam, H., Firdaus, M., Rifa'i, M., Ekaputri, I.D., Mahmiah,, 2025. The characterization of blue shark (*Prionace glauca*) cartilage potential as nature-derived drug material. IOP Conf. Ser. Earth Environ. Sci. 1755-1307. 1473 (1), 012049. doi:10.1088/1755-1315/1473/1/012049.

Ahmad, A., Ahsan, H., 2020. Lipid-based formulations in cosmeceuticals and biopharmaceuticals. Biomed. Dermatol. 2398-8460. 4 (1). doi:10.1186/s41702-020-00062-9.

Ahmad, U., Akhtar, J., (Eds.), 2023. Cosmetic Products and Industry: New Advances and Applications. IntechOpen, Erscheinungsort Nicht Ermittelbar.

Ahmmed, M.K., Carne, A., Bunga, S., Tian, H. (Sabrina), Bekhit, A.E.D.A., 2021. Lipidomic signature of Pacific lean fish species head and skin using gas chromatography and nuclear magnetic resonance spectroscopy. Food Chem. 18737072. 365. Available from: www.elsevier.com/locate/foodchem. doi:10.1016/j.foodchem.2021.130637.

Akanno, A., Guzmán, E., Ortega, F., Rubio, R.G., 2020. Behavior of the water/vapor interface of chitosan solutions with an anionic surfactant: effect of polymer-surfactant interactions. Phys. Chem. Chem. Phys. 14639076. 22 (40), 23360–23373. Available from: http://pubs.rsc.org/en/journals/journal/cp. doi:10.1039/d0cp02470h.

Akbaş, A., Kılınç, F., Şener, S., Hayran, Y., 2023. Vitamin D levels in patients with seborrheic dermatitis. Revista da Associação Médica Brasileira. 1806-9282. 69 (7). doi:10.1590/1806-9282.20230022.

Al Hajj, W., Salla, M., Krayem, M., Khaled, S., Hassan, H.F., Khatib, S.E., 2024. Hydrolyzed collagen: exploring its applications in the food and beverage industries and assessing its impact on human health—a comprehensive review. Heliyon. 24058440. 10 (16). Available from: https://www.sciencedirect.com/science/journal/24058440. doi:10.1016/j.heliyon.2024.e36433.

Al-Atif, H., 2022. Collagen supplements for aging and wrinkles: a paradigm shift in the field of dermatology and cosmetics. Dermatol. Pract. Concept. 2160-9381. 12 (1), e2022018. doi:10.5826/dpc.1201a18.

Al-Nimry, S., Dayah, A.A., Hasan, I., Daghmash, R., 2021. Cosmetic, biomedical and pharmaceutical applications of fish gelatin/hydrolysates. Mar. Drugs. 1660-3397. 19 (3), 145. doi:10.3390/md19030145.

Alfaro, A.D.T., Balbinot, E., Weber, C.I., Tonial, I.B., Machado-Lunkes, A., 2015. Fish gelatin: characteristics, functional properties, applications and future potentials. Food Eng. Rev. 18667929. 7 (1), 33–44. Available from: http://www.springer.com/life+sci/food+science/journal/12393. doi:10.1007/s12393-014-9096-5.

Alfutaimani, A.S., Alharbi, N.K., Alahmari, A.S., Alqabbani, A.A., Aldayel, A.M., 2024. Exploring the landscape of lipid nanoparticles (LNPs): a comprehensive review of LNPs types and biological sources of lipids. Int. J. Pharm. X. 25901567. 8. Available from: https://www.sciencedirect.com/science/journal/25901567. doi:10.1016/j.ijpx.2024.100305.

Allard, R., Malak, N.A., Huc, A., 2003. Collagen Product Containing Collagen of Marine Origin with a Low Odor and Preferably with Improved Mechanical Properties, and its Use in the Form of Cosmetic or Pharmaceutical Compositions or Products, https://patents.google.com/patent/US6660280B1/en.

Alves, A., Marques, A., Martins, E., Silva, T., Reis, R., 2017. Cosmetic potential of marine fish skin collagen. Cosmetics. 2079-9284. 4 (4), 39. doi:10.3390/cosmetics4040039.

Alves, A., Sousa, E., Kijjoa, A., Pinto, M., 2020. Marine-derived compounds with potential use as cosmeceuticals and nutricosmetics. Molecules. 1420-3049. 25 (11), 2536. doi:10.3390/molecules25112536.

Aranaz, I., Acosta, N., Civera, C., Elorza, B., Mingo, J., Castro, C., Gandía, M., Caballero, A.H., 2018. Cosmetics and cosmeceutical applications of chitin, chitosan and their derivatives. Polymers. 2073-4360. 10 (2), 213. doi:10.3390/polym10020213.

Ashraf, S.A., Adnan, M., Patel, M., Siddiqui, A.J., Sachidanandan, M., Snoussi, M., Hadi, S., 2020. Fish-based bioactives as potent nutraceuticals: exploring the therapeutic perspective of sustainable food from the sea. Mar. Drugs. 16603397. 18 (5). Available from: https://www.mdpi.com/1660-3397/18/5/265. doi:10.3390/md18050265.

Atef, M., Ojagh, S.M., 2017. Health benefits and food applications of bioactive compounds from fish byproducts: a review. J. Funct. Foods. 17564646. 35, 673–681. doi:10.1016/j.jff.2017.06.034.

Awuchi, C.G., Chukwu, C.N., Iyiola, A.O., Noreen, S., Morya, S., Adeleye, A.O., Twinomuhwezi, H., Leicht, K., Mitaki, N.B., Okpala, C.O.R., 2022. Bioactive compounds and therapeutics from fish: revisiting their suitability in functional foods to enhance human wellbeing. Biomed. Res. Int. 23146141. 2022. Available from: http://www.hindawi.com/journals/biomed/. doi:10.1155/2022/3661866.

Azarian, M.H., Sutapun, W., 2022. Biogenic calcium carbonate derived from waste shells for advanced material applications: a review. Front. Mater. 22968016. 9. Available from: https://www.journal.frontiersin.org/journal/materials. doi:10.3389/fmats.2022.1024977.

Badilli, U., Inal, O., 2025. Current approaches in cosmeceuticals: peptides, biotics and marine biopolymers. Polymers. 2073-4360. 17 (6), 798. doi:10.3390/polym17060798.

Balami, S., Sharma, A., Karn, R., 2019. Significance of nutritional value of fish for human health. Malaysian J. Halal Res. 2616-1923. 2 (2), 32–34. doi:10.2478/mjhr-2019-0012.

Barba, F.J., Lorenzo, J.M. ((Eds.)), 2020. Aquaculture and By-products: Challenges and Opportunities in the Use of Alternative Protein Sources and Bioactive Compounds. Academic Press/Imprint of Elsevier, Amsterdam, The Netherlands.

Barh, D., Azevedo, V., 2018. Omics Technologies and Bio-Engineering: Vol. 2: Towards Improving Quality of Life. Elsevier, India, pp. 1–420. Available from http://www.sciencedirect.com/science/book/9780128158708. doi:10.1016/C2017-0-04064-8.

Beaumont, M., Blachier, F., 2020. Amino acids in intestinal physiology and health. In: Wu, G., Ed., Amino Acids in Nutrition and Health: Amino Acids in Systems Function and Health. Springer International Publishing, Cham, pp. 1–20.

Bergmann, W., Feeney, R.J., 1950. The isolation of a new thymine pentoside from sponges. J. Am. Chem. Soc. 15205126. 72 (6), 2809–2810. doi:10.1021/ja01162a543.

Bidleman, T.F., Andersson, A., Brugel, S., Ericson, L., Haglund, P., Kupryianchyk, D., Lau, D.C.P., Liljelind, P., Lundin, L., Tysklind, A., Tysklind, M., 2019. Bromoanisoles and methoxylated bromodiphenyl ethers in macroalgae from Nordic coastal regions. Environ. Sci. Process. Impacts. 20507895. 21 (5), 881–892. Available from: http://pubs.rsc.org/en/journals/journal/em. doi:10.1039/c9em00042a.

Bojarska, J., 2020. Amino acids and short peptides as anti-aging “Superfood”. Int. J. Nutr. Sci. 5 (1), 1039.

Bose, V.B.S.C., Balaganesan, V., Govindaraj, G., Veerichetty, V., 2023. Cellular antioxidant and cytotoxic activity of astaxanthin and ellagic acid on UV irradiated skin melanoma cells and gel formulation. Mater. Today Proc. 22147853. doi:10.1016/j.matpr.2023.08.209.

Brotherton, C.A., Balskus, E.P., 2015. Shedding light on sunscreen biosynthesis in zebrafish. eLife. 2050084X. 4 (May), 1–3. Available from: http://elifesciences.org/content/elife/4/e07961full.pdf. doi:10.7554/eLife.07961.

Brunt, E.G., Burgess, J.G., 2018. The promise of marine molecules as cosmetic active ingredients. Int. J. Cosmet. Sci. 0142-5463. 40 (1), 1–15. doi:10.1111/ics.12435.

Caballero, B., Trugo, L.C., Finglas, P.M., 2003. Encyclopedia of Food Sciences and Nutrition. Academic Press, Amsterdam New York.

Cadar, E., Pesterau, A.M., Prasacu, I., Ionescu, A.M., Pascale, C., Dragan, A.M.L., Sirbu, R., Tomescu, C.L., 2024. Marine antioxidants from marine collagen and collagen peptides with nutraceuticals applications: a review. Antioxidants. 20763921. 13 (8). Available from: www.mdpi.com/journal/antioxidants. doi:10.3390/antiox13080919.

Caffrey, C., Leamy, A., O'Sullivan, E., Zabetakis, I., Lordan, R., Nasopoulou, C., 2023. Cardiovascular diseases and marine oils: a focus on omega-3 polyunsaturated fatty acids and polar lipids. Mar. Drugs. 1660-3397. 21 (11), 549. doi:10.3390/md21110549.

Calder, P.C., 2012. Mechanisms of action of (n-3) fatty acids. J. Nutr. 00223166. 142 (3), 592S. doi:10.3945/jn.111.155259.

Calder, P.C., 2015. Marine omega-3 fatty acids and inflammatory processes: effects, mechanisms and clinical relevance. Biochim. Biophys. Acta Mol. Cell Biol. Lipids. 18792618. 1851 (4), 469–484. Available from: www.elsevier.com/locate/bbalip. doi:10.1016/j.bbalip.2014.08.010.

Cantoresi, F., Caserini, M., Bidoli, A., Maggio, F., Marino, R., Carnevale, C., Sorgi, P., Palmieri, R., 2014. Randomized controlled trial of a water-soluble nail lacquer based on hydroxypropyl-chitosan (HPCH), in the management of nail psoriasis. Clin. Cosmet. Investig. Dermatol. 11787015. 7, 185–190. Available from: http://www.dovepress.com/getfile.php?fileID=20238. doi:10.2147/CCID.S61659.

Carella, F., Esposti, L.D., Adamiano, A., Iafisco, M., 2021. The use of calcium phosphates in cosmetics, state of the art and future perspectives. Materials. 1996-1944. 14 (21), 6398. doi:10.3390/ma14216398.

Carrasqueira, J., Bernardino, S., Bernardino, R., Afonso, C., 2025. Marine-derived polysaccharides and their potential health benefits in nutraceutical applications. Mar. Drugs. 1660-3397. 23 (2), 60. doi:10.3390/md23020060.

Caruso, G., Floris, R., Serangeli, C., Di Paola, L., 2020. Fishery wastes as a yet undiscovered treasure from the sea: biomolecules sources, extraction methods and valorization. Mar. Drugs. 1660-3397. 18 (12), 622. doi:10.3390/md18120622.

Casadidio, C., Peregrina, D.V., Gigliobianco, M.R., Deng, S., Censi, R., Di Martino, P., 2019. Chitin and chitosans: characteristics, eco-friendly processes, and applications in cosmetic science. Mar. Drugs. 16603397. 17 (6). Available from: https://www.mdpi.com/1660-3397/17/6/369/pdf. doi:10.3390/md17060369.

Castrogiovanni, P., Trovato, F., Loreto, C., Nsir, H., Szychlinska, M., Musumeci, G., 2016. Nutraceutical supplements in the management and prevention of osteoarthritis. Int. J. Mol. Sci. 1422-0067. 17 (12), 2042. doi:10.3390/ijms17122042.

Catala, A.E., 2017. Fatty Acids. IntechOpen.

Chaiwong, N., Leelapornpisid, P., Jantanasakulwong, K., Rachtanapun, P., Seesuriyachan, P., Sakdatorn, V., Leksawasdi, N., Phimolsiripol, Y., 2020. Antioxidant and moisturizing properties of carboxymethyl chitosan with different molecular weights. Polymers. 2073-4360. 12 (7), 1445. doi:10.3390/polym12071445.

Chavda, V.P., Acharya, D., Hala, V., Daware, S., Vora, L.K., 2023. Sunscreens: a comprehensive review with the application of nanotechnology. J. Drug Deliv. Sci. Technol. 17732247. 86. Available from: http://www.editionsdesante.fr/category.php?id_category=48. doi:10.1016/j.jddst.2023.104720.

Chen, K., Guo, B., Luo, J., 2017. Quaternized carboxymethyl chitosan/organic montmorillonite nanocomposite as a novel cosmetic ingredient against skin aging. Carbohydr. Polym. 01448617. 173, 100–106. doi:10.1016/j.carbpol.2017.05.088.

Chen, T., Hou, H., 2016. Protective effect of gelatin polypeptides from Pacific cod (*Gadus macrocephalus*) against UV irradiation-induced damages by inhibiting inflammation and improving transforming growth factor-β/Smad signaling pathway. J. Photochem. Photobiol. B. 10111344. 162, 633–640. doi:10.1016/j.jphotobiol.2016.07.038.

Chen, T., Hou, H., Lu, J., Zhang, K., Li, B., 2016. Protective effect of gelatin and gelatin hydrolysate from salmon skin on UV irradiation-induced photo-aging of mice skin. J. Ocean Univ. China. 19935021. 15 (4), 711–718. Available from: http://www.springerlink.com/content/1672-5182. doi:10.1007/s11802-016-2953-5.

Chen, Y., Jin, H., Yang, F., Jin, S., Liu, C., Zhang, L., Huang, J., Wang, S., Yan, Z., Cai, X., Zhao, R., Fangmiao, Y., Yang, Z., Ding, G., Tang, Y., 2019. Physicochemical, antioxidant properties of giant croaker (*Nibea japonica*) swim bladders collagen and wound healing evaluation. Int. J. Biol. Macromol. 01418130. 138, 483–491. doi:10.1016/j.ijbiomac.2019.07.111.

Chotphruethipong, L., Sukketsiri, W., Aluko, R.E., Sae-leaw, T., Benjakul, S., 2021. Effect of hydrolyzed collagen from defatted Asian sea bass (*Lates calcarifer*) skin on fibroblast proliferation, migration and antioxidant activities. J. Food Sci. Technol. 09758402. 58 (2), 541–551. Available from: http://www.springerlink.com/content/121580/. doi:10.1007/s13197-020-04566-4.

Ciavatta, M.L., Lefranc, F., Vieira, L.M., Kiss, R., Carbone, M., van Otterlo, W.A.L., Lopanik, N.B., Waeschenbach, A., 2020. The phylum Bryozoa: from biology to biomedical potential. Mar. Drugs. 16603397. 18 (4). Available from: https://www.mdpi.com/1660-3397/18/4/200/pdf. doi:10.3390/md18040200.

Cohen, G., Jakus, J., Portillo, M., Gvirtz, R., Ogen-Shtern, N., Silberstein, E., Ayzenberg, T., Rozenblat, S., 2023. In vitro, ex vivo, and clinical evaluation of anti-aging gel containing EPA and CBD. J. Cosmet. Dermatol. 1473-2130. 22 (11), 3047–3057. doi:10.1111/jocd.15815.

Coppola, D., Lauritano, C., Esposito, F.P., Riccio, G., Rizzo, C., Pascale, D.D., 2021. Fish waste: from problem to valuable resource. Mar. Drugs. 1660-3397. 19 (2), 116. doi:10.3390/md19020116.

Danby, S.G., Andrew, P.V., Taylor, R.N., Kay, L.J., Chittock, J., Pinnock, A., Ulhaq, I., Fasth, A., Carlander, K., Holm, T., Cork, M.J., 2022. Different types of emollient cream exhibit diverse physiological effects on the skin barrier in adults with atopic dermatitis. Clin. Exp. Dermatol. 13652230. 47 (6), 1154–1164. Available from: http://onlinelibrary.wiley.com/journal/10.1111/(ISSN)1365-2230. doi:10.1111/ced.15141.

Das, P., Dutta, A., Panchali, T., Khatun, A., Kar, R., Das, T.K., Phoujdar, M., Chakrabarti, S., Ghosh, K., Pradhan, S., 2024. Advances in therapeutic applications of fish oil: a review. Meas. Food. 27722759. 13, 100142. doi:10.1016/j.meafoo.2024.100142.

Davinelli, S., Nielsen, M.E., Scapagnini, G., 2018. Astaxanthin in skin health, repair, and disease: a comprehensive review. Nutrients 10, 522.

Deng, L., Wang, B., Wenying, L., Han, Z., Chen, S., Wang, H., 2022. Bacterial cellulose reinforced chitosan-based hydrogel with highly efficient self-healing and enhanced antibacterial activity for wound healing. Int. J. Biol. Macromol. 01418130. 217, 77–87. doi:10.1016/j.ijbiomac.2022.07.017.

Deng, Y., Huang, L., Zhang, C., Xie, P., Cheng, J., Wang, X., Liu, L., 2020. Skin-care functions of peptides prepared from Chinese quince seed protein: sequences analysis, tyrosinase inhibition and molecular docking study. Ind. Crops Prod. 09266690. 148, 112331. doi:10.1016/j.indcrop.2020.112331.

Desai, S.J., Prickril, B., Rasooly, A., 2018. Mechanisms of phytonutrient modulation of cyclooxygenase-2 (COX-2) and inflammation related to cancer. Nutr. Cancer. 15327914. 70 (3), 350–375. Available from: http://www.tandfonline.com/toc/hnuc20/current. doi:10.1080/01635581.2018.1446091.

Di Landro, A., Cazzaniga, S., Parazzini, F., Ingordo, V., Cusano, F., Atzori, L., Cutrì, F.T., Musumeci, M.L., Zinetti, C., Pezzarossa, E., Bettoli, V., Caproni, M., Scocco, G.L., Bonci, A., Bencini, P., Naldi, L., 2012. Family history, body mass index, selected dietary factors, menstrual history, and risk of moderate to severe acne in adolescents and young adults. J. Am. Acad. Dermatol. 10976787. 67 (6), 1129–1135. doi:10.1016/j.jaad.2012.02.018.

Dutta, S., Kumar, S.P.J., Banerjee, R., 2023. A comprehensive review on astaxanthin sources, structure, biochemistry and applications in the cosmetic industry. Algal Res. 74, 103168.

Eckes, M., Dove, S., Siebeck, U.E., Grutter, A.S., 2015. Fish mucus versus parasitic gnathiid isopods as sources of energy and sunscreens for a cleaner fish. Coral Reefs. 07224028. 34 (3), 823–833. Available from: https://www.link.springer.de/link/service/journals/00338/index.htm. doi:10.1007/s00338-015-1313-z.

Edgley, D.E., Carruthers, M., Gabagambi, N.P., Saxon, A.D., Smith, A.M., Joyce, D.A., Vernaz, G., Santos, M.E., Turner, G.F., Genner, M.J., 2024. Lateral line system diversification during the early stages of ecological speciation in cichlid fish. BMC Ecol. Evol. 14726785. 24 (1). Available from: https://bmcecolevol.biomedcentral.com/. doi:10.1186/s12862-024-02214-5.

Elbialy, Z.I., Atiba, A., Abdelnaby, A., Al-Hawary, I.I., Elsheshtawy, A., El-Serehy, H.A., Abdel-Daim, M.M., Fadl, S.E., Assar, D.H., 2020. Collagen extract obtained from Nile tilapia (*Oreochromis niloticus* L.) skin accelerates wound healing in rat model via up regulating VEGF, bFGF, and α-SMA genes expression. BMC Vet. Res. 17466148. 16 (1), 352. doi:10.1186/s12917-020-02566-2.

Elhiss, S., Hamdi, A., Chahed, L., Boisson-Vidal, C., Majdoub, H., Bouchemal, N., Laschet, J., Kraiem, J., Cerf, D.L., Maaroufi, R.M., Chaubet, F., Mansour, M.B., 2024. Hyaluronic acid from bluefin tuna by-product: structural analysis and pharmacological activities. Int. J. Biol. Macromol. 01418130. 264 (Pt 1), 130424. doi:10.1016/j.ijbiomac.2024.130424.

Eren, B., Tanrıverdi, S.T., Aydın Köse, F., Özer, Ö., 2019. Antioxidant properties evaluation of topical astaxanthin formulations as anti-aging products. J. Cosmet. Dermatol. 1473-2130. 18 (1), 242–250. doi:10.1111/jocd.12665.

Fang, Q., Guo, S., Zhou, H., Han, R., Wu, P., Han, C., 2017. Astaxanthin protects against early burn-wound progression in rats by attenuating oxidative stress-induced inflammation and mitochondria-related apoptosis. Sci. Rep. 7, 41440.

Fernández-Peña, L., Guzmán, E., 2020. Physicochemical aspects of the performance of hair-conditioning formulations. Cosmetics. 2079-9284. 7 (2), 26. doi:10.3390/cosmetics7020026.

Fernando, I.P.S., Jayawardena, T.U., Wu, J., 2023. Marine proteins and peptides: production, biological activities, and potential applications. Food Innov. Adv. 2836774X. 2 (2), 69–84. Available from: https://www.maxapress.com/article/doi/10.48130/FIA-2023-0009. doi:10.48130/FIA-2023-0009.

Ferreira, M.S., Resende, D.I.S.P., Lobo, J.M.S., Sousa, E., Almeida, I.F., 2021. Marine ingredients for sensitive skin: market overview. Mar. Drugs. 16603397. 19 (8). Available from: https://www.mdpi.com/1660-3397/19/8/464/pdf. doi:10.3390/MD19080464.

Fonseca, S., Amaral, M.N., Reis, C.P., Custódio, L., 2023. Marine natural products as innovative cosmetic ingredients. Mar. Drugs. 16603397. 21 (3). Available from: http://www.mdpi.com/journal/marinedrugs. doi:10.3390/md21030170.

Formisano, E., Proietti, E., Borgarelli, C., Pisciotta, L., 2023. Psoriasis and vitamin D: a systematic review and meta-analysis. Nutrients. 2072-6643. 15 (15), 3387. doi:10.3390/nu15153387.

Franco, W., Arazo, M.C.R., Benavides, S., 2023. Recent advances in the encapsulation of marine phenolic compounds. In: Perez Correa, J.R., Mateos, R., Dominguez, H. (Eds.), Marine Phenolic Compounds: Science and Engineering. Elsevier, Chile, pp. 239–264. Available from: https://www.sciencedirect.com/book/9780128235898. doi:10.1016/B978-0-12-823589-8.00011-X.

Fu, Y., Chongyang, L., Wang, Q., Gao, R., Cai, X., Wang, S., Zhang, Y., 2022. The protective effect of collagen peptides from bigeye tuna (*Thunnus obesus*) skin and bone to attenuate UVB-induced photoaging via MAPK and TGF-β signaling pathways. J. Funct. Foods. 17564646. 93, 105101. doi:10.1016/j.jff.2022.105101.

Gacesa, R., Lawrence, K.P., Georgakopoulos, N.D., Yabe, K., Dunlap, W.C., Barlow, D.J., Wells, G., Young, A.R., Long, P.F., 2018. The mycosporine-like amino acids porphyra-334 and shinorine are antioxidants and direct antagonists of Keap1-Nrf2 binding. Biochimie. 61831638. 154, 35–44. Available from: www.elsevier.com/locate/biochimie. doi:10.1016/j.biochi.2018.07.020.

Galasso, C., Corinaldesi, C., Sansone, C., 2017. Carotenoids from marine organisms: biological functions and industrial applications. Antioxidants. 2076-3921. 6 (4), 96. doi:10.3390/antiox6040096.

Ganguly, A., Ian, C.K., Sheshala, R., Sahu, P.S., Al-Waeli, H., Meka, V.S., 2017. Application of diverse natural polymers in the design of oral gels for the treatment of periodontal diseases. J. Mater. Sci. Mater. Med. 15734838. 28 (3). Available from: www.wkap.nl/journalhome.htm/0957-4530. doi:10.1007/s10856-017-5852-4.

Gao, H., Nan, W., Wang, N., Jie, L., Sun, J., Peng, Q., 2022a. Chitosan-based therapeutic systems and their potentials in treatment of oral diseases. Int. J. Biol. Macromol. 01418130. 222 (Pt B), 3178–3194. doi:10.1016/j.ijbiomac.2022.10.090.

Gao, Q., Shang, Y., Zhou, W., Deng, S., Peng, C., 2022b. Marine collagen peptides: a novel biomaterial for the healing of oral mucosal ulcers. Dent. Mater. J. 0287-4547. 41 (6), 850–859. doi:10.4012/dmj.2021-323.

Ghalamara, S., Brazinha, C., Silva, S., Pintado, M., 2024. Valorization of fish processing by-products: biological and functional properties of bioactive peptides. Curr. Food Sci. Technol. Rep. 2662-8473. 2 (4), 393–409. doi:10.1007/s43555-024-00045-5.

Ghannoum, M.A., Long, L., Isham, N., Bulgheroni, A., Setaro, M., Caserini, M., Palmieri, R., Mailland, F., 2015. Ability of hydroxypropyl chitosan nail lacquer to protect against dermatophyte nail infection. Antimicrob. Agents Chemother. 0066-4804. 59 (4), 1844–1848. doi:10.1128/aac.04842-14.

Ghareeb, M.A., Tammam, M.A., El-Demerdash, A., Atanasov, A.G., 2020. Insights about clinically approved and preclinically investigated marine natural products. Curr. Res. Biotechnol. 25902628. 2, 88–102. Available from: https://www.journals.elsevier.com/current-research-in-biotechnology/. doi:10.1016/j.crbiot.2020.09.001.

Golovach, I., Rekalov, D., Akimov, O.Y., Kostenko, H., Kostenko, V., Mishchenko, A., Solovyova, N., Kostenko, V., 2023. Molecular mechanisms and potential applications of chondroitin sulphate in managing post-traumatic osteoarthritis. Reumatologia. 20849834. 61 (5), 395–407. Available from: https://www.termedia.pl/Journals. doi:10.5114/reum/172211.

González-Serrano, D.J., Hadidi, M., Varcheh, M., Jelyani, A.Z., Moreno, A., Lorenzo, J.M., 2022. Bioactive peptide fractions from collagen hydrolysate of common carp fish byproduct: antioxidant and functional properties. Antioxidants. 20763921. 11 (3). Available from: https://www.mdpi.com/2076-3921/11/3/509/pdf. doi:10.3390/antiox11030509.

Guertler, A., Neu, K., Lill, D., Clanner-Engelshofen, B., French, L.E., Reinholz, M., 2024. Exploring the potential of omega-3 fatty acids in acne patients: a prospective intervention study. J. Cosmet. Dermatol. 14732165. 23 (10), 3295–3304. Available from: http://onlinelibrary.wiley.com/journal/10.1111/(ISSN)1473-2165. doi:10.1111/jocd.16434.

Guzmán, E., Ortega, F., Rubio, R.G., 2022. Chitosan: a promising multifunctional cosmetic ingredient for skin and hair care. Cosmetics. 20799284. 9 (5). Available from: www.mdpi.com/journal/cosmetics. doi:10.3390/cosmetics9050099.

Haq, M., Suraiya, S., Ahmed, S., Chun, B.-S., 2021. Phospholipids from marine source: extractions and forthcoming industrial applications. J. Funct. Foods. 17564646. 80, 104448. doi:10.1016/j.jff.2021.104448.

He, J., Zhang, J., Yingjie, X., Yigang, M., Guo, X., 2022. The structural and functional differences between three species of fish scale gelatin and pigskin gelatin. Foods. 2304-8158. 11 (24), 3960. doi:10.3390/foods11243960.

Henseler, 2023. Investigating the Effects of Argireline in a Skin Serum Containing Hyaluronic Acids on Skin Surface Wrinkles Using the Visia® Complexion Analysis Camera System for Objective Skin Analysis. GMS Interdisciplinary Plastic and Reconstructive Surgery DGPW, 12. doi:10.3205/iprs000179.

Hesse, G.W., 1979. Chronic zinc deficiency alters neuronal function of hippocampal mossy fibers. Science. 00368075. 205 (4410), 1005–1007. doi:10.1126/science.224456.

Holick, M.F., 2007. Vitamin D deficiency. N. Engl. J. Med. 0028-4793. 357 (3), 266–281. doi:10.1056/nejmra070553.

Honrado, A., Rubio, S., Antonio Beltrán, J., Calanche, J., 2022. Fish by-product valorization as source of bioactive compounds for food enrichment: characterization, suitability and shelf life. Foods. 2304-8158. 11 (22), 3656. doi:10.3390/foods11223656.

Hou, H., Bafang, L., Zhang, Z., Xue, C., Guangli, Y., Wang, J., Bao, Y., Lin, B., Sun, J., Peng, Z., Shiwei, S., 2012. Moisture absorption and retention properties, and activity in alleviating skin photodamage of collagen polypeptide from marine fish skin. Food Chem. 03088146. 135 (3), 1432–1439. doi:10.1016/j.foodchem.2012.06.009.

Hu, X., Song, L., Huang, L., Zheng, Q., Rongmin, Y., 2012. Antitumor effect of a polypeptide fraction from *Arca subcrenata* in vitro and in vivo. Mar. Drugs. 1660-3397. 10 (12), 2782–2794. doi:10.3390/md10122782.

Huang, T.H., Wang, P.W., Yang, S.C., Chou, W.L., Fang, J.Y., 2018. Cosmetic and therapeutic applications of fish oil's fatty acids on the skin. Mar. Drugs. 16603397. 16 (8). Available from: http://www.mdpi.com/1660-3397/16/8/256/pdf. doi:10.3390/md16080256.

Husein El Hadmed, H., Castillo, R.F., 2016. Cosmeceuticals: peptides, proteins, and growth factors. J. Cosmet. Dermatol. 14732165. 15 (4), 514–519. Available from: http://onlinelibrary.wiley.com/journal/10.1111/(ISSN)1473-2165. doi:10.1111/jocd.12229.

Ikarashi, N., Kon, R., Nagoya, C., Ishikura, A., Sugiyama, Y., Takahashi, J., Sugiyama, K., 2020. Effect of astaxanthin on the expression and activity of aquaporin-3 in skin in an in-vitro study. Life. 2075-1729. 10 (9), 193. doi:10.3390/life10090193.

Imokawa, G., 2019. The xanthophyll carotenoid astaxanthin has distinct biological effects to prevent the photoaging of the skin even by its postirradiation treatment. Photochem. Photobiol. 0031-8655. 95 (2), 490–500. doi:10.1111/php.13039.

Ito, N., Seki, S., Ueda, F., 2018. The protective role of astaxanthin for UV-induced skin deterioration in healthy people—a randomized, double-blind, placebo-controlled trial. Nutrients. 2072-6643. 10 (7), 817. doi:10.3390/nu10070817.

Ivic, M., Slugan, A., Leskur, D., Rusic, D., Perisin, A.S., Modun, D., Durdov, T., Bozic, J., Vukovic, D., Bukic, J., 2024. Efficacy and safety assessment of topical omega fatty acid product in experimental model of irritant contact dermatitis: randomized controlled trial. Appl. Sci. 2076-3417. 14 (15), 6423. doi:10.3390/app14156423.

Jerosch, J., 2011. Effects of glucosamine and chondroitin sulfate on cartilage metabolism in OA: outlook on other nutrient partners especially omega-3 fatty acids. Int. J. Rheumatol. 1687-9260. 2011, 1–17. doi:10.1155/2011/969012.

Jiang, D., Zhenzhen, H., Liu, F., Zhang, R., Duo, B., Jianjie, F., Cui, Y., Mei, L., 2014. Heavy metals levels in fish from aquaculture farms and risk assessment in Lhasa, Tibetan Autonomous Region of China. Ecotoxicology. 0963-9292. 23 (4), 577–583. doi:10.1007/s10646-014-1229-3.

Jimbo, N., Kawada, C., Nomura, Y., 2016. Optimization of dose of collagen hydrolysate to prevent UVB-irradiated skin damage. Biosc. Biotechnol. Biochem. 0916-8451. 80 (2), 356–359. doi:10.1080/09168451.2015.1086258.

Jimenez-Champi, D., Romero-Orejon, F.L., Muñoz, A.M., Ramos-Escudero, F., 2024. The revalorization of fishery by-products: types, bioactive compounds, and food applications. Int. J. Food Sci. 23145765. 2024. Available from: http://www.hindawi.com/journals/ijfs/. doi:10.1155/2024/6624083.

Joy, J.M., Padmaprakashan, A., Pradeep, A., Paul, P.T., Mannuthy, R.J., Mathew, S., 2024. A review on fish skin-derived gelatin: elucidating the gelatin peptides—preparation, bioactivity, mechanistic insights, and strategies for stability improvement. Foods. 23048158. 13 (17). Available from: www.mdpi.com/journal/foods. doi:10.3390/foods13172793.

Kageyama, H., Waditee-Sirisattha, R., Antioxidative,, 2019. Anti-inflammatory, and anti-aging properties of mycosporine-like amino acids: molecular and cellular mechanisms in the protection of skin-aging. Mar. Drugs. 1660-3397. 17 (4), 222. doi:10.3390/md17040222.

Kandyliari, A., Mallouchos, A., Papandroulakis, N., Golla, J.P., Lam, T.K.T., Sakellari, A., Karavoltsos, S., Vasiliou, V., Kapsokefalou, M., 2020. Nutrient composition and fatty acid and protein profiles of selected fish by-products. Foods. 23048158. 9 (2). Available from: https://www.mdpi.com/2304-8158/9/2/190. doi:10.3390/foods9020190.

Kang, H.K., Lee, H.H., Seo, C.H., Park, Y., 2019. Antimicrobial and immunomodulatory properties and applications of marine-derived proteins and peptides. Mar. Drugs. 16603397. 17 (6). Available from: https://www.mdpi.com/1660-3397/17/6/350/pdf. doi:10.3390/md17060350.

Kang, J.W., Hyun, S.H., Kim, H.M., Park, S.Y., Lee, J.A., Lee, I.C., Bae, J.S., 2024. The effects of fucoidan-rich polysaccharides extracted from *Sargassum horneri* on enhancing collagen-related skin barrier function as a potential cosmetic product. J. Cosmet. Dermatol. 14732165. 23 (4), 1365–1373. Available from: http://onlinelibrary.wiley.com/journal/10.1111/(ISSN)1473-2165. doi:10.1111/jocd.16108.

Kim, S.-K., 2013. Marine Proteins and Peptides: Biological Activities and Applications. John Wiley & Sons Inc, Chichester, West Sussex, UK.

Kim, S.-K.E., 2023. Marine Biochemistry: Applications. CRC Press, Boca Raton, FL.

Kim, S.K., Karadeniz, F., 2012. Biological importance and applications of squalene and squalane. Adv. Food Nutr. Res. 65, 223–233. Available from http://www.elsevier.com/wps/find/bookdescription.cws_home/704624/description#description. doi:10.1016/B978-0-12-416003-3.00014-7.

Klimaszewska, E., Seweryn, A., Ogorzałek, M., Nizioł-Łukaszewska, Z., Wasilewski, T., 2019. Reduction of irritation potential caused by anionic surfactants in the use of various forms of collagen derived from marine sources in cosmetics for children. Tenside Surfact. Deterg. 2195-8564. 56 (3), 180–187. doi:10.3139/113.110616.

Koch, C., Sures, B., 2018. Environmental concentrations and toxicology of 2,4,6-tribromophenol (TBP). Environ. Pollut. 02697491. 233, 706–713. doi:10.1016/j.envpol.2017.10.127.

Kodali, D., Hembrick-Holloman, V., Gunturu, D.R., Samuel, T., Jeelani, S., Rangari, V.K., 2022. Influence of fish scale-based hydroxyapatite on forcespun polycaprolactone fiber scaffolds. ACS Omega. 24701343. 7 (10), 8323–8335. Available from: https:www.pubs.acs.org/journal/acsodf. doi:10.1021/acsomega.1c05593.

Komatsu, T., Sasaki, S., Manabe, Y., Hirata, T., Sugawara, T., Slominski, A.T., 2017. Preventive effect of dietary astaxanthin on UVA-induced skin photoaging in hairless mice. PLOS ONE. 1932-6203. 12 (2), e0171178. doi:10.1371/journal.pone.0171178.

Kuang, C.Y., Mohtar, N.F., 2018. Effects of different soaking time on the extraction of gelatin from shortfin scad (*Decapterus macrosoma*) heads. JEB 39, 888–894. doi:10.22438/jeb/39/5(SI)/11.

Kumari, S., Annamareddy, S.H.K., Abanti, S., Rath, P.K., 2017. Physicochemical properties and characterization of chitosan synthesized from fish scales, crab and shrimp shells. Int. J. Biol. Macromol. 18790003. 104, 1697–1705. Available from: www.elsevier.com/locate/ijbiomac. doi:10.1016/j.ijbiomac.2017.04.119.

Kundam, D.N., Okpunyi Acham, I., Tartenger Girgih, A., 2018. Bioactive compounds in fish and their health benefits. Asian Food Sci. J. 25817752. 4 (4), 1–14. doi:10.9734/afsj/2018/41803.

Lall, S.P., Kaushik, S.J., 2021. Nutrition and metabolism of minerals in fish. Animals. 20762615. 11 (9). Available from: https://www.mdpi.com/2076-2615/11/9/2711/pdf. doi:10.3390/ani11092711.

Latreille, J., Kesse-Guyot, E., Malvy, D., Andreeva, V., Galan, P., Tschachler, E., Hercberg, S., Guinot, C., Ezzedine, K., 2013. Association between dietary intake of n-3 polyunsaturated fatty acids and severity of skin photoaging in a middle-aged Caucasian population. J. Dermatol. Sci. 09231811. 72 (3), 233–239. doi:10.1016/j.jdermsci.2013.07.006.

Lawrence, K.P., Gacesa, R., Long, P.F., Young, A.R., 2018. Molecular photoprotection of human keratinocytes in vitro by the naturally occurring mycosporine-like amino acid palythine. Br. J. Dermatol. 00070963. 178 (6), 1353–1363. doi:10.1111/bjd.16125.

Lee, D.U., Kim, S.C., Choi, D.Y., Jung, W.K., Moon, M.J., 2023. Basic amino acid-mediated cationic amphiphilic surfaces for antimicrobial pH monitoring sensor with wound healing effects. Biomater. Res. 20557124. 27 (1). Available from: https://biomaterialsres.biomedcentral.com/. doi:10.1186/s40824-023-00355-0.

Lee, S., Koo, M.H., Han, D.W., Kim, I.C., Lee, J.H., Kim, J.H., Sultana, R., Kim, S.Y., Youn, U.J., Kim, J.H., 2022. Comparison of fatty acid contents and MMP-1 inhibitory effects of the two Antarctic fish, *Notothenia rossii* and *Champsocephalus gunnari*. Molecules. 14203049. 27 (14). Available from: http://www.mdpi.com/journal/molecules. doi:10.3390/molecules27144554.

Lei, T., Lin, Y., Pei, Y., Sun, H., Guo, C., 2025. Applications of elastin in cosmetics: prospects and challenges. Cosmetics. 2079-9284. 12 (1), 18. doi:10.3390/cosmetics12010018.

Lens, M., 2025. Phospholipid-based vesicular systems as carriers for the delivery of active cosmeceutical ingredients. Int. J. Mol. Sci. 1422-0067. 26 (6), 2484. doi:10.3390/ijms26062484.

Li, C., Fu, Y., Dai, H., Wang, Q., Gao, R., Zhang, Y., 2022. Recent progress in preventive effect of collagen peptides on photoaging skin and action mechanism. Food Sci. Hum. Wellness. 22134530. 11 (2), 218–229. doi:10.1016/j.fshw.2021.11.003.

Liu, Y., Mao, J., Guo, Z., Yufang, H., Wang, S., 2022. Polyvinyl alcohol/carboxymethyl chitosan hydrogel loaded with silver nanoparticles exhibited antibacterial and self-healing properties. Int. J. Biol. Macromol. 01418130. 220, 211–222. doi:10.1016/j.ijbiomac.2022.08.061.

Liu, Y., Shang, J., Chen, Y., Feng, X., 2025. Potential applications of chitosan in seborrheic dermatitis and other skin diseases: a comprehensive review. Clin. Cosmet. Investig. Dermatol. 11787015. 18, 533–542. Available from: https://www.dovepress.com/article/download/100872. doi:10.2147/CCID.S504778.

Liu, Z., Zhao, N., Liang, L., Menggeng, L., Nie, X., Wang, Y., Liu, Q., Zhou, Q., Shu, P., 2024. Evaluation of the anti-aging potential of acetyl tripeptide-30 citrulline in cosmetics. Int. J. Pharm. 03785173. 663, 124557. doi:10.1016/j.ijpharm.2024.124557.

Loftsson, T., Ilievska, B., Asgrimsdottir, G.M., Ormarsson, O.T., Stefansson, E., 2016. Fatty acids from marine lipids: biological activity, formulation and stability. J. Drug Deliv. Sci. Technol. 17732247. 34, 71–75. Available from: http://www.editionsdesante.fr/category.php?id_category=48. doi:10.1016/j.jddst.2016.03.007.

Loh, X.J., Young, D.J., Guo, H., Tang, L., Wu, Y.L., Zhang, G., Tang, C., Ruan, H., 2021. Pearl powder—an emerging material for biomedical applications: a review. Materials. 19961944. 14 (11). Available from: https://www.mdpi.com/1996-1944/14/11/2797/pdf. doi:10.3390/ma14112797.

Lønne, G.K., Gammelsæter, R., Haglerød, C., 2013. Composition characterization and clinical efficacy study of a salmon egg extract. Int. J. Cosmet. Sci. 0142-5463. 35 (5), 515–522. doi:10.1111/ics.12071.

Lopes, D., Rey, F., Leal, M.C., Lillebø, A.I., Calado, R., Domingues, M.R., 2021. Bioactivities of lipid extracts and complex lipids from seaweeds: current knowledge and future prospects. Mar. Drugs. 16603397. 19 (12). Available from: https://www.mdpi.com/1660-3397/19/12/686/pdf. doi:10.3390/md19120686.

López-Álvarez, M., González, P., Serra, J., Fraguas, J., Valcarcel, J., Vázquez, J.A., 2020. Chondroitin sulfate and hydroxyapatite from *Prionace glauca* shark jaw: physicochemical and structural characterization. Int. J. Biol. Macromol. 18790003. 156, 329–339. Available from: www.elsevier.com/locate/ijbiomac. doi:10.1016/j.ijbiomac.2020.04.010.

Lu, J., Hou, H., Fan, Y., Yang, T., Bafang, L., 2017. Identification of MMP-1 inhibitory peptides from cod skin gelatin hydrolysates and the inhibition mechanism by MAPK signaling pathway. J. Funct. Foods. 17564646. 33, 251–260. doi:10.1016/j.jff.2017.03.049.

Lu, W.Y., Li, H.J., Li, Q.Y., Wu, Y.C., 2021. Application of marine natural products in drug research. Bioorg. Med. Chem. 14643391. 35. Available from: http://www.journals.elsevier.com/bioorganic-and-medicinal-chemistry/. doi:10.1016/j.bmc.2021.116058.

Maia Campos, P.M.B.G., Franco, R.S.B., Kakuda, L., Cadioli, G.F., Costa, G.M.D., Bouvret, E., 2021. Oral supplementation with hydrolyzed fish cartilage improves the morphological and structural characteristics of the skin: a double-blind, placebo-controlled clinical study. Molecules. 14203049. 26 (16). Available from: https://www.mdpi.com/1420-3049/26/16/4880/pdf. doi:10.3390/molecules26164880.

Malmvärn, A., Marsh, G., Kautsky, L., Athanasiadou, M., Bergman, Å., Asplund, L., 2005. Hydroxylated and methoxylated brominated diphenyl ethers in the red algae *Ceramium tenuicorne* and blue mussels from the Baltic sea. Environ. Sci. Technol. 0013-936X. 39 (9), 2990–2997. doi:10.1021/es0482886.

Manel, S., Guerin, P.E., Mouillot, D., Blanchet, S., Velez, L., Albouy, C., Pellissier, L., 2020. Global determinants of freshwater and marine fish genetic diversity. Nat. Commun. 20411723. 11 (1). Available from: http://www.nature.com/ncomms/index.html. doi:10.1038/s41467-020-14409-7.

Marques, I., Botelho, G., Guiné, R., 2019. Comparative study on nutritional composition of fish available in Portugal. Nutr. Food Sci. 0034-6659. 49 (5), 925–941. doi:10.1108/nfs-11-2018-0311.

Márquez-Balbás, G., Sánchez-Regaña, M., Millet, U., 2011. Study on the use of omega-3 fatty acids as a therapeutic supplement in treatment of psoriasis. Clin. Cosmet. Investig. Dermatol. 1178-7015. 4, 73. doi:10.2147/CCID.S17220.

Martins, E., Castro, P., Ribeiro, A.B., Pereira, C.F., Casanova, F., Vilarinho, R., Moreira, J., Ramos, Ó.L., 2024. Bleached hair as standard template to insight the performance of commercial hair repair products. Cosmetics. 20799284. 11 (5). Available from: www.mdpi.com/journal/cosmetics. doi:10.3390/cosmetics11050150.

Martins, E., Reis, R.L., Silva, T.H., 2023. In vivo skin hydrating efficacy of fish collagen from Greenland halibut as a high-value active ingredient for cosmetic applications. Mar. Drugs. 16603397. 21 (2). Available from: http://www.mdpi.com/journal/marinedrugs. doi:10.3390/md21020057.

Mata-Sotres, J.A., Marques, V.H., Barba, D., Braga, A., Araújo, B., Viana, M.T., Rombenso, A.N., 2021. Increasing dietary SFA:MUFA ratio with low levels of LC-PUFA affected lipid metabolism, tissue fatty acid profile and growth of juvenile California Yellowtail (*Seriola dorsalis*). Aquaculture. 00448486. 543. Available from: http://www.journals.elsevier.com/aquaculture/. doi:10.1016/j.aquaculture.2021.737011.

Mateos, R., Ricardo Pérez-Correa, J., Domínguez, H., 2020. Bioactive properties of marine phenolics. Mar. Drugs. 1660-3397. 18 (10), 501. doi:10.3390/md18100501.

Medeiros, L.H.C., Vasconcelos, B.M.F., Silva, M.B., Souza-Junior, A.A., Chavante, S.F., Andrade, G.P.V., 2021. Chondroitin sulfate from fish waste exhibits strong intracellular antioxidant potential. Braz. J. Med. Biol. Res. 1414-431X. 54 (10). doi:10.1590/1414-431x2020e10730.

Meephansan, J., Rungjang, A., Yingmema, W., Deenonpoe, R., Ponnikorn, S., 2017. Effect of astaxanthin on cutaneous wound healing. Clin. Cosmet. Investig. Dermatol. 10, 259–265.

Mititelu, M., Stanciu, G., Drăgănescu, D., Ioniță, A.C., Neacşu, S.M., Dinu, M., Stefan-van Staden, R.-I., Moroşan, E., 2022. Mussel Shells, a valuable calcium resource for the pharmaceutical industry. Mar. Drugs. 1660-3397. 20 (1), 25. doi:10.3390/md20010025.

Mogobe, O., Mosepele, K., Masamba, W.R.L., 2015. Essential mineral content of common fish species in Chanoga, Okavango Delta, Botswana. Afr. J. Food Sci. 1996-0794. 9 (9), 480–486. doi:10.5897/AJFS2015.1307.

Mohamed, A.E., Elgammal, W.E., Ibrahim, A.G., Dawaba, H.M., Nossier, E.S., Dawaba, A.M., 2025. Thiadiazole chitosan conjugates as a novel cosmetic ingredient for rinse-off hair conditioners: design, formulation, characterization and in silico-molecular docking studies. BMC Chem. 2661801X. 19 (1). Available from: https://bmcchem.biomedcentral.com/. doi:10.1186/s13065-025-01404-6.

Molina-Ramírez, C., Mazo, P., Zuluaga, R., Gañán, P., Álvarez-Caballero, J., 2021. Characterization of chitosan extracted from fish scales of the Colombian endemic species *Prochilodus magdalenae* as a novel source for antibacterial starch-based films. Polymers. 2073-4360. 13 (13), 2079. doi:10.3390/polym13132079.

Monti, D., Tampucci, S., Paganini, V., Burgalassi, S., Chetoni, P., Galván, J., Celandroni, F., Ghelardi, E., 2022. Ciclopirox hydroxypropyl chitosan (CPX-HPCH) nail lacquer and breathable cosmetic nail polish: in vitro evaluation of drug transungual permeation following the combined application. Life. 2075-1729. 12 (6), 801. doi:10.3390/life12060801.

Morganti, P., Palombo, M., Tishchenko, G., Yudin, V., Guarneri, F., Cardillo, M., Ciotto, P.D., Carezzi, F., Morganti, G., Fabrizi, G., 2014. Chitin-hyaluronan nanoparticles: a multifunctional carrier to deliver anti-aging active ingredients through the skin. Cosmetics. 2079-9284. 1 (3), 140–158. doi:10.3390/cosmetics1030140.

Morsy, R., Ali, S.S., El-Shetehy, M., 2017. Development of hydroxyapatite-chitosan gel sunscreen combating clinical multidrug-resistant bacteria. J. Mol. Struct. 00222860. 1143, 251–258. Available from: www.elsevier.com/inca/publications/store/5/0/0/8/5/0/index.htt. doi:10.1016/j.molstruc.2017.04.090.

Mota, S., Rego, L., Sousa, E., Cruz, M.T., Almeida, I.M.D., 2025. Usage frequency and ecotoxicity of skin depigmenting agents. Pharmaceuticals. 14248247. 18 (3). Available from: https://www.mdpi.com/journal/pharmaceuticals. doi:10.3390/ph18030368.

Mourão, P.A., Vilanova, E., Soares, P.A., 2018. Unveiling the structure of sulfated fucose-rich polysaccharides via nuclear magnetic resonance spectroscopy. Curr. Opin. Struct. Biol. 1879033X. 50, 33–41. Available from: http://www.elsevier.com/locate/sbi. doi:10.1016/j.sbi.2017.10.011.

Murakami, H., Shimbo, K., Inoue, Y., Takino, Y., Kobayashi, H., 2012. Importance of amino acid composition to improve skin collagen protein synthesis rates in UV-irradiated mice. Amino Acids. 0939-4451. 42 (6), 2481–2489. doi:10.1007/s00726-011-1059-z.

Astaxanthin Collagen All-in-One Gel, n.d. https://www.dhccare.com/astaxanthin-collagen-all-in-one-gel.html.

CosIng—Cosmetics—GROWTH - European Commission, n.d. https://ec.europa.eu/growth/tools-databases/cosing/details/74131.

Cropure Orange Roughy—Croda, n.d. https://cosmetics.specialchem.com/product/i-croda-cropure-orange-roughy.

InstantPeelTM Exfoliant, n.d. https://earthenskincare.com/products/instant-peel-exfoliant.

Marine Bioactive Peptides: Anti-Photoaging Mechanisms and Potential Skin Protective Effects, n.d. https://www.mdpi.com/1467-3045/46/2/63.

Nutricoll Natural Marine Collagen Powder - Chitinor, n.d. https://cosmetics.specialchem.com/product/i-chitinor-seagarden-nutricoll-natural-marine-collagen-powder.

Peptides in Cosmetics: from Pharmaceutical Breakthroughs to Skincare Innovations, n.d. https://www.mdpi.com/2079-9284/12/3/107.

Premium High-Purity Marine Collagen Peptides | Thala, n.d. https://www.thalaingredients.com/thalacol/.

Proximate composition of New Zealand Marine Finfish and Shellfish, n.d. https://www.fao.org/4/ae581e/ae581e09.htm#bm9.

Smart and Sustainable Hair Products Based on Chitin-Derived Compounds, n.d. https://www.mdpi.com/2079-9284/8/1/20.

Usage of Synthetic Peptides in Cosmetics for Sensitive Skin, n.d. https://www.mdpi.com/1424-8247/14/8/702.

Zellulin® ZelluGEN 10% Solution - Avant, n.d. https://cosmetics.specialchem.com/product/i-avant-zellulin-zellugen-10-solution.

Nasopoulou, C., Psani, E., Sioriki, E., Demopoulos, C.A., Zabetakis, I., 2013. Evaluation of sensory and *in vitro* cardio protective properties of sardine (*Sardina pilchardus*): the effect of grilling and brining. Food Nutr. Sci. 2157-944X. 04 (09), 940–949. doi:10.4236/fns.2013.49122.

Nasopoulou, C., Tsoupras, A.B., Karantonis, H.C., Demopoulos, C.A., Zabetakis, I., 2011. Fish polar lipids retard atherosclerosis in rabbits by down-regulating PAF biosynthesis and up-regulating PAF catabolism. Lipids Health Dis. 1476511X. 10. doi:10.1186/1476-511X-10-213.

Nerhus, I., Markhus, M.W., Nilsen, B.M., Øyen, J., Maage, A., Ødegård, E.R., Midtbø, L.K., Frantzen, S., Kögel, T., Graff, I.E., Lie, Ø., Dahl, L., Kjellevold, M., 2018. Iodine content of six fish species, Norwegian dairy products and hen's egg. Food Nutr. Res. 1654-661X. 62 (0). doi:10.29219/fnr.v62.1291.

Ngandjui, Y.A.T., Kereeditse, T.T., Kamika, I., Madikizela, L.M., Msagati, T.A.M., 2024. Nutraceutical and medicinal importance of marine molluscs. Mar. Drugs. 16603397. 22 (5). Available from: http://www.mdpi.com/journal/marinedrugs. doi:10.3390/md22050201.

Nguyen, S., Escudero, C., Sediqi, N., Smistad, G., Hiorth, M., 2017. Fluoride loaded polymeric nanoparticles for dental delivery. Eur. J. Pharm. Sci. 09280987. 104, 326–334. doi:10.1016/j.ejps.2017.04.004.

Nigam, S.K., Kunkel, G., Prescott, S.M., 1996. Platelet-activating Factor and Related Lipid Mediators 2: Roles in Health and Disease. Springer, Boston, MA.

Nikolakopoulou, Z., Shaikh, M.H., Dehlawi, H., Michael-Titus, A.T., Parkinson, E.K., 2013. The induction of apoptosis in pre-malignant keratinocytes by omega-3 polyunsaturated fatty acids docosahexaenoic acid (DHA) and eicosapentaenoic acid (EPA) is inhibited by albumin. Toxicol. Lett. 18793169. 218 (2), 150–158. doi:10.1016/j.toxlet.2013.01.021.

Nimisha, A.S., 2024. Exploring marine-derived bioactives for innovative cosmeceutical applications: a review. J. Appl. Nat. Sci. 2231-5209. 16 (2), 478–494. doi:10.31018/jans.v16i2.5433.

Nip, J., Hermanson, K., Lee, J., 2025. n-3 PUFAs docosahexaenoic acid and eicosapentaenoic acid are effective natural pro-resolution ingredients for topical skin applications. Int. J. Cosmet. Sci. 0142-5463. 47 (5), 820–826. doi:10.1111/ics.13068.

Nitulescu, G., Lupuliasa, D., Adam-Dima, I., Nitulescu, G.M., 2023. Ultraviolet filters for cosmetic applications. Cosmetics. 20799284. 10 (4). Available from: www.mdpi.com/journal/cosmetics. doi:10.3390/cosmetics10040101.

Niu, T., Xuan, R., Jiang, L., Wei, W., Zhen, Z., Song, Y., Hong, L., Zheng, K., Zhang, J., Qingshan, X., Tan, Y., Yan, X., Chen, H., 2018. Astaxanthin induces the Nrf2/HO-1 antioxidant pathway in human umbilical vein endothelial cells by generating trace amounts of ROS. J. Agric. Food Chem. 0021-8561. 66 (6), 1551–1559. doi:10.1021/acs.jafc.7b05493.

Ntohogian, S., Gavriliadou, V., Christodoulou, E., Nanaki, S., Lykidou, S., Naidis, P., Mischopoulou, L., Barmpalexis, P., Nikolaidis, N., Bikiaris, D.N., 2018. Chitosan nanoparticles with encapsulated natural and UF-purified annatto and saffron for the preparation of UV protective cosmetic emulsions. Molecules. 1420-3049. 23 (9), 2107. doi:10.3390/molecules23092107.

Nurilmala, M., Suryamarevita, H., Hizbullah, H.H., Jacoeb, A.M., Ochiai, Y., 2022. Fish skin as a biomaterial for halal collagen and gelatin. Saudi J. Biol. Sci. 1319562X. 29 (2), 1100–1110. Available from: http://www.ksu.edu.sa/sites/Colleges/CollegeofScinces/BotanyDepartment/SJBS/Default.aspx. doi:10.1016/j.sjbs.2021.09.056.

Oda, Y., Zhang, Q., Matsunaga, S., Fujita, M.J., Sakai, R., 2017. Two new mycosporine-like amino acids LC-343 and mycosporine-ethanolamine from the micronesian marine sponge *Lendenfeldia chondrodes*. Chem. Lett. 13480715. 46 (8), 1272–1274. Available from: http://www.journal.csj.jp/doi/pdf/10.1246/cl.170490. doi:10.1246/cl.170490.

Oliver, J.M., Ross, E.L., Frank, E.K., 1994. The discovery of marine natural products with therapeutic potential. In: Gullo, V.P. (Ed.), Discovery of Novel Natural Products with Therapeutic Potential. Elsevier, pp. 109–174.

Ozogul, F., Cagalj, M., Šimat, V., Ozogul, Y., Tkaczewska, J., Hassoun, A., Kaddour, A.A., Kuley, E., Rathod, N.B., Phadke, G.G., 2021. Recent developments in valorisation of bioactive ingredients in discard/seafood processing by-products. Trends Food Sci. Technol. 09242244. 116, 559–582. Available from: http://www.elsevier.com/wps/find/journaldescription.cws_home/601278/description#description. doi:10.1016/j.tifs.2021.08.007.

Panayiotou, A., Samartzis, D., Nomikos, T., Fragopoulou, E., Karantonis, H.C., Demopoulos, C.A., Zabetakis, I., 2000. Lipid fractions with aggregatory and antiaggregatory activity toward platelets in fresh and fried cod (*Gadus morhua*): correlation with platelet-activating factor and atherogenesis. J. Agric. Food Chem. 00218561. 48 (12), 6372–6379. doi:10.1021/jf000701f.

Papadopoulou, S.N.A., Adamantidi, T., Kranas, D., Cholidis, P., Anastasiadou, C., Tsoupras, A., 2025a. A comprehensive review on the valorization of bioactives from marine animal by-products for health-promoting, biofunctional cosmetics. Mar. Drugs. 16603397. 23 (8). Available from: https://www.mdpi.com/journal/marinedrugs. doi:10.3390/md23080299.

Papadopoulou, S.N.A., Anastasiou, E.A., Adamantidi, T., Ofrydopoulou, A., Letsiou, S., Tsoupras, A., 2025b. A comprehensive review on the beneficial roles of vitamin D in skin health as a bio-functional ingredient in nutricosmetic, cosmeceutical, and cosmetic applications. Appl. Sci. 2076-3417. 15 (2), 796. doi:10.3390/app15020796.

Papikinou, M.A., Pavlidis, K., Cholidis, P., Kranas, D., Adamantidi, T., Anastasiadou, C., Tsoupras, A., 2024. Marine fungi bioactives with anti-inflammatory, antithrombotic and antioxidant health-promoting properties against inflammation-related chronic diseases. Mar. Drugs. 16603397. 22 (11). Available from: http://www.mdpi.com/journal/marinedrugs. doi:10.3390/md22110520.

Park, J.H., Yeo, I.J., Han, J.H., Suh, J.W., Lee, H.P., Hong, J.T., 2018. Anti-inflammatory effect of astaxanthin in phthalic anhydride-induced atopic dermatitis animal model. Exp. Dermatol. 27, 378–385.

Park, J.H., Yeo, I.J., Jang, J.S., Kim, K.C., Park, M.H., Lee, H.P., Han, S.-B., Hong, J.T., 2019. Combination effect of titrated extract of *Centella asiatica* and astaxanthin in a mouse model of phthalic anhydride-induced atopic dermatitis. Allergy Asthma Immunol. Res. 11, 548.

Park, J.I., Lee, J.E., Shin, H.J., Song, S., Lee, W.K., Hwang, J.S., 2017. Oral administration of glycine and leucine dipeptides improves skin hydration and elasticity in UVB-irradiated hairless mice. Biomol. Ther. 20054483. 25 (5), 528–534. Available from: http://www.biomolther.org/journal/download_pdf.php?doi=10.4062/biomolther.2017.089. doi:10.4062/biomolther.2017.089.

Park, K., Kim, W., Kim, H.Y., 2014. Optimal lamellar arrangement in fish gills. Proc. Natl. Acad. Sci. U. S. A. 10916490. 111 (22), 8067–8070. Available from: http://www.pnas.org/content/111/22/8067.full.pdf+html. doi:10.1073/pnas.1403621111.

Parolini, C., 2020. Marine n-3 polyunsaturated fatty acids: efficacy on inflammatory-based disorders. Life Sci. 00243205. 263, 118591. doi:10.1016/j.lfs.2020.118591.

Parolini, C., 2024. The role of marine n-3 polyunsaturated fatty acids in inflammatory-based disease: the case of rheumatoid arthritis. Mar. Drugs. 1660-3397. 22 (1), 17. doi:10.3390/md22010017.

Paththuwe Arachchi, M.J.P., Subash, A., Bamigbade, G.B., Abdin, M., Ulla, N., Ayyash, M., 2025. Fish byproducts as a sustainable source of glycosaminoglycans: extraction processes, food applications, nutraceutical advancements, and challenges. Trends Food Sci. Technol. 09242244. 159. Available from: https://www.sciencedirect.com/science/journal/09242244. doi:10.1016/j.tifs.2025.104963.

Patruno, C., Napolitano, M., Argenziano, G., Peris, K., Ortoncelli, M., Girolomoni, G., Offidani, A., Ferrucci, S.M., Amoruso, G.F., Rossi, M., et al., 2021. Dupilumab therapy of atopic dermatitis of the elderly: a multicentre, real-life study. J. Eur. Acad. Dermatol. Venereol. 35, 958–964.

Peng, Z., Gao, J., Weimin, S., Cao, W., Zhu, G., Qin, X., Zhang, C., Qi, Y., 2022. Purification and identification of peptides from oyster (*Crassostrea hongkongensis*) protein enzymatic hydrolysates and their anti-skin photoaging effects on UVB-irradiated HaCaT cells. Mar. Drugs. 1660-3397. 20 (12), 749. doi:10.3390/md20120749.

Pereira, L., Cotas, J., 2023. Therapeutic potential of polyphenols and other micronutrients of marine origin. Mar. Drugs. 1660-3397. 21 (6), 323. doi:10.3390/md21060323.

Piccirillo, C., Rocha, C., Tobaldi, D.M., Pullar, R.C., Labrincha, J.A., Ferreira, M.O., Castro, P.M.L., Pintado, M.M.E., 2014. A hydroxyapatite–Fe_2O_3 based material of natural origin as an active sunscreen filter. J. Mater. Chem. B. 2050-750X. 2 (36), 5999–6009. doi:10.1039/C4TB00984C.

Pilkington, S.M., Watson, R.E.B., Nicolaou, A., Rhodes, L.E., 2011. Omega-3 polyunsaturated fatty acids: photoprotective macronutrients. Exp. Dermatol. 16000625. 20 (7), 537–543. doi:10.1111/j.1600-0625.2011.01294.x.

Pintea, A., Manea, A., Pintea, C., Vlad, R.A., Bîrsan, M., Antonoaea, P., Rédai, E.M., Ciurba, A., 2025. Peptides: emerging candidates for the prevention and treatment of skin senescence: a review. Biomolecules. 2218273X. 15 (1). Available from: http://www.mdpi.com/journal/biomolecules. doi:10.3390/biom15010088.

Prajaputra, V., Isnaini, N., Maryam, S., Ernawati, E., Deliana, F., Haridhi, H.A., Fadli, N., Karina, S., Agustina, S., Nurfadillah, N., Arisa, I.I., Desiyana, L.S., Bakri, T.K., 2024. Exploring marine collagen: sustainable sourcing, extraction methods, and cosmetic applications. S. Afr. J. Chem. Eng. 10269185. 47, 197–211. Available from: https://www.journals.elsevier.com/south-african-journal-of-chemical-engineering/. doi:10.1016/j.sajce.2023.11.006.

Prihanto, A.A., Nurdiani, R., Bagus, A.D., 2019. Production and characteristics of fish protein hydrolysate from parrotfish (*Chlorurus sordidus*) head. PeerJ. 2167-8359. 7 (12), e8297. doi:10.7717/peerj.8297.

Rafatullah, M., Siddiqui, M.R., Khan, M.A., Kapoor, R.T., 2024. Multidisciplinary Applications of Marine Resources: A Step Towards Green and Sustainable Future Multidisciplinary Applications of Marine Resources: A Step Towards Green and Sustainable Future. Springer Nature, Malaysia, pp. 1–441. Available from https://link.springer.com/book/9789819750573. doi:10.1007/978-981-97-5057-3.

Rahman, A., Rehmani, R., Pirvu, D.G., Huang, S.M., Puri, S., Arcos, M., 2024. Unlocking the therapeutic potential of marine collagen: a scientific exploration for delaying skin aging. Mar. Drugs. 16603397. 22 (4). Available from: http://www.mdpi.com/journal/marinedrugs. doi:10.3390/md22040159.

Rajabimashhadi, Z., Gallo, N., Salvatore, L., Lionetto, F., 2023. Collagen derived from fish industry waste: progresses and challenges. Polymers. 2073-4360. 15 (3), 544. doi:10.3390/polym15030544.

Ramadhany, Y.F., Achmad, H., Khairunnisa, P., Mardiana, M., 2018. The efficacy of chitosan toothpaste based white shrimp (Litopenaeus vannamei) to decrease streptococcus mutans colonies in children with early childhood caries. In: Mandasari, M., Maharani, D.A., Kusdhany, L., Wimardhani, Y.S., Kiswanjaya, B., Idrus, E., Yavuz, I., Kulkarni, G.(K.), Callea, M., Jain, A. (Eds.), Proceedings of the 11th International Dentistry Scientific Meeting (IDSM 2017). Atlantis Press, Jakarta, Indonesia.

Raman, M., Gopakumar, K., 2018. Fish collagen and its applications in food and pharmaceutical industry: a review. EC Nutr. 13 (12), 752–767.

Rasal, P.B., Khajure, K.A., 2024. Marine-derived products for cosmeceuticals: a comprehensive review. Int. J. Sci. Res. Technol. doi:10.5281/zenodo.14092144.

Rathod, N.B., Elabed, N., Punia, S., Ozogul, F., Kim, S.K., Rocha, J.M., 2023. Recent developments in polyphenol applications on human health: a review with current knowledge. Plants. 22237747. 12 (6). Available from: www.mdpi.com/journal/plants. doi:10.3390/plants12061217.

Redfern, S., Dermiki, M., Fox, S., Lordan, R., Shiels, K., Saha, S.K., Tsoupras, A., Zabetakis, I., 2021. The effects of cooking salmon sous-vide on its antithrombotic properties, lipid profile and sensory characteristics. Food Res. Int. 09639969. 139, 109976. doi:10.1016/j.foodres.2020.109976.

Reilly, D.M., Lozano, J., 2021. Skin collagen through the lifestages: importance for skin health and beauty. Plast. Aesthet. Res. 23496150. 8. Available from: https://oaepublishstorage.blob.core.windows.net/31d21692-1f43-4888-b39d-c1c25032fcda/3863.pdf. doi:10.20517/2347-9264.2020.153.

Rejinold, N.S., Choi, G., Choy, J.H., 2021. Chitosan hybrids for cosmeceutical applications in skin, hair and dental care: an update. Emerg. Mater. 2522574X. 4 (5), 1125–1142. Available from: https://www.springer.com/journal/42247. doi:10.1007/s42247-021-00280-9.

Resende, D.I.S.P., Ferreira, M.S., Sousa-Lobo, J.M., Sousa, E., Almeida, I.F., 2021. Usage of synthetic peptides in cosmetics for sensitive skin. Pharmaceuticals. 14248247. 14 (8). Available from: https://www.mdpi.com/1424-8247/14/8/702/pdf. doi:10.3390/ph14080702.

Rocha, M.S., Marques, C.F., Carvalho, A.C., Martins, E., Ereskovsky, A., Reis, R.L., Silva, T.H., 2024. The characterization and cytotoxic evaluation of *Chondrosia reniformis* collagen isolated from different body parts (ectosome and choanosome) envisaging the development of biomaterials. Mar. Drugs. 16603397. 22 (2). Available from: http://www.mdpi.com/journal/marinedrugs. doi:10.3390/md22020055.

Rosic, N., 2019. Mycosporine-like amino acids: making the foundation for organic personalised sunscreens. Mar. Drugs. 1660-3397. 17 (11), 638. doi:10.3390/md17110638.

Rotter, A., Varamogianni-Mamatsi, D., Pobirk, A.Z., Matjaž, M.G., Cueto, M., Díaz-Marrero, A.R., Jónsdóttir, R., Sveinsdóttir, K., Catalá, T.S., Romano, G., Guler, B.A., Atak, E., Zrimec, M.B., Bosch, D., Deniz, I., Gaudêncio, S.P., Grigalionyte-Bembič, E., Klun, K., Zidar, L., Rius, A.C., Baebler, Š., Lukić Bilela, L., Rinkevich, B., Mandalakis, M., 2024. Marine cosmetics and the blue bioeconomy: from sourcing to success stories. iScience. 25890042. 27 (12). Available from: https://www.sciencedirect.com/science/journal/25890042. doi:10.1016/j.isci.2024.111339.

Salvatore, L., Gallo, N., Natali, M.L., Campa, L., Lunetti, P., Madaghiele, M., Blasi, F.S., Corallo, A., Capobianco, L., Sannino, A., 2020. Marine collagen and its derivatives: versatile and sustainable bio-resources for healthcare. Mater. Sci. Eng. C. 18730191. 113. Available from: https://www.journals.elsevier.com/materials-science-and-engineering-c. doi:10.1016/j.msec.2020.110963.

Saranya, R., Jayapriya, J., Tamil Selvi, A., 2018. Purification, characterization, molecular modeling and docking study of fish waste protease. Int. J. Biol. Macromol. 01418130. 118 (Pt A), 569–583. doi:10.1016/j.ijbiomac.2018.06.119.

Shahidi, F.E., 2010. Maximising the Value of Marine By-products. Woodhead, Cambridge Boca Raton, FL.

Shalaby, M., Agwa, M., Saeed, H., Khedr, S.M., Morsy, O., El-Demellawy, M.A., 2020. Fish scale collagen preparation, characterization and its application in wound healing. J. Polym. Environ. 15728919. 28 (1), 166–178. Available from: http://www.kluweronline.com/issn/1566-2543/. doi:10.1007/s10924-019-01594-w.

Shibuya, S., Ozawa, Y., Toda, T., Watanabe, K., Tometsuka, C., Ogura, T., Koyama, Y.-I., Shimizu, T., 2014. Collagen peptide and vitamin C additively attenuate age-related skin atrophy in Sod1-deficient mice. Biosci. Biotechnol. Biochem. 0916-8451. 78 (7), 1212–1220. doi:10.1080/09168451.2014.915728.

Siahaan, E.A., Agusman, R.P., Shin, K.H., Kim, S.K., 2022. Potential cosmetic active ingredients derived from marine by-products. Mar. Drugs. 16603397. 20 (12). Available from: http://www.mdpi.com/journal/marinedrugs. doi:10.3390/md20120734.

Šimat, V., Rathod, N., Čagalj, M., Hamed, I., Mekinić, I.G., 2022. Astaxanthin from crustaceans and their byproducts: a bioactive metabolite candidate for therapeutic application. Mar. Drugs. 1660-3397. 20 (3), 206. doi:10.3390/md20030206.

Sinha, R., Häder, D.P., 2020. Natural Bioactive Compounds: Technological Advancements. Elsevier, India, pp. 1–479. Available from https://www.elsevier.com/books/natural-bioactive-compounds/sinha/978-0-12-820655-3. doi:10.1016/B978-0-12-820655-3.01001-6.

Sionkowska, A., Adamiak, K., Musiał, K., Gadomska, M., 2020. Collagen based materials in cosmetic applications: a review. Materials. 1996-1944. 13 (19), 4217. doi:10.3390/ma13194217.

Sionkowska, A., Kaczmarek, B., Michalska, M., Lewandowska, K., Grabska, S., 2017. Preparation and characterization of collagen/chitosan/hyaluronic acid thin films for application in hair care cosmetics. Pure Appl. Chem. 1365-3075. 89 (12), 1829–1839. doi:10.1515/pac-2017-0314.

Solano, F., 2020. Metabolism and functions of amino acids in the skin. In: Wu, G., Ed., Amino Acids in Nutrition and Health: Amino Acids in Systems Function and Health. Springer International Publishing, Cham, pp. 187–199.

Sotelo, C.G., Blanco, M., Ramos, P., Vázquez, J.A., Perez-Martin, R.I., 2021. Sustainable sources from aquatic organisms for cosmeceuticals ingredients. Cosmetics. 20799284. 8 (2). Available from: https://www.mdpi.com/2079-9284/8/2/48/pdf. doi:10.3390/cosmetics8020048.

Sousa, R.O., Alves, A.L., Carvalho, D.N., Martins, E., Oliveira, C., Silva, T.H., Reis, R.L., 2020. Acid and enzymatic extraction of collagen from Atlantic cod (*Gadus morhua*) swim bladders envisaging health-related applications. J. Biomater. Sci. Polym. Ed. 15685624. 31 (1), 20–37. Available from: http://www.tandfonline.com/loi/tbsp20. doi:10.1080/09205063.2019.1669313.

Subhan, F., Hussain, Z., Tauseef, I., Shehzad, A., Wahid, F., 2021. A review on recent advances and applications of fish collagen. Crit. Rev. Food Sci. Nutr. 1040-8398. 61 (6), 1027–1037. doi:10.1080/10408398.2020.1751585.

Sugibayashi, K., Yusuf, E., Todo, H., Dahlizar, S., Sakdiset, P., Arce, F.J., See, G.L., 2019. Halal cosmetics: a review on ingredients, production, and testing methods. Cosmetics. 20799284. 6 (3). Available from: www.mdpi.com/journal/cosmetics. doi:10.3390/cosmetics6030037.

Suleria, H., Osborne, S., Masci, P., Gobe, G., 2015. Marine-based nutraceuticals: an innovative trend in the food and supplement industries. Mar. Drugs. 1660-3397. 13 (10), 6336–6351. doi:10.3390/md13106336.

Sun, L., Zhang, Y., Zhuang, Y., 2013. Antiphotoaging effect and purification of an antioxidant peptide from tilapia (*Oreochromis niloticus*) gelatin peptides. J. Funct. Foods. 17564646. 5 (1), 154–162. doi:10.1016/j.jff.2012.09.006.

Suresh, P.V., Kudre, T.G., Johny, L.C., 2018. Sustainable valorization of seafood processing by-product/discard. In: Singhania, R.R., Agarwal, R.A., Kumar, R.P., Sukumaran, R.K., Eds., Waste to Wealth. Springer Singapore, Singapore, pp. 111–139.

Suuronen, P., Gilman, E., 2020. Monitoring and managing fisheries discards: new technologies and approaches. Mar. Policy. 0308597X. 116, 103554. doi:10.1016/j.marpol.2019.103554.

Tałałaj, U., Uścinowicz, P., Bruzgo, I., Surażyński, A., Zaręba, I., Markowska, A., 2019. The effects of a novel series of KTTKS analogues on cytotoxicity and proteolytic activity. Molecules. 1420-3049. 24 (20), 3698. doi:10.3390/molecules24203698.

Teixeira, C.M., Coelho, M.P., Gil, M.M., Pita, C., Silva, P.M., 2024. Changing the way we look to fisheries' discards. Reg. Stud. Mar. Sci. 23524855. 71. Available from: https://www.sciencedirect.com/science/journal/23524855. doi:10.1016/j.rsma.2024.103434.

Thy, L.T.M., Duy, H.K., Dat, N.M., 2025. Applications of lecithin in emulsion stabilization and advanced delivery systems in cosmetics: a mini-review. Results Surf. Interfaces. 26668459. 19. Available from: https://www.sciencedirect.com/science/journal/26668459. doi:10.1016/j.rsurfi.2025.100543.

Tkaczewska, J., Morawska, M., Kulawik, P., Zając, M., 2018. Characterization of carp (*Cyprinus carpio*) skin gelatin extracted using different pretreatments method. Food Hydrocoll. 0268005X. 81, 169–179. doi:10.1016/j.foodhyd.2018.02.048.

Topuz, O.K., Aygün, T., Alp, A.C., Yatmaz, H.A., Torun, M., Yerlikaya, P., 2021. Characterization and emulsifying properties of aquatic lecithins isolated from processing discard of rainbow trout fish and its eggs. Food Chem. 18737072. 339. Available from: www.elsevier.com/locate/foodchem. doi:10.1016/j.foodchem.2020.128103.

Traverso, F., Aicardi, S., Bozzo, M., Zinni, M., Amaroli, A., Galli, L., Candiani, S., Vanin, S., Ferrando, S., 2024. New insights into geometric morphometry applied to fish scales for species identification. Animals. 2076-2615. 14 (7), 1090. doi:10.3390/ani14071090.

Tsoupras, A., Brummell, C., Kealy, C., Vitkaitis, K., Redfern, S., Zabetakis, I., 2022. Cardio-protective properties and health benefits of fish lipid bioactives; the effects of thermal processing. Mar. Drugs. 1660-3397. 20 (3), 187. doi:10.3390/md20030187.

Tsoupras, A., Lordan, R., Demuru, M., Shiels, K., Saha, S., Nasopoulou, C., Zabetakis, I., 2018. Structural elucidation of Irish organic farmed salmon (*Salmo salar*) polar lipids with antithrombotic activities. Mar. Drugs. 1660-3397. 16 (6), 176. doi:10.3390/md16060176.

Tsoupras, A., Lordan, R., Shiels, K., Saha, S.K., Nasopoulou, C., Zabetakis, I., 2019a. In vitro antithrombotic properties of salmon (*Salmo salar*) phospholipids in a novel food-grade extract. Mar. Drugs. 16603397. 17 (1). Available from: https://www.mdpi.com/1660-3397/17/1/62/pdf. doi:10.3390/md17010062.

Tsoupras, A., O'Keeffe, E., Lordan, R., Redfern, S., Zabetakis, I., 2019b. Bioprospecting for antithrombotic polar lipids from salmon, herring, and boarfish by-products. Foods. 2304-8158. 8 (9), 416. doi:10.3390/foods8090416.

Ucak, İ., Nayik, G.A., 2022. PUFA and MUFA. In: Kour, J., Nayik, G.A. (Eds.), Nutraceuticals and Health Care. Elsevier, pp. 199–215.

Urbi, Z., Azmi, N.S., Ming, L.C., Hossain, M.S., 2022. A concise review of extraction and characterization of chondroitin sulphate from fish and fish wastes for pharmacological application. Curr. Issues Mol. Biol. 14673045. 44 (9), 3905–3922. Available from: https://www.mdpi.com/journal/cimb. doi:10.3390/cimb44090268.

Urrea-Victoria, V., Hernández, A.R., Castellanos, L., Alves, I.A., Novoa, D.M.A., 2025. The role of mycosporine-like amino acids in skin care formulations: a patent review (2014–2024). Photochem. Photobiol. Sci. 14749092. 24 (5), 847–861. Available from: https://www.springer.com/journal/43630. doi:10.1007/s43630-025-00717-8.

Valcarcel, J., Hermida-Merino, C., Piñeiro, M.M., Hermida-Merino, D., Vázquez, J.A., 2021. Extraction and characterization of gelatin from skin by-products of seabream, seabass and rainbow trout reared in aquaculture. Int. J. Mol. Sci. 14220067. 22 (22). Available from: https://www.mdpi.com/1422-0067/22/22/12104/pdf. doi:10.3390/ijms222212104.

van Hoogevest, P., Fahr, A., 2019. Phospholipids in cosmetic carriers. In: Cornier, J., Keck, C.M., Van de Voorde, M., Eds., Nanocosmetics: From Ideas to Products. Springer International Publishing, Cham, pp. 95–140.

Vázquez, J.A., Meduíña, A., Durán, A.I., Nogueira, M., Fernández-Compás, A., Pérez-Martín, R.I., Rodríguez-Amado, I., 2019. Production of valuable compounds and bioactive metabolites from by-products of fish discards using chemical processing, enzymatic hydrolysis, and bacterial fermentation. Mar. Drugs. 16603397. 17 (3). Available from: https://www.mdpi.com/1660-3397/17/3/139/pdf. doi:10.3390/md17030139.

Vázquez, J.A., Rodríguez-Amado, I., Montemayor, M.I., Fraguas, J., González, M.P.D., Murado, M.A., 2013. Chondroitin sulfate, hyaluronic acid and chitin/chitosan production using marine waste sources: characteristics, applications and eco-friendly processes: a review. Mar. Drugs. 16603397. 11 (3), 747–774. Available from: http://www.mdpi.com/1660-3397/11/3/747/pdf. doi:10.3390/md11030747.

Veeruraj, A., Liu, L., Zheng, J., Jianping, W., Arumugam, M., 2019. Evaluation of astaxanthin incorporated collagen film developed from the outer skin waste of squid *Doryteuthis singhalensis* for wound healing and tissue regenerative applications. Mater. Sci. Eng. C. 09284931. 95, 29–42. doi:10.1016/j.msec.2018.10.055.

Velissaridou, A., Panoutsopoulou, E., Prokopiou, V., Tsoupras, A., 2024. Cardio-protective-promoting properties of functional foods inducing HDL-cholesterol levels and functionality. Nutraceuticals. 1661-3821. 4 (4), 469–502. doi:10.3390/nutraceuticals4040028.

Venkatesan, J., Anil, S., Kim, S.K., Shim, M.S., 2017. Marine fish proteins and peptides for cosmeceuticals: a review. Mar. Drugs. 16603397. 15 (5). Available from: http://www.mdpi.com/1660-3397/15/5/143/pdf. doi:10.3390/md15050143.

Verma, M., Gahlot, N., Singh, S.S.J., Rose, N.M., 2021. UV protection and antibacterial treatment of cellulosic fibre (cotton) using chitosan and onion skin dye. Carbohydr. Polym. 01448617. 257. Available from: http://www.elsevier.com/wps/find/journaldescription.cws_home/405871/description#description. doi:10.1016/j.carbpol.2020.117612.

Vílchez, C., Forján, E., Cuaresma, M., Bédmar, F., Garbayo, I., Vega, J.M., 2011. Marine carotenoids: biological functions and commercial applications. Mar. Drugs. 16603397. 9 (3), 319–333. Available from: http://www.mdpi.com/1660-3397/9/3/319/pdf. doi:10.3390/md9030319.

Wada, N., Sakamoto, T., Matsugo, S., 2015. Mycosporine-like amino acids and their derivatives as natural antioxidants. Antioxidants. 2076-3921. 4 (3), 603–646. doi:10.3390/antiox4030603.

Waditee-Sirisattha, R., Kageyama, H., 2021. Protective effects of mycosporine-like amino acid-containing emulsions on UV-treated mouse ear tissue from the viewpoints of antioxidation and antiglycation. J. Photochem. Photobiol. B. 10111344. 223, 112296. doi:10.1016/j.jphotobiol.2021.112296.

Wang, C.H., Doan, C.T., Nguyen, V.B., Nguyen, A.D., Wang, S.L., 2019. Reclamation of fishery processing waste: a mini-review. Molecules. 14203049. 24 (12). Available from: https://www.mdpi.com/1420-3049/24/12/2234/pdf. doi:10.3390/molecules24122234.

Wang, L., Jayawardena, T.U., Hyun, J., Wang, K., Fu, X., Xu, J., Gao, X., Park, Y., Jeon, Y.J., 2023. Antioxidant and anti-photoaging effects of a fucoidan isolated from *Turbinaria ornata*. Int. J. Biol. Macromol. 18790003. 225, 1021–1027. Available from: www.elsevier.com/locate/ijbiomac. doi:10.1016/j.ijbiomac.2022.11.164.

Wang, L., Jiang, Y., Wang, X., Zhou, J., Cui, H., Weidong, X., Yuanqing, H., Haile, M., Gao, R., 2018. Effect of oral administration of collagen hydrolysates from *Nile tilapia* on the chronologically aged skin. J. Funct. Foods. 17564646. 44, 112–117. doi:10.1016/j.jff.2018.03.005.

Wang, W., Xue, C., Mao, X., 2020. Chitosan: structural modification, biological activity and application. Int. J. Biol. Macromol. 01418130. 164, 4532–4546. doi:10.1016/j.ijbiomac.2020.09.042.

Wang, X., 2021. Natural bioactive compounds from fish. In: Sinha, R.P., Häder, D.-P. (Eds.), Natural Bioactive Compounds. Elsevier, pp. 393–408.

Wang, X., Wu, J., 2019. Modulating effect of fatty acids and sterols on skin aging. J. Funct. Foods. 17564646. 57, 135–140. doi:10.1016/j.jff.2019.04.011.

Waszkielewicz, A.M., Mirosław, K., 2024. Peptides and their mechanisms of action in the skin. Appl. Sci. 2076-3417. 14 (24), 11495. doi:10.3390/app142411495.

Wauquier, F., Boutin-Wittrant, L., Bouvret, E., Faouder, J.L., Roux, V., Macian, N., Pickering, G., Wittrant, Y., 2022. Benefits of circulating human metabolites from fish cartilage hydrolysate on primary human dermal fibroblasts, an ex vivo clinical investigation for skin health applications. Nutrients. 2072-6643. 14 (23), 5027. doi:10.3390/nu14235027.

Wu, G., 2020. Amino acids in nutrition and health: amino acids in systems function and health. Adv. Exp. Med. Biol. 1265. doi:10.1007/978-3-030-45328-2.

Wu, Q., Cheng, N., Fang, D., Wang, H., Rahman, F.-U., Hao, H., Zhang, Y., 2024. Recent advances on application of polysaccharides in cosmetics. J. Dermatol. Sci. Cosmet. Technol. 2950306X. 1 (1), 100004. doi:10.1016/j.jdsct.2024.100004.

Xhauflaire-Uhoda, E., Fontaine, K., Piérard, G.E., 2008. Kinetics of moisturizing and firming effects of cosmetic formulations. Int. J. Cosmet. Sci. 0142-5463. 30 (2), 131–138. doi:10.1111/j.1468-2494.2008.00436.x.

Xia, E., Zhu, X., Gao, X., Jindong, N., Guo, H., 2021. Antiaging potential of peptides from underused marine bioresources. Mar. Drugs. 1660-3397. 19 (9), 513. doi:10.3390/md19090513.

Xie, J.-J., Chen, X., Niu, J., Wang, J., Wang, Y., Liu, Q.-Q., 2017. Effects of astaxanthin on antioxidant capacity of golden pompano (*Trachinotus ovatus*) in vivo and in vitro. Fish. Aquat. Sci. 2234-1757. 20 (1). doi:10.1186/s41240-017-0052-1.

Xie, P.-J., Huang, L.-X., Zhang, C.-H., Ding, S.-S., Deng, Y.-J., Wang, X.-J., 2018. Skin-care effects of dandelion leaf extract and stem extract: antioxidant properties, tyrosinase inhibitory and molecular docking simulations. Ind. Crops Prod. 09266690. 111, 238–246. doi:10.1016/j.indcrop.2017.10.017.

Yang, H., Zhang, Q., Zhang, B., Zhao, Y., Wang, N., 2023. Potential active marine peptides as anti-aging drugs or drug candidates. Mar. Drugs. 1660-3397. 21 (3), 144. doi:10.3390/md21030144.

Yang, M., Zhou, M., Song, L., 2020. A review of fatty acids influencing skin condition. J. Cosmet. Dermatol. 1473-2130. 19 (12), 3199–3204. doi:10.1111/jocd.13616.

Yang, Y., McClements, D.J., 2013. Vitamin E bioaccessibility: influence of carrier oil type on digestion and release of emulsified α-tocopherol acetate. Food Chem. 18737072. 141 (1), 473–481. Available from: www.elsevier.com/locate/foodchem. doi:10.1016/j.foodchem.2013.03.033.

Yoshimura, T., Manabe, C., Nagumo, J.-I., Nagahama, T., Sato, T., Murakami, S., 2023. Taurine accelerates the synthesis of ceramides and hyaluronic acid in cultured epidermis and dermal fibroblasts. Exp. Ther. Med. 1792-0981. 26 (5). doi:10.3892/etm.2023.12211.

Yuan, Q., Shi, X., Haiqiong, M., Yao, Y., Zhang, B., Zhao, L., 2024. Recent progress in marine chondroitin sulfate, dermatan sulfate, and chondroitin sulfate/dermatan sulfate hybrid chains as potential functional foods and therapeutic agents. Int. J. Biol. Macromol. 01418130. 262 (Pt 1), 129969. doi:10.1016/j.ijbiomac.2024.129969.

Yushuang, L., Yang, L., Sijia, W., Chen, J., Lin, H., 2022. Structural, functional, rheological, and biological properties of the swim bladder collagen extracted from grass carp (*Ctenopharyngodon idella*). LWT. 00236438. 153, 112518. doi:10.1016/j.lwt.2021.112518.

Zamora-Sillero, J., Gharsallaoui, A., Prentice, C., 2018. Peptides from fish by-product protein hydrolysates and its functional properties: an overview. Mar. Biotechnol. 1436-2228. 20 (2), 118–130. doi:10.1007/s10126-018-9799-3.

Zasada, M., Budzisz, E., 2019. Retinoids: active molecules influencing skin structure formation in cosmetic and dermatological treatments. Adv. Dermatol. Allergol. 1642-395X. 36 (4), 392–397. doi:10.5114/ada.2019.87443.

Zhang, Y., Sun, Q., Liu, S., Wei, S., Xia, Q., Hongwu, J., Deng, C., Hao, J., 2021. Extraction of fish oil from fish heads using ultra-high pressure pretreatment prior to enzymatic hydrolysis. Innov. Food Sci. Emerg. Technol. 14668564. 70, 102670. doi:10.1016/j.ifset.2021.102670.

Zhang, Z., Wang, J., Ding, Y., Dai, X., Yong, L., 2011. Oral administration of marine collagen peptides from Chum Salmon skin enhances cutaneous wound healing and angiogenesis in rats. J. Sci. Food Agric. 0022-5142. 91 (12), 2173–2179. doi:10.1002/jsfa.4435.

Zhao, Y., Wang, C., Zou, B., Lin, F., Ren, S., Zhang, X., 2023. Design and evaluation of tretinoin fatty acid vesicles for the topical treatment of psoriasis. Molecules. 1420-3049. 28 (23), 7868. doi:10.3390/molecules28237868.

Zheng, X., Yanyu, D., Zhong, R., Zhu, Y., Jiang, H., Liang, P., Shi, F., 2025. Effect of extraction solvents on the lipid profiles and volatile compounds of fish roe phospholipids. Food Chem. 03088146. 476, 143444. doi:10.1016/j.foodchem.2025.143444.

Zhuang, Y., Sun, L., 2011. Preparation of reactive oxygen scavenging peptides from tilapia (*Oreochromis niloticus*) skin gelatin: optimization using response surface methodology. J. Food Sci. 17503841. 76 (3), C483. Available from: http://onlinelibrary.wiley.com/journal/10.1111/(ISSN)1750-3841. doi:10.1111/j.1750-3841.2011.02108.x.

Zúñiga-López, C.M., Márquez-Pérez, K., Argueta-Figueroa, L., Bautista-Hernández, M.A., Torres-Rosas, R., 2024. Chitosan for the treatment of inflammation of the oral mucosa: a systematic review. Medicina Oral Patología Oral y Cirugia Bucal. 16986946. 29 (1), e9. doi:10.4317/medoral.25987.

Chapter 23

Insects

Vassiliki Chrysikopoulou, Konstantinos Pavlidis, Evgenia Lamprianidou, and Alexandros Tsoupras
Hephaestus Laboratory, School of Chemistry, Faculty of Sciences, Democritus University of Thrace, Kavala University Campus, Kavala, Greece

1 Introduction

Natural bioactive ingredients are becoming increasingly sought after for the formulation and enhancement of countless products, particularly in the cosmetics industry. In particular, over the past decade, there has been an increased demand for renewable bioingredients, which has driven the pharmaceutical and cosmetics industries to continually offer innovative products to consumers. Undoubtedly, cosmetics have become an essential part of our daily lives, and the cosmetics market has experienced rapid growth, while products based on natural ingredients are now in high demand from both consumers and manufacturers.

Cosmetic formulations containing bioactive compounds with protective benefits and therapeutic functions can deliver highly desirable results for consumers, hydrating and rejuvenating the skin (Ngoc et al., 2023). For this purpose, both known and promising potential sources of bioactive compounds are constantly being investigated for their potential use in the cosmetic and pharmaceutical industries. Sources of natural bioactive compounds include a variety of organisms, such as animals, plants, and microorganisms.

Another source of bioactive compounds has emerged in recent years: insect farming, which represents a promising solution for the production of proteins, lipids, alkaloids, and terpenoids, imparting impressive effects to the products in which they are incorporated (Bioactive Compounds from Hermetia Illucens Larvae as Natural Ingredients for Cosmetic Application, n.d.). The extraction of natural bioactive compounds from insect cultures offers advantages such as reduced greenhouse gas emissions, low environmental costs, large-scale industrial production, and the ability to be fed and maintained using organic waste, requiring less water and food compared to other sources, such as animals and plants. Insects also possess natural defense mechanisms, and thus the substances they produce typically have strong antimicrobial properties, which are utilized in cosmetic formulations, for example, to combat acne (Bulet and Stöcklin, 2005).

2 Materials and methods

The information analyzed in this review was collected through searches using various research tools, such as *Google Scholar*, as well as publisher research databases, such as *Science Direct*, *ACS journals*, *MDPI*, and *Web of Science databases*, in combination with bibliographic sources and social research networks such as *Research Gate*. From all these sources, research articles, bibliographic reviews, etc. were accessed that mention the role of various bioactive compounds derived from insects in industrial cosmetics for the mitigation and control of skin pathologies and their impact on health, stability, safety, and side effects. The time frame of the review was set at 2020–2026.

3 Insects as a source of biofunctional cosmetic ingredients

3.1 Distribution of cosmetically relevant insect species

Insect classification follows a Linnaean hierarchy that is now being reshaped by large-scale phylogenomic data. Traditional morphology-based schemes recognize almost 30 orders, with Coleoptera, Diptera, Lepidoptera, and Hymenoptera comprising the "big four" holometabolan groups, together containing over 75% of described insect species (Février and Barraclough, 2025).

Biofunctional Cosmetics for Health. https://doi.org/10.1016/B978-0-443-27500-5.00019-8

Coleoptera, also known as beetles, represent the most speciose animal order, with nearly 400,000 described species and many more that still remain unnamed (Cai et al., 2022). Phylogenomic analysis refining beetle evolution and classification revealed a Carboniferous origin of the crown group and a Paleozoic emergence of all modern suborders (Cai et al., 2022). Furthermore, the suborder Adephaga, which includes ground and aquatic beetles, diversified in the mid-Permian, and its crown split at the end-Permian (Baca et al., 2021). Within Polyphaga, the most diverse suborder, genomic data reveal that plant-feeding beetles radiated after the acquisition of bacterial and fungal lignocellulose-degrading enzymes via horizontal gene transfer (McKenna et al., 2019). Longhorn beetles, also known as *Chrysomeloidea*, are an example of resolving deep splits with mitochondrial genome analysis and are dated with the origin of the super-family to the late Jurassic, while their diversification is linked to the early-Cretaceous angiosperm radiation.

Diptera, also known as flies, rank among the most species-rich insect orders. A comprehensive catalog of Moroccan Diptera listed roughly over 3000 species in 948 genera, highlighting the order's taxonomic breadth in the Mediterranean North African transition zone (Kettani et al., 2022). There are similar studies in Chile and Indonesian islands like Wallace, which collectively portray Diptera as a globally distributed, ecologically pivotal order that provides a foundational context for examining the distribution of cosmetically relevant insect species (Barahona-Segovia et al., 2024; Hudiwaku et al., 2021).

Lepidoptera represent one of the most speciose insect orders, with contemporary DNA-barcode surveys revealing extensive diversity across contrasting biogeographic realms. In Crete, a comprehensive effort generated sequences confirming 1230 species in 62 families and genetically verifying 724 of them (Huemer et al., 2025). The study also documented 112 unnamed barcode clusters, which are likely to conceal additional taxa (Huemer et al., 2025).

Hymenoptera, encompassing bees, wasps, ants, and related lineages, similarly display a globally extensive but underexplored species diversity. Global assessments of bee diversity highlight substantial taxonomic evidence, estimating 3771–5230 undescribed bee species worldwide, with especially large gaps in Asia and Africa, implying that current lists capture only a fraction of the actual diversity (Dorey et al., 2026).

Cosmetically relevant insects, which may include cochineal (*Dactylopius coccus*), honey bee families, silk moth (*Bombyx mori*), and lac insects (*Kerria lacca*), are distributed across distinct biogeographic zones, thus shaping their availability for the cosmetics industry. Cochineal insects are native to tropical and subtropical regions. They thrive on *Opuntia cacti* in arid to semiarid habitats of Central America, Mexico, and parts of South Africa, and have been introduced to other warm zones for commercial cultivation (Vakte and Sonawane, 2024). Furthermore, honey bees (*Apidae,* excluding *Apis mellifera*) are dominant in the United States, where 1081 wild bee species span families like *Andrenidae, Halictidae, Megachilidae,* and others (Guzman et al., 2024). Moreover, silk moths, historically domesticated in East Asia, are now reared primarily in China, India, and South-East Asian countries, where mulberry (*Morus* spp.) plantations provide the sole larval food sources (Fan et al., 2024). Lac insects, another source of natural resin and pigment, inhabit tropical and subtropical forests of India, Thailand, and southern China. Their abundance is directly linked to the distribution of cultivated host trees and is supported by the high genetic and phylogenetic diversity reported for insect assemblages in cultivated vegetation across China (Fan et al., 2024).

3.2 Bioactive compounds derived from insects with cosmetic potential

3.2.1 Phenolic compounds

Phenolic compounds are a diverse group of secondary metabolites, characterized by one or more aromatic rings bearing hydroxyl groups. These compounds are widely recognized for their antioxidant, antiinflammatory, and antithrombotic activities, which makes them highly relevant for dermatological and cosmetic applications (Chrysikopoulou et al., 2025).

Recent studies indicate that edible insects contain a variety of phenolic compounds, either synthesized indirectly through metabolic pathways or accumulated from plant-based diets consumed during development. The phenolic profile of insects is therefore strongly influenced by species, diet, and environmental conditions (Huemer et al., 2025; Torres-Castillo and Olazarán-Santibáñez, 2023). Further studies have managed to identify several phenolic acids and flavonoids in insect extracts. For instance, extracts from *Acheta domesticus*, which is the house cricket, were shown to contain 4-hydroxybenzoic acid, p-coumaric acid, ferulic acid, and syringic acid. All of these acids have exhibited significant antioxidant activity, scavenging free radicals in 2,2-diphenyl-1-picrylhydrazyl (DPPH) and 2,2'-azino-bis(3-ethylbenzothiazoline-6-sulfonic acid (ABTS) assays as well (Nino et al., 2021b). In addition, flavonoids such as quercetin, luteolin, kaempferol, and isovitexin have also been reported in edible insects like the buffalo worm (*Alphitobius diaperinus*) (Purkiewicz et al., 2025).

Biological activities of insect-derived phenolic compounds are mainly attributed to their ability to neutralize reactive oxygen species (ROS) and modulate signaling pathways linked to oxidative stress and inflammation (Nino et al., 2021a; Chrysikopoulou et al., 2025). Since oxidative stress plays a central role in skin aging, inflammation, and UV-induced damage, these compounds may be significant for cosmetic applications. Experimental studies have also demonstrated that phenolic extracts from insects, such as yellow mealworm (YMW) (*Tenebrio molitor*), exhibit significant antioxidant activity, highlighting their potential as natural ingredients for cosmetic formulations (Muñoz-Seijas et al., 2025).

3.2.2 Carotenoids

Carotenoids are a class of lipophilic tetraterpenoid pigments, commonly found in nature, where they contribute to different biological functions and to coloration (Elmaidomy et al., 2026). In insects, carotenoids are of particular interest as bioactive compounds due to their antioxidant, photoprotective, and antiinflammatory properties, which are crucial for cosmetic applications (Elmaidomy et al., 2026).

In contrast to plants or microorganisms, insects cannot synthesize carotenoids de novo and therefore acquire them through their diet (Maoka et al., 2021). Similar to phenolic content, the carotenoid profile of insects is highly variable and depends strongly on species, developmental stage, and feeding substrate. A recent study demonstrates that the carotenoid composition of insects directly reflects that of their diet, as shown in *Musca domestica*, where larval feed composition determined carotenoid accumulation in adult insects (Lahmi et al., 2024). A range of carotenoids has been identified in insects, including lutein, β-carotene, β-cryptoxanthin, and zeaxanthin, which are commonly derived from plant sources (Maoka, 2020). Furthermore, specific insect species contain unique carotenoid derivatives or modified structures, reflecting their metabolomic transformation after dietary intake (Maoka et al., 2021).

Carotenoids are not only responsible for pigmentation but also for protection against oxidative stress or involvement in certain signaling pathways (Tan et al., 2020). In the cosmetics field, the biological activities of carotenoids are primarily attributed to their conjugated double-bond system, which enables efficient quenching of singlet oxygen and scavenging of free radicals. Their antioxidant activity is highly important in skincare, preventing aging, inflammation, or cellular damage (Elmaidomy et al., 2026). Therefore insect-derived carotenoids may contribute further to eco-friendly and circular economy-based cosmetic ingredients.

3.2.3 Volatile fatty acids

Volatile fatty acids (VFAs), commonly referring to short-chain fatty acids such as palmitic acid, myristic acid, and oleic acid, represent a relevant bioactive source of insect-derived lipids (Franco et al., 2022). These compounds may be produced either from endogenous metabolic processes or from microbial activity. Although studies specifically addressing VFAs in insect cosmetics are still limited, they show potential in innovative cosmetic formulations (Franco et al., 2022).

In insect-derived lipid extracts, short-chain fatty acids are often part of free fatty acids that requires removal during refining processes. Specifically, certain processes like degumming and neutralization are necessary to reduce free fatty acid content to improve stability and other properties (Franco et al., 2022; Kolobe et al., 2023). Moreover, the fatty acid profile of insects, including the proportion of free and short-chain fatty acids (FAs), is highly dependent on species, developmental stage, and feeding substrate (Franco et al., 2022; Palupi et al., 2025).

3.2.4 Phospholipids

Phospholipids (PLs) are a major class of polar lipids in insects and play a fundamental role in maintaining cell membrane structure and function. In contrast to VFAs, PLs are more studied and characterized in edible insects and have attracted increasing attention. Compositional analyses have demonstrated that insect lipids contain PLs, including classes such as phosphatidylcholine, phosphatidylethanolamine, phosphatidylinositol, phosphatidylserine, and sphingomyelin (SM) (Kolobe et al., 2023).

Recent analytical studies further confirm that multiple PL species are present in insects, with phosphatidylcholine often being a dominant fraction in edible insects (Ochiai and Komiya, 2021). Furthermore, another research study has highlighted that the PL fraction of insects is particularly enriched in polyunsaturated fatty acids. For example, a recent study investigated lipid classes across several edible insect species, showing that PLs contain the highest polyunsaturated fatty acids (PUFA) content compared to other classes (Perez-Santaescolastica et al., 2023). These fatty acids are strongly associated with antiinflammatory activity and the maintenance of skin barrier integrity, making them really valuable for cosmetic formulations (Nicolaou and Kendall, 2024; Sawada et al., 2021). Another advancement in this field is the identification of insects as a novel source of lecithin, a PL-rich material widely used in cosmetics. Lecithin can successfully be extracted from black soldier flies and YMWs, revealing a complex profile of glycerophospholipids and SM, with compositional differences compared to plant-derived lecithin, including higher levels of sphingolipids (Li et al., 2024). In conclusion, insect-derived PLs are promising agents for sustainable cosmetics.

3.2.5 Terpenoids

The environment and plants inevitably interact with insects, resulting in the emission of volatile organic compounds. These compounds include terpenoids, emitted volatile organic compounds, which are extremely useful for mediating communication between this natural system and beneficial species, with the aim of maintaining the food balance. They also play an important role in alleviating abiotic and biotic stress. In general, a huge diversity of terpenes and terpenoids has been created, both in insects and in plants, due to their constant interactions (Fig. 23.1) (Boncan et al., 2020). Terpenes occur naturally in insects and greatly influence their behavior. It is reported that >50 pheromones based on terpenes and terpenoids have been identified in >52 insect species, across various insect orders, such as Coleoptera, Blattodea, Hemiptera, Lepidoptera, Diptera, Hymenoptera, etc. (Yang et al., 2025). Due to their diverse structures and derivatives, terpenes are being researched for various commercial applications. They possess and offer a powerful package of actions, including antimicrobial, antiviral, antiallergic, antiinflammatory, antipyretic, immunomodulatory, and antispasmodic effects. In dermatology and cosmetics, due to these exceptional properties, terpenes and terpenoids are used as ingredients in skin care products. Their role in mitigating skin inflammation, which can result from both bacterial and viral infections, as well as other pathogenic factors such as psoriasis and acne, has been highlighted, acting as natural substitutes for conventional pharmaceutical interventions used to combat the aforementioned conditions, which often cause undesirable side effects (Trepa et al., 2024). By interfering with mechanisms such as protein kinase inhibition, proinflammatory cytokine expression inhibition, and other mechanisms involved in inflammatory processes, terpenoid compounds are effective in combating skin inflammation (Yang et al., 2025; Trepa et al., 2024).

3.2.6 Alkaloids

Alkaloids are a diverse group of natural phytochemical compounds that control plant growth and provide biological and medicinal effects (Faisal et al., 2023). Insect-derived alkaloids represent a class of natural products that contain nitrogen and provide signaling functions and antimicrobial properties in insects (Seabrooks and Hu, 2017). The literature review identified the involvement of various alkaloid compounds in health applications, providing potent antiinflammatory, anticancer, and antimicrobial properties. In the insect kingdom, with regard to alkaloids, particular research emphasis is placed on piperidine alkaloids such as solenopsin A, which is a rich bioactive component of the venom of *Solenopsis invicta*, a species of ant native to South America that has recently established itself in Europe (Dioguardi et al., 2024). These alkaloids are the most promising, as they have shown strong activity against *Candida auris* biofilms, utilizing antiinflammatory and antimicrobial actions. Although alkaloids are not yet established ingredients in industrial cosmetic products, their

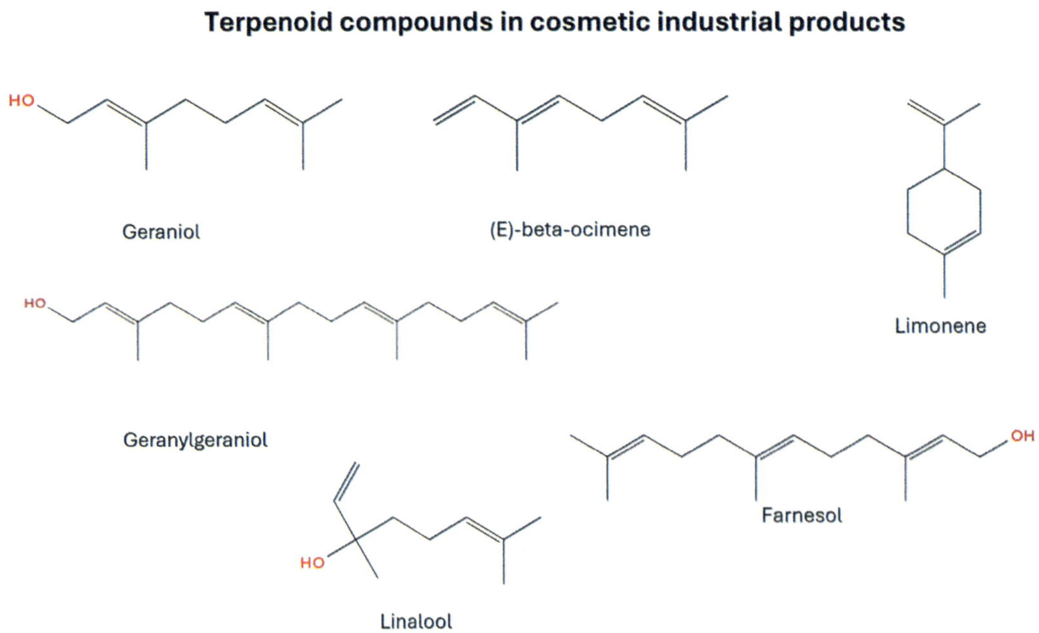

FIG. 23.1 Representative terpenoid compounds of particular importance in cosmetic industrial products, contributing significantly to skin care. Terpenoids such as limonene, (E)-β-ocimene, and geranylgeraniol, due to their aromatic and antioxidant properties, contribute to the fragrance, care, and hygiene of the skin when incorporated into cosmetic products. *(Source: Structures were obtained from Molview.org).*

biological actions make them promising candidates for research in the cosmetics industry. The experimentally strong action of solenopsins against *C. auris* biofilms could indicate remarkable and valuable data for study in their application in cosmetic ingredients, such as in products concerned with skin surface hygiene, scalp hygiene, and various other formulations. However, their application requires extensive regulatory and toxicological evaluations (Honorato et al., 2024).

3.2.7 Bee venom and other defensive secretions

Bee venom (BV) is a toxin secreted from the stingers of worker bees and is currently used to treat skin conditions such as vitiligo, psoriasis, and acne (El-Wahed et al., 2021). BV is a complex secretion consisting of enzymes, peptides, and bioactive molecules such as phospholipase A2, adolapin, melittin (MLT), and apamin, which work together to give this substance its various biological activities (An et al., 2018). Extensive studies have been conducted on the suppression of proinflammatory signaling pathways, particularly the nuclear factor kappa B pathway, which regulates inflammatory cytokines such as TNF-α, IL-1β, and IL-6. It has also been shown that BV affects the signaling of mitogen-activated protein kinase, which includes pathways with a significant impact on cell proliferation and inflammatory responses.

BV is used to a relatively small extent in commercial cosmetic preparations, such as face masks, demonstrating various therapeutic uses in pathological conditions and various clinical therapeutic studies, including psoriasis. The therapeutic use of BV, according to reports, extends to conditions such as atopic dermatitis, common acne, alopecia, vitiligo, psoriasis, wound healing, and other pathological conditions (Fig. 23.2). BV is noted for its antimicrobial, antiinflammatory, and regenerative effects on the skin, specifically suppressing inflammatory mediators associated with atopic dermatitis and acne. Along with its advantages, it also presents challenges and concerns regarding its use due to immune system reactions. Allergic reactions are the biggest challenge preventing the use of BV in therapeutic applications on a continuous basis. It is constantly emphasized that side effects due to BV, such as local irritation, anaphylaxis, and various allergic reactions, should be approached with caution so that various factors, such as dosage, evaluation, and safety, become increasingly clear regarding this therapeutic defensive secretion of bees (El-Wahed et al., 2021).

According to the clinical study by Han et al., the introduction of BV into serum has been studied for the treatment and improvement of facial wrinkles in people whose skin had been damaged by sunlight. The study provided impressive results, as 12 weeks after treatment, wrinkle analysis showed significant reductions in the total surface area of wrinkles, their depth, and their number, highlighting the antiwrinkle potential of BV as a topical cosmetic ingredient. The findings of this

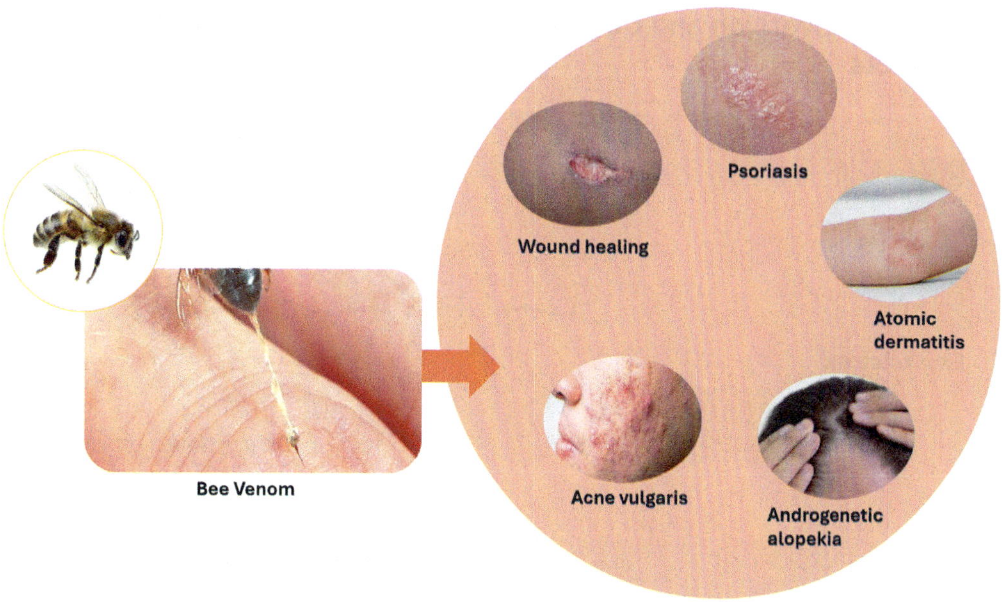

FIG. 23.2 Dermatological and cosmetic applications of bee venom. This biological toxin has been investigated for its antimicrobial and antiinflammatory properties, demonstrating its contribution to combating and mitigating various skin conditions, such as wound healing, psoriasis, atopic dermatitis, androgenetic alopecia, and acne. *(Source: From the open-access published article of El-Wahed, A.A.A., Khalifa, S.A.M., Elashal, M.H., Musharraf, S.G., Saeed, A., Khatib, A., Tahir, H.E., Zou, X., Naggar, Y.A., Mehmood, A., Wang, K., El-Seedi, H.R., 2021. Cosmetic applications of bee venom. Toxins. 20726651. 13 (11). Available from: https://www.mdpi.com/2072-6651/13/11/810/pdf. https://doi.org/10.3390/toxins13110810).*

study are very important, as they provide direct human evidence of the use of BV in cosmetic formulations with antiaging properties, suggesting that it may affect the degradation pathways of the dermal matrix resulting from ultraviolet radiation, promoting skin regeneration (Han et al., 2015).

3.2.8 Chitin and chitosan from insect exoskeletons

Chitin and chitosan are among the most abundant natural polysaccharides and key structural components of the insect exoskeleton, providing protection and enhanced mechanical properties and durability. In the cosmetics industry, chitin and chitosan have attracted interest due to their biocompatibility, lack of toxicity, biodegradability, and functionality, making them sustainable natural ingredients for dermatological applications and cosmetic products (Fig. 23.3). Chitin derived from insects has lower allergenicity and risk of inducing side effects compared to traditional crustacean sources used in dermatological products. Especially when derived from insect farming by-products (e.g., mealworms), chitin aligns with the principles of the circular economy and promotes the production of green and biofunctional cosmetics (Rinaudo, 2006; Zhu et al., 2016). In insects, chitin forms a large part of the exoskeleton of the cuticle, which is replaced by a new cuticle, and is also found in the internal structures of insects. Chitin is also associated with the protection of the intestinal epithelium in many insect species and various other invertebrates, enhancing protection against microbial invasion, and is of great importance as a renewable resource for the pharmaceutical industry (Merzendorfer, 2006).

Chitosan is a polysaccharide derived from chitin through deacetylation and has attracted the attention of both the academic community and the cosmetics industry due to its properties. Chitosan possesses a wide range of important properties that are highly sought after in cosmetic formulations, as it acts as a natural humectant and moisturizer for the skin (Fig. 23.3). One of its most important properties is its antimicrobial action, which is related to its ability to interact with microbial cell membranes, utilizing ionic interactions due to its cationic nature, and it reduces the need for preservatives in the formulation of cosmetic products. Consequently, chitosan is a promising candidate for use in antiacne and preservative-free products, as well as in hair care formulations where microbial control is essential.

Although chitosan is not a very popular ingredient in cosmetics compared to otherpolymers, such as hyaluronic acid (HA) and collagen, more and more cosmetic products containing chitosan are being introduced to the market due to its multiple beneficial properties. Chitosan, as well as some of its derivatives—in cases where it is not used in its pure form—has been approved by the FDA and the EU. A key function of chitosan is that it binds water, hydrating the skin and modifying its rheology, creating a hydrophilic film that prevents water loss (Fig. 23.3) (Kulka and Sionkowska, 2023).

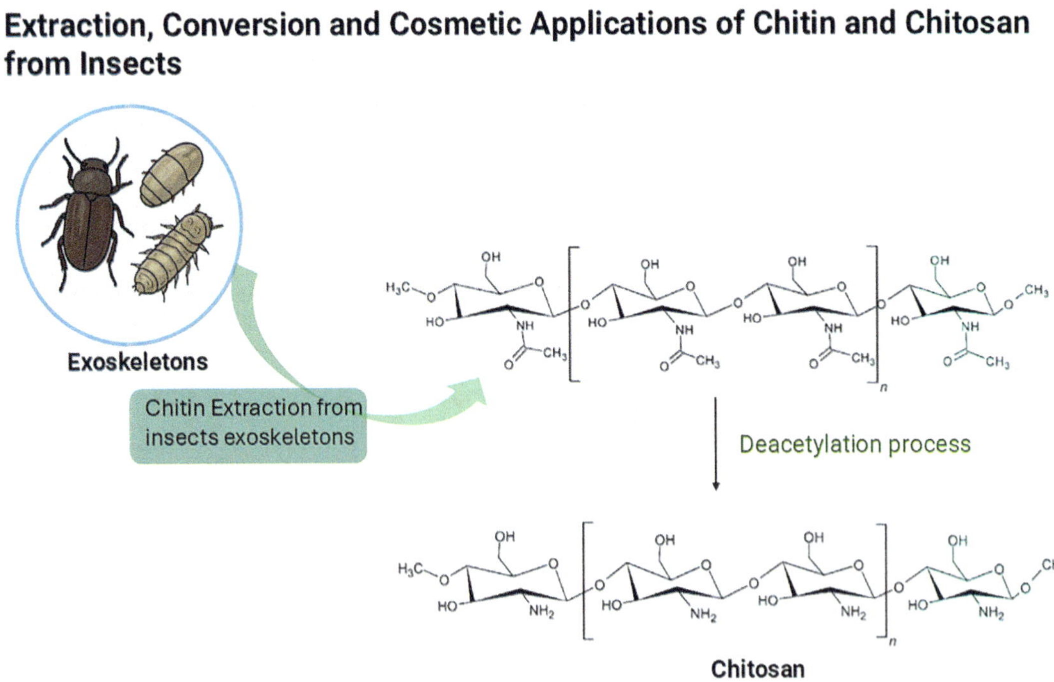

FIG. 23.3 Extraction, conversion, and cosmetic applications of chitosan from insects. *(Source: Created with the open-access free platform of BioRender. com; accessed 23 March 2026).*

4 Experimental evidence from cosmetic and dermatological research

4.1 Phenolic compounds

Phenolic compounds are widely acknowledged for their diverse physiological activities, such as antibacterial, antioxidant, antiinflammatory, and anticancer properties (Kim et al., 2024). Kim et al. investigated solvent fractions obtained from *Allomyrina dichotoma larvae* extract (ADLE) to evaluate fractions with enhanced antioxidant and antiphotoaging activity based on solvent polarity and to compare the inhibitory effects on UVB-induced skin aging using the identified fractions. The study demonstrated that ADLE reduced intracellular ROS levels, indicating significant antioxidant activity. Moreover, the ethyl acetate fraction of ADLE inhibited the expression of MMP-1/AP-1, which are involved in collagen degradation during photoaging, demonstrating a collagen-restoring effect. Overall, their findings highlighted that ADLE may represent a promising natural source of phenolic-rich bioactives for antiphotoaging cosmetic applications (Kim et al., 2024).

4.2 Carotenoids

Carotenoids play a crucial role in animals and plants, and numerous studies have confirmed their anticancer, antiinflammatory, antibacterial, antidiabetic, and neuroprotective properties (Liu et al., 2024).

In the study by Liu et al., the potential of natural sericin containing carotenoids, derived from the yellow-red cocoons of *B. mori*, for cosmetic applications is explored. The physicochemical and antimicrobial properties of this carotenoid-enriched sericin were compared with those of white cocoon sericin. The results demonstrated that natural sericin containing carotenoids exhibited superior antibacterial activity, anticancer properties, cytocompatibility, and antioxidant activity compared to white cocoon sericin. These findings suggest that natural sericin with carotenoids offers greater potential for cosmetic applications than the commonly used white cocoon sericin (Liu et al., 2024).

4.3 Proteins/peptides

In the field of proteins and peptides, edible insect extracts have shown promising potential for antiaging applications in cosmetic research (Yeerong et al., 2021). For example, sericin has been found to offer biocompatibility, biodegradability, antiinflammatory, antioxidant, antibacterial, UV protection, antiaging, antityrosinase, and anticancer effects. It also promotes skin regeneration and collagen production, making it an ideal ingredient for sensitive skin and a highly sought-after addition to antiaging skincare products (Dragojlov et al., 2025).

In an experimental study by Yeerong et al. on six Thai edible insects (*B. mori*, *Omphisa fuscidentalis*, *Euconocephalus* sp., *Patanga succincta*, *A. domesticus*, and *Lethocerus indicus*), aqueous, ethanolic, and hexane extracts were compared for their protein content, antioxidant and antiaging activity, and irritation potential to confirm their safety for topical application. The results showed that the aqueous extracts of most insects had higher protein content compared to the ethanolic extracts. Similar results were observed for antioxidant activities, where the aqueous extracts exhibited significant radical scavenging and ferric-reducing abilities. Moreover, aqueous extracts of most insects demonstrated the highest anticollagenase activities, followed by ethanolic extracts and hexane extracts, respectively. Overall, the aqueous extract of A. domesticus exhibited the highest antioxidant, anticollagenase, and antielastase activities without causing irritation in both HET-CAM and clinical studies, resulting in its further usage as a cosmeceutical active ingredient for antiwrinkle skin care (Yeerong et al., 2021).

In another study by *Dragojlov* et al., a protein derived from *B. mori* silkworm cocoons, silk sericin, was extracted and then blended with gelatin to enhance mechanical strength and stability, resulting in robust films suitable for cosmetic applications. Precisely, the created films were used as eye patches and were tested by 20 participants to examine their efficacy in enhancing skin hydration, elasticity, and smoothness. The eye patches exhibited water-soluble properties due to the hydrophilicity of sericin, which enhanced the interaction of the patches with the skin and improved skin smoothness and elasticity. These findings provide insights into the potential benefits of electro-infused membranes for skin health and appearance.

4.4 Unsaturated fatty acids

Insect-derived oils are particularly noteworthy for their rich composition of beneficial fatty acids, including oleic, palmitic, linoleic, and linolenic acids, and have potential applications in skincare products, mainly due to the presence of omega-3, 6, and 9 fatty acids (Boonmee and Chittrakorn et al., 2026; Almeida et al., 2022). In addition, omega-3 (ω-3) and omega-6 (ω-6) FAs have been reported to reduce inflammation and can play a significant role in formulations aimed at inflammatory skin diseases such as atopic dermatitis or psoriasis (Almeida et al., 2022).

A study by *Boonmee* et al. examined house crickets (*A. domesticus*), black soldier fly larvae (BSFL) (*Hermetia illucens*), and silkworms (*B. mori*) and investigated the effects of high pressure processing (HPP) at 200–600 MPa for 5 min or ultrasonication (UL) at 37 kHz for 5–15 min, followed by dehydration and extraction using supercritical carbon dioxide (SC-CO_2) or solvent extraction pretreatments on microbial load reduction, proximate composition, and structural changes of the insect samples. High levels of omega-6 and omega-9 fatty acids were observed, along with minor but potentially nutritionally meaningful amounts of omega-3 fatty acids. Notably, the oil derived from BSFL exhibited the highest concentration of lauric acid, known for its antimicrobial properties. Moreover, the fatty acid profiles of the three edible insect oils also revealed significant amounts of C16:0, C18:1c9, and C18:2, which are known for their health benefits, highlighting the potential of insect oils not only as nutraceuticals but also as ingredients in cosmetic formulations (Boonmee and Chittrakorn et al., 2026).

Another article by Almeida et al. investigated different extraction methods (decoction, microwaves, maceration, and ultrasound), using water, acetone, and *n*-hexane as extraction solvents, to evaluate the yields of the BSFL lipid extracts, as well as their lipid profile. Their results showed that lipid extracts, highly rich in lauric acid, had a limited antioxidant performance; however, none of them exhibited toxicity at the concentrations applied in the tests with the *Artemia salina* model, making them promising for pharmaceutical and cosmetic applications and with good prospects for biocompatibility with skin (Almeida et al., 2022).

4.5 Phospholipids

Li et al. examined two insect species, BSFL (*H. illucens*) and YMW (*T. molitor*) to extract lecithin and evaluate the lipid profile, specifically PLs. They found that insect lecithin contained SM, which was absent in soy lecithin. Besides, insect lecithin showed a higher percentage of the "other" PLs compared to soy lecithin. Overall, a total of 47 glycerophospholipid and SM molecules were identified, some of which were bioactive compounds, such as FAHFA and ceramide, providing it with the potential for nutritional application. However, it should be further investigated to determine whether it is suitable for cosmeceutical applications (Li et al., 2024).

4.6 BV and venom-derived bioactives

As the skin ages, there is an increased risk of infections, chronic wounds, and various types of dermatitis, such as atopic dermatitis (Tanuğur Samancı and Kekeçoğlu, 2022). For this reason, many products that prevent and treat skin aging have become popular, including BV as an antiwrinkle agent and an antiaging agent (Orrù et al., 2025; Zhao et al., 2025).

In the study by Zhao et al., the antiaging effects of BV and its main component, MLT, were evaluated by analyzing skin tissue sections and conducting an in vivo study using a mouse model treated with D-galactose to induce aging. The results showed the production of HA and hydroxyproline in mouse skin, an increase in collagen synthesis, and regulation of the expression of genes associated with collagen formation (Col1a1 and Col3a1) as well as inflammatory factors (IL-1β and IL-10) after treatment with BV and MLT. Overall, these bioactives may alleviate skin aging in mice by inhibiting inflammation, promoting collagen synthesis, and regulating glucose, protein, and lipid metabolism, highlighting the potential applicability of BV and MLT in skin aging treatments and cosmetic products (Zhao et al., 2025).

In a study comparing the BV from four different Apis species (*Apis cerana*, *Apis florea*, *Apis dorsata*, and *A. mellifera*), significant differences were observed in the antioxidant properties and irritation potential of the venoms. Specifically, the extract from *A. dorsata* demonstrated the highest antioxidant activity, showing good potential for applications in conditions related to oxidation (ROS, such as superoxide radical (O_2) and hydrogen peroxide (H_2O_2), which are markers of oxidative stress), making it useful for antiaging properties. Furthermore, the study revealed that *A. dorsata* venom exhibited no irritation at concentrations lower than 0.1 mg/mL, making it an ideal candidate for topical cosmetic formulations (Somwongin et al., 2018).

In another study, Orrù et al. investigated the antioxidant activity of honeybee venom (HBV) and its components using the DPPH method and showed that its radical scavenging activity is strongly influenced by both the solvent and the pH. The authors found that water and PBS-based systems were more suitable than organic solvents such as methanol or ethanol. Moreover, their research further demonstrates that mildly acidic pH (pH 5–6) enhances the antioxidant activity of HBV, which overlaps with the natural pH of the skin, showing that it may be important for the development of HBV-based cosmetic formulations (Orrù et al., 2025).

Particularly noteworthy is a clinical study conducted by Mi Han et al., who investigated the effects of BV serum on people with facial wrinkles. The results were evident after the eighth week, while after the 12th week, significant differences were observed in the number, area, and depth of the wrinkles. These findings suggest that HBV serum may be a promising cosmeceutical for the treatment of wrinkles, as the irritant effect of the venom is negligible (Han et al., 2015).

Samancı and Kekeçoğlu examined a prototype skincare product containing BV, propolis, honey, beeswax, and royal jelly and indicated that it did not alter its appearance for up to 90 days. The antioxidant capacity of the prototype was found to be 86.72%, which may be related to the presence of BV and propolis, making it consistent with the literature findings for cosmetic products. According to the dermatological analysis of 10 volunteers aged between 21 and 65 years, no adverse reactions were observed on their skin due to BV. In addition, the product exhibited antiwrinkle properties and improved skin elasticity, highlighting its potential suitability for cosmeceutical formulations (Tanuğur Samancı and Kekeçoğlu, 2022).

4.7 Shell-derived compounds: Chitin, chitosan, and derivatives

In recent years, the use of insects as key ingredients in cosmetic products has grown rapidly. Recently, drug carriers that enhance the topical action of active compounds have received a lot of attention, and chitin is one of them (Zainol Abidin et al., 2023). Chitosan, selected in research by Zainol Abidin et al., is derived from an insect, specifically *Oryctes rhinoceros*, a common invasive beetle of coconut. The insect was utilized to create chitosan–gold nanoparticles (CCG-NPs) loaded with curcumin. The results showed that the synthesized CCG-NP is a stable, spherical, nano-sized, nontoxic, and homogeneous solution and hence has very high potential in cosmeceutical applications (Zainol Abidin et al., 2023).

5 Commercial cosmetic products containing insect-derived bioactive ingredients

Commercial cosmetic products that are already on the market incorporate insect-derived bioactives, illustrating how these promising agents can be used in cosmetic formulations.

Bee-derived bioactives from honey, propolis, royal-jelly, and bee-venom are the main examples. These appear in antiaging serums, revitalizing skincare products, acne treatments, and moisturizers. Specifically, these products claim to stimulate collagen production while providing antimicrobial, antioxidant, soothing, and antiaging effects (Borse, 2024). Furthermore, natural colorants such as carminic acid from cochineal insects are used in lipsticks and blushes, providing a stable red pigment that replaces synthetic dyes (Borse, 2024). Another insect-derived bioactive used in cosmetic products is silk proteins like sericin and fibroin extracted from silk moths, which are marketed for their hydration and repair benefits in skincare, especially in premium face creams (Borse, 2024).

Another commonly used insect-derived bioactive is lipids from the black-soldier fly (*H. illucens*). These lipid bioactives are promising in the cosmetic industry as eco-friendly emollients. More specifically, the oil, rich in lauric, palmitic, linoleic, and oleic acids, is formulated in different products like lotions, soaps, and emulsion delivery systems that enhance the function of the skin barrier and antioxidant activity (Almeida et al., 2020, 2024; Jessica et al., 2025). Specifically, lipid nanoparticles from BSFL have also been used for atopic dermatitis treatment, showing great potential for cosmeceuticals (Almeida et al., 2024). Furthermore, chitin and chitosan nanoparticles from *O. rhinoceros* and other species of beetles demonstrated great potential for curcumin delivery systems, with similar performance to commercial chitosan, introducing another nontoxic insect-derived bioactive for cosmeceutical applications (Zainol Abidin et al., 2023). Last but not least, aqueous extracts of house cricket demonstrate antioxidant activity, with nonirritant properties and inhibition of collagenase, and are supported as eco-friendly antiaging agents (Yeerong et al., 2021). Together, these studies document the growing potential of insect-based bioactives, already incorporated in commercial cosmetic formulations.

6 Future directions and challenges in insect-based cosmetic ingredients

6.1 Future perspectives

Insects are emerging as sustainable and efficient alternative sources of biofunctional ingredients for cosmetic applications. As aforementioned, they are indeed a novel, rich, alternative animal natural source of bioactive compounds such as peptides, lipids, chitin, and antioxidants, which exhibit moisturizing, antiaging, antimicrobial, and skin repair properties. Compared to conventional animal-derived ingredients, insect-based resources require fewer inputs, generate lower environmental impact, and align with circular economy principles by valorizing organic waste streams. Their biochemical diversity also offers novel functionalities, opening opportunities for innovative formulations targeting skin health and protection. Future perspectives focus on optimizing extraction technologies, ensuring safety and regulatory acceptance, improving insect culturing methodologies and safety, and enhancing consumer perception. As research advances, insect-derived ingredients are expected to play a key role in the development of sustainable, high-performance cosmeceuticals.

6.2 Limitations

While this study provides useful information on the health-promoting properties and bioactivities of insect-derived compounds, there are several limitations that should be noted. Initially, information regarding safety and toxicity is limited, and the possibility of allergic reactions to insect extracts with long-term use is unknown, even though natural ingredients are considered safer than synthetic ones. Due to the limited clinical data, there is a noticeable barrier to the cosmetic use of insect-based ingredients. Furthermore, another limitation concerns the origin of the bioactive ingredients, as it is not easy to ascertain whether the insects themselves contain the bioactive ingredients or whether they are derived from their diet or microbiota.

7 Conclusions

Compounds derived from insects and used in cosmetic formulations represent a new avenue for the production of next-generation cosmetics, combining sustainability with efficacy and providing consumers with enhanced benefits in their skincare and treatment routines. Insects appear to function as a production plant for diverse molecules, such as alkaloids, terpenoids, and peptides, which provide antimicrobial, antiaging, moisturizing, and other desirable effects that address ongoing cosmetic needs, filling significant gaps in this field. Aligning insect farming with the circular economy is also a major advantage for scaling up this facility to an industrial level. However, the transition of these compounds from laboratory research to clinical trials requires caution, particularly regarding allergic reactions and various adverse effects. Future research should focus on clinical and toxicological evaluations to fully elucidate the potential adverse effects that insect-derived bioactive compounds may cause, as well as their full functionality. Given this premise and ongoing research, insects are expected to play a significant role in the development and research of cosmetic and pharmaceutical products.

References

Bioactive compounds from *Hermetia illucens* larvae as natural ingredients for cosmetic application, n.d. MDPI. Available from: https://www.mdpi.com/2218-273X/10/7/976. (Accessed 24 March 2026).

Almeida, C., Rijo, P., Rosado, C., 2020. Bioactive compounds from *Hermetia illucens* larvae as natural ingredients for cosmetic application. Biomolecules. 2218-273X. 10 (7), 976. doi:10.3390/biom10070976.

Almeida, C., Murta, D., Nunes, R., Rolim Baby, A., Fernandes, Â., Barros, L., Rijo, P., Rosado, C., 2022. Characterization of lipid extracts from the *Hermetia illucens* larvae and their bioactivities for potential use as pharmaceutical and cosmetic ingredients. Heliyon. 24058440. 8 (5), e09455. doi:10.1016/j.heliyon.2022.e09455.

Almeida, C., Roque, R., Vieira, J., Júlio, A., Saraiva, N., Pereira-Leite, C., Rosado, C., 2024. Lipid extract from Black Soldier Fly larvae: a high value excipient for solid lipid nanoparticles tailored to tackle atopic dermatitis. Int. J. Pharm. 03785173. 667 (Pt B), 124929. doi:10.1016/j.ijpharm.2024.124929.

An, H., Kim, J., Kim, W., Gwon, M., Gu, H.M., Jeon, M.J., Han, S., Pak, S.C., Lee, C., Park, I.S., Park, K., 2018. Therapeutic effects of bee venom and its major component, melittin, on atopic dermatitis in vivo and in vitro. Br. J. Pharmacol. 175. Available from https://bpspubs.onlinelibrary.wiley.com/doi/10.1111/bph.14487?utm_source=chatgpt.com.

Baca, S.M., Gustafson, G.T., Alexander, A.M., Gough, H.M., Toussaint, E.F.A., 2021. Integrative phylogenomics reveals a Permian origin of *Adephaga beetles*. Syst. Entomol. 13653113. 46 (4), 968–990. Available from: http://onlinelibrary.wiley.com/journal/10.1111/(ISSN)1365-3113. doi:10.1111/syen.12506.

Barahona-Segovia, R.M., Madriz, R.I., González, C.R., de Souza Amorim, D., 2024. An update on the knowledge and general understanding of the Chilean Diptera diversity. Zootaxa. 11755334. 5518 (1), 1–87. Available from: https://mapress.com/zt/issue/view/zootaxa.5518.1. doi:10.11646/zootaxa.5518.1.1.

Boncan, D.A.T., Tsang, S.S.K., Li, C., Lee, I.H.T., Lam, H.M., Chan, T.F., Hui, J.H.L., 2020. Terpenes and terpenoids in plants: interactions with environment and insects. Int. J. Mol. Sci. 14220067. 21 (19), 1–19. Available from: https://www.mdpi.com/1422-0067/21/19/7382/pdf. doi:10.3390/ijms21197382.

Boonmee, N., Chittrakorn, S., et al., 2026. Effects of high pressure and ultrasonication pretreatments and supercritical carbon dioxide extraction on physico-chemical properties of edible insect oils—Boonmee—2024. J. Food Process Eng. 24. Available from https://onlinelibrary.wiley.com/doi/10.1111/jfpe.14781.

Borse, S.R., 2024. Exploring the role of insects in cosmetic industry: bioactive compounds and extraction techniques: a comprehensive review. Int. J. Entomol. Res. 9 (12), 166–170.

Bulet, P., Stöcklin, R., 2005. Insect antimicrobial peptides: structures, properties and gene regulation. Protein Pept. Lett. 09298665. 12 (1), 3–11. doi:10.2174/0929866053406011.

Cai, C., Tihelka, E., Giacomelli, M., Lawrence, J.F., Ślipiński, A., Kundrata, R., Yamamoto, S., Thayer, M.K., Newton, A.F., Leschen, R.A.B., Gimmel, M.L., Lü, L., Engel, M.S., Bouchard, P., Huang, D., Pisani, D., Donoghue, P.C.J., 2022. Integrated phylogenomics and fossil data illuminate the evolution of beetles. R. Soc. Open Sci. 2054-5703. 9 (3). doi:10.1098/rsos.211771.

Chrysikopoulou, V., Rampaouni, A., Koutsia, E., Ofrydopoulou, A., Mittas, N., Tsoupras, A., 2025. Anti-inflammatory, antithrombotic and antioxidant efficacy and synergy of a high-dose vitamin C supplement enriched with a low dose of bioflavonoids. Nutrients. 20726643. 17 (16). Available from: http://www.mdpi.com/journal/nutrients/. doi:10.3390/nu17162643.

Dioguardi, M., Cantore, S., Sovereto, D., Sanesi, L., Martella, A., Almasri, L., Musella, G., Muzio, L.L., Ballini, A., 2024. Therapeutic potential of *Solenopsis invicta* venom: a scoping review of its bioactive molecules, biological aspects, and health applications. Biomolecules. 2218-273X. 14 (12), 1499. doi:10.3390/biom14121499.

Dorey, J.B., Gilpin, A.M., Johnston, N.P., Esquerré, D., Hughes, A.C., Ascher, J.S., Orr, M.C., 2026. Estimating global bee species richness and taxonomic gaps. Nat. Commun. 20411723. 17 (1). Available from: https://www.nature.com/ncomms/. doi:10.1038/s41467-026-69029-4.

Dragojlov, I., Aad, R., Ami, D., Mangiagalli, M., Natalello, A., Vesentini, S., 2025. Silk sericin-based electrospun nanofibers forming films for cosmetic applications: preparation, characterization, and efficacy evaluation. Molecules. 14203049. 30 (3). Available from: http://www.mdpi.com/journal/molecules. doi:10.3390/molecules30030715.

Elmaidomy, A.H., Zayed, A., Abbas, G.M., Badr, N.H., Bringmann, G., Wu, J., Abdelmohsen, U.R., 2026. Exploring natural colorants from plants to insects: chemistry, functions, and modern uses. RSC Adv. 20462069. 16 (8), 7097–7119. Available from: http://pubs.rsc.org/en/journals/journal/ra. doi:10.1039/d5ra09252c.

El-Wahed, A.A.A., Khalifa, S.A.M., Elashal, M.H., Musharraf, S.G., Saeed, A., Khatib, A., Tahir, H.E., Zou, X., Naggar, Y.A., Mehmood, A., Wang, K., El-Seedi, H.R., 2021. Cosmetic applications of bee venom. Toxins. 20726651. 13 (11). Available from: https://www.mdpi.com/2072-6651/13/11/810/pdf. doi:10.3390/toxins13110810.

Faisal, S., Badshah, S.L., Kubra, B., Emwas, A.H., Jaremko, M., 2023. Alkaloids as potential antivirals. A comprehensive review. Nat. Prod. Bioprospect. 21922209. 13 (1). Available from: https://www.springer.com/journal/13659. doi:10.1007/s13659-022-00366-9.

Fan, H., Liu, T., Chen, Y., Liao, Z., Chen, J., Hu, Y., Qiao, G., Wei, F., 2024. Geographical patterns and determinants of insect biodiversity in China. Sci. China Life Sci. 1869-1889. 67 (6), 1255–1265. Available from: https://www.springer.com/journal/11427. doi:10.1007/s11427-023-2483-0.

Février, P.J., Barraclough, T.G., 2025. Do the "big four" orders of insects comprise evolutionarily significant higher taxa with coherent patterns of selection on protein-coding genes? Evol. Lett. 20563744. 9 (3), 355–366. Available from: https://academic.oup.com/evlett. doi:10.1093/evlett/qraf005.

Franco, A., Salvia, R., Scieuzo, C., Schmitt, E., Russo, A., Falabella, P., 2022. Lipids from insects in cosmetics and for personal care products. Insects. 2075-4450. 13 (1), 41. doi:10.3390/insects13010041.

Guzman, L.M., Elle, E., Morandin, L.A., Cobb, N.S., Chesshire, P.R., McCabe, L.M., Hughes, A., Orr, M., M'Gonigle, L.K., 2024. Impact of pesticide use on wild bee distributions across the United States. Nat. Sustain. 23989629. 7 (10), 1324–1334. Available from: https://www.nature.com/natsustain/. doi:10.1038/s41893-024-01413-8.

Han, S.M., Hong, I.P., Woo, S.O., Chun, S.N., Park, K.K., Nicholls, Y.M., Pak, S.C., 2015. The beneficial effects of honeybee-venom serum on facial wrinkles in humans. Clin. Interv. Aging. 11781998. 10, 1587–1592. Available from: https://www.dovepress.com/getfile.php?fileID=27317. doi:10.2147/CIA.S84940.

Honorato, L., Bonilla, J.J.A., da Silva, L.R., Kornetz, J., Zamith-Miranda, D., Valdez, A., Nosanchuk, J., Fox, E., Nimrichter, L., 2024. *Alkaloids solenopsins* from fire ants display in vitro and in vivo activity against the yeast *Candida auris*. Virulence. 2150-5594. 15 (1). doi:10.1080/21505594.2024.2413329.

Hudiwaku, S., Himawan, T., Rizali, A., 2021. Diversity and species composition of fruit flies (Diptera: tephritidae) in Lombok Island, Indonesia. Biodiversitas. 20854722. 22 (10), 4608–4616. Available from: https://smujo.id/biodiv/article/download/8957/5225. doi:10.13057/biodiv/d221054.

Huemer, P., Berggren, K., Aarvik, L., Rennwald, E., Hausmann, A., Segerer, A., Staffoni, G., Mærk Aspaas, A., Trichas, A., Hebert, P.D.N., 2025. Extensive DNA barcoding of Lepidoptera of Crete (Greece) reveals significant taxonomic and faunistic gaps and supports the first comprehensive checklist of the island's fauna. Insects. 2075-4450. 16 (5), 438. doi:10.3390/insects16050438.

Jessica, A., Aina, S., Rahayu, R., Agustin, R., 2025. Prepupae OIL for cosmetic application and anti-hyaluronidase activity-nanoemulsions of black soldier fly (*Hermetia illucens*). Int. J. Appl. Pharm. 09757058. 17 (1), 8–14. Available from: https://journals.innovareacademics.in/index.php/ijap/article/download/54048/31582. doi:10.22159/ijap.2025.v17s1.02.

Kettani, K., Ebejer, M.J., Ackland, D.M., Bächli, G., Barraclough, D., Barták, M., Tolrá, M.C., Černý, M., Cerretti, P., Chandler, P., Dakki, M., Daugeron, C., De Jong, H., Dils, J., Disney, H., Droz, B., Evenhuis, N., Gatt, P., Graciolli, G., Grichanov, I.Y., Haenni, J.P., Hauser, M., Himmi, O., Macgowan, I., Mathieu, B., Mouna, M., Munari, L., Nartshuk, E.P., Negrobov, O.P., Oosterbroek, P., Pape, T., Pont, A.C., Popov, G.V., Rognes, K., Skuhravá, M., Skuhravý, V., Speight, M., Tomasovic, G., Trari, B., Tschorsnig, H.P., Vala, J.C., Tschirnhaus, M.V., Wagner, R., Whitmore, D., Woźnica, A.J., Zatwarnicki, T., Zwick, P., 2022. Catalogue of the Diptera (Insecta) of Morocco—an annotated checklist, with distributions and a bibliography. ZooKeys. 13132970. 1094, 1–466. Available from: https://goto.arphahub.com/download/pdf/62644. doi:10.3897/zookeys.1094.62644.

Kim, K., Park, E.Y., Baek, D.J., Lee, C.S., Oh, Y.S., 2024. Antiphotoaging effects of solvent fractions isolated from *Allomyrina dichotoma* larvae extract. Biochem. Biophys. Rep. 24055808. 38. Available from: https://www.sciencedirect.com/science/journal/24055808. doi:10.1016/j.bbrep.2024.101660.

Kolobe, S.D., Manyelo, T.G., Malematja, E., Sebola, N.A., Mabelebele, M., 2023. Fats and major fatty acids present in edible insects utilised as food and livestock feed. Vet. Anim. Sci. 2451943X. 22. Available from: www.journals.elsevier.com/veterinary-and-animal-science. doi:10.1016/j.vas.2023.100312.

Kulka, K., Sionkowska, A., 2023. Chitosan based materials in cosmetic applications: a review. Molecules. 14203049. 28 (4). Available from: http://www.mdpi.com/journal/molecules. doi:10.3390/molecules28041817.

Lahmi, L.O., Harari, A., Shaish, A., Tsurim, I., 2024. The carotenoid composition of larvae feed is reflected in adult house fly (*Musca domestica*) body. Insects. 20754450. 15 (7). Available from: http://www.mdpi.com/journal/insects. doi:10.3390/insects15070521.

Li, A., Dewettinck, K., Verheust, Y., Van de Walle, D., Raes, K., Diehl, B., Tzompa-Sosa, D.A., 2024. Edible insects as a novel source of lecithin: extraction and lipid characterization of black soldier fly larvae and yellow mealworm. Food Chem. 03088146. 452, 139391. doi:10.1016/j.foodchem.2024.139391.

Liu, S., Zhang, Q., Zhou, H., Zhang, B., Yu, M., Wang, Y., Liu, Y., Chai, C., 2024. The potential of natural carotenoids-containing sericin of the domestic silkworm *Bombyx mori*. Int. J. Mol. Sci. 14220067. 25 (7). Available from: http://www.mdpi.com/journal/ijms. doi:10.3390/ijms25073688.

Maoka, T., 2020. Carotenoids as natural functional pigments. J. Nat. Med. 18610293. 74 (1). Available from: http://www.springerlink.com/content/1861-0293/. doi:10.1007/s11418-019-01364-x.

Maoka, T., Kawase, N., Hironaka, M., Nishida, R., 2021. Carotenoids of hemipteran insects, from the perspective of chemo-systematic and chemical ecological studies. Biochem. Syst. Ecol. 03051978. 95, 104241. doi:10.1016/j.bse.2021.104241.

McKenna, D.D., Shin, S., Ahrens, D., Balke, M., Beza-Beza, C., Clarke, D.J., Donath, A., Escalona, H.E., Friedrich, F., Letsch, H., Liu, S., Maddison, D., Mayer, C., Misof, B., Murin, P.J., Niehuis, O., Peters, R.S., Podsiadlowski, L., Pohl, H., Scully, E.D., Yan, E.V., Zhou, X., Ślipiński, A., Beutel, R.G., 2019. The evolution and genomic basis of beetle diversity. Proc. Natl. Acad. Sci. U. S. A. 10916490. 116 (49), 24729–24737. Available from: https://www.pnas.org/content/pnas/116/49/24729.full.pdf. doi:10.1073/pnas.1909655116.

Merzendorfer, H., 2006. Insect chitin synthases: a review. J. Comp. Physiol. B, Biochem. Syst. Environ. Physiol. 01741578. 176 (1), 1–15. doi:10.1007/s00360-005-0005-3.

Muñoz-Seijas, N., Fernandes, H., Fernández, B., Domínguez, J.M., Salgado, J.M., 2025. Eco-friendly technologies for obtaining antioxidant compounds and protein hydrolysates from edible insect Tenebrio molitor beetles. Food Chem. 18737072. 464. Available from: https://www.sciencedirect.com/science/journal/03088146. doi:10.1016/j.foodchem.2024.141726.

Ngoc, L.T.N., Moon, J.Y., Lee, Y.C., 2023. Insights into bioactive peptides in cosmetics. Cosmetics. 20799284. 10 (4). Available from: www.mdpi.com/journal/cosmetics. doi:10.3390/cosmetics10040111.

Nicolaou, A., Kendall, A.C., 2024. Bioactive lipids in the skin barrier mediate its functionality in health and disease. Pharmacol. Ther. 01637258. 260, 108681. doi:10.1016/j.pharmthera.2024.108681.

Nino, M.C., Reddivari, L., Osorio, C., Kaplan, I., Liceaga, A.M., 2021a. Insects as a source of phenolic compounds and potential health benefits. J. Insects Food Feed. 2352-4588. 7 (7), 1077–1087. doi:10.3920/jiff2020.0113.

Nino, M.C., Reddivari, L., Ferruzzi, M.G., Liceaga, A.M., 2021b. Targeted phenolic characterization and antioxidant bioactivity of extracts from edible acheta domesticus. Foods. 23048158. 10 (10). Available from: https://www.mdpi.com/2304-8158/10/10/2295/pdf. doi:10.3390/foods10102295.

Ochiai, M., Komiya, Y., 2021. Detection of edible insect derived phospholipids with polyunsaturated fatty acids by thin-layer chromatography, gas chromatography, and enzymatic methods. J. Food Compos. Anal. 08891575. 99, 103869. doi:10.1016/j.jfca.2021.103869.

Orrù, A., Pittau, B., Pettinau, F., 2025. Shedding light on the antioxidant activity of bee venom using a 2,2-diphenyl-1-picrylhydrazyl assay in a detergent-based buffer. Molecules. 14203049. 30 (3). Available from: http://www.mdpi.com/journal/molecules. doi:10.3390/molecules30030640.

Palupi, E., Nasir, S.Q., Jayanegara, A., Susanto, I., Ismail, A., Iwansyah, A.C., Setiawan, B., Sulaeman, A., Rizal, M., Damanik, M., Filianty, F., 2025. Meta-analysis on the fatty acid composition of edible insects as a sustainable food and feed. Future Foods. 26668335. 11, 100529. doi:10.1016/j.fufo.2024.100529.

Perez-Santaescolastica, C., de Pril, I., van de Voorde, I., Fraeye, I., 2023. Fatty acid and amino acid profiles of seven edible insects: focus on lipid class composition and protein conversion factors. Foods. 23048158. 12 (22). Available from: www.mdpi.com/journal/foods. doi:10.3390/foods12224090.

Purkiewicz, A., Karabulut, G., Tańska, M., Ivanišová, E., Harangozo, Ľ., Starowicz, M., Pietrzak-Fiećko, R., Łozowicka, B., Kaczyński, P., Goksen, G., 2025. Compositional analysis of amino acids, fatty acids, minerals, and aroma compounds in buffalo worm (*Alphitobius diaperinus*) larval powder and recovery of bioactive compounds via ultrasound-assisted extraction. Food Chem. X. 25901575. 32, 103262. doi:10.1016/j.fochx.2025.103262.

Rinaudo, M., 2006. Chitin and chitosan: properties and applications. Prog. Polym. Sci. 00796700. 31 (7), 603–632. doi:10.1016/j.progpolymsci.2006.06.001.

Sawada, Y., Saito-Sasaki, N., Nakamura, M., 2021. Omega 3 fatty acid and skin diseases. Front. Immunol. 16643224. 11. Available from: https://www.frontiersin.org/journals/immunology#. doi:10.3389/fimmu.2020.623052.

Seabrooks, L., Hu, L., 2017. Insects: an underrepresented resource for the discovery of biologically active natural products. Acta Pharm. Sin. B. 22113843. 7 (4), 409–426. Available from: http://www.elsevier.com/wps/find/journaldescription.cws_home/725753/description#description. doi:10.1016/j.apsb.2017.05.001.

Somwongin, S., Chantawannakul, P., Chaiyana, W., 2018. Antioxidant activity and irritation property of venoms from Apis species. Toxicon. 18793150. 145, 32–39. Available from: www.elsevier.com/locate/toxicon. doi:10.1016/j.toxicon.2018.02.049.

Tan, K., Zhang, H., Lim, L.S., Ma, H., Li, S., Zheng, H., 2020. Roles of carotenoids in invertebrate immunology. Front. Immunol. 16643224. 10. Available from: https://www.frontiersin.org/journals/immunology#. doi:10.3389/fimmu.2019.03041.

Tanuğur Samancı, A.E., Kekeçoğlu, M., 2022. Development of a cream formulation containing bee venom and other bee products. J. Cosmet. Dermatol. 14732165. 21 (10), 4913–4920. Available from: http://onlinelibrary.wiley.com/journal/10.1111/(ISSN)1473-2165. doi:10.1111/jocd.14891.

Torres-Castillo, J.A., Olazarán-Santibáñez, F.E., 2023. Insects as source of phenolic and antioxidant entomochemicals in the food industry. Front. Nutr. 2296861X. 10. Available from: https://www.journal.frontiersin.org/journal/nutrition. doi:10.3389/fnut.2023.1133342.

Trepa, M., Sułkowska-Ziaja, K., Kała, K., Muszyńska, B., 2024. Therapeutic potential of fungal terpenes and terpenoids: application in skin diseases. Molecules. 14203049. 29 (5). Available from: http://www.mdpi.com/journal/molecules. doi:10.3390/molecules29051183.

Vakte, S.R., Sonawane, C.P., 2024. Cochineal insects (*Dactylopius coccus*) in cosmetics: an overview of taxonomy, composition, extraction methods, applications, and regulatory perspectives. Int. J. Entomol. Res. 9 (10), 148–153. Available fromhttps://www.entomologyjournals.com/assets/archives/2024/vol9issue10/9286.pdf.

Yang, J.C., Zhang, J.P., Wu, C.Y., Bai, Y., Guedes, R.N.C., Dewer, Y., Li, F.Q., Zang, L.S., 2025. Diversity and role of volatile terpene and terpenoid pheromones in insects. J. Econ. Entomol. 1938291X. 118 (1), 9–18. Available from: https://academic.oup.com/jee/issue. doi:10.1093/jee/toae271.

Yeerong, K., Sriyab, S., Somwongin, S., Punyoyai, C., Chantawannakul, P., Anuchapreeda, S., Prommaban, A., Chaiyana, W., 2021. Skin irritation and potential antioxidant, anti-collagenase, and anti-elastase activities of edible insect extracts. Sci. Rep. 20452322. 11 (1). Available from: www.nature.com/srep/index.html. doi:10.1038/s41598-021-02382-0.

Zainol Abidin, N.A., Kormin, F., Abidin, N.A.Z., Bakar, M.F.A., Moujdin, I.A., 2023. Synthesis and characterization of curcumin-chitosan loaded gold nanoparticles by *Oryctes rhinoceros*' chitin for cosmeceutical application. Molecules. 14203049. 28 (4). Available from: http://www.mdpi.com/journal/molecules. doi:10.3390/molecules28041799.

Zhao, H., Liu, M., Chen, L., Gong, Y., Ma, W., Jiang, Y., 2025. Study on the effect of bee venom and its main component melittin in delaying skin aging in mice. Int. J. Mol. Sci. 14220067. 26 (2). Available from: http://www.mdpi.com/journal/ijms. doi:10.3390/ijms26020742.

Zhu, K.Y., Merzendorfer, H., Zhang, W., Zhang, J., Muthukrishnan, S., 2016. Biosynthesis, turnover, and functions of chitin in insects. Annu. Rev. Entomol. 00664170. 61, 177–196. Available from: http://arjournals.annualreviews.org/loi/ento. doi:10.1146/annurev-ento-010715-023933.

Chapter 24

Dairy and dairy by-products

Athina Velissaridou, Theodora Adamantidi, Anna Ofrydopoulou, and Alexandros Tsoupras
Hephaestus Laboratory, School of Chemistry, Faculty of Sciences, Democritus University of Thrace, Kavala University Campus, Kavala, Greece

1 Introduction

There is a long history of using dairy products for both esthetic and therapeutic purposes, extending across centuries and cultures. Since antiquity, people have recognized the beneficial properties of milk and its by-products for body care and disease treatment. Milk, in particular, was regarded not only as a nutritious food but also as a sacred substance symbolizing purity, fertility, and well-being. Its smooth texture, softness, and whiteness were associated with the ideal image of healthy, youthful skin, contributing to its gradual popularity as a beauty treatment, especially among the upper classes. From ancient Egypt and Rome to medieval times and Renaissance Europe, milk and its derivatives became an indispensable part of women's beauty rituals and natural medicine, paving the way for their modern use in the natural cosmetics industry (Walker, 2000).

The most commonly used dairy derivatives in cosmetic formulations include milk, yogurt, butter, and fermented products such as kefir. Each provides a distinct chemical composition that contributes to skin care and overall health. At first, milk, a rich source of lactose, proteins, lipids, vitamins, and minerals, is widely applied in both liquid and powder form (Kazimierska and Kalinowska-Lis, 2021). The milk protein fraction, mainly consisting of caseins and whey proteins, exhibits antioxidant, antimicrobial, and antiinflammatory properties, helping reduce acne-related inflammation and improving skin appearance. Amino acids such as methionine, proline, and threonine play crucial roles in collagen synthesis, enhancing skin elasticity and accelerating wound healing. Milk-derived peptides further reduce oxidative stress through their free radical scavenging activity (Mehra et al., 2021; Park, 2009). Moreover, milk lipids strengthen the skin barrier, preserve hydration, and restore elasticity, while carbohydrates, particularly lactose, contribute additional moisturizing effects (Bertin et al., 2008; Fluhr et al., 2008). Finally, vitamins, including tocopherol and retinol, provide antioxidant, photoprotective, and regenerative abilities, synergizing with other milk bioactives to maintain skin integrity and resilience (Kazimierska and Kalínowska-Lis, 2021; Chan et al., 2017a).

Although milk is the main source of bioactive compounds used in cosmetics, its derivatives, and more specifically yogurt, cheese, butter, and kefir, are also of considerable cosmetic value. Yogurt combines the nutritional richness of milk with fermentation benefits. During lactic fermentation, lactose is converted to lactic acid, producing numerous microbial metabolites that define yogurt's unique properties. Lactic acid enhances the moisturizing and brightening effects beyond those of milk, while live lactic acid bacteria (LAB) and their metabolites balance the skin microbiome and reinforce the skin barrier (Ichimura, 2024; Nagaoka, 2019; Cheng, 2010; Kimoto-Nira et al., 2014). Following yogurt's potential, butter, the lipid-rich fraction of milk, contains fatty acids, triglycerides, and phospholipids at higher concentrations than milk itself. Its mono- and polyunsaturated fatty acids promote hydration and skin barrier repair, while its fat-soluble antioxidants strengthen its protective and regenerative functions (Lee et al., 2020; Pădureţ, 2021; Krakowska-Sieprawska et al., 2025). In addition, cheese during its fermentation and ripening process develops a rich profile of peptides, amino acids, lipids, and microbial metabolites linked to collagen stimulation, improved skin elasticity, and enhanced hydration and barrier function (Fernandes et al., 2025). Finally, kefir is a fermented beverage produced by the synergistic activity of LAB and yeasts. Rich in proteins, peptides, lipids, and diverse fermentation-derived bioactives (e.g., microbial metabolites, sugars, organic acids), it demonstrates great antimicrobial, wound healing, and immunoregulatory effects, making it a promising cosmetic agent (Vieira et al., 2021; Azizi et al., 2021; Huseini et al., 2012).

The appeal of milk and its derivatives in cosmetics has historically been linked to their esthetic properties, including smoothness, soft feeling, moisturizing, and soothing effects, alongside their symbolic association with purity and vitality. In recent decades, scientific advancements have clarified the molecular mechanisms underlying these long-observed benefits, facilitating

Biofunctional Cosmetics for Health. https://doi.org/10.1016/B978-0-443-27500-5.00024-1

their systematic incorporation into cosmetic formulations (Ichimura, 2024; Nagaoka, 2019; Cheng, 2010; Kimoto-Nira et al., 2014). The successful utilization of dairy bioactives in cosmetics strongly depends on the extraction and isolation techniques employed, which vary from conventional (e.g., enzymatic hydrolysis, fermentation) to green, innovative technologies [e.g., ultrasound-assisted extraction (UAE)] that have further improved the efficiency, selectivity, yield, and sustainability of the process (Mathews et al., 2024). Despite their wide acceptance, dairy-based ingredients in cosmetics must be evaluated for their safety, particularly in relation to allergenicity. Advances in purification techniques and hydrolyzed protein fractions have helped minimize their allergenic potential, thereby enhancing the safety profile of dairy-derived cosmetics (He et al., 2025).

The cosmetic industry has already incorporated dairy derivatives into a range of commercial products. Milk powders and hydrolyzed proteins are commonly used in moisturizing creams and antiaging formulations (Kazimierska and Kalinowska-Lis, 2021), whereas yogurt, cheese, and kefir extracts are integrated into face masks and probiotic-enriched skincare lines (Yeom et al., 2011; Ningsih and Eka Putra, 2025). Furthermore, butter-derived lipids are employed in emollient creams, lip balms, and body butters, highlighting their versatility (Panchal et al., 2021).

Novel dermatological and biochemical studies have unraveled the roles of specific dairy components. For instance, proteomic and lipidomic analyses have detailed the interactions and functionality of milk proteins and lipid fractions in biological and chemical processes (Augustyniak et al., 2023). Milk-derived peptides have been correlated with antioxidant mechanisms and the regulation of inflammatory pathways, while lipid fractions enhance moisture retention and skin integrity. Such findings provide a molecular explanation for the soothing and regenerative properties once known only through empirical use. Fermented products such as yogurt, cheese, and kefir add further value, as they are rich in lactic acid, exopolysaccharides (EPSs) (produced by LAB), and microbial metabolites that improve hydration and skin regeneration. Modern scientific methods enable the quantification and validation of these effects, allowing their reliable translation into cosmetic applications (Augustyniak et al., 2023; Cosentino et al., 2025; Faraz, 2020).

Considering the consumer demand for "clean beauty," shifting consumer expectations have reinforced this trend. Today's cosmetic consumers actively seek innovative products that combine the appeal of natural ingredients with scientifically proven efficacy. Industry standards also demand evidence-based claims, pushing for the integration of dairy bioactives into formulations supported by rigorous data. Advances in extraction technologies and delivery systems have further enabled the targeted, safe, and effective incorporation of dairy-derived compounds into skincare. This evolution marks a shift from traditional applications to science-driven cosmetics, ensuring not only sustainable efficacy and safety but also consumer trust (Augustyniak et al., 2023; Cosentino et al., 2025; Faraz, 2020). In this review, the extraction methods, bioactive components, health-promoting properties, and cosmetic applications of dairy-based cosmetics are discussed. The key highlights of this review are summarized in Fig. 24.1.

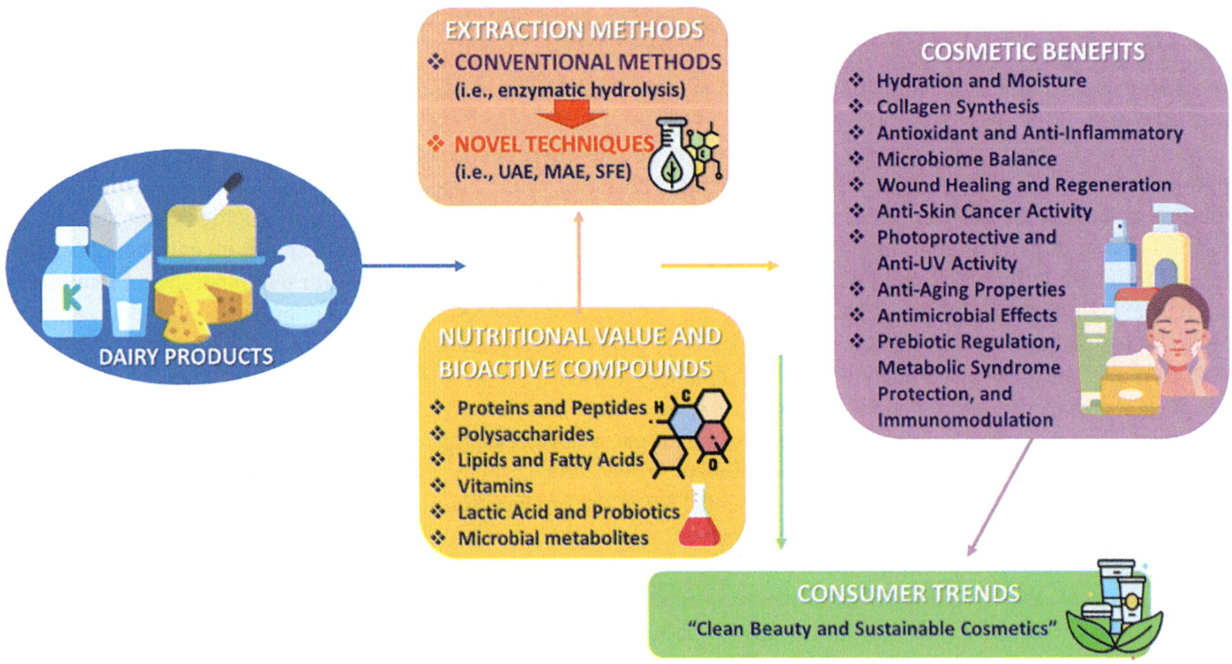

FIG. 24.1 Dairy bioactives extraction methods, pharmacological properties, and cosmetic applications. *(Source: Parts of this figure were obtained from the free open-access platform https://www.flaticon.com/ (Accessed 19 September 2025).)*

2 Extraction methods for bioactives from dairy products and factors affecting the extraction yield

2.1 Extraction methods of bioactives from dairy products

The extraction of bioactive compounds from dairy products is a crucial step for their application in cosmetic formulations, as it directly affects the purity, yield, and integrity of the isolated components. Considering the structural diversity of dairy-derived molecules, ranging from proteins and peptides to lipids, vitamins, and minerals, no single universally applicable extraction technique exists. Instead, a wide array of conventional and advanced processes has been developed. The choice of the extraction method depends on multiple factors, including the type and stability of the target compound, the required degree of purity, and broader considerations, including the cost, sustainability, and industrial applicability. Ultimately, extraction techniques and their underlying mechanisms are essential for the successful utilization of dairy bioactives in cosmetology (Bisht et al., 2025; Granato et al., 2022).

Conventional techniques such as maceration, distillation, acid precipitation, membrane filtration, and solvent extraction form the foundation of dairy bioactive recovery. Their importance lies in their simplicity, reproducibility, and long history of industrial use, ensuring technical reliability and regulatory acceptance (Bisht et al., 2025; Granato et al., 2022). Maceration relies on solvent exposure (aqueous, alcoholic, or mixed) to leach soluble compounds from a substrate (Mathews et al., 2024). It is a mild technique that minimizes damage to fragile bioactives but suffers from long extraction times, low yields, and high solvent consumption (Farooq et al., 2021; Andrade et al., 2025; Nighojkar et al., 2019). Distillation separates volatile compounds based on differences in boiling points under relatively mild conditions and is classified into membrane, vacuum, and steam distillation (Hausmann et al., 2011; Gontarek-Castro and Castro-Muñoz, 2024). Nevertheless, distillation may subject the substrates to high temperatures, increasing the degradation risk of heat-sensitive components (i.e., vitamins, peptides) (Altay et al., 2024; Moejes et al., 2015). Steam and vacuum distillation reduce thermal stress and are mainly applied to recover volatile fractions, such as aromatic compounds and fat-soluble molecules in dairy products (Altay et al., 2024; Mottram and Elmore, 2003; Berk, 2018).

Another conventional method, acid precipitation, is widely used for protein fractionation, for instance, separating casein from whey proteins at specific pH values [usually lowering the pH via the addition of inorganic acids (HCl) or organic acids (lactic or acetic acid)] (Neelima et al., 2013; Chen et al., 2023). This technique enables the recovery of whey-derived peptides like β-lactoglobulin, α-lactalbumin (α-LA), lactoferrin, glycomacropeptide (GMP), and immunoglobulins, as well as other secondary bioactive fractions, such as phospholipids and growth factors produced during acid hydrolysis (Rocafi et al., 2011), with high antioxidant, antimicrobial, skin-beneficial, metabolic health, and immunomodulatory value (Rusu et al., 2009; Etzel, 2004). Following this, membrane-based filtration [microfiltration (MF), ultrafiltration (UF), nanofiltration (NF)] provides gentler, selective separation based on pore size or molecular weight, while preserving the structural integrity of proteins and peptides (Kumar et al., 2013). MF is mostly used as the first step to remove bacteria, somatic cells, and fat globules, an approach widely used to produce high-quality whey protein isolates enriched in β-lactoglobulin, α-LA, and lactoferrin. Furthermore, UF further refines the separation, whereas NF provides an extra selectivity layer, retaining peptides and larger proteins while allowing partial passage of minerals and small organic acids. Using MF, UF, and NF sequentially drives the precise composition definition of dairy fractions, ensuring maximum recovery and bioactivity of the compounds (Akbache et al., 2009; Ho, 2007). Finally, solvent extraction is applied to recover lipophilic compounds such as conjugated linoleic acid (CLA), phospholipids, fat-soluble vitamins A and D, and carotenoids (Castro-Gómez et al., 2014; Schweigert et al., 2000; Barakat et al., 2015), using chloroform, methanol, hexane, or petroleum solvents (Cheng et al., 2019; Nunes and Torres, 2010). Although effective, it poses challenges related to solvent residues and sustainability. Thus currently, ethanol is the preferred "green" solvent (Chemat et al., 2012).

Rising global interest in dairy-derived bioactive compounds for cosmetic use has led both research and industry to an increased demand for innovative technologies for the retrieval and utilization of these substances. Advanced extraction methods have been developed to overcome the limitations of conventional technologies, providing greater selectivity, efficiency, and sustainability. These include UAE, microwave-assisted extraction (MAE), enzyme-assisted extraction (EAE), supercritical fluid extraction (SFE), pulsed electric field extraction (PEF), pressurized liquid extraction (PLE), and electrodialysis (ED) (Bisht et al., 2025; Granato et al., 2022).

At first, the UAE method enhances mass transfer via cavitation, thermal, and mechanical effects, improving yields while minimizing solvent use. UAE reduces extraction times, minimizes solvent consumption, and sustains thermosensitive agents from degradation (Călinescu et al., 2021; Chemat et al., 2017), promoting the solubility and mobility of targeted molecules and easing their diffusion into the solvent (Qiu et al., 2020; Wen et al., 2018; Tiwari, 2015). However, excessive exposure may degrade sensitive bioactives (Yang et al., 2017; Ding et al., 2021). Polyphenol extraction by UAE is very effective, yielding higher concentrations compared to conventional methods (Mehmood et al., 2019; Kwaw et al.,

2018), whereas polysaccharides revealed increased solubility and bioavailability through UAE (Kang et al., 2019; Xu et al., 2018). Following this, MAE couples microwave energy with solvents, achieving rapid heating, improved extraction yields (Camel, 2000; Teo et al., 2013; Medina et al., 2015), and efficient extraction of lipids, triglycerides, phospholipids, minor lipid molecules (e.g., sterols), and bioactive peptides (Solaberrieta et al., 2022; Dos Santos Venâncio Costa and Bragagnolo, 2017; ElKhori et al., 2007). It is particularly useful for dairy lipidomics and toxin analysis but remains limited in large-scale dairy applications (Campaniello et al., 2024). Moreover, EAE utilizes hydrolytic enzymes to selectively release bound molecules under mild conditions (Dominiak et al., 2014; Shen et al., 2023), using mainly cellulases, hemicellulases, and pectinases (for plant media), as well as proteases and lipases (for protein- and lipid-based matrices) (Jeevan Kumar et al., 2017; Kumar and Tingirikari, 2023). EAE provides higher selectivity than UAE and MAE, improving the yields of whey peptides (WP), proteins, and lipids (Gao et al., 2023), and allowing the effective recovery of major and minor bioactives, as well as taste and flavor agents in dairy products (Dominiak et al., 2014; Sutay Kocabaş et al., 2022).

SFE, usually with supercritical CO_2 (Krishnegowda et al., 2021), allows the recovery of lipids, vitamins, and volatile fractions at low temperatures, preserving thermolabile compounds (Krishnegowda et al., 2021; Sprick et al., 2019) and providing high selectivity and yields (Sánchez-Camargo et al., 2014; Björklund and Sparr-Eskilsson, 2005). It is especially effective for fatty acids, cholesterol, and fat-soluble vitamins (Krishnegowda et al., 2021; Macías et al., 2014; Singh et al., 2018), as well as linoleic acid, vitamins (A and E), and aromatic compounds from dairy products (Macías et al., 2014; Berg et al., 2000; Larráyoz et al., 2000). Furthermore, PLE is an effective alternative for extracting bioactives and nutritious components from dairy (Castro-Gómez et al., 2014; Acquavia et al., 2025). PLE applies high pressure and moderate heat to accelerate extraction (Alvarez-Rivera et al., 2019; Sun et al., 2012), enabling the recovery of both polar and nonpolar molecules, such as lipids, vitamins, and proteins (Castro-Gómez et al., 2014; Carabias-Martínez et al., 2005; Teixeira et al., 2024; Chatzimitakos et al., 2024). PEF, on the contrary, is capable of increasing cell membrane permeability through applied electroporation, operating at low temperatures. Hence, thermal degradation of heat-sensitive compounds is kept to a minimum (Cavalcanti et al., 2023). PEF improves the release of flavonoids and essential oils in plants (Grzelka et al., 2025; Genovese et al., 2023). As for dairy products, PEF enhances the release of milk fat globule membrane (MFGM) phospholipids and sphingolipids (Yang et al., 2021; Mehta et al., 2025), as well as the extraction of whey proteins and peptides like lactoferrin and immunoglobulins (Šalaševičius et al., 2021; Madureira et al., 2007). Finally, ED uses alternating cation-exchange membranes and anion-exchange membranes under electric current to selectively remove ions from one solution and concentrate them in another (Bazinet, 2005; Ozel et al., 2022). ED is especially useful for the removal of salts and metals, the isolation of charged peptides and proteins, and, thus, the whey demineralization process (Dufton et al., 2018; Ozel et al., 2022).

Following extraction, the precise identification and quantification of dairy-derived bioactives are achieved through advanced analytical platforms. Techniques, including high-performance liquid chromatography (HPLC) and ultra-high-performance liquid chromatography, as well as gas and liquid chromatography–mass spectrometry (GC–MS and LC–MS), are routinely applied to characterize key dairy components, such as proteins, peptides, fatty acids, and minor metabolites (Barakat et al., 2015; Chatzimitakos et al., 2024; Yen et al., 2015; Poveda et al., 2008). In recent years, metabolomics approaches combined with chemometric tools have enhanced the resolution, reproducibility, and overall profiling of dairy extracts, ensuring quality control, batch-to-batch consistency, and the authentication of dairy-based nutraceutical and cosmetic products (Teo et al., 2013; Nielsen et al., 2024). Table 24.1 provides indicative experimental studies and review examples of each extraction technique utilized for dairy product bioactive extraction.

2.2 Factors affecting the extraction yield of dairy product extracts

The extraction of bioactive compounds from dairy products and their derivatives faces unique challenges compared to other matrices, such as plants, due to the complex composition, structural diversity, and high sensitivity of dairy biomolecules. Many of the most valuable bioactive dairy components, such as lactoferrin and immunoglobulins, are particularly thermo-sensitive and prone to chemical or oxidative degradation (Liu et al., 2022b). Prolonged or excessive heating can simultaneously lead to protein denaturation and aggregation, peptide hydrolysis, and oxidation of unsaturated fatty acids, ultimately compromising both yield and functional activity. Likewise, numerous bioactives derived from dairy products are sensitive to extreme pH values, while others undergo photooxidation and autooxidation upon exposure to light or oxygen, as seen in fat-soluble vitamins, including vitamins A, D, E, and K (Fanelli et al., 1985; Clarke et al., 2021; Pérez Núñez et al., 2024).

The yield and efficiency of extracting bioactive substances from dairy products largely depend on a constellation of physicochemical, technological, and operational factors. Both the particle size and the pretreatment of the raw material play a decisive role. Reducing protein aggregate size and fat globules increases the surface area, facilitating solvent penetration and enhancing mass transfer rates. Nevertheless, excessive particle size reduction or aggressive pretreatments can trigger

TABLE 24.1 Indicative examples of each extraction method used for dairy product bioactive extraction.

Extraction method	Extractant and yield[a]	Conditions	Analysis method	Analytes[a]	References
Maceration	• Aqueous or aqueous ethanol solutions that offer moderate yields of soluble proteins, small peptides, and vitamins (low method selectivity)	• Room temperature or mild warming • Long contact times (hours to days) • Sample-to-solvent ratio is rather large	• Maceration is often coupled with HPLC, LC–MS, and other spectrophotometric techniques	• Soluble peptides, amino acids, water-soluble vitamins, and simple antioxidants are most often extracted at moderate-to-low yields	(Kamal et al., 2021)
Distillation [simultaneous distillation extraction (SDE)] in semihard Spanish goat cheese	• Solvents: extraction with dichloromethane and camphor as an internal standard • Nd recovery yield	• For SDE, the extracts were concentrated under nitrogenous steam to 100 μL • GC–MS was used (helium carrier gas at 24 cm/sec, 100°C)	• SDE: 10 g of cheese and 2 mL of dichloromethane were used for SDE, along with 90 μL of camphor as an internal standard (nitrogenous steam) • The organic extracts of cheeses were then subjected to GC–MS analysis of volatile composition and olfactometry	• 50 volatile compounds were identified • Short-chain fatty acids contributed the most to the aroma, especially acids (84%) and 3-methylbutanoic acid, ketones (10%), lactones (2.5%, e.g., δ-decalactone), ethyl esters of hexanoic and dodecanoic acid (1.4%), benzenes (1% e.g., phenylacetaldehyde, 1-hexanol), <1% alcohols, <1% aldehydes, and <1% furans (GC-MS) • Principal component analysis (PCA) revealed a good correlation between sensory attributes and specific volatile agents	(Poveda et al., 2008)
Acid precipitation (novel method using phosphate precipitation)	• Cow, goat, porcine, and transgenic pig milk were utilized • Phosphate salt and a freeze–thaw procedure • >90% recovery	• 0.2 mL of 1 M sodium phosphate buffer at various pH values • (5.8–8.0) was added to 0.8 mL of cow, goat, and porcine milk • Frozen at 20°C, 1 h • Thaw: 7600 × g, 10 min	• A phosphate salt and a freeze–thaw method were applied to obtain a casein-free whey protein fraction • Milk was mixed with the phosphate, frozen completely, thawed, and centrifuged to obtain the whey fraction and the casein pellet	• This fraction contained >90% yield, with a slight loss of bioactivity of the target protein • Recombinant human factor IX and hirudin from the transgenic pig milk were purified • Efficient pretreatment approach before chromatographic purification of milk • Separation of milk caseins under neutral or weakly acidic conditions	(Yen et al., 2015)
Membrane filtration [using UF in a plate-and-frame (PF)] in bovine skim milk for obtaining the highest possible milk protein concentration (MPC)	• Ultrafiltration membrane with PF • Final total solids (TS) recovery: 26.83%, 29.92%, and 34.24% for PF_{22}, PF_{50}MS, and PF_{50}HS, respectively	• UF: operated between 4°C and 9°C through four parallel loops, at 400 kPa • PF: The feed was further concentrated at 22°C (~30% TS) and at a high temperature of 50°C • UF carried on until the pressure drop reached 900 kPa for PF_{22} and PF_{50}HS and for PF_{50}MS until 30% TS was achieved	• Three replicates of UF skim milk were concentrated under four different PF settings: feed, 22°C, 50°C for medium solids, and 50°C for high solids (PF_{22}, PF_{50}MS, and PF_{50}HS, respectively)	• The average permeate flux and final TS were notably higher for the treatments conducted at 50°C compared to 22°C • Permeate fluxes of 8.76, 10.50, and 11.18 L/m^2h and 26.83%, 29.92%, and 34.24% for PF_{22}, PF_{50}MS, and PF_{50}HS, respectively • The apparent viscosity of the final retentates was 577, 1513, and 12,805 cP at a constant shear rate of 100 1/s for PF_{22}, PF_{50}MS, and PF_{50}HS, respectively • Standard plate count increased in the high-temperature PF retentates, and the overall process was ideal for improving the MPC • Nd-specific proteins or bioactives	(Mishra et al., 2025)

Continued

TABLE 24.1 Indicative examples of each extraction method used for dairy product bioactive extraction — cont'd

Extraction method	Extractant and yield[a]	Conditions	Analysis method	Analytes[a]	References
Solvent extraction [using the liquid biphasic flotation (LBF)] in expired milk	• Solvents: ethanol and dipotassium hydrogen phosphate • Recovery yield: 94.97% and separation efficiency: 86.289%	• Optimized conditions: 80% concentration of ethanol as the top phase, 150 g/L dipotassium hydrogen phosphate, and 10% (w/v) milk as the bottom phase (pH 9.15), at 7.5-min flotation and 25 cc/min	• Following the LBF system preparation, expired milk was stored in a refrigerator (2°C) to reduce bacterial activity • A 15-mL mixture of salt/milk was used as the top phase, and 15 mL of pure alcohol as the bottom phase in LBF • The LBF mixture settled for 30 s, and then the two layers were formed, pipetted, and tested for proteins	• Milk proteins: 13.64 mg/mL • The scale-up of the experiment by 40 times (to ensure commercialization) led to a recovery yield of 78.92% and a separation efficiency of 85.62% • Nd-specific proteins or bioactives	(Tham et al., 2019)
Ultrasound-assisted extraction (UAE) for kefir fermentation	• Ultrasonic sound wave effect on kefir fermentation time • Nd total yield/recovery	• UAE: 5 min continuous, 22 mm probe, 24 kHz, 400 W, and 30% amplitude	• Microbiological analysis, pH measurement, and titratable acidity (% lactic acid) were also performed	• Fermentation time was decreased by 1 h by the UAE applied in kefir fermentation • UAE improved exopolysaccharide (EPS) production rates (1.32 ± 0.02 to 1.51 ± 0.21 g/kg) and lactic acid production rates (0.14 to 0.58 ± 0.03%), but it did not affect the quality of EPS and lactic acid	(Düven et al., 2021)
Microwave-assisted extraction (MAE) [using microwave vacuum drying (MVD)] in pasteurized cream	• Microwaves were utilized for cream homogenization • Reconstitution yielded a TS content of ~43%	• Cream was diluted to 36 ± 0.3% TS with pasteurized skim milk to achieve a desirable fat content of 30% • Heated at 65°C–67°C and homogenized at 1.8, 3.5, 5.3, or 7 MPa in the first pass and 3.5 MPa in the second pass (optimal: 7/3.5 MPa) • Evaporation: 65°C–70°C (20–25 kPa)	• Dehydrated cream microstructure, color, and free fat were evaluated via scanning electron microscopy (SEM), colorimetry, and solvent extraction • Effects of homogenization and functionality were also investigated via confocal laser scanning microscopy, color, particle sizing, and texture analysis	• Reconstituted MVD cream whipped faster, was more cohesive, and firmer when two-step homogenization at 7/3.5 MPa was used • Fat globules in this cream were covered by phospholipids, which explained its similar function compared with pasteurized cream • Reconstituted MVD could potentially be utilized in cheese, butter, or ice cream • The cream can be evaporated to TS levels higher than those of skim milk • Nd specific bioactives	(Dumpler and Moraru, 2024)
Enzyme-assisted extraction (EAE) for the extraction of aflatoxin M_1 (AFM_1) from 24 different cheese samples	• EAE using proteolytic enzymes, pepsin, or pepsin–pancreatin • Solvent: HCl • The pepsin–HCl method was employed as the best method, along with the HPLC technique, and offered 96.3%, 95.4%, and 95.5% recovery at 0.25, 0.50, and 1.00 μg/kg spiking levels	• The pH was adjusted to 7.4 ± 0.2 with 1 M NaOH (3–5 mL) and 40 mL of pancreatin solution, and stirred at 37°C (3 h and 45 min) • The mixture was centrifuged at 11,700 × g for 10 min at 4°C and filtered through a folded filter paper	• 300 g of cheese portions were collected and kept at −20°C, and an aliquot of the sample extract (30 mL) was purified using an IA column • After purification through an immunoaffinity column, AFM_1 is analyzed via HPLC-FLD • EAE was compared with the standard chloroform (CH) extraction technique	• Extraction efficacy of the EAE methods was independent of the ripening time of the cheese • CH was not able to fully recover AFM_1 from ripened cheese • The pepsin–HCl method was the best for AFM_1 extraction, being simpler, avoiding solvent evaporation, dissolution, and partition in a separating funnel, as well as providing higher recoveries, a comparable limit of detection (LOD) and quantitation (LOQ), and more accurate results • The pepsin–HCl method does not use chlorinated solvents and is considered green	(Pietri et al., 2016)

Supercritical fluid extraction (SFE) with CO_2 from whey protein phospholipid (PL) concentrate (WPPC)	• SFE-CO_2 with ethanol as the co-solvent for PL enrichment, with HPLC and thin-layer chromatography • Highest amount of extracted PL: 26.26 g/100 g of fat	• 41.4 MPa and 60°C were the optimal conditions • Optimal SFE condition for a concentrated PL lipid fraction: 35.0 MPa, 40°C, and 15% ethanol co-solvent	• SFE-CO_2 was performed first, followed by SFE with ethanol as the co-solvent in the second stage • For the second stage: A 3 × 3 × 2 factorial design with several extraction pressures, temperatures, and ethanol concentrations was used to evaluate the extraction efficacy, the total PL, and the best proportion of each PL from the solids collected	• Total PLs extracted from WPPC were notably affected by ethanol concentration but were insignificantly affected by pressure and temperature conditions • High concentrations of sphingomyelin (11.07 g/100 g of fat), phosphatidylcholine (10.07 g/100 g of fat), and phosphatidylethanolamine (7.2 g/100 g of fat) were recovered, which accounted for 2–3 times more than conventional solvent extraction with ethanol • Exhausted solids after SFE were enriched with denatured protein (72% on a dry basis), with significantly higher water-holding capacity and emulsifying ability than untreated WPPC	(Sprick et al., 2019b)
Pulsed field electric extraction (PEF) for the structural analysis of milk fat globule membrane (MFGM)	• PEF was employed • Increased cream overrun by up to 69% using low-intensity PEF • PEF processing conditions (9, 15, and 21 kV/cm for 66 μs) resulted in notably higher fat yields (97.3%–97.4%)	• Cream volume /L milk was optimized by the low PEF intensity • Overrun and cream stability were optimized during whipping for 20 and 60 s, respectively, at 15,000 rpm using a high-shear mixer	• Low-temperature (9°C–12°C) PEF was analyzed in milk before cream separation at different intensities (9–27 kV/cm, 66 μs, 16–28 kJ/L) • Untreated and PEF-treated milk and obtained cream, were assessed for fat, protein, casein, lactose, and TS content, as well as particle size distribution • Sodium dodecyl sulfate–polyacrylamide gel electrophoresis (SDS–PAGE) was also utilized	• Cream volume/L milk was most efficiently increased by 31% at the low PEF intensity compared to untreated milk and cream • Overrun and stability were improved by the lowest and highest PEF intensities, achieving up to 69% enlarged overrun and up to 22% higher stability, respectively • SDS–PAGE results for the cream revealed noticeably different bands for some of the protein components, with structural changes in MFGM-, whey-, and phosphoproteins • Intense bands of xanthine oxidase, xanthine dehydrogenase, butyrophilin, bovine serum albumin, adipophilin, and glycoproteins PAS6/7 were observed at 21 kV/cm • PEF led to the reconfiguration of the cream matrix due to the different interactions	(Walkling-Ribeiro et al., 2024)
Electrodialysis (ED) [bipolar membrane ED (EDBM)] for the electroacidification of skim milk	• Sodium sulfate, sodium hydroxide in the form of pellets, and 65% w/w nitric acid were utilized • TS: 13.39 ± 1.31%, 5°C • Nd total recovery	• EBDM experiments were conducted at a constant voltage of 6.0 V (1 V/cell pair) • Constant circulation flow rates of diluate, concentrate, and electrolyte solutions were set to 70 ± 2 L/h and 55 ± 1 L/h, respectively (with a linear flow velocity of 16 ± 5 cm/s)	• The effect of temperatures 5°C–30°C was assessed • Ion transport during electroacidification by bipolar membranes (BMs) coupled with cation-exchange membranes (CMs) was also evaluated • BMs' and CMs' properties, EDBM performance, and parameters,mass flux (J), capacity (C_F), specific energy consumption (E), and current efficiency (η), were calculated	• Skim milk pH was decreased by ~14.3% through the proton ions generated due to a water-splitting reaction in the bipolar interface region • At low temperatures, 5°C and 10°C, Ca^{2+}, an important mineral in milk processing, has a higher mobility in total flux through the CM compared to higher temperatures • The highest TS: 13.39 ± 1.31%, total Ca^{2+}: 33.40 ± 1.34%, total K^+: 41.29 ± 0.83%, total P: 11.99 ± 0.56%, lactose: 9.48 ± 3.70%, and total protein contents: 11.04 ± 1.06% were observed at 5°C • The highest ash: 29.39 ± 0.68%, ash on a dry basis: 25.98 ± 0.57%, total Mg^{2+}: 35.36 ± 0.92%, and total Cl^-: 15.09 ± 0.14% were observed at 10°C, whereas the highest total SO_4^{2-}: 20.60 ± 0.19% was observed at 15°C • EDBM can be used for the electroacidification of skim milk with minimal loss of its protein and lactose value	(Merkel et al., 2024)

[a] *Nd stands for "Not defined." Yield: % and Analytes: % of the total content or concentration, if retrievable.*

degradation reactions, loss of conformational integrity, or even complete inactivation of bioactivity (Drăghici-Popa et al., 2023). Extraction conditions, including temperature, pressure, pH, and duration, critically affect both yield and compound stability. Mild processing parameters promote the efficient diffusion and solubilization of bioactives, whereas harsh conditions, such as elevated temperatures, may cause oxidation, irreversible denaturation, or chemical transformation of sensitive agents (Nielsen et al., 2024; Karrar et al., 2022).

The choice of extraction solvents is also a determining factor in maintaining bioactivity. Polar solvents, including water or hydroalcoholic mixtures, are widely applied for extracting hydrophilic components, such as polyphenols, proteins, and peptides, while nonpolar solvents are required for lipophilic molecules, such as fatty acids, carotenoids, and fat-soluble vitamins. Solvent polarity, dielectric constant, and potential for hydrogen bonding may also influence extraction selectivity and recovery rates. However, strong interactions of solvents with proteins and lipids can promote complex formation, aggregation, or precipitation, ultimately reducing both extraction yield and compound bioactivity (Kamal et al., 2023; Watanabe et al., 2022). Therefore careful optimization of solvent systems and extraction parameters is crucial to strike a balance between efficiency and the preservation of the functional activity of bioactive molecules in dairy-derived extracts.

3 Nutritional composition and bioactive profile of dairy product extracts

3.1 Nutritional composition of dairy product extracts

The nutritional composition of dairy products varies considerably depending on the type, processing, and fermentation, yet all provide a unique profile of macronutrients, micronutrients, and functional biomolecules. A plethora of proteins, peptides, lipid fractions, carbohydrates, fatty acids, vitamins, minerals, and microbial metabolites are observed in dairy products, offering many benefits, including antiinflammatory, antioxidant, antimicrobial, and several other properties (González et al., 2019; Hess et al., 2021; Bordoni et al., 2017). Milk, most commonly from cows or goats, remains the cornerstone of dairy nutrition, with cow's milk being rich in casein and whey proteins, while goat's milk contains slightly higher short- and medium-chain fatty acids (SCFAs) (Prosser, 2021; Stergiadis et al., 2019; Ceballos et al., 2009; Lambrini et al., 2020; Turkmen, 2017; Gupta et al., 2016; Collard and McCormick, 2021; Yasmin et al., 2012). Kefir, a fermented milk drink usually originating from cows, adds further value as it comprises not only milk nutrients but also a wide variety of bioactive fermentation metabolites that support gut and skin health (Gul et al., 2015; Oliveira et al., 2019; La Torre et al., 2024; Hew et al., 2023; Farag et al., 2020; Yilmaz-Ersan et al., 2018; Satir and Guzel-Seydim, 2016).

Butter, mainly composed of milk fat, provides concentrated amounts of saturated fatty acids (SFAs) and fat-soluble vitamins (e.g., A, D, E, K), thereby enhancing its protective structural potential in both nutrition and cosmetics (Vioque-Amor et al., 2023; Jinjarak et al., 2006; Cheng et al., 2023; Thorning et al., 2017; Hae-Soo et al., 2013). Moreover, cheeses represent a highly diverse group, with their contents depending on processing and maturation. More specifically, they are classified as soft (e.g., cream cheese), semihard (e.g., cheddar), and hard cheeses (e.g., Parmesan), while cottage cheese also stands out (Pozzobon and Pozzobon, 2019; Ahmed, 2016; Garrett, 1943; Manuelian et al., 2017; Hordofa, 2018; Albayrak, 2023; Sadvari et al., 2024; Kabelová et al., 2009; Abellán et al., 2012; Campos et al., 2025; Gille et al., 2018; Park et al., 2017; O'Brien and O'Connor, 2004; Sant'Ana et al., 2013; Kontodimos et al., 2023; Kawęcka and Pasternak, 2022; Innosa et al., 2020; Rampazzo et al., 2022). Finally, yogurt, whether cow- or goat-derived, combines the base nutrients of milk, containing high amounts of lactic acid and fermentation-derived bioactives (Wang et al., 2023; Ibrahim et al., 2021; Terzioğlu et al., 2023; Pappa et al., 2024; Teixeira et al., 2022; Mohammed et al., 2022; Hernandez and Park, 2014; Tremblay and Panahi, 2017; El-Abbadi et al., 2014; Khan et al., 2020; Fu et al., 2017; D'Andrea et al., 2023; Melse-Boonstra, 2020; Gille and Schmid, 2015). Table 24.2 represents a summary of the most common dairy products, milk, cheese, butter, yogurt, and kefir, highlighting their nutritional and, therefore, industrial value.

3.2 Bioactive profile of dairy product extracts

Dairy products are not only recognized as rich sources of essential macronutrients such as proteins, fats, and carbohydrates, but they also harbor a wide spectrum of bioactive compounds that extend their value beyond basic nutrition. These compounds, derived from the intrinsic components of milk and from microbial and biochemical transformations that occur during fermentation and processing, contribute to a range of functional health-promoting properties, potentially making them useful in cosmetic product formulation (Nielsen et al., 2024; Kontodimos et al., 2023). Among them, polysaccharides such as MFGMs or EPSs, protein-derived bioactives (e.g., lactoferrin, casein, and whey derivatives), microbial metabolites and bacteriocins, phospholipids and sphingolipids, sterols (e.g., cholesterol), CLA, phytoestrogens (mainly derived from the diet of the animal the dairy product is made from), organic acids (e.g., lactic or acetic acid), volatile compounds like

TABLE 24.2 Most important nutritional values of the most common dairy products.

Nutritional profile[a]	**Milk** (Prosser, 2021; Stergiadis et al., 2019; Ceballos et al., 2009; Lambrini et al., 2020; Turkmen, 2017; Getaneh et al., 2016; Collard and McCormick, 2021; Yasmin et al., 2012)		**Kefir** (Gul et al., 2015; Oliveira et al., 2019; La Torre et al., 2024; Hew et al., 2023; Farag et al., 2020; Yilmaz-Ersan et al., 2018; Satir and Guzel-Seydim, 2016)	**Butter** (Vioque-Amor et al., 2023; Jinjarak et al., 2006; Cheng et al., 2023; Thorning et al., 2017; Hae-Soo et al., 2013)	**Cheese** (Pozzobon and Pozzobon, 2019; Ahmed, 2016; Garrett, 1943; Manuelian et al., 2017; Hordofa, 2018; Albayrak, 2023; Sadvari et al., 2024; Kabelová et al., 2009; Abellán et al., 2012; Campos et al., 2025; Gille et al., 2018; Park et al., 2017; O'Brien and O'Connor, 2004; Sant'Ana et al., 2013; Kontodimos et al., 2023; Kawęcka and Pasternak, 2022; Innosa et al., 2020; Rampazzo et al., 2022)					**Yogurt** (Wang et al., 2023; Ibrahim et al., 2021; Terzioğlu et al., 2023; Pappa et al., 2024; Teixeira et al., 2022; Mohammed et al., 2022; Hernandez and Park, 2014; Tremblay and Panahi, 2017; El-Abbadi et al., 2014; Khan et al., 2020; Fu et al., 2017; D'Andrea et al., 2023; Melse-Boonstra, 2020; Gille and Schmid, 2015)	
	Cow milk (whole)	Goat milk (whole)	Cow kefir	Cow butter	Soft cow cheese	Semihard cow cheese	Hard cow cheese	Goat cheese	Cottage cow cheese	Cow yogurt	Goat yogurt
Total proteins	2.82%–3.27%	2.82%–3.48%	5.80 ± 0.10%	~0.5 g (traces)	15.66 ± 0.88–19.73 ± 1.54 g/100 g	24.82 ± 1.79–29.69 ± 1.48 g/100 g	27.67 ± 1.19–34.21 ± 1.60 g/100 g	15.78 ± 0.82–17.79 ± 1.22 g/100 g	3.41% (10.34–11.12 g/100 g)	2.89–4.25 ± 0.03%	3.18–5.04 ± 0.03%
Casein	2.14 g/100 g of milk	2.55 g/100 g of milk	+	+	+	+	+	+	+	+	+
Whey proteins	17.35 g/100 g of protein	17.30 g/100 g of protein	+	+	+	+	+	+	+	+	+
Total ash	0.65%–0.70%	0.75%–0.86%	0.73 ± 0.11%	0.09%–0.15%	1.0%–2.73%	2.31 ± 0.13–4.9%	3.4%–4.3%	2.26 ± 0.31–3.90 ± 0.06 g/100 g	0.76%–1.22%	0.39–0.82 ± 0.01%	0.59–0.87 ± 0.02%
Total fat	3.42%–3.49%	3.58%–5.23%	2.15 ± 0.05%	Solid: 37.27 ± 0.63–84.35 ± 0.38%	16.11 ± 1.32–27.65 ± 2.15 g/100 g	24.50 ± 3.87–29.58 ± 1.28 g/100 g	27.89 ± 1.18–33.50 ± 2.22 g/100 g	16.44 ± 0.73–17.12 ± 0.46 g/100 g	3.55%	2.02–4.55 ± 0.05%	2.10–4.77 ± 0.04%
Total amount of polyunsaturated fatty acids (PUFAs)	25.56%–27.3% of FAs	25.3%–25.67% of FAs	66.6 ± 4.1%/fermented milk	3.09 ± 0.11–3.72 ± 0.04% of FAs	0.67 ± 0.08–1.34 ± 0.25% of FAs	1.15 ± 0.26–1.37 ± 0.20% of FAs	1.25 ± 0.13–1.70 ± 0.20% of FAs	5.39 ± 0.24% of FAs	0.003–0.123 g/100 g	3.19 ± 0.04 mg/100 g	5.16 ± 0.01 mg/100 g
Total amount of monounsaturated fatty acids (MUFAs)	3.20%–3.97% of FAs	4.08%–4.38% of FAs	506.4 ± 34.8%/fermented milk	19.00 ± 0.11–24.11 ± 0.07% of FAs	4.25 ± 0.38–7.17 ± 0.48% of FAs	6.65 ± 1.01–7.66 ± 0.76% of FAs	7.36 ± 0.82–8.54 ± 0.40% of FAs	26.53 ± 0.47% of FAs	0.079–0.778 g/100 g	34.07 ± 0.01 mg/100 g	28.15 ± 0.02 mg/100 g
Total amount of saturated fatty acids (SFAs)	68.8%–71.24% of FAs	70.3%–70.42% of FAs	655.2 ± 34.3%/fermented milk	72.79 ± 0.18–77.28 ± 0.15% of FAs	10.31 ± 0.81–17.63 ± 1.24% of FAs	15.35 ± 2.49–18.90 ± 0.88% of FAs	17.72 ± 2.44–19.54 ± 2.17% of FAs	68.08 ± 0.67% of FAs	0.169–1.718 g/100 g	62.74 ± 0.04 mg/100 g	66.69 ± 0.03 mg/100 g

Continued

TABLE 24.2 Most important nutritional values of the most common dairy products — cont'd

Nutritional profile[a]		Milk (Prosser, 2021; Stergiadis et al., 2019; Ceballos et al., 2009; Lambrini et al., 2020; Turkmen, 2017; Getaneh et al., 2016; Collard and McCormick, 2021; Yasmin et al., 2012)		**Kefir** (Gul et al., 2015; Oliveira et al., 2019; La Torre et al., 2024; Hew et al., 2023; Farag et al., 2020; Yilmaz-Ersan et al., 2018; Satir and Guzel-Seydim, 2016)	**Butter** (Vioque-Amor et al., 2023; Jinjarak et al., 2006; Cheng et al., 2023; Thorning et al., 2017; Hae-Soo et al., 2013)	**Cheese** (Pozzobon and Pozzobon, 2019; Ahmed, 2016; Garrett, 1943; Manuelian et al., 2017; Hordofa, 2018; Albayrak, 2023; Sadvari et al., 2024; Kabelová et al., 2009; Abellán et al., 2012; Campos et al., 2025; Gille et al., 2018; Park et al., 2017; O'Brien and O'Connor, 2004; Sant'Ana et al., 2013; Kontodimos et al., 2023; Kawęcka and Pasternak, 2022; Innosa et al., 2020; Rampazzo et al., 2022)					**Yogurt** (Wang et al., 2023; Ibrahim et al., 2021; Terzioğlu et al., 2023; Pappa et al., 2024; Teixeira et al., 2022; Mohammed et al., 2022; Hernandez and Park, 2014; Tremblay and Panahi, 2017; El-Abbadi et al., 2014; Khan et al., 2020; Fu et al., 2017; D'Andrea et al., 2023; Melse-Boonstra, 2020; Gille and Schmid, 2015)	
		Cow milk (whole)	Goat milk (whole)	Cow kefir	Cow butter	Soft cow cheese	Semihard cow cheese	Hard cow cheese	Goat cheese	Cottage cow cheese	Cow yogurt	Goat yogurt
Total essential amino acids		1298.36 mg/100 g milk	1639.84 mg/100 g milk	70–634 ± 16 mg/100 g kefir	+	Total free amino acids: ~23.0–43.5 g/kg	Total free amino acids: ~52.9–96.9 g/kg	Total free amino acids: ~71.6 g/kg	Total free amino acids: ~82.43–83.03 mg/100 g	+	Essential/Total amino acid ratio: 53.55%	Essential/Total amino acid ratio: 51.66%
Total nonessential amino acids		1522.58 mg/100 g milk	1840.15 mg/100 g milk	134–991 ± 19 mg/100 g kefir	+					+		
Lactose		4.13%–4.90%	4.27%–4.52%	6.18 ± 0.49%	2.93–5.93%	LOD	LOD	LOD	4.1%–4.4%	4.93%	Carbohydrate/Lactose: 3.02%–7.14%	Carbohydrate/Lactose: 3.29%–6.20%
Total solids (TS)		11.36%	13.57%	11.41%–11.67%	0.75 ± 0.23–3.90 ± 0.34%	18— >60%	58%–69%	>60%	12.2 g/100 g	7.72–22.80%	15.25 ± 0.11%	15.59 ± 0.10%
Minerals	Potassium (K)	2.037 g/kg	1.528 g/kg	1120 ± 29 μg/g	24.0 mg/100 g	0.30 ± 0.07–1.77 ± 0.31 mg/g	1.11 ± 0.16–1.61 ± 0.30 mg/g	1.59 ± 0.10–2.11 ± 0.41 mg/100 g	1.77 ± 0.11 mg/100 g	104–137 mg/100 g	136.87 ± 0.51 mg/100 g	187.33 ± 0.48 mg/100 g
	Phosphorus (P)	0.908 g/kg	0.986 g/kg	1760 ± 28 μg/g	24.0 mg/100 g	1.93 ± 0.22–2.40 ± 0.26 mg/g	3.77 ± 0.15–4.02 ± 0.37 mg/g	4.12 ± 0.16–4.76 ± 0.29 mg/100 g	1.08 ± 0.06 mg/100 g	159–190 mg/100 g	85.33 ± 0.01 mg/100 g	92.33 ± 0.21 mg/100 g
	Magnesium (Mg)	0.113 g/kg	0.144 g/kg	111 ± 7 μg/g	2.00 mg/100 g	0.10 ± 0.01–0.14 ± 0.03 mg/g	0.21 ± 0.01–0.24 ± 0.02 mg/g	0.25 ± 0.01–0.29 ± 0.02 mg/100 g	0.07 ± 0.00 mg/100 g	8–11 mg/100 g	13.33 ± 0.52–60.5 ± 0.1 mg/100 g	13.73 ± 0.48–68.8 ± 1.3 mg/100 g
	Sodium (Na)	0.377 g/kg	0.354 g/kg	479 ± 8 μg/g	11.0 mg/100 g	1.63 ± 0.36–7.19 ± 1.26 mg/g	2.89 ± 2.22–8.03 ± 0.83 mg/g	4.85 ± 0.61–7.00 ± 1.10 mg/100 g	2.25 ± 0.52 mg/100 g	315–372 mg/100 g	47.48 mg/100 g	44.94 mg/100 g
	Calcium (Ca)	1.128 g/kg	1.066 g/kg	1020 ± 19 μg/g	15.0–24.0 mg/100 g	2.84 ± 0.40–3.26 ± 0.39 mg/g	6.33 ± 0.46–7.11 ± 0.85 mg/g	6.96 ± 0.32–8.45 ± 0.61 mg/100 g	0.64 ± 0.02 mg/100 g	83–86 mg/100 g	120.33 ± 0.14–134.2 ± 1.7 mg/100 g	125.67 ± 0.11–133.4 ± 2.7 mg/100 g

	Zinc (Zn)	3.416 g/kg	2.889 g/kg	14 ± 1 μg/g	0.09 mg/100 g	14.28 ± 2.35–18.75 ± 2.23 μg/g	26.94 ± 2.72–31.07 ± 3.37 μg/g	30.63 ± 1.73–36.59 ± 2.81 μg/100 g	2.79 ± 0.14 μg/100 g	0.4–0.47 mg/100 g	0.37 ± 0.31–1.1 ± 0.04 mg/100 g	0.32 ± 0.21–1.1 ± 0.01 mg/100 g
		0.035 g/kg	0.070 g/kg	<LOQ	Traces	0.14 ± 0.06–0.26 ± 0.04 μg/g	0.40 ± 0.07–1.66 ± 2.95 μg/g	0.35 ± 0.05–8.54 ± 2.28 μg/100 g	0.23 ± 0.02 μg/100 g	Traces	0.72 mg/100 g	0.99 mg/100 g
	Iodine (I)	0.363 g/kg	0.673 g/kg	<LOQ	Traces	Traces	Traces	Traces	Traces	Traces	<LOQ	<LOQ
	Iron (Fe)	0.214 g/kg	0.216 g/kg	6.7 ± 0.2 μg/g	0.02 mg/100 g	0.66 ± 0.11–1.33 ± 1.70 μg/g	1.40 ± 0.72–2.23 ± 0.22 μg/g	1.21 ± 0.45–1.77 ± 0.91 μg/100 g	0.73 ± 0.15 μg/100 g	0.07–0.15 mg/100 g	0.37 ± 0.42 mg/100 g	0.32 ± 0.49 mg/100 g
Vitamins	Vitamin A	21.0–126 IU/100 g	39.0–185 IU/100 g	3.56 ± 0.19 mg/100 g	2499 IU/100 g	40–345 μg/100 g	165–350 μg/100 g	270–345 μg/100 g	288–407 μg/100 g	2–37 μg/100 g	8.45 ± 1.04–55.17 ± 0.08 μg/100 g	11.84 ± 0.47 — < 70 μg/100 g
	Vitamin B_1	0.038–0.045 mg/100 g	0.048–0.068 mg/100 g	0.052 ± 0.006 mg/100 g	0.005 mg/100 g	0.02–0.05 μg/100 g	0.03–0.05 μg/100 g	~0.03 μg/100 g	~0.07 mg/100 g	0.023–0.027 mg/100 g	~0.01–0.21 mg/100 g	~0.02–0.06 mg/100 g
	Vitamin B_2	0.162 mg/100 g	0.138 mg/100 g	0.151 ± 0.02 mg/100 g	0.034 mg/100 g	0.13–0.65 μg/100 g	0.30–0.53 μg/100 g	0.28–0.44 μg/100 g	0.38–0.68 mg/100 g	0.163–0.226 mg/100 g	~0.04–0.21 mg/100 g	~0.05–0.15 mg/100 g
	Vitamin B_3	0.084 mg/100 g	0.277 mg/100 g	0.159 ± 0.02 mg/100 g	0.042 mg/100 g	0.06–0.96 μg/100 g	0.04–0.11 μg/100 g	0.10–0.12 μg/100 g	0.43–1.15 mg/100 g	0.099–0.144 mg/100 g	~0.02–0.50 mg/100 g	~0.05–0.60 mg/100 g
	Vitamin B_5	0.314 mg/100 g	0.310 mg/100 g	+	0.110 mg/100 g	0.25–0.71 μg/100 g	0.29–0.51 μg/100 g	0.31–0.43 μg/100 g	0.19–0.68 mg/100 g	+	~0.02–0.20 mg/100 g	~0.02–0.25 mg/100 g
	Vitamin B_6	0.038–0.045 mg/100 g	0.038–0.045 mg/100 g	0.024 ± 0.006 mg/100 g	0.003 mg/100 g	0.03–0.13 μg/100 g	Traces—0.13 μg/100 g	0.08–0.13 μg/100 g	0.06–0.25 μg/100 g	0.016–0.046 μg/100 g	~0.01–0.06 mg/100 g	~0.01–0.06 mg/100 g
	Vitamin B_7	2.00 μg/100 g	1.50 μg/100 g	+	Traces	1.6–7.6 μg/100 g	1.4–4.0 μg/100 g	2.3–3.3 μg/100 g	+	+	Traces	Traces
	Vitamin B_9	5.00 mg/100 g	1.00 mg/100 g	+	3.00 μg/100 g	11–102 μg/100 g	12–56 μg/100 g	12–18 μg/100 g	+	9–12 μg/100 g	~5.00–20.00 μg/100 g	~5.0–25.0 μg/100 g
	Vitamin B_{12}	0.357 μg/100 g	0.065 μg/100 g	+	0.170 μg/100 g	0.3–2.1 μg/100 g	0.9–2.1 μg/100 g	0.9–1.9 μg/100 g	12.5 ± 15.8 ng/100 g	0.43–0.46 μg/100 g	~0.10–0.60 μg/100 g	~0.05–0.40 μg/100 g
	Vitamin C	2.00–6.68 mg ascorbic acid/100 mL	2.00–5.48 mg ascorbic acid/100 mL	0.43 ± 0.02 mg/ascorbic acid per 100 g	Traces	Traces	Traces	Traces	Traces	Traces	<LOQ	Traces—2.0 mg/100 g
	Vitamin D	0.70 IU/g fat	0.70 IU/g fat	+	0.90 μg/100 g	0.03–0.50 μg/100 g	Traces—0.26 μg/100 g	0.21–0.25 μg/100 g	0.40–0.50 μg/100 g	Traces—0.1 μg/100 g	<LOQ	Traces—0.50 μg/100 g

Continued

TABLE 24.2 Most important nutritional values of the most common dairy products— cont'd

Nutritional profile[a]		Milk (Prosser, 2021; Stergiadis et al., 2019; Ceballos et al., 2009; Lambrini et al., 2020; Turkmen, 2017; Getaneh et al., 2016; Collard and McCormick, 2021; Yasmin et al., 2012)		Kefir (Gul et al., 2015; Oliveira et al., 2019; La Torre et al., 2024; Hew et al., 2023; Farag et al., 2020; Yilmaz-Ersan et al., 2018; Satir and Guzel-Seydim, 2016)	Butter (Vioque-Amor et al., 2023; Jinjarak et al., 2006; Cheng et al., 2023; Thorning et al., 2017; Hae-Soo et al., 2013)	Cheese (Pozzobon and Pozzobon, 2019; Ahmed, 2016; Garrett, 1943; Manuelian et al., 2017; Hordofa, 2018; Albayrak, 2023; Sadvari et al., 2024; Kabelová et al., 2009; Abellán et al., 2012; Campos et al., 2025; Gille et al., 2018; Park et al., 2017; O'Brien and O'Connor, 2004; Sant'Ana et al., 2013; Kontodimos et al., 2023; Kawęcka and Pasternak, 2022; Innosa et al., 2020; Rampazzo et al., 2022)					Yogurt (Wang et al., 2023; Ibrahim et al., 2021; Terzioğlu et al., 2023; Pappa et al., 2024; Teixeira et al., 2022; Mohammed et al., 2022; Hernandez and Park, 2014; Tremblay and Panahi, 2017; El-Abbadi et al., 2014; Khan et al., 2020; Fu et al., 2017; D'Andrea et al., 2023; Melse-Boonstra, 2020; Gille and Schmid, 2015)	
		Cow milk (whole)	Goat milk (whole)	Cow kefir	Cow butter	Soft cow cheese	Semihard cow cheese	Hard cow cheese	Goat cheese	Cottage cow cheese	Cow yogurt	Goat yogurt
	Vitamin E	0.041–0.226 mg/100 g	0.121 mg/100 g	0.018–0.025 mg/100 g	20.0–184.0 μg/100 mL	0.02–1.00 μg/100 g	0.39–0.78 μg/100 g	0.55–0.70 μg/100 g	0.18–0.26 mg/100 g	0.01–0.08 mg/100 g	0.07 ± 0.01–0.22 ± 0.03 mg/100 g	0.02–0.20 mg/100 g
		38.1 ± 8.6 μg/100 g	+	10.2 ± 0.3 μg/100 g	7.00 μg/100 g	~40–55 μg/100 g	~80–150 μg/100 g	~282 μg/100 g	~1.80–2.50 μg/100 g	Traces	~0.5–2.0 μg/100 g	~0.5–3.0 μg/100 g
Calories (energy)		60–64 kcal/100 g	60–70 kcal/100 g	46–50 kcal/100 g	747 kcal/100 g	~ 289–433 kcal/100 g	~300–400 kcal/100 g	~370— >400 kcal/100 g	~264–452 kcal/100 g	72–103 kcal/100 g	56–106 kcal/100 g	57 kcal/100 g

[a]*The "+" stands for indications that the nutrient exists, but no exact content information was retrieved. The "–" stands for nonretrievable information.*

alcohols, aldehydes, ketones, or esters, and bioactive peptides are predominantly detected in dairy products, followed by smaller or trace amounts of terpenes, flavonoids (primarily isoflavones), carotenoids (mainly β-carotene), and phenolic acids/polyphenols. Each one of these major classes of interest imparts antioxidant, antimicrobial, antiinflammatory, and immunomodulatory effects that depend on the type (e.g., milk, kefir, butter, cheese, or yogurt), origin (e.g., cow, goat), and processing, fermentation, and ripening method of the dairy product (Nielsen et al., 2024; Kontodimos et al., 2023).

Fermented dairy products, such as kefir (Vieira et al., 2021; Gul et al., 2015; La Torre et al., 2024; Farag et al., 2020), ripened cheeses (Santiago-López et al., 2018; Do Nascimento Rangel et al., 2023; Jonnala et al., 2021; Ni et al., 2020; Fernández-García et al., 2008; Kuhnle et al., 2008), and yogurt (Kuhnle et al., 2008; Ibeagha-Awemu et al., 2009; Liu et al., 2024; Papaioannou et al., 2021), are especially enriched in secondary metabolites formed by microbial activity, including EPSs, bacteriocins, organic acids, alcohols, aldehydes, and ketones. These molecules not only shape the sensory characteristics of dairy but also enhance their biological activity by modulating gut microbiota, improving digestive health, and providing antimicrobial defense. Similarly, lipid-derived compounds, such as CLA and sphingolipids, are consistently present in ruminant-derived products, offering well-documented cardioprotective and antiinflammatory roles. Finally, plant-derived metabolites, such as phytoestrogens, phenolic acids, and flavonoids, may also appear in trace but significant amounts, often transferred from the animal's diet, further adding to the complexity of the dairy bioactive matrix (Farag et al., 2020; Ni et al., 2020; Papaioannou et al., 2021).

Milk (Acquavia et al., 2025; Stergiadis et al., 2019; Biadała and Konieczny, 2018; ALKaisy et al., 2023; Perna et al., 2018; Rocchetti et al., 2022; Park and Nam, 2015) and butter (Vioque-Amor et al., 2023; Jinjarak et al., 2006; Hae-Soo et al., 2013; Lopez et al., 2017), although being less complex than fermented dairy, remain important carriers of bioactive agents. Milk, whether from cows or goats, contains various peptides with antimicrobial and antihypertensive properties, immunoglobulins, lactoferrins, and oligosaccharides that support gut and immune health. Butter, being fat-rich, is particularly notable for its lipid-derived bioactives such as CLA, sphingomyelin, SCFAs, and fat-soluble vitamins (A, D, E, K), which collectively contribute to cardiovascular health, immune modulation, antiinflammatory effects, and skin-protective functions. These products act as primary dietary sources of lipophilic antioxidants and lipids, presenting both nutritional value and bioactivity (Nielsen et al., 2024; Kontodimos et al., 2023).

Table 24.3 provides a comprehensive overview of the major classes of bioactive compounds reported in different dairy products, including whole cow and goat milk, kefir, butter, soft, semihard, hard, and cottage cheeses, as well as cow and goat yogurt. For each class, representative examples are listed alongside their presence or absence in each dairy product, as well as their documented biological activities. Fig. 24.2 illustrates the main bioactives of each class found in milk, kefir, butter, cheese, and yogurt dairy products.

4 Dairy product extracts in cosmetics and cosmeceuticals: A review of their skin health-promoting properties and their antiskin disease value

Dairy-derived bioactives, including proteins, peptides, vitamins, and antioxidants, contribute to antiinflammatory responses, oxidative stress reduction, tumor suppression, enhanced skin hydration, photoprotection, antiaging effects, antimicrobial defense, and immune modulation. These combined actions highlight the potential of dairy products as natural ingredients for skin care and overall health promotion (Yeom et al., 2011; Ningsih and Eka Putra, 2025; Khan et al., 2019; da Gama et al., 2018; Bhosale et al., 2019). The numerous health-promoting activities of dairy product extracts are discussed in the following subsections, while an overview of their health-promoting activities and potential cosmetic value is depicted in Fig. 24.3.

4.1 Antioxidant activity of dairy product extracts

Milk and its derivatives contain a wide range of natural antioxidants that contribute to protection against oxidative stress. These include proteins and peptides, amino acids, vitamins, and enzymes, which act independently or synergistically (Bielecka et al., 2022). Caseins and whey proteins account for approximately 80% and 20% of the total milk proteins, respectively, and are therefore the main contributors to the antioxidant activity of milk (El-Sayed and Awad, 2019; Milk protein for improved metabolic health: a review of the evidence | Nutrition & Metabolism, n.d.). Their activity is highly correlated with their amino acid content, such as methionine, cysteine, and tyrosine, which can neutralize free radicals and chelate metals. The sequence and structure of these proteins and peptides also play a crucial role in determining their antioxidant capacity (Barac et al., 2019). Fat-soluble vitamins, particularly vitamins A and E, further enhance antioxidant protection by scavenging free radicals and inhibiting lipid peroxidation in the MFGM (Mukesh et al., 2014; Rashad et al., 2011). In addition, dairy products are rich in protein-modulated enzymatic systems such as catalase and glutathione

TABLE 24.3 Bioactive compounds identified in the most common dairy product extracts.

Compound class and reported biological activity	Compound (examples)	Dairy product[a]									
		Milk (Acquavia et al., 2025; Stergiadis et al., 2019; Biadała and Konieczny, 2018; ALKaisy et al., 2023; Perna et al., 2018; Rocchetti et al., 2022; Park and Nam, 2015)		**Kefir (Vieira et al., 2021; Gul et al., 2015; La Torre et al., 2024; Farag et al., 2020)**	**Butter (Vioque-Amor et al., 2023; Jinjarak et al., 2006; Hae-Soo et al., 2013; Lopez et al., 2017)**	**Cheese (Santiago-López et al., 2018; Do Nascimento Rangel et al., 2023; Jonnala et al., 2021; Ni et al., 2020; Fernández-García et al., 2008; Kuhnle et al., 2008)**				**Yogurt (Kuhnle et al., 2008; Ibeagha-Awemu et al., 2009; Liu et al., 2024; Papaioannou et al., 2021)**	
		Cow	**Goat**	**Cow**	**Cow**	**Soft**	**Semihard**	**Hard**	**Cottage**	**Cow**	**Goat**
Poly- and oligosaccharides • Prebiotic, skin hydration, and immunomodulation	Milk oligosaccharides, exopolysaccharides (EPSs) (e.g., from kefir: kefiran), and milk fat globule membranes (MFGMs)	+	+	+/ (Strong EPS presence)	+/ (Mainly MFGMS)	+	+	+	+	+/ (Strong EPS presence)	+/ (Strong EPS presence)
Protein-derived bioactives • Antimicrobial, iron binding, antiinflammatory, antioxidant, wound healing, and collagen modulating	Lactoferrin, lactoperoxidase, β-lactoglobulin, α-lactalbumin, and immunoglobulins Casein proteins: β-, κ-, αs1-, and αs2-casein Whey proteins	+	+	+/ (Increased during fermentation)	+/ (Traces mainly concentrated in the butter's water-in-oil emulsion's < 1% milk solids component)	+	+	+	+	+	+
Microbial metabolites/bacteriocins • Antimicrobial and immunomodulatory	Nisin-type peptides, bacteriocins, and exopolysaccharides	+/ (Traces)	+/ (Traces)	+/ (Mainly bacteriocins)	-	+	+	+	+	+	+
Carotenoids and fat-soluble pigments • Antioxidant and antiaging	Carotenoids (e.g., β-carotene and lutein)	+	+/ (Goats convert it to vitamin A)	+/ (Concentrated)	+	+	+	+	+	+/ (Traces)	+/ (Traces)
Phospholipids and sphingolipids • Cell-membrane stabilization, skin barrier support, and antiinflammatory	Phosphatidylcholine and sphingomyelin	+	+	+/ (MFGM remnants)	+/ (MFGM remnants)	+	+	+	+	+/ (High)	+/ (High)

Phenolic acids (hydroxycinnamic and hydroxybenzoic acids) • Antioxidant, antiinflammatory, ultraviolet (UV)-protective, and radical scavenging	• Hydroxybenzoic acids: p-hydroxybenzoic acid, gallic acid, protocatechuic acid, syringic acid, vanillic acid, and gentisic acid • Hydroxycinnamic acids: ferulic acid, caffeic acid, cinnamic acid, and *p*-coumaric acid	+/ (Traces mainly through the diet)	+/ (Traces mainly through the diet)	+/ (Can be concentrated/modified)	+/ (Traces)	+/ (Low)	+/ (Low)	+/ (Low)	+/ (Low)	+/ (Low)	+/ (Low)
Flavonoids and flavonoid derivatives • Antioxidant, radical scavenging, anti-inflammatory, and antimicrobial	• Flavonoids: Catechin, epicatechin, rutin, quercetin, and kaempferol • Plant isoflavones (e.g., daidzein, genistein, glycitein, formononetin, and naringenin)	Traces mainly through the diet	Traces mainly through the diet	+/ (mainly plant isoflavones)	–/ (Traces)	+/ (low)	+/ (low)	+/ (low)	+/ (low)	+	+
Terpenes and terpenoids • Antioxidant, radical scavenging, anti-inflammatory, and antimicrobial	• Terpenes: (e.g., limonene, α-pinene, and *p*-cymene) • Terpenoids: limonene oxide, carvacrol, and geraniol	+	+	+/ (Traces)	+	+	+	+	+	+	+
Sterols • Antiinflammatory, membrane, and skin barrier support	• Cholesterol, animal sterol lipids, and minor phytosterols	+	+	+	+/ (High)	+	+	+	+	+	+
Phytoestrogens • Estrogenic or antiestrogenic effects, antioxidant properties, bone metabolism, cardiovascular health, anticancer benefits, and skin health	• Plant lignans (e.g., secoisolariciresinol, matairesinol, hydroxymatairesinol, and lariciresinol) • Mammalian lignans (e.g., enterolactone and enterodiol) • Coumestans (e.g., coumestrol)	+	+	+/ (Mainly lignans)	–/ (Traces)	+	+	+	+	+	+
Conjugated linoleic acid (CLA) • Antioxidant, antiadipogenic, antiinflammatory, and skin barrier support	• *Cis*-9, *trans*-11 CLA (ruminant)	+	+	+	+	+	+	+	+	+	+

Continued

TABLE 24.3 Bioactive compounds identified in the most common dairy product extracts— cont'd

Compound class and reported biological activity	Compound (examples)	Dairy product[a]									
		Milk (Acquavia et al., 2025; Stergiadis et al., 2019; Biadała and Konieczny, 2018; ALKaisy et al., 2023; Perna et al., 2018; Rocchetti et al., 2022; Park and Nam, 2015)		**Kefir** (Vieira et al., 2021; Gul et al., 2015; La Torre et al., 2024; Farag et al., 2020)	**Butter** (Vioque-Amor et al., 2023; Jinjarak et al., 2006; Hae-Soo et al., 2013; Lopez et al., 2017)	**Cheese** (Santiago-López et al., 2018; Do Nascimento Rangel et al., 2023; Jonnala et al., 2021; Ni et al., 2020; Fernández-García et al., 2008; Kuhnle et al., 2008)				**Yogurt** (Kuhnle et al., 2008; Ibeagha-Awemu et al., 2009; Liu et al., 2024; Papaioannou et al., 2021)	
		Cow	Goat	Cow	Cow	Soft	Semihard	Hard	Cottage	Cow	Goat
Organic acids and sulfur compounds • Antimicrobial, metabolic effects, keratolytic/skin exfoliant (lactic acid), and wound healing support (butyric acid)	• Lactic acid, acetic acid, butyric acid, pyruvic acid, citric acid, lactate, acetate, pyruvate, succinate, fumarate, and propionate • Sulfur Compounds (dimethylsulfone)	+	+	+/ (high lactic and acetic acid amounts)	+	+	+	+	+	+	+
Other (volatile or not) secondary metabolites • Sensory attributes, antimicrobial properties, and antiinflammatory characteristics formed during fermentation and ripening	• Alcohols (e.g., ethanol, mannitol, phenylethyl alcohol, 3-methyl-butanol, and glycerol) • Phenolic lactones (e.g., δ-caprolactone, δ-octalactone), • Ketones (e.g., diacetyl, acetoin, acetone, 2-butanone, 2-heptanone, and 2-nonanone) • Aldehydes (e.g., acetaldehyde, hexanal, nonanal, octanal, 2,3-butanedione) • Esters (e.g., ethyl acetate, ethyl decanoate, ethyl hexanoate)	+	+	+/ (mainly alcohols and acetaldehydes)	+	+	+	+	+	+	+

[a]*The "+" indicates that the nutrient exists, even in trace amounts. The "–" indicates that the nutrient does not exist.*

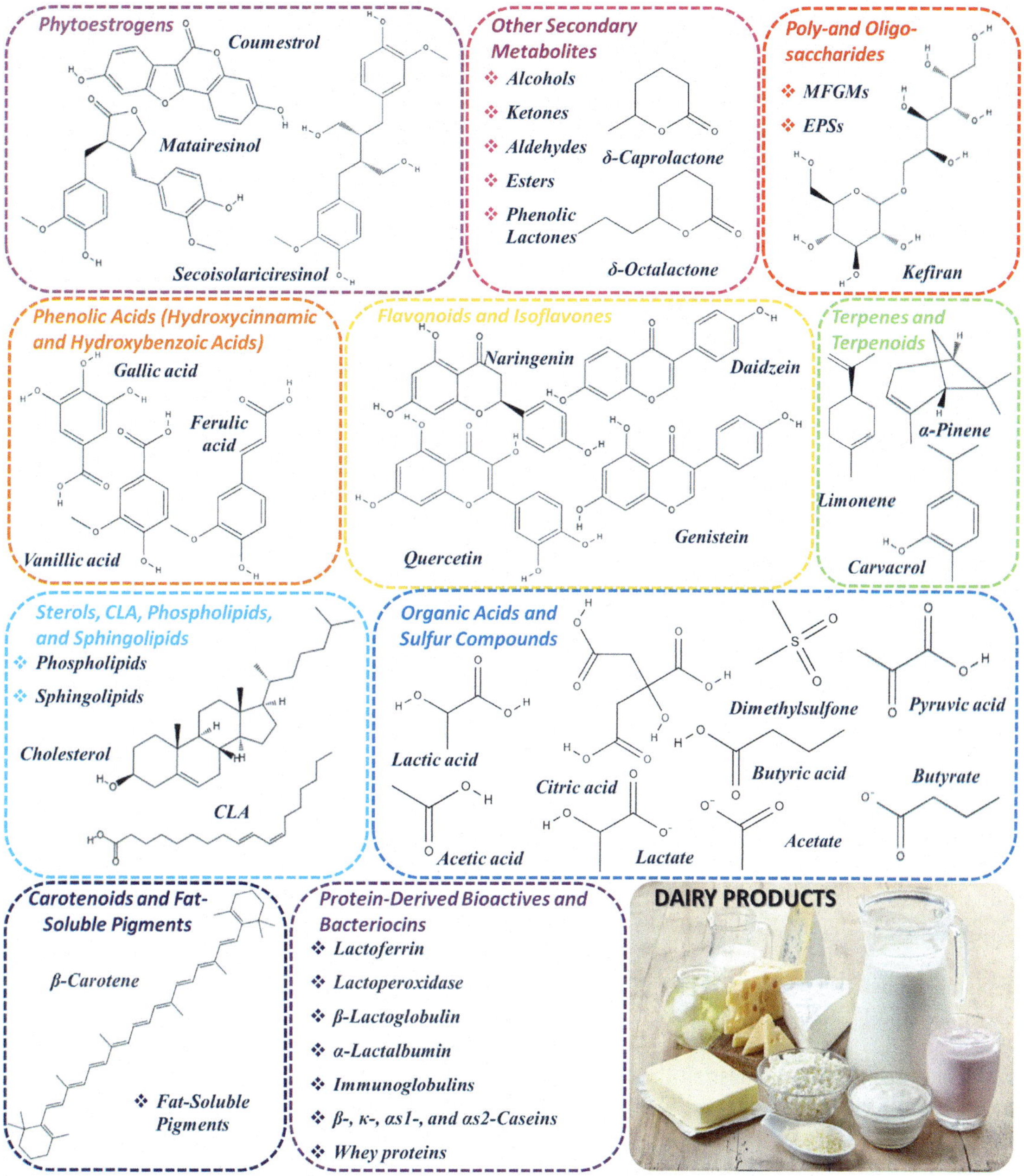

FIG. 24.2 Structural Illustration of the predominant bioactives in dairy product extracts. *(Source: Parts of this figure were obtained from the free open-access platforms: https://www.molview.org/ and https://unsplash.com/ (Accessed 19 September 2025).)*

peroxidase, which are essential for neutralizing superoxide anion radicals and reactive oxygen species (ROS) (Bielecka et al., 2022).

Oxidative stress is a key driver of premature skin aging and damage, and therefore the natural antioxidant compounds in milk and dairy products may play a protective role in maintaining skin health. More specifically, dairy product antioxidants with high antioxidant activity, including whey proteins, caseins, minerals, vitamin E, carotenoids, ascorbic acid, and enzymes, are being proposed as agents with great potential in balancing genetics-, age-, metabolism-, physical activity-, high metabolic load-, and dietary imbalances-related free radicals that trigger oxidative stress-induced diseases (Khan et al., 2019). Furthermore, ROS generated by ultraviolet (UV) radiation, environmental pollutants, and cellular metabolism accelerate collagen degradation, impair barrier function, and trigger inflammation. Bioactives from dairy have been shown to counteract these effects by enhancing skin hydration, supporting structural integrity, and strengthening cellular defenses (Tranchida et al., 2025; Papaccio et al., 2022; Lim et al., 2022).

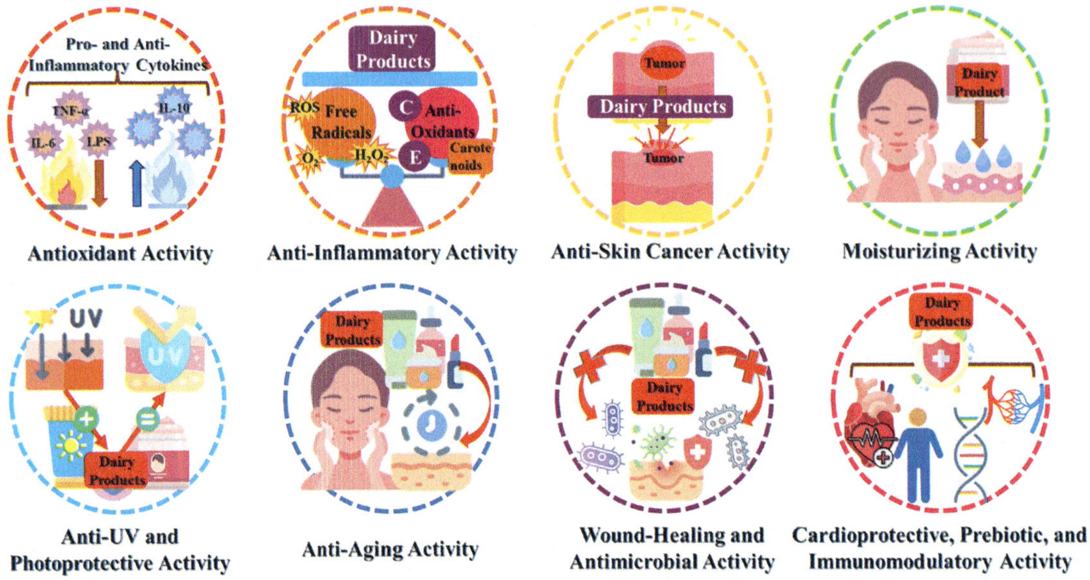

FIG. 24.3 Overview of the health-promoting activities and potential cosmetic value of dairy bioactives. *IL-6* and *IL-10*, interleukins 6 and 10; *LPS*, lipopolysaccharides; *TNF-α*, tumor necrosis factor α; *UV*, ultraviolet (radiation). *(Source: Parts of this figure were obtained from the free open-access platform https://www.flaticon.com/ (Accessed 19 September 2025).)*

Sik et al. (2023) recently published a holistic review regarding the antioxidant and polyphenol content of several dairy products, including raw milk, ricotta, and cottage cheese, as well as sweet and acid whey produced either by cows or goats. The total phenolic content (TPC) of raw milk ranged from 420.34 to 490.72 mg gallic acid equivalents (GAE)/100 mL, and the total antioxidant capacity was found to be between 8.95 and 28.72 mg ascorbic acid equivalents (AAE)/100 mL. For cottage cheeses, polyphenols ranged between 32.29 and 124.29 mg GAE/100 mL, and antioxidant values were between 14.12 and 16.38 mg AAE/100 mL. Ricotta cheeses from different types of cow milk, on the contrary, revealed antioxidant values of 10.84–15.93 mg AAE/100 mL and a polyphenol content of 10.55–19.01 mg GAE/100 mL. Marked differences were recorded for both TPC and total antioxidant capacity of sweet and sour whey, which revealed 32.29–124.29 mg GAE/100 mL and 43.50–98.03 mg GAE/100 mL values regarding their polyphenolic content, as well as 10.85–197.55 mg AAE/100 mL and 13.28–158.69 mg AAE/100 mL antioxidant capacity, respectively. In this research, it was finally concluded that dairy products from different breeds and species may exhibit significant quality differences, while whey may hold great antioxidant potential for future cosmetics, probably due to their high free radical scavenger content (Sik et al., 2023).

Yilmaz-Ersan et al. (2018), comparing the antioxidant capacity of cow and ewe kefirs, demonstrated that the mean TPC was significantly elevated during the storage periods, while heat-treated cow milk used for kefir manufacture showed the highest TPC (152.14 mg GAE/100 mL). In addition, the 1,1-diphenyl-2-picrylhydrazyl radical (DPPH) inhibition, 2,2-azinobis (3-ethylbenzothiazoline-6-sulfonic acid) (ABTS), and ferric reducing antioxidant power (FRAP) assays exhibited varying values depending on the starter culture and milk type. During fermentation, the DPPH values were 1.68 mg for ewe kefir from kefir grains (E-GR) and 9.05 mg TE/100 mL for ewe kefir from starter culture (E-CS), respectively, whereas DPPH values of 3.99 and 9.57 mg TE/100 mL were reported for cow kefir from kefir grains (C-GR) and cow kefir from starter culture (C-CS). Similarly, ABTS values were 11.34 and 32.93 mg TE/100 mL for E-GR and E-CS, respectively, and 10.25 and 22.44 mg TE/100 mL for C-GR and C-CS, respectively. Regarding the FRAP assay, E-GR and E-CS revealed 5.09 and 15.27 mg TE/100 mL, while C-GR and C-CS revealed 145.00 and 12.34 mg TE/100 mL, respectively. Finally, the vitamin E and β-carotene content was similar in all kefir samples during storage. These findings hold great promise for the health-promoting and antioxidant potential of dairy products, highlighting their potential cosmetic value, as well as the need for more in vivo studies to further evaluate such hypotheses (Yilmaz-Ersan et al., 2018).

Shori (2013) investigated the antioxidant potential of soy-enriched cow's and camel's milk yogurts, along with LAB viability and TPC. Fermentation was carried out with *Glycine max* L. soybeans, and antioxidant activity through the DPPH assay, TPC, and viable colony counts (VCC) of *Lactobacillus* spp. and *Streptococcus thermophilus* were assessed over 21 days of refrigerated storage. Both yogurts showed increased TPC (day 0:149.59 ± 1.8 and day 7:111.44 ± 2.8 μg GAE/mL for soybean–camel milk yogurt, in contrast to day 0:60.04 ± 0.01 and day 7:55.22 ± 0.01 μg GAE/mL for plain-camel milk yogurt and day 21:43.17 ± 1.2 μg GAE/mL for the soybean–cow milk yogurt), with soy-camel yogurt containing twice the phenolic content of plain camel yogurt in the first week. Antioxidant capacity rose significantly in both products, early in cow's yogurt and during the first week in camel's yogurt. VCC increased by 10% for *Lactobacillus* spp. in cow's yogurt and 30% in camel's yogurt, while *S. thermophilus* counts were consistently higher in cow's yogurt. Moreover, the highest antioxidant activity was found on day 0 for soybean-cow milk yogurt (61.76 ± 2.2%) and day 7 for soybean–camel milk yogurt (53.16 ± 0.1%). These findings highlight the antioxidant potential of fermented dairy products and demonstrate how plant enrichment can further reinforce their bioactivity and potentially, cosmetic value (Shori, 2013).

Oxidative stress is also a central mechanism in skin inflammation, cellular dysfunction, and tissue injury. Glutathione, the primary intracellular antioxidant, plays a critical role in maintaining redox balance and protecting skin integrity. Recently, a pilot clinical study evaluated whether oral supplementation with a nondenatured bioactive whey protein isolate, previously shown to elevate glutathione levels, could reduce oxidative stress in patients with psoriasis *vulgaris* (Prussick et al., 2013). Seven participants received 20 g/day of whey protein isolate for 3 months alongside their regular treatments. Clinical outcomes, assessed using the Psoriasis Area and Severity Index and photographic documentation, revealed marked improvements in skin lesions, including reduced redness, scaling, and thickness. These preliminary results suggest that this isolate may enhance antioxidant defenses and mitigate oxidative damage in the skin, underscoring the therapeutic potential of dairy-derived proteins and warranting further investigation in larger, controlled trials (Prussick et al., 2013).

4.2 Antiinflammatory activity of dairy product extracts

Inflammation is a key factor in the pathogenesis of several skin disorders, including acne, dermatitis, and eczema. The bioactive components naturally present in milk and its derivatives have been shown to possess antiinflammatory properties, potentially alleviating skin irritation and improving skin barrier function. Casein and whey proteins, in particular, release bioactive peptides during fermentation and digestion that can regulate immune responses by suppressing proinflammatory cytokines such as tumor necrosis factor α (TNF-α), interleukin 6 (IL-6), and IL-1β (Masoomikarimi and Salehi, 2022). In addition, MFGM components, including phospholipids and glycoproteins, exhibit antiinflammatory effects, supporting barrier integrity and reducing skin irritation (Kazimierska and Kalinowska-Lis, 2021; Kim et al., 2010). Fat-soluble vitamins A, D, and E further contribute by regulating immune responses and maintaining skin homeostasis (Chan et al., 2017). Clinical studies strengthen this evidence, highlighting that milk and its fermented products, enriched in bioactive peptides and metabolites, exert beneficial effects on inflammatory skin conditions (Hess et al., 2021; Bordoni et al., 2017).

A systematic overview of the effects of dairy consumption on systemic inflammation and its related diseases revealed that consuming dairy products did not adversely affect the biomarkers of low-grade systemic inflammation [e.g., C-reactive protein (CRP), TNF-α and its receptor, and monocyte chemotactic protein-1 (MCP-1)]. In addition, the inflammatory scores of markers like adiponectin, B-lymphocytes, basophils, CRP, IL-1β, IL-4, IL-5, IL-6, IL-8, IL-13, macrophages, monocytes, neutrophils, TNF-α, and the vascular cell adhesion molecule 1 (VCAM-1) were lower in dairy-based diets, with similar results observed for both low- and high-fat dairy foods. Fermented dairy foods significantly lowered inflammation biomarkers in contrast to their nonfermented counterparts, whereas dairy food consumption led to a weakly antiinflammatory effect in individuals without a sensitivity or allergy to dairy foods (Hess et al., 2021).

Several key inflammatory/immunoregulatory pathways are modulated by dairy consumption. At first, milk-derived casein hydrolyzates were shown to suppress TNF-α-induced nuclear factor κB (NF-κB) activation in endothelial cells in a peroxisome proliferator-activated receptor γ-dependent manner, inhibiting MCP-1 and IL-8 expression. Meta-analyses of dairy consumption confirm reductions in CRP, IL-6, TNF-α, and MCP-1 markers among adults (Moosavian et al., 2020). In addition, dairy consumption is correlated with adhesion molecule expression modulation, as it can lower inflammatory VCAM-1, intercellular adhesion molecule 1, and E-selectin expression (Marcone et al., 2015). Whey and casein peptide hydrolysates could also suppress IL-6, TNF-α, and IL-1β upon lipopolysaccharide (LPS) stimulation in RAW 264.7 macrophage cells, offering systemic cytokine modulation (Dalaka et al., 2024). Regarding toll-like receptor (TLR) signaling, intact and mildly hydrolyzed whey proteins activated TLR-2, 3, 5, and 9 in reporter cell lines, whereas casein hydrolysates inhibited TLR-5 and TLR-9 signaling (Kiewiet et al., 2017).

Interestingly, in abdominally obese adults, whey, casein, and medium-chain SFAs from milk modulated adipokine signaling (including adiponectin, leptin, and MCP-1), positively influencing low-grade inflammation in adipose tissue in obese or metabolic syndrome (MS) contexts (Bohl et al., 2016). Milk bioactive peptides, such as αS2-casein, have suppressed the Janus kinase (JAK)/signal transducer and activator of transcription 3 (STAT3) signaling pathway phosphorylation, while CLA, abundant in milk fat, notably downregulated the IL-6/JAK2/STAT3 signaling, particularly in colon inflammation and cancer models (Rohmah et al., 2015). Finally, whey proteins can activate Akt signaling in keratinocytes and fibroblasts, contributing to skin repair and antioxidant defense, while β-lactoglobulin peptides may inhibit phosphoinositide 3-kinase

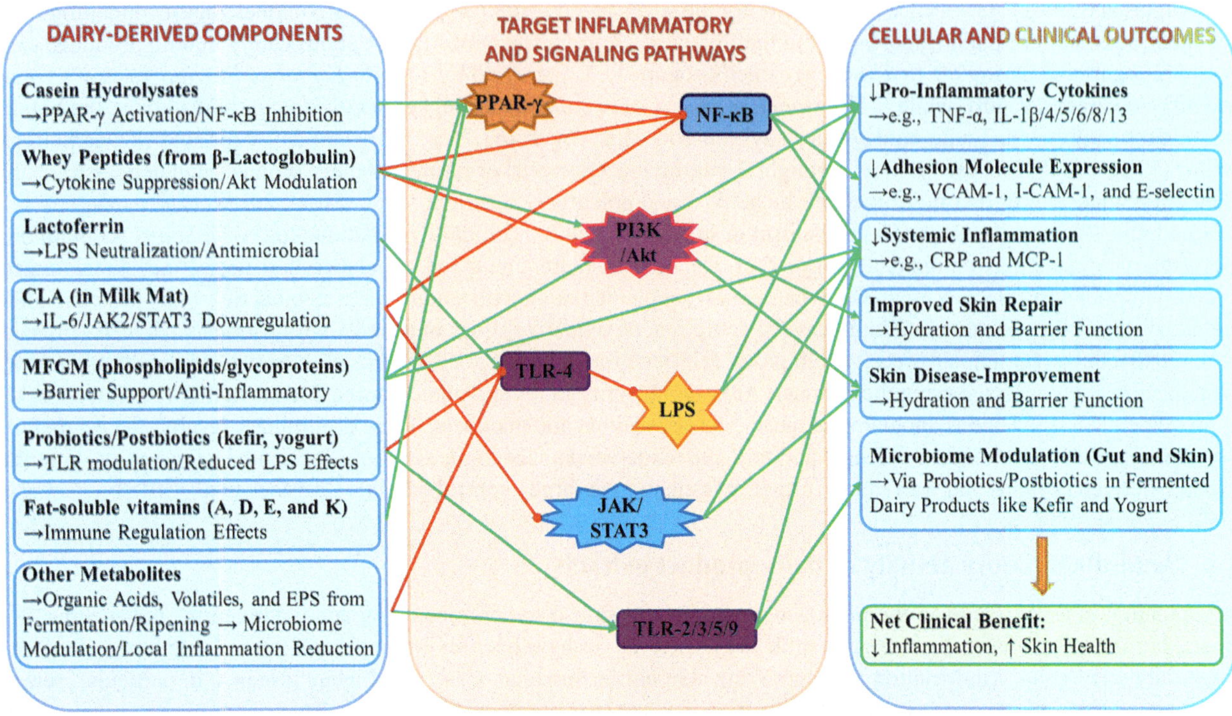

FIG. 24.4 Mechanistic overview of the inflammatory signaling modulation by dairy-derived bioactives. *(Source: Parts of this figure were obtained from the free open-access platform https://www.flaticon.com/ (Accessed 19 September 2025).)*

(PI3K) phosphorylation, and casein/whey hydrolysates can notably reduce LPS-induced cytokine release, modulating the NF-κB signaling. Fig. 24.4 provides a mechanistic overview of how dairy bioactives target inflammatory and signaling pathways, leading to positive cellular and clinical outcomes (Sik et al., 2023; Sun et al., 2024).

Chan et al. conducted a randomized, placebo-controlled clinical trial to evaluate the efficacy of lactoferrin in combination with vitamin E and zinc for the treatment of moderate acne *vulgaris*. A total of 168 participants received capsules containing 100 mg of lactoferrin, 11 IU of vitamin E, and 5 mg of zinc daily for 3 months, while the placebo group received starch capsules. The intervention group showed a significant reduction in total acne lesions, with a 14.5% decrease by week 2 and up to 28.5% by week 10. Comedone reduction reached 32.5%, while inflammatory lesions decreased by 44% compared with the placebo. Improvements in smear grade were also observed by week 12, though no further significant changes occurred at trial completion. These findings demonstrate that twice-daily administration of lactoferrin with vitamin E and zinc can notably reduce acne lesions, offering a safe, natural approach to acne management (Chan et al., 2017).

Another placebo-controlled clinical trial investigated the effects of whey powder combined with a spray-dried water extract of field dodder in adults with moderate-to-severe atopic dermatitis over 15 days. Assessments were conducted at baseline, after treatment, and 15 days postdiscontinuation (follow-up). By the end of the follow-up period, the intervention group experienced a significant increase in skin moisture and elasticity compared with the placebo. Itching was markedly reduced after 15 days, with further improvements noted during follow-up. While pigmentation changes did not significantly differ between groups, the intervention group showed a gradual decrease over time. In addition, no significant alterations in skin pH or sebum production were observed. Overall, short-term supplementation with whey powder improved skin elasticity, reduced itching, and enhanced overall skin appearance, revealing the vast potential of dairy products in providing a natural alternative to skin-related cosmetics and potentially managing inflammatory skin conditions (Mehrbani et al., 2015).

4.3 Antiskin cancer activity of dairy product extracts

Growing scientific interest in dairy-derived bioactive compounds has unveiled their potent role in managing chronic conditions, including cancer. Melanoma, a type of skin cancer, stands out as the most aggressive form due to its high metastatic ability and resistance to conventional therapies (Patel et al., 2021). The primary cause of melanoma is UV radiation, which induces DNA damage in skin cells, although genetic predisposition also plays a crucial role. Recent research indicates that dairy product extracts, particularly those enriched with peptides, lipids, and antioxidants, exhibit significant anticancer action through multiple mechanisms, including oxidative stress regulation, suppression of proinflammatory signaling, and modulation of immune system responses (Rodríguez-Alcalá et al., 2017; Flis et al., 2025a, 2025b; Parodi, 2001).

Emerging insights further emphasize the complex bidirectional relationship between cancer and thrombosis (cancer-associated thrombosis), which represents a leading cause of morbidity and mortality among cancer patients (Tsoupras et al., 2024). While malignancies are known to induce hyperoxygenation through the release of prothrombotic agents, platelet activation, and endothelial dysfunction, coagulation processes themselves appear to facilitate cancer progression (Xulu and Augustine, 2022; Liao et al., 2023). Microclots can shield circulating tumor cells from immune surveillance, thereby enhancing metastatic potential, while the thrombosis-associated proinflammatory and hypoxic microenvironment promotes angiogenesis and tumor growth. Although thrombosis does not directly cause carcinogenesis, it plays a critical role in maintaining tumor growth and enhancing metastatic capacity (Pavlovic et al., 2023; Tsantes et al., 2024). Considering that hypercoagulability and thrombotic events are often linked to cancer progression and metastasis, dairy-derived agents may reduce platelet aggregation and modulate coagulation cascades, highlighting an additional therapeutic avenue of significant clinical interest (Lordan and Zabetakis, 2017; Lordan et al., 2017).

A 2019 study evaluated the antithrombotic and hypocholesterolemic properties of milk fermented with specific *Lactococcus lactis* strains, both before and after simulated gastrointestinal digestion (SGD). The experimental design involved fermentation with three distinct *L. lactis* strains (Lc-571, Lc-572, and Lc-600), followed by the preparation of <3 kDa water-soluble fractions (WSF) for analysis. Antithrombotic activity was assessed through thrombi-induced fibrin polymerization, while anticoagulant potential, micellar cholesterol solubility, and bile acid-binding capacity were also examined. The results demonstrated strain-specific effects on bioactivities: milk WSFs fermented with Lc-572 had strong antithrombotic action (0.049 mg/mL) and pronounced hypocholesterolemic effects, including a 55% reduction in micellar cholesterol solubility and a 27% increase in bile acid binding. Lc-571 milk primarily conferred antithrombotic activity (0.045 mg/mL), whereas its Lc-600 counterpart mainly showed hypocholesterolemic effects, with 31.4% inhibition of micellar cholesterol solubility and 70% bile acid binding. Importantly, these bioactivities remained stable after simulated digestion, indicating that the functional properties were resistant to gastrointestinal conditions and likely bioavailable. Collectively, these findings suggest that fermented milk containing specific *L. lactis* strains may provide functional ingredients capable of reducing thrombosis and cholesterol, thus contributing to cardiovascular and oncological health (Rendon-Rosales et al., 2019).

Hwang et al. investigated the anticarcinogenic properties of CLA, focusing on its role in tumor promotion in mouse skin. Using HR-1 hairless mice, the researchers topically applied the *cis*-9, *trans*-11 CLA isomer (9*Z*, 11*E*-CLA) and induced tumor promotion with 12-O-tetradecanoyl-phorbol-13-acetate (TPA, 10 nmol). Tumor-promoting activity was evaluated via cyclooxygenase-2 (COX-2) expression, a key enzyme upregulated in carcinogenesis, and NF-κB signaling, as well as upstream pathways, including IκB kinase (IKK), PI3K–Akt, and mitogen-activated protein kinases (MAPKs) (extracellular signal-regulated kinases (ERKs) and *p38*). The results revealed that 9*Z*, 11*E*-CLA significantly suppressed TPA-induced COX-2 expression by inhibiting NF-κB activation. Mechanistically, CLA prevented IκBα phosphorylation and degradation, thereby blocking NF-κB nuclear translocation and DNA binding. Moreover, CLA reduced the phosphorylation of ERK, *p38* MAPK, and Akt, indicating broad modulation of proinflammatory and tumor-promoting signaling. Further analysis showed that 9*Z*, 11*E*-CLA attenuated the phosphorylation and catalytic activity of IKKα/β, a critical upstream regulator of NF-κB. Co-treatment with the IKKβ-specific inhibitor SC-514 confirmed that IKK suppression mediated reductions in Akt and NF-κB activation, as well as COX-2 expression. Taken together, these findings demonstrate that 9*Z*, 11*E*-CLA inhibits tumor promoter-induced COX-2 expression by blocking the IKK/NF-κB and PI3K–Akt pathways in vivo. This mechanistic evidence supports the antitumor-promoting and antiinflammatory potential of CLA as a bioactive, dairy-derived compound, particularly in skin cancer prevention (Hwang et al., 2007).

4.4 Moisturizing properties of dairy product extracts

Maintaining adequate skin hydration is a fundamental aspect of dermatological health, directly influencing skin barrier integrity, elasticity, and overall resilience against risk factors such as microorganisms and environmental stressors. Beyond conventional moisturizers, natural bioactives derived from dairy products have gained increasing attention for their potential to enhance skin hydration. Among these, dairy proteins and lipids are particularly important, as they provide structural and functional components that can efficiently interact with the skin barrier and regulate skin hydration processes (Ahn et al., 2022a; Augustyniak et al., 2023). Dairy lipids, especially phospholipids and ceramide precursors, may strengthen the lipid matrix of the *stratum corneum*, reducing transepidermal water loss (TEWL) and improving skin hydration. Meanwhile, dairy proteins, including casein and whey fractions, exhibit moisturizing properties by binding water molecules and enhancing the skin's natural moisturizing factor (Davoodi et al., 2016).

Sweet whey, a cheese by-product, is recognized for its antioxidant and antiinflammatory properties, primarily attributed to its high content of bioactive peptides derived from whey proteins. To explore its cosmetic potential, Sobkowska et al. conducted an in vivo study assessing the moisturizing effects of sweet whey baths and wet wraps on human skin. Thirteen healthy adult women without dermatological disorders participated in the trial. Each underwent sweet whey baths (65 g dissolved in 935 g of water) applied to the inner forearm for 20 min, while whey-soaked wet wraps were applied to the left cheek. A control group underwent the same procedure with tap water. The results revealed that whey baths significantly improved skin barrier function compared to tap water, demonstrating a notable reduction in TEWL. On the facial skin, enhanced hydration was observed, surpassing the effects seen on the forearm. No significant alterations in melanin content, skin pH, or erythema were detected, suggesting that the treatment preserved the natural skin balance. These findings support sweet whey as an effective natural moisturizing ingredient capable of reducing TEWL and strengthening the skin barrier (Sobkowska et al., 2021).

In a 2024 randomized, placebo-controlled, double-blind clinical trial, the effects of a cosmetic cream enriched with 15% lyophilized sheep colostrum on skin hydration and overall skin quality were evaluated in 52 women aged 40–70 years. Participants applied either the colostrum-enriched cream or a placebo for 8 weeks. Skin hydration was measured using a corneometer, while TEWL was assessed as an indicator of barrier function. Additional parameters, such as skin elasticity, sebum production, erythema, and skin tone, were also monitored. The results showed a significant improvement in skin hydration in the colostrum group, with an increase of 15.2 units (35.9–51.1), whereas the placebo group exhibited only a minor, nonsignificant change. TEWL values indicated improved barrier function, and increased skin elasticity suggested enhanced firmness. These effects were attributed to the bioactive components of sheep colostrum, including immunoglobulins, lactoferrin, growth factors, and milk peptides. Participants also reported subjective improvements, such as greater softness, reduced redness, and decreased sensitivity. Collectively, these outcomes highlight their potential as effective moisturizing and skin-rejuvenating agents (Kazimierska et al., 2024).

4.5 Anti-UV and photoprotective properties of dairy product extracts

UV radiation is one of the primary environmental factors responsible for accelerated skin aging, DNA damage, and oxidative and inflammatory stress in skin cells (Chen et al., 2021; Liu et al., 2019). Recent research has demonstrated that bioactive compounds naturally found in milk, particularly peptides released from casein and whey proteins, possess photoprotective properties (Xie et al., 2022). These peptides exert antioxidant and antiinflammatory effects, helping neutralize UV-produced ROS. Milk proteins, lipids, and specific amino acids, such as tryptophan and tyrosine, are also capable of directly absorbing UV radiation, contributing to the skin's natural photoprotection (Ahn et al., 2022a; Biter et al., 2019; Fohely et al., 2021). Moreover, vitamins present in milk reinforce UV-protective effects by scavenging free radicals and preventing lipid peroxidation (Ambagaspitiya et al., 2024; Ahn et al., 2022b). Clinical and preclinical studies support the notion that milk-derived peptides and compounds enhance the skin's tolerance to UV damage by increasing its antioxidant capacity and improving skin hydration.

A 2022 clinical study investigated the photoprotective effects of sphingomyelin-rich milk phospholipids against UVB-induced skin damage in a hairless mouse model. The mice were divided into five groups: one receiving a saline solution without UVB exposure, one exposed to UVB with saline treatment, and three intervention groups exposed to UVB radiation while receiving low (50 mg/kg, ML), medium (100 mg/kg, MM), or high (150 mg/kg, MH) doses of milk phospholipids daily for 3 months. In the control group, UVB exposure caused visible erythema, wrinkle formation, and increased skin thickness and roughness. In contrast, the intervention groups showed markedly reduced skin alterations, with the MH group exhibiting the strongest suppression of erythema and wrinkle depth. UVB exposure significantly reduced skin moisture and increased TEWL, while phospholipid supplementation preserved hydration and decreased TEWL. Moreover, UVB exposure downregulated hyaluronic acid (HA)-synthesizing enzymes (HAS), leading to reduced skin tissue HA levels, whereas phospholipid supplementation restored HA levels by reactivating HAS. These results indicate that sphingomyelin-rich milk phospholipids exert broad photoprotective effects, alleviating UVB-induced symptoms, improving hydration, and restoring skin barrier integrity dose-dependently, with the greatest efficacy observed at higher doses (Ahn et al., 2022b).

Kimura et al. (2014) further examined the protective effects of orally administered WP against chronic UVB-caused skin aging in male hairless melanin-deficient mice. Four groups were included: a control group without UVB exposure or supplementation, and two treatment groups receiving WP orally twice daily at 200 and 400 mg/kg for 17 weeks. The mice's back skin was exposed to 36–180 mJ/cm^2 UVB radiation three times a week to induce photoaging. UVB exposure significantly increased skin thickness, promoted wrinkle formation, and reduced elasticity. WP administration counteracted these changes, dose-dependently, with the 400 mg/kg dose providing the strongest protection. Biomarker analyses revealed that UVB exposure elevated matrix metalloproteinases (MMP-2, pro-MMP-9), vascular endothelial growth factor, the proliferation marker Ki-67, and oxidative DNA damage marker 8-hydroxy-2-deoxyguanosine. WP treatment inhibited these markers, thereby preventing collagen degradation, DNA damage, and excessive angiogenesis. In addition, WP supplementation could maintain type IV collagen integrity and decrease oxidative stress-associated damage. These findings indicate the significant photoprotective potential of WP through the modulation of proaging signaling pathways, supporting their application in skin care and cosmetics (Kimura et al., 2014).

A more recent 2024 clinical study evaluated the effects of whey protein supplementation like yak whey protein (YWP) on UV-induced skin photoaging and gut microbiota regulation in hairless mice. The mice were exposed to a controlled combination of UVA and UVB radiation and divided into five groups: a negative control group (sterile water), a UVR-exposed control group (UVR, sterile water), and three treatment groups receiving low-dose YWP [YWP-L, 200 mg/kg body weight (BW)], medium-dose YWP (YWP-M, 400 mg/kg BW), or high-dose YWP (YWP-H, 800 mg/kg BW). YWP supplementation notably reduced wrinkle formation, minimized dehydration, and improved skin barrier integrity compared to UVR-only controls. Biochemical analyses revealed potent antioxidant effects, as YWP decreased oxidative stress skin biomarkers and proinflammatory cytokine levels, including IL-1α, IL-6, and TNF-α. YWP also inhibited MMP-1, 3, and 12 expression, hence promoting the preservation of type I and III collagen and elastin fibers. In addition, YWP modulated gut microbiota composition, increasing beneficial bacterial populations such as *Lachnospiraceae* NK4A136, unclassified *Clostridiales*, and *Alistipes*. Collectively, these results demonstrate that YWP exerts UV-protective, antiinflammatory, and antioxidant effects, while enhancing collagen integrity and skin resilience, making whey proteins highly promising bioactives for dermocosmetic applications (Wang et al., 2024).

4.6 Antiaging activity of dairy product extracts

Dairy extracts have gained considerable attention for their potential role in preserving skin firmness and structure. Numerous environmental factors, including UV radiation and pollutants, as well as intrinsic physiological processes, contribute to premature skin aging by accelerating collagen degradation and impairing skin barrier function (Bocheva et al., 2023; D'Orazio et al., 2013; Tang et al., 2024). Milk and its derivatives are rich in bioactive compounds that promote collagen synthesis and overall skin health, as demonstrated by a growing body of clinical evidence. More specifically, colostrum, milk ceramides (waxy lipid molecules), and fractions of fermented dairy products have been shown to enhance skin hydration, improve elasticity, and reduce wrinkle formation (Ahn et al., 2022b; Playford and Weiser, 2021; Arslan et al., 2021).

Ahn et al. (2024) conducted a randomized, placebo-controlled clinical trial to evaluate the effects of oral milk ceramide supplementation on skin health, focusing on hydration, elasticity, and periorbital wrinkle reduction. Sixty healthy women aged 30–35 years participated in this 12-week intervention. The treatment group received 600 mg/day of milk ceramides, while the control group received a taste- and appearance-matched placebo. At the study's conclusion, the intervention group showed a significant increase in skin hydration and elasticity compared to the placebo group. Notably, digital imaging assessments confirmed a reduction in the depth and severity of eye wrinkles. TEWL was also reduced in the intervention group, reflecting improved barrier function. Profilometric analysis further revealed enhanced smoothness and reduced skin roughness. These findings confirm that oral supplementation with milk ceramides can effectively reduce wrinkle formation and improve key parameters of skin quality, serving as potential active ingredients in future commercial antiwrinkle creams and serums (Ahn et al., 2024).

Another study investigated the effects of bovine milk on collagen production and its potential antiaging properties in human skin fibroblasts. Fibroblasts were cultured and exposed to varying concentrations of commercial bovine milk, followed by measurements of cell proliferation and collagen-associated gene expression. The results showed that bovine milk substantially stimulated collagen type I synthesis, increasing fibroblast proliferation by approximately 2.3-fold at an effective concentration (EC_{50}) of 2.5% milk. Mechanistic analysis revealed that this effect was mediated through the activation of the STAT6 signaling pathway, and pharmacological inhibition of STAT6 abolished collagen production. The study concluded that bovine milk agents can enhance collagen synthesis via STAT6 signaling, underlining its potential application in antiaging skincare products and reinforcing the broader utility of milk-derived ingredients in promoting skin health (Kippenberger et al., 2015).

4.7 Wound healing and antimicrobial activity of dairy product extracts

Certain dairy components have demonstrated potent therapeutic properties in wound healing and antimicrobial defense. Among these are lactoferrin, immunoglobulins, and lipids, bioactive compounds able to promote tissue regeneration, enhance collagen synthesis, and modulate immune responses, all of which are critical processes in wound repair. In addition, dairy-derived compounds possess a broad spectrum of antimicrobial properties. For example, lactoferrin is known to bind iron, inhibit bacterial proliferation, and prevent viral spread, while milk peptides can disrupt microbial membranes and block pathogen adherence (Kell et al., 2020; Guha et al., 2021; Mohanty et al., 2016). Recent clinical studies into dairy-based topical formulations provide growing evidence of accelerated wound closure, strong antimicrobial defense, and improved skin recovery (Soutelino et al., 2024).

Brück et al. (2003) evaluated the benefits of milk-derived proteins on intestinal infection resistance in newborn rhesus macaques. Subjects were divided into four feeding groups from birth to 5 months: breastfed, fed with powdered milk, or powdered milk supplemented with either GMP or α-LA. Weekly blood and rectal samples were collected to monitor microbial composition, and at 4.5 months, all groups underwent oral provocation with 10^8 units of *Escherichia coli* O127. Significant differences emerged: breastfed and α-LA-supplemented infants exhibited no diarrhea, suggesting a protective effect, whereas GMP-supplemented infants experienced periodic diarrhea, and the control group developed acute diarrhea. Fecal smear analysis confirmed that diet affected the colonic microbiome, both before and after infection, with α-LA diminishing *E. coli* colonies and enhancing host resistance (Brück et al., 2003).

In a 2022 experimental study, researchers developed lactoferrin-enriched cheddar cheese to combine the nutritional and antimicrobial effects of whey protein with a widely consumed product. Cheeses were fortified with lactoferrin at 5, 10, 15, and 20 mg/100 g (T1–T4) and aged for 3 months. The results revealed that lactoferrin did not negatively affect the compositional or sensory properties but conferred clear antimicrobial activity. T3 and T4 groups demonstrated significantly decreased microbial counts (6.51 and 6.21 log CFU/mL, respectively) compared to the control (7.9 log CFU/mL). Furthermore, lactoferrin antioxidant activity also increased with lactoferrin concentration, with T4 reaching 78.82% compared to 45.79% in the control. Compositional analysis confirmed no alterations in fatty acid profiles, organoleptic quality, or oxidative stability, supporting the feasibility of functionalizing cheddar cheese with lactoferrin (Adnan et al., 2023).

Mudgil et al. (2022) further investigated the antifungal effects of whey and casein hydrolysates from camel and cow milk against clinically relevant *Candida* species. Hydrolysates were prepared using alcalase and protease for different durations (2, 4, and 6 h). While intact casein proteins showed no activity against *Candida albicans*, certain hydrolysates exhibited remarkable antifungal potency. Camel casein hydrolysate (2 h) achieved 93.69% inhibition against *C. albicans*, followed by cow casein hydrolysate treated with protease (81.66%), both outperforming fluconazole (76.92%). Against *Candida krusei*, several 2–6-h hydrolysates and cow whey hydrolysate (6 h, alcalase) exceeded fluconazole efficacy. For *Candida parapsilosis*, however, only the 4- and 6-h hydrolysates showed moderate inhibition (19.31% and 23.82%, respectively), which were lower than fluconazole (29.86%) (Mudgil et al., 2022).

4.8 Other health-promoting benefits of dairy product extracts

Beyond the basic benefits of dairy-derived components, recent research has revealed a wider spectrum of bioactive properties with significant implications for both skin and overall health. These include prebiotic effects, immune system regulation, and cardiovascular and metabolic benefits. Although still in the early stages, experimental and clinical findings broaden the role of dairy bioactive substances from simple protective agents to multifunctional determinants of systemic and dermatological wellness (González et al., 2019; Geniselli da Silva et al., 2024).

Modern dietary habits, characterized by a high intake of ultra-processed foods and frequent antibiotic use, inevitably disrupt the gut microbiome. Fermented dairy products represent a natural, food-based strategy for restoring microbial balance, as they provide probiotics and metabolites that reinforce intestinal barrier integrity and regulate immune responses (González et al., 2019; Geniselli da Silva et al., 2024). Clinical and preclinical studies have shown that regular consumption of fermented dairy products improves microbial diversity, increases SCFA levels, and reduces cardiometabolic risk markers such as low-density lipoprotein (LDL) cholesterol and fasting glucose (Companys et al., 2020). Öneş et al. (2025) conducted a controlled clinical trial to assess the effects of daily kefir consumption on the gut microbiome, body composition, and athletic performance in professional female soccer players. Twenty-one athletes were divided into two groups and assigned either to consume 200 mL/day of kefir or maintain their usual diet. At the end of the trial, the intervention group showed a significant increase in microbial diversity, with notable rises in *Akkermansia muciniphila* and *Faecalibacterium prausnitzii*, gut bacteria associated with improved energy metabolism and antiinflammatory activity. These microbial alterations correlated positively with enhanced athletic performance, improved body composition, and higher dietary fiber and protein intake (Öneş et al., 2025).

Several milk proteins also exert strong immunomodulatory effects essential for maintaining health. For instance, lactoferrin binds free iron, creating an unfavorable environment for pathogenic bacterial growth while simultaneously regulating cytokine production to balance pro- and antiinflammatory responses. Lysozyme, in contrast, directly targets bacterial cell walls, enhancing antimicrobial defense (Kell et al., 2020; Ferraboschi et al., 2021). Together, these proteins support both innate and adaptive immunity by stimulating macrophages and T-cell responses, thereby strengthening host defenses.

Through these mechanisms, they not only reduce susceptibility to infections but also regulate inflammatory pathways, ultimately preventing skin barrier impairment due to chronic inflammation (Séverin and Wenshui, 2005; Krissansen, 2007). Rusu et al. (2009) conducted an in vitro study to evaluate the direct and indirect effects of cow's milk serum-purified whey protein extract (WPE) on neutrophil functions, which are central to innate immunity. Using acid precipitation and MF, researchers obtained an 85% protein white powder. HPLC analysis revealed β-lactoglobulin (370 μg/mg), α-LA (25 μg/mg), lactoferrin (14 μg/mg), and bovine serum albumin (13 μg/mg) as the main components. Human blood neutrophils pretreated with WPE for 24 h were then assessed for their natural immune functions. Although WPE did not exert direct effects, pretreatment significantly enhanced neutrophil chemotaxis, superoxide production, degranulation, and phagocytosis dose-dependently in response to *N*-formyl-methionine-leucine-phenylalanine. β-Lactoglobulin and α-LA were the main active components, with GMP amplifying their effects. These findings suggest that WPE may prime neutrophils, improving their responsiveness to subsequent stimulation and thus enhancing innate immune defenses (Rusu et al., 2009).

MS is defined as a cluster of interrelated metabolic abnormalities, including obesity, elevated blood pressure, hyperglycemia, high triglycerides, and low high-density lipoprotein (HDL) cholesterol levels. Individuals with MS have a significantly increased risk of developing cardiovascular diseases (CVDs), such as coronary artery disease, type II diabetes, and stroke. MS reflects a state of chronic low-grade inflammation coupled with insulin resistance, contributing to endothelial dysfunction, atherogenesis, and lipid metabolism impairment. Epidemiological studies consistently demonstrate that MS predisposes individuals to higher CVD incidence, making its prevention and management a global public health priority. Dairy product consumption has been linked to a reduced risk of MS (Pfeuffer and Schrezenmeir, 2007). Dairy proteins contain bioactive peptides capable of regulating blood pressure, improving insulin sensitivity, and modulating inflammatory pathways. Fermented dairy provides probiotics and prebiotics that beneficially shape gut microbiota, influencing systemic metabolism and cardiometabolic health (Mena-Sánchez et al., 2019).

Interestingly, in a 2021 clinical trial, the effects of probiotic kefir on physiological and biochemical markers in MS individuals were investigated. Forty-eight MS patients were assigned either to consume kefir and curd (1.6 mL/kg for men, 1.0 mL/kg for women) for 12 weeks or to receive a placebo. The kefir group showed significant improvements in multiple cardiometabolic parameters: reductions in blood pressure, fasting glucose, LDL-cholesterol, non-HDL cholesterol, triglycerides, and oxidized-LDL cholesterol, alongside increases in HDL-cholesterol. In addition, kefir intake was associated with a reduction in the estimated 10-year CVD risk (da Silva Ghizi et al., 2021). Similarly, Bellikci-Koyu et al. (2022) examined daily probiotic kefir consumption on anthropometric, biochemical, and inflammatory markers in MS patients. Participants consumed either 180 mL/day of probiotic kefir or unfermented milk for 3 months. The kefir group showed a 4% increase in serum apolipoprotein A1 concentrations, while the milk group experienced a 2.4% decrease. Among participants with baseline LDL-cholesterol levels above 130 mg/dL, kefir intake reduced serum LDL-cholesterol and apolipoprotein B concentrations by 7.6% and 5.4%, respectively, though differences relative to the milk group were not statistically significant. Both groups revealed reductions in systolic and diastolic blood pressure. Importantly, kefir also led to significant decreases in inflammatory and cardiovascular risk biomarkers, including IL-6, IL-10, and homocysteine (Bellikci-Koyu et al., 2022).

5 Dairy product extract applications in natural cosmetic formulations

Dairy product extracts, rich in bioactive proteins, peptides, and growth factors, are gaining increasing attention in the development of natural cosmetics. Their unique composition provides multiple benefits for skin health, including hydration, antioxidant protection, antiinflammatory activity, and stimulation of collagen synthesis. These properties are increasingly harnessed through the incorporation of dairy-derived ingredients into cosmetic formulations, where they function both as active agents and as natural enhancers of skin texture and resilience. The primary aim of these formulations is to utilize the functional potential of milk peptides, whey proteins, and other dairy-derived compounds to strengthen the skin barrier, promote moisture retention, and deliver antiaging and protective effects, all while remaining suitable for sensitive skin and aligned with clean-label product trends (Yeom et al., 2011; Ningsih and Eka Putra, 2025; Collard and McCormick, 2021; da Gama et al., 2018; Bhosale et al., 2019; Suganya and Anuradha, 2017; Gupta et al., 2016; Burnett et al., 2022).

5.1 Skin care-based applications of dairy product extracts

The focus of skin-care applications involving dairy product extracts lies in delivering concentrated bioactives through topical vehicles such as creams, serums, and hydrogels. These delivery systems ensure that key proteins, peptides, and growth factors remain stable and biologically active upon application, enabling targeted effects on hydration, elasticity, and overall skin health. By integrating dairy-derived bioactives into natural cosmetic formulations, researchers and product developers can harness the combined moisturizing, antioxidant, and regenerative properties of milk components, offering an evidence-based approach to effective, natural cosmetics for functional and sustainable skincare (Yeom et al., 2011; Ningsih and Eka Putra, 2025; Collard and McCormick, 2021; da Gama et al., 2018; Bhosale et al., 2019; Suganya and Anuradha, 2017; Gupta et al., 2016; Burnett et al., 2022).

Incorporating dairy-derived bioactive peptides into topical formulations represents a cutting-edge approach in modern skincare, merging the multifunctional properties of milk proteins with advanced delivery systems. Milk peptides, typically generated through enzymatic hydrolysis of casein and β-lactoglobulin, display a wide range of biological activities, including antioxidant, antiinflammatory, and antiaging effects (Pei et al., 2025). These features make them ideal for enhancing skin health, improving elasticity, and combating visible signs of aging. Hydrogels enriched with milk peptides and whey proteins are particularly promising carriers due to their biocompatibility, structural versatility, and ability to provide a controlled and sustained release of bioactives. Produced via physical, chemical, or enzymatic cross-linking methods, such hydrogels stabilize and protect the peptides while facilitating their penetration into deeper skin layers (Ito et al., 2020).

Recent studies have demonstrated that milk protein-based hydrogels hold considerable potential in biomedical fields such as tissue regeneration and wound healing (Huang et al., 2024; Hu et al., 2022). Although primarily explored in therapeutic contexts, their unique properties of hydration, controlled bioactive delivery, and excellent biocompatibility also position them as powerful tools for cosmetic innovation. In skincare, peptide-enriched hydrogels can be incorporated into creams, serums, and facial masks to support collagen and elastin production, reduce wrinkle depth, enhance hydration and barrier function, and soothe irritation and redness. Importantly, the use of dairy by-products such as whey for peptide extraction aligns with sustainability and circular economy principles, reinforcing their value not only in advancing cosmetic science but also in promoting ethical and eco-conscious product development in cosmetic industries (Pei et al., 2025).

5.2 Hair care-based applications of dairy product extracts

Incorporating milk-derived proteins, such as caseins and whey proteins, along with their enzymatic hydrolysates, into shampoos and conditioners represents an evidence-based strategy to improve hair strength, manageability, and shine. These effects are achieved through a dual mechanism: the formation of a substantively deposited film on the hair surface and peptide-mediated repair of structural damage. Milk proteins and their derived peptides and amino acids, including α-LA, β-lactoglobulin, and lactoferrin, are already recognized and widely used in cosmetics. When applied in a conditioned form, they adhere to the cuticle, forming a thin protective layer while simultaneously delivering amino acids and small peptides that repair surface damage to hair fibers (Kazimierska and Kalinowska-Lis, 2021; Hu: Scalable milk-derived whey protein hydrogel as, n.d.). Hydrolyzed milk proteins, particularly low-molecular-weight oligopeptides, are especially advantageous in rinse-off and leave-in formulations due to their enhanced ability to penetrate the cortex and bind strongly to damaged areas. This mechanism underlies improvements in tensile strength, reduced protein loss after chemical treatment, and boosted wet and dry combability. Controlled studies on dyed and chemically oxidized hair further demonstrate that conditioners enriched with hydrolyzed milk proteins reduce protein loss and improve combability and mechanical resistance, validating their benefits in color/chemically treated hair (da Gama et al., 2018; Tinoco et al., 2022).

Functionally, hydrolyzed milk proteins act as antistatic agents, film formers, and humectants. Ingredient authorities and suppliers consistently classify them as established hair conditioning actives, and Cosmetic Ingredient Review (CIR) assessments confirm their safety for topical use. Recent biomaterials research highlights the versatility of casein, which can form robust, food-grade protective coatings, such as tannic acid/casein photopolymerized films, increasing tensile strength by up to 20% while maintaining elasticity. These findings suggest that milk protein-based systems can serve not only as everyday conditioners but also as advanced protective treatments (Kyung et al., 2025). From a formulation standpoint, product performance depends strongly on factors, including molecular weight distribution, hydrolysis degree, concentration, and pH, as well as co-ingredients such as silicones, cationic polymers, and surfactants that influence deposition and film formation (Kyung et al., 2025). Hydrolyzed milk proteins are typically used at low concentrations and are generally regarded as safe, but formulators must still consider stability testing, microbiological control, and potential allergenicity in sensitive consumers. Importantly, using whey and other dairy by-products as peptide sources supports circular economy objectives, adding sustainability value to hair care products while reducing waste from the food industry (Kazimierska and Kalinowska-Lis, 2021; Tinoco et al., 2022).

5.3 Soothing and barrier repair formulations

Dairy-derived bioactives, particularly milk peptides and whey proteins, are gaining broad recognition for their role in soothing sensitive skin and restoring impaired barrier function, making them highly relevant for dermatological conditions such as atopic dermatitis. These compounds provide antiinflammatory, antioxidant, and antimicrobial effects while supporting epidermal repair. Hydrolyzed milk peptides, due to their small molecular size, can modulate inflammatory pathways, diminish redness and irritation, and stimulate ceramide synthesis and lipid organization in the *stratum corneum*. This helps decrease TEWL and enhances skin hydration (Nielsen et al., 2024). Whey-derived components, such as lactoferrin and immunoglobulins, further strengthen these effects by modulating the skin microbiome and reducing colonization by microbes that exacerbate dermatitis symptoms. Clinical and preclinical studies further support that partially hydrolyzed whey-based formulas improve skin barrier integrity, reduce the incidence of atopic dermatitis in high-risk populations, and regulate the expression of hydration-related genes in keratinocytes (Holvoet et al., 2021; Nicolaou et al., 2022).

Advances in biomaterials science add further value, demonstrating that hydrogels constructed from dairy proteins serve as biocompatible delivery systems capable of controlled peptide release while maintaining a moist microenvironment conducive to barrier repair. From a formulation standpoint, dairy bioactives can be combined synergistically with well-established barrier-supporting agents such as ceramides, HA, and panthenol, creating highly effective products for sensitive and atopic skin. In addition, their derivation from whey and other dairy by-products aligns with circular economy principles, transforming food industry waste into high-value cosmetic actives. This dual functionality of therapeutic efficacy and sustainability positions dairy-derived peptides and proteins as promising candidates for next-generation soothing and barrier repair skincare formulations (Pei et al., 2025; Park et al., 2019).

5.4 Examples from commercial products using dairy product extracts

A variety of cosmetic formulations incorporate dairy-derived bioactive compounds, reflecting both their multifunctional properties and their long-standing use in traditional skincare. Commercial examples range from cow, goat, and donkey milk creams and cleansers, valued for their moisturizing and soothing effects, to hydrolyzed milk proteins and WP utilized in shampoos, conditioners, and serums for hair strengthening, repair, and enhanced shine. Recently, ingredients derived from yogurt, kefir, buttermilk, and cheese by-products have been introduced into topical applications, offering antioxidant, antiinflammatory, and microbiome-modulating benefits, while supporting circular economy principles by valorizing dairy industry residues and waste (Yeom et al., 2011; Ningsih and Eka Putra, 2025; da Gama et al., 2018; Bhosale et al., 2019; Bhatia, 2022). Table 24.4 introduces indicative cases of commercial milk and dairy-based cosmetic products, highlighting their purpose and properties.

5.5 Discussion of safety and regulatory considerations for dairy product extracts use in cosmetic applications

The use of dairy-derived extracts in cosmetic formulations offers functional benefits such as moisturization, barrier reinforcement, and enhanced nutritional value. However, their incorporation raises important safety and regulatory considerations. Toxicological and clinical data generally support the safety of dairy proteins, including caseins and whey-derived fractions, at concentrations used in cosmetics. The CIR expert panel has confirmed the safety of these ingredients under current usage conditions, with no evidence of irritation, hypersensitivity, or mutagenicity in standard tests. For example, hydrolyzed casein caused no irritation in human patch studies at concentrations up to 30%, and systemic absorption from topical application is negligible compared to dietary exposure (Burnett, 2017). Nonetheless, allergenicity remains the primary safety concern. Caseins, α-LA, and β-lactoglobulin are well-known allergens, and while dermal exposure generally presents a lower risk, immunoglobulin E-mediated reactions in sensitized individuals cannot be excluded. Both the CIR and toxicological reviews highlight that consumers with milk and dairy allergies may experience adverse reactions, emphasizing the need for transparent labeling (Burnett et al., 2022).

In the European Union, cosmetic safety is governed by Regulation (EC) No 1223/2009, which enforces a "safe by design" principle. Each product must undergo a cosmetic product safety report, including toxicological profiles, systemic exposure assessments, and the calculation of a margin of safety. The Scientific Committee on Consumer Safety requires the evaluation of irritation, sensitization, genotoxicity, repeated dose toxicity, and toxico-kinetics, with special attention to protein allergens. The animal by-products regulation (EC) No 1069/2009 prohibits raw material sourcing (the use of Category 1 and 2 high-risk materials in cosmetics), allowing only the use of Category 3 materials from animals fit for human consumption in cosmetics (European Commission, Health and Consumer Protection Directorate-General, 2005).

In the United States, cosmetics fall under the Federal Food, Drug, and Cosmetic Act. Unlike the EU, premarket approval is not required by the Food and Drug Administration (FDA), except for color additives. Section 601 prohibits adulterated or misbranded products, placing responsibility for safety on manufacturers. The FDA also maintains a list of prohibited and restricted ingredients, which does not include dairy proteins (Prohibited & Restricted Ingredients in Cosmetics, 2024; HF Program, n.d.). Furthermore, many milk-derived proteins are classified as "generally recognized as safe" (GRAS) for food

TABLE 24.4 Examples of cosmetic products made from dairy-derived bioactives.

Cosmetic product	Cosmetic use	Dairy ingredient	Beneficial impact	References
Bodyfarm—Donkey Milk Anti-Wrinkle and Nourishing Day Cream	Day face cream	Donkey milk	Antioxidant and antiaging impact improves skin elasticity and notably reduces face wrinkles	(Greek Islands, n.d.)
Aphrodite Skin Care—Peptide Advanced Anti-Wrinkle Day Cream	Day antiwrinkle cream	Olive oil, donkey milk, and biopeptides	Skin moisturizing, wrinkle-reducing, and skin firmness-improving cream	Peptide Advanced Anti-Wrinkle Day Cream—Aphrodite Skin Care (n.d.)
Korres—Donkey Milk Protein Strengthening Face Cream, 40 mL	Day face cream	Donkey milk proteins + vitamins B and E.	Skin nourishing and moisturizing	Korres Mediterranean Donkey Milk Protein Strengthening Face Cream, 40 ml (n.d.)
Morfose—Milk Therapy Creamy Milk Shampoo	Hair shampoo	Hydrolyzed milk protein	Deep moisturization, enhanced hair growth, and softness enhancement	(Morfose Milk Therapy Creamy Milk Shampoo, n.d.)
Kallos Cosmetics—Keratin Regenerating Shampoo with Keratin and Milk Protein	Hair shampoo	Hydrolyzed milk protein and keratin	Strengthening and restoring damaged hair structure	(KJMN Sampon Keratinnal és Tejproteinnel—Kallos Cosmetics, n.d.)
Plaggoona—MEDIPEEL$^+$ Red Lacto-Collagen Barrier Firming Cream	Face cream	Fermented milk	Skin moisturizing, cleansing, and firming properties	(Medi-Peel Red Lacto Collagen Barrier Firming Cream, 80 ml, n.d.)
Nayelle—Prebiotic Skincare Line	Face creams/masks/serums/oils	Goat milk kefir-derived probiotics	Enhancing collagen and hyaluronic acid production while reducing redness	(The Benefits of Kefir in Skin Care—What is Kefir and Its Benefit for Skin, n.d.)
Kefirko—Organic Soap Made from Fresh Kefir	Organic soap for hair and body care	Kefir-derived skincare bioactives	Cleansing effect, skin-nourishing, for sensitive skin and dry skin types	(COSMETICS, n.d.)
Korres—Smart Yogurt Super Serum with Probiotics and Greek Yogurt Skincare Line	Face serum/gel cream/intense cream/face mask	Greek yogurt and oat extract/ginger/chia oil/shea butter, and other bioactives	Skin moisturizing, redness alleviation for sensitive skin or dry skin, and in-depth skin healing	(no date a)
Korres—Yogurt Lip Balm—Suncare Protection, Sun Protection Factor (SPF) 20	Lip balm for suncare protection	Greek yogurt, balsam oil, and vitamin E	Deep hydration, nourishment, and sun protection	(Yoghurt Lip balm—Suncare Protection SPF 20, n.d.)
Surnaturel Cosmetics—Cow's Milk Butter Cream 50 mL	Face cream	Cow's milk butter	Deep hydration, moisturization, and skin nourishment	(Surnat Cosmet, n.d.)
Skinaz—Mozzarella Cheese Cream	Face cream and lotion	Mozzarella, quark cheese, and shea butter	Brightening, skin-moisturizing, and wrinkle-improving cream	(SKINAZ Mozzarella Cheese Cream | Ingredients & Benefits, n.d.)

use, indirectly supporting their cosmetic safety profile, though GRAS does not replace cosmetic-specific risk assessment (GRAS Notices, n.d.).

Labeling requirements are central to consumer protection in both jurisdictions. In the EU, Article 19 of Regulation (EC) No. 1223/2009 mandates ingredient listing under the International Nomenclature of Cosmetic Ingredients. Proteins such as casein, hydrolyzed milk, or sodium caseinate must be explicitly declared, an important safeguard for milk-allergic consumers (Regulation—1223/2009—EN—Cosmetic Products Regulation—EUR-Lex, n.d.). The CIR expert panel has specifically noted that milk-derived proteins may pose an allergenic risk to sensitized individuals, even when used topically, and has, therefore, recommended transparent labeling to prevent consumers from coming into contact with potential allergens (Burnett, 2017). Similarly, in the United States, 21 CFR Part 701.3 requires ingredients to be listed in descending order of predominance by weight (Cosmetic Labeling, n.d.). Both CIR and toxicological reviews stress transparent labeling to minimize allergen exposure risks (Burnett et al., 2022). Beyond labeling, Good Manufacturing Practice (GMP) requirements further safeguard product safety. In the EU, Article 8 of Regulation (EC) No 1223/2009 enforces GMP compliance, typically demonstrated via ISO 22716:2007 (ISO, n.d.; Regulation (EC) No 1223/2009 of the European Parliament and of the Council of 30 November 2009 on cosmetic products (recast) (Text with EEA relevance), 2009). This ensures vast quality management, microbial safety testing, and protein hydrolysis profile verification, all particularly important for dairy-derived ingredients prone to variability or contamination (Burnett et al., 2022; Regulation (EC) No 1223/2009 of the European Parliament and of the Council of 30 November 2009 on cosmetic products (recast) (Text with EEA relevance), 2009). In theUnited States, GMP is not legally mandated, but FDA guidance exists (Commissioner O of the Draft Guidance for Industry: Cosmetic Good Manufacturing Practices 2024, n.d.; Commissioner O of the Good Manufacturing Practice (GMP) Guidelines/Inspection Checklist for Cosmetics, n.d.). Many US manufacturers voluntarily adopt ISO 22716:2007 to align with global standards (European Commission, Health and Consumer Protection Directorate-General, 2005).

Taken together, safety assessments, transparent labeling, and GMP compliance create a comprehensive framework for managing the risks of allergenicity, contamination, and variability associated with dairy-derived cosmetic ingredients. While the EU system emphasized premarket regulatory control, the United States mainly relies on the manufacturer's accountability and postmarket enforcement. Both frameworks ultimately converge on ensuring consumer safety through accurate labeling and adherence to quality standards.

6 Incorporation and encapsulation delivery systems of dairy product extracts for several applications

Dairy-derived bioactive compounds are of increasing interest, not only in cosmetics but also in food, beverages, and pharmaceuticals. However, their incorporation into formulations presents challenges related to instability, poor solubility, and sensitivity to degradation during processing and manufacturing. For instance, milk-derived proteins and peptides may undergo enzymatic hydrolysis in the gastrointestinal tract, while molecules such as lactoferrin and CLA are prone to oxidative degradation. To overcome these challenges, advanced encapsulation and delivery systems have been developed to improve bioavailability, stability, and targeted release (Yeom et al., 2011; Ningsih and Eka Putra, 2025; Bhosale et al., 2019; Suganya and Anuradha, 2017; Gupta et al., 2016; Bhatia, 2022).

Microencapsulation and nanoencapsulation are the most widely applied approaches for incorporating dairy- or plant-derived bioactives. In these techniques, compounds are entrapped within protective carrier matrices, usually composed of proteins, polysaccharides, or lipids (Costa et al., 2023). Microencapsulation typically yields larger capsules that act as physical barriers, protecting sensitive molecules during food processing and storage. This method is commonly used to stabilize probiotics, antimicrobial peptides, and fat-soluble vitamins in dairy products. On the contrary, nanoencapsulation operates on the nanometer scale (1–1000 nm) using nanocarriers such as protein nanoparticles, liposomes, or naturally occurring casein micelles. Their high surface area-to-volume ratio enhances solubility, stability, and bioavailability, while enabling controlled release triggered by pH, enzymatic activity, or temperature changes. Casein micelles, for example, naturally encapsulate hydrophobic molecules such as vitamin D or CLA, improving their solubility and absorption in aqueous environments (Suganya and Anuradha, 2017). Recent advances in nanotechnology have also enabled the fortification of dairy products with nanostructured functional ingredients, including nanopeanut sprout, nanochitosan, and nanoginseng extracts, integrated into milk, yogurt, and cheese. These are formulated as nanopowders or nanoemulsions, which show superior dispersibility, solubility, and bioavailability compared to conventional powders. Nanocalcium, for instance, has been studied as a fortifying ingredient in dairy, demonstrating higher biocompatibility and absorption efficacy than standard calcium supplements (Kwak et al., 2014).

Casein micelles are natural nanocarriers of particular interest, as they represent ~80% of bovine milk proteins. Composed of αS1-, αS2-, β-, and κ-caseins stabilized by calcium phosphate, micelles are amphiphilic, enabling them to encapsulate both hydrophobic compounds (e.g., vitamins, lipophilic peptides) and hydrophilic bioactives (e.g., minerals, therapeutic peptides) (Głąb and Boratyński, 2017; Zahariev et al., 2023). κ-Casein, located on the micelle surface, also provides steric stabilization, preventing aggregation and facilitating the controlled release under specific physiological conditions, such as pH variation or enzymatic digestion (Głąb and Boratyński, 2017). In functional dairy applications, casein micelles improve the delivery of fat-soluble vitamins and lipids (e.g., vitamin D, CLA), probiotics, and antimicrobial peptides, shielding them from enzymatic degradation and guaranteeing their high bioactivity and effectiveness at the intended site of action (Sadiq et al., 2021).

Liposomes are another versatile encapsulation system composed of one or more phospholipid bilayers surrounding an aqueous core. Their structural similarity to biological membranes enables the encapsulation of both hydrophilic and hydrophobic compounds, facilitating efficient cellular transport and protection against degradation (Bhosale et al., 2019; Narvekar et al., 2012). Liposomes release encapsulated compounds by fusing with cell membranes, making them highly relevant in dermatological and cosmetic applications. For example, milk-derived peptides delivered via liposomes can enhance skin hydration, reduce inflammation, and provide antimicrobial protection (Liu et al., 2022a; Zeng et al., 2021; Li et al., 2021). Liposome-based delivery also allows the adjustment of release kinetics by modifying lipid composition, vesicle size, or surface charge, while prolonging the shelf life of bioactives in dairy (Marsanasco and Alonso, 2022; Rudzińska et al., 2024).

At this point, the significance of nanoemulsions in cosmetic production must be discussed as well. Nanoemulsions are colloidal dispersions of immiscible liquids, typically oil-in-water or water-in-oil, with droplet sizes of 20–200 nm. Their extremely small droplet size confers a large surface area, enhancing the solubility, stability, and bioavailability of encapsulated molecules (Gupta et al., 2016). In gastrointestinal delivery, nanoemulsions improve the absorption of lipophilic nutrients by promoting micelle formation at the intestinal mucosa. Release profiles can be tuned by modifying droplet composition, emulsifier type, and interfacial properties (Niu et al., 2020). Nanoemulsions are especially effective in protecting hydrophobic bioactives like omega-3 fatty acids, CLA, vitamins A, D, E, and K, and antioxidant peptides against oxidation and degradation (Kaptan, 2024). Fortification of dairy products like yogurt and functional beverages with nanoemulsions has been shown to enhance nutrient bioavailability and health benefits, while efficiently reducing the required dosage compared to conventional formulations (Rao et al., 2023).

Encapsulation and delivery technologies, including microencapsulation, casein micelles, liposomes, and nanoemulsions, have transformed the use of dairy-derived bioactives in functional foods, nutraceuticals, pharmaceuticals, and cosmetics. These systems provide protection from degradation, enhance solubility and stability parameters, and allow controlled, targeted release. Their adaptability enables customized formulations addressing nutritional, therapeutic, or cosmetic needs, underlining their critical role in translating the inherent health benefits of dairy bioactives into commercially viable applications (Yeom et al., 2011; Ningsih and Eka Putra, 2025; Bhosale et al., 2019; Suganya and Anuradha, 2017; Gupta et al., 2016; Bhatia, 2022).

7 Limitations, challenges, and future perspectives

Bioactive compounds derived from dairy products have gained significant attention within the cosmetic industry due to their moisturizing, antioxidant, and antiinflammatory benefits. However, their incorporation into formulations poses challenges, with allergenicity being the primary concern. Milk and dairy proteins, particularly casein and whey, are well-known allergens and may elicit immune reactions in sensitive individuals, even upon topical application. Thus the presence of allergenic ingredients in skincare products raises issues of consumer safety and regulatory compliance. To address this, cosmetics manufacturers are required to conduct rigorous safety assessments and may employ hydrolyzed or chemically modified protein forms, which reduce allergenicity while maintaining bioactivity. Clear labeling of dairy-derived agents also remains essential to ensure transparency, consumer trust, and informed decision-making (Aguilar-Toalá et al., 2022; Afzal et al., 2024).

Another important aspect lies in the stability of bioactive substances during formulation and storage. Proteins and peptides are sensitive to environmental factors such as pH, temperature, and oxidation, which may cause transubstantiation or loss of bioactivity over time. To counter this, formulators must adopt strategies such as co-formulation with stabilizing agents or the use of controlled-release systems, ensuring functional integrity preservation throughout the product's shelf life (Aguilar-Toalá et al., 2022; Afzal et al., 2024). Formulation challenges arise as protein-ingredient interactions with surfactants, emulsifiers, or preservatives may cause precipitation, denaturation, or loss of activity, limiting the flexibility in product development (Yeom et al., 2011; Bhosale et al., 2019; Suganya and Anuradha, 2017; Gupta et al., 2016; Bhatia, 2022). Moreover, the scalability and cost of extracting, purifying, and stabilizing bioactive peptides remain barriers when compared with synthetic or plant-based alternatives, despite advances in whey valorization.

Shifting consumer values further complicates the integration of dairy-derived bioactives into cosmetic formulations. The growing demand for vegan and cruelty-free products has redefined the beauty and cosmetics industry, with some consumers actively avoiding animal-derived ingredients regardless of their safety or efficacy (Runte et al., 2024). Brands must therefore balance scientific efficacy with ethical transparency by communicating sourcing practices, environmental commitments, or by offering plant-based alternatives. This approach helps maintain both consumer trust and brand credibility (Bhatia, 2022; Perret et al., 2025). Beyond the rising demand for vegan and cruelty-free cosmetics, certain populations may reject dairy-based products due to lactose intolerance concerns or dietary/religious restrictions, such as kosher and halal requirements (Bhatia, 2022; Perret et al., 2025).

On the contrary, the valorization of dairy by-products presents exciting opportunities for innovation and sustainability. Whey, a by-product of cheese manufacturing, is rich in proteins, peptides, and other bioactives with proven moisturizing, antioxidant, and antiinflammatory effects (Luparelli et al., 2025). Advanced processing methods, including protein fractionation and concentration, allow for the recovery of bioactives that remain suitable and biologically active in cosmetic formulations. For example, whey protein isolate (WPI)-based bioactive peptide-stabilized nanoemulsions have revealed stability under diverse processing conditions, ensuring consistent functional performance (Adjonu et al., 2023). Incorporating whey-derived ingredients not only enhances product efficacy but also supports sustainability by reducing waste and promoting circular economy principles (Zandona et al., 2021).

In addition to allergenicity, stability concerns, and evolving consumer preferences, several other limitations must be considered when incorporating dairy-derived bioactives into cosmetics. One key issue is microbial contamination, as proteins and peptides can serve as nutrient sources for microbes if preservation and GMP standards are not strictly maintained (Wong et al., 2000; Michalek et al., 2019). Moreover, batch-to-batch variability in dairy extracts, driven by differences in animal diet, breed, and processing methods, can affect the reproducibility of bioactivity and product consistency (Aguilar-Toalá et al., 2022; Afzal et al., 2024).

Overall, despite the fact that dairy-derived compounds hold strong potential for cosmetic innovation, their use is constrained by allergenicity, stability issues, and evolving consumer preferences. Nonetheless, the valorization of dairy by-products offers a sustainable pathway forward. Future progress will depend on advances in protein modification, stabilization technologies, ethical sourcing, and circular economy integration to ensure the development of safe, effective, and environmentally responsible dairy-based cosmetic products.

8 Conclusions

Dairy-derived bioactive compounds exhibit multifunctional properties directly relevant to cosmetic science. Their antioxidant, antiinflammatory, antimicrobial, moisturizing, and regenerative activities contribute to skin hydration, elasticity, and barrier restoration, thereby validating their traditional use with modern biochemical and clinical evidence. The extraction of these compounds is feasible using a wide range of techniques. While conventional methods remain useful, advanced approaches such as UAE, EAE, and SFE offer superior efficiency, selectivity, and bioactivity preservation. These methods align with sustainability goals by minimizing both solvent use and industrial waste. Importantly, the valorization of dairy by-products, such as whey, is crucial for advancing circular economy practices, transforming residues into valuable cosmetic agents.

Despite promising evidence, most existing research emphasizes the health benefits of dairy extracts through oral consumption, with comparatively limited systematic investigations into their topical effects in cosmetic applications. To bridge this gap, further in vitro, in vivo, and clinical studies are required to clarify skin mechanisms of action, optimize formulation strategies, ensure long-term safety, and confirm efficacy under real-life conditions. Dairy extracts represent a unique combination of bioactive richness, extraction feasibility, and sustainability, making them highly promising candidates for next-generation natural cosmetics. By addressing current research gaps and prioritizing dermatological validation, these compounds can evolve into cornerstone agents for safe, effective, and eco-friendly cosmetic products.

Acknowledgments

The authors would like to thank the School of Chemistry in the Faculty of Sciences at Democritus University of Thrace for their continuous support.

Conflicts of interest

The authors declare no conflicts of interest.

Author contributions

A.T. was involved in conceptualization, methodology, validation, supervision, and project administration. A.T., A.V., and T.A. were involved in investigation, writing—review and editing, and visualization. All authors software and writing—original draft preparation and have read and agreed to the published version of the manuscript.

Funding

This research received no external funding.

References

Regulation (EC) No 1223/2009 of the European Parliament and of the Council of 30 November 2009 on Cosmetic Products (recast) (Text with EEA Relevance), No. 342, 2009.

Prohibited & Restricted Ingredients in Cosmetics, 2024.

Abellán, A., Cayuela, J.M., Pino, A., Martínez-Cachá, A., Salazar, E., Tejada, L., 2012. Free amino acid content of goat's milk cheese made with animal rennet and plant coagulant. J. Sci. Food Agric. 10970010. 92 (8), 1657–1664. doi:10.1002/jsfa.5528.

Acquavia, M.A., Villone, A., Rubino, R., Bianco, G., 2025. A comprehensive review of milk components: recent developments on extraction and analysis methods. Molecules. 1420-3049. 30 (9), 1994. doi:10.3390/molecules30091994.

Adjonu, R., Doran, G., Torley, P., Agboola, S., 2023. Stability of whey protein bioactive peptide-stabilised nanoemulsions: effect of pH, ions, heating and freeze–thawing. Int. J. Food Sci. Technol. 0950-5423. 58 (4), 1787–1794. doi:10.1111/ijfs.16292.

Adnan, A., Nadeem, M., Ahmad, M.H., Tayyab, M., Khan, M.K., Imran, M., Iqbal, A., Rahim, M.A., Awuchi, C.G., 2023. Effect of lactoferrin supplementation on composition, fatty acids composition, lipolysis and sensory characteristics of cheddar cheese. Int. J. Food Prop. 15322386. 26 (1), 437–452. Available from: https://www.tandfonline.com/loi/ljfp20. doi:10.1080/10942912.2023.2166953.

Afzal, A., Afzaal, M., Saeed, F., Shah, Y.A., Raza, M.A., Khan, M.H., Asghar, A., Akram, N., Ateeq, H., Asres, D.T., 2024. Milk protein based encapsulation of probiotics and other food material: comprehensive review. Int. J. Food Prop. 15322386. 27 (1), 245–262. Available from: https://www.tandfonline.com/loi/ljfp20. doi:10.1080/10942912.2024.2304283.

Aguilar-Toalá, J.E., Quintanar-Guerrero, D., Liceaga, A.M., Zambrano-Zaragoza, M.L., 2022. Encapsulation of bioactive peptides: a strategy to improve the stability, protect the nutraceutical bioactivity and support their food applications. RSC Adv. 2046-2069. 12 (11), 6449–6458. doi:10.1039/d1ra08590e.

Ahmed, I., 2016. Comparative study of cottage cheese prepared from various sources of milk. Proc. Pak. Acad. Sci. 53, 269–282.

Ahn, Y., Kim, M.G., Choi, Y.J., Lee, S.J., Suh, H.J., Jo, K., 2022b. Photoprotective effects of sphingomyelin-containing milk phospholipids in ultraviolet B–irradiated hairless mice by suppressing nuclear factor-κB expression. J. Dairy Sci. 15253198. 105 (3), 1929–1939. Available from: http://www.elsevier.com/wps/find/journaldescription.cws_home/721317/description#description. doi:10.3168/jds.2021-21192.

Ahn, Y., Kim, M.G., Jo, K., Hong, K.B., Suh, H.J., 2022a. Effects of sphingomyelin-containing milk phospholipids on skin hydration in UVB-exposed hairless mice. Molecules. 14203049. 27 (8). Available from: https://www.mdpi.com/1420-3049/27/8/2545/pdf. doi:10.3390/molecules27082545.

Ahn, Y., Suh, H.J., Hong, K.-B., Choi, Y., Lee, S.J., Jung, E.-J., 2024. Oral intake of milk ceramides improves skin hydration, elasticity, and wrinkles around the eyes: a 12-week, randomized, double-blind, placebo-controlled trial. J. Funct. Foods. 17564646. 113, 106008. doi:10.1016/j.jff.2024.106008.

Akbache, A., Lamiot, E., Moroni, O., Turgeon, S., Gauthier, S.F., Pouliot, Y., 2009. Use of membrane processing to concentrate TGF-β2 and IGF-I from bovine milk and whey. J. Membr. Sci. 03767388. 326 (2), 435–440. doi:10.1016/j.memsci.2008.10.026.

Albayrak, A., 2023. Some properties of semi-hard cheese made from cow's and goat's milk. Harranziraat. 2587-1358. 27 (2), 265–276. doi:10.29050/harranziraat.1195205.

ALKaisy, Q.H., Al-Saadi, J.S., AL-Rikabi, A.K.J., Altemimi, A.B., Hesarinejad, M.A., Abedelmaksoud, T.G., 2023. Exploring the health benefits and functional properties of goat milk proteins. Food Sci. Nutr. 20487177. 11 (10), 5641–5656. Available from: onlinelibrary.wiley.com/journal/10.1002/%28ISSN%292048-7177 . doi:10.1002/fsn3.3531.

Altay, Ö., Köprüalan Aydın, Ö., Öner, H.B., Filiz, Ö., Ertekin, F.K., 2024. Principles of distillation process. In: Jafari, S.M., Malekjani, N. (Eds.), Mass Transfer Operations in the Food Industry: Unit Operations and Processing Equipment in the Food Industry. Elsevier, Turkey, pp. 45–81. Available from: https://www.sciencedirect.com/book/9780128195369. doi:10.1016/B978-0-12-819536-9.00008-4.

Alvarez-Rivera, G., Bueno, M., Ballesteros-Vivas, D., Mendiola, J.A., Ibañez, E., 2019. Pressurized liquid extraction. In: Poole, C.F. (Ed.), Liquid-Phase Extraction. Elsevier, Spain, pp. 375–398. Available from: https://www.sciencedirect.com/science/book/9780128169117. doi:10.1016/B978-0-12-816911-7.00013-X.

Ambagaspitiya, S.S., Appuhamillage, G.A., Dassanayake, R.S., 2024. Impact of vitamin D on ultraviolet-induced photoaging and skin diseases. Explor. Med. 26923106. 5 (3), 363–383. Available from: https://www.explorationpub.com/Journals/em/Article/1001226. doi:10.37349/emed.2024.00225.

Andrade, T.A., Fetzer, D.E.L., Dos Passos, N.H.M., Ambye-Jensen, M., 2025. Maceration and fractionation technologies in a demonstration-scale green biorefinery: proteins, sugars, and lipids extraction and energy efficiency. Ind. Crops Prod. 09266690. 223. Available from: https://www.sciencedirect.com/science/journal/09266690. doi:10.1016/j.indcrop.2024.120142.

Arslan, A., Duman, H., Kaplan, M., Uzkuç, H., Bayraktar, A., Ertürk, M., Alkan, M., Frese, S.A., Duar, R.M., Henrick, B.M., Karav, S., 2021. Determining total protein and bioactive protein concentrations in bovine colostrum. J. Vis. Exp. 1940-087X. 2021 (178). doi:10.3791/63001.

Augustyniak, A., Gottardi, D., Giordani, B., Gaffey, J., Mahon, H.M., 2023. Dairy bioactives and functional ingredients with skin health benefits. J. Funct. Foods. 17564646. 104, 105528. doi:10.1016/j.jff.2023.105528.

Azizi, N.F., Kumar, M.R., Yeap, S.K., Abdullah, J.O., Khalid, M., Omar, A.R., Osman, M.A., Mortadza, S.A.S., Alitheen, N.B., 2021. Kefir and its biological activities. Foods. 23048158. 10 (6). Available from: https://www.mdpi.com/2304-8158/10/6/1210/pdf. doi:10.3390/foods10061210.

Barac, M., Pesic, M., Zilic, S., Smiljanic, M., Ignjatovic, I.S., Vucic, T., Kostic, A., Milincic, D., 2019. The influence of milk type on the proteolysis and antioxidant capacity of white-brined cheese manufactured from high-heat-treated milk pretreated with chymosin. Foods. 2304-8158. 8 (4), 128. doi:10.3390/foods8040128.

Barakat, I.S.A., Hammouri, M.K., Habib, I., 2015. Simultaneous determination of vitamins A and D3 in dairy products by liquid chromatography-tandem mass spectrometry (LC-MS/MS). IOP Conf. Ser. Mater. Sci. Eng. 1757-8981. 92 (1), 012020. doi:10.1088/1757-899x/92/1/012020.

Bazinet, L., 2005. Electrodialytic phenomena and their applications in the dairy industry: a review. Crit. Rev. Food Sci. Nutr. 1040-8398. 45 (4), 307–326. doi:10.1080/10408690490489279.

Bellikci-Koyu, E., Sarer-Yurekli, B.P., Karagozlu, C., Aydin-Kose, F., Ozgen, A.G., Buyuktuncer, Z., 2022. Probiotic kefir consumption improves serum apolipoprotein A1 levels in metabolic syndrome patients: a randomized controlled clinical trial. Nutr. Res. 18790739. 102, 59–70. Available from: www.elsevier.com/locate/nutres. doi:10.1016/j.nutres.2022.02.006.

Berg, H., Turner, C., Dahlberg, L., Mathiasson, L., 2000. Determination of food constituents based on SFE: applications to vitamins A and E in meat and milk. J. Biochem. Biophys. Methods. 0165022X. 43 (1-3), 391–401. doi:10.1016/s0165-022x(00)00063-4.

Berk, Z., 2018. Distillation. Elsevier BV, pp. 329–351. doi:10.1016/b978-0-12-812018-7.00013-0.

Bertin, C., Zunino, H., Lanctin, M., Stamatas, G.N., Camel, E., Robert, C., Issachar, N., 2008. Combined retinol–lactose–glycolic acid effects on photoaged skin: a double-blind placebo-controlled study. Int. J. Cosmet. Sci. 0142-5463. 30 (3), 175–182. doi:10.1111/j.1468-2494.2008.00441.x.

Bhatia, D.M., 2022. Consumer behaviour towards green cosmetics: the literature signifying a shift towards circularity and sustainability. Int. J. Sci. Res. Eng. Manag. 25823930. 06 (07). doi:10.55041/ijsrem15374.

Bhosale, S., Fulpagare, Y., Desale, R., 2019. Nanoliposomes: applications in food and dairy industry. Int. J. Adv. Res. Biol. Sci. 6 (11), 79–84.

Biadała, A., Konieczny, P., 2018. Goat's milk-derived bioactive components—a review. Mljekarstvo. 18464025. 68 (4), 239–253. Available from: https://hrcak.srce.hr/file/303651. doi:10.15567/mljekarstvo.2018.0401.

Bielecka, M., Cichosz, G., Czeczot, H., 2022. Antioxidant, antimicrobial and anticarcinogenic activities of bovine milk proteins and their hydrolysates—a review. Int. Dairy J. 09586946. 127, 105208. doi:10.1016/j.idairyj.2021.105208.

Bisht, A., Sahu, S.C., Kumar, A., Maqsood, S., Barwant, M.M., Jaiswal, S.G., 2025. Recent advances in conventional and innovative extraction techniques for recovery of high-added value compounds for food additives and nutraceuticals. Food Phys. 29500699. 2, 100047. doi:10.1016/j.foodp.2025.100047.

Biter, A.B., Pollet, J., Chen, W.H., Strych, U., Hotez, P.J., Bottazzi, M.E., 2019. A method to probe protein structure from UV absorbance spectra. Anal. Biochem. 10960309. 587. Available from: http://www.elsevier.com/inca/publications/store/6/2/2/7/8/1/index.htt. doi:10.1016/j.ab.2019.113450.

Björklund, E., Sparr-Eskilsson, C., 2005. Extraction | Supercritical Fluid Extraction. Elsevier BV, pp. 597–604. doi:10.1016/b0-12-369397-7/00691-9.

Bocheva, G., Slominski, R.M., Slominski, A.T., 2023. Environmental air pollutants affecting skin functions with systemic implications. Int. J. Mol. Sci. 1422-0067. 24 (13), 10502. doi:10.3390/ijms241310502.

Bohl, M., Bjørnshave, A., Gregersen, S., Hermansen, K., 2016. Whey and casein proteins and medium-chain saturated fatty acids from milk do not increase low-grade inflammation in abdominally obese adults. Rev. Diabet. Stud. 1613-6071. 13 (2-3), 148–157. doi:10.1900/RDS.2016.13.148.

Bordoni, A., Danesi, F., Dardevet, D., Dupont, D., Fernandez, A.S., Gille, D., Dos Santos, C.N., Pinto, P., Re, R., Rémond, D., Shahar, D.R., Vergères, G., 2017. Dairy products and inflammation: a review of the clinical evidence. Crit. Rev. Food Sci. Nutr. 15497852. 57 (12), 2497–2525. Available from: www.tandf.co.uk/journals/titles/10408398.asp. doi:10.1080/10408398.2014.967385.

Brück, W.M., Kelleher, S.L., Gibson, G.R., Nielsen, K.E., Chatterton, D.E.W., Lönnerdal, B., 2003. rRNA probes used to quantify the effects of glycomacropeptide and α-lactalbumin supplementation on the predominant groups of intestinal bacteria of infant rhesus monkeys challenged with enteropathogenic *Escherichia coli*. J. Pediatr. Gastroenterol. Nutr. 37 (3), 273–280. doi:10.1097/00005176-200309000-00014.

Burnett, C.L., 2017. Safety Assessment of Milk Proteins and Protein Derivatives as Used in Cosmetics. Cosmetic Ingredient Review.

Burnett, C.L., Bergfeld, W.F., Belsito, D.V., Hill, R.A., Klaassen, C.D., Liebler, D.C., Marks, J.G., Shank, R.C., Slaga, T.J., Snyder, P.W., Heldreth, B., 2022. Safety assessment of bovine milk proteins and protein derivatives as used in cosmetics. Int. J. Toxicol. 1091-5818, 1092874X. 41 (2_suppl), 43S–56S. Available from: https://journals.sagepub.com/doi/10.1177/10915818221098137. doi:10.1177/10915818221098137.

Călinescu, I., Vinatoru, M., Ghimpețeanu, D., Lavric, V., Mason, T.J., 2021. A new reactor for process intensification involving the simultaneous application of adjustable ultrasound and microwave radiation. Ultrason. Sonochem. 13504177. 77, 105701. doi:10.1016/j.ultsonch.2021.105701.

Camel, V., 2000. Microwave-assisted solvent extraction of environmental samples. TrAC Trends Anal. Chem. 01659936. 19 (4), 229–248. doi:10.1016/s0165-9936(99)00185-5.

Campaniello, M., Nardelli, V., Zianni, R., Tomaiuolo, M., Miedico, O., Iammarino, M., Mentana, A., 2024. Microwave-assisted extraction/UHPLC-Q-orbitrap-MS-based lipidomic workflow for comprehensive study of lipids in soft cheese. Foods. 2304-8158. 13 (7), 1033. doi:10.3390/foods13071033.

Campos, B.M., Moreira-Leite, B.S., Salgado, A., Ramalho, E., Marmelo, I., Malfeito-Ferreira, M., de Sousa, P.H.M., Henriques, A., Noronha, J.P., Diniz, M.S., Mata, P., 2025. Development of innovative Mediterranean-style semi-hard goat's cheese supplemented with seaweeds (*Palmaria palmata* and *Ulva* sp.) and its characterization. Appl. Sci. 2076-3417. 15 (15), 8232. doi:10.3390/app15158232.

Carabias-Martínez, R., Rodríguez-Gonzalo, E., Revilla-Ruiz, P., Hernández-Méndez, J., 2005. Pressurized liquid extraction in the analysis of food and biological samples. J. Chromatogr. A. 00219673. 1089 (1-2), 1–17. doi:10.1016/j.chroma.2005.06.072.

Castro-Gómez, M.P., Rodriguez-Alcalá, L.M., Calvo, M.V., Romero, J., Mendiola, J.A., Ibañez, E., Fontecha, J., 2014. Total milk fat extraction and quantification of polar and neutral lipids of cow, goat, and ewe milk by using a pressurized liquid system and chromatographic techniques. J. Dairy Sci. 00220302. 97 (11), 6719–6728. doi:10.3168/jds.2014-8128.

Cavalcanti, R.N., Balthazar, C.F., Margalho, L.P., Freitas, M.Q., Sant'Ana, A.S., Cruz, A.G., 2023. Pulsed electric field-based technology for microbial inactivation in milk and dairy products. Curr. Opin. Food Sci. 22147993. 54. Available from: http://www.journals.elsevier.com/current-opinion-in-food-science/. doi:10.1016/j.cofs.2023.101087.

Ceballos, L.S., Morales, E.R., de la Torre Adarve, G., Castro, J.D., Martínez, L.P., Sampelayo, M.R.S., 2009. Composition of goat and cow milk produced under similar conditions and analyzed by identical methodology. J. Food Compos. Anal. 08891575. 22 (4), 322–329. doi:10.1016/j.jfca.2008.10.020.

Chan, H., Chan, G., Santos, J., Dee, K., Co, J.K., 2017. A randomized, double-blind, placebo-controlled trial to determine the efficacy and safety of lactoferrin with vitamin E and zinc as an oral therapy for mild to moderate acne vulgaris. Int. J. Dermatol. 13654632. 56 (6), 686–690. Available from: http://onlinelibrary.wiley.com/journal/10.1111/(ISSN)1365-4632. doi:10.1111/ijd.13607.

Chatzimitakos, T., Athanasiadis, V., Kotsou, K., Mantiniotou, M., Kalompatsios, D., Makrygiannis, I., Bozinou, E., Lalas, S.I., 2024. Optimization of pressurized liquid extraction (PLE) parameters for extraction of bioactive compounds from *Moringa oleifera* leaves and bioactivity assessment. Int. J. Mol. Sci. 1422-0067. 25 (9), 4628. doi:10.3390/ijms25094628.

Chemat, F., Rombaut, N., Sicaire, A.G., Meullemiestre, A., Fabiano-Tixier, A.S., Abert-Vian, M., 2017. Ultrasound assisted extraction of food and natural products. Mechanisms, techniques, combinations, protocols and applications. A review. Ultrason. Sonochem. 18732828. 34, 540–560. Available from: www.elsevier.com/inca/publications/store/5/2/5/4/5/1. doi:10.1016/j.ultsonch.2016.06.035.

Chemat, F., Vian, M.A., Cravotto, G., 2012. Green extraction of natural products: concept and principles. Int. J. Mol. Sci. 14220067. 13 (7), 8615–8627. Available from: http://www.mdpi.com/1422-0067/13/7/8615/pdf. doi:10.3390/ijms13078615.

Chen, G.Q., Qu, Y., Gras, S.L., Kentish, S.E., 2023. Separation technologies for whey protein fractionation. Food Eng. Rev. 18667929. 15 (3), 438–465. Available from: https://www.springer.com/journal/12393. doi:10.1007/s12393-022-09330-2.

Chen, J., Liu, Y., Zhao, Z., Qiu, J., 2021. Oxidative stress in the skin: impact and related protection. Int. J. Cosmet. Sci. 14682494. 43 (5), 495–509. Available from: http://onlinelibrary.wiley.com/journal/10.1111/(ISSN)1468-2494. doi:10.1111/ics.12728.

Cheng, H., 2010. Volatile flavor compounds in yogurt: a review. Crit. Rev. Food Sci. Nutr. 1040-8398. 50 (10), 938–950. doi:10.1080/10408390903044081.

Cheng, S., Rathnakumar, K., Martínez-Monteagudo, S.I., 2019. Extraction of dairy phospholipids using switchable solvents: a feasibility study. Foods. 2304-8158. 8 (7), 265. doi:10.3390/foods8070265.

Cheng, S., Wei, L., Shimin, W., Yuxing, G., Wang, C., Xie, S., Juan, W., Chen, X., Cheong, L.-Z., 2023. Functional butter for reduction of consumption risk and improvement of nutrition. Grain Oil Sci. Technol. 25902598. 6 (4), 172–184. doi:10.1016/j.gaost.2023.09.001.

Clarke, H.J., McCarthy, W.P., O'sullivan, M.G., Kerry, J.P., Kilcawley, K.N., 2021. Oxidative quality of dairy powders: influencing factors and analysis. Foods. 23048158. 10 (10). Available from: https://www.mdpi.com/2304-8158/10/10/2315/pdf. doi:10.3390/foods10102315.

Collard, K.M., McCormick, D.P., 2021. A nutritional comparison of cow's milk and alternative milk products. Acad. Pediatr. 18762867. 21 (6), 1067–1069. Available from: http://www.elsevier.com/wps/find/authored_newsitem.cws_home/companynews05_01099. doi:10.1016/j.acap.2020.12.007.

Companys, J., Pla-Pagà, L., Calderón-Pérez, L., Llauradó, E., Solà, R., Pedret, A., Valls, R.M., 2020. Fermented dairy products, probiotic supplementation, and cardiometabolic diseases: a systematic review and meta-analysis. Adv. Nutr. 21618313. 11 (4), 834–863. doi:10.1093/advances/nmaa030.

Cosentino, C., Paolino, R., Tarricone, S., Valentini, V., Rragni, M., Freschi, P., 2025. Cosmetics industry as a promising opportunity for donkey breeding: consumer acceptability of a cosmetic cream based on milk from the martina franca breed. J. Anim. Plant Sci. 10187081. 35 (2), 584–591. doi:10.36899/japs.2025.2.0049.

Cosmetic Labeling, n.d. 21 CFR Part 701. Available from: https://www.ecfr.gov/current/title-21/part-701.

COSMETICS, n.d. Available from: https://kefirko.com/product-category/cosmetics/.

Costa, R.O.D.A., Passos, T.S., Silva, E.M.D.S., Dos Santos, N.C.S., de A. Morais, A.H., 2023. Encapsulated peptides and proteins with an effect on satiety. Nanomaterials. 2079-4991. 13 (7), 1166. doi:10.3390/nano13071166.

D'Andrea, A.E., Kinchla, A.J., Nolden, A.A., 2023. A comparison of the nutritional profile and nutrient density of commercially available plant-based and dairy yogurts in the United States. Front. Nutr. 2296861X. 10. Available from: https://www.journal.frontiersin.org/journal/nutrition. doi:10.3389/fnut.2023.1195045.

D'Orazio, J., Jarrett, S., Amaro-Ortiz, A., Scott, T., 2013. UV Radiation and the Skin. Int. J. Mol. Sci. 1422-0067. 14 (6), 12222–12248. doi:10.3390/ijms140612222.

da Gama, R.M., França-Stefoni, S.A., Sá-Dias, T.C., Bedin, V., Baby, A.R., Velasco, M.V.R., 2018. Protective effect of conditioner agents on hair treated with oxidative hair dye. J. Cosmet. Dermatol. 14732165. 17 (6), 1090–1095. Available from: http://onlinelibrary.wiley.com/journal/10.1111/(ISSN)1473-2165. doi:10.1111/jocd.12484.

da Silva Ghizi, A.C., de Almeida Silva, M., de Andrade Moraes, F.S., da Silvada Silvada Silva, C.L., Endringer, D.C., Scherer, R., Lenz, D., de Lima, E.M., Brasil, G.A., Maia, J.F., Souza Bissoli, N., de Andrade, T.U., 2021. Kefir improves blood parameters and reduces cardiovascular risks in patients with metabolic syndrome. PharmaNutrition. 22134344. 16, 100266. doi:10.1016/j.phanu.2021.100266.

Dalaka, E., Stefos, G.C., Politis, I., Theodorou, G., 2024. Evaluation of in vitro antihypertensive and anti-inflammatory properties of dairy by-products. Appl. Sci. 2076-3417. 14 (16), 6885. doi:10.3390/app14166885.

Davoodi, S.H., Shahbazi, R., Esmaeili, S., Sohrabvandi, S., Mortazavian, A.M., Jazayeri, S., Taslimi, A., 2016. Health-related aspects of milk proteins. Iran. J. Pharm. Res. 17266890. 15 (3), 573–591. Available from http://ijpr.sbmu.ac.ir/article_1897_41b4a50aecfd13c75d768b304005889c.pdf.

Ding, Y., Haile, M., Wang, K., Azam, S.M.R., Wang, Y., Zhou, J., Wenjuan, Q., 2021. Ultrasound frequency effect on soybean protein: acoustic field simulation, extraction rate and structure. LWT. 00236438. 145, 111320. doi:10.1016/j.lwt.2021.111320.

Do Nascimento Rangel, A.H., de Araújo Bezerra, D.A.F.V., Sales, D.C., de Oliveira Moura Araújo, E., de Lucena, L.M., Lúcia Figueiredo Porto, A., Viviane Ubaldo Mesquita Véras, Í., Lacerda, A.F., Vaz Di Mambro Ribeiro, C., Anaya, K., 2023. An overview of the occurrence of bioactive peptides in different types of cheeses. Foods. 2304-8158. 12 (23), 4261. doi:10.3390/foods12234261.

Dominiak, M., Søndergaard, K.M., Wichmann, J., Vidal-Melgosa, S., Willats, W.G.T., Meyer, A.S., Mikkelsen, J.D., 2014. Application of enzymes for efficient extraction, modification, and development of functional properties of lime pectin. Food Hydrocoll. 0268005X. 40, 273–282. Available from: https://www.journals.elsevier.com/food-hydrocolloids. doi:10.1016/j.foodhyd.2014.03.009.

Dos Santos Venâncio Costa, D., Bragagnolo, N., 2017. Development and validation of a novel microwave assisted extraction method for fish lipids. Eur. J. Lipid Sci. Technol. 1438-7697. 119 (3). doi:10.1002/ejlt.201600108.

Drăghici-Popa, A.M., Boscornea, A.C., Brezoiu, A.M., Tomas, Ş.T., Pârvulescu, O.C., Stan, R., 2023. Effects of extraction process factors on the composition and antioxidant activity of blackthorn (*Prunus spinosa* L.) fruit extracts. Antioxidants. 20763921. 12 (10). Available from: www.mdpi.com/journal/antioxidants. doi:10.3390/antiox12101897.

Dufton, G., Mikhaylin, S., Gaaloul, S., Bazinet, L., 2018. How electrodialysis configuration influences acid whey deacidification and membrane scaling. J. Dairy Sci. 00220302. 101 (9), 7833–7850. doi:10.3168/jds.2018-14639.

Dumpler, J., Moraru, C.I., 2024. Microwave vacuum drying of dairy cream: processing, reconstitution, and whipping properties of a novel dairy product. J. Dairy Sci. 15253198. 107 (2), 774–789. Available from: https://www.sciencedirect.com/science/journal/00220302. doi:10.3168/jds.2023-23657.

Düven, G., Kumcuoğlu, S., Kışla, D., 2021. Ultrasonication-assisted kefir production and its effect on fermentation time and EPS production. Food Biosci. 22124292. 42, 101059. doi:10.1016/j.fbio.2021.101059.

El-Abbadi, N.H., Dao, M.C., Meydani, S.N., 2014. Yogurt: role in healthy and active aging. Am. J. Clin. Nutr. 00029165. 99 (5), 1263S. doi:10.3945/ajcn.113.073957.

El-Sayed, M., Awad, S., 2019. Milk bioactive peptides: antioxidant, antimicrobial and anti-diabetic activities. Adv. Biochem. 2329-0870. 7 (1), 22. doi:10.11648/j.ab.20190701.15.

ElKhori, S., Paré, J.R.J., Bélanger, J.M.R., Pérez, E., 2007. The microwave-assisted process (MAPTM1): extraction and determination of fat from cocoa powder and cocoa nibs. J. Food Eng. 02608774. 79 (3), 1110–1114. doi:10.1016/j.jfoodeng.2006.01.089.

Etzel, M.R., 2004. Manufacture and use of dairy protein fractions. J. Nutr. 00223166. 134 (4), 996S. doi:10.1093/jn/134.4.996s.

European Commission, Health and Consumer Protection Directorate-General, 2005. Risk of Ingredients Deriving from Category 1-Material and Category 2-Material as Defined in Regulation 1774/2002 in Cosmetic Products.

Fanelli, A.J., Burlew, J.V., Gabriel, M.K., 1985. Protection of milk packaged in high density polyethylene against photodegradation by fluorescent light. J. Food Prot. 0362028X. 48 (2), 112–117. doi:10.4315/0362-028x-48.2.112.

Farag, M.A., Jomaa, S.A., El-Wahed, A.A., El-Seedi, H.R., 2020. The many faces of kefir fermented dairy products: quality characteristics, flavour chemistry, nutritional value, health benefits, and safety. Nutrients. 2072-6643. 12 (2), 346. doi:10.3390/nu12020346.

Faraz, A., 2020. Role of camel milk in beauty products. FARMER REFORMERA. 2519-7835. 5 (9).

Farooq, S., Mir, S.A., Shah, M.A., Manickavasagan, A., 2021. Extraction techniques. In: Mir, S.A., Manickavasagan, A., Shah, M.A. (Eds.), Plant Extracts: Applications in the Food Industry. Academic Press, pp. 23–37. Available from: https://www.sciencedirect.com/book/9780128224755. doi:10.1016/B978-0-12-822475-5.00005-3.

Fernandes, J., Gomes, S., Reboredo, F.H., Pintado, M.E., Amaral, O., Dias, J., Alvarenga, N., 2025. Clean label approaches in cheese production: where are we? Foods. 23048158. 14 (5). Available from: www.mdpi.com/journal/foods. doi:10.3390/foods14050805.

Fernández-García, E., Imhof, M., Schlichtherle-Cerny, H., Bosset, J.O., Nuñez, M., 2008. Terpenoids and benzenoids in La Serena cheese made at different seasons of the year with a *Cynara cardunculus* extract as coagulant. Int. Dairy J. 09586946. 18 (2), 147–157. doi:10.1016/j.idairyj.2007.08.007.

Ferraboschi, P., Ciceri, S., Grisenti, P., 2021. Applications of lysozyme, an innate immune defense factor, as an alternative antibiotic. Antibiotics. 2079-6382. 10 (12), 1534. doi:10.3390/antibiotics10121534.

Flis, Z., Molik, E., Ptak, A., Szatkowski, P., 2025b. Natural bioactive compounds in sheep milk: potential biomedical applications. Curr. Issues Mol. Biol. 1467-3045. 47 (6), 456. doi:10.3390/cimb47060456.

Flis, Z., Ptak, A., Szatkowski, P., Czauderna, M., Molik, E., 2025a. Bioactive compounds in sheep milk: the therapeutic potential of CLA, lactoferrin, and orotic acid in skin cancer treatment. J. Anim. Feed Sci. 1230–1388. doi:10.22358/jafs/203559/2025.

Fluhr, J.W., Darlenski, R., Surber, C., 2008. Glycerol and the skin: holistic approach to its origin and functions. Br. J. Dermatol. 0007-0963. 159 (1), 23–34. doi:10.1111/j.1365-2133.2008.08643.x.

Fohely, F., Sabarna, K., Suardi, N., 2021. A comparative study of the effects of X-radiation and gamma-radiation on structural characteristics of raw milk protein (study case of goat's milk). ECS J. Solid State Sci. Technol. 28, 7–24.

Fu, X., Harshman, S.G., Shen, X., Haytowitz, D.B., Karl, J.P., Wolfe, B.E., Booth, S.L., 2017. Multiple vitamin K forms exist in dairy foods. Curr. Dev. Nutr. 24752991. 1 (6), e000638. doi:10.3945/cdn.117.000638.

Gao, Y., Guo, M., Wang, D., Zhao, D., Wang, M., 2023. Advances in extraction, purification, structural characteristics and biological activities of hemicelluloses: a review. Int. J. Biol. Macromol. 01418130. 225, 467–483. doi:10.1016/j.ijbiomac.2022.11.099.

Garrett, O.F., 1943. The calcium and phosphorus content of commercially made cottage cheese. J. Dairy Sci. 00220302. 26 (4), 305–308. doi:10.3168/jds.s0022-0302(43)92722-5.

Geniselli da Silva, V.G., Tonkie, J.N., Clémence Roy, N., Smith, N.W., Wall, C., Kruger, M.C., Mullaney, J.A., McNabb, W.C., 2024. The effect of complementary foods on the colonic microbiota of weaning infants: a systematic review. Crit. Rev. Food Sci. Nutr. 1040-8398. 1–16. doi:10.1080/10408398.2024.2439036.

Genovese, J., Stručić, M., Serša, I., Novickij, V., Rocculi, P., Miklavčič, D., Mahnič-Kalamiza, S., Kranjc, M., 2023. PEF treatment effect on plant tissues of heterogeneous structure no longer an enigma: MRI insights beyond the naked eye. Food Chem. 03088146. 405, 134892. doi:10.1016/j.foodchem.2022.134892.

Getaneh, G., Mebrat, A., Wubie, A., Kendie, H., 2016. Review on goat milk composition and its nutritive value. J. Nutr. Health Sci. 23939060. 3 (4). doi:10.15744/2393-9060.3.401.

Gille, D., Schmid, A., 2015. Vitamin B12 in meat and dairy products. Nutr. Rev. 0029-6643. 73 (2), 106–115. doi:10.1093/nutrit/nuu011.

Gille, D., Walther, B., Badertscher, R., Bosshart, A., Brügger, C., Brühlhart, M., Gauch, R., Noth, P., Vergères, G., Egger, L., 2018. Detection of lactose in products with low lactose content. Int. Dairy J. 09586946. 83, 17–19. doi:10.1016/j.idairyj.2018.03.003.

Głąb, T.K., Boratyński, J., 2017. Potential of casein as a carrier for biologically active agents. Top. Curr. Chem. 23648961. 375 (4). Available from: http://www.springer.com/chemistry/journal/41061. doi:10.1007/s41061-017-0158-z.

Gontarek-Castro, E., Castro-Muñoz, R., 2024. Membrane distillation assisting food production processes of thermally sensitive food liquid items: a review. Crit. Rev. Food Sci. Nutr. 1040-8398. 64 (18), 6073–6086. doi:10.1080/10408398.2022.2163223.

González, S., Fernández-Navarro, T., Arboleya, S., Reyes-Gavilán, C.G.D.L., Salazar, N., Gueimonde, M., 2019. Fermented dairy foods: impact on intestinal microbiota and health-linked biomarkers. Front. Microbiol. 1664302X. 10 (MAY). Available from: https://www.frontiersin.org/journals/microbiology#. doi:10.3389/fmicb.2019.01046.

Granato, D., Carocho, M., Barros, L., Zabetakis, I., Mocan, A., Tsoupras, A., Cruz, A.G., Pimentel, T.C., 2022. Implementation of sustainable development goals in the dairy sector: perspectives on the use of agro-industrial side-streams to design functional foods. Trends Food Sci. Technol. 09242244. 124, 128–139. doi:10.1016/j.tifs.2022.04.009.

GRAS Notices, n.d. Available from: https://www.hfpappexternal.fda.gov/scripts/fdcc/index.cfm?set=GRASNotices.

Greek Islands, n.d. Bodyfarm Donkey Milk. Anti-Wrinkle & Nourishing Day Cream 50 ml. Available from: https://greekislandsstore.gr/en/product/bodyfarm-donkey-milk-anti-wrinkle-nourishing-day-cream-50ml/.

Grzelka, K., Matkowski, A., Chodaczek, G., Jaśpińska, J., Pawlikowska-Bartosz, A., Słupski, W., Lechniak, D., Szumacher-Strabel, M., Olorunlowu, S., Szulc, K., Cieślak, A., Ślusarczyk, S., 2025. Pulsed electric field (PEF) treatment results in growth promotion, main flavonoids extraction, and phytochemical profile modulation of *Scutellaria baicalensis* Georgi roots. Int. J. Mol. Sci. 1422-0067. 26 (1), 100. doi:10.3390/ijms26010100.

Guha, S., Sharma, H., Deshwal, G.K., Rao, P.S., 2021. A comprehensive review on bioactive peptides derived from milk and milk products of minor dairy species. Food Prod. Process. Nutr. 26618974. 3 (1). Available from: https://www.springer.com/journal/43014. doi:10.1186/s43014-020-00045-7.

Gul, O., Mortas, M., Atalar, I., Dervisoglu, M., Kahyaoglu, T., 2015. Manufacture and characterization of kefir made from cow and buffalo milk, using kefir grain and starter culture. J. Dairy Sci. 00220302. 98 (3), 1517–1525. doi:10.3168/jds.2014-8755.

Gupta, A., Eral, H.B., Hatton, T.A., Doyle, P.S., 2016. Nanoemulsions: formation, properties and applications. Soft Matter. 17446848. 12 (11), 2826–2841. Available from: http://pubs.rsc.org/en/journals/journal/sm. doi:10.1039/c5sm02958a.

Hae-Soo, K., Palanivel, G., Al, M.M., 2013. Butter, Ghee, and Cream Products Milk and Dairy Products in Human Nutrition: Production, Composition and Health. Wiley, South Korea, pp. 390–411. Available from https://onlinelibrary.wiley.com/doi/book/10.1002/9781118534168. doi:10.1002/9781118534168.ch18.

Hausmann, A., Sanciolo, P., Vasiljevic, T., Ponnampalam, E., Quispe-Chavez, N., Weeks, M., Duke, M., 2011. Direct contact membrane distillation of dairy process streams. Membranes. 2077-0375. 1 (1), 48–58. doi:10.3390/membranes1010048.

He, M., Jun, H., Deng, J., Chen, X., Liu, C., Olatunji, O.J., Suttikhana, I., Ashaolu, T.J., 2025. Cow milk allergy: its clinical aspects, mechanisms, and innovative mitigation strategies beyond enzymatic hydrolysis. J. Funct. Foods. 17564646. 130, 106933. doi:10.1016/j.jff.2025.106933.

Hernandez, K., Park, Y.W., 2014. Evaluation of 20 macro and trace mineral concentrations in commercial goat milk yogurt and its cow milk counterpart. Food Nutr. Sci. 2157-944X. 05 (10), 889–895. doi:10.4236/fns.2014.510098.

Hess, J.M., Stephensen, C.B., Kratz, M., Bolling, B.W., 2021. Exploring the links between diet and inflammation: dairy foods as case studies. Adv. Nutr. 21565376. 12, 1–13. Available from: http://advances.nutrition.org/. doi:10.1093/advances/nmab108.

Hew, J., Shafie, S., Sulaiman, N., 2023. Proximate composition and antimicrobial activity of kefir produced from cow's and almond milk. J. Trop. Life Sci. 20875517. 13 (2), 287–296. doi:10.11594/jtls.13.02.06.

HF Program, n.d. Summary of Color Additives for Use in the United States in Foods, Drugs, Cosmetics, and Medical Devices.

Ho, C.C., 2007. Membranes for Bioseparations Bioprocessing for Value-Added Products from Renewable Resources. Elsevier, United States, pp. 163–183. Available from http://www.sciencedirect.com/science/book/9780444521149. doi:10.1016/B978-044452114-9/50008-6.

Holvoet, S., Nutten, S., Dupuis, L., Donnicola, D., Bourdeau, T., Hughes-Formella, B., Simon, D., Simon, H.-U., Carvalho, R.S., Spergel, J.M., Koletzko, S., Blanchard, C., 2021. Partially hydrolysed whey-based infant formula improves skin barrier function. Nutrients. 2072-6643. 13 (9), 3113. doi:10.3390/nu13093113.

Hordofa, B.B., 2018. Acidification process and properties of soft cheese made from cow milk using different starter cultures. Afr. J. Food Sci. Technol. 21415455. 09 (02). doi:10.14303/ajfst.2018.229.

Hu, Z., Cao, W., Shen, L., Sun, Z., Kang, Y., Zhu, Q., Ren, T., Zhang, L., Zheng, H., Gao, C., Yong, H., Guo, C., Zhu, Y., Ren, D., 2022. Scalable milk-derived whey protein hydrogel as an implantable biomaterial. ACS Appl. Mater. Interfaces. 1944-8244. 14 (25), 28501–28513. doi:10.1021/acsami.2c02361.

Hu: scalable Milk-Derived Whey Protein Hydrogel As. Available from: https://scholar.google.com/scholar_lookup?journal=ACS%20Appl%20Mater%20Interfaces&title=Scalable%20milk-derived%20whey%20protein%20hydrogel%20as%20an%20implantable%20biomaterial&author=Z.%20Hu&author=W.%20Cao&author=L.%20Shen&volume=14&publication_year=2022&pages=28501-28513&pmid=35703017&doi=10.1186/s40824-023-00346-1&.

Huang, Y., Zhu, Q., Zhu, Y., Valencak, T.G., Han, Y., Ren, T., Guo, C., Ren, D., 2024. Rapid UV photo-cross-linking of α-lactalbumin hydrogel biomaterial to enable wound healing. ACS Omega. 24701343. 9 (1), 401–412. Available from: https://www.pubs.acs.org/journal/acsodf. doi:10.1021/acsomega.3c05793.

Huseini, H.F., Rahimzadeh, G., Fazeli, M.R., Mehrazma, M., Salehi, M., 2012. Evaluation of wound healing activities of kefir products. Burns. 18791409. 38 (5), 719–723. doi:10.1016/j.burns.2011.12.005.

Hwang, D.M., Kundu, J.K., Shin, J.W., Lee, J.C., Lee, H.J., Surh, Y.J., 2007. Cis-9,trans-11-Conjugated linoleic acid down-regulates phorbol ester-induced NF-κB activation and subsequent COX-2 expression in hairless mouse skin by targeting IκB kinase and PI3K-Akt. Carcinogenesis. 14602180. 28 (2), 363–371. doi:10.1093/carcin/bgl151.

Ibeagha-Awemu, E.M., Liu, J.R., Zhao, X., 2009. Bioactive Components in Yogurt Products Bioactive Components in Milk and Dairy Products. Wiley-Blackwell, Canada, pp. 235–250. Available from http://onlinelibrary.wiley.com/book/10.1002/9780813821504. doi:10.1002/9780813821504.ch9.

Ibrahim, A., Naufalin, R., Muryatmo, E., Dwiyanti, H., 2021. Comparative study between cow and goat milk yogurt based on composition and sensory evaluation. IOP Conf. Ser. Earth Environ. Sci. 1755-1307. 746 (1), 012001. doi:10.1088/1755-1315/746/1/012001.

Ichimura, T., 2024. Yogurt Production, Vol. 2851. Springer Science and Business Media LLC, pp. 63–74. doi:10.1007/978-1-0716-4096-8_5.

Innosa, D., Ianni, A., Faccia, M., Martino, C., Grotta, L., Saletti, M.A., Pomilio, F., Martino, G., 2020. Physical, nutritional, and sensory properties of cheese obtained from goats fed a dietary supplementation with olive leaves. Animals. 2076-2615. 10 (12), 2238. doi:10.3390/ani10122238.

ISO, n.d. ISO 22716:2007. Available from: https://www.iso.org/standard/36437.html. (Accessed 14 September 2025).

Ito, S., Hirobe, S., Kuwabara, Y., Nagao, M., Saito, M., Quan, Y.S., Kamiyama, F., Fujisawa, T., Okada, N., 2020. Immunogenicity of milk protein-containing hydrophilic gel patch for epicutaneous immunotherapy for milk allergy. Pharm. Res. 1573904X. 37 (3). Available from: www.wkap.nl/journalhome.htm/0724-8741. doi:10.1007/s11095-019-2728-y.

Jeevan Kumar, S.P., Kumar, G.V., Dash, A., Scholz, P., Banerjee, R., 2017. Sustainable green solvents and techniques for lipid extraction from microalgae: a review. Algal Res. 22119264. 21, 138–147. doi:10.1016/j.algal.2016.11.014.

Jinjarak, S., Olabi, A., Jiménez-Flores, R., Walker, J.H., 2006. Sensory, functional, and analytical comparisons of whey butter with other butters. J. Dairy Sci. 00220302. 89 (7), 2428–2440. doi:10.3168/jds.s0022-0302(06)72316-5.

Jonnala, B.R.Y., McSweeney, P.L.H., Cotter, P.D., Zhong, S., Sheehan, J.J., Kopec, R.E., 2021. Comparison of the carotenoid profiles of commonly consumed smear-ripened cheeses. LWT. 00236438. 135. Available from: https://www.journals.elsevier.com/lwt. doi:10.1016/j.lwt.2020.110241.

Kabelová, I., Dvořáková, M., Čížková, H., Dostálek, P., Melzoch, K., 2009. Determination of free amino acids in cheeses from the Czech market. Czech J. Food Sci. 12121800. 27 (3), 143–150. doi:10.17221/1415-cjfs.

Kamal, H., Ali, A., Cheng Foh, L., 2023. Green solvent processing: effect of type of solvent on extraction and quality of protein from dairy and non-dairy expired milk products. Food Chem. 03088146. 400, 133988. doi:10.1016/j.foodchem.2022.133988.

Kamal, H., Le, C.F., Salter, A.M., Ali, A., 2021. Extraction of protein from food waste: an overview of current status and opportunities. Compr. Rev. Food Sci. Food Saf. 15414337. 20 (3), 2455–2475. Available from: http://onlinelibrary.wiley.com/journal/10.1111/(ISSN)1541-4337. doi:10.1111/1541-4337.12739.

Kang, Q., Chen, S., Shufang, L., Wang, B., Liu, X., Hao, L., Jike, L., 2019. Comparison on characterization and antioxidant activity of polysaccharides from *Ganoderma lucidum* by ultrasound and conventional extraction. Int. J. Biol. Macromol. 01418130. 124, 1137–1144. doi:10.1016/j.ijbiomac.2018.11.215.

Kaptan, B., 2024. Use of nanoemulsion technology in dairy industry. Turk. J. Agric. Food Sci. Technol. 2148-127X. 12 (s2), 2415–2428. doi:10.24925/turjaf.v12is2.2415-2428.6953.

Karrar, E., Ahmed, I.A.M., Manzoor, M.F., Wei, W., Sarpong, F., Wang, X., 2022. Lipid-soluble vitamins from dairy products: extraction, purification, and analytical techniques. Food Chem. 18737072. 373. Available from: www.elsevier.com/locate/foodchem. doi:10.1016/j.foodchem.2021.131436.

Kawęcka, A., Pasternak, M., 2022. Nutritional and dietetic quality of milk and traditional cheese made from the milk of native breeds of sheep and goats. J. Appl. Anim. Res. 0971-2119. 50 (1), 39–46. doi:10.1080/09712119.2021.2020125.

Kazimierska, K., Erkiert-Polguj, A., Kalinowska-Lis, U., 2024. The efficacy of a cosmetic preparation containing sheep colostrum on mature skin: a randomized placebo-controlled double-blind study. Appl. Sci. 2076-3417. 14 (7), 2862. doi:10.3390/app14072862.

Kazimierska, K., Kalinowska-Lis, U., 2021. Milk proteins—their biological activities and use in cosmetics and dermatology. Molecules. 1420-3049. 26 (11), 3253. doi:10.3390/molecules26113253.

Kell, D.B., Heyden, E.L., Pretorius, E., 2020. The biology of lactoferrin, an iron-binding protein that can help defend against viruses and bacteria. Front. Immunol. 1664-3224. 11. doi:10.3389/fimmu.2020.01221.

Khan, I.T., Nadeem, M., Imran, M., Khalique, A., 2020. Impact of post fermentation cooling patterns on fatty acid profile, lipid oxidation and antioxidant features of cow and buffalo milk set yoghurt. Lipids Health Dis. 1476-511X. 19 (1). doi:10.1186/s12944-020-01263-1.

Khan, I.T., Nadeem, M., Imran, M., Ullah, R., Ajmal, M., Jaspal, M.H., 2019. Antioxidant properties of milk and dairy products: a comprehensive review of the current knowledge. Lipids Health Dis. 1476511X. 18 (1). Available from: http://www.lipidworld.com/home/. doi:10.1186/s12944-019-0969-8.

Kiewiet, M.B.G., Dekkers, R., Gros, M., Joost van Neerven, R.J., Groeneveld, A., de Vos, P., Faas, M.M., Yin, H.H., 2017. Toll-like receptor mediated activation is possibly involved in immunoregulating properties of cow's milk hydrolysates. PLoS One. 1932-6203. 12 (6), e0178191. doi:10.1371/journal.pone.0178191.

Kim, J., Ko, Y., Park, Y.K., Kim, N.I., Ha, W.K., Cho, Y., 2010. Dietary effect of lactoferrin-enriched fermented milk on skin surface lipid and clinical improvement of acne vulgaris. Nutrition. 08999007. 26 (9), 902–909. Available from: www.elsevier.com/locate/nut. doi:10.1016/j.nut.2010.05.011.

Kimoto-Nira, H., Nagakura, Y., Kodama, C., Shimizu, T., Okuta, M., Sasaki, K., Koikawa, N., Sakuraba, K., Suzuki, C., Suzuki, Y., 2014. Effects of ingesting milk fermented by *Lactococcus lactis* H61 on skin health in young women: a randomized double-blind study. J. Dairy Sci. 00220302. 97 (9), 5898–5903. doi:10.3168/jds.2014-7980.

Kimura, Y., Sumiyoshi, M., Kobayashi, T., 2014. Whey peptides prevent chronic ultraviolet B radiation–induced skin aging in melanin-possessing male hairless mice. J. Nutr. 00223166. 144 (1), 27–32. doi:10.3945/jn.113.180406.

Kippenberger, S., Zöller, N., Kleemann, J., Müller, J., Kaufmann, R., Hofmann, M., Bernd, A., Meissner, M., Valesky, E., Picardo, M., 2015. STAT6-Dependent collagen synthesis in human fibroblasts is induced by bovine milk. PLoS One. 1932-6203. 10 (7), e0131783. doi:10.1371/journal.pone.0131783.

Kontodimos, I., Chatzimanoli, E., Kasapidou, E., Basdagianni, Z., Karatzia, M.-A., Amanatidis, M., et al, 2023. Characterization of bioactive compounds and element content in goat milk and cheese products. Biol. Life Sci. Forum. 26, 98. doi:https://doi.org/10.3390/Foods2023-15131

Krakowska-Sieprawska, A., Walczak-Skierska, J., Ludwiczak, A., Białczak, D., Pomastowski, P., 2025. Compositional dynamics of lipid and phospholipid profiles during milk transport and processing: implications for butter quality and stability. ACS Food Sci. Technol. 2692-1944. 5 (5), 1858–1868. doi:10.1021/acsfoodscitech.4c01074.

Krishnegowda, R., Ravindra, M.R., Sharma, M., 2021. Application of supercritical fluid extraction for extraction or enrichment of phospholipids in egg and dairy products: a review. J. Food Process Eng. 0145-8876. 44 (6). doi:10.1111/jfpe.13692.

Krissansen, G.W., 2007. Emerging health properties of whey proteins and their clinical implications. J. Am. Coll. Nutr. 15411087. 26 (6), 713–723. doi:10.1080/07315724.2007.10719652.

Kuhnle, G.G.C., Dell'Aquila, C., Aspinall, S.M., Runswick, S.A., Mulligan, A.A., Bingham, S.A., 2008. Phytoestrogen content of foods of animal origin: dairy products, eggs, meat, fish, and seafood. J. Agric. Food Chem. 0021-8561. 56 (21), 10099–10104. doi:10.1021/jf801344x.

Kumar, P., Sharma, N., Ranjan, R., Kumar, S., Bhat, Z.F., Jeong, D.K., 2013. Perspective of membrane technology in dairy industry: a review. Asian-Australas. J. Anim. Sci. 19765517. 26 (9), 1347–1358. Available from: http://www.ajas.info/. doi:10.5713/ajas.2013.13082India.

Kumar, V., Tingirikari, J.M.R., 2023. Degree of methylation: a key to the functional properties of low methylated pectin derived from pectin rich agrowaste. Food Biosci. 22124292. 56, 103386. doi:10.1016/j.fbio.2023.103386.

Kwak, H.-S., Mijan, M.A., Ganesan, P., 2014. Chapter 11 - Application of nanomaterials, nano- and microencapsulation to milk and dairy products. In: Kwak, H.-S. (Ed.), Nano- and Microencapsulation for Foods. Wiley and Sons, pp. 273–300. Available from: https://www.wiley.com/remtitle.cgi?isbn=1118292332. doi:10.1002/9781118292327.ch11.

Kwaw, E., Ma, Y., Tchabo, W., Apaliya, M.T., Sackey, A.S., Wu, M., Xiao, L., 2018. Impact of ultrasonication and pulsed light treatments on phenolics concentration and antioxidant activities of lactic-acid-fermented mulberry juice. LWT. 00236438. 92, 61–66. Available from: https://www.journals.elsevier.com/lwt. doi:10.1016/j.lwt.2018.02.016.

Kyung, S., Koh, W.G., Lee, H.J., 2025. A photo-crosslinked casein-tannic acid system for enhanced hair protection: a green chemistry approach. Polymers. 20734360. 17 (12). Available from: http://www.mdpi.com/journal/polymers. doi:10.3390/polym17121585.

La Torre, C., Caputo, P., Cione, E., Fazio, A., 2024. Comparing nutritional values and bioactivity of kefir from different types of animal milk. Molecules. 1420-3049. 29 (11), 2710. doi:10.3390/molecules29112710.

Lambrini, K., Aikaterini, F., Konstantinos, K., Christos, I., Ioanna, P.V., Areti, T., 2020. Milk nutritional composition and its role in human health. J. Pharm. Pharmacol. 23282150. 9 (1). doi:10.17265/2328-2150/2021.01.002.

Larráyoz, P., Ibáñez, F.C., Ordóñez, A.I., Torre, P., Barcina, Y., 2000. Evaluation of supercritical fluid extraction as sample preparation method for the study of Roncal cheese aroma. Int. Dairy J. 09586946. 10 (11), 755–759. doi:10.1016/s0958-6946(00)00109-6.

Lee, K., Kim, A., Hong, K.B., Suh, H.J., Jo, K., 2020. Preparation and characterization of a polar milk lipid-enriched component from whey powder. Food Sci. Anim. Resour. 26360780. 40 (2), 209–220. Available from: https://www.kosfaj.org/archive/view_article?pid=kosfa-40-2-209. doi:10.5851/kosfa.2020.e5.

Li, C., Zhang, Y., Wan, Y., Wang, J., Lin, J., Zhiming, L., Huang, P., 2021. STING-activating drug delivery systems: design strategies and biomedical applications. Chin. Chem. Lett. 10018417. 32 (5), 1615–1625. doi:10.1016/j.cclet.2021.01.001.

Liao, K., Zhang, X., Liu, J., Teng, F., Yingcheng, H., Cheng, J., Yang, Q., Zhang, W., Xie, Y., Guo, D., Cao, G., Yanmei, X., Huang, B., Wang, X., 2023. The role of platelets in the regulation of tumor growth and metastasis: the mechanisms and targeted therapy. MedComm. 2688-2663. 4 (5). doi:10.1002/mco2.350.

Lim, H.W., Kohli, I., Ruvolo, E., Kolbe, L., Hamzavi, I.H., 2022. Impact of visible light on skin health: the role of antioxidants and free radical quenchers in skin protection. J. Am. Acad. Dermatol. 10976787. 86 (3), S27. Available from: http://www.elsevier.com/inca/publications/store/6/2/3/3/7/0/index.htt. doi:10.1016/j.jaad.2021.12.024.

Liu, N., Matsumura, H., Kato, T., Ichinose, S., Takada, A., Namiki, T., Asakawa, K., Morinaga, H., Mohri, Y., De Arcangelis, A., Geroges-Labouesse, E., Nanba, D., Nishimura, E.K., 2019. Stem cell competition orchestrates skin homeostasis and ageing. Nature. 0028-0836. 568 (7752), 344–350. doi:10.1038/s41586-019-1085-7.

Liu, P., Chen, G., Zhang, J., 2022a. A review of liposomes as a drug delivery system: current status of approved products, regulatory environments, and future perspectives. Molecules. 1420-3049. 27 (4), 1372. doi:10.3390/molecules27041372.

Liu, Y.H., Liu, T.T., Niu, J.Q., Zhang, X.S., Xu, W.S., Song, S., Wang, Z., 2024. Characterization of phospholipidome in milk, yogurt and cream, and phospholipid differences related to various dairy processing methods. Food Chem. 18737072. 454. Available from: https://www.sciencedirect.com/science/journal/03088146. doi:10.1016/j.foodchem.2024.139733.

Liu, Y., Hettinga, K., Liu, D., Zhang, L., Zhou, P., 2022b. Current progress of emerging technologies in human and animals' milk processing: retention of immune-active components and microbial safety. Compr. Rev. Food Sci. Food Saf. 1541-4337. 21 (5), 4327–4353. doi:10.1111/1541-4337.13019.

Lopez, C., Blot, M., Briard-Bion, V., Cirié, C., Graulet, B., 2017. Butter serums and buttermilks as sources of bioactive lipids from the milk fat globule membrane: differences in their lipid composition and potentialities of cow diet to increase n-3 PUFA. Food Res. Int. 09639969. 100 (Pt 1), 864–872. doi:10.1016/j.foodres.2017.08.016.

Lordan, R., Tsoupras, A., Zabetakis, I., 2017. Phospholipids of animal and marine origin: structure, function, and anti-inflammatory properties. Molecules. 1420-3049. 22 (11), 1964. doi:10.3390/molecules22111964.

Lordan, R., Zabetakis, I., 2017. Invited review: the anti-inflammatory properties of dairy lipids. J. Dairy Sci. 00220302. 100 (6), 4197–4212. doi:10.3168/jds.2016-12224.

Luparelli, A., Trisciuzzi, D., Schirinzi, W.M., Caputo, L., Smiriglia, L., Quintieri, L., Nicolotti, O., Monaci, L., 2025. Whey proteins and bioactive peptides: advances in production, selection and bioactivity profiling. Biomedicines. 2227-9059. 13 (6), 1311. doi:10.3390/biomedicines13061311.

Macías, D.S., Castro, N., Argüello, A., Flores, R.J., 2014. Supercritical fluid extraction application on dairy products and by-products. In: Handbook on Supercritical Fluids: Fundamentals, Properties and Applications. Nova Science Publishers, Inc., Ecuador, pp. 281–300. Available from: https://api.semanticscholar.org/CorpusID:220622519.

Madureira, A.R., Pereira, C.I., Gomes, A.M.P., Pintado, M.E., Malcata, F.X., 2007. Bovine whey proteins—overview on their main biological properties. Food Res. Int. 09639969. 40 (10), 1197–1211. doi:10.1016/j.foodres.2007.07.005.

Manuelian, C.L., Currò, S., Penasa, M., Cassandro, M., De Marchi, M., 2017. Characterization of major and trace minerals, fatty acid composition, and cholesterol content of Protected Designation of Origin cheeses. J. Dairy Sci. 00220302. 100 (5), 3384–3395. doi:10.3168/jds.2016-12059.

Marcone, S., Haughton, K., Simpson, P.J., Belton, O., Fitzgerald, D.J., 2015. Milk-derived bioactive peptides inhibit human endothelial-monocyte interactions via PPAR-γ dependent regulation of NF-κB. J. Inflamm. 1476-9255. 12 (1), 1. doi:10.1186/s12950-014-0044-1.

Marsanasco, M., Alonso, S. del V., 2022. Stability of bioactive compounds in liposomes after pasteurisation and storage of functional chocolate milk. Int. J. Food Sci. Technol. 0950-5423. 57 (1), 361–369. doi:10.1111/ijfs.15420.

Masoomikarimi, M., Salehi, M., 2022. Modulation of the immune system promotes tissue regeneration. Mol. Biotechnol. 1073-6085. 64 (6), 599–610. doi:10.1007/s12033-021-00430-8.

Mathews, A., Arbal, A.V., Kaarunya, A., Jha, P.K., Le-Bail, A., Rawson, A., 2024. Conventional Vs Modern Extraction Techniques in the Food Industry. Elsevier BV, pp. 97–146. doi:10.1016/b978-0-12-819516-1.00013-2.

Medina, A.L., da Silva, M.A.O., de Sousa Barbosa, H., Arruda, M.A.Z., Marsaioli, A., Bragagnolo, N., 2015. Rapid microwave assisted extraction of meat lipids. Food Res. Int. 09639969. 78, 124–130. Available from: www.elsevier.com/inca/publications/store/4/2/2/9/7/0. doi:10.1016/j.foodres.2015.10.028.

Mehmood, A., Ishaq, M., Zhao, L., Yaqoob, S., Safdar, B., Nadeem, M., Munir, M., Wang, C., 2019. Impact of ultrasound and conventional extraction techniques on bioactive compounds and biological activities of blue butterfly pea flower (*Clitoria ternatea* L.). Ultrason. Sonochem. 13504177. 51, 12–19. doi:10.1016/j.ultsonch.2018.10.013.

Mehra, R., Singh, R., Nayan, V., Buttar, H.S., Kumar, N., Kumar, S., Bhardwaj, A., Kaushik, R., Kumar, H., 2021. Nutritional attributes of bovine colostrum components in human health and disease: a comprehensive review. Food Biosci. 22124292. 40, 100907. doi:10.1016/j.fbio.2021.100907.

Mehrbani, M., Choopani, R., Fekri, A., Mehrabani, M., Mosaddegh, M., Mehrabani, M., 2015. The efficacy of whey associated with dodder seed extract on moderate-to-severe atopic dermatitis in adults: a randomized, double-blind, placebo-controlled clinical trial. J. Ethnopharmacol. 03788741. 172, 325–332. doi:10.1016/j.jep.2015.07.003.

Mehta, B.M., Mutkule, S.N., Hebishy, E., Datta, N., 2025. Milk sphingolipids as functional components. Acad. Nutr. Diet. 3067-1345. 2 (2). doi:10.20935/acadnutr7694.

Melse-Boonstra, A., 2020. Bioavailability of micronutrients from nutrient-dense whole foods: zooming in on dairy, vegetables, and fruits. Front. Nutr. 2296-861X. 7. doi:10.3389/fnut.2020.00101.

Mena-Sánchez, G., Becerra-Tomás, N., Babio, N., Salas-Salvadó, J., 2019. Dairy product consumption in the prevention of metabolic syndrome: a systematic review and meta-analysis of prospective cohort studies. Adv. Nutr. 21618313. 10 (suppl_2), S144. doi:10.1093/advances/nmy083.

Merkel, A., Rudolph-Schöpping, G., Suwal, S., Lipnizki, F., Lillevang, S.K., Ahrné, L., 2024. Application of bipolar membrane electrodialysis for acidification of skim milk. A comprehensive study on process performance and effects on ion-exchange membranes. J. Membr. Sci. 03767388. 694, 122429. doi:10.1016/j.memsci.2024.122429.

Michalek, I.M., John, S.M., Dos Santos, F.L.C., 2019. Microbiological contamination of cosmetic products—observations from Europe, 2005–2018. J. Eur. Acad. Dermatol. Venereol. 0926-9959. 33 (11), 2151–2157. doi:10.1111/jdv.15728.

Mishra, A., Salunke, P., Sunkesula, V., Metzger, L.E., 2025. Manufacture of high-solids milk protein concentrate retentate using plate-and-frame membrane filtration system at low and high temperatures. J. Dairy Sci. 15253198. 108 (5), 4785–4795. Available from: https://www.sciencedirect.com/science/journal/00220302. doi:10.3168/jds.2024-25472.

Moejes, S., Guzmán, M.R., Hanemaaijer, J., Barrera, K.H., Feenstra, L., van Boxtel, T., 2015. Membrane distillation for milk concentration. In: 29th EFFoST International Conference Proceedings, 10–12 November 2015, Athens, Greece.

Mohammed, P.A.E.I., Elgasim, P.E.A., Basheer, P.E.O., 2022. Physicochemical, minerals and fatty acids of yoghurt as affected by milk source. Int. J. Innov. Sci. Eng. Technol. 9, 24–38.

Mohanty, D., Jena, R., Choudhury, P.K., Pattnaik, R., Mohapatra, S., Saini, M.R., 2016. Milk derived antimicrobial bioactive peptides: a review. Int. J. Food Prop. 15322386. 19 (4), 837–846. Available from: www.tandf.co.uk/journals/titles/10942912.asp. doi:10.1080/10942912.2015.1048356.

Moosavian, S.P., Rahimlou, M., Saneei, P., Esmaillzadeh, A., 2020. Effects of dairy products consumption on inflammatory biomarkers among adults: a systematic review and meta-analysis of randomized controlled trials. Nutr. Metab. Cardiovasc. Dis. 15903729. 30 (6), 872–888. Available from: http://www.elsevier.com/wps/find/journaldescription.cws_home/704955/description#description. doi:10.1016/j.numecd.2020.01.011.

Mottram, D.S., Elmore, J.S., 2003. Sensory Evaluation | Aroma. Elsevier BV, pp. 5174–5180. doi:10.1016/b0-12-227055-x/01068-3.

Mudgil, P., AlMazroui, M., Redha, A.A., Kilari, B.P., Srikumar, S., Maqsood, S., 2022. Cow and camel milk-derived whey and casein protein hydrolysates demonstrated effective antifungal properties against selected Candida species. J. Dairy Sci. 15253198. 105 (3), 1878–1888. Available from: http://www.elsevier.com/wps/find/journaldescription.cws_home/721317/description#description. doi:10.3168/jds.2021-20944.

Mukesh, M., Mann, S., Shandilya, U.K., Kumar, P., Mohanty, A., 2014. Determination of antioxidant capacity and free radical scavenging activity of milk from native cows (*Bos indicus*), exotic cows (*Bos taurus*), and riverine buffaloes (*Bubalus bubalis*) across different lactation stages. Int. J. Dairy Sci. Process. 23791578, 66–70. doi:10.19070/2379-1578-1600013.

Commissioner O of the Draft Guidance for Industry: cosmetic Good Manufacturing Practices 2024, n.d. Available from: https://www.fda.gov/regulatory-information/search-fda-guidance-documents/draft-guidance-industry-cosmetic-good-manufacturing-practices.

Commissioner O of the Good Manufacturing Practice (GMP) Guidelines/Inspection Checklist for Cosmetics, n.d.

KJMN Sampon Keratinnal és Tejproteinnel—Kallos Cosmetics, n.d. Available from: https://kallos.com/products/kjmn-sampon-keratinnal-es-tejproteinnel.

Korres Mediterranean Donkey Milk Protein Strengthening Face Cream 40 ml, n.d. Available from: https://epharmadora.com/cosmetics/face/day-creams/korres-mediterranean-donkey-milk-protein-strengthening-face-cream-40ml.

Medi-Peel Red Lacto Collagen Barrier Firming Cream, 80ml, n.d. Available from: https://plaggona-skincare.com/products/medi-peel-red-lacto-peptide-collagen-barrier-cream-80-ml.

Milk Protein for Improved Metabolic Health: a Review of the Evidence | nutrition & Metabolism, n.d. Available from: https://nutritionandmetabolism.biomedcentral.com/articles/10.1186/1743-7075-10-46.

Morfose Milk Therapy Creamy Milk Shampoo, n.d. Available from: https://morfose.eu/en/product/morfose-milk-therapy-creamy-milk-shampoo/.

Peptide Advanced Anti-Wrinkle Day Cream - Aphrodite Skin Care, n.d. Available from: https://www.aphroditeusa.com/peptide-advanced-anti-wrinkle-day-cream/.

Regulation - 1223/2009 - EN - Cosmetic Products Regulation - EUR-Lex, n.d. Available from: https://eur-lex.europa.eu/legal-content/EN/TXT/?uri=CELEX%3A32009R1223.

The Benefits of Kefir in Skin Care—What is Kefir and Its Benefit for Skin, n.d. Available from: https://nayelle.com/benefits-kefir-skin-care/?srsltid=AfmBOoo8S5CzflsF96bAwISdgShyVlGIHNqeLz179xvGEMXGOvPMK11I.

Yoghurt Lip Balm—Suncare Protection SPF 20, n.d. Available from: https://gr.korres.com/products/lipcarelip-balm-yoghurt-suncare-protection-spf20?srsltid=AfmBOoqfZ1KZOEHTe-iptL4y0zSHG2Zo5CDUNiI6VNGQBu6LZ16FnJSo.

Nagaoka, S., 2019. Yogurt production. In: Kanauchi, M. (Ed.), Lactic Acid Bacteria. In: Methods in Molecular Biology, vol. 1887. Springer New York. pp. 45–54. Available from: https://www.springer.com/series/7651. doi:10.1007/978-1-4939-8907-2_5.

Narvekar, M., Xue, H.Y., Wong, H.L., 2012. A novel hybrid delivery system: polymer-oil nanostructured carrier for controlled delivery of highly lipophilic drug all-trans-retinoic acid (ATRA). Int. J. Pharm. 18733476. 436 (1-2), 721–731. doi:10.1016/j.ijpharm.2012.07.042.

Neelima, R.S., Rajput, Y.S., Mann, B., 2013. Chemical and functional properties of glycomacropeptide (GMP) and its role in the detection of cheese whey adulteration in milk: a review. Dairy Sci. Technol. 1958-5586. 93 (1), 21–43. doi:10.1007/s13594-012-0095-0.

Ni, Q., Gasperi, F., Aprea, E., Betta, E., Bergamaschi, M., Tagliapietra, F., Schiavon, S., Bittante, G., 2020. The volatile organic compound profile of ripened cheese is influenced by crude protein shortage and conjugated linoleic acid supplementation in the cow's diet. J. Dairy Sci. 00220302. 103 (2), 1377–1390. doi:10.3168/jds.2019-16495.

Nicolaou, N., Pancheva, R., Karaglani, E., Sekkidou, M., Marinova-Achkar, M., Popova, S., Tzaki, M., Kapetanaki, A., Iacovidou, N., Boutsikou, T., Iliodromiti, Z., Papaevangelou, V., Sardeli, O., Xepapadaki, P., Papathoma, E., Thijs-Verhoeven, I., Kudla, U., Ulfman, L.H., Schaafsma, A., Manios, Y., 2022. The risk reduction effect of a nutritional intervention with a partially hydrolyzed whey-based formula on cow's milk protein allergy and atopic dermatitis in high-risk infants within the first 6 months of life: the Allergy Reduction Trial (A.R.T.), a multicenter double-blinded randomized controlled study. Front. Nutr. 2296-861X. 9. doi:10.3389/fnut.2022.863599.

Nielsen, S.D.H., Liang, N., Rathish, H., Kim, B.J., Lueangsakulthai, J., Koh, J., Qu, Y., Schulz, H.J., Dallas, D.C., 2024. Bioactive milk peptides: an updated comprehensive overview and database. Crit. Rev. Food Sci. Nutr. 15497852. 64 (31), 11510–11529. Available from: https://www.tandfonline.com/loi/bfsn20. doi:10.1080/10408398.2023.2240396.

Nighojkar, A., Patidar, M.K., Nighojkar, S., 2019. Pectinases: Production and Applications for Fruit Juice Beverages. Elsevier BV, pp. 235–273. doi:10.1016/b978-0-12-815259-1.00008-2.

Ningsih, Y.D.P., Eka Putra, D., 2025. Value chain and added value in goat milk-based enterprise: a case study of Kefir Jember. J. Supply Chain Entrep. 3090-563X. 1 (1), 13–19. doi:10.64268/josce.v1i1.5.

Niu, Z., Acevedo-Fani, A., McDowell, A., Barnett, A., Loveday, S.M., Singh, H., 2020. Nanoemulsion structure and food matrix determine the gastrointestinal fate and in vivo bioavailability of coenzyme Q10. J. Control. Release. 18734995. 327, 444–455. Available from: www.elsevier.com/locate/jconrel. doi:10.1016/j.jconrel.2020.08.025.

Nunes, J.C., Torres, A.G., 2010. Fatty acid and CLA composition of Brazilian dairy products, and contribution to daily intake of CLA. J. Food Compos. Anal. 08891575. 23 (8), 782–789. doi:10.1016/j.jfca.2010.03.023.

O'Brien, N.M., O'Connor, T.P., 2004. Nutritional aspects of cheese. Cheese: Chem. Phys. Microbiol. 1, 573–581. Available from http://www.sciencedirect.com/science/bookseries/1874558X. doi:10.1016/S1874-558X(04)80083-6.

Oliveira, A.P.D., Santos, G.A.D., Nomura, C.S., Naozuka, J., 2019. Elemental chemical composition of products derived from kefir fermented milk. J. Food Compos. Anal. 08891575. 78, 86–90. Available from: http://www.elsevier.com/inca/publications/store/6/2/2/8/7/8/index.htt. doi:10.1016/j.jfca.2019.02.005.

Öneş, E., Zavotçu, M., Nisan, N., Baş, M., Sağlam, D., 2025. Effects of Kefir consumption on gut microbiota and athletic performance in professional female soccer players: a randomized controlled trial. Nutrients. 2072-6643. 17 (3), 512. doi:10.3390/nu17030512.

Ozel, B., McClements, D.J., Arikan, C., Kaner, O., Oztop, M.H., 2022. Challenges in dried whey powder production: quality problems. Food Res. Int. 09639969. 160, 111682. doi:10.1016/j.foodres.2022.111682.

Pădureț, S., 2021. The effect of fat content and fatty acids composition on color and textural properties of butter. Molecules. 1420-3049. 26 (15), 4565. doi:10.3390/molecules26154565.

Panchal, B., Truong, T., Prakash, S., Bansal, N., Bhandari, B., 2021. Influence of emulsifiers and dairy ingredients on manufacturing, microstructure, and physical properties of butter. Foods. 2304-8158. 10 (5), 1140. doi:10.3390/foods10051140.

Papaccio, F., D'Arino, A., Caputo, S., Bellei, B., 2022. Focus on the contribution of oxidative stress in skin aging. Antioxidants. 2076-3921. 11 (6), 1121. doi:10.3390/antiox11061121.

Papaioannou, G., Kosma, I., Badeka, A.V., Kontominas, M.G., 2021. Profile of volatile compounds in dessert yogurts prepared from cow and goat milk, using different starter cultures and probiotics. Foods. 2304-8158. 10 (12), 3153. doi:10.3390/foods10123153.

Pappa, E.C., Kondyli, E., Pappas, A.C., Kyriakaki, P., Zoidis, E., Papalamprou, L., Karageorgou, A., Simitzis, P., Goliomytis, M., Tsiplakou, E., Georgiou, C.A., 2024. Physicochemical characteristics of commercially available Greek yoghurts. Dairy. 2624862X. 5 (3), 436–450. Available from: https://www.mdpi.com/journal/dairy. doi:10.3390/dairy5030034.

Park, J., Choi, J.H., Kim, S., Jang, I., Jeong, S., Lee, J.Y., 2019. Micropatterned conductive hydrogels as multifunctional muscle-mimicking biomaterials: graphene-incorporated hydrogels directly patterned with femtosecond laser ablation. Acta Biomater. 18787568. 97, 141–153. Available from: http://www.journals.elsevier.com/acta-biomaterialia. doi:10.1016/j.actbio.2019.07.044.

Park, Y.W., 2009. Bioactive Components in Milk and Dairy Products. Wiley. doi:10.1002/9780813821504.

Park, Y.W., Jeanjulien, C., Siddique, A., 2017. Factors affecting sensory quality of goat milk cheeses: a review. Adv. Dairy Res. 2329888X. 05 (03). doi:10.4172/2329-888X.1000185.

Park, Y.W., Nam, M.S., 2015. Bioactive peptides in milk and dairy products: a review. Korean J. Food Sci. Anim. Resour. 2234246X. 35 (6), 831–840. Available from: http://www.kosfa.kr/journal.do?method=currentIssue&journalSeq=J000033&menuId=0201&introMenuId=0201. doi:10.5851/kosfa.2015.35.6.831.

Parodi, P.W., 2001. Cow's milk components with anti-cancer potential. Aust. J. Dairy Technol. 56, 65–73.

Patel, M., Eckburg, A., Gantiwala, S., Hart, Z., Dein, J., Lam, K., Puri, N., 2021. Resistance to molecularly targeted therapies in melanoma. Cancers. 2072-6694. 13 (5), 1115. doi:10.3390/cancers13051115.

Pavlovic, D., Niciforovic, D., Markovic, M., Papic, D., 2023. Cancer-associated thrombosis: epidemiology, pathophysiological mechanisms, treatment, and risk assessment. Clin. Med. Insights Oncol. 1179-5549. 17. doi:10.1177/11795549231220297.

Pei, J., Zhu, Q., Zhu, Y., Guo, C., Valencak, T.G., Tang, S.Y., Ren, T., Ren, D., 2025. Milk protein-based hydrogels: development and biomedical applications. Biomater. Transl. 2096112X. 6 (2), 127–150. Available from: https://www.biomat-trans.com/EN/2096-112X/home.shtml. doi:10.12336/bmt.24.00071.

Pérez Núñez, I., Díaz, R., Quiñones, J., Martínez, A., Velázquez, L., Huaiquipán, R., Tapia, D., Muñoz, A., Valdés, M., Sepúlveda, N., Paz, E., 2024. Molecular characteristics and processing technologies of dairy products from non-traditional species. Molecules. 1420-3049. 29 (22), 5427. doi:10.3390/molecules29225427.

Perna, A., Simonetti, A., Grassi, G., Gambacorta, E., 2018. Effect of αS1-casein genotype on phenolic compounds and antioxidant activity in goat milk yogurt fortified with *Rhus coriaria* leaf powder. J. Dairy Sci. 00220302. 101 (9), 7691–7701. doi:10.3168/jds.2018-14613.

Perret, J.K., Velázquez, A.G., Mehn, A., 2025. Green cosmetics—the effects of package design on consumers' willingness-to-pay and sustainability perceptions. Sustainability. 2071-1050. 17 (6), 2581. doi:10.3390/su17062581.

Pfeuffer, M., Schrezenmeir, J., 2007. Milk and the metabolic syndrome. Obes. Rev. 1467-7881. 8 (2), 109–118. doi:10.1111/j.1467-789x.2006.00265.x.

Pietri, A., Fortunati, P., Mulazzi, A., Bertuzzi, T., 2016. Enzyme-assisted extraction for the HPLC determination of aflatoxin M1 in cheese. Food Chem. 03088146. 192, 235–241. doi:10.1016/j.foodchem.2015.07.006.

Playford, R.J., Weiser, M.J., 2021. Bovine colostrum: its constituents and uses. Nutrients. 20726643. 13 (1), 1–24. Available from: https://www.mdpi.com/2072-6643/13/1/265/pdf. doi:10.3390/nu13010265.

Poveda, J.M., Sánchez-Palomo, E., Pérez-Coello, M.S., Cabezas, L., 2008. Volatile composition, olfactometry profile and sensory evaluation of semi-hard Spanish goat cheeses. Dairy Sci. Technol. 19585594. 88 (3), 355–367. doi:10.1051/dst:2007021.

Pozzobon, V., Pozzobon, C., 2019. Cottage cheese in a diet—a review. Nutr. Food Sci. 0034-6659. 49 (6), 1265–1274. doi:10.1108/nfs-03-2019-0073.

Prosser, C.G., 2021. Compositional and functional characteristics of goat milk and relevance as a base for infant formula. J. Food Sci. 17503841. 86 (2), 257–265. Available from: http://onlinelibrary.wiley.com/journal/10.1111/(ISSN)1750-3841. doi:10.1111/1750-3841.15574.

Prussick, R., Prussick, L., Gutman, J., 2013. Psoriasis improvement in patients using glutathione-enhancing, nondenatured whey protein isolate: a pilot study. J. Clin. Aesthet. Dermatol. 19412789. 6 (10), 23–26. Available from http://jcadonline.epubxp.com/i/191151.

Qiu, L., Zhang, M., Chitrakar, B., Bhandari, B., 2020. Application of power ultrasound in freezing and thawing processes: effect on process efficiency and product quality. Ultrason. Sonochem. 13504177. 68, 105230. doi:10.1016/j.ultsonch.2020.105230.

Rampazzo, G., Zironi, E., Pagliuca, G., Gazzotti, T., 2022. Analysis of cobalamin (Vit B12) in ripened cheese by ultra-high-performance liquid chromatography coupled with mass spectrometry. Foods. 2304-8158. 11 (18), 2745. doi:10.3390/foods11182745.

Rao, S., Radhakrishnan, P., Valiathan, S., Supriya, M., 2023. Rosehip oil nanoemulsion as a stable delivery system for omega-3 fatty acids to enhance the nutritional value of yogurt. Food Chem. Adv. 2772753X. 3, 100545. doi:10.1016/j.focha.2023.100545.

Rashad, M.M., Mahmoud, A.E., Abdou, H.M., Nooman, M.U., 2011. Improvement of nutritional quality and antioxidant activities of yeast fermented soybean curd residue. Afr. J. Biotechnol. 16845315. 10 (28), 5504–5513. Available from http://www.academicjournals.org/AJB/PDF/pdf2011/20Jun/Rashad%20et%20al.pdf.

Rendon-Rosales, M.Á., Torres-Llanez, M.J., González-Córdova, A.F., Hernández-Mendoza, A., Mazorra-Manzano, M.A., Vallejo-Cordoba, B., 2019. In vitro antithrombotic and hypocholesterolemic activities of milk fermented with specific strains of *Lactococcus lactis*. Nutrients. 20726643. 11 (9). Available from: https://www.mdpi.com/2072-6643/11/9/2150/pdf. doi:10.3390/nu11092150.

Rocafi, A., Lamiot, E., Moroni, O., Turgeon, S.L., Gauthier, S.F., Pouliot, Y., 2011. Effect of milk thermal history on the recovery of TGF-β2 by acid precipitation of whey protein concentrates. Dairy Sci. Technol. 19585594. 91 (5), 615–627. doi:10.1007/s13594-011-0041-6.

Rocchetti, G., Ghilardelli, F., Mosconi, M., Masoero, F., Gallo, A., 2022. Occurrence of polyphenols, isoflavonoids, and their metabolites in milk samples from different cow feeding regimens. Dairy. 2624-862X. 3 (2), 314–325. doi:10.3390/dairy3020024.

Rodríguez-Alcalá, L.M., Castro-Gómez, M.P., Pimentel, L.L., Fontecha, J., 2017. Milk fat components with potential anticancer activity—a review. Biosci. Rep. 15734935. 37 (6). Available from: http://www.bioscirep.org/content/37/6/BSR20170705.full-text.pdf. doi:10.1042/BSR20170705.

Rohmah, R.N., Hardiyanti, F., Fatchiyah, F., 2015. Inhibition on JAK-STAT3 signaling transduction cascade is taken by bioactive peptide alpha-S2 casein protein from goat Ethawah breed milk. Acta Inform. Med. 19865988. 23 (4), 233–238. Available from: http://www.ejmanager.com/mnstemps/6/6-1438265539.pdf?t=1444469595. doi:10.5455/aim.2015.23.233-238.

Rudzińska, M., Grygier, A., Knight, G., Kmiecik, D., 2024. Liposomes as carriers of bioactive compounds in human nutrition. Foods. 2304-8158. 13 (12), 1814. doi:10.3390/foods13121814.

Runte, M., Guth, J.N., Ammann, J., 2024. Consumers' perception of plant-based alternatives and changes over time. A linguistic analysis across three countries and ten years. Food Qual. Prefer. 09503293. 113, 105057. doi:10.1016/j.foodqual.2023.105057.

Rusu, D., Drouin, R., Pouliot, Y., Gauthier, S., Poubelle, P.E., 2009. A bovine whey protein extract can enhance innate immunity by priming normal human blood neutrophils. J. Nutr. 15416100. 139 (2), 386–393. Available from: http://jn.nutrition.org/cgi/reprint/139/2/386. doi:10.3945/jn.108.098459Canada.

Sadiq, U., Gill, H., Chandrapala, J., 2021. Casein micelles as an emerging delivery system for bioactive food components. Foods. 2304-8158. 10 (8), 1965. doi:10.3390/foods10081965.

Sadvari, V.Y., Shevchenko, L.V., Slobodyanyuk, N.M., Furman, S.V., Lisohurska, D.V., Lisohurska, O.V., 2024. Chemical composition of craft hard cheeses from raw goat milk during the ripening process. Regul. Mech. Biosyst. 25202588. 15 (4), 666–673. Available from: https://medicine.dp.ua/index.php/med/article/view/1045. doi:10.15421/022496.

Šalaševičius, A., Uždavinytė, D., Visockis, M., Ruzgys, P., Šatkauskas, S., 2021. Effect of pulsed electric field (PEF) on bacterial viability and whey protein in the processing of raw milk. Appl. Sci. 2076-3417. 11 (23), 11281. doi:10.3390/app112311281.

Sánchez-Camargo, A.P., Mendiola, J.A., Ibáñez, E., Herrero, M., 2014. Supercritical Fluid Extraction. Elsevier BV. doi:10.1016/b978-0-12-409547-2.10753-x.

Sant'Ana, A.M.S., Bezerril, F.F., Madruga, M.S., Batista, A.S.M., Magnani, M., Souza, E.L., Queiroga, R.C.R.E., 2013. Nutritional and sensory characteristics of Minas fresh cheese made with goat milk, cow milk, or a mixture of both. J. Dairy Sci. 00220302. 96 (12), 7442–7453. doi:10.3168/jds.2013-6915.

Santiago-López, L., Aguilar-Toalá, J.E., Hernández-Mendoza, A., Vallejo-Cordoba, B., Liceaga, A.M., González-Córdova, A.F., 2018. Invited review: bioactive compounds produced during cheese ripening and health effects associated with aged cheese consumption. J. Dairy Sci. 15253198. 101 (5), 3742–3757. Available from: http://www.elsevier.com/wps/find/journaldescription.cws_home/721317/description#description. doi:10.3168/jds.2017-13465.

Satir, G., Guzel-Seydim, Z.B., 2016. How kefir fermentation can affect product composition? Small Rumin. Res. 09214488. 134, 1–7. Available from: www.elsevier.com/inca/publications/store/5/0/3/3/1/7/index.htt. doi:10.1016/j.smallrumres.2015.10.022.

Schweigert, F.J., Hurtienne, A., Bathe, K., 2000. Improved extraction procedure for carotenoids from human milk. Int. J. Vitam. Nutr. Res. 03009831. 70 (3), 79–83. Available from: http://www.medcontent.ch/content/0300-9831. doi:10.1024/0300-9831.70.3.79.

Séverin, S., Wenshui, X., 2005. Milk biologically active components as nutraceuticals: review. Crit. Rev. Food Sci. Nutr. 1040-8398. 45 (7-8), 645–656. doi:10.1080/10408690490911756.

Shen, L., Pang, S., Zhong, M., Sun, Y., Qayum, A., Liu, Y., Rashid, A., Baoguo, X., Liang, Q., Haile, M., Ren, X., 2023. A comprehensive review of ultrasonic assisted extraction (UAE) for bioactive components: principles, advantages, equipment, and combined technologies. Ultrason. Sonochem. 13504177. 101, 106646. doi:10.1016/j.ultsonch.2023.106646.

Shori, A.B., 2013. Antioxidant activity and viability of lactic acid bacteria in soybean-yogurt made from cow and camel milk. J. Taibah Univ. Sci. 16583655. 7 (4), 202–208. Available from: https://www.tandfonline.com/journals/tusc20. doi:10.1016/j.jtusci.2013.06.003.

Sik, B., Buzás, H., Kapcsándi, V., Lakatos, E., Daróczi, F., Székelyhidi, R., 2023. Antioxidant and polyphenol content of different milk and dairy products. J. King Saud Univ. Sci. 10183647. 35 (7), 102839. doi:10.1016/j.jksus.2023.102839.

Singh, S.K., Pavan, M.S., Sai Prasanna, N., Kant, R., 2018. Applications of super critical fluid extraction in milk and dairy industry: a review. J. Food Process. Technol. 21577110. 9 (12). doi:10.4172/2157-7110.1000769.

SKINAZ Mozzarella Cheese Cream | ingredients & Benefits. Available from: https://www.hwahae.com/en/products/SKINAZ-Mozzarella-Cheese-Cream/1735259.

Sobkowska, D., Micek, I., Urbańska, M., Seraszek-Jaros, A., Nowak, G., Zaprutko, L., Czajkowski, R., Adamski, Z., Gornowicz-Porowska, J., 2021. The effects of baths and wet wraps with a sweet whey solution on the level of hydration and barrier function of the epidermis. Adv. Dermatol. Allergol. 1642-395X. 38 (5), 798–803. doi:10.5114/ada.2021.110078.

Solaberrieta, I., Mellinas, A.C., Espagnol, J., Hamzaoui, M., Jiménez, A., Carmen Garrigós, M., 2022. Valorization of tomato seed by-products as a source of fatty acids and bioactive compounds by using advanced extraction techniques. Foods. 2304-8158. 11 (16), 2408. doi:10.3390/foods11162408.

Soutelino, M.E.M., de Oliveira Silva, A.C., Rocha, R.D.S., 2024. Natural antimicrobials in dairy products: benefits, challenges, and future trends. Antibiotics. 2079-6382. 13 (5), 415. doi:10.3390/antibiotics13050415.

Sprick, B., Linghu, Z., Amamcharla, J.K., Metzger, L.E., Smith, J.S., 2019. Selective extraction of phospholipids from whey protein phospholipid concentrate using supercritical carbon dioxide and ethanol as a co-solvent. J. Dairy Sci. 00220302. 102 (12), 10855–10866. doi:10.3168/jds.2019-16419.

Stergiadis, S., Nørskov, N.P., Purup, S., Givens, I., Lee, M.R.F., 2019. Comparative nutrient profiling of retail goat and cow milk. Nutrients. 20726643. 11 (10). Available from: https://www.mdpi.com/2072-6643/11/10/2282/pdf. doi:10.3390/nu11102282.

Suganya, V., Anuradha, V., 2017. Microencapsulation and nanoencapsulation: a review. Int. J. Pharm. Clin. Res. 0975-1556. 9 (3). doi:10.25258/ijpcr.v9i3.8324.

Sun, H., Xusheng, G., Yunkai, L., Wang, A., 2012. Application of accelerated solvent extraction in the analysis of organic contaminants, bioactive and nutritional compounds in food and feed. J. Chromatogr. A. 00219673. 1237, 1–23. doi:10.1016/j.chroma.2012.03.003.

Sun, Y., Xiujuan, L., Jiang, Z., Haiyan, L., Wei, S., 2024. Goat milk exerts anxiolytic and anti-depressive effects through modulating JAK/STAT3 and p-Akt/CREB signaling pathways in chronic unpredictable mild stress mice. J. Funct. Foods. 17564646. 116, 106170. doi:10.1016/j.jff.2024.106170.

Surnat Cosmet, n.d. Cow's Milk Butter. Available from: https://surnaturelcosmetics.com/en/products/beurre-de-lait-de-vache-format-decouverte.

Sutay Kocabaş, D., Lyne, J., Ustunol, Z., 2022. Hydrolytic enzymes in the dairy industry: applications, market and future perspectives. Trends Food Sci. Technol. 09242244. 119, 467–475. doi:10.1016/j.tifs.2021.12.013.

Tang, X., Yang, T., Daojiang, Y., Xiong, H., Zhang, S., 2024. Current insights and future perspectives of ultraviolet radiation (UV) exposure: friends and foes to the skin and beyond the skin. Environ. Int. 01604120. 185, 108535. doi:10.1016/j.envint.2024.108535.

Teixeira, J.L.D.P., Baptista, D.P., Orlando, E.A., Gigante, M.L., Pallone, J.A.L., 2022. Effect of processing on the bioaccessibility of essential minerals in goat and cow milk and dairy products assessed by different static in vitro digestion models. Food Chem. 18737072. 374. Available from: www.elsevier.com/locate/foodchem. doi:10.1016/j.foodchem.2021.131739.

Teixeira, R.F., Araujo, T.R., Oliveira, D.D., Zielinski, A.A.F., 2024. Unveiling the potential of pressurized liquid extraction for recovering protein fractions from broken black beans: insights into thermal and structural properties. Food Hydrocoll. 0268005X. 149. Available from: https://www.sciencedirect.com/science/journal/0268005X. doi:10.1016/j.foodhyd.2023.109649.

Teo, C.C., Chong, W.P.K., Ho, Y.S., 2013. Development and application of microwave-assisted extraction technique in biological sample preparation for small molecule analysis. Metabolomics. 15733890. 9 (5), 1109–1128. doi:10.1007/s11306-013-0528-7.

Terzioğlu, M.E., Bakırcı, İ., Oz, E., Brennan, C.S., Huppertz, T., Amarowicz, R., Khan, M.R., Elobeid, T., Aadil, R.M., Oz, F., 2023. Comparison of camel, buffalo, cow, goat, and sheep yoghurts in terms of various physicochemical, biochemical, textural and rheological properties. Int. Dairy J. 09586946. 146. Available from: www.elsevier.com/inca/publications/store/4/0/5/8/6/0/index.htt. doi:10.1016/j.idairyj.2023.105749.

Tham, P.E., Ng, Y.J., Sankaran, R., Khoo, K.S., Chew, K.W., Yap, Y.J., Malahubban, M., Zakry, F.A.A., Show, P.L., 2019. Recovery of protein from dairy milk waste product using alcohol-salt liquid biphasic flotation. Processes. 22279717. 7 (12). Available from: https://www.mdpi.com/2227-9717/7/12/875. doi:10.3390/PR7120875.

Thorning, T.K., Bertram, H.C., Bonjour, J.-P., de Groot, L., Dupont, D., Feeney, E., Ipsen, R., Lecerf, J.M., Mackie, A., McKinley, M.C., Michalski, M.-C., Rémond, D., Risérus, U., Soedamah-Muthu, S.S., Tholstrup, T., Weaver, C., Astrup, A., Givens, I., 2017. Whole dairy matrix or single nutrients in assessment of health effects: current evidence and knowledge gaps. Am. J. Clin. Nutr. 19383207. 105 (5), 1033–1045. http://ajcn.nutrition.org/content/105/5/1033.full.pdf+html. doi:10.3945/ajcn.116.151548.

Tinoco, A., Martins, M., Cavaco-Paulo, A., Ribeiro, A., 2022. Biotechnology of functional proteins and peptides for hair cosmetic formulations. Trends Biotechnol. 01677799. 40 (5), 591–605. doi:10.1016/j.tibtech.2021.09.010.

Tiwari, B.K., 2015. Ultrasound: a clean, green extraction technology. TrAC Trends Anal. Chem. 01659936. 71, 100–109. doi:10.1016/j.trac.2015.04.013.

Tranchida, N., Molinari, F., Franco, G.A., Cordaro, M., Di Paola, R., 2025. Potential role of dietary antioxidants during skin aging. Food Sci. Nutr. 20487177. 13 (5). Available from: onlinelibrary.wiley.com/journal/10.1002/%28ISSN%292048-7177. doi:10.1002/fsn3.70231.

Tremblay, A., Panahi, S., 2017. Yogurt consumption as a signature of a healthy diet and lifestyle. J. Nutr. 00223166. 147 (7), 1476S. doi:10.3945/jn.116.245522.

Tsantes, A.G., Petrou, E., Tsante, K.A., Sokou, R., Frantzeskaki, F., Domouchtsidou, A., Chaldoupis, A.E., Fortis, S.P., Piovani, D., Nikolopoulos, G.K., Iacovidou, N., Bonovas, S., Samonis, G., Tsantes, A.E., 2024. Cancer-associated thrombosis: pathophysiology, laboratory assessment, and current guidelines. Cancers. 2072-6694. 16 (11), 2082. doi:10.3390/cancers16112082.

Tsoupras, A., Adamantidi, T., Finos, M.A., Philippopoulos, A., Detopoulou, P., Tsopoki, I., Kynatidou, M., Demopoulos, C.A., 2024. Re-assessing the role of platelet activating factor and its inflammatory signaling and inhibitors in cancer and anti-cancer strategies. Front. Biosci. Landmark. 27686698. 29 (10). Available from: https://www.imrpress.com/journal/FBL/29/10. doi:10.31083/j.fbl2910345.

Turkmen, N., 2017. The nutritional value and health benefits of goat milk components. In: Watson, R.R., Collier, R.J., Preedy, V.R. (Eds.), Nutrients in Dairy and Their Implications for Health and Disease. Academic Press, pp. 441–449. Available from: https://www.sciencedirect.com/science/book/9780128097625. doi:10.1016/B978-0-12-809762-5.00035-8.

Vieira, C.P., Rosario, A.I.L.S., Lelis, C.A., Rekowsky, B.S.S., Carvalho, A.P.A., Rosário, D.K.A., Elias, T.A., Costa, M.P., Foguel, D., Conte-Junior, C.A., 2021. Bioactive compounds from kefir and their potential benefits on health: a systematic review and meta-analysis. Oxid. Med. Cell. Longev. 19420994. 2021. Available from: http://www.hindawi.com/journals/oximed/. doi:10.1155/2021/9081738.

Vioque-Amor, M., Gómez-Díaz, R., Río-Celestino, M.D., Avilés-Ramírez, C., 2023. Butter from different species: composition and quality parameters of products commercialized in the South of Spain. Animals. 2076-2615. 13 (22), 3559. doi:10.3390/ani13223559.

Walker, H., 2000. Milk—beyond the dairy. In: Proceedings of the Oxford Symposium on Food and Cookery 1999. Prospect Books, Totnes, Devon, England, pp. 1–384.

Walkling-Ribeiro, M., Jacob, T., Ahrné, L., 2024. Impact of pulsed electric field intensity on the cream separation efficiency from bovine milk and physico-chemical properties of the cream. Food Res. Int. 09639969. 180, 114074. doi:10.1016/j.foodres.2024.114074.

Wang, D., Zhou, Y., Zhao, J., Ren, C., Yan, W., 2024. Oral yak whey protein can alleviate UV-induced skin photoaging and modulate gut microbiota composition. Foods. 2304-8158. 13 (16), 2621. doi:10.3390/foods13162621.

Wang, L., Tao, W., Zhang, Y., Yang, K., Yuting, H., Deng, K., Liang, C., Yachun, G., 2023. Comparative studies on the nutritional and physicochemical properties of yoghurts from cows', goats', and camels' milk powder. Int. Dairy J. 09586946. 138, 105542. doi:10.1016/j.idairyj.2022.105542.

Watanabe, Y., Hirokawa, M., Furukawa, A., Kawasaki, L., Takumi, H., Masuyama, A., 2022. Improvements in extraction yield by solid phase lipid extraction from liquid infant formula and human milk, and the fatty acid distribution in milk TAG analyzed by joint JOCS/AOCS official method Ch 3a-19. Front. Nutr. 2296-861X. 9. doi:10.3389/fnut.2022.970837.

Wen, C., Zhang, J., Zhang, H., Dzah, C.S., Zandile, M., Duan, Y., Ma, H., Luo, X., 2018. Advances in ultrasound assisted extraction of bioactive compounds from cash crops—a review. Ultrason. Sonochem. 18732828. 48, 538–549. Available from: www.elsevier.com/inca/publications/store/5/2/5/4/5/1. doi:10.1016/j.ultsonch.2018.07.018.

Wong, S., Street, D., Delgado, S.I., Klontz, K.C., 2000. Recalls of foods and cosmetics due to microbial contamination reported to the U.S. Food and Drug Administration. J. Food Prot. 0362028X. 63 (8), 1113–1116. Available from: http://www.ingentaconnect.com/content/iafp/jfp. doi:10.4315/0362-028X-63.8.1113.

Xie, Y., Wang, J., Zheng, L., Luan, Y., Mingyi, L., Peng, X., Xiao, S., Zhang, S., 2022. Damage prevention effect of milk-derived peptides on UVB irradiated human foreskin fibroblasts and regulation of photoaging related indicators. Food Res. Int. 09639969. 161, 111798. doi:10.1016/j.foodres.2022.111798.

Xu, Y., Guo, Y., Duan, S., Wei, H., Liu, Y., Wang, L., Huo, X., Yang, Y., 2018. Effects of ultrasound irradiation on the characterization and bioactivities of the polysaccharide from blackcurrant fruits. Ultrason. Sonochem. 13504177. 49, 206–214. doi:10.1016/j.ultsonch.2018.08.005.

Xulu, K.R., Augustine, T.N., 2022. Targeting platelet activation pathways to limit tumour progression: current state of affairs. Pharmaceuticals. 1424-8247. 15 (12), 1532. doi:10.3390/ph15121532.

Yang, S., Suwal, S., Andersen, U., Otte, J., Ahrné, L., 2021. Effects of pulsed electric field on fat globule structure, lipase activity, and fatty acid composition in raw milk and milk with different fat globule sizes. Innov. Food Sci. Emerg. Technol. 14668564. 67, 102548. doi:10.1016/j.ifset.2020.102548.

Yang, X., Yunliang, L., Suyun, L., Oladejo, A.O., Wang, Y., Huang, S., Zhou, C., Wang, Y., Mao, L., Zhang, Y., Haile, M., Xiaofei, Y., 2017. Effects of multi-frequency ultrasound pretreatment under low power density on the enzymolysis and the structure characterization of defatted wheat germ protein. Ultrason. Sonochem. 13504177. 38, 410–420. doi:10.1016/j.ultsonch.2017.03.001.

Yasmin, A., Huma, N., Butt, M.S., Zahoor, T., Yasin, M., 2012. Seasonal variation in milk vitamin contents available for processing in Punjab, Pakistan. J. Saudi Soc. Agric. Sci. 1658077X. 11 (2), 99–105. doi:10.1016/j.jssas.2012.01.002.

Yen, C.H., Lin, Y.S., Tu, C.F., 2015. A novel method for separation of caseins from milk by phosphates precipitation. Prep. Biochem. Biotechnol. 15322297. 45 (1), 18–32. Available from: www.tandf.co.uk/journals/titles/10826068.asp. doi:10.1080/10826068.2013.877030.

Yeom, G., Yun, D.M., Kang, Y.W., Kwon, J.S., Kang, I.O., Kim, S.Y., 2011. Clinical efficacy of facial masks containing yoghurt and *Opuntia humifusa* raf (F-YOP). J. Cosmet. Sci. 15257886. 62 (5), 505–514.

Yilmaz-Ersan, L., Ozcan, T., Akpinar-Bayizit, A., Sahin, S., 2018. Comparison of antioxidant capacity of cow and ewe milk kefirs. J. Dairy Sci. 00220302. 101 (5), 3788–3798. doi:10.3168/jds.2017-13871.

Zahariev, N., Draganova, M., Zagorchev, P., Pilicheva, B., 2023. Casein-based nanoparticles: a potential tool for the delivery of daunorubicin in acute lymphocytic leukemia. Pharmaceutics. 1999-4923. 15 (2), 471. doi:10.3390/pharmaceutics15020471.

Zandona, E., Blažić, M., Režek Jambrak, A., 2021. Whey utilisation: sustainable uses and environmental approach. Food Technol. Biotechnol. 13342606. 59 (2), 147–161. Available from: http://www.ftb.com.hr/. doi:10.17113/ftb.59.02.21.6968.

Zeng, H., Yujie, Q., Zhang, Z., Liu, C., Peng, W., Zhang, Y., 2021. Nanomaterials toward the treatment of Alzheimer's disease: recent advances and future trends. Chin. Chem. Lett. 10018417. 32 (6), 1857–1868. Available from: https://www.iso.org/standard/36437.html. doi:10.1016/j.cclet.2021.01.014.

Section V

Sustainable inorganic bioactive ingredients from natural resources

Chapter 25

Natural minerals and metal ions

Kalliopi Ladomenou, Maria-Chrysanthi Kafentzi, and Ida Bogdani
Hephaestus Laboratory, School of Chemistry, Faculty of Sciences, Democritus University of Thrace, Kavala, Greece

1 Introduction: Natural cosmetics and inorganic bioactives

Consumer demand for clean, sustainable, and biobased products has catalyzed a global shift in the cosmetics sector toward natural ingredients and transparent supply chains (Goyal and Jerold, 2021). Over the last decade, "natural" has matured from a marketing claim into a design principle that integrates safety, efficacy, and life-cycle thinking across sourcing, manufacturing, and end of use. Within this movement, inorganic materials, natural minerals, and essential metal ions play indispensable roles in both conventional cosmetics and emerging biofunctional formulations.

In this chapter, "natural cosmetics" refers to formulations prioritizing ingredients of natural origin and minimal processing (Dini and Laneri, 2021); "organic" denotes compliance with certified agricultural standards governing cultivation and processing (Brito et al., 2022); and "biofunctional" highlights ingredients that provide measurable biological benefits, for example, antioxidative protection, barrier repair, photoprotection, antimicrobial activity, or wound support, beyond purely esthetic effects (Goyal and Jerold, 2021)

Minerals and metal ions contribute to functional performance and formulation architecture. Clays and silicates regulate rheology, oil control, and sensorial feel while enabling adsorptive detoxification. Zeolites and volcanic minerals extend this with ion-exchange and molecular-sieving behavior (Sarruf et al., 2024). Metal oxides, notably titanium dioxide (TiO_2) and zinc oxide (ZnO), underpin broad-spectrum ultraviolet (UV) protection via reflection and scattering, while iron oxides deliver stable pigmentation and visible-light shielding in color products (Araki and Baby, 2025). Marine-derived salts, such as magnesium (Mg)- and potassium (K)-rich, are associated with soothing and remineralizing effects in spa and dermocosmetic applications. Many of these materials exhibit bio-interactive properties that situate them at the interface of cosmetics and cosmeceuticals.

Unlike single-molecule actives, minerals sourced from geological or marine deposits exhibit compositional variability and may contain trace contaminants such as lead (Pb), cadmium (Cd), arsenic (As), mercury (Hg), nickel (Ni), chromium (Cr), cobalt (Co), or crystalline impurities (e.g., quartz) if not properly specified and purified. Extraction and processing can also impose environmental and social burdens. Consequently, risk management requires end-to-end control: responsible sourcing, technical specifications (purity, particle size, crystalline phase), validated analytical testing [e.g., inductively coupled plasma mass spectrometry (ICP-MS), inductively coupled plasma-optical emission spectrometry (ICP-OES), atomic absorption spectroscopy (AAS)], and toxicological assessment appropriate to use conditions (dermal, periorbital, lip, rinse-off vs. leave-on).

Sustainable use of inorganics combines ethical supply chains (auditing of mica, talc, iron oxide pigments), green extraction (phytomining, bioleaching), circularity (waste valorization, marine and geothermal brines), and regulatory frameworks that harmonize definitions of natural origin and set boundaries for contaminants. At the product level, safety is ensured through specification-driven ingredient qualification, Good Manufacturing Practice, and exposure-based risk assessment that considers particle size (including nanoforms), solubility/ion release, photoreactivity, and ecotoxicity for rinse-off products.

This chapter is organized into eight sections. Section 2 surveys natural mineral-based cosmetic ingredients, including clays and silicates, zeolites and volcanic materials, metal oxides, and Dead Sea/marine minerals, linking their structure to cosmetic functions and sustainability concerns. Section 3 examines essential metal ions, highlighting their roles in photoprotection, antimicrobial defense, wound healing, antiaging, and regenerative applications. Section 4 explores plant-derived compounds and their complexes with metal ions, emphasizing bioactivity, chelation, nanoparticle (NP) synthesis, and formulation challenges. Section 5 discusses sustainability and green sourcing, covering responsible mining, phytomining, bioleaching, marine and geothermal resources, waste valorization, and regulatory frameworks. Section 6 addresses toxicological risks and heavy metal contamination, outlining contaminants, toxic effects, regulations, analytical techniques,

Biofunctional Cosmetics for Health. https://doi.org/10.1016/B978-0-443-27500-5.00004-6

and mitigation strategies. Section 7 highlights emerging formulation trends, including hybrid mineral–biopolymer systems, smart delivery technologies, eco-designed nanocosmetics, and personalized mineral supplementation. Finally, Section 8 provides conclusions, synthesizing key insights and outlining future directions for safe, sustainable, and biofunctional cosmetic innovations.

2 Natural mineral-based cosmetic ingredients

Minerals have been part of beauty and skincare rituals for centuries, from ancient Egyptian kohl to modern clay masks. In contemporary formulations, they enhance texture, stability, and color while also providing measurable benefits to skin health. Increasingly, research highlights how these natural materials support regenerative and protective functions, making them a bridge between traditional beauty practices and cosmeceutical science (Carretero and Pozo, 2010; Lopez-Galindo et al., 2007). The following sections review four important categories of natural mineral-based cosmetic ingredients: clays and silicates, zeolites and volcanic minerals, metal oxides, and Dead Sea and marine minerals, with emphasis on their cosmetic relevance.

2.1 Clays and silicates

Clays are among the best-known natural minerals in cosmetics, used since antiquity for cleansing, healing, and beautification. Their layered structures and fine particle sizes give them a strong absorptive capacity, making them ideal for removing excess oil, toxins, and impurities from the skin. Montmorillonite, kaolinite, and illite, for example, are staples in facial masks and topical formulations, where they provide purifying and mattifying effects (Carretero, 2002; Sandri et al., 2016).

Beyond cleansing, clays also support skin health in more complex ways. Studies show that their ion-exchange ability and mineral content can promote wound healing and tissue repair, offering cosmeceutical benefits beyond surface-level purification (Moraes et al., 2017; Sandri et al., 2016; Viseras et al., 2021). In practical terms, this means clay masks and compresses may not only refresh the complexion, but also help calm inflammation and support regeneration in sensitive or damaged skin (Moraes et al., 2017).

Silicates are vital for their functional role in formulations. Talc, for instance, is valued for its smooth feel and oil-absorbing properties in powders and foundations, while hydrated magnesium silicates improve product spreadability and stability. It has been shown that silicates do more than act as "inert" fillers: they can interact with active molecules, modifying their release and enhancing efficacy (Carretero and Pozo, 2010).

With clays and silicates, the cosmetic industry faces a delicate balance. Their natural abundance and multifunctionality make them indispensable, but ensuring sustainability and safety requires responsible mining practices and rigorous purification.

2.2 Zeolites and volcanic minerals

Zeolites, a family of crystalline aluminosilicates, are gaining popularity in skincare because of their remarkable ability to trap and exchange ions (Souza et al., 2023). Their porous, cage-like structures allow them to act as molecular sieves, capturing heavy metals, toxins, and pollutants while simultaneously releasing beneficial ions, such as calcium and magnesium. This makes zeolites particularly attractive in detoxifying masks, deodorants, and oral care products, where purification is a key function.

Volcanic minerals also play a distinct role in cosmetics. Volcanic ash, pumice, and basalt-derived materials are rich in silica and trace elements, lending themselves to exfoliation and remineralization. Volcanic ash, in particular, is commonly used in scrubs and masks for its ability to gently remove dead skin cells while revitalizing the skin's surface. Recent work highlighted volcanic ash as a sustainable filler in biocomposites, underscoring its potential as an eco-friendly cosmetic raw material (Aliotta et al., 2023).

Innovation is also reshaping the use of these minerals. In another research study, it was demonstrated that gold-decorated zeolite nanocomposites produced antiaging and skin-lightening effects, suggesting that functionalized mineral carriers can enhance antioxidant activity and improve skin tone (Lee et al., 2023). Such findings point to a future where zeolites and volcanic minerals are not just base ingredients but active cosmeceutical tools.

2.3 Metal oxides

Metal oxides are among the most important natural minerals in modern cosmetics, particularly in sunscreens and color products. Zinc oxide and titanium dioxide are well-known as physical UV filters. Unlike chemical sunscreens that absorb radiation, these oxides scatter and reflect harmful UV rays, providing broad-spectrum protection. Their nanoscale versions offer transparency while maintaining efficacy, an advantage for wearable daily sunscreens (Bwatanglang et al., 2022; Pan et al., 2021).

Zinc oxide also brings additional skin benefits. It has antimicrobial, antiinflammatory, and soothing properties, making it suitable for acne-prone, irritated, or sensitive skin (Gupta et al., 2014). Banerjee and Samanta evaluated the safety of zinc oxide in sunscreens, concluding that while generally safe, risk assessments should carefully consider particle size and solubility to avoid unintended systemic absorption (Banerjee and Samanta, 2022).

Recent studies suggest zinc-based compounds may play a role in regenerative and antiaging treatments. Zhang et al. (2022a) reported that spindle-like zinc silicate NPs accelerated burn wound healing by stimulating angiogenesis, while another study by Chen et al. (2025a) showed that zinc silicate-loaded microneedle patches reduced oxidative stress and boosted collagen synthesis. These findings highlight the growing overlap between sun protection, therapeutic skincare, and regenerative dermatology.

Other oxides also contribute to cosmetics (Pan et al., 2021). Iron oxides are widely used as pigments in foundations and color cosmetics, offering a safe alternative to synthetic dyes. Magnesium oxide and cerium oxide are being explored for their antioxidant and soothing properties (Lansdown, 1995). Also, the potential of combining silver with zinc or other metal oxides in nail care applications for their antifungal properties has been reported (Pereira et al., 2014). In addition, titanium dioxide has been reported to exhibit antimicrobial effects against several bacteria and fungi (Serov et al., 2024).

2.4 Dead Sea and marine minerals

Marine-derived minerals, particularly those from the Dead Sea, have become iconic in cosmeceuticals. Dead Sea muds and salts are exceptionally rich in magnesium, potassium, calcium, and bromide, elements known to soothe irritation, detoxify skin, and strengthen the barrier function. They are widely used in masks, scrubs, and spa therapies, often marketed for their ability to improve hydration, elasticity, and inflammatory skin conditions such as psoriasis (Mourelle et al., 2021).

Seawater itself is another valuable resource. Naturally containing magnesium, sodium, potassium, and trace elements, it has been incorporated into hydrating sprays and soothing skincare products for its revitalizing effects (Couteau and Coiffard, 2020). Algal extracts further expand this marine toolkit. Seaweeds, for example, accumulate minerals alongside polysaccharides and antioxidants, delivering moisturizing and protective benefits (Couteau and Coiffard, 2020; Mourelle et al., 2021). Microalgal peloids are also gaining recognition for their dual mineral-organic composition, offering novel applications in wellness and cosmetic treatments (Mourelle et al., 2021).

The appeal of these marine ingredients lies not only in their efficacy but also in their alignment with consumers' interest in natural, "blue beauty" formulations.

3 Metal ions and their cosmetic functions

Essential metal ions play dynamic roles in skin physiology and cosmetic performance. Acting as cofactors, signaling mediators, and structural agents, they support processes ranging from photoprotection and antimicrobial defense to wound healing and antiaging. This section examines zinc, copper, magnesium, calcium, iron, silver, gold, potassium, selenium, and manganese, highlighting both their biological mechanisms and their applications in cosmetic formulations.

3.1 Introduction

The role of metal ions in maintaining skin health is both ancient and modern. For centuries, topical zinc ointments, copper vessels, and magnesium-rich baths have been used in traditional remedies to treat skin ailments. Today, advances in dermatological science have clarified why such practices were effective: metal ions act as enzymatic cofactors, regulate signaling cascades, and participate in structural tissue repair. In cosmetics, their functions extend from photoprotection and antimicrobial activity to wound healing and antiaging effects (Gupta et al., 2014). At the same time, rising awareness of sustainability has brought attention to the sourcing of these elements.

3.2 Zinc

Zinc is often considered the workhorse among dermatological metals. Its therapeutic use in acne and inflammatory dermatoses is well-documented (Gupta et al., 2014). Beyond therapy, zinc is fundamental to regeneration. Recent studies demonstrate that zinc, particularly when combined with magnesium, accelerates wound closure by promoting angiogenesis and epithelialization (Yang et al., 2023).

When incorporated into natural polymers such as chitosan, zinc ions enhance antibacterial and antiinflammatory effects, while simultaneously stimulating fibroblast migration and keratinocyte activity (Mutlu et al., 2022). Modern biomaterials have pushed this further: zinc-based metal-organic frameworks show both antibacterial and antiinflammatory properties (Chen et al., 2022), and zinc ferrite NPs have been shown to inhibit bacterial proliferation while promoting tissue repair (Haghniaz et al., 2021). Earlier clinical work on hydrocolloid dressings containing zinc oxide also confirmed faster epithelial regrowth, highlighting zinc's longstanding role in wound healing (Ågren et al., 1993).

Zinc's cosmetic role extends to photoprotection. Zinc oxide is among the most reliable UV filters available, providing broad-spectrum protection. Nanostructured ZnO has even been explored in textiles, functioning as both a UV barrier and a gas sensor (Subbiah et al., 2018). Encapsulation strategies, such as ZnO-loaded colloidosomes, enhance UV protection efficiency while reducing irritation (Jia et al., 2025). Given ecological concerns, reef-safe formulations combining ZnO with organic filters have been designed (Battistin et al., 2022). Recent studies suggest ZnO NPs also influence cellular communication by promoting migrasome formation, underscoring their bioactivity beyond UV defense (Li et al., 2025).

3.3 Copper

Copper plays a central role in angiogenesis, collagen cross-linking, and antioxidant defense, making it especially relevant in wound healing and rejuvenating cosmetics. Collagen-rich dermal matrices releasing both copper and zinc ions promote the programmed healing of diabetic wounds, supporting vascularization and balanced remodeling (Chen et al., 2025b). Chitin sponges modified with copper and polyphenols similarly demonstrated antibacterial, antioxidant, and provascularization activity, supporting scarless healing in burn models (Li et al., 2021b). Hydrogels incorporating copper ions with antimicrobial peptides or polyphenols further enhance antibacterial defense while reducing oxidative stress (Hu et al., 2023; Yao et al., 2025).

Beyond wound healing, copper is strongly associated with skin rejuvenation. The tripeptide glycyl-L-histidyl-L-lysine-Cu^{2+} enhances proteoglycan and glycosaminoglycan synthesis, leading to improved elasticity and a reduction of fine lines (Siméon et al., 2000). On a structural level, copper guides elastin fiber assembly, mimicking natural extracellular matrix organization (Kothapalli and Ramamurthi, 2009). In severe burns, CuCS/Cur dressings have even supported neutralized regeneration by promoting the recovery of nerve-related dermal structures (Zhang et al., 2024).

3.4 Magnesium

Magnesium, abundant in marine environments, is closely linked to barrier function and antiinflammatory activity. Its longstanding use is illustrated by magnesium-rich Dead Sea salts in eczema and psoriasis care. Contemporary studies confirm its synergy with zinc in accelerating wound closure, collagen maturation, and tissue regeneration (Yang et al., 2023).

Biodegradable scaffolds embedding magnesium meshes within collagen–chitosan structures represent an innovative approach, as they not only provide structural integrity and antibacterial protection but also allow for gradual ion release during repair (Guo et al., 2025). Research on magnesium alloys has also explored their anticorrosive and self-healing properties, with potential adaptation to future dermatological applications (Oni et al., 2025).

3.5 Calcium

Calcium is fundamental to keratinocyte differentiation and epidermal barrier renewal. Delivery systems based on hydroxyapatite microspheres have been developed to release calcium gradually, thereby stimulating keratinocyte activity through calcium-motor protein pathways and promoting hydration and repair (Liu et al., 2025).

Calcium signaling is also implicated in skin pathology. Calcium release-activated calcium channels have been identified as therapeutic targets in allergic and inflammatory skin diseases (Yan et al., 2019). Marine-derived calcium salts, often used in spa therapies, are known to improve hydration and reinforce the skin barrier, making them a longstanding component of cosmetic practices.

3.6 Iron

While iron is most familiar in cosmetics as iron oxides used in pigments, bioactive iron materials are gaining attention for their therapeutic functions. Zero-valent iron in alginate hydrogels has been shown to promote rapid hemostasis and antibacterial action (Han et al., 2025). Iron-based self-gelling powders prepared from chitosan derivatives also seal wounds effectively while stimulating repair (Hu et al., 2025). Iron-containing hydrogels remodel energy metabolism and regulate redox balance, significantly accelerating diabetic wound healing (Jin et al., 2026). Composites incorporating both iron and selenium have demonstrated multifunctional benefits, combining antibacterial, antioxidant, and regenerative activities (Bhardwaj et al., 2025). More experimental applications, such as multifunctional iron coordination networks for self-healing "e-skins," suggest that iron-based systems could expand into novel cosmetic technologies (Zhang et al., 2022a).

3.7 Silver

Silver has a long history as an antimicrobial, but nanosilver has made it particularly attractive in contemporary cosmetics. Green-synthesized silver NPs demonstrate strong antibacterial and antibiofilm activity, as well as tyrosinase inhibition, making them promising in skin-whitening and antiacne products (Kaliappan et al., 2025). In regenerative medicine, AgNP-loaded hydrogels enhance diabetic wound closure by suppressing infection and oxidative stress. Silk fibroin composites incorporating silver-gallic acid NPs have shown similarly improved healing outcomes (Han et al., 2025). Embedding silver NPs within γ-cyclodextrin frameworks increases their stability and antimicrobial efficacy while reducing environmental risk (Alotaibi et al., 2023).

3.8 Gold

Gold, once included in cosmetics for prestige alone, is now valued for its functional contributions. Gold NPs synthesized from Panax ginseng leaves improve antioxidant capacity, moisture retention, and whitening effects in keratinocyte models (Jiménez-Pérez et al., 2018). In advanced formulations, gold–curcumin nanohybrids have demonstrated antibacterial and antibiofilm effects when activated by photosonotherapy, suggesting use in infected wounds and implants (Jiménez-Pérez et al., 2018). Analytical studies have confirmed the presence of ultratrace levels of gold in some commercial products (Zawisza et al., 2022). While these findings underscore gold's appeal, safety evaluations caution that nanogold, like nanosilver, requires careful monitoring to avoid long-term accumulation or irritation (Pulit-Prociak et al., 2019).

3.9 Potassium

Potassium is essential for osmotic balance and mitochondrial function. Recent studies indicate that modulation of mitochondrial potassium channels has antiaging effects, including enhanced energy metabolism and protection against oxidative damage (Lewandowska et al., 2024). Potassium-rich marine salts are widely incorporated into spa-based cosmetic treatments, where they are associated with skin revitalization and hydration.

3.10 Selenium

Selenium contributes to the skin's antioxidant defense by supporting enzymes such as glutathione peroxidase. Its combination with iron in Fe/Se nanocomposites has demonstrated dual antibacterial and antioxidant effects, accelerating wound healing in experimental models (Bhardwaj et al., 2025). This dual action highlights selenium's potential in next-generation antioxidant-rich cosmetic formulations.

3.11 Manganese

Manganese functions as a cofactor for antioxidant enzymes such as superoxide dismutase, thereby protecting skin cells from oxidative stress (Fu et al., 2025). Although manganese is less widely used in formulations compared with zinc or copper, its role in oxidative balance makes it an emerging candidate for antiaging skin care (Grujicic and Allen, 2025). In a study, Hussain and Goldberg (2007) assessed a facial serum containing a manganese glycyl-L-histidyl-L-lysine complex to improve the appearance of cutaneous photoaging (Hussain and Goldberg, 2007).

4 Plant-derived compounds and metal ion complexes

Plant-derived compounds contribute bioactivity and selectivity to cosmetic formulations, often through metal chelation and complexation. Rich in polyphenols, flavonoids, and peptides, these natural ligands enhance antioxidant defense, modulate metal absorption, and support novel NP synthesis. This section explores the mineral content of plants, the bioactivity of extracts, chelation properties, challenges of extraction, and the development of phytomediated metal-based NPs.

4.1 Minerals in plants

Extensive research has been conducted on the trace essential and nontoxic elements in various plants. Variations in elemental composition across species and plant parts provide valuable insights into their nutritional and biomedical relevance. Among the most investigated sources are *Camellia sinensis*, *Moringa oleifera*, and Spirulina, each showing distinct mineral compositions. An analysis of tea samples derived from *C. sinensis*, encompassing green, black, and instant varieties, revealed potassium as the predominant metal. Substantial levels of calcium, magnesium, and aluminum were also detected, whereas manganese was present in comparatively lower amounts (Fernández-Cáceres et al., 2001). Leaves of the *M. oleifera* plant have higher levels of sodium, calcium, manganese, and potassium compared to other parts. In contrast, the stem bark of the plant is rich in potassium, calcium, magnesium, and iron, while the seeds contain higher amounts of copper, magnesium, and zinc (Vinodkumar et al., 2025). Spirulina, the blue–green algae, is another well-recognized mineral source, which contains significant amounts of potassium, phosphorus, calcium, iron, sodium, magnesium, zinc, cobalt, manganese, and selenium in its composition (Podgórska-Kryszczuk, 2024). *Cucurbitaceae* seeds, including those from *Citrullus lanatus* (watermelon), *Cucumis melo* (melon), and *Cucurbita pepo* (pumpkin), are rich in essential minerals, with concentrations varying across species, highlighting their suitability as cosmetic ingredients (Sousa et al., 2025). Calcium is particularly abundant in *C. melo*, while magnesium and potassium are found in high levels in both *C. melo* and *C. pepo*. Zinc is notably present in *C. melo*, and iron is prominent in *C. lanatus*. In addition, these seeds contain trace elements such as cobalt, aluminum, and manganese.

4.2 Bioactivity of plant extracts

Many plants have antimicrobial activities due to various active principles, secondary metabolites, or phytochemicals like tannins, polyphenols, flavonoids, and many other organic constituents (Rahman et al., 2021). Polyphenol-rich extracts are promising cosmetic agents, as they mitigate oxidative stress, delay skin aging, and, when applied topically, provide antioxidant defense, reduce UV-induced damage, inhibit dermal proteinases, and exert antimicrobial and anticancer effects (Farhan, 2024). Among these, green tea extracts are particularly noteworthy, as they exhibit efficient skin penetration, enhance hydration, reduce UV-induced erythema and inflammation, and contribute to the improvement of skin texture (Luo et al., 2024).

The activity of plant-derived compounds often results from forming a protective film on the skin and directly interacting with pollutants through chelation. For example, a multicomponent powder from standardized polyphenol-rich extracts has been shown to attenuate skin damage induced by metal deposition from air pollution (Giacomelli et al., 2018). In addition, it has been suggested that tannins, especially condensed tannins, may serve as potential regulators of metal absorption, helping to prevent the accumulation of toxic levels (Zhang et al., 2022c).

4.3 Metal chelation and complexes

A key characteristic of plant-derived compounds intended for industrial applications is their specificity and selectivity toward particular metals. While certain plant-derived compounds exhibit this property, the majority display low selectivity, binding indiscriminately to multiple metals (Nobahar et al., 2021). The properties of both ligands and metals contribute to the formation of molecules with markedly enhanced activity, as chelation typically amplifies biological efficacy (Abdalla and Aly, 2025). Numerous plant-derived metal-ion complexes exert antioxidative, antiinflammatory, anticancer, and other beneficial effects (Mucha et al., 2021). Kostyuk and coworkers demonstrated for the first time that complexed flavonoids exhibit a significantly lower degree of oxidation compared to their free counterparts (Kostyuk et al., 2004). In addition, a strong correlation has been reported between polyphenols' antioxidative activity and their affinity for Fe^{II} ions, suggesting that the suppression of the Fenton reaction is most probably caused by chelation of the ion (Miličević and Raos, 2016). Moreover, tannins are excellent chelators of metals such as iron(III), aluminum, and copper. Each ferric ion can bind several tannin molecules simultaneously, being able to bind to at least three o-dihydroxyphenyl groups. In a research study, it has been reported that tannin, in combination with metal salts, can be successfully used for hair dyeing (Sargsyan et al., 2020). Also, metal-chelating peptides can block the production of free radicals and have certain antioxidant activity. By chelating with metal ions, peptides can change the physical position of transition metals and hinder the interaction between metals, lipids, and peroxides, thus realizing antioxidation (Lu and Dong, 2022).

4.4 Challenges

Extraction and purification of plant-derived compounds are often challenging, costly, and dependent on large amounts of organic solvents that may harm the environment. More sustainable, low-cost approaches focus on using fewer processing steps, readily available plants, or plant byproducts from other industries. However, the stability and efficiency of these bioactive constituents can be compromised under extreme temperatures, varying pH conditions, or in the presence of certain chemical agents.

4.5 Plant-mediated metal-based NPs

Green synthesis of NPs using plants has gained attention due to their availability, low cost, and rich phytoconstituents. The integration of phytocompounds with metal nanoparticles (MNPs) has emerged as a promising strategy in biomedical and cosmetic applications. By combining the bioactive properties of plant-derived compounds with the unique physical and chemical characteristics of MNPs, phyto-MNPs exhibit enhanced functionalities. Phyto-MNPs, particularly those of silver, gold, zinc, and copper, have gained attention for skin care. A key feature of phyto-AuNPs is their ability to enhance the sun protection factor (SPF), making them effective UV protectors or boosters in sunscreen formulations, thanks to their remarkable photostability (Gubitosa et al., 2018). Furthermore, the demonstrated antioxidant and antiaging properties of phyto-AgNPs (Jiménez Pérez et al., 2017), together with the notable anticancer and antioxidant activities of phyto-CuONPs (Rehana et al., 2017), highlight their potential for application in cosmetic formulations. Also, phyto-ZnONPs have attracted significant attention in cosmetic products, such as creams, lotions, and other formulations, due to their capability to block both UVA and UVB rays and increase the SPF (Sonia et al., 2017). Moreover, they function as antioxidants that penetrate the skin, support cellular repair, act as natural preservatives, and exhibit broad-spectrum antibacterial and antifungal activity.

The main challenge for phyto-MNPs in dermopharmaceutical and cosmetic use is the lack of standardized dosing (Paiva-Santos et al., 2021). Understanding their biological mechanisms, controlling production and stability, and establishing safe doses are essential. Once standardized, phyto-MNPs can be incorporated into formulations like lotions, gels, and creams, followed by thorough toxicological testing, in vitro and in vivo studies, and eventually clinical trials, paving the way for their use in cosmetics.

4.6 Conclusion

Plant-based materials represent an increasingly important component of cosmetic formulations. Owing to their biocompatibility and environmental favorability, they are gaining prominence as alternatives to synthetic agents. Future research should emphasize sustainable sourcing, stability testing, standardized formulation, optimized processing, rigorous safety assessment, and regulatory frameworks to fully harness their cosmetic potential.

5 Sustainability and green sourcing

The sourcing of minerals and metal ions raises important ethical and environmental considerations. This section discusses responsible mining, phytomining, bioleaching, marine and geothermal resources, waste valorization, and the regulatory frameworks that guide sustainable practices.

The cosmetics industry is increasingly committed to minimizing environmental and social impacts throughout the product life cycle, from raw material extraction to consumer use. As demand for "green" and "clean" beauty grows, sourcing practices for minerals and plant-derived ingredients must ensure efficacy, safety, and traceability. A critical concern is the presence of toxic metals. For example, US FDA surveys showed that eye shadows, blushes, and compact powders often contain higher heavy metal levels than other categories, largely due to mineral-based pigments and fillers. This underlines the need for sustainable sourcing and purification strategies. This section reviews key approaches: responsible mining, phytomining, bioleaching, marine resources, geothermal fluids, waste valorization, and regulatory frameworks (Fig. 25.1).

5.1 Responsible mining and sustainable mining

Mining can have severe environmental and social consequences. Mica mining in India illustrates these risks, with health hazards, water and soil contamination, waste accumulation, unsafe workplaces, and even child labor (Treyman et al., 2024; Schwartz et al., 2021). Comparable concerns exist in palm oil production, where deforestation drives biodiversity loss and climate change (Martins and Marto, 2023). Responsible mining emphasizes minimizing impacts, ensuring worker safety, protecting communities, and fostering transparency. Two frameworks dominate: (1) improving extraction and processing methods in line with environmental principles and (2) embedding circularity by reintegrating mined materials into the economy (Gorman and Dzombak, 2018; Wall et al., 2017). For cosmetics, this implies auditing supply chains (mica, talc, iron oxides), while ensuring ethical labor and ecological rehabilitation.

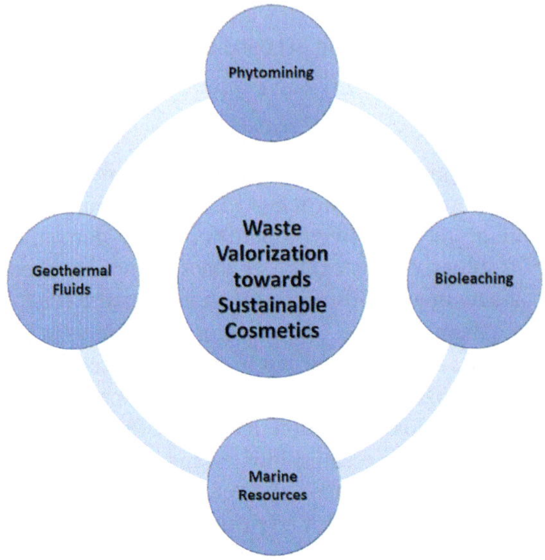

FIG. 25.1 Sustainable mineral sourcing pathways: Phytomining, bioleaching, marine/geothermal, and waste valorization toward sustainable cosmetics.

Also, conventional mining is being replaced or supplemented by greener approaches such as phytomining, bioleaching, and recovery from marine and agricultural resources, ensuring that cosmetic applications remain not only effective but also environmentally responsible.

5.2 Phytomining

Phytomining employs hyperaccumulator plants to extract metals from low-grade ores, industrial wastes, or contaminated soils (Akinbile et al., 2023). These plants can store metal concentrations 10–100 times higher than nonaccumulating species. After harvest and incineration, metal-rich ash is processed to yield valuable elements. Currently, over 700 hyperaccumulator species have been identified, with nickel being the most commonly accumulated (523 species), followed by copper, cobalt, manganese, zinc, and selenium (Reeves et al., 2018). While natural hyperaccumulation of precious metals (e.g., gold, platinum) remains rare, certain plants produce metabolites such as cyanide or thiourea derivatives that facilitate induced uptake (Akinbile and Mbohwa, 2025). For cosmetics, phytomining offers low-impact access to metals such as zinc, copper, or manganese without extensive mining.

5.3 Bioleaching

Bioleaching uses bacteria or fungi to extract metals from ores by oxidizing mineral substrates (Bosecker, 1997). Depending on the mineral and environmental conditions, microorganisms can operate through direct enzymatic interactions or indirect oxidation via metabolite production. Industrial-scale bioleaching largely relies on *Thiobacillus* spp., while fungi such as *Aspergillus* and *Penicillium* species are effective in mobilizing base metals (Dusengemungu et al., 2021; Saldaña et al., 2023). For the cosmetic industry, bioleaching represents a biocompatible extraction method that reduces the need for harsh chemicals and energy-intensive processes, aligning with green chemistry principles.

5.4 Marine resources

The ocean is a vast reservoir of minerals. Three major types of marine deposits have attracted attention: polymetallic manganese nodules, cobalt-rich crusts, and seafloor massive sulfides. These resources provide manganese, iron, cobalt, nickel, zinc, and rare earth elements, often in higher concentrations than terrestrial ores (Wang et al., 2024; Ochromowicz et al., 2021). In parallel, biological marine sources such as seaweeds are gaining importance in cosmetics. Seaweeds accumulate macro- and trace elements, including sodium, potassium, zinc, and magnesium, and are classified into green (Chlorophyta), brown (Ochrophyta), and red (Rhodophyta) algae (Premarathna et al., 2022). Extracts from red and brown algae, rich in minerals and polysaccharides, are widely used for hydration and skin barrier reinforcement. Seawater itself is a valuable source of magnesium, calcium, potassium, and sodium, which confer soothing and revitalizing effects on the skin (Guillerme et al., 2017). However, sustainable harvesting is crucial to prevent overexploitation of marine resources. Controlled collection and eco-friendly processing methods allow companies to tap into the therapeutic potential of marine minerals while preserving fragile ecosystems.

5.5 Geothermal fluids

Geothermal fluids, formed through interactions between water and host rocks, can be enriched in valuable metals such as lithium, cesium, rubidium, zinc, and rare earths (Gallup, 1998; Harper et al., 1992). With proper extraction methods, geothermal systems could provide dual benefits: renewable energy generation and recovery of critical raw materials. For cosmetics, geothermal brines represent an emerging sustainable source of mineral salts used in spa therapies and skin-care products. Silica-rich volcanic systems often yield lithium, cesium, and rubidium, while saline chloride-rich systems are enriched in iron, zinc, and other base metals (Bourcier et al., 2005).

5.6 Valorization of waste

Waste valorization is a rapidly advancing field, converting industrial, agricultural, and consumer waste into secondary raw materials. Global mining generates an estimated 282.5 billion tons of waste annually, containing recoverable metals such as copper, zinc, and iron (Akinbile and Mbohwa, 2025). Agrowastes also present valuable opportunities, as eggshells are rich in calcium carbonate (Yadav et al., 2021). By recovering minerals from waste, the cosmetic sector can embrace circular economy principles, reducing dependence on virgin mining.

5.7 Regulatory framework

Regulations and certifications play a decisive role in steering cosmetics toward sustainability. Concerns about heavy metal contamination (e.g., cadmium, nickel, rubidium) and ethical issues, such as animal testing, have pushed companies to adopt green chemistry principles in product design (Bom et al., 2019; Franca and Ueno, 2020). International certification schemes, including USDA Organic (United States), JAS (Japan), and Canada Organic, as well as standards such as COSMOS and Natrue, define criteria for natural and organic raw materials. Furthermore, ISO 16128 (parts 1 and 2) provides a framework for quantifying natural origin content, ensuring transparency in product labeling (Lee and Kwon, 2022). Together, these frameworks enhance consumer trust and incentivize industries to adopt sustainable sourcing.

6 Toxicological risks and heavy metal contamination

While natural minerals and metals provide valuable cosmetic functions, they also pose risks if contaminated with toxic elements. Heavy metals such as rubidium, cadmium, arsenic, mercury, nickel, chromium, and cobalt can enter formulations through raw materials, processing, or packaging. This section reviews common contaminants, their toxicological effects, regulatory frameworks, analytical detection techniques, and mitigation strategies to ensure product safety.

6.1 Heavy metal contaminants

The increased use of cosmetics has raised concerns about product safety due to potential heavy metal contamination. Commonly detected contaminants in several cosmetic products have been summarized (Abed et al., 2024) (Fig. 25.2). These metals often enter through contaminated raw materials such as pigments, mineral-based substances, or plant extracts; environmental exposure during sourcing; or contamination from manufacturing equipment and packaging (Borowska and Brzóska, 2015). As clays are naturally sourced, they often contain impurities such as quartz, feldspar, or even trace heavy

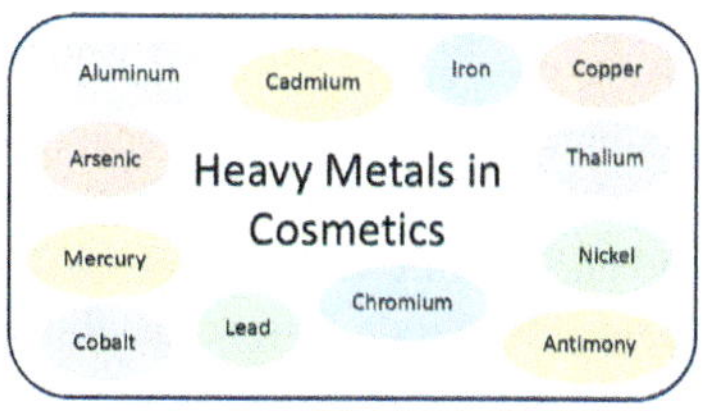

FIG. 25.2 Commonly detected heavy metals in cosmetic products: Aluminum, antimony, arsenic, cadmium, chromium, cobalt, copper, iron, mercury, nickel, lead, and thallium.

metals. If used unrefined, they can pose health risks (Sarruf et al., 2024). In the case of cosmetic clays, Carretero and Pozo (2010) likewise noted the paradox: while they offer well-documented therapeutic effects, careless sourcing and use could expose consumers to toxic elements (Carretero and Pozo, 2010).

In certain cases, they become a part of cosmetic products intentionally in the form of pigments, preservatives, UV filters, as well as antiperspirant, antifungal, and antibacterial agents (Arshad et al., 2020). For example, cadmium is widely recognized for its role in pigments, with its compounds commonly used to produce yellow, orange, and red colors (Raza-Naqvi et al., 2022). Also, mercury is commonly used in skin-lightening creams for its melanin-inhibiting properties (Gyamfi et al., 2023) and as a preservative in other cosmetics, such as hand and body creams and lotions (Pramanik et al., 2021).

6.2 Toxic effects

Prolonged use of cosmetics may cause a range of adverse health effects due to the presence of toxic metals. Recently, researchers have detected dangerous levels of heavy metals, including chromium, manganese, nickel, cobalt, cadmium, and lead, in lipsticks, often exceeding limits set by Health Canada and the FDA (Saah et al., 2024). Heavy metals in cosmetics can affect health mainly through skin absorption or accidental ingestion. Chromium, copper, and cadmium were particularly high, posing risks such as skin irritation, neurotoxicity, kidney and liver damage, bone demineralization, and carcinogenic effects. Lead levels also raised concerns, especially for children and pregnant women (Saah et al., 2024). The WHO classifies mercury among the top ten chemicals of major public health concern due to its severe toxic effects, including skin damage, kidney injury, neurological disorders, and bioaccumulation (Ho et al., 2017). Moreover, dyes (such as those in eye shadows) may contain chromium and nickel, which can cause contact blepharitis (Kicińska and Kowalczyk, 2025). Mercury is highly toxic, linked to bone demineralization, kidney dysfunction, brain damage, reproductive failure, and poisoning; thus its use must remain within FDA-defined limits. Even at low levels, cadmium and other toxic heavy metals in cosmetics pose potential health risks, as they accumulate in biological systems over time (Safavi et al., 2019). Lastly, aluminum may cause gene instability, alter gene expression, or enhance oxidative stress (Sanajou et al., 2021).

6.3 Regulations and limits

The use of heavy metals in cosmetics is restricted or prohibited in many countries; however, permissible limits vary, hindering the establishment of universal regulations (Gyamfi et al., 2024). For instance, the allowable limit for Pb is 1.0 and 10 mg/kg for the FDA and Health Canada, respectively (Health Canada, 2011; US FDA, 2018), while many developing countries lack legislation governing the import, distribution, and use of cosmetic products. To resolve this, efforts have been made to establish regulatory frameworks. In cosmetic clays, the importance of setting strict compositional and technical specifications has been documented, including purification and particle size control (Lopez-Galindo et al., 2007).

Also, in the EU, the cosmetic regulatory framework is provided by Regulation (EC) No. 1223/2009 of the European Commission, which has overall responsibility for cosmetic legislation (Anonymous, 2009). Annex II of the Cosmetics Regulation (EC) No. 1223/2009 lists the heavy metals and their derivatives that are prohibited, and Annex III lists those that are restricted. In addition, specific positive lists of substances are provided for various ingredient categories, including colorants, preservatives, and UV filters (Annexes IV, V, and VI, respectively). These toxicological concerns highlight the importance of accurate, reliable techniques to determine metal levels in cosmetic products.

6.4 Analytical techniques

Several processing methods have been developed to isolate heavy metals from cosmetic products before spectroscopic analysis. The most applicable methods are dry digestion, wet digestion, solid-phase microextraction, and chelation solvent extraction (Papadopoulos et al., 2022). Four instrumental techniques predominate to quantify heavy metals in cosmetic products (Gyamfi et al., 2024). Flame atomic absorption spectroscopy (FAAS), graphite furnace atomic absorption spectroscopy (GFAAS), inductively coupled plasma-optical emission spectrometry (ICP-OES), and inductively coupled plasma mass spectrometry (ICP-MS) are among the most reliable methods for the detection and analytical control of heavy metals. FAAS is commonly applied for heavy metal determination due to its precision, cost-effectiveness, and ease of operation, while also offering high selectivity and minimal matrix interference. In a research study, a modified solid-phase extraction method was developed using functionalized Fe_3O_4 NPs to quantify lead and cadmium in lipsticks, eye shadows, and eyeliners (Ebrahimzadeh et al., 2013). The approach, combined with FAAS, showed high recovery, repeatability, and minimal interference from other metals. The levels of lead, cadmium, and arsenic in four common cosmetic products were detected using GFAAS (Saadatzadeh et al., 2019). This method combines excellent detection limits with the ability to run unattended, enhancing its overall practicality.

ALqadami et al. (2013) developed a sensitive ICP-OES method for detecting arsenic, cadmium, bismuth (Bi), lead, titanium, and mercury in whitening creams (ALqadami et al., 2013). ICP-OES is capable of simultaneous multielement analysis, which makes the technique widely used in laboratories handling large sample sets. In another study, the concentration of silver, barium, bismuth, cadmium, lead, strontium (Sr), and thallium (Tl) was determined by the ICP-MS technique in 94 eye shadows after pretreatment of the samples (Pawlaczyk et al., 2021). ICP-MS demonstrates exceptional multi-element capabilities and is capable of performing isotopic analysis. In addition, the technique can accurately measure analytes at trace and ultra-trace concentrations (Gyamfi et al., 2024). Sensitive methods for detecting mercury in cosmetics have been developed, underlining the ongoing risk of contamination in poorly regulated markets (Wang et al., 2012). As mercury easily becomes gaseous, other studies proposed a method for rapid mercury detection in cosmetic products. The samples were analyzed directly using a Mercury Analyzer without further preparation (Houmine et al., 2025; Saadatzadeh et al., 2019).

6.5 Mitigation strategies

Mitigating heavy metals in cosmetics requires a combination of regulatory, material, and technological strategies. Regulatory frameworks should establish and harmonize strict limits for metals in raw materials and finished products, supported by routine monitoring using validated analytical techniques and traceability. Moreover, manufacturers should prioritize the use of high-purity raw materials, such as clays, pigments, and herbal extracts. In addition, adopting green chemistry principles by replacing metal-based additives with safer alternatives helps reduce contamination in cosmetic products. Collaboration among regulators, industry, and academia is also essential to enforce quality assurance and guarantee the safety and quality of finished products. Finally, transparent labeling practices, coupled with increased public awareness, are crucial for empowering consumers to make thoughtful decisions about their cosmetic purchases.

7 Emerging trends in formulations

Looking forward, innovation in cosmetic science is reshaping the use of minerals and metals. This section highlights hybrid mineral–biopolymer systems, smart delivery technologies, eco-designed nanocosmetics, and personalized mineral supplementation as next-generation strategies. The cosmetic industry is evolving rapidly, with innovative formulations integrating natural minerals, metal ions, and plant-derived compounds into multifunctional systems. Emerging designs now combine sustainability with advanced efficacy, targeting both performance and eco-responsibility.

7.1 Hybrid systems

Hybrid materials that combine metals with organic compounds offer unique advantages. Examples include metal–polyphenol networks (Lin et al., 2024), clay–biopolymer composites (Zeggai et al., 2024), and other multifunctional nanohybrids (Sharma et al., 2023). These systems integrate the stability and functionality of inorganic components with the biocompatibility of natural polymers, improving bioactivity, stability, and controlled release. For instance, metal–polyphenol networks have been reported to enhance antioxidant capacity and provide UV protection, while clay-biopolymer composites act as detoxifying and remineralizing agents. Moreover, organic–inorganic hybrids derived from natural plant dyes are gaining interest in cosmetics. For example, color-tunable curcumin–palygorskite hybrid pigments have been developed, where the observed color variations result from the coordination of different metal ions (Cu^{2+}, Zn^{2+}, Mg^{2+}, Al^{3+}, and Fe^{3+}) with the surface silanol groups of palygorskite (Li et al., 2021a).

7.2 Smart delivery systems

Responsive delivery technologies are reshaping cosmeceuticals (Kim, 2025). pH-responsive clays, redox-sensitive metal complexes, and thermosensitive gels enable controlled release of active ingredients in response to local skin conditions. Such systems have been designed to protect bioactives, optimize their pharmacokinetic profiles, facilitate passage across biological barriers, and improve intracellular penetration and targeted distribution (Ahmed et al., 2022). Thus they improve therapeutic outcomes, minimize irritation, and enhance bioavailability. For example, redox-responsive zinc or copper complexes can deliver antioxidant effects precisely under oxidative stress conditions.

7.3 Nanocosmetics

Nanotechnology continues to expand in cosmetics, with eco-designed NPs offering controlled penetration, improved stability, and multifunctional activity (Piluk et al., 2024). Nanoparticles of zinc oxide, silver, gold, and titanium dioxide are particularly studied for sunscreens, antiaging, and antimicrobial applications. To address safety concerns, recent approaches emphasize green synthesis, biodegradable coatings, and safe-by-design strategies. For instance, reef-safe ZnO NPs (Battistin et al., 2022) or biodegradable gold nanocarriers (Cao et al., 2016) represent examples of how nanotechnology can meet both regulatory and consumer expectations.

7.4 Personalized mineral supplementation

The convergence of cosmetics and nutrition has given rise to nutricosmetics, where oral supplementation complements topical application (Pandey et al., 2024). Minerals such as zinc, selenium, and magnesium are increasingly formulated into dietary supplements that support skin health from within. Personalized approaches, supported by digital health platforms and skin diagnostics, enable tailored mineral supplementation strategies. This integration reflects a broader shift toward holistic, preventive skin care.

8 Conclusions

Natural minerals and metal ions, including those derived from plants, provide versatile functions in cosmetics. Yet, their natural origin does not automatically guarantee safety, making vigilance regarding heavy metal contamination and ecological impact essential. Sustainability, safety, and functionality must go hand in hand to ensure that biofunctional cosmetics contribute positively to both consumer health and environmental well-being.

Looking forward, innovation will likely center on hybrid systems, eco-designed nanomaterials, and sustainable sourcing practices that align efficacy with responsibility. Regulatory frameworks and consumer awareness will further drive industry transformation, ensuring transparency and trust. By integrating traditional knowledge with modern science, next-generation cosmetic formulations can achieve a balance between natural inspiration and technological advancement.

References

Abdalla, E.M., Aly, S.A., 2025. Using Coordination Compounds as Antioxidants. IntechOpen. doi:10.5772/intechopen.1005817.

Abed, M.S., Moosa, A.A., Alzuhairi, M.A., 2024. Heavy metals in cosmetics and tattoos: a review of historical background, health impact, and regulatory limits. J. Hazard. Mater. Adv. 13, 100390. doi:10.1016/j.hazadv.2023.100390.

Ågren, M.S., Franzén, L., Chvapil, M., 1993. Effects on wound healing of zinc oxide in a hydrocolloid dressing. J. Am. Acad. Dermatol. 29, 221–227. doi:10.1016/0190-9622(93)70172-P.

Ahmed, I.A., Mikail, M.A., Zamakshshari, N.H., Mustafa, M.R., Hashim, N.M., Othman, R., 2022. Trends and challenges in phytotherapy and phytocosmetics for skin aging. Saudi J. Biol. Sci. 1319562X. 29 (8). Available from http://www.ksu.edu.sa/sites/Colleges/CollegeofScinces/BotanyDepartment/SJBS/Default.aspx. doi:10.1016/j.sjbs.2022.103363.

Akinbile, B.J., Makhubela, B.C.E., Ambushe, A.A., 2023. Phytomining of valuable metals: status and prospective-a review. Int. J. Environ. Anal. Chem. 103, 3913–3933. doi:10.1080/03067319.2021.1917557.

Akinbile, B.J., Mbohwa, C., 2025. Incorporating hyperaccumulating plants in phytomining, remediation and resource recovery: recent trends in the African region—a review. RSC Sustain. 27538125. 3 (4), 1652–1671. Available from https://www.rsc.org/journals-books-databases/about-journals/rsc-sustainability/#scope. doi:10.1039/d5su00021a.

Aliotta, L., Gigante, V., Lazzeri, A., 2023. Volcanic ash as filler in biocomposites: an example of circular economy in volcanic areas. Sustain. Mater. Technol. 37, e00660. doi:10.1016/j.susmat.2023.e00660.

Alotaibi, H., Chung, E., Chung, S.H., Ren, G., Singh, V., Huang, J., 2023. Sustainable γ-cyclodextrin frameworks containing ultra-fine silver nanoparticles with enhanced antimicrobial efficacy. Carbohydr. Polym. 01448617. 304, 120516. doi:10.1016/j.carbpol.2022.120516.

ALqadami, A., Abdalla, M., ALOthman, Z., Omer, K., 2013. Application of solid phase extraction on multiwalled carbon nanotubes of some heavy metal ions to analysis of skin whitening cosmetics using ICP-AES. Int. J. Environ. Res. Public Health. 1660-4601. 10 (1), 361–374. doi:10.3390/ijerph10010361.

Anonynous, 2009. Regulation (EC) No 1223/2009 of the European parliament and of the council. Off. J. Eur. Union 342, 59–209.

Araki, S.M., Baby, A.R., 2025. New perspectives on titanium dioxide and zinc oxide as inorganic UV filters: advances, safety, challenges, and environmental considerations. Cosmetics. 20799284. 12 (2). Available from www.mdpi.com/journal/cosmetics. doi:10.3390/cosmetics12020077.

Arshad, H., Mehmood, M.Z., Shah, M.H., Abbasi, A.M., 2020. Evaluation of heavy metals in cosmetic products and their health risk assessment. Saudi Pharm. J. 13190164. 28 (7), 779–790. Available from http://www.sciencedirect.com/science/journal/13190164. doi:10.1016/j.jsps.2020.05.006.

Banerjee, T., Samanta, A., 2022. 4 - Metal oxides for cosmetics and sunscreens. In: Mondal, K. (Ed.), Metal Oxides for Biomedical and Biosensor Applications. Elsevier, pp. 119–135. ISBN: 9780128230336. doi:10.1016/B978-0-12-823033-6.00002-8.

Battistin, M., Pascalicchio, P., Tabaro, B., Hasa, D., Bonetto, A., Manfredini, S., Baldisserotto, A., Scarso, A., Ziosi, P., Brunetta, A., Brunetta, F., Vertuani, S., 2022. A safe-by-design approach to "Reef Safe" sunscreens based on ZnO and organic UV filters. Antioxidants. 2076-3921. 11 (11), 2209. doi:10.3390/antiox11112209.

Bhardwaj, D., Chawla, V., Gupta, A., Dhiman, A., Singh, Y., Agrawal, G., 2025. Fe/Se nanocomposite-loaded chitosan/alginate films for wound healing. Int. J. Biol. Macromol. 01418130. 306 (Pt 3), 141626. doi:10.1016/j.ijbiomac.2025.141626.

Bom, S., Jorge, J., Ribeiro, H.M., Marto, J., 2019. A step forward on sustainability in the cosmetics industry: a review. J. Clean. Prod. 09596526. 225, 270–290. doi:10.1016/j.jclepro.2019.03.255.

Borowska, S., Brzóska, M.M., 2015. Metals in cosmetics: implications for human health. J. Appl. Toxicol. 10991263. 35 (6), 551–572. Available from http://onlinelibrary.wiley.com/journal/10.1002/(ISSN)1099-1263. doi:10.1002/jat.3129.

Bosecker, K., 1997. Bioleaching: metal solubilization by microorganisms. FEMS Microbiol. Rev. 1574-6976. 20 (3-4), 591–604. doi:10.1111/j.1574-6976.1997.tb00340.x.

Bourcier, W., Lin, M., Nix, G., 2005. Recovery of minerals and metals from geothermal fluids. In: 2003 SME Annual Meeting, Cincinnati, OH, United States. Available from: https://www.osti.gov/servlets/purl/883558.

Brito, T.P., De Souza-esquerdo, V.F., Borsatto, R.S., 2022. State of the art on research about organic certification: a systematic literature review. Org. Agr 12, 177–190. doi:10.1007/s13165-022-00390-6.

Bwatanglang, I.B., Obulapuram, P.K., Mohammad, F., Albalawi, A.N., Chavali, M., Al-Lohedan, H.A., Ibrahim, T., 2022. Metal oxide-involved photocatalytic technology in cosmetics and beauty products. In: Sagadevan, S., Podder, J., Mohammad, F. (Eds.), Metal Oxides for Optoelectronics and Optics-Based Medical Applications. Elsevier Science Ltd, Nigeria, pp. 301–337. Available from: https://www.sciencedirect.com/book/9780323858243. doi:10.1016/B978-0-323-85824-3.00002-6.

Cao, M., Jiayang, L., Tang, J., Chen, C., Zhao, Y., 2016. Gold nanomaterials in consumer cosmetics nanoproducts: analyses, characterization, and dermal safety assessment. Small. 1613-6810. 12 (39), 5488–5496. doi:10.1002/smll.201601574.

Carretero, M.I., 2002. Clay minerals and their beneficial effects upon human health. A review. Appl. Clay Sci. 01691317. 21 (3-4), 155–163. doi:10.1016/S0169-1317(01)00085-0.

Carretero, M.I., Pozo, M., 2010. Clay and non-clay minerals in the pharmaceutical and cosmetic industries Part II. Active ingredients. Appl. Clay Sci. 01691317. 47 (3-4), 171–181. doi:10.1016/j.clay.2009.10.016.

Chen, F.Z., Zhang, Z.W.B., Li, Q.F., Tan, P.C., Chang, J., Zhou, S.B., 2025a. Zinc silicate-loaded microneedle patch reduces reactive oxygen species production and enhances collagen synthesis for ultraviolet B-induced skin repair. Biomater. Res. 20557124. 29. Available from https://spj.science.org/doi/10.34133/bmr.0175. doi:10.34133/bmr.0180.

Chen, L., Zeng, S., Jiang, Z., Huang, C., Zhang, H., Liu, X., Liu, B., Wen, Q., Zhou, H., Shi, P., Liu, K., Yang, L., 2025b. Collagen-rich porcine acellular dermal matrix-eggshell membrane sponge promotes programmed healing of diabetic wounds through the sustained release of Cu2+/Zn2+. Int. J. Biol. Macromol. 310, 143545. doi:10.1016/j.ijbiomac.2025.143545.

Chen, Y., Cai, J., Liu, D., Liu, S., Lei, D., Zheng, L., Wei, Q., Gao, M., 2022. Zinc-based metal organic framework with antibacterial and anti-inflammatory properties for promoting wound healing. Regen. Biomater. 2056-3418. 9. doi:10.1093/rb/rbac019.

Couteau, C., Coiffard, L., 2020. Phycocosmetics and other marine cosmetics, specific cosmetics formulated using marine resources. Mar. Drugs. 1660-3397. 18 (6), 322. doi:10.3390/md18060322.

Dini, I., Laneri, S., 2021. The new challenge of green cosmetics: natural food ingredients for cosmetic formulations. Molecules. 1420-3049. 26 (13), 3921. doi:10.3390/molecules26133921.

Dusengemungu, L., Kasali, G., Gwanama, C., Mubemba, B., 2021. Overview of fungal bioleaching of metals. Environ. Adv. 26667657. 5, 100083. doi:10.1016/j.envadv.2021.100083.

Ebrahimzadeh, H., Moazzen, E., Amini, M.M., Sadeghi, O., 2013. Pyridine-2,6-diamine-functionalized Fe3O4 nanoparticles as a novel sorbent for determination of lead and cadmium ions in cosmetic samples. Int. J. Cosmet. Sci. 14682494. 35 (2), 176–182. doi:10.1111/ics.12023.

Farhan, M., 2024. The promising role of polyphenols in skin disorders. Molecules. 1420-3049. 29 (4), 865. doi:10.3390/molecules29040865.

Fernández-Cáceres, P.L., Martín, M.J., Pablos, F., González, A.G., 2001. Differentiation of tea (*Camellia sinensis*) varieties and their geographical origin according to their metal content. J. Agric. Food Chem. 00218561. 49 (10), 4775–4779. doi:10.1021/jf0106143.

Franca, C.C.V., Ueno, H.M., 2020. Green cosmetics: perspectives and challenges in the context of green chemistry. Desenvolv. Meio Ambient. 21769109. 53, 133–150. Available from https://revistas.ufpr.br/made/article/view/62322/40588. doi:10.5380/dma.v53i0.62322.

Fu, Y., Sun, H., Jin, Y., Cheng, S., Yanyi, W., Liu, C., Fan, L., Juqun, X., Shixin, L., Zhang, L., 2025. Self-assembled antioxidant enzyme-mimicking hydrogel: targeting oxidative stress and macrophage organization for improving degenerated intervertebral discs. Mater. Today Bio. 25900064. 31, 101586. doi:10.1016/j.mtbio.2025.101586.

Gallup, D.L., 1998. Geochemistry of geothermal fluids and well scales, and potential for mineral recovery. Ore Geol. Rev. 01691368. 12 (4), 225–236. Available from http://www.sciencedirect.com/science/journal/01691368. doi:10.1016/S0169-1368(98)00004-3.

Giacomelli, L., Togni, S., Meneghin, M., Eggenhöffner, R., Maramaldi, G., 2018. In vivo validation of the multicomponent powder (Vitachelox®) against the deposition of polluting ions. Clin. Cosmet. Invest. Dermatol. 1178-7015. 11, 109–113. doi:10.2147/CCID.S156324.

Gorman, M.R., Dzombak, D.A., 2018. A review of sustainable mining and resource management: transitioning from the life cycle of the mine to the life cycle of the mineral. Resour. Conserv. Recycl. 18790658. 137, 281–291. Available from www.elsevier.com/locate/resconrec. doi:10.1016/j.resconrec.2018.06.001.

Goyal, N., Jerold, F., 2021. Biocosmetics: technological advances and future outlook. Environ. Sci. Pollut. Res. 30, 25148–25169. doi:10.1007/s11356-021-17567-3.

Grujicic, J., Allen, A.R., 2025. Manganese superoxide dismutase: structure, function, and implications in human disease. Antioxidants. 2076-3921. 14 (7), 848. doi:10.3390/antiox14070848.

Gubitosa, J., Rizzi, V., Lopedota, A., Fini, P., Laurenzana, A., Fibbi, G., Fanelli, F., Petrella, A., Laquintana, V., Denora, N., Comparelli, R., Cosma, P., 2018. One pot environmental friendly synthesis of gold nanoparticles using *Punica granatum* juice: a novel antioxidant agent for future dermatological and cosmetic applications. J. Colloid Interface Sci. 00219797. 521, 50–61. doi:10.1016/j.jcis.2018.02.069.

Guillerme, J.-B., Couteau, C., Coiffard, L., 2017. Applications for marine resources in cosmetics. Cosmetics 4, 35. doi:10.3390/cosmetics4030035.

Guo, S., Yang, M., Zhilang, X., Liming, G., Changdao, M., Defu, L., 2025. Sandwich-like chitosan/collagen barrier membrane with passivated magnesium mesh as the skeleton. Int. J. Biol. Macromol. 01418130. 308 (Pt 3), 142590. doi:10.1016/j.ijbiomac.2025.142590.

Gupta, M., Mahajan, V.K., Mehta, K.S., Chauhan, P.S., 2014. Zinc therapy in dermatology: a review. Dermatol. Res. Pract. 16876113. 2014. Available from https://onlinelibrary.wiley.com/journal/3029. doi:10.1155/2014/709152.

Gyamfi, O., Aboko, J., Ankapong, E., Marfo, J.T., Awuah-Boateng, N.Y., Agyei, V., Sarpong, K., Dartey, E., 2023. Heavy metals in local and imported cosmetics in Ghana and their health risk assessment. Cogent Public Health. 2770-7571. 10 (1). doi:10.1080/27707571.2023.2217693.

Gyamfi, O., Aboko, J., Ankapong, E., Marfo, J.T., Awuah-Boateng, N.Y., Sarpong, K., Dartey, E., 2024. A systematic review of heavy metals contamination in cosmetics. Cutan. Ocul. Toxicol. 15569535. 43 (1), 5–12. Available from http://www.tandfonline.com/loi/icot20. doi:10.1080/15569527.2023.2268197.

Haghniaz, R., Rabbani, A., Vajhadin, F., Khan, T., Kousar, R., Khan, A.R., Montazerian, H., Iqbal, J., Libanori, A., Kim, H.J., Wahid, F., 2021. Anti-bacterial and wound healing-promoting effects of zinc ferrite nanoparticles. J. Nanobiotechnol. 14773155. 19 (1). Available from http://www.jnanobiotechnology.com/start.asp. doi:10.1186/s12951-021-00776-w.

Han, J., Meng, Q., Xue, S., Wenxuan, S., Jiannan, W., 2025. Silk fibroin methacryloyl hydrogel loaded with silver-gallic acid nanoparticles for enhanced diabetic wound healing. Int. J. Biol. Macromol. 01418130. 307 (Pt 4), 142108. doi:10.1016/j.ijbiomac.2025.142108.

Harper, R.T., Thain, I.A., Johnston, J.H., 1992. Towards the efficient utilization of geothermal resources. Geothermics 21, 641–651. doi:10.1016/0375-6505(92)90017-4.

Health Canada, 2011. Consumer Product Safety: Draft Guidance on Heavy Metal Impurities in Cosmetics. Government of Canada.

Ho, Y.B., Abdullah, N.H., Hamsan, H., Tan, E.S.S., 2017. Mercury contamination in facial skin lightening creams and its health risks to user. Regul. Toxicol. Pharmacol. 10960295. 88, 72–76. Available from http://www.elsevier.com/inca/publications/store/6/2/2/9/3/9/index.htt. doi:10.1016/j.yrtph.2017.05.018.

Houmine, S., Hamri, H.E., Jouhadi, Z., Bouchahta, H., Fekhaoui, M., 2025. Determination of mercury content in skin lightening cosmetics products using a direct mercury analyser. Cutan. Ocul. Toxicol. 1556-9527. 44 (3), 281–289. doi:10.1080/15569527.2025.2511717.

Hu, X., Zhang, H., Cheng, H., Hu, H.J., Tang, S., Zhong, B.H., Li, Y.C., Lan, L.M., Chen, Y., Song, K., Jiang, G.B., 2025. Iron-based driven chitosan quaternary ammonium salt self-gelling powder: sealing uncontrollable bleeding and promoting wound healing. Int. J. Biol. Macromol. 18790003. 300. Available from https://www.sciencedirect.com/science/journal/01418130. doi:10.1016/j.ijbiomac.2025.140330.

Hu, Y., Xiong, Y., Zhu, Y., Zhou, F., Liu, X., Chen, S., Zhanpeng, L., Shaohai, Q., Chen, L., 2023. Copper-epigallocatechin gallate enhances therapeutic effects of 3D-printed dermal scaffolds in mitigating diabetic wound scarring. ACS Appl. Mater. Interfaces. 1944-8244. 15 (32), 38230–38246. doi:10.1021/acsami.3c04733.

Hussain, M., Goldberg, D.J., 2007. Topical manganese peptide in the treatment of photodamaged skin. J. Cosmet. Laser Ther. 14764180. 9 (4), 232–236. doi:10.1080/14764170701704668.

Jia, J., Liu, R.K., Sun, Q., Wang, J.X., 2025. Multifunctional ZnO-loaded colloidosomes with multiple synergies as a UV filter. ACS Appl. Mater. Interfaces. 19448252. 17 (1), 2271–2280. Available from http://pubs.acs.org/journal/aamick. doi:10.1021/acsami.4c18007.

Jiménez Pérez, Z.E., Mathiyalagan, R., Markus, J., Kim, Y.J., Kang, H.M., Abbai, R., Seo, K.H., Wang, D., Soshnikova, V., Yang, D.C., 2017. Ginseng-berry-mediated gold and silver nanoparticle synthesis and evaluation of their in vitro antioxidant, antimicrobial, and cytotoxicity effects on human dermal fibroblast and murine melanoma skin cell lines. Int. J. Nanomed. 11782013. 12, 709–723. Available from https://www.dovepress.com/getfile.php?fileID=34996. doi:10.2147/IJN.S118373.

Jiménez-Pérez, Z.E., Singh, P., Kim, Y.J., Mathiyalagan, R., Kim, D.H., Lee, M.H., Yang, D.C., 2018. Applications of Panax ginseng leaves-mediated gold nanoparticles in cosmetics relation to antioxidant, moisture retention, and whitening effect on B16BL6 cells. J. Ginseng Res. 12268453. 42 (3), 327–333. Available from http://www.journals.elsevier.com/journal-of-ginseng-research/. doi:10.1016/j.jgr.2017.04.003.

Jin, C., Lin, Y.-Z., Zhang, R.-Y., Zhang, D.-P., Xue, K.-K., Jie, X., Jiang, X.-Q., Han, L.-J., Liu, L.-Y., Shi, Y.-F., Jin, M.-Q., Miu, J.-S., Ying-feng, L., Cai, L.-Y., Lin, Z., Yang, L., Xiao, J., 2026. A multifunctional hydrogel promotes diabetic wound healing by remodeling iron balance and energy metabolism. Biomaterials. 01429612. 326, 123640. doi:10.1016/j.biomaterials.2025.123640.

Kaliappan, K., Nagarajan, P., Jayabalan, J., Pushparaj, H., Elumalai, S., Paramanathan, B., Manickam, V., Jang, H.T., Mani, G., 2025. Systematic antimicrobial, biofilm, free radical inhibition and tyrosinase inhibition assessments of efficient green silver nanoparticles from the aqueous root extract of Cyphostemma adenocaule (CA). RSC Pharmaceutics. 2976-8713. 2 (1), 147–162. doi:10.1039/d4pm00173g.

Kicińska, A., Kowalczyk, M., 2025. Health risks from heavy metals in cosmetic products available in the online consumer market. Sci. Rep. 2045-2322. 15 (1). doi:10.1038/s41598-024-83477-2.

Kim, J., 2025. Smart nanocarriers in cosmeceuticals through advanced delivery systems. Biomimetics. 23137673. 10 (4). Available from www.mdpi.com/journal/biomimetics. doi:10.3390/biomimetics10040217.

Kostyuk, V.A., Potapovich, A.I., Strigunova, E.N., Kostyuk, T.V., Afanas'ev, I.B., 2004. Experimental evidence that flavonoid metal complexes may act as mimics of superoxide dismutase. Arch. Biochem. Biophys. 00039861. 428 (2), 204–208. doi:10.1016/j.abb.2004.06.008.

Kothapalli, C.R., Ramamurthi, A., 2009. Copper nanoparticle cues for biomimetic cellular assembly of crosslinked elastin fibers. Acta Biomater. 17427061. 5 (2), 541–553. Available from http://www.journals.elsevier.com/acta-biomaterialia. doi:10.1016/j.actbio.2008.09.004.

Lansdown, A.B.G., 1995. Physiological and toxicological changes in the skin resulting from the action and interaction of metal ions. Crit. Rev. Toxicol. 10408444. 25 (5), 397–462. doi:10.3109/10408449509049339.

Lee, J., Kwon, K.H., 2022. Future perspective safe cosmetics: focused on associated with ISO natural organic index. J. Cosmet. Dermatol. 14732165. 21 (12), 6619–6627. Available from http://onlinelibrary.wiley.com/journal/10.1111/(ISSN)1473-2165. doi:10.1111/jocd.15398.

Lee, S., Lee, G., Jeon, G., Lee, H., Park, S., Sohn, Y., Park, Y., Ryu, S., 2023. Anti-aging and lightening effects of Au-decorated zeolite-based biocompatible nanocomposites in epidermal delivery systems. J. Funct. Biomater. 2079-4983. 14 (2), 66. doi:10.3390/jfb14020066.

Lewandowska, J., Kalenik, B., Wrzosek, A., Szewczyk, A., 2024. Redox regulation of mitochondrial potassium channels activity. Antioxidants. 2076-3921. 13 (4), 434. doi:10.3390/antiox13040434.

Li, A., Yang, C., Zhang, L., 2025. Zinc oxide nanoparticles promote migrasomes formation. J. Hazard. Mater. 490, 137792. doi:10.1016/j.jhazmat.2025.137792.

Li, S., Mu, B., Yan, P., Kang, Y., Wang, Q., Wang, A., 2021a. Incorporation of different metal ion for tuning color and enhancing antioxidant activity of curcumin/palygorskite hybrid materials. Front. Chem. 9, 760941. doi:10.3389/fchem.2021.760941.

Li, Z., Huang, X., Lin, L., Jiao, Y., Zhou, C., Liu, Z., 2021b. Polyphenol and Cu2+ surface-modified chitin sponge synergizes with antibacterial, antioxidant and pro-vascularization activities for effective scarless regeneration of burned skin. Chem. Eng. J. 419, 129488. doi:10.1016/j.cej.2021.129488.

Lin, Z., Liu, H., Richardson, J.J., Xu, W., Chen, J., Zhou, J., Caruso, F., 2024. Metal-phenolic network composites: from fundamentals to applications. Chem. Soc. Rev. 14604744. 53 (22), 10800–10826. Available from http://pubs.rsc.org/en/journals/journal/cs. doi:10.1039/d3cs00273j.

Liu, S., Song, L., Huang, S., Liu, Z., Xu, Y., Wang, Z., Qiu, H., Wang, J., Chen, Z., Xiao, Y., Wang, H., Zhu, X., Zhang, K., Zhang, X., Lin, H., 2025. Hydroxyapatite microspheres encapsulated within hybrid hydrogel promote skin regeneration through the activation of calcium signaling and motor protein pathway. SSRN. 15565068. Available from https://www.ssrn.com/index.cfm/en/. doi:10.2139/ssrn.5142587.

Lopez-Galindo, A., Viseras, C., Cerezo, P., 2007. Compositional, technical and safety specifications of clays to be used as pharmaceutical and cosmetic products. Appl. Clay Sci. 36, 51–63. doi:10.1016/j.clay.2006.06.016.

Lu, W., Dong, C., 2022. Research progress of metal chelating peptides. Food Health. 2815-9179. 4 (4), 19. doi:10.53388/fh20221101019.

Luo, Q., Luo, L., Zhao, J., Wang, Y., Luo, H., 2024. Biological potential and mechanisms of Tea's bioactive compounds: an Updated review. J. Adv. Res. 20901232. 65, 345–363. doi:10.1016/j.jare.2023.12.004.

Martins, A.M., Marto, J.M., 2023. A sustainable life cycle for cosmetics: from design and development to post-use phase. Sustain. Chem. Pharm. 23525541. 35. Available from http://www.journals.elsevier.com/sustainable-chemistry-and-pharmacy. doi:10.1016/j.scp.2023.101178.

Miličević, A., Raos, N., 2016. Modelling of protective mechanism of iron(II)-polyphenol binding with OH-related molecular descriptors. Croatica Chemica Acta. 00111643. 89 (4). doi:10.5562/cca2996.

Moraes, J.D.D., Bertolino, S.R.A., Cuffini, S.L., Ducart, D.F., Bretzke, P.E., Leonardi, G.R., 2017. Clay minerals: properties and applications to dermocosmetic products and perspectives of natural raw materials for therapeutic purposes—a review. Int. J. Pharm. 18733476. 534 (1-2), 213–219. Available from www.elsevier.com/locate/ijpharm. doi:10.1016/j.ijpharm.2017.10.031.

Mourelle, M.L., Gómez, C.P., Legido, J.L., 2021. Microalgal peloids for cosmetic and wellness uses. Mar. Drugs 19, 666. doi:10.3390/md19120666.

Mucha, P., Skoczyńska, A., Małecka, M., Hikisz, P., Budzisz, E., 2021. Overview of the antioxidant and anti-inflammatory activities of selected plant compounds and their metal ions complexes. Molecules. 1420-3049. 26 (16), 4886. doi:10.3390/molecules26164886.

Mutlu, N., Liverani, L., Kurtuldu, F., Galusek, D., Boccaccini, A.R., 2022. Zinc improves antibacterial, anti-inflammatory and cell motility activity of chitosan for wound healing applications. Int. J. Biol. Macromol. 18790003. 213, 845–857. Available from www.elsevier.com/locate/ijbiomac. doi:10.1016/j.ijbiomac.2022.05.199.

Nobahar, A., Carlier, J.D., Miguel, M.G., Costa, M.C., 2021. A review of plant metabolites with metal interaction capacity: a green approach for industrial applications. BioMetals. 15728773. 34 (4), 761–793. Available from www.wkap.nl/journalhome.htm/0966-0844. doi:10.1007/s10534-021-00315-y.

Ochromowicz, K., Aasly, K., Kowalczuk, P., 2021. Recent advancements in metallurgical processing of marine minerals. Minerals 11, 1437. doi:10.3390/min11121437.

Oni, B.A., Tomomewo, O.S., Evro, S., Misiani, A.N., Sanni, S.E., 2025. A review of anticorrosive, superhydrophobic and self-healing properties of coating-composites as corrosion barriers on magnesium alloys: recent advances, challenges and future directions. J. Magnes. Alloy. 22139567. 13 (6), 2435–2469. Available from https://www.sciencedirect.com/science/journal/22139567. doi:10.1016/j.jma.2025.05.013.

Paiva-Santos, A.C., Herdade, A.M., Guerra, C., Peixoto, D., Pereira-Silva, M., Zeinali, M., Mascarenhas-Melo, F., Paranhos, A., Veiga, F., 2021. Plant-mediated green synthesis of metal-based nanoparticles for dermopharmaceutical and cosmetic applications. Int. J. Pharm. 18733476. 597. Available from www.elsevier.com/locate/ijpharm. doi:10.1016/j.ijpharm.2021.120311.

Pan, S., Goudoulas, T.B., Jeevanandam, J., Tan, K.X., Chowdhury, S., Danquah, M.K., 2021. Therapeutic applications of metal and metal-oxide nanoparticles: dermato-cosmetic perspectives. Front. Bioeng. Biotechnol. 22964185. 9. Available from http://journal.frontiersin.org/journal/bioengineering-and-biotechnology#archive. doi:10.3389/fbioe.2021.724499.

Pandey, A.S., Bawiskar, D., Wagh, V., 2024. Nanocosmetics and skin health: a comprehensive review of nanomaterials in cosmetic formulations. Cureus. doi:10.7759/cureus.52754.

Papadopoulos, A., Assimomytis, N., Varvaresou, A., 2022. Sample preparation of cosmetic products for the determination of heavy metals. Cosmetics 9, 21. doi:10.3390/cosmetics9010021.

Pawlaczyk, A., Gajek, M., Balcerek, M., Szynkowska-Jóźwik, M.I., 2021. Determination of metallic impurities by ICP-MS technique in eyeshadows purchased in Poland. Part I. Molecules. 1420-3049. 26 (21), 6753. doi:10.3390/molecules26216753.

Pereira, L., Dias, N., Carvalho, J., Fernandes, S., Santos, C., Lima, N., 2014. Synthesis, characterization and antifungal activity of chemically and fungal-produced silver nanoparticles against Trichophyton rubrum. J. Appl. Microbiol. 13645072. 117 (6), 1601–1613. doi:10.1111/jam.12652.

Piluk, T., Faccio, G., Letsiou, S., Liang, R., Freire-Gormaly, M., 2024. A critical review investigating the use of nanoparticles in cosmetic skin products. Environ. Sci. Nano. 20518161. 11 (9), 3674–3692. Available from http://pubs.rsc.org/en/journals/journal/en. doi:10.1039/d4en00489b.

Podgórska-Kryszczuk, I., 2024. Spirulina—an invaluable source of macro- and micronutrients with broad biological activity and application potential. Molecules. 1420-3049. 29 (22), 5387. doi:10.3390/molecules29225387.

Pramanik, S., Kumar, M., Qureshi, A., 2021. Mercury in skin-care products in India and consumer exposure risks. Regul. Toxicol. Pharmacol. 121, 104870. doi:10.1016/j.yrtph.2021.104870.

Premarathna, A.D., Tuvikene, R., Fernando, P.H.P., Adhikari, R., Perera, M.C.N., Ranahewa, T.H., Howlader, M.M., Wangchuk, P., Jayasooriya, A.P., Rajapakse, R.P.V.J., 2022. Comparative analysis of proximate compositions, mineral and functional chemical groups of 15 different seaweed species. Sci. Rep. 20452322. 12 (1). Available from https://www.nature.com/srep/. doi:10.1038/s41598-022-23609-8.

Pulit-Prociak, J., Grabowska, A., Chwastowski, J., Majka, T.M., Banach, M., 2019. Safety of the application of nanosilver and nanogold in topical cosmetic preparations. Colloids Surf. B Biointerfaces. 09277765. 183, 110416. doi:10.1016/j.colsurfb.2019.110416.

Rahman, M.M., Rahaman, M.S., Islam, M.R., Hossain, M.E., Mithi, F.M., Ahmed, M., Saldías, M., Akkol, E.K., Sobarzo-Sánchez, E., 2021. Multifunctional therapeutic potential of phytocomplexes and natural extracts for antimicrobial properties. Antibiotics. 20796382. 10 (9). Available from https://www.mdpi.com/2079-6382/10/9/1076/pdf. doi:10.3390/antibiotics10091076.

Raza-Naqvi, S.A., Idrees, F., Sherazi, T.A., Anjum-Shahzad, S., Ul-Hassan, S., Ashraf, N., 2022. Toxicology of heavy metals used in cosmetics. J. Chil. Chem. Soc. 0717-9707. 67 (3), 5615–5622. doi:10.4067/s0717-97072022000305615.

Reeves, R.D., Baker, A.J.M., Jaffré, T., Erskine, P.D., Echevarria, G., van der Ent, A., 2018. A global database for plants that hyperaccumulate metal and metalloid trace elements. New Phytol. 14698137. 218 (2), 407–411. Available from http://www.wiley.com/bw/editors.asp?ref=0028-646X&site=1. doi:10.1111/nph.14907.

Rehana, D., Mahendiran, D., Kumar, R.S., Rahiman, A.K., 2017. Evaluation of antioxidant and anticancer activity of copper oxide nanoparticles synthesized using medicinally important plant extracts. Biomed. Pharmacother. 19506007. 89, 1067–1077. Available from www.elsevier.com/locate/biomedpharm. doi:10.1016/j.biopha.2017.02.101.

Saadatzadeh, A., Afzalan, S., Zadehdabagh, R., Tishezan, L., Najafi, N., Seyedtabib, M., Noori, S.M.A., 2019. Determination of heavy metals (lead, cadmium, arsenic, and mercury) in authorized and unauthorized cosmetics. Cutan. Ocul. Toxicol. 15569535. 38 (3), 207–211. Available from http://www.tandfonline.com/loi/icot20. doi:10.1080/15569527.2019.1590389.

Saah, S.A., Boadi, N.O., Sakyi, P.O., Smith, E.Q., 2024. Human health risks of lead, cadmium, and other heavy metals in lipsticks. Heliyon. 24058440. 10 (23). Available from https://www.sciencedirect.com/science/journal/24058440. doi:10.1016/j.heliyon.2024.e40576.

Safavi, S., Najarian, R., Rasouli-Azad, M., Masoumzadeh, S., Ghaderi, A., Eghtesadi, R., 2019. A narrative review of heavy metals in cosmetics; health risks. Int. J. Pharm. Res. 09752366. 11 (4), 182–190. Available from http://www.ijpronline.com/Default.aspx. doi:10.31838/ijpr/2019.11.04.031.

Saldaña, M., Jeldres, M., Madrid, F.M.G., Gallegos, S., Salazar, I., Robles, P., Toro, N., 2023. Bioleaching modeling—a review. Materials. 1996-1944. 16 (10), 3812. doi:10.3390/ma16103812.

Sanajou, S., Şahin, G., Baydar, T., 2021. Aluminium in cosmetics and personal care products. J. Appl. Toxicol. 41, 1704–1718. doi:10.1002/jat.4228.

Sandri, G., Bonferoni, M.C., Rossi, S., Ferrari, F., Aguzzi, C., Viseras, C., Caramella, C., 2016. Clay minerals for tissue regeneration, repair, and engineering. Wound Healing Biomater. 2, 385–402. Available from http://www.sciencedirect.com/science/book/9781782424567. doi:10.1016/B978-1-78242-456-7.00019-2.

Sargsyan, L., Vill, V., Hippe, T., 2020. Investigations of vegetable tannins as hair dyes and their interactions with pre-bleached hair fibres. Int. J. Cosmet. Sci. 42, 320–327. doi:10.1111/ics.12624.

Sarruf, F.D., Contreras, V.J.P., Martinez, R.M., Velasco, M.V.R., Baby, A.R., 2024. The scenario of clays and clay minerals use in cosmetics/dermocosmetics. Cosmetics. 20799284. 11 (1). Available from www.mdpi.com/journal/cosmetics. doi:10.3390/cosmetics11010007.

Schwartz, F.W., Lee, S., Darrah, T.H., 2021. A review of the scope of artisanal and small-scale mining worldwide, poverty, and the associated health impacts. GeoHealth 5, e2020GH000325. doi:10.1029/2020GH000325.

Serov, D.A., Gritsaeva, A.V., Yanbaev, F.M., Simakin, A.V., Gudkov, S.V., 2024. Review of antimicrobial properties of titanium dioxide nanoparticles. Int. J. Mol. Sci. 14220067. 25 (19). Available from http://www.mdpi.com/journal/ijms. doi:10.3390/ijms251910519.

Sharma, A., Agarwal, P., Sebghatollahi, Z., Mahato, N., 2023. Functional nanostructured materials in the cosmetics industry: a review. ChemEngineering. 2305-7084. 7 (4), 66. doi:10.3390/chemengineering7040066.

Siméon, A., Wegrowski, Y., Bontemps, Y., Maquart, F.X., 2000. Expression of glycosaminoglycans and small proteoglycans in wounds: modulation by the tripeptide-copper complex glycyl-L-histidyl-L-lysine-Cu2+. J. Invest. Dermatol. 0022202X. 115 (6), 962–968. Available from http://www.nature.com/jid/index.html. doi:10.1046/j.1523-1747.2000.00166.x.

Sonia, S., Linda Jeeva Kumari, H., Ruckmani, K., Sivakumar, M., 2017. Antimicrobial and antioxidant potentials of biosynthesized colloidal zinc oxide nanoparticles for a fortified cold cream formulation: a potent nanocosmeceutical application. Mater. Sci. Eng. C. 09284931. 79, 581–589. doi:10.1016/j.msec.2017.05.059.

Sousa, C., Moutinho, C.G., Carvalho, M., Matos, C., Vinha, A.F., 2025. Transforming by-products into functional resources: the potential of Cucurbitaceae family seeds in cosmetics. Seeds. 26741024. 4 (3). Available from https://www.mdpi.com/journal/seeds. doi:10.3390/seeds4030036.

Souza, I., García-Villén, F., Viseras, C., Pergher, S., 2023. Zeolites as ingredients of medicinal products. Pharmaceutics. 1999-4923. 15 (5), 1352. doi:10.3390/pharmaceutics15051352.

Subbiah, D.K., Mani, G.K., Babu, K.J., Das, A., Rayappan, J.B.B., 2018. Nanostructured ZnO on cotton fabrics—a novel flexible gas sensor & UV filter. J. Clean. Prod. 09596526. 194, 372–382. doi:10.1016/j.jclepro.2018.05.110.

Treyman, M., Bezdudnaya, A., Razumovsky, V., Smirnov, R., Nurmurodov, T., 2024. Research, control and greening of mica mining processes in the regions. E3S Web Conf. 2267-1242. 525, 02001. doi:10.1051/e3sconf/202452502001.

US FDA, 2018. Chapter 9: federal food, drug & cosmetic act on hazardous chemicals in cosmetics. In: Food and Drugs. Subchapter VI : Cosmetics.

Vinodkumar, T., Dinesh, T., Ghosh, K., Ilavarasan, R., 2025. A comprehensive analysis of minerals in *Moringa oleifera* leaves, seeds, stem bark, and ash using inductively coupled plasma-optical emission spectroscopy (ICP-OES). Discov. Chem. 3005-1193. 2 (1). doi:10.1007/s44371-025-00115-0.

Viseras, C., Sánchez-Espejo, R., Palumbo, R., Liccardi, N., García-Villén, F., Borrego-Sánchez, A., Massaro, M., Riela, S., López-Galindo, A., 2021. Clays in cosmetics and personal-care products. Clays Clay Miner. 0009-8604. 69 (5), 561–575. doi:10.1007/s42860-021-00154-5.

Wall, F., Rollat, A., Pell, R.S., 2017. Responsible sourcing of critical metals. Elements 13, 313–318. doi:10.2138/gselements.13.5.313.

Wang, X., Qin, W., Maolin, L., Liu, X., Cheng, Y., Chen, S., Yang, C., 2024. Mineralogy of deep-sea manganese nodules and advances in extraction technology of valuable elements from manganese nodules. Metals. 2075-4701. 14 (12), 1359. doi:10.3390/met14121359.

Wang, Y., Yang, H., Pschenitza, M., Niessner, R., Yuan, L., Knopp, D., Deng, A., 2012. Highly sensitive and specific determination of mercury(II) ion in water, food and cosmetic samples with an ELISA based on a novel monoclonal antibody. Anal. Bioanal. Chem. 1618-2642. 403 (9), 2519–2528. doi:10.1007/s00216-012-6052-1.

Yadav, V.K., Yadav, K.K., Tirth, V., Gnanamoorthy, G., Gupta, N., Algahtani, A., Islam, S., Choudhary, N., Modi, S., Jeon, B.H., 2021. Extraction of value-added minerals from various agricultural, industrial and domestic wastes. Materials. 19961944. 14 (21). Available from https://www.mdpi.com/1996-1944/14/21/6333/pdf. doi:10.3390/ma14216333.

Yan, S., Chen, W., Zhang, Y., Jie, L., Chen, X., 2019. Calcium release-activated calcium modulator 1 as a therapeutic target in allergic skin diseases. Life Sci. 00243205. 228, 152–157. doi:10.1016/j.lfs.2019.05.001.

Yang, F., Xue, Y., Wang, F., Guo, D., Yunjiao, H., Zhao, X., Yan, F., Yuqian, X., Xia, D., Liu, Y., 2023. Sustained release of magnesium and zinc ions synergistically accelerates wound healing. Bioact. Mater. 2452199X. 26, 88–101. doi:10.1016/j.bioactmat.2023.02.019.

Yao, J., Xiao, L., Lin, M., Han, Z., Wang, X., Guo, J., Bing, W., Xia, J., 2025. Bifunctional copper ion/melittin incorporated hydrogel with antimicrobial and antioxidant capabilities for infected skin wound healing. Mater. Des. 02641275. 250, 113631. doi:10.1016/j.matdes.2025.113631.

Zawisza, B., Sitko, R., Gagor, A., 2022. Determination of ultra-trace gold in cosmetics using aluminum-magnesium layered double hydroxide/graphene oxide nanocomposite. Talanta 245, 123460. doi:10.1016/j.talanta.2022.123460.

Zeggai, F.Z., Touahra, F., Labied, R., Lerari, D., Chebout, R., Bachari, K., 2024. Biopolymers-clay Nanocomposites: Synthesis Pathways, Properties, and Applications. IntechOpen. doi:10.5772/intechopen.114879.

Zhang, H., Ma, W., Ma, H., Qin, C., Chen, J., Wu, C., 2022a. Spindle-like zinc silicate nanoparticles accelerating innervated and vascularized skin burn wound healing. Adv. Healthc. Mater. 21922659. 11 (10). Available from http://onlinelibrary.wiley.com/journal/10.1002/(ISSN)2192-2659. doi:10.1002/adhm.202102359.

Zhang, L., Zhang, H., Tang, L., Hu, X., Xu, M., 2022c. Isolation, characterization, antioxidant activity, metal-chelating activity, and protein-precipitating capacity of condensed tannins from plum (*Prunus salicina*) fruit. Antioxidants 11, 714. doi:10.3390/antiox11040714.

Zhang, Z., Chang, D., Zeng, Z., Yuze, X., Jing, Y., Fan, C., Yang, C., Chang, J., 2024. CuCS/Cur composite wound dressings promote neuralized skin regeneration by rebuilding the nerve cell "factory" in deep skin burns. Mater. Today Bio. 25900064. 26, 101075. doi:10.1016/j.mtbio.2024.101075.

Chapter 26

Exploring natural carbon in biofunctional cosmetics

Ioanna Koumentakou, Alexandros Tsoupras, and George Z. Kyzas
Hephaestus Laboratory, School of Chemistry, Faculty of Sciences, Democritus University of Thrace, Kavala University Campus, Kavala, Greece

1 Introduction

Due to rising customer demand for customized, innovative, and scientifically based products, the cosmetics business has experienced phenomenal expansion in recent decades (Salvioni et al., 2021). Since Raymond Reed defined the term "cosmetics" in 1961, the cosmetic field has evolved far beyond its initial focus on beauty enhancement. These days, cosmetics include multipurpose products designed to enhance skin tone, texture, and general health (Dubey et al., 2022). In addition, according to international regulations, cosmetics are defined as substances or combinations that are applied to the human body's external parts, such as the skin, hair, lips, nails, and mucous membranes, for purposes like cleaning, scenting, protecting, or altering appearance (Anastasiou et al., 2024).

Cosmetic companies are under pressure to implement environmentally responsible practices due to concerns about pollution, ecological destruction, and possible safety (Grădinaru et al., 2022). These concerns are amplified in today's digital environment, where reputational risks spread rapidly. To stay competitive and reliable, brands are consequently moving toward eco-conscious innovation and sustainability-centered business models (Sudha et al., 2018).

Natural carbon materials have become a very attractive path for biofunctional cosmetics within this larger sustainability agenda (Singh, 2021). High surface area, adjustable porosity, and exceptional adsorption capacity are only a few of the distinctive physicochemical characteristics of carbon materials, including activated carbon (AC) and carbon nanostructures (Budiman et al., 2024). These qualities make them appealing for developing cosmetic formulations, as well as for biological and environmental applications (Ngoc et al., 2023b).

The revolutionary importance of carbon nanomaterials, such as graphene, nanotubes, and polymer-based carbon nanocomposites, in improving cosmetic goods has been highlighted by recent advances in material science (Manikandan et al., 2021). Enhancing stability, facilitating the regulated release of active ingredients, and extending product efficacy can help formulations meet customer expectations for longevity and performance (Chatzimitakos et al., 2020).

However, there are difficulties in using carbon nanoparticles in cosmetics (Budiman et al., 2024). The possible environmental effects of widespread use are major concerns, as is ensuring these materials are safe and biocompatible to protect consumer health and comply with legal requirements (Petric, 2021). The rate at which natural carbon compounds can transition from laboratory invention to widely used cosmetic applications will depend on how effectively these issues are addressed through thorough research and testing (Murugan et al., 2024).

This chapter examines the role of natural carbon in biofunctional cosmetics, emphasizing its properties, applications, benefits, and limitations. By exploring how carbon materials can lead innovation in cosmetic formulations, this study underscores their potential to reshape the industry's future, merging performance, sustainability, and consumer trust into the next generation of cosmetic solutions.

2 Carbon materialws for cosmetic applications

2.1 Production of carbon from biomass

Biomass-derived carbon has been highlighted as a sustainable and alternative solution to conventional carbon sources, offering significant potential for developing advanced and environmentally friendly materials (Zhou et al., 2022). Because

Biofunctional Cosmetics for Health. https://doi.org/10.1016/B978-0-443-27500-5.00003-4

of their abundance, affordability, and high carbon content, municipal wastes, forestry by-products, and agricultural residues are increasingly used as renewable precursors for carbon synthesis (Shams et al., 2015). Biomass can be converted into a variety of carbon compounds, such as AC, carbon nanofibers (CNFs), and even carbon nanotubes (CNTs), using methods like pyrolysis, hydrothermal carbonization, and chemical activation (Gayathiri et al., 2022). Surface area, porosity, and shape are among the physicochemical characteristics of the resultant carbon that are highly dependent on the kind of biomass and processing parameters, allowing for customized design for specific uses (Abuelnoor et al., 2021). Furthermore, it is possible to integrate the natural heteroatoms found in biomass, such as oxygen, nitrogen, and sulfur, into the produced carbon to enhance surface functionality, wettability, and catalytic activity (Malini et al., 2023). In line with the ideas of green chemistry and the circular economy, this sustainable approach not only reduces dependency on fossil fuel-based feedstocks but also adds value to industrial and agricultural wastes (Yin et al., 2023). Carbon synthesized from biomass presents opportunities to create environmentally friendly functional chemicals in the cosmetics industry, combining sustainability and effectiveness.

2.2 Carbon materials

2.2.1 Activated carbon

AC has attracted growing attention in the cosmetics industry due to its unique pore structure, high surface area, and versatile surface chemistry (Budiman et al., 2024). Because of its physicochemical characteristics, AC may effectively adsorb pollutants, toxins, and excess sebum from the skin while also enhancing the stability and safety of cosmetic compositions. Through physical adsorption and chemical interactions, AC can act as a catalyst to increase the reactivity of active chemicals, like whitening agents, in addition to its cleansing properties, thus enhancing product performance (Lan et al., 2023). As agricultural and municipal waste materials offer plentiful, affordable, and environmentally benign carbon precursors, biomass-derived AC has become a more viable option for cosmetic applications (Guo et al., 2017). AC synthesized from biomass presents a variety of morphologies, from sheet-like structures to hierarchical porous networks, depending on the biomass source and synthesis circumstances. These morphologies have a direct impact on the adsorption behavior and functional efficiency of A—C (Singh et al., 2018). The AC application in biofunctional cosmetics is further expanded by adding heteroatoms like oxygen, nitrogen, and sulfur, which improve surface wettability and add electroactive sites (Cherusseri and Kar, 2016; Guo et al., 2017). Because of these characteristics and properties, AC is positioned as a multipurpose substance that promotes skin cleaning and fits the industry's increasing focus on sustainability, innovation, and consumer safety (Sinha et al., 2020).

2.3 Carbon nanotubes

CNTs represent a novel class of nanomaterials with promising applications in the cosmetics field due to their exceptional structural and functional properties (Kizil et al., 2024). CNTs are cylindrical carbon allotropes, which can be single-walled carbon nanotubes (SWCNTs) , made up of a single graphene layer rolled into a tube, or multiwalled carbon nanotubes (MWCNTs), composed of multiple concentric graphitic shells with a typical interlayer spacing of approximately 0.34 nm (Bikiaris et al., 2022). CNTs can reach lengths of several μm and diameters of 1–100 nm (Rennhofer and Zanghellini, 2021). They help improve cosmetic products because of their exceptional mechanical, electrical, and optical qualities, enormous surface area, and exceptionally high aspect ratio (Zhou et al., 2021). Specifically, CNTs can enhance cosmetic formulation stability, provide unique textural qualities, and enable the controlled administration of active chemicals (Angelopoulou et al., 2022). These properties are potentially useful for decorative cosmetics, such as lipsticks and mascaras, where improved adherence, durability, and performance are highly desirable (Fytianos et al., 2020). Recent developments have demonstrated that CNTs may also be produced from various biomass sources, including lignocellulosic waste, agricultural wastes, and other renewable carbon-rich precursors (Zhou et al., 2022).

2.3.1 Graphene-based materials

Graphene-based materials have recently attracted growing interest in cosmetics due to their exceptional physicochemical properties and versatility (Faruque et al., 2021). Graphene, the fundamental structural unit of graphite, consists of a single layer of sp^2-hybridized carbon atoms arranged in a two-dimensional hexagonal lattice (Faruque et al., 2021).

This unique structure imparts excellent characteristics, such as high mechanical strength, improved electrical and thermal conductivity, large surface area, optical transparency, and chemical stability. Beyond these properties, graphene derivatives, such as graphene oxide (GO) and reduced graphene oxide (rGO), offer tunable surface chemistries (Fig. 26.1), nanoporous architectures, and enhanced dispersibility in aqueous and polymeric systems, which make them highly adaptable for cosmetic formulations (Bikiaris et al., 2022; Kavian et al., 2023). In particular, graphene's high adsorption capacity and antimicrobial

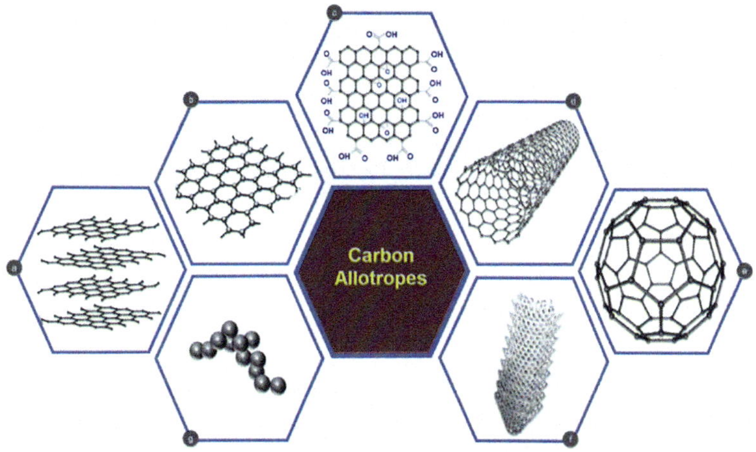

FIG. 26.1 Graphene-based materials: (A) graphite, (B) graphene, (C) graphene oxide, (D) carbon nanotubes, (E) fullerene, (F) carbon nanofibers, (G) carbon dot. *(From Faruque, M.A.A., Syduzzaman, M., Sarkar, J., Bilisik, K., Naebe, M., 2021. A review on the production methods and applications of graphene-based materials. Nanomaterials. 20794991. 11 (9). Available from: https://www.mdpi.com/2079-4991/11/9/2414/pdf. doi:10.3390/nano11092414.)*

efficacy support its use in skin purification products, while its ability to facilitate controlled release and stabilization of active ingredients enhances the performance and stability of biofunctional cosmetics (Luo et al., 2018). Graphene and its derivatives can be produced from various biomass sources, such as peanut shells (Purkait et al., 2017), coconut shells (Sun et al., 2013), wheat straw, tea tree plants (Zhou et al., 2016), and camphor leaves (*Cinnamomum camphora*) (Shams et al., 2015).

2.4 Fullerene

Fullerenes, the third allotropic form of carbon after graphite and diamond, are unique cage-like molecules composed entirely of carbon atoms arranged in spherical, ellipsoidal, or cylindrical architectures (Lens, 2009; Benn et al., 2011). Among them, C_{60} and C_{70} are the most widely studied for cosmetic applications due to their remarkable antioxidant properties and ability to scavenge reactive oxygen species (ROS) (Mousavi et al., 2017). Since oxidative stress plays a central role in skin aging, fullerenes have been incorporated into cosmetic formulations such as sunscreens, skin-whitening agents, and antiaging products to improve skin protection and rejuvenation (Kato et al., 2010). The first commercial application was the water-soluble polyvinylpyrrolidone (PVP)–fullerene complex, marketed as "Radical Sponge," which highlighted their potential as radical quenching ingredients (Lens, 2011). Beyond their antioxidant activity, fullerenes and their derivatives exhibit diverse biological activities, including antimicrobial, antiviral, neuroprotective, and cytoprotective effects (Robles et al., 2024). However, despite these promising attributes, concerns remain regarding their potential cytotoxicity and ability to induce cell dysfunction, emphasizing the need for careful safety assessments and regulatory oversight.

2.5 Carbon dots

A novel category of carbon compounds is the carbon dots (C-dots), which are smaller than 10 nm (Zaib et al., 2023). C-dots consist of a large amount of carbon and a small amount of other elements (H, N, and O) present on the surface (Kurian and Paul, 2021). The structure of C-dots is characterized by a graphite core (sp^2 hybridized carbon) and an amorphous carbon shell. C-dots exhibit high water solubility, photoluminescence properties, biocompatibility, low toxicity, and high chemical stability (Lin et al., 2021). Their nanosize and surface functional groups enable customized interactions with biomolecules and other materials, which are primarily responsible for these characteristics.

Several studies on the synthesis of C-dots from plant-based ingredients have produced C-dots that enhance their attractiveness in cosmetic applications by inheriting desirable properties like antioxidant qualities, skin-soothing effects, and compatibility with different formulations (Li et al., 2022; Ashok Kumar et al., 2023).

The use of C-dots synthesized from plant extracts offers a fresh way to combine natural chemicals and nanotechnology (Moon et al., 2020; Centeno et al., 2021). Utilizing the inherent qualities of plant-based precursors, C-dots can acquire favorable characteristics such as skin-soothing effects, antioxidant qualities, and compatibility with different formulations, which highlight their attractiveness in cosmetic applications (Ngoc et al., 2023a). C-dots generated from plant extracts are regarded as innovative components because of their intrinsic biodegradability, renewability, and potential to support the growing trend of green chemistry in the cosmetics sector (Marseille, 2023).

TABLE 26.1 Cosmetics incorporating carbon-based products (Singh, 2021).

Company	Cosmetic product
A! Absolute!	Magnetic Nail Lacquer
Boots	No7 Stay Perfect Eye Shadow
Bourjois	Liner Feutre Eyeliner
butter London	Nail Polish
butter London	Patent Shine Nail Lacquer
CoverGirl	Intensify Me Liquid Eyeliner
Jesse's Girl Cosmetics	Liquid Eyeliner
L'Oréal Paris	Infallible Never Fail Liquid Eyeliner
Max Factor	False Lash Effect 24 h Bold Volume Mascara; Masterpiece Glide & Define Liquid Eye Liner
OPI Brazil	Nail Lacquer Collection
Prestige	My Biggest Lashes Mascara
RevitaLash	Volumizing Mascara
Revlon	ColorStay Liquid Eye Pen.
SensatioNail	Gel Nail Polish
Surya Brasil	Natural Nail Polish

2.6 Carbon-based cosmetic products

A wide range of items designed for particular skin or body parts is included in the category of cosmetics. Similarly, carbon-based compounds are used in various personal care products, each of which meets specific requirements. Commercial cosmetics that use carbon-based compounds are shown in Table 26.1.

3 Carbon-based materials in skin care cosmetic products

Over the past decade, significant progress has been made in exploring carbon-based additives as functional ingredients in skincare formulations, particularly due to their unique physicochemical properties.

3.1 Cleanser cosmetic products

Carbon-based materials have been increasingly incorporated into cleanser formulations due to their exceptional adsorption capacity and detoxifying properties. AC, in particular, has been widely utilized in facial cleansers and masks because of its high surface area, which effectively removes impurities, pollutants, and excess sebum from the skin surface (Budiman et al., 2024; Ganjoo et al., 2023). By binding oil, dirt, and toxins, AC provides deep pore cleansing, reduces pore visibility, and improves skin texture, making it especially suitable for oily and acne-prone skin (Syarif et al., 2023). Similarly, CNFs demonstrate even higher oil-absorbing potential, offering enhanced control of sebum production compared to traditional cosmetic ingredients . Recent studies have also highlighted the use of bamboo-derived carbon in biodegradable cleansing masks, where its combination with polymers such as PVP significantly improves adsorption performance, surpassing that of commercial cleansing products (Liu and Zhang, 2022).

3.2 Antioxidant products

Carbon-based materials have demonstrated remarkable antioxidant potential, making them highly attractive for incorporation into cosmetic formulations designed to counteract oxidative skin damage and premature aging. Among them, carbon dots (CDs) have emerged as multifunctional antioxidants capable of efficiently scavenging ROS, thereby protecting skin cells from oxidative stress-induced senescence and preserving skin vitality (Qu, 2019; He et al., 2021). Their antiradical activity has been demonstrated through comparative assays using standard nitrogen-centered radicals such as 1,1-diphenyl-2-picrylhydrazyl (DPPH ·). The primary scavenging mechanism involves hydrogen atom transfer from surface functional groups, carboxyl (–COOH), hydroxyl (–OH), and amino (–NH_2/–NH–), to DPPH ·, resulting in its reduction to DPPH–H (Fig. 26.2) (Ngoc et al., 2023b). Beyond delaying wrinkle formation, CDs also help maintain barrier function, and their

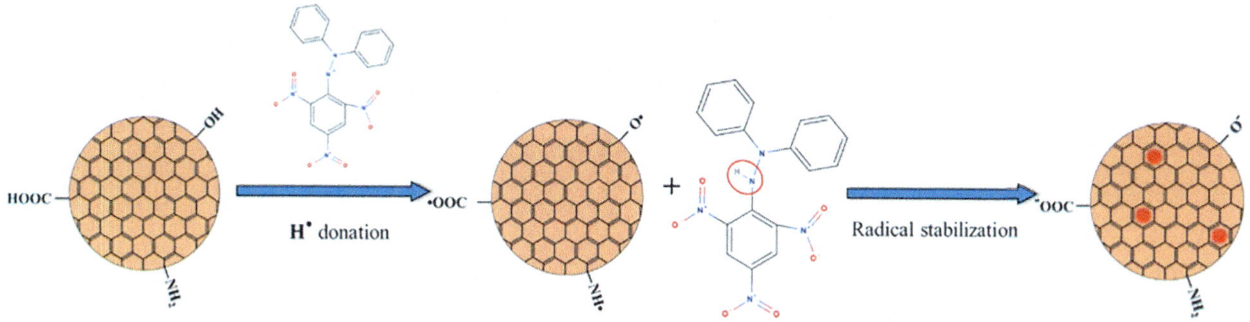

FIG. 26.2 Antioxidant effects of CDs. Mechanisms of antioxidant activity of CDs. *(From Ngoc, L.T.N., Moon, J.Y., Lee, Y.C., 2023b. Plant extract-derived carbon dots as cosmetic ingredients. Nanomaterials 20794991. 13 (19). Available from: https://www.mdpi.com/journal/nanomaterials. doi:10.3390/nano13192654.)*

antioxidant efficiency can be further enhanced through surface functionalization (Li, 2020). Recent advances in carbon quantum dots (CQDs), such as tannic acid-derived CQDs synthesized via microwave-assisted pyrolysis, have shown excellent radical scavenging activity, achieving over 80% free radical inhibition at very low concentrations (Son et al., 2021). Moreover, CDs incorporated into temperature-sensitive hydrogel systems demonstrated superior photothermal antioxidant activity, highlighting their versatility in advanced cosmetic formulations (Wang et al., 2024).

Graphene-based nanomaterials also exhibit strong antioxidant properties. Both GO and rGO have been reported to possess free radical scavenging capabilities, with applications in wound healing and antiaging skin care, where oxidative balance is critical (Priyadarsini et al., 2018). Comparative studies have shown that few-layer graphene (FLG) exhibits higher ROS scavenging activity than GO despite its lower surface area, suggesting that pristine sp^2 carbon domains on basal planes play a dominant role over hydroxyl or hydroquinone groups in radical neutralization (Qiu et al., 2014). In addition, Pan et al. reported that GO displayed a DPPH scavenging rate exceeding 90% at 50 μg/mL, outperforming rGO due to its higher oxidation degree (Pan et al., 2025). Furthermore, Hsin-Yu Chou et al. demonstrated that CNTs and GO nanoribbons (GONRs) can regulate melanin production by mitigating oxidative stress. GONRs exhibit enhanced antioxidative performance in both intracellular and extracellular models (Chou et al., 2020). Moreover, fullerenes represent another extensively studied class of carbon antioxidants in cosmetics (Dugan et al., 2001). Their unique cage-like structure enables them to accept multiple electrons and effectively quench singlet oxygen and other ROS, resulting in notable antiaging and antiwrinkle benefits (Ikeda, 2012). Clinical studies with fullerene derivatives, such as LipoFullerene, have shown improved wrinkle reduction and skin elasticity (Dugan et al., 2001). Romero Robles et al. further confirmed the antioxidant potential of fullerene (C60) formulations in dermal fibroblast cultures, where fullerenol incorporation significantly reduced ROS production at both 0.2% and 0.5% concentrations (Robles et al., 2024). Interestingly, the radical scavenging ability of nanodiamonds (NDs) and fullerenes was found to be significantly enhanced under ultraviolet (UV) irradiation, in contrast to vitamin C, which decreased in efficacy under the same conditions (Lin et al., 2019).

3.3 Sun protection

UV radiation represents one of the most significant environmental stressors for the skin. While the ozone layer filters ultraviolet-C (UVC) and part of ultaviolet-B (UVB), the remaining UVB and ultaviolet-A (UVA) rays reach the Earth's surface and contribute to erythema, photoaging, and the development of skin cancers such as melanoma (Budiman et al., 2024). Sunscreens are commonly evaluated by their sun protection factor (SPF) and ultraviolet protection factor, but many conventional filters suffer from issues such as photoinstability, skin irritation, or limited spectral coverage (Stan and Ania, 2022). In this context, carbon-based nanomaterials have attracted growing interest as multifunctional agents capable of providing broad UV protection, high stability, and additional biological benefits.

CNTs were among the first carbon nanomaterials investigated for photoprotection. Their strong UV absorption arises from the π-conjugated CC bonds within their tubular structure, which dissipates the energy of incident radiation (Swapna et al., 2017). Comparative studies have shown that SWCNTs are more effective absorbers than MWCNTs, owing to their higher surface area and fewer structural defects (Mahmoudifard and Safi, 2012). When incorporated into cosmetic emulsions, CNTs significantly enhanced SPF values, with 2% MWCNT-containing formulations reaching SPF levels above 30, highlighting their potential as powerful UV absorbers (Bikiaris et al., 2022).

Furthermore, graphene-based nanomaterials provide another promising avenue. GO and rGO block UV radiation and exert antioxidant and biological protective effects. For example, GO has been shown to protect fibroblasts against

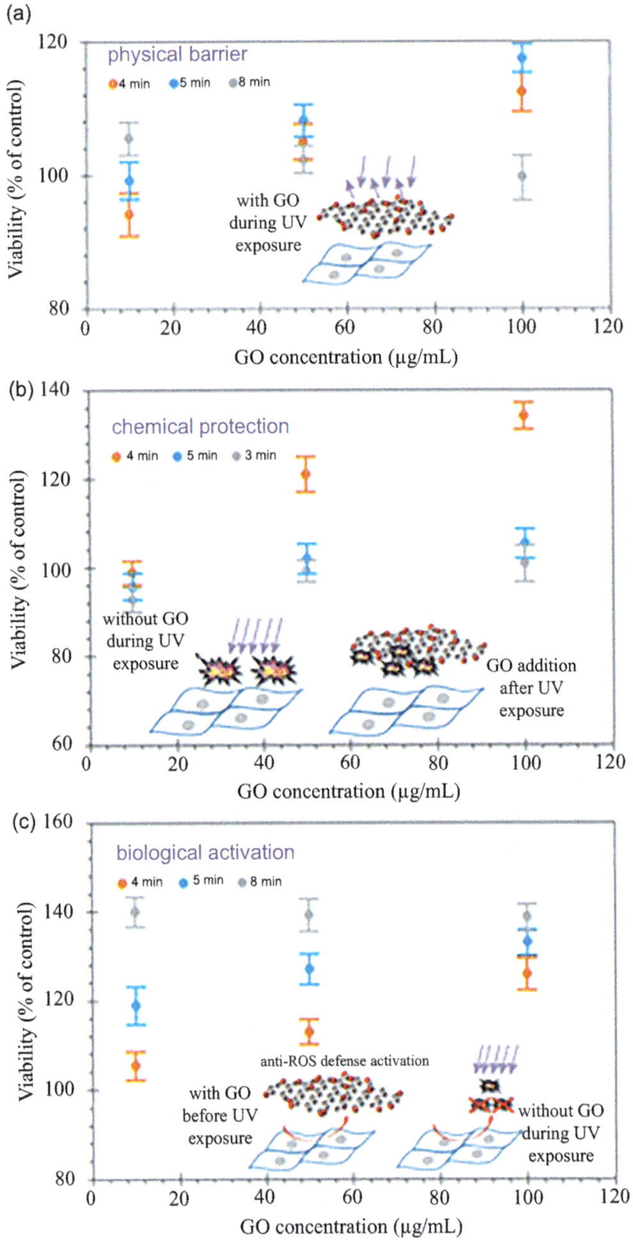

FIG. 26.3 Effect of UV irradiation duration and GO concentration on 3T3 fibroblast proliferation. GO acts as (A) a physical barrier, (B) a chemical antioxidant protector, and (C) a biological activator. *(Data from Bolibok, P., Roszek, K., Wiśniewski, M., 2018. Graphene oxide-mediated protection from photodamage. J. Phys. Chem. Lett. 19487185. 9 (12), 3241–3244. Available from: https://pubs.acs.org/journal/jpclcd. doi:10.1021/acs.jpclett.8b01349, copyright ACS.)*

UVB-induced damage through a combination of physical shielding, radical scavenging, and the activation of endogenous antioxidant defenses. In emulsions, GO contributes to moderate SPF enhancement, while FLG demonstrates stronger ROS scavenging despite its smaller surface area, underscoring the importance of sp^2 carbon domains in photoprotection (Fig. 26.3) (Bolibok et al., 2018). Fullerenes, particularly C60 and its derivatives, are among the most extensively studied carbon antioxidants for photoprotection. Lin et al. (2019) demonstrated that aqueous dispersions of NDs and C60 exhibited SPF values of 1.88 and 6.41, respectively, with minimal spectral shifts after prolonged irradiation, confirming their stability as UV filters. In another study, Kato et al. (2014) reported that fullerene derivatives (C60/PVP, C60/Sqn) suppressed UV/TiO_2-induced phototoxicity in keratinocytes by reducing ROS generation and lipid peroxidation. More recently, hybrid nanomaterials offer further promise. AC combined with silver nanoparticles (AgNPs), synthesized using *Usnea undulata* extract, functioned as a broad-spectrum UVA + UVB blocker with favorable protection indices (Nguyen et al., 2024).

Similarly, graphene–TiO_2 composites have been reported to stabilize organic UV filters, reducing photocatalytic degradation and improving sunscreen durability (Bartoszewska et al., 2023). Several studies have shown that CQDs exhibited outstanding anti-UV application results and good compatibility in polymers (Negi et al., 2025). One study prepared CQDs and polyvinyl alcohol (PVA) composite emulsion with strong fluorescence under UV radiation to confirm the potential applications of CQDs as UV absorbers in antiaging polymers and skin sunscreen. The sun protection performance was evaluated in vivo under industry-standard testing conditions using samples of PVA and CQDs@PVA emulsions. Under irradiation equivalent to one minimal erythema dose (MED), skin areas treated with the PVA emulsion alone showed a progressive increase in erythema with rising radiation intensities. In contrast, no erythema was observed on skin coated with the CQDs@PVA emulsion, even after exposure to five MEDs, demonstrating its superior photoprotective efficacy (Hu et al., 2019). Moreover, Nuntahirun et al. prepared green-synthesized CQDs derived from tea and alpha-hydroxy acids as the co-precursors, including gluconic acid (GA), citric acid, and tartaric acid. They then prepared the solution and emulsion, adding them. All CDs exhibited strong UV absorption with SPF ranges of 1.1–1.8 for solutions and 1.1–2.5 for emulsions, especially in the UVB and UVC regions, with GA-CDs having the highest UV absorption (Nuntahirun et al., 2023). More recently, Xu et al. synthesized nitrogen-doped carbon dots with full-spectrum UV absorption, achieving SPF > 50 and PFA++++ ratings in transparent films while maintaining > 93% visible light transmittance.

4 Antiinflammatory and antibacterial cosmetic products

Inflammation and microbial imbalance are two major contributors to compromised skin health, which is often linked to premature aging, acne, and environmental damage. Carbon-based nanomaterials are increasingly being investigated as multifunctional ingredients in cosmetic formulations because they combine antioxidant, antiinflammatory, and antibacterial effects within a single system.

CDs exhibit promising antibacterial actions since interactions between their positively charged surface and negatively charged bacterial membranes can destabilize membranes and cause rupture. Doping CDs with heteroatoms such as nitrogen, sulfur, and boron showed significantly enhanced bactericidal activity by generating ROS and causing electrostatic disruption of bacterial membranes (Saravanan et al., 2024). In addition, green-synthesized CDs derived from natural sources such as anthocyanin-rich plants (e.g., blackberries and purple potatoes), coffee residues, and medicinal herbs have demonstrated broad-spectrum antimicrobial effects against *Escherichia coli, Staphylococcus aureus*, and *Candida albicans*, achieving inhibition rates of up to 99% (Macedo et al., 2025). These materials have also been incorporated into cosmetic and hygiene formulations, including soaps and cleansing solutions, effectively eliminating bacteria and protecting against skin infections. Interestingly, two patents have been identified for healing agents. One proposes a CD photocatalyst to be used in the preparation of an antibacterial product that promotes the healing of wounds caused by *S. aureus* infections (CN109550049-B). The second is a disruptive innovation in the field of chronic wound healing developed by a Chinese nanomaterials company (Beijing Zhongke East Asia Nano Material Technology Co. Ltd.) using low-temperature plasma technology. The scientists synthesized CDs in the wound itself, promoting the conversion of the infecting bacteria into CDs with antibacterial and antibiofilm properties. The researchers reported biological safety and low bacterial resistance (CN115317517-A) (Macedo et al., 2025). In addition to their antibacterial activity, CDs have demonstrated strong antiinflammatory effects. Ngoc et al. explained that CDs scavenge ROS, preventing oxidative stress-induced activation of inflammatory pathways such as NF-κB and MAPK, which are commonly triggered by UV irradiation and pollutants. This activity translates into reduced expression of proinflammatory cytokines, including TNF-α, IL-1, and IL-6, thereby helping to preserve collagen synthesis and protect against premature skin aging (Ngoc et al., 2023b). Moreover, hybrid systems that combine carbon materials with metallic nanoparticles have also shown promise. For instance, AgNPs synthesized via *U. undulata* extract and immobilized on AC (AgNPs/AC) inhibited the growth of common pathogens such as *Escherichia coli, Staphylococcus aureus, Bacillus cereus*, and *Pseudomonas aeruginosa* with minimum inhibitory concentrations as low as 10 μg/mL (Nguyen et al., 2024). Moreover, graphene-based nanomaterials exhibit potent antibacterial activity, which arises from their unique physicochemical properties and interactions with microbial cell structures (Olborska et al., 2020). Liu et al. investigated the antibacterial mechanisms of four graphene derivatives, graphite (Gt), graphite oxide (GtO), GO, and rGO, against *E. coli* (Liu et al., 2011). Their findings revealed that several factors influence antibacterial efficiency, including material size, solubility, dispersion stability, concentration, and surface chemistry. Smaller graphene sheets with higher densities of oxygen-containing functional groups showed stronger interactions with bacterial membranes, resulting in membrane penetration, oxidative stress, and accelerated bacterial cell death. GO exhibited the highest antibacterial activity, followed by rGO, Gt, and GtO. The materials also induced oxidative damage to key cellular components such as lipids, proteins, DNA, and glutathione, with rGO demonstrating the strongest glutathione oxidation capacity.

Complementary results were reported by Pulingam et al., who examined the antibacterial behavior of GO against both Gram-positive (*S. aureus, Enterococcus faecalis*) and Gram-negative (*E. coli, P. aeruginosa*) bacteria. The antibacterial effect of GO was found to depend on concentration, exposure duration, and bacterial morphology. For Gram-positive bacteria, inactivation occurred primarily through a cell-trapping or wrapping mechanism, whereas Gram-negative bacteria were inactivated by direct membrane disruption (Pulingam et al., 2019). Due to its excellent antimicrobial activity, GO has been added to emulsion and hydrogel-based skin care products to avoid microbial infections. A topical hydrogel treatment based on a polymeric network of gelatin–PVA–hyaluronic acid encapsulating a GO nanoconjugate, on which AgNPs have been grown by Jorge Luis Patarroyo et al., presenting 100% bacterial growth inhibition (Patarroyo et al., 2022). In another study, GO-based nanocarriers were integrated into a green neem oil emulsion and exhibited substantial antibacterial activity (inhibition zones of 39 ± 0.02 mm against *Staphylococcus epidermidis*) and considerable antifungal activity against *C. albicans* (inhibition zone of 43 ± 0.13 mm) (Al-Zuhairy et al., 2025).

5 Carbon-based materials in hair cosmetic products

Carbon-based materials have also been used in hair care formulations, owing to their exceptional adsorption capacity, chemical versatility, and ability to improve both scalp health and cosmetic performance. AC and related nanomaterials are increasingly incorporated into shampoos and conditioners to remove pollutants, excess sebum, and chemical residues from the scalp, thereby promoting a cleaner environment that supports healthy hair growth. Their strong adsorption properties allow the elimination of impurities and residues from styling products or environmental contaminants, making them particularly beneficial for oily hair types and individuals living in urban or polluted environments (Budiman et al., 2024). Specifically, AC was added to a shampoo formulation made from natural ingredients, which showed effective removal of dust, toxic substances, and dandruff from hair (Divya, 2019). Moreover, CNFs have also been introduced into shampoo formulations for oil control. Their high surface area and controlled adsorption behavior enable efficient removal of excess scalp oil without darkening the hair fibers, leaving hair clean, soft, and lightweight. This targeted oil-regulation capability offers an advantage over conventional surfactants that can sometimes over-strip natural oils and irritate the scalp (Manikandan et al., 2021). Several studies have also explored the application of CNTs as hair colorants and functional additives. Huang et al. described the incorporation of CNTs, either chemically functionalized or physically modified, into hair colorant compositions to enhance their affinity for hair fibers. The nanoscale dimensions and high surface-area-to-volume ratio of CNTs enable close interaction with keratin fibers, providing more durable coloration and uniform coverage (Carrasco-Marin, 2005). Peptide-based CNT colorants, formed by the coupling of a hair-binding peptide to the nanotube surface, created diblock compositions and increased the affinity to hair through covalent conjugation (Huang et al., 2005).

More recently, graphene-based materials such as GO and rGO have gained significant attention as innovative, nonreactive hair dyes. GO and rGO can be dispersed in water without the need for toxic solvents or oxidizing agents, providing a safer and more environmentally friendly alternative to conventional dyes. When applied by brushing or spraying, these graphene-based formulations can impart a range of shades from brown to black that remain stable after repeated washing. The unique two-dimensional structure of graphene sheets, with an apparent thickness of about 1 nm and lateral dimensions up to several micrometers, allows them to form smooth, flexible, and adherent coatings on hair fibers. Upon partial reduction, GO transforms into rGO, which darkens due to its increased optical absorption, yielding long-lasting coloration (Luo et al., 2018). In addition to color enhancement, graphene-based dyes can impart new optical, electrical, and thermal properties to hair, potentially improving antistatic behavior, heat resistance, and overall cosmetic performance. GO was also combined with chitosan to produce a hair formulation that gave it brown to black colors and demonstrated a durable effect, resisting multiple shampooings, antistatic, and heat dissipation (Luo et al., 2018).

6 Carbon-based materials in eye cosmetic products

Carbon nanomaterials have long been associated with eye cosmetics, both in traditional formulations and in modern nanotechnology-based products. Professor Maheshwar Sharon from the Indian Institute of Technology (IIT) Bombay investigated the composition of kaajal, a traditional Indian eye cosmetic, and revealed through scanning electron microscopy that the soot obtained from burning mustard oil consists of a network of CNTs and nanoparticles with diameters below 50 nm. The tubular morphology of CNTs was found to prevent mechanical irritation to the eyes, explaining the comfort and safety associated with traditional kaajal use (Singh, 2021).

Another study presented the development of carbon nanobuds, a hybrid nanostructure combining the unique properties of CNTs and fullerenes. These materials consist of CNTs covalently bonded to fullerene-like "buds," yielding a structure that merges the flexibility and conductivity of CNTs with the spherical geometry and chemical reactivity of fullerenes.

Carbon nanobuds exhibit excellent field emission characteristics, making them suitable for incorporation in cosmetic formulations such as mascaras and lipsticks, where uniform dispersion, adhesion, and optical properties are critical (Fytianos et al., 2020). Their unique hybrid structure offers enhanced pigment stability and potential for novel textural and esthetic effects.

Carbon black has been powdered in cosmetic products, providing a deep black coloration characteristic of eyeliners, mascaras, and eyeshadows. Under the European Union's Regulation No. 1223/2009/EC, carbon black is listed in Annex IV as an approved cosmetic colorant with a maximum authorized concentration of 10% in nano form. Carbon black is one of the most widely used pigments in decorative eye products due to its strong color intensity, stability, and ease of formulation (Balwierz et al., 2023).

7 Carbon-based materials in oral care cosmetic products

Carbon-based materials, particularly AC and CNFs, have demonstrated promising utility in oral cosmetics and hygiene products. AC can remove impurities and neutralize odors due to its strong adsorption properties, resulting in fresher breath and cleaner tooth surfaces (Agrawal et al., 2018). Effectiveness of toothpaste from activated charcoal as teeth whitening: A systematic literature review. CNFs have also been investigated as gentle yet effective agents for dental care applications. According to Singh et al., CNF incorporation into toothpaste formulations produced a nonacidic, pH-balanced, sulfate-free product capable of whitening teeth and supporting gum health without causing enamel abrasion. Owing to their softness and chemical inertness, CNFs act as passive polishing agents that enhance brightness while maintaining safety for daily oral use (Singh, 2021).

8 Carbon-based materials in lip care cosmetic products

In lip care formulations, carbon-based nanomaterials such as CDs have opened new avenues for enhancing moisture retention and sensory properties. Dong et al. reported the synthesis of fluorescent carbon dots derived from carmine cochineal (Car-CDs), which exhibited exceptional hygroscopic and moisture-preserving capabilities. When incorporated into moisturizing lipsticks, these Car-CDs significantly improved long-lasting hydration while maintaining low toxicity and excellent optical stability. The relationship between the structural features of Car-CDs and their moisture retention performance was elucidated, revealing that surface functional groups play a key role in water-binding capacity (Dong et al., 2021).

9 Toxicity of carbon-based materials in cosmetic products

As carbon-based materials become increasingly incorporated into cosmetic formulations, from skin and hair care to color cosmetics, it is essential to evaluate their safety and potential toxicological effects critically. While these materials offer unique properties such as adsorption, antioxidation, and photoprotection, their nanoscale size and chemical reactivity raise important questions regarding long-term human and environmental safety.

The US Food and Drug Administration classifies CNFs as harmless when used externally, although inhalation should be strictly avoided, as airborne fibers may induce pulmonary inflammation and fibrosis (Singh, 2021). Similarly, studies on CNTs indicate that toxicity depends strongly on their physicochemical characteristics, including size, shape, surface functionalization, and aggregation state. Shorter, functionalized CNTs tend to be less toxic than longer, unmodified ones. Pulmonary exposure, primarily an occupational hazard, remains the most significant risk, with evidence of lung inflammation, granuloma formation, and fibrosis in high-dose animal studies (Santos et al., 2019).

CDs are among the most extensively studied nanocarbons for cosmetics, and most reports indicate excellent biocompatibility. For example, Chatzimitakos et al. demonstrated that CDs derived from *Dunaliella salina microalgae* were nontoxic to cells even at 100–600 μg/mL concentrations and protected eukaryotic cells from UV-induced damage (Chatzimitakos et al., 2020). Numerous in vitro studies have confirmed that plant extract-derived CDs, including those from broccoli, tannic acid, and carmine cochineal, maintain over 80%–100% cell viability at concentrations up to 500 μg/mL, indicating low cytotoxicity. In vivo assessments using zebrafish embryos also revealed high survival rates (>85%) and hatching rates, while mammalian studies showed no organ damage after prolonged exposure (Ngoc et al., 2023b).

Nevertheless, CD toxicity is negligible and depends on particle size, surface charge, and aggregation. For example, smaller CDs (10–20 nm) tend to be more toxic than larger ones (40–100 nm), while CDs that aggregate in the culture medium are more toxic than those that remain dispersed (Macedo et al., 2025). For cosmetic use, manufacturers must therefore ensure consistent production quality, evaluate skin irritation and sensitization through standardized assays (e.g.,

Draize and local lymph node tests), and comply with cosmetic regulatory standards (Dos Santos et al., 2024). Moreover, fullerenes, including C_{60} and its derivatives, have shown both promise and controversy. Although used in antioxidant and antiaging cosmetics, several studies have reported potential biological effects such as oxidative stress, inflammation, and cytotoxicity at high concentrations. The increasing use of fullerene-containing cosmetics also raises environmental concerns, as these molecules can enter aquatic ecosystems through rinse-off products. Graphene-based materials, including GO and rGO, have also been scrutinized for safety. While GO generally exhibits good biocompatibility, high concentrations (20–50 mg/mL) can impair cellular functions by 20%–50%. Some studies have shown that graphene particles can translocate to internal organs such as the liver, lungs, and kidneys, potentially causing inflammation or oxidative damage. In addition, prolonged exposure to GO has even been linked to ocular opacity in animal models. The method of graphene reduction plays a critical role in its safety profile, chemical reduction using hydrazine poses toxicity risks, whereas "green" reduction using plant extracts or ascorbic acid is considered safer but still requires optimization for large-scale production (Dos Santos et al., 2024).

Carbon black (CI 77266) remains one of the most widely used colorants in eye and lip cosmetics. Although concerns about PAH residues and possible carcinogenicity have been raised, evidence indicates that these compounds cannot be released under normal skin application conditions. However, animal inhalation studies have shown potential for gene mutations and chronic lung inflammation. At the same time, epidemiological data among workers chronically exposed to airborne carbon black suggest increased rates of keratosis and precancerous lesions. Consequently, the International Agency for Research on Cancer (IARC) classifies carbon black as a Group 2B "possible human carcinogen." However, it is considered safe for dermal application in cosmetics when inhalation exposure is prevented (Balwierz et al., 2023).

Toxicity in carbon-based materials is highly dependent on size, morphology, chemical composition, surface coatings, and exposure route. In general, dermal exposure to carbon nanomaterials used in cosmetics appears to pose minimal acute risk, whereas inhalation remains the primary safety concern, particularly during the manufacturing or handling of nanopowders. To ensure consumer safety, rigorous quality control and standardized toxicological testing, including in vitro cytotoxicity, genotoxicity, and long-term in vivo studies, are essential.

The growing focus on environmental sustainability has encouraged the development of biomass-derived carbon materials as greener and safer alternatives. Agricultural and forestry residues are now used as carbon sources to produce AC, CNFs, and even CNTs through eco-friendly processes such as hydrothermal carbonization and pyrolysis. These bioderived carbons often exhibit improved surface chemistry and lower impurity levels, aligning with green chemistry and circular economy principles (Zhou et al., 2022).

10 Conclusions

Incorporating carbon-based materials into cosmetics signifies a major paradigm shift toward sustainability, multifunctionality, and technological sophistication in the beauty industry. This study shows that natural and synthetic carbon forms—ranging from AC to advanced nanostructures like CNTs, graphene, fullerenes, and carbon dots—offer unmatched opportunities for performance enhancement and eco-innovation. Their exceptional adsorption, antioxidative, antimicrobial, and photoprotective properties enable formulations that beautify, protect, and rejuvenate the skin and hair. Moreover, developing biomass-derived carbon materials presents a sustainable path that aligns with circular economy principles by utilizing agricultural and forestry residues as renewable precursors. This approach minimizes waste, reduces dependence on fossil-based sources, and supports green chemistry practices.

However, the full potential of carbon nanomaterials can only be realized through rigorous safety evaluation and responsible innovation. Despite generally favorable dermal compatibility, nanoscale carbon particles may pose health and environmental risks, particularly through inhalation or uncontrolled release into ecosystems. Thus comprehensive toxicity testing, standardized characterization, and transparent regulatory oversight are crucial for ensuring safe consumer use. Equally important is optimizing synthesis methods to achieve consistency, purity, and eco-friendliness at an industrial scale.

Future research should focus on integrating carbon nanomaterials with natural bioactives to create synergistic cosmetic systems capable of targeted delivery, sustained release, and enhanced efficacy. In addition, adopting "green nanotechnology" approaches—such as plant-based synthesis and biodegradable carrier systems—will strengthen consumer trust and meet the rising demand for clean, ethical beauty. Ultimately, carbon's versatility makes it a key enabler in transforming the cosmetic industry toward a model that harmonizes scientific innovation with environmental stewardship. Carbon-based materials are poised to define the next generation of biofunctional cosmetics and drive progress toward a more responsible and high-performing beauty future by bridging functionality, safety, and sustainability.

References

Abuelnoor, N., AlHajaj, A., Khaleel, M., Vega, L.F., Abu-Zahra, M.R.M., 2021. Activated carbons from biomass-based sources for CO2 capture applications. Chemosphere 18791298. 282. Available from: https://www.elsevier.com/locate/chemosphere. doi:10.1016/j.chemosphere.2021.131111.

Agrawal, P., Panda, S., Mishra, S.R., 2018. A review on activated charcoal tooth paste. World J. Pharm. Res. 7, 478. doi:10.20959/wjpr20189-12132.

Al-Zuhairy, S.A.K.S., Elhabal, S.F., Elrefai, M.F.M., Hababeh, S., Nelson, J., Fady, M., Elzohairy, N.A., Ewedah, T.M., Mousa, I.S., Hamdan, A.M.E., 2025. Polylactic-co-glycolic acid/alginate/neem oil-reduced graphene oxide as a pH-sensitive nanocarrier for hesperidin drug delivery: antimicrobial and acute otitis media assessments. Pharmaceuticals 14248247. 18 (3). Available from: https://www.mdpi.com/journal/pharmaceuticals. doi:10.3390/ph18030381.

Anastasiou, E.A., et al., 2024. Nanostructured materials in industrial applications, personal care, and health care: a cosmetic approach. Ref. Module Mater. Sci. Eng. doi:10.1016/B978-0-323-95486-0.00087-9.

Angelopoulou, P., Giaouris, E., Gardikis, K., 2022. Applications and prospects of nanotechnology in food and cosmetics preservation. Nanomaterials 20794991. 12 (7). Available from: https://www.mdpi.com/2079-4991/12/7/1196/pdf. doi:10.3390/nano12071196.

Ashok Kumar, S., Dheeraj Kumar, M., Saikia, M., Renuga Devi, N., Subramania, A., 2023. A review on plant derived carbon quantum dots for bio-imaging. Mater. Adv. 2633-5409. 4 (18), 3951–3966. doi:10.1039/d3ma00254c.

Balwierz, R., Biernat, P., Jasińska-Balwierz, A., Siodłak, D., Kusakiewicz-Dawid, A., Kurek-Górecka, A., Olczyk, P., Ochędzan-Siodłak, W., 2023. Potential carcinogens in makeup cosmetics. Int. J. Environ. Res. Public Health 16604601. 20 (6). Available from: https://www.mdpi.com/journal/ijerph. doi:10.3390/ijerph20064780.

Bartoszewska, M., Adamska, E., Kowalska, A., Grobelna, B., 2023. Novelty cosmetic filters based on nanomaterials composed of titanium dioxide nanoparticles. Molecules 14203049. 28 (2). Available from: https://www.mdpi.com/journal/molecules. doi:10.3390/molecules28020645.

Benn, T.M., Westerhoff, P., Herckes, P., 2011. Detection of fullerenes (C60 and C70) in commercial cosmetics. Environ. Pollut. 02697491. 159 (5), 1334–1342. doi:10.1016/j.envpol.2011.01.018.

Bikiaris, N.D., Koumentakou, I., Lykidou, S., Nikolaidis, N., 2022. Innovative skin product O/W emulsions containing lignin, multiwall carbon nanotubes and graphene oxide nanoadditives with enhanced sun protection factor and UV stability properties. Appl. Nano 26733501. 3 (1), 1–15. Available from: https://www.mdpi.com/journal/applnano. doi:10.3390/applnano3010001.

Bolibok, P., Roszek, K., Wiśniewski, M., 2018. Graphene oxide-mediated protection from photodamage. J. Phys. Chem. Lett. 19487185. 9 (12), 3241–3244. Available from: https://pubs.acs.org/journal/jpclcd. doi:10.1021/acs.jpclett.8b01349.

Budiman, I., Amirta, R., Yuliansyah, B.A.W., Fatriasari, W., 2024. Activated Carbon for Cosmetics Applications Biomass-Based Cosmetics: Research Trends and Future Outlook. Springer Nature, Indonesia, pp. 217–237. Available from: https://link.springer.com/book/10.1007/978-981-97-1908-2. doi:10.1007/978-981-97-1908-2_10.

Carrasco-Marin, F., 2005. Hair coloring and cosmetic compositions comprising carbon nanotubes. J. Phys. Chem. B 107 (12), 199–202.

Centeno, L., Romero-García, J., Alvarado-Canché, C., Carlos Gallardo-vega, G.T.-P., Díaz Barriga-castro, E., Edgar, N.C.-Á., Ledezma-Pérez, A., de León, A., 2021. Green synthesis of graphene quantum dots from *Opuntia* sp. extract and their application in phytic acid detection. Sens. Bio-Sens. Res. 22141804. 32, 100412. doi:10.1016/j.sbsr.2021.100412.

Chatzimitakos, T.G., Kasouni, A., Troganis, A., Leonardos, I., Tzovenis, I., Ntzouvaras, A., Stalikas, C., 2020. Carbon nanodots synthesized from dunaliella salina as sun protection filters. C. 2311-5629. 6 (4), 69. doi:10.3390/c6040069.

Cherusseri, J., Kar, K.K., 2016. Hierarchical carbon nanopetal/polypyrrole nanocomposite electrodes with brush-like architecture for supercapacitors. Phys. Chem. Chem. Phys. Accessed: Oct. 07, 2025. [Online]. Available from: https://pubs.rsc.org/en/content/articlehtml/2016/cp/c6cp00150e. doi:10.1039/C6CP00150E.

Chou, H.Y., Wang, H.M.D., Kuo, C.H., Lu, P.H., Wang, L., Kang, W., Sun, C.L., 2020. Antioxidant graphene oxide nanoribbon as a novel whitening agent inhibits microphthalmia-associated transcription factor-related melanogenesis mechanism. ACS Omega 24701343. 5 (12), 6588–6597. Available from: https://pubs.acs.org/journal/acsodf. doi:10.1021/acsomega.9b04316.

Divya, K.H., 2019. Studies on the addition of activated charcoal in herbal shampoo. Glob. J. Res. Eng. 19 (C2), 15–20. Available from: https://engineeringresearch.org/index.php/GJRE/article/view/1968.

Dong, et al., 2021. Fluorescent carbon dots with excellent moisture retention capability for moisturizing lipstick. J. Nanobiotechnol. 19. doi:10.1186/S12951-021-01029-6.

Dos Santos, F.K.F., Júnior, A.A.M.P., Filho, A.L.N., Fonseca, C.J.N., Isidorio, D.K.M., Araújo, F.D.A., Oliveira, P.H.A., Júnior, V.F.D.V., 2024. Graphene and natural products: a review of antioxidant properties in graphene oxide reduction. Int. J. Mol. Sci. 14220067. 25 (10). Available from: https://www.mdpi.com/journal/ijms. doi:10.3390/ijms25105182.

Dubey, S.K., Dey, A., Singhvi, G., Pandey, M.M., Singh, V., Kesharwani, P., 2022. Emerging trends of nanotechnology in advanced cosmetics. Colloids Surf. B Biointerfaces 18734367. 214. Available from: https://www.elsevier.com/locate/colsurfb. doi:10.1016/j.colsurfb.2022.112440.

Dugan, L.L., Lovett, E.G., Quick, K.L., Lotharius, J., Lin, T.T., O'Malley, K.L., 2001. Fullerene-based antioxidants and neurodegenerative disorders. Parkinsonism Relat. Disord. 13538020. 7 (3), 243–246. doi:10.1016/s1353-8020(00)00064-x.

Faruque, M.A.A., Syduzzaman, M., Sarkar, J., Bilisik, K., Naebe, M., 2021. A review on the production methods and applications of graphene-based materials. Nanomaterials. 20794991. 11 (9). Available from: https://www.mdpi.com/2079-4991/11/9/2414/pdf. doi:10.3390/nano11092414.

Fytianos, G., Rahdar, A., Kyzas, G.Z., 2020. Nanomaterials in cosmetics: recent updates. Nanomaterials 20794991. 10 (5). Available from: https://www.mdpi.com/2079-4991/10/5/979/pdf. doi:10.3390/nano10050979.

Ganjoo, R., Sharma, S., Kumar, A., Daouda, M.M.A., 2023. Activated Carbon: Fundamentals, Classification, and Properties. Royal Society of Chemistry (RSC), pp. 1–22. doi:10.1039/bk9781839169861-00001.

Gayathiri, M., Thiruchelvi Pulingam, K.T.L., Sudesh, K., 2022. Activated carbon from biomass waste precursors: factors affecting production and adsorption mechanism. Chemosphere. 00456535. 294, 133764. doi:10.1016/j.chemosphere.2022.133764.

Grădinaru, C., Obadă, D.R., Grădinaru, I.A., Dabija, D.C., 2022. Enhancing sustainable cosmetics brand purchase: a comprehensive approach based on the sor model and the triple bottom line. Sustainability 14 (21), 14118. doi:10.3390/SU142114118.

Guo, N., Li, M., Sun, X., Wang, F., Yang, R., 2017. Tremella derived ultrahigh specific surface area activated carbon for high performance supercapacitor. Mater. Chem. Phys. 02540584. 201, 399–407. Available from: https://www.journals.elsevier.com/materials-chemistry-and-physics. doi:10.1016/j.matchemphys.2017.08.054.

He, Z., Xu, Q., Newland, B., Foley, R., Lara-Sáez, I., Curtin, J.F., Wang, W., 2021. Reactive oxygen species (ROS): utilizing injectable antioxidative hydrogels and ROS-producing therapies to manage the double-edged sword. J. Mater. Chem. B 20507518. 9 (32), 6326–6346. Available from: https://pubs.rsc.org/en/journals/journal/tb. doi:10.1039/d1tb00728a.

Hu, G., Lei, B., Jiao, X., Wu, S., Zhang, X., Zhuang, J., Liu, X., Hu, C., Liu, Y., 2019. Synthesis of modified carbon dots with performance of ultraviolet absorption used in sunscreen. Opt. Express 10944087. 27 (5), 7629–7641. Available from: https://www.osapublishing.org/oe/abstract.cfm?uri=oe-27-5-7629. doi:10.1364/OE.27.007629.

Huang, X., Kobos, R., Xu, G., 2005. Peptide-based carbon nanotube hair colorants and their use in hair colorant and cosmetic compositions. WO2005117537.

Ikeda, A., 2012. Clinical evaluation of fullerene-containing cosmetics for wrinkle improvement. J. Clin. Biochem. Nutr. 51 (3), 193–198.

Kato, S., Aoshima, H., Saitoh, Y., Miwa, N., 2014. Fullerene-C60 derivatives prevent UV-irradiation/TiO 2-induced cytotoxicity on keratinocytes and 3D-skin tissues through antioxidant actions. J. Nanosci. Nanotechnol. 15334899. 14 (5), 3285–3291. Available from: https://docserver.ingentaconnect.com/deliver/connect/asp/15334880/v14n5/s1.pdf?expires=1396932523&id=77794639&titleid=4286&accname=Elsevier+BV&checksum=D7E37FA8E36B3F21BA26ADB84FE0F2FB. doi:10.1166/jnn.2014.8719.

Kato, S., Taira, H., Aoshima, H., Saitoh, Y., Miwa, N., 2010. Clinical evaluation of fullerene-C 60 dissolved in squalane for anti-wrinkle cosmetics. J. Nanosci. Nanotechnol. 15334880. 10 (10), 6769–6774. doi:10.1166/jnn.2010.3053.

Kavian, M., Ghani, M., Raoof, J.B., 2023. Polyoxometalate/reduced graphene oxide composite stabilized on the inner wall of a stainless steel tube as a sorbent for solid-phase microextraction of some parabens followed by quantification via high-performance liquid chromatography. Microchem. J. 0026265X. 187. Available from: https://www.elsevier.com/inca/publications/store/6/2/0/3/9/1. doi:10.1016/j.microc.2023.108413.

Kizil, N., Erbilgin, D., Basaran, E., Yola, M.L., Yilmaz, E., Marouch, S., Soylak, M., 2024. Determination of rhodamine B in cosmetics, candy, water, and plastic by a novel multiwalled carbon nanotube (MWCNT)@zinc oxide@magnetite nanocomposite for magnetic solid-phase extraction (MSPE) with spectrophotometric detection. Anal. Lett. 1532236X. 57 (7), 1182–1196. Available from: https://www.tandf.co.uk/journals/titles/00032719.asp. doi:10.1080/00032719.2023.2243353.

Kurian, M., Paul, A., 2021. Recent trends in the use of green sources for carbon dot synthesis–A short review. Carbon Trends. 26670569. 3, 100032. doi:10.1016/j.cartre.2021.100032.

Lan, J., Wang, B., Bo, C., Gong, B., Ou, J., 2023. Progress on fabrication and application of activated carbon sphere in recent decade. J. Ind. Eng. Chem. 22345957. 120, 47–72. Available from: https://www.sciencedirect.com/science/journal/1226086X. doi:10.1016/j.jiec.2022.12.045.

Lens, M., 2009. Use of fullerenes in cosmetics. Recent Pat. Biotechnol. 3 (2), 118–123. doi:10.2174/187220809788700166.

Lens, M., 2011. Recent progresses in application of fullerenes in cosmetics. Recent Pat. Biotechnol. 18722083. 5 (2), 67–73. Available from: https://www.eurekaselect.com/650/journal/recent-patents-biotechnology. doi:10.2174/187220811796365707.

Li, H., 2020. Surface functionalization of carbon dots enhances antioxidant activity for biomedical and cosmetic use. Nano Res. 13 (12), 3165–3177.

Li, L., Han, Y., Wang, L., Jiang, W., Zhao, H., 2022. Dye plants derived carbon dots for flexible secure printing. Nanomaterials 20794991. 12 (18). Available from: https://www.mdpi.com/journal/nanomaterials. doi:10.3390/nano12183168.

Lin, Q., Xu, R.H.J.X., Yang, N., Karim, A.A., Loh, X.J., Zhang, K., 2019. UV protection and antioxidant activity of nanodiamonds and fullerenes for sunscreen formulations. ACS Appl. Nano Mater. 25740970. 2 (12), 7604–7616. Available from: https://pubs.acs.org/journal/aanmf6. doi:10.1021/acsanm.9b01698.

Lin, X., Xiong, M., Zhang, J., Chen, H., Xiaoming, M., Zhang, H., Kuang, Y., Yang, M., Huang, Q., 2021. Carbon dots based on natural resources: synthesis and applications in sensors. Microchem. J. 0026265X. 160, 105604. doi:10.1016/j.microc.2020.105604.

Liu, S., Zeng, T.H., Hofmann, M., Burcombe, E., Wei, J., Jiang, R., Kong, J., Chen, Y., 2011. Antibacterial activity of graphite, graphite oxide, graphene oxide, and reduced graphene oxide: membrane and oxidative stress. ACS Nano. 1936086X. 5 (9), 6971–6980. doi:10.1021/nn202451x.

Liu, W.-Y., Zhang, C.-H., 2022. Bamboo-derived carbon composites for biodegradable facial cleansing masks. Mater. Sci. Eng. C 134, 112643.

Luo, C., Zhou, L., Chiou, K., Huang, J., 2018. Multifunctional graphene hair dye. Chem 24519294. 4 (4), 784–794. Available from: https://www.cell.com/chem/home. doi:10.1016/j.chempr.2018.02.021.

Macedo, T.M., Paulo, Í.S., Dusi, R.G., Magalhães, A.O., Ferreira, E.S., de Freitas Espeleta, A., Lucchese, A.M., 2025. Innovations in dermocosmetics: carbon dot applications on human skin. MRS Commun. 21596867. 15 (6), 1352–1361. Available from: https://www.springer.com/journal/43579. doi:10.1557/s43579-025-00808-8.

Mahmoudifard, M., Safi, M., 2012. Novel study of carbon nanotubes as UV absorbers for the modification of cotton fabric. J. Text. Inst. 17542340. 103 (8), 893–899. doi:10.1080/00405000.2011.622461.

Malini, K., Selvakumar, D., Kumar, N.S., 2023. Activated carbon from biomass: preparation, factors improving basicity and surface properties for enhanced CO_2 capture capacity – a review. J. CO2 Util. 22129820. 67, 102318. doi:10.1016/j.jcou.2022.102318.

Manikandan, N., Suresh, K.V.P., Siva, M.S., Rathis, G., Vishnu, S.K., Shabariganesh, T.K., 2021. Carbon nanotubes and their properties-The review. Mater. Today Proc. 22147853. 47, 4682–4685. https://www.sciencedirect.com/journal/materials-today-proceedings. doi:10.1016/j.matpr.2021.05.543.

Marseille, M., 2023. The prospect use of carbon dots in skin care. Accessed: Oct. 07, 2025. [Online]. Available from: https://scholarship.miami.edu/esploro/outputs/graduate/The-Prospect-Use-of-Carbon-Dots/991031825106102976.

Moon, J.Y., Ngoc, L.T.N., Chae, M., Tran, V.V., Lee, Y.C., 2020. Effects of microwave-assisted *Opuntia humifusa* extract in inhibiting the impacts of particulate matter on human keratinocyte skin cell. Antioxidants 20763921. 9 (4). Available from: https://www.mdpi.com/2076-3921/9/4/271/pdf. doi:10.3390/antiox9040271.

Mousavi, S.Z., Nafisi, S., Maibach, H.I., 2017. Fullerene nanoparticle in dermatological and cosmetic applications. Nanomedicine. 15499642. 13 (3), 1071–1087. doi:10.1016/j.nano.2016.10.002.

Murugan, B., Sagadevan, S., Moharana, S., 2024. Polymer-based carbon nanocomposite materials for cosmetic and packaging applications. Eng. Mater. 3404, 205–222. Available from: https://www.springer.com/series/4288. doi:10.1007/978-981-97-6329-0_9.

Negi, R., Pandey, A., Upadhye, V.J., Berdimurodov, E., Jain, B., Singh, S., 2025. Anti-aging properties and utilization of carbon quantum dots in cosmetics. In: Jayakumar, A., Sabarish, R., Kim, J.T., Parameswaranpillai, J. (Eds.), Carbon Quantum Dots from Natural Sources: Properties, Development, and Emerging Applications. CRC Press, Boca Raton, pp. 140–164. ISBN: 9781003437857. doi:10.1201/9781003437857-9.

Ngoc, L.T.N., Moon, J.Y., Lee, Y.C., 2023a. Antioxidants for improved skin appearance: intracellular mechanism, challenges and future strategies. Int. J. Cosmet. Sci. 14682494. 45 (3), 299–314. Available from: https://onlinelibrary.wiley.com/journal/10.1111/(ISSN)1468-2494. doi:10.1111/ics.12848.

Ngoc, L.T.N., Moon, J.Y., Lee, Y.C., 2023b. Plant extract-derived carbon dots as cosmetic ingredients. Nanomaterials 20794991. 13 (19). Available from: https://www.mdpi.com/journal/nanomaterials. doi:10.3390/nano13192654.

Nguyen, T.T.T., Nguyen, M.T.L., Nguyen, T.K.N., Huynh, H.T., Le, M.N., Le, P.H., 2024. Antibacterial and photoprotective activities of silver nanoparticles of lichen extract loaded in activated carbon. Lett. Appl. NanoBioSci. 22846808. 13 (1). Available from: https://nanobioletters.com/wp-content/uploads/2023/08/LIANBS131.011.pdf. doi:10.33263/LIANBS131.011.

Nuntahirun, P., Hanchaina, R., Ratchatacharoensak, A., Supjaroenpisan, M., Suptawornkul, S., Wang, Y., Kangsamaksin, T., Paoprasert, P., 2023. Development of carbon dots synthesized from green tea and alpha-hydroxyl acids with enhanced antioxidant activity, photostability and UV protection properties. ChemistrySelect 23656549. 8 (46). Available from: https://onlinelibrary.wiley.com/journal/10.1002/(ISSN)2365-6549. doi:10.1002/slct.202302541.

Olborska, A., Janas-Naze, A., Kaczmarek, Ł., Warga, T., Halin, D.S.C., 2020. Antibacterial effect of graphene and graphene oxide as a potential material for fiber finishes. Autex Res. J. 14709589. 20 (4), 506–516. Available from: https://www.degruyter.com/view/j/aut. doi:10.2478/aut-2020-0009.

Pan, X., Yu, R., Wu, J., Liang, J., Huang, W., Huang, R., Li, W., Xie, Y., Zhao, Y., Huang, Y., Wu, J., Xie, J., Chen, Z., Zhang, L., Wu, M., Fang, Y., Hu, R., Zhang, J., 2025. Two—Dimensional materials as antioxidants and sunscreen agents in cosmetics. Braz. J. Phys. 16784448. 55 (4). Available from: https://www.springer.com/journal/13538. doi:10.1007/s13538-025-01813-x.

Patarroyo, J.L., Cifuentes, J., Muñoz, L.N., Cruz, J.C., Reyes, L.H., 2022. Novel antibacterial hydrogels based on gelatin/polyvinyl-alcohol and graphene oxide/silver nanoconjugates: formulation, characterization, and preliminary biocompatibility evaluation. Heliyon 24058440. 8 (3). Available from: https://www.journals.elsevier.com/heliyon/. doi:10.1016/j.heliyon.2022.e09145.

Petric, D., 2021. Review of toxic chemicals in cosmetics. ScienceOpen. doi:10.14293/S2199-1006.1.SOR-.PPKO7OD.V1.

Priyadarsini, S., Mohanty, S., Mukherjee, S., Basu, S., Mishra, M., 2018. Graphene and graphene oxide as nanomaterials for medicine and biology application. J. Nanostruct. Chem. 21938865. 8 (2), 123–137. Available from: https://www.springer.com/journal/40097. doi:10.1007/s40097-018-0265-6.

Pulingam, T., Thong, K.L., Ali, M.E., Appaturi, J.N., Dinshaw, I.J., Ong, Z.Y., Leo, B.F., 2019. Graphene oxide exhibits differential mechanistic action towards Gram-positive and Gram-negative bacteria. Colloids Surf. B Biointerfaces 18734367. 181, 6–15. Available from: https://www.elsevier.com/locate/colsurfb. doi:10.1016/j.colsurfb.2019.05.023.

Purkait, T., Singh, G., Singh, M., Kumar, D., Dey, R.S., 2017. Large area few-layer graphene with scalable preparation from waste biomass for high-performance supercapacitor. Sci. Rep. 20452322. 7 (1). Available from: https://www.nature.com/srep/index.html. doi:10.1038/s41598-017-15463-w.

Qiu, Y., Wang, Z., Owens, A.C.E., Kulaots, I., Chen, Y., Kane, A.B., Hurt, R.H., 2014. Antioxidant chemistry of graphene-based materials and its role in oxidation protection technology. Nanoscale 20403372. 6 (20), 11744–11755. Available from: https://pubs.rsc.org/en/journals/journal/nr. doi:10.1039/c4nr03275f.

Qu, D., 2019. Antioxidant and anti-inflammatory properties of carbon dots for skincare applications. ACS Appl. Mater. Interfaces 11 (33), 30690–30699.

Rennhofer, H., Zanghellini, B., 2021. Dispersion state and damage of carbon nanotubes and carbon nanofibers by ultrasonic dispersion: a review. Nanomaterials 20794991. 11 (6). Available from: https://www.mdpi.com/2079-4991/11/6/1469/pdf. doi:10.3390/nano11061469.

Robles, R., Itzel, Y., Carrillo, Z., Valeria, V., Trinidad, S., 2024. 22nd LACCEI International Multi-Conference for Engineering, Education, and Technology: Sustainable Engineering for a Diverse, Equitable, and Inclusive Future at the Service of Education, Research, and Industry for a Society 5.0, 17–19 July 2024, San Jose, Csta Rica. pp. 1–9. doi:10.18687/LACCEI2024.1.1.324.

Salvioni, L., Morelli, L., Ochoa, E., Labra, M., Fiandra, L., Palugan, L., Prosperi, D., Colombo, M., 2021. The emerging role of nanotechnology in skincare. Adv. Colloid Interface Sci. 00018686. 293, 102437. doi:10.1016/j.cis.2021.102437.

Santos, A.C., Panchal, A., Rahman, N., Pereira-Silva, M., Pereira, I., Veiga, F., Lvov, Y., 2019. Evolution of hair treatment and care: prospects of nanotube-based formulations. Nanomaterials 20794991. 9 (6). Available from: https://www.mdpi.com/2079-4991/9/6/903/pdf. doi:10.3390/nano9060903.

Saravanan, A., Das, P., Maruthapandi, M., Aryal, S., Michaeli, S., Mastai, Y., Luong, J.H.T., Gedanken, A., 2024. Heteroatom co-doping (N, NS, NB) on carbon dots and their antibacterial and antioxidant properties. Surf. Interfaces. 24680230. 46, 103857. doi:10.1016/j.surfin.2024.103857.

Shams, S.S., Zhang, L.S., Hu, R., Zhang, R., Zhu, J., 2015. Synthesis of graphene from biomass: a green chemistry approach. Mater. Lett. 18734979. 161, 476–479. Available from: https://www.journals.elsevier.com/materials-letters/. doi:10.1016/j.matlet.2015.09.022.

Singh, A., 2021. Carbon Nanofiber in Cosmetics Carbon Nanofibers: Fundamentals and Applications. Wiley, India, pp. 341–363. Available from: https://onlinelibrary.wiley.com/doi/book/10.1002/9781119769149. doi:10.1002/9781119769149.ch14.

Singh, S.K., Prakash, H., Akhtar, M.J., Kar, K.K., 2018. Lightweight and high-performance microwave absorbing heteroatom-doped carbon derived from chicken feather fibers. ACS Sustain. Chem. Eng. 21680485. 6 (4), 5381–5393. Available from: https://pubs.acs.org/journal/ascecg. doi:10.1021/acssuschemeng.8b00183.

Sinha, P., Banerjee, S., Kar, K.K., 2020. Characteristics of activated carbon. Springer Ser. Mater. Sci. 300, 125–154. Available from: https://www.springer.com/series/856?changeHeader. doi:10.1007/978-3-030-43009-2_4.

Son, M.H., Park, S.W., Jung, Y.K., 2021. Antioxidant and anti-aging carbon quantum dots using tannic acid. Nanotechnology 13616528. 32 (41). Available from: https://iopscience.iop.org/article/10.1088/1361-6528/ac027b. doi:10.1088/1361-6528/ac027b.

Stan, C.S., Ania, M.C.C., 2022. Carbon nanomaterials as solar UV protectors targeting applications ranging from paints/varnishes to pharma/cosmetic products. LE STUDIUM Multidiscip. J. 6 (6), 27–33. doi:10.34846/LE-STUDIUM.237.01.FR.04-2022.

Sudha, P.N., Sangeetha, K., Vijayalakshmi, K., Barhoum, A., 2018. Nanomaterials history, classification, unique properties, production and market. In: Barhoum, A., Makhlouf, A.S.H. (Eds.), Emerging Applications of Nanoparticles and Architectural Nanostructures: Current Prospects and Future Trends. Elsevier Inc., India, pp. 341–384. Available from: https://www.sciencedirect.com/science/book/9780323512541. doi:10.1016/B978-0-323-51254-1.00012-9.

Sun, L., Tian, C., Li, M., Meng, X., Wang, L., Wang, R., Yin, J., Fu, H., 2013. From coconut shell to porous graphene -like nanosheets for high-power supercapacitors. J. Mater. Chem. A Accessed: Oct. 07, 2025. [Online]. Available from: https://pubs.rsc.org/en/content/articlehtml/2013/ta/c3ta10897j. doi:10.1039/C3TA10897J.

Swapna, M.S., Beryl, C., Reshma, S.S., Chandran, V., Vishnu, V.S., Radhamany, P.M., Sankararaman, S., 2017. Ultraviolet protection action of carbon nanoparticles in leaves. BioNanoScience 21911649. 7 (4), 583–587. Available from: https://www.springerlink.com/content/2191-1630. doi:10.1007/s12668-017-0454-7.

Syarif, F.H., Alma'sum, N.R., Saputra, R.P., Ratiani, S.I., Rizkita, A.D., 2023. Review of green synthesis: activated charcoal to reduce sebum levels in oily facial skin. Proceeding International Conference on Religion, Science and Education, Vol. 2, pp. 605–609. Accessed: Oct. 07, 2025. [Online]. Available from: https://sunankalijaga.org/prosiding/index.php/icrse/article/view/971.

Wang, H., Sun, S., Zhao, Y., Wang, P., Zhou, Y., Sun, H., Yang, J., Cheng, K., Li, S., Lin, H., 2024. Carbon dots with integrated photothermal antibacterial and heat-enhanced antioxidant properties for diabetic wound healing. Small 16136829. 20 (45). Available from: https://onlinelibrary.wiley.com/journal/10.1002/(ISSN)1613-6829. doi:10.1002/smll.202403160.

Yin, Q., Li, X., Yong, X., Sha, P., Zhang, Q., Dong, H., Sui, J., Jianhua, Y., Liyan, Y., Dong, L., 2023. An environmentally friendly process to derive N/O/S-codoped porous carbon from biomass waste with high yield for high performance supercapacitor. Diam. Relat. Mater. 09259635. 134, 109798. doi:10.1016/j.diamond.2023.109798.

Zaib, M., Arshad, A., Khalid, S., Shahzadi, T., 2023. One pot ultrasonic plant mediated green synthesis of carbon dots and their application invisible light induced dye photocatalytic studies: a kinetic approach. Int. J. Environ. Anal. Chem. 10290397. 103 (17), 5063–5081. Available from: https://www.tandf.co.uk/journals/titles/03067319.asp. doi:10.1080/03067319.2021.1934463.

Zhou, H., Luo, D., Chen, D., Tan, X., Bai, X., Liu, Z., Yang, X., Liu, W., 2021. Current advances of nanocarrier technology-based active cosmetic ingredients for beauty applications. Clin. Cosmet. Investig. Dermatol. 11787015. 14, 867–887. Available from: https://www.dovepress.com/getfile.php?fileID=71642. doi:10.2147/CCID.S313429.

Zhou, H., Zhang, J., Amiinu, I.S., Zhang, C., Liu, X., Tu, W., Pan, M., Mu, S., 2016. Transforming waste biomass with an intrinsically porous network structure into porous nitrogen-doped graphene for highly efficient oxygen reduction. Phys. Chem. Chem. Phys. Accessed: Oct. 07, 2025. [Online]. Available from: https://pubs.rsc.org/en/content/articlehtml/2016/cp/c6cp00174b. doi:10.1039/C6CP00174B.

Zhou, Y., Jiajun, H., Chen, R., Xiaodong, L., 2022. Recent advances in biomass-derived graphene and carbon nanotubes. Mater. Today Sustain. 25892347. 18, 100138. doi:10.1016/j.mtsust.2022.100138.

Section VI

Natural bioactives for environmentally friendly cosmetic and nutricosmetic packaging

Chapter 27

Utilization of biodegradable and environmentally friendly natural bioactives for cosmetic and nutricosmetic packaging

Ioanna Koumentakou, Alexandros Tsoupras, and George Z. Kyzas
Hephaestus Laboratory, School of Chemistry, Faculty of Sciences, Democritus University of Thrace, Kavala University Campus, Kavala, Greece

1 Introduction

The cosmetics market has presented a significant economic impact in recent years and is expected to increase further in the next few years, which is attributed to the development of new, innovative, and effective formulations (Grădinaru et al., 2022). The increase in population and the global encouragement of self-care and self-control have led to a rise in the consumption of cosmetic products among women and men. A study indicated that the German cosmetic market is expected to generate EUR 33.4 billion in sales, an 8.4% rise over 2022. A Chinese report showed that men's cosmetic products have proliferated by nearly 3000%, increasing by 30% in 2020. Moreover, the global cosmetics market was worth roughly USD 507.8 billion by 2018 and is expected to reach USD 758.4 billion by 2025 (Packaging waste statistics—Statistics Explained—Eurostat, n.d.).

Beyond the economic impact, in recent years, particular importance has been given to the environmental impact of increased cosmetic product consumption. The Worldwide Fund for Nature presented an article stating that human activity is depleting natural resources more quickly than nature can regenerate, and people's decisions today will define the chances of our next generation (Swetha et al., 2023). It is necessary to develop sustainability to guarantee sufficient resources for the survival of future generations. In this scenario, the continuous growth of the cosmetic industry and its high consumption of natural resources represent a major field requiring a long-term vision to manage sustainability, covering a product's whole lifecycle and, consequently, all supply chain participants (Defruyt and Sander, 2019).

The beauty and cosmetic industry uses enormous amounts of packaging and mostly depends on esthetic appeal and sensory experience to draw clients. By 2028, this field's revenue is expected to reach USD 129 billion (Swetha et al., 2023), indicating its importance and impact. Packaging is crucial in cosmetic products because it confines and safeguards products and guarantees their durability, quality, and safety (Marano et al., 2022). Plastic packages are the most commonly used in cosmetic products because they are inexpensive, lightweight, long-lasting, and efficiently shield products from gases and moisture. However, it is the most critical environmental pollutant in the cosmetic sector. Only around 2% of plastic packaging is recycled back into new packaging materials, is synthesized using fossil fuels, and does not biodegrade (Sylvester, 2024). Most of it ends up in the environment or landfills, where it may linger for hundreds of years (Revenue of the cosmetics industry worldwide| Statista, n.d.). It was noted that the European Union generated a staggering 79.3 million tons of rubbish in 2020, with each person producing 177.2 kg of packaging waste.

In this path, eco-friendly initiatives are indirectly supported by high-quality packaging. To support Sustainable Development Goal 12 of the UN, which promotes responsible consumption and production, the global scientific community, designers, and manufacturers focus on developing more ecologically friendly packaging materials. Nowadays, customers are more drawn to companies that use ethical business practices and have a green-sustainable vision, resulting in natural ingredient items and eco-friendly packaging becoming more popular (Amberg and Fogarassy, 2019). To meet these requirements, numerous cosmetic companies are incorporating recyclable, reusable, or biodegradable materials into their packaging lines (Table 27.1) (Versino et al., 2023).

Biofunctional Cosmetics for Health. https://doi.org/10.1016/B978-0-443-27500-5.00027-7

TABLE 27.1 Cosmetic companies that use sustainable packaging.

Cosmetic company	Sustainable packaging
L'Oréal	Paper/cardboard, reduce by 20% the intensity of the quantity of packaging used for products.
Caudalie	Collect and recycle the same amount of plastic they use yearly from beaches.
la Roche-Poche	Paper tube and a significantly smaller cap for tube products, reducing the use of plastic.
Avène	93% of packaging is recyclable.
Estée Lauder	High content of postconsumer recycled materials is used for their bottles.
Origins	Use of 30% recycled material and cardboard in its packaging.
Kjaer weis	Refillable metal palettes, sustainable shipping materials, compostable/recyclable packaging elements.
Bioten	All face cream boxes are certified by the FSC, the Forest Stewardship Council, and are made of paper.
Riman Korea	New packaging made with naturally derived materials: polylactic acid (PLA)-polyhydroxyalkanoate (PHA) composite.
CJ Olive Young	Uses eco-friendly packaging made from an amorphous PHA/PLA blend.

Nevertheless, conventional recycling of cosmetic packaging is challenging because cosmetic formulations frequently leave greasy or sticky residues within containers. On the contrary, the reusability of packaging poses risks due to the growth of microorganisms and the stability of the packaging material, casting doubt on the quality of the product and the safety of the end consumer. As a result, research on new biodegradable materials is gaining popularity, and environmentally friendly cosmetic packages are being developed (Saha et al., 2020).

Therefore the present literature review analyzes the state-of-the-art methods for producing new biodegradable materials used in the cosmetic sector, delving deeper into their properties, environmental performance, risks, and potential to replace traditional plastics.

2 Characteristics of packaging for cosmetic products

Cosmetic packaging mostly depends on esthetic appeal and promotion to draw clients. However, their primary role is to safeguard the safety and quality of the formulation and provide stability over its shelf life, as environmental conditions significantly impact cosmetic products' stability, efficacy, and appearance (Cinelli et al., 2019). Therefore compatibility, barrier qualities, safety regulations, and esthetic concerns must all be considered when choosing packaging materials. One of the most critical factors in cosmetic packaging is the material's barrier performance, or its capacity to stop or reduce the flow of light, moisture, and gases and to withstand chemical reactions with the product. Many cosmetic formulations include complex mixes of active chemicals, natural extracts, oils, and perfumes, which are sensitive to changes in temperature, light (remarkably UV light), oxygen, and water vapor (Del Greco et al., 2024). These may lead to microbial contamination, color changes, hydrolysis, or oxidative deterioration. In the literature, some standard critical thresholds regarding cosmetic packaging requirements to avoid the above alterations (Table 27.2) are referenced.

However, beyond the usual critical thresholds, each cosmetic product has unique packaging requirements based on its distribution conditions, intended use, and formulation properties (A Text Book of Pharmaceutics for I Year Diploma in Pharmacy—Βιβλία Google, 2024). The stability and functionality of the packed product can be affected by several variables, including closure methods, color additives, resin formulation, and container composition. Therefore thorough stability tests must be conducted to assess interactions between the formulation and the packaging under various environmental conditions. Some of its phases include conceptual planning, material selection, prototype, validation, and ongoing quality control (Jenita et al., 2025). In addition to providing convenience without sacrificing integrity, packaging needs to be sturdy enough to safeguard the product during handling, storage, and distribution (The Science and Technology of Flexible Packaging: Multilayer Films from—Barry A. Morris—Βιβλία Google, n.d.). Systems like breakable caps, shrink bands, or sealed closures that let customers spot tampering are essential deterrents against fraud and contamination.

As the packaging sector develops further, the cosmetic industry must balance ensuring product safety with achieving sustainability goals, especially with the emergence of eco-conscious design principles (Rosette et al., 2012).

TABLE 27.2 Standard critical thresholds regarding cosmetic packaging requirements.

Environmental factor	Typical critical thresholds/exposure limits	Main degradation effects on cosmetics	References
Oxygen (O_2)	Sensitive above 0.1%–1% O_2 inside container; oxidation rate doubles with every 10°C increase	Oxidation of oils, vitamins (A, C, E), and pigments, leading to color change, rancidity, and efficacy loss	(Swetha et al., 2023; Dayan and Kromidas, 2011; Jacobsen et al., 2017)
Water vapor (H_2O)	Deterioration when moisture absorption >3%–5%, WVTR > 5 $g/m^2 \cdot$ day destabilizes emulsions	Phase separation, viscosity change, microbial growth	(Resimović et al., 2022; Saha et al., 2020)
Ultraviolet (UV) and visible light	Exposure to 280–400 nm UV for >10–20 h causes measurable degradation	Photodegradation of natural extracts and essential oils, fragrance instability	(Cinelli et al., 2019; Dayan and Kromidas, 2011)
Temperature variations	Degradation above 40°C or below 5°C, shelf life halves per 10°C rise	Oxidation, melting, viscosity loss, microbial growth	(Packaging waste statistics—Statistics Explained—Eurostat, n.d.; Garba and Garba, 2023)
Migration between product and packaging	Migration limits < 10 mg/dm^2 (EU Regulation No. 10/2011)	Contamination with plasticizers or monomers, absorption of oils into packaging walls	(Versino et al., 2023; Del Greco et al., 2024)

3 Biodegradable plastic for cosmetic packaging

The cosmetic packaging, long dependent on petroleum-derived polymers, is seeking sustainable alternatives that meet both product performance standards and environmental objectives (Cinelli et al., 2019). In response to these constraints, modified biobased and biodegradable polymers have emerged. These innovative polymers combine mechanical strength, chemical resistance, and biodegradability to protect sensitive beauty formulations. The most commonly used biopolymers for cosmetic packaging are polylactic acid (PLA), polyhydroxyalkanoates (PHAs), and polysaccharide-based materials such as cellulose, starch, and chitosan derivatives. These materials can be used for both rigid and flexible packaging applications and provide versatility for various cosmetic products (Dayan and Kromidas, 2011). Common cosmetics-based plastics include PLA, biopolyethylene, and biopolyethylene terephthalate.

Because they are derived from renewable resources like plant oils, sugarcane, or maize starch, they function comparably to their conventional equivalents while reducing dependency on fossil fuels. The cosmetics sector already uses these polymers to package liquid formulations, lipsticks, lotions, and creams (Mifsud et al., 2023).

However, cosmetic packaging has specific technological requirements because of cosmetic items' inherent qualities. Formulations frequently contain natural oils, volatile chemicals, and reactive substances that are susceptible to temperature, light, and oxygen. To protect the cosmetic formulation from external factors, the manufacturing industry incorporates additives into biobased packaging materials (Kumar and Gupta, 2012). For instance, UV-light stabilizers are especially crucial for transparent or translucent packaging since they shield the product from photoactivated deterioration. In addition, processing aids, catalysts, and antioxidants have been added to improve the packaging material's processability and long-term stability. Pigments and colors can also be added to enhance visual appeal (Gabor and Tita, 2012).

Another key consideration in cosmetic packaging is plasticizers, which improve flexibility and ductility in bioplastic materials. However, their selection must be carefully made to minimize oxygen and water vapor transmission between the product and its container. The migration of additives or other chemical components from the packaging to the product can alter the formulation's chemistry, reduce its effectiveness, and affect its quality (Drobac et al., 2020). Conversely, the diffusion of product components into the packaging can weaken the material's mechanical resistance and durability. This two-way migration poses challenges for ensuring both product integrity and packaging lifespan (Santos et al., 2025).

The growing global demand for bioplastic packaging reflects the cosmetic industry's commitment to reducing its environmental footprint. Biodegradable and compostable polymers offer distinct advantages over conventional petroleum-based plastics, which lack recyclability and persist in the environment for centuries. Biopolymer-based packaging, on the contrary, can contribute to a circular economy, as these materials are designed to return safely to nature through composting or biodegradation (Cinelli et al., 2019).

3.1 Polylactic acid

PLA is one of the most popular polymers for packaging, including in the cosmetics industry, with 140,000 tons of global PLA production per year, because it is made from renewable resources and is a biodegradable polymer. PLA, as a viable alternative to petrochemical-based polymers, will help reduce environmental problems. PLA exhibits competitive mechanical properties, good heat stability, biocompatibility, high processability, and a renewable origin, making it a desirable substitute for polymers derived from petroleum (Bikiaris et al., 2023). In addition, the production process of PLA offers several benefits compared to other biopolymers. First, the lactide monomer is synthesized from lactic acid, which is obtained through the fermentation of renewable resources such as corn, cassava starch, and potato. Furthermore, the production and use of PLA save energy, reduce the volume of landfills, enable the fabrication of compostable hybrid paper-plastic packaging, and allow for modification with other materials to optimize physical properties. D-Lactic acid and L-lactic acid are two optical isomers of lactic acid that are commonly used in the manufacturing industry to produce PLA with different properties (Fig. 27.1). A homopolymer of poly(L-lactic acid) and a copolymer of poly(D, L-lactic acid) are the two most common industrial forms of PLA (Balla et al., 2021).

Because PLA is a thermoplastic polymer, it can be produced using standard plastic manufacturing methods like injection molding, blow molding, extrusion, and thermoforming. It softens when heated and hardens when cooled. Depending on its crystallinity, PLA can be either amorphous or semicrystalline; the latter has better mechanical strength and stiffness (Koumentakou et al., 2024). Semicrystalline PLA usually has an elongation at break of around 4%, a tensile modulus of about 3 GPa, and a tensile strength of between 50 and 70 MPa. Its melting temperature (T_m) is between 150°C and 180°C, its glass transition temperature (T_g) is between 50°C and 60°C, and its crystallization temperature (T_c) is between 90°C and 140°C. Because of its mechanical and thermal properties, PLA is especially well-suited for rigid cosmetic containers, including bottles, pots, and jars (Balla et al., 2021).

However, the main drawbacks of PLA are its brittleness and slow crystallization rate, which can cause deformation or decreased stability, particularly when heated (Cojocaru et al., 2022). To overcome these limitations, the research community focuses on PLA modification using physical or chemical methods to improve the material's characteristics, such as its fundamental mechanical and thermal characteristics, and to function as an antibacterial and antioxidant (De et al., 2015). Common PLA modification techniques include adding nucleation agents, thermal annealing treatment, and blending treatment. To reduce PLA's high cost, one of the various modification techniques is material blending with less expensive materials (Yang et al., 2015). In addition, using eco-friendly materials for PLA co-blending modification is a practical way to preserve the benefits of PLA degradability (Tang et al., 2020). Graphene and reduced graphene oxide have also been used as fillers in PLA matrices at different concentrations to manufacture nanocomposite films with enhanced barrier qualities and strong mechanical resistance (Ivanov et al., 2019). Furthermore, it has been demonstrated that the aromatic rings of lignin nanoparticles enhance PLA's mechanical and thermal characteristics. Particularly in the case of PLA, the performance of the finished PLA nanocomposite packaging products can be enhanced by the lignin nanoparticles' antibacterial and antioxidant properties, as well as their UV protection and reduced water sorption capacity (Cavallo et al., 2021).

In a similar way, PLA has been mixed with other polymers, such as poly(butylene adipate-co-terephthalate) (PBAT), to improve its toughness and elasticity, resulting in materials more suited for applications requiring greater flexibility (Ding et al., 2018). Nowadays, PLA has also been reinforced with biobased ingredients, such as cellulose nanofibers and cellulose nanocrystals, to produce green nanocomposites with enhanced mechanical, thermomechanical, and barrier properties. It has been reported that nanocellulose–PLA films can be voluntarily recycled and reprocessed into packaging films without undergoing substantial quality changes (Ahankari et al., 2021).

In addition, nanoclays have been incorporated into the PLA matrix via different techniques like solvent casting, melt blending, and in situ polymerization to improve the properties of PLA. The most widely used clays to produce PLA nanocomposite packages are organic montmorillonite (MMT), bentonite, and halloysite nanotubes (HNTs) (Jawaid et al., n.d.).

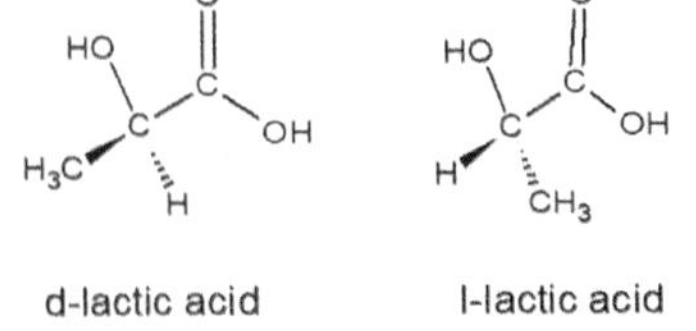

FIG. 27.1 Lactic acid stereoisomers. *(Data from Tümer, E.H., Erbil, H.Y., 2021. Extrusion-based 3D printing applications of PLA composites: a review. Coatings 11 (4), 390. doi:10.3390/COATINGS11040390.)*

It has been noted that PLA reinforced with nanoclays presents enhanced mechanical and thermal properties, improved barrier performance, and accelerated biodegradation. However, a small amount of nanoclays needs to be added to the PLA packaging materials to improve mechanical properties due to the incompatibility between the hydrophobic PLA polymer matrix and the hydrophilic nanoclays (Jawaid et al., n.d.). Another key requirement for cosmetic packaging is maintaining high barrier properties against oxygen, water vapor, and ultraviolet (UV) light. PLA naturally provides a better UV barrier than low-density polyethylene (Oliver-Ortega et al., 2021; Bala et al., 2022). Still, its gas and moisture barrier performance can be further improved by incorporating inorganic fillers such as layered silicates or MMT. Even at low concentrations (1–5 wt%), these nanoclays can significantly enhance the overall mechanical and barrier properties by creating a more tortuous path for gas diffusion (Bikiaris et al., 2023). The degree of improvement depends on the dispersion and compatibility of the clay within the polymer matrix. The FP7 BioBeauty Project in Europe investigated the potential of PLA–nanoclay nanocomposites for use in cosmetics. Extrusion and injection molding were used to fabricate tubes and pots, and the materials' cytotoxicity and cutaneous safety were assessed (Connolly et al., 2019). The findings confirmed the safety of non-organophilic clays (such as sodium-based clays) for cosmetic applications by showing that they were biocompatible and did not have mutagenic consequences (Akshaykranth et al., 2025). Cosmetic formulations packed in PLA nanocomposites showed stability for up to 20 days, according to studies of accelerated oxidation, which varied depending on the thickness and nanoclay content of the PLA-based packaging (Oliver-Ortega et al., 2021).

For high-temperature uses, such as hot liquid filling, PLA and polycarbonate (PC) blends have shown increased thermal and mechanical resistance above the PLA glass transition temperature. The toughness and elastic modulus of these blends can be further increased by reinforcing them with cellulose acetate or cellulosic fibers. Depending on the level of cellulose acetylation, PLA/cellulose acetate blends provide a completely biodegradable substitute for PLA/PC composites, which are only partially biodegradable due to the presence of PC. Recent developments in PLA reinforced with plasticized cellulose acetate have shown great promise for rigid cosmetic packaging by exhibiting increased toughness while retaining a high Young's modulus (Gigante et al., 2022).

Despite its advantages, PLA is prone to hydrolytic degradation, especially in the presence of moisture, oils, or ethanol, common components in cosmetic formulations. The molecular weight of PLA and its mechanical integrity rapidly decline when hydrolysis breaks down its ester linkages (Elsawy et al., 2017). Studies have shown that exposure to formulations, including water or alcohol can accelerate hydrolysis, which may impact the packaged product's shelf life. Although PLA maintains enough stability for the majority of cosmetic applications, to improve PLA's long-term endurance, researchers have considered coating it with barrier layers that are resistant to moisture or mixing it with hydrophobic substances (Tripathi et al., 2021). For instance, biodegradable nanocomposites were prepared by incorporating modified nanocellulose fibers into the PLA matrix and then applied to the paper surface via a cast-coating process, reducing the water vapor transmission rate (WVTR) of paper (Song et al., 2014).

Metal oxides have also been used as additive agents to improve the thermal stability, toughness, optical properties, tensile strength, etc., of PLA packaging, while also imparting antimicrobial and antiviral activities (Mulla et al., 2021). Among them, TiO_2 and ZnO metal oxides are the most widely used to fabricate PLA-based packages with antimicrobial capacity against a wide range of microorganisms, such as *Escherichia coli*, *Pseudomonas aeruginosa*, and *Staphylococcus aureus* (Ghozali et al., 2020). PLA-based packaging firmly addresses the cosmetics sector's sustainability objectives. Strong mechanical performance, biodegradability, and renewable sourcing are combined with the possibility of plasticization, mixing, and nanocomposite reinforcement modification (Biswal, 2024). PLA is one of the most promising biobased materials for next-generation green cosmetic packaging, balancing environmental responsibility, safety, and functionality, with further study needed to enhance its toughness, barrier performance, and hydrolytic resistance.

4 Polyhydroxyalkanoates

Among biodegradable polymers, PHAs attract interest because of their promising qualities, including excellent biodegradability in different environments, not just in composting plants, and versatility. PHAs can, in fact, be prepared and processed for use in a wide range of products, such as films, adhesives, packaging, molded goods, paper coatings, nonwoven textiles, and performance additives (Bugnicourt et al., 2014). PHA polymers are naturally formed by microorganisms during biomass growth. The most common and well-characterized member of the PHAs family is poly(3-hydroxybutyrate) (PHB), a homopolymer of 3-hydroxybutyrate (Fig. 27.2).

PHAs are biodegradable thermoplastics that have emerged as a promising alternative to fossil-based plastics for packaging, driven by EU directives that require all plastic packaging to be reusable or recyclable by 2030. Commercially available copolymers of hydroxybutyrate and hydroxyvalerate, such as poly(β-hydroxybutyrate-co-β-hydroxyvalerate) (PHBV),

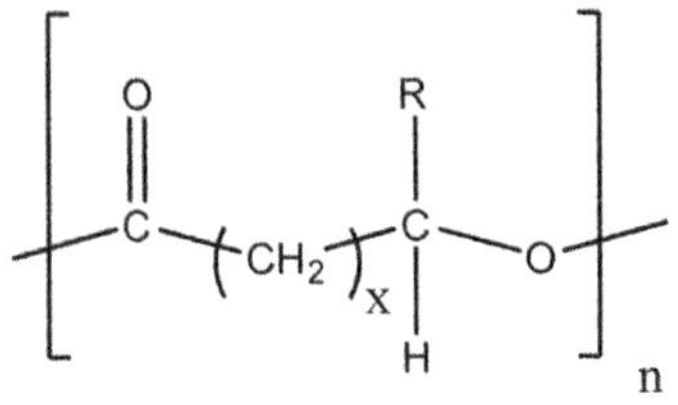

FIG. 27.2 A monomeric unit of polyhydroxyalkanoate. *(Data from Cinelli, P., Coltelli, M.B., Signori, F., Morganti, P., Lazzeri, A., 2019. Cosmetic packaging to save the environment: future perspectives. Cosmetics. 20799284. 6 (2). Available from https://res.mdpi.com/cosmetics/cosmetics-06-00026/article_deploy/cosmetics-06-00026.pdf?filename=&attachment=1. https://doi.org/10.3390/COSMETICS6020026.)*

have good mechanical and thermoplastic qualities comparable to polypropylene (PP). PHB is utilized in flexible intermediate bulk containers and bulk shrink packaging for food packaging (Jabeen et al., 2015). Although PHAs offer inherent biodegradability, their high production cost—up to 300× that of PP—and limited mechanical performance hinder large-scale adoption. Reinforcing PHAs with natural vegetal fiber fillers (cellulose, hemicellulose, lignin) can lower material costs, improve stiffness, and tailor barrier properties. The fiber composition dictates interfacial adhesion (Cazón et al., 2020). For instance, cellulose provides high strength but is hydrophobic, while hemicellulose is hydrophilic and reduces adhesion. Pretreatments such as mechanical grinding, enzymatic cleaning, alkaline washing, or plasma exposure modify fiber surface chemistry, enhancing fiber-matrix bonding and stress transfer. Mechanical tests showed that adding ≤30 wt% fibers raises Young's modulus from 10 to 24,000 MPa, yet elongation at break often drops below 7 % due to reduced matrix ductility. Tensile strength typically remains close to the neat polymer, with optimal values around 20–30 MPa. However, excessive fiber loading (>30 wt%) creates agglomerates acting as stress concentrators with lower strength. Incorporating plasticizers into the PHAs matrix reduces Young's modulus (Muthuraj et al., 2017). In a composite of PHBV/thermoplastic polyurethane–cellulose, where three different additives were used, the compatibilization between fiber and matrix was enhanced, and the viscosity of the films increased, but Young's modulus decreased compared with the PHBV controls (Sánchez-Safont et al., 2018). Adding ZnO nanoparticles to PHB and PHBV improved the biopolymers' vapor barrier capacity and increased their crystallinity, thermal stability, Young's modulus, tensile strength, and impact strength. In addition, both Gram-positive and Gram-negative bacteria were susceptible to their antibacterial action. It was also found that the migration levels of the composites in polar and nonpolar simulants were within the bounds of current packaging material regulations (Díez-Pascual, 2017). Bruzaud and Bourmaud studied solution-cast combinations of PHBV and an organically modified MMT (OMMT) at loadings of 1%, 2.5%, and 5%, the usual range where the advantages of adding nanofillers are expected. In this experiment, elongation at break dropped while tensile strength and modulus increased as the OMMT level increased (Bruzaud and Bourmaud, 2007).

PHAs are more favorable than PLA for application in contact with skin because of certain features, such as their incredibly high biocompatibility (Chen et al., 2014) and reduced greenhouse gas emissions (Yu and Chen, 2008), even if PLA is now less expensive and produced on a larger scale. Moreover, PHAs are also highly biodegradable, as they can be broken down by a variety of aerobic and anaerobic microorganisms, including bacteria, cyanobacteria, and fungi, in a variety of settings, including soil, fresh water, industrial and residential compost, and marine ecosystems, both as raw materials (Deroiné et al., 2014) and as a polymeric matrix in biocomposites (Seggiani et al., 2018). Because of these characteristics, PHA-based materials are promising for cosmetic packaging applications.

5 Polysaccharides

The most common polysaccharides in cosmetic packaging are by-products of starch and cellulose. Furthermore, because of their antibacterial qualities, chitosan and chitin have lately been used as active packaging. Packaging materials based on polysaccharides must be inexpensive, readily available, and provide certain functional or particular qualities. Polysaccharide-based biodegradable packaging products are well known for effectively blocking the flow of gases like CO_2 and O_2. The great gas barrier qualities are crucial for preventing solvent penetration in formulations that could lead to toxicity or quality loss, or for delaying the loss of organic vapors (aroma compounds) during storage.

6 Cellulose

Cellulose is the most abundant renewable polymer on Earth and has been extensively utilized as a raw material for developing biodegradable cosmetic packaging products. Its popularity stems from its chemical stability, nontoxicity, low cost, renewability, and biocompatibility, all of which make it an ideal candidate for sustainable packaging, including cosmetic

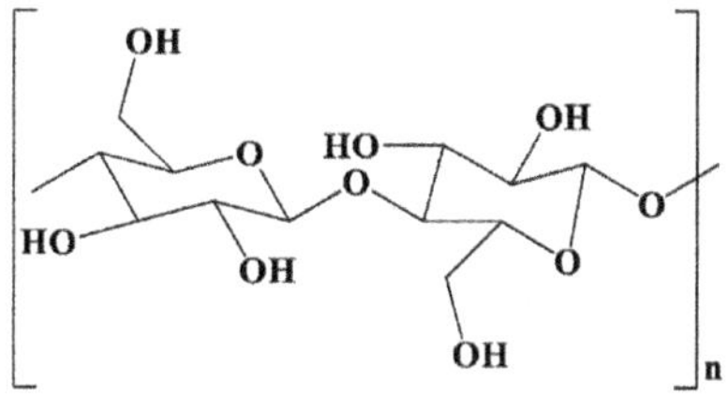

FIG. 27.3 Structure of cellulose. *(Data from Aziz, T., Farid, A., Haq, F., Kiran, M., Ullah, A., Zhang, K., Li, C., Ghazanfar, S., Sun, H., Ullah, R., Ali, A., Muzammal, M., Shah, M., Akhtar, N., Selim, S., Hagagy, N., Samy, M., Jaouni, S.K.A., 2022. A review on the modification of cellulose and its applications. Polymers. 20734360. 14 (15). Available from https://www.mdpi.com/journal/polymers. doi:10.3390/polym14153206.)*

applications (Liu et al., 2021). Cellulose can be extracted from various plant-based sources, such as wood, cotton, hemp, and agricultural residues, as well as from microbial and marine organisms like bacteria and tunicates (Sirviö et al., 2013).

Structurally, cellulose is a linear polysaccharide consisting of repeating units of anhydroglucose ($(C_6H_{10}O_5)n$) linked by β(1→4) glycosidic bonds (Fig. 27.3). The number of glucose units per chain varies depending on the source (Thakur, 2014). Because of its extensive network of intra- and intermolecular hydrogen bonds, cellulose exhibits high crystallinity and poor solubility in most solvents, especially polar ones, such as water.

Several methods have been studied to dissolve cellulose to make preparing biodegradable films or polymers for packaging cosmetics easier. Among these are ionic liquids, LiCl/*N,N*-dimethylacetamide, alkali/urea systems, molten inorganic salt hydrates (such as $ZnCl_2 \cdot 4H_2O$, $LiI \cdot 2H_2O$, and LiBr), tetra-butylammonium fluoride/dimethyl sulfoxide combinations, and NaOH/thiourea solutions (Lindman et al., 2010; Wang et al., 2016). Aqueous transition metal complexes with nitrous ligands are used in more advanced dissolution techniques because they may efficiently break hydrogen bonds and encourage cellulose solvation before film formation.

In addition to its structural and chemical benefits, cellulose has great organoleptic and sensory qualities, such as color, odor, and taste neutrality, which make it ideal for materials that come into contact with cosmetics.

Moreover, cellulose is lightweight and, unlike heavier synthetic polymers, helps reduce packaging waste. Furthermore, notable barrier qualities of cellulose-based films also reduce the movement of gases, moisture, lipids, and solutes, increasing product shelf life and maintaining quality (Wang et al., 2020). According to a study by Wang et al., multilayer cellulose structures achieved enhanced resistance and water repellency while increasing tensile strength by up to four times. The prepared films showed a 93% reduction in WVTR and a contact angle of 113 degrees, indicating strong hydrophobic behavior (Wang et al., 2021).

Despite being biodegradable and renewable, pure cellulose films frequently exhibit brittleness and a high sensitivity to moisture. By adding proteins to cellulose matrices, the hydroxyl groups of cellulose and the amino or carboxyl groups of proteins form intermolecular hydrogen bonds, strengthening the film's structure and enhancing its tensile strength, elasticity, and moisture-repellent qualities. For example, adding soy protein isolate to cellulose resulted in a roughly 35% increase in tensile strength and a nearly 25% decrease in water vapor permeability, suggesting improved mechanical and barrier performance (Xiao et al., 2021). Similarly, the preparation of a dense, three-dimensional polymeric network in gelatin-cellulose nanofiber composites has demonstrated improved moisture resistance and thermal stability (Leite et al., 2024).

Furthermore, cellulose can be functionalized through blending with metal nanoparticles such as silver (Ag), copper (Cu), titanium dioxide (TiO_2), and zinc oxide (ZnO). The resulting nanocomposites exhibit strong antimicrobial and antioxidant properties, which are essential for active packaging systems that inhibit microbial growth and prolong product shelf life (Cazón and Vázquez, 2021). The nanoparticles disrupt microbial membranes, generate reactive oxygen species, and interfere with enzymatic activity.

However, the direct incorporation of nanoparticles raises safety concerns due to the potential migration of metal ions into packaged products, which can lead to risks of bioaccumulation or toxicity.

7 Starch

Starch is one of the most commonly used natural biopolymers for sustainable and cosmetic packaging due to its capacity to form films, biodegradability, and renewable nature (Fig. 27.4) (Gabor and Tita, 2012). Glucose monomers are organized into two structurally different polysaccharides, amylose and amylopectin, to form starch, which is widely available from a variety of botanical sources such as wheat, maize, potatoes, rice, and legumes (Wróblewska-Krepsztul et al., 2018). Depending on the source of the starch, the ratio of these two components changes, which affects the material's mechanical performance, water sensitivity, and crystallinity (Pokhrel, 2015).

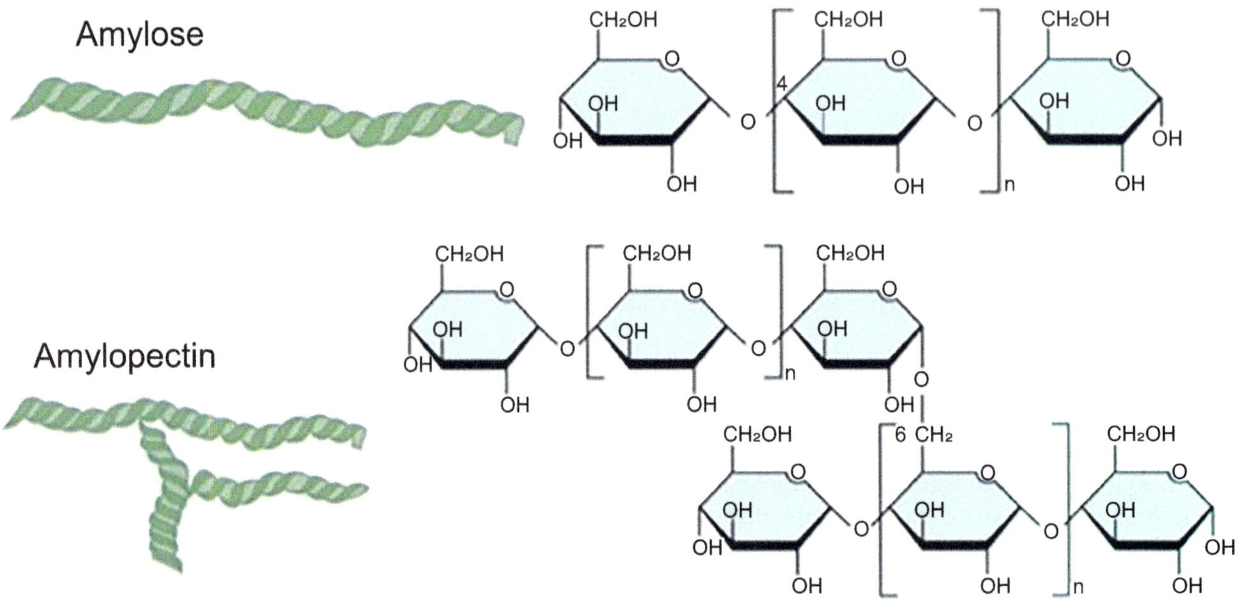

FIG. 27.4 Chemical illustration of starch structure. *(Data from Pedreiro, S., Figueirinha, A., Silva, A.S., Ramos, F., 2021. Bioactive edible films and coatings based in gums and starch: phenolic enrichment and foods application. Coatings 11 (11), 1393. doi:10.3390/COATINGS11111393.)*

Since starch is a biopolymer, it satisfies many of the basic requirements for environmentally friendly packaging materials, including being nontoxic, renewable, affordable, and easily processed, as well as having good compatibility with other biopolymers (López et al., 2008). However, brittleness, high water permeability, and poor thermal stability are some intrinsic drawbacks of native starch. Starch can be modified chemically, physically, or biochemically, or by combining these methods to overcome these problems and customize its qualities for packaging uses (Masina et al., 2017). Such modifications enhance its functionality as a thickener, gelling agent, binder, adhesive, and film-forming material (Haroon et al., 2016).

According to the modification mechanism, chemically modified starches are typically divided into two types (Korma, 2016):

1. Branching modifications, which include acid-modified, oxidized, and pregelatinized starches, where the degree of polymer branching or depolymerization is altered, and
2. Substitution modifications, involving cross-linking or copolymerization with other molecules to introduce new functional groups. Among these, substituted starches, such as starch acetates, are most commonly employed for film fabrication because they form stable, transparent, and mechanically resistant gels upon drying (Mohamad Yazid et al., 2018). Incorporating acetate groups not only enhances the stability and transparency of the films but also slows down retrogradation and aging processes, improving long-term performance (Tian et al., 2018).

Plasticizers, usually glycerol or other low-molecular-weight hydrophilic substances like sucrose, glucose, fructose, amino acids, and water, are added to starch-based films to improve their extensibility and flexibility to alleviate their brittleness (Niranjana Prabhu and Prashantha, 2018).

Thermoplastic starch (TPS), a type of starch that is frequently used in coating and film production, is synthesized when it is plasticized and heated to high temperatures. The degree of plasticization has a significant impact on TPS's mechanical strength and moisture sensitivity (Zuo et al., 2015). TPS-based coatings enhance barrier performance, decrease gas and moisture transfer, and strengthen the mechanical integrity of the end product (Versino et al., 2016). Casting and extrusion are common manufacturing processes for starch-based films, enabling homogeneous film creation and scalability (Das et al., 2013).

Despite these developments, starch's low tensile strength, high gas permeability, and poor water resistance make it unsuitable for direct application in cosmetic packaging (Marichelvam et al., 2019). Dialdehyde starch (DAS), which interacts with hydroxyl groups to synthesize a more cohesive and uniform polymer network, is one cross-linking approach that researchers have used to solve these issues (Keshk et al., 2019). The resulting starch/DAS composites exhibit better mechanical strength, homogeneity of film, and moisture management. For example, starch/DAS films demonstrated greater water solubility (4%–8%), tensile strength (2–3 MPa), and higher moisture content (7%–12%) than starch/silica blends (moisture content, MC ~11%–14%, water solubility, WS ~8%–19%, tensile strength, TS ~0.5–0.7 MPa) (Oluwasina et al., 2021). In addition, DAS possesses antibacterial and antiviral properties due to its reactive carbonyl groups, which also contribute to improved antioxidant function and reduced moisture absorption (Bajer and Burkowska-But, 2022). The properties of these composites can be further enhanced by incorporating bioactive organic acids such as caffeic or quinic acid, which provide antioxidants and antibacterial protection while improving film elasticity and stiffness (Bajer, 2024).

In recent years, starch has also been effectively combined with other biodegradable polymers to create a synergistic balance between environmental friendliness and mechanical strength. Significant improvements in properties have been demonstrated by composites such as PLA/starch (Yusoff et al., 2021), PBAT/starch (Fourati et al., 2018), polyvinyl alcohol (PVA)/TPS (Heidarian et al., 2017), chitosan/starch (Xu et al., 2005), and polycaprolactone/starch (Wu, 2003). PLA/starch blends, for example, exhibit better stiffness and processability; however, compatibilizers such as silane coupling agents or maleic anhydride are sometimes required to reduce phase separation (Yusoff et al., 2021). PVA/TPS composites demonstrate higher water resistance and tensile strength due to intermolecular hydrogen bonding (Fourati et al., 2018), whereas PBAT/starch films provide excellent toughness and elongation, making them ideal for flexible cosmetic packaging (Heidarian et al., 2017). Similarly, chitosan/starch films combine chitosan's antibacterial properties with starch's film-forming ability, offering both mechanical and bioactive functionality, which makes them perfect for active cosmetic packaging (Lozano-Navarro et al., 2018).

A further technique to improve starch performance is to add nanoscale fillers. Mechanical strength, thermal stability, and barrier qualities are greatly enhanced by the addition of nanoclays (MMT) (Campos-Requena et al., 2017), bentonite (Sarkar et al., 2021), HNTs, nanosilica (SiO_2) (Liu et al., 2018), and metal oxides (TiO_2, ZnO) (López et al., 2015). For example, the network structure formed by combining nanosilica and corn starch prevented the water molecules from dissolving and improved the film's water resistance.

Similarly, films manufactured from thermoplastic starch can be enhanced with a natural and safe mineral filler, such as talc, to create a synthetic bionanocomposite that is suitable for cosmetic packaging and has improved functional properties, such as low water vapor and oxygen permeability (López et al., 2015). In a different study, the starch matrix was reinforced (1086 MPa) by hydrogen bonding with cellulose nanofibers or lignocellulosic fillers, increasing stiffness and decreasing water absorption (Lendvai et al., 2017).

8 Chitosan

Chitin is a natural polysaccharide found in the cell walls of fungi and yeasts, as well as in the exoskeletons of crustaceans, insects, and marine organisms such as crabs, shrimps, and mollusks. Chitosan, its deacetylated derivative, is the second most prevalent biopolymer in nature (Kulka and Sionkowska, 2023). The degree of deacetylation, which controls the solubility and physicochemical characteristics of chitin and chitosan, is the primary structural difference between the two (Cinelli et al., 2019). Chitosan, with a degree of deacetylation greater than 50%, is soluble in acidic environments due to the protonation of amino groups. The molecular weight, crystallinity, and biological activity of the resultant chitosan are strongly influenced by the chitin supply, reaction parameters, and processing circumstances (Rachtanapun et al., 2024).

Chitosan is a cationic polymer that has been investigated for its multifunctional performance in active packaging. The molecular weight and degree of deacetylation control its physicochemical behavior (Kodolova-Chukhontseva et al., 2023). It dissolves in aqueous solutions below pH ~6 due to the protonation of its amino groups, whereas higher pH and/or high molecular weight promote hydrogen-bonded aggregation and crystallinity. The bioactivity of chitosan is supported by these modifiable characteristics (Thambiliyagodage et al., 2023). Furthermore, chitosan exhibits antibacterial activity due to electrostatic interactions between the protonated $-NH_3^+$ groups of chitosan and negatively charged microbial envelopes, leading to membrane breakdown and leakage. The characteristic groups of chitosan are also responsible for its antioxidant activity, as the amino and hydroxyl groups in chitosan contribute hydrogen and electrons to quench radicals and bind pro-oxidant metals (Souza et al., 2020).

Due to these characteristics of chitosan, the cosmetic packaging industry has paid close attention to combining chitosan and its derivatives with other biopolymers or active ingredients to fabricate edible films and biodegradable packaging materials (Kulka and Sionkowska, 2023).

Blending chitosan with other biopolymers, including riboflavin, pullulan derivatives, agarose, starch, and gelatin, has been shown in studies to significantly increase biological activity, mechanical strength, and barrier qualities. Chitosan/agarose and chitosan/starch films showed improved flexibility, water vapor resistance, and antibacterial activity compared to pure chitosan film (Jridi et al., 2014). However, chitosan/gelatin composites demonstrated stronger tensile strength and UV-barrier capacity (Hu et al., 2016).

Furthermore, adding useful chemicals like riboflavin provided potent UV defense and antibacterial action without sacrificing transparency (Su et al., 2021).

Nanobiocomposite films with improved mechanical and functional qualities for cosmetic packaging have been produced by incorporating nanotechnology into chitosan-based materials (Aranaz et al., 2018). Despite favorable antibacterial and film-forming properties, the mechanical constraints of chitosan films prevent wider industrial adoption. To overcome these problems, adding nanoparticles to the chitosan matrix has proven to be a successful tactic (El-Araby et al., 2023). Studies have shown that embedding metal oxide nanoparticles such as MgO, TiO_2 (Anaya-Esparza et al., 2020), and ZnO (Tabassum et al., 2024) within chitosan or carboxymethyl chitosan matrices significantly improves tensile strength, thermal stability, water resistance, and UV barrier performance, while also enhancing antibacterial and antioxidant properties. For instance, MgO and TiO_2 nanoparticles confer excellent antimicrobial efficacy and structural reinforcement (De Silva et al., 2017), whereas ZnO nanoparticles combined with plant extracts or gallic acid provide synergistic antibacterial and antioxidant activities (Tabassum et al., 2024).

9 "Green" packaging and microbial risks

Cosmetic packaging fulfills several vital functions, including maintaining the stability and effectiveness of the product, as well as guaranteeing user ease and visual attractiveness (Dayan and Kromidas, 2011). In recent years, the cosmetics industry has pursued "green" or eco-friendly packaging options due to the increased focus on sustainability. Although this shift is in line with environmental goals, it presents a number of physicochemical and microbiological difficulties that need to be carefully considered when developing new products (Nazir et al., 2025).

Eco-friendly packaging materials, which are usually synthesized from renewable resources or are biodegradable, are beneficial in decreasing the environmental impact from a sustainability standpoint (Cinelli et al., 2019). These materials might, however, have poorer barrier qualities than conventional petrochemical polymers, making cosmetic formulations more vulnerable to external elements, including moisture, oxygen, and microbiological intrusion (Rosette et al., 2012).

Microbial contamination remains one of the most significant risks associated with cosmetic packaging, particularly when the container design facilitates product exposure (da Silva et al., 2025). Packaging types such as wide-mouth jars or tubs, favored for their convenience and luxury appeal, allow repeated contact with fingers or applicators, actions that can introduce microorganisms and biological debris. Conversely, airless pumps, aerosol systems, and single-use formats provide greater protection by minimizing exposure to the external environment and microbial contamination (Del Greco et al., 2024).

Another critical factor in microbiological risk control is consumer behavior. Contamination risk is significantly increased by actions, including diluting products with tap water, refilling empty containers, combining incompatible formulations, and leaving packages open (Perret et al., 2025). Though frequently outside the manufacturer's control, packaging design that deters misuse, such as by using nonrefillable formats, tamper-evident closures, or restricted dispensing systems, can positively impact these behaviors.

Microbial stability is also affected by material selection in environmentally friendly packaging. In cosmetic packaging, biopolymers like cellulose, starch, chitosan, PLA, and PHAs are increasingly used. Some of these materials are hydrophilic, which might increase moisture transmission and compromise product preservation systems, despite their low toxicity and biodegradability (Almeida et al., 2021). Furthermore, some biobased materials may have chemical interactions with cosmetic formulations that change the effectiveness of preservatives or speed up the degradation rate. Testing for compatibility between the product formulation and the packaging substrate is therefore essential (Dayan and Kromidas, 2011). Accelerated aging under regulated temperature and humidity settings is commonly used in stability evaluations to assess microbiological safety and physical integrity throughout the intended shelf life.

To ensure consumer protection while advancing green packaging initiatives, a comprehensive risk assessment framework should be applied during the design and validation stages (Rosette et al., 2012). This includes evaluating microbial ingress potential, preservative system robustness, and the integrity of sealing mechanisms under realistic conditions of use and storage. Moreover, integrating antimicrobial agents or surface modifications (e.g., metal oxide nanoparticles such as ZnO or TiO_2) into biopolymer matrices has been explored as a strategy to enhance microbial resistance (Kim et al., 2022); however, such approaches must be balanced against potential migration, toxicity, and regulatory constraints (da Silva et al., 2025).

10 Limitations and future perspectives

Most research on sustainable or biodegradable packaging has been conducted in the food sector, where concerns, including material performance, preservation effectiveness, and regulatory compliance, have received the majority of attention (Cinelli et al., 2019). On the contrary, the cosmetics packaging industry is still largely unstudied, while facing similar issues with consumer safety, product stability, and environmental sustainability. This imbalance highlights a crucial knowledge gap regarding the behavior of biodegradable materials in the particular physicochemical and microbiological circumstances connected to cosmetic compositions (Morel et al., 2024).

Furthermore, limited research has been conducted on the effects of environmental factors, such as temperature, humidity, and light exposure, on the structural and barrier qualities of biodegradable materials used in cosmetics (Vrabič-Brodnjak and Jestratijević, 2024). Accelerated and real-time stability testing, coupled with advanced analytical methods, should be implemented to establish standardized protocols for assessing the durability and safety of green packaging systems in cosmetics (D'Adamo et al., 2024).

Interdisciplinary collaborations integrating environmental science, toxicology, and cosmetic formulation technology are necessary to address the limited studies on cosmetic packaging. Potential chemical interactions, leachables, or biodegradation by-products that might compromise consumer safety or alter product composition would be identified with the aid of these efforts (Abubakar and Mina, 2024). Furthermore, cross-sector comparisons between research on food and cosmetic packaging may also yield insightful methodological information and hasten the creation of sturdy, biodegradable, and functionally stable cosmetic packaging (Kaestner et al., 2023).

Future research should therefore prioritize the systematic investigation of biodegradable packaging for cosmetic applications, particularly focusing on stability over time and during actual product use. Unlike food products, cosmetics often contain complex emulsions, natural oils, surfactants, and active ingredients that can interact chemically with packaging materials. Such interactions may compromise the mechanical integrity of the packaging. Long-term studies evaluating formulation-packaging compatibility, migration behavior, and degradation kinetics under realistic storage and consumer-use conditions are needed to ensure sustainability and safety.

11 Conclusions

Transitioning to global sustainable solutions, including cosmetic packaging, is crucial in reducing petroleum-based plastic waste. Biodegradable and biobased materials such as PLA, PHAs, and polysaccharides such as cellulose, starch, and chitosan have emerged as promising candidates, combining environmental benefits with functionality suitable for cosmetic packaging applications. These polymers are biodegradable, biocompatible, and reduce carbon emissions compared to conventional plastics. However, they still face challenges such as brittleness, sensitivity to moisture, poor barrier qualities, and the possibility of active ingredients or additives migrating into formulations. Studies have shown that combining biopolymers with fillers such as metal oxides, cellulose nanofibers, lignin nanoparticles, or nanoclays can significantly improve their mechanical, thermal, and antibacterial properties, providing a pathway to secure and efficient "green" packaging options. However, long-term stability, formulation-packaging compatibility, and microbiological contamination remain significant issues for consumer safety and regulatory compliance. The systematic assessment of biodegradation kinetics, degradation behavior, and interaction mechanisms between cosmetic formulations and packaging substrates under real storage and usage conditions should be the top priority of future studies. To overcome present constraints, interdisciplinary cooperation across material science, microbiology, and cosmetic chemistry will be essential.

References

A Text Book of Pharmaceutics for I Year Diploma in Pharmacy - Βιβλία Google, 2024. Available from: https://books.google.gr/books?hl=el&lr=&id=71UrEQAAQBAJ&oi=fnd&pg=PA67&dq=Yanamadala,+P.+K.+. (Accessed 20 October 2025).

Abubakar, S., Mina, E.A., 2024. The effect of branding and packaging of locally made cosmetic products on the buying decision of customers. a case study of cosmetic products in rivers state. Indonesian Annu. Conf. Ser. 3, 150–157. Available from: https://ojs.literacyinstitute.org/index.php/iacseries/article/view/1518.

Ahankari, S.S., Subhedar, A.R., Bhadauria, S.S., Dufresne, A., 2021. Nanocellulose in food packaging: a review. Carbohydr. Polym. 01448617. 255. Available from http://www.elsevier.com/wps/find/journaldescription.cws_home/405871/description#description. doi:10.1016/j.carbpol.2020.117479.

Akshaykranth, A., Ajayan, J., Anitha, N., 2025. Development of biodegradable PLA/Nanoclay/ZnO polymer films for future industrial packaging applications. Results Surf. Interfaces 26668459. 19, 100518. doi:10.1016/j.rsurfi.2025.100518.

Almeida, T., Silvestre, A.J.D., Vilela, C., Freire, C.S.R., 2021. Bacterial nanocellulose toward green cosmetics: recent progresses and challenges. Int. J. Mol. Sci. 14220067. 22 (6), 1–25. Available from https://www.mdpi.com/1422-0067/22/6/2836/pdf. doi:10.3390/ijms22062836.

Amberg, N., Fogarassy, C., 2019. Green consumer behavior in the cosmetics market. Resources. 20799276. 8 (3). Available from https://res.mdpi.com/d_attachment/resources/resources-08-00137/article_deploy/resources-08-00137.pdf. doi:10.3390/resources8030137.

Anaya-Esparza, L.M., Ruvalcaba-Gómez, J.M., Maytorena-Verdugo, C.I., González-Silva, N., Romero-Toledo, R., Aguilera-Aguirre, S., Pérez-Larios, A., Montalvo-González, E., 2020. Chitosan-tio2: a versatile hybrid composite. Materials. 19961944. 13 (4). Available from https://www.mdpi.com/journal/materials. doi:10.3390/ma13040811.

Aranaz, I., Acosta, N., Civera, C., Elorza, B., Mingo, J., Castro, C., Gandía, M.D.L.L., Caballero, A.H., 2018. Cosmetics and cosmeceutical applications of chitin, chitosan and their derivatives. Polymers. 20734360. 10 (2). Available from http://www.mdpi.com/2073-4360/10/2/213/pdf. doi:10.3390/polym10020213.

Bajer, D., 2024. Eco-friendly, biodegradable starch-based packaging materials with antioxidant features. Polymers 16 (7), 958. doi:10.3390/POLYM16070958.

Bajer, D., Burkowska-But, A., 2022. Innovative and environmentally safe composites based on starch modified with dialdehyde starch, caffeine, or ascorbic acid for applications in the food packaging industry. Food Chem. 03088146. 374, 131639. doi:10.1016/j.foodchem.2021.131639.

Bala, A., Arfelis, S., Oliver-Ortega, H., Méndez, J.A., 2022. Life cycle assessment of PE and PP multi film compared with PLA and PLA reinforced with nanoclays film. J. Clean. Prod. 09596526. 380. Available from https://www.journals.elsevier.com/journal-of-cleaner-production. doi:10.1016/j.jclepro.2022.134891.

Balla, E., et al, 2021. Poly(lactic Acid): a versatile biobased polymer for the future with multifunctional properties—from monomer synthesis, polymerization techniques and molecular weight increase to PLA applications. Polymers 13 (11), 1822. doi:10.3390/POLYM13111822.

Bikiaris, N.D., Koumentakou, I., Samiotaki, C., Meimaroglou, D., Varytimidou, D., Karatza, A., Kalantzis, Z., Roussou, M., Bikiaris, R.D., Papageorgiou, G.Z., 2023. Recent advances in the investigation of poly(lactic acid) (PLA) nanocomposites: incorporation of various nanofillers and their properties and applications. Polymers. 2073-4360. 15 (5), 1196. doi:10.3390/polym15051196.

Biswal, T., 2024. Recent progress in PLA-based composite and their application to biomedical and cosmetic fields. In: Jana, S. (Ed.), Biopolymers in Pharmaceutical and Food Applications: Vol. 1. Wiley, India, pp. 497–530. Available from: https://onlinelibrary.wiley.com/doi/book/10.1002/9783527848133/. doi:10.1002/9783527848133.ch23.

Bruzaud, S., Bourmaud, A., 2007. Thermal degradation and (nano)mechanical behavior of layered silicate reinforced poly(3-hydroxybutyrate-co-3-hydroxyvalerate) nanocomposites. Polym. Test. 01429418. 26 (5), 652–659. doi:10.1016/j.polymertesting.2007.04.001.

Bugnicourt, E., Cinelli, P., Lazzeri, A., Alvarez, V., 2014. Polyhydroxyalkanoate (PHA): review of synthesis, characteristics, processing and potential applications in packaging. Express Polym. Lett. 1788618X. 8 (11), 791–808. doi:10.3144/expresspolymlett.2014.82.

Campos-Requena, V.H., Rivas, B.L., Pérez, M.A., Figueroa, C.R., Figueroa, N.E., Sanfuentes, E.A., 2017. Thermoplastic starch/clay nanocomposites loaded with essential oil constituents as packaging for strawberries. In vivo antimicrobial synergy over *Botrytis cinerea*. Postharvest Biol. Technol. 09255214. 129, 29–36. Available from. www.elsevier.com/inca/publications/store/5/0/3/3/1/3/index.htt. doi:10.1016/j.postharvbio.2017.03.005.

Cavallo, E., Xiaoyan, H., Luzi, F., Dominici, F., Cerrutti, P., Bernal, C., Foresti, M.L., Torre, L., Puglia, D., 2021. UV Protective, antioxidant, antibacterial and compostable polylactic acid composites containing pristine and chemically modified lignin nanoparticles. Molecules. 1420-3049. 26 (1), 126. doi:10.3390/molecules26010126.

Cazón, P., Vázquez, M., 2021. Bacterial cellulose as a biodegradable food packaging material: a review. Food Hydrocoll. 0268005X. 113, 106530. doi:10.1016/j.foodhyd.2020.106530.

Cazón, P., Velázquez, G., Vázquez, M., 2020. Regenerated cellulose films combined with glycerol and polyvinyl alcohol: effect of moisture content on the physical properties. Food Hydrocoll. 0268005X. 103, 105657. doi:10.1016/j.foodhyd.2020.105657.

Chen, Y., Tsai, Y.H., Chou, I.N., Tseng, S.H., Wu, H.S., 2014. Application of biodegradable polyhydroxyalkanoates as surgical films for ventral hernia repair in mice. J. Polym. Sci. 16879430. 2014. Available from http://www.hindawi.com/journals/ijps/. doi:10.1155/2014/789681.

Cinelli, P., Coltelli, M.B., Signori, F., Morganti, P., Lazzeri, A., 2019. Cosmetic packaging to save the environment: future perspectives. Cosmetics. 20799284. 6 (2). Available from https://res.mdpi.com/cosmetics/cosmetics-06-00026/article_deploy/cosmetics-06-00026.pdf?filename=&attachment=1. doi:10.3390/COSMETICS6020026.

Cojocaru, V., Frunzaverde, D., Miclosina, C.O., Marginean, G., 2022. The influence of the process parameters on the mechanical properties of PLA specimens produced by fused filament fabrication—a review. Polymers. 20734360. 14 (5). Available from https://www.mdpi.com/2073-4360/14/5/886/pdf. doi:10.3390/polym14050886.

Connolly, M., Zhang, Y., Brown, D.M., Ortuño, N., Jordá-Beneyto, M., Stone, V., Fernandes, T.F., Johnston, H.J., 2019. Novel polylactic acid (PLA)-organoclay nanocomposite bio-packaging for the cosmetic industry; migration studies and in vitro assessment of the dermal toxicity of migration extracts. Polym. Degrad. Stab. 01413910. 168, 108938. doi:10.1016/j.polymdegradstab.2019.108938.

D'Adamo, I., Gastaldi, M., Giacalone, R., Kazancoglu, Y., 2024. A strategic and social analytics model for sustainable packaging in the cosmetic industry. Supply Chain Anal. 29498635. 8. Available from https://www.sciencedirect.com/journal/supply-chain-analytics. doi:10.1016/j.sca.2024.100090.

da Silva, J.D., Silva, F.A.M., Rodrigues, C.F., 2025. Microbial contamination in cosmetic products. Cosmetics 12 (5), 198. doi:10.3390/COSMETICS12050198.

Das, D.K., Dutta, H., Mahanta, C.L., 2013. Development of a rice starch-based coating with antioxidant and microbe-barrier properties and study of its effect on tomatoes stored at room temperature. LWT. 00236438. 50 (1), 272–278. doi:10.1016/j.lwt.2012.05.018.

Dayan, N., Kromidas, L., 2011. Formulating, Packaging, and Marketing of Natural Cosmetic Products Formulating, Packaging, and Marketing of Natural Cosmetic Products. John Wiley and Sons, United States, Available from http://onlinelibrary.wiley.com/book/10.1002/9781118056806. doi:10.1002/9781118056806.

De Silva, R.T., Mantilaka, M.M.M.G.P.G., Ratnayake, S.P., Amaratunga, G.A.J., de Silva, K.M.N., 2017. Nano-MgO reinforced chitosan nanocomposites for high performance packaging applications with improved mechanical, thermal and barrier properties. Carbohydr. Polym. 01448617. 157, 739–747. Available from. http://www.elsevier.com/wps/find/journaldescription.cws_home/405871/description#description. doi:10.1016/j.carbpol.2016.10.038.

De, O.A.G., Teixeira, V.G., Da, S.A.L.N., De, S.A.M.F., 2015. An investigation of crystallization and rheological behaviors of PLA/HDPE/Nano-$CaCO_3$ composites by experimental design. AIP Conf. Proc. 15517616. http://scitation.aip.org/content/aip/proceeding/aipcp1664. doi:10.1063/1.4918390.

Defruyt and Sander, 2019. Towards a New Plastics Economy. Available from: http://journals.openedition.org/factsreports, Special Issue 19, pp. 78–81, http://journals.openedition.org/factsreports/5369. (Accessed 13 October 2025).

Del Greco, A., Bani, M., Rampoldi, G., Ardenghi, S., Galli, P., Strepparava, M.G., Russo, S., 2024. Re-evaluating beauty: attitudes and perceptions of eco-friendly packaging in beauty care products—a systematic review. Sustain. Prod. Consum. 23525509. 52, 458–468. Available from. https://www.sciencedirect.com/science/journal/23525509. doi:10.1016/j.spc.2024.11.011.

Deroiné, M., Duigou, A.L., Corre, Y.M., Gac, P.Y.L., Davies, P., César, G., Bruzaud, S., 2014. Seawater accelerated ageing of poly(3-hydroxybutyrate-co-3-hydroxyvalerate). Polym. Degrad. Stab. 01413910. 105 (1), 237–247. doi:10.1016/j.polymdegradstab.2014.04.026.

Díez-Pascual, A.M., 2017. Biodegradable Food Packaging Nanocomposites Based on ZnO-reinforced Polyhydroxyalkanoates. Elsevier BV, pp. 185–221. doi:10.1016/b978-0-12-804302-8.00006-6.

Ding, Y., Lu, B., Wang, P., Wang, G., Ji, J., 2018. PLA-PBAT-PLA tri-block copolymers: effective compatibilizers for promotion of the mechanical and rheological properties of PLA/PBAT blends. Polym. Degrad. Stab. 01413910. 147, 41–48. doi:10.1016/j.polymdegradstab.2017.11.012.

Drobac, J., Alivojvodic, V., Maksic, P., Stamenovic, M., Mansour, G., Tzetzis, D., Kyratsis, P., 2020. Green face of packaging—sustainability issues of the cosmetic industry packaging. MATEC Web Conf. 2261-236X. 318, 01022. doi:10.1051/matecconf/202031801022.

El-Araby, A., Janati, W., Ullah, R., Ercisli, S., Errachidi, F., 2023. Chitosan, chitosan derivatives, and chitosan-based nanocomposites: eco-friendly materials for advanced applications (a review). Front. Chem. 22962646. 11. Available from http://journal.frontiersin.org/journal/chemistry. doi:10.3389/fchem.2023.1327426.

Elsawy, M.A., Kim, K.H., Park, J.W., Deep, A., 2017. Hydrolytic degradation of polylactic acid (PLA) and its composites. Renew. Sustain. Energy Rev. 18790690. 79, 1346–1352. Available from. https://www.journals.elsevier.com/renewable-and-sustainable-energy-reviews. doi:10.1016/j.rser.2017.05.143.

Fourati, Y., Tarrés, Q., Mutjé, P., Boufi, S., 2018. PBAT/thermoplastic starch blends: effect of compatibilizers on the rheological, mechanical and morphological properties. Carbohydr. Polym. 01448617. 199, 51–57. Available from. http://www.elsevier.com/wps/find/journaldescription.cws_home/405871/description#description. doi:10.1016/j.carbpol.2018.07.008.

Gabor, D., Tita, O., 2012. Biopolymers used in food packaging: a review. Acta Univ. Cibiniensis Ser. E Food Technol. 2344150X. 16 (2), 3–19. Available from http://saiapm.ulbsibiu.ro/rom/cercetare/ACTA_E/AUCFT2012_II_3_19.pdf.

Garba, A.I., Garba, A.I., 2023. Food preservation packaging. Food Process. Packag. Technol. Recent Adv. doi:10.5772/INTECHOPEN.110043.

Ghozali, M., Fahmiati, S., Triwulandari, E., Restu, W.K., Farhan, D., Wulansari, M., Fatriasari, W., 2020. PLA/metal oxide biocomposites for antimicrobial packaging application. Polym.-Plast. Technol. Mater. 2574089X. 59 (12), 1332–1342. Available from https://www.tandfonline.com/loi/lpte21. doi:10.1080/25740881.2020.1738475.

Gigante, V., Aliotta, L., Coltelli, M.B., Lazzeri, A., 2022. Mechanical response of reactive extruded biocomposites based on recycled poly(lactic acid) (R-PLA)/recycled polycarbonate (R-PC) and cellulosic fibers with different aspect ratios. Macromol. 26736209. 2 (4), 509–521. Available from https://www.mdpi.com/journal/macromol. doi:10.3390/macromol2040032.

Grădinaru, C., Obadă, D.-R., Grădinaru, I.-A., Dabija, D.-C., 2022. Enhancing sustainable cosmetics brand purchase: a comprehensive approach based on the SOR model and the triple bottom line. Sustainability 2071-1050. 14 (21), 14118. doi:10.3390/su142114118.

Haroon, M., Wang, L., Yu, H., Abbasi, N.M., Abdin, Z.-U., Saleem, M., Khan, R.U., Ullah, R.S., Chen, Q., Wu, J., 2016. Chemical modification of starch and its application as an adsorbent material. RSC Adv. 20462069. 6 (82), 78264–78285. Available from http://pubs.rsc.org/en/journals/journalissues. doi:10.1039/c6ra16795k.

Heidarian, P., Behzad, T., Sadeghi, M., 2017. Investigation of cross-linked PVA/starch biocomposites reinforced by cellulose nanofibrils isolated from aspen wood sawdust. Cellulose. 1572882X. 24 (8), 3323–3339. doi:10.1007/s10570-017-1336-4.

Hu, Z., Hong, P., Liao, M., Kong, S., Huang, N., Chunyan, O., Sidong, L., 2016. Preparation and characterization of chitosan—agarose composite films. Materials. 1996-1944. 9 (10), 816. doi:10.3390/ma9100816.

Ivanov, E., Kotsilkova, R., Xia, H., Chen, Y., Donato, R.K., Donato, K., Godoy, A.P., Di Maio, R., Silvestre, C., Cimmino, S., Angelov, V., 2019. PLA/Graphene/MWCNT composites with improved electrical and thermal properties suitable for FDM 3D printing applications. Appl. Sci. 2076-3417. 9 (6), 1209. doi:10.3390/app9061209.

Jabeen, N., Majid, I., Nayik, G.A., Yildiz, F., 2015. Bioplastics and food packaging: a review. Cogent Food Agric. 2331-1932. 1 (1), 1117749. doi:10.1080/23311932.2015.1117749.

Jacobsen, C., Paiva-Martins, F., Schwarz, K., 2017. Lipid oxidation and antioxidants in food. Eur. J. Lipid Sci. Technol. 14389312. 119 (6). Available from http://www3.interscience.wiley.com/journal/69502350/home. doi:10.1002/ejlt.201700170.

Jawaid, M., El, A., Qaiss, K., Bouhfid, R., n.d. Engineering Materials Nanoclay Reinforced Polymer Composites Nanocomposites and Bionanocomposites. Available from: http://www.springer.com/series/4288.

Jenita, J.J.L., Rathore, S.S., Manjula, D., Barnabas, W., 2025. Packaging, Container, and Closure of Ophthalmic Products Complex Ophthalmic Dosage Forms: Advances in Biomedical Applications and Future Perspectives. Springer Science+Business Media, India, pp. 355–392. doi:10.1007/978-981-96-6306-4_12.

Jridi, M., Hajji, S., Ayed, H.B., Lassoued, I., Mbarek, A., Kammoun, M., Souissi, N., Nasri, M., 2014. Physical, structural, antioxidant and antimicrobial properties of gelatin-chitosan composite edible films. Int. J. Biol. Macromol. 18790003. 67, 373–379. Available from. www.elsevier.com/locate/ijbiomac. doi:10.1016/j.ijbiomac.2014.03.054.

Kaestner, L., Scope, C., Neumann, N., Woelfel, C., 2023. Sustainable circular packaging design: a systematic literature review on strategies and applications in the cosmetics industry. Proc. Des. Soc. 3, 3265–3274.

Keshk, S.M.A.S., El-Zahhar, A.A., Haija, M.A., Bondock, S., 2019. Synthesis of a magnetic nanoparticles/dialdehyde starch-based composite film for food packaging. Starch/Staerke. 1521379X. 71 (1-2). Available from http://onlinelibrary.wiley.com/journal/10.1002/(ISSN)1521-379X. doi:10.1002/star.201800035.

Kim, I., Viswanathan, K., Kasi, G., Thanakkasaranee, S., Sadeghi, K., Seo, J., 2022. ZnO Nanostructures in active antibacterial food packaging: preparation methods, antimicrobial mechanisms, safety issues, future prospects, and challenges. Food Rev. Int. 15256103. 38 (4), 537–565. Available from www.tandf.co.uk/journals/titles/87559129.asp. doi:10.1080/87559129.2020.1737709.

Kodolova-Chukhontseva, V.V., Rozova, E.Y., Dresvyanina, E.N., Nashchekina, Y.A., Dobrovol'skaya, I.P., Vlasova, E.N., Bystrov, S.G., Popova, E.N., Maslennikova, T.P., Yudin, V.E., Morganti, P., 2023. New composite materials based on chitosan films reinforced with chitin nanofibrils for cosmetic application. Cosmetics. 20799284. 10 (2). Available from www.mdpi.com/journal/cosmetics. doi:10.3390/cosmetics10020051.

Korma, S.A., 2016. Chemically modified starch and utilization in food stuffs. Int. J. Nutr. Food Sci. 5 (4), 264. doi:10.11648/J.IJNFS.20160504.15.

Koumentakou, I., Michopoulou, A., Noordam, M.J., Terzopoulou, Z., Bikiaris, D.N., 2024. 3D-printed scaffolds for tissue engineering applications using thermosensitive hydrogels based on biopolymer blends. J. Mater. Sci. 15734803. 59 (20), 9021–9041. Available from https://www.springer.com/journal/10853. doi:10.1007/s10853-024-09707-0.

Kulka, K., Sionkowska, A., 2023. Chitosan based materials in cosmetic applications: a review. Molecules. 14203049. 28 (4). Available from http://www.mdpi.com/journal/molecules. doi:10.3390/molecules28041817.

Kumar, S., Gupta, S.K., 2012. Applications of biodegradable pharmaceutical packaging materials: a review. Middle East J. Sci. Res. 19998147. 12 (5), 699–706. Available from http://www.idosi.org/mejsr/mejsr12(5)12/16.pdf. doi:10.5829/idosi.mejsr.2012.12.5.63241India.

Leite, L.S.F., Gars, M.L., Azeredo, H.M.C., Moreira, F.K.V., Mattoso, L.H.C., Bras, J., 2024. Insights into the effect of carboxylated cellulose nanocrystals on mechanical and barrier properties of gelatin films for flexible packaging applications. Int. J. Biol. Macromol. 18790003. 280. Available from https://www.sciencedirect.com/science/journal/01418130. doi:10.1016/j.ijbiomac.2024.135726.

Lendvai, L., Apostolov, A., Karger-Kocsis, J., 2017. Characterization of layered silicate-reinforced blends of thermoplastic starch (TPS) and poly(butylene adipate-co-terephthalate). Carbohydr. Polym. 01448617. 173, 566–572. Available from. http://www.elsevier.com/wps/find/journaldescription.cws_home/405871/description#description. doi:10.1016/j.carbpol.2017.05.100.

Lindman, B., Karlström, G., Stigsson, L., 2010. On the mechanism of dissolution of cellulose. J. Mol. Liq. 01677322. 156 (1), 76–81. doi:10.1016/j.molliq.2010.04.016.

Liu, Y., Ahmed, S., Sameen, D.E., Wang, Y., Lu, R., Dai, J., Li, S., Qin, W., 2021. A review of cellulose and its derivatives in biopolymer-based for food packaging application. Trends Food Sci. Technol. 09242244. 112, 532–546. Available from. http://www.elsevier.com/wps/find/journaldescription.cws_home/601278/description#description. doi:10.1016/j.tifs.2021.04.016.

Liu, Y., Fan, L., Mo, X., Yang, F., Pang, J., 2018. Effects of nanosilica on retrogradation properties and structures of thermoplastic cassava starch. J. Appl. Polym. Sci. 10974628. 135 (2). Available from http://onlinelibrary.wiley.com/journal/10.1002/(ISSN)1097-4628. doi:10.1002/app.45687.

López, O.V., Castillo, L.A., García, M.A., Villar, M.A., Barbosa, S.E., 2015. Food packaging bags based on thermoplastic corn starch reinforced with talc nanoparticles. Food Hydrocoll. 0268005X. 43, 18–24. Available from. https://www.journals.elsevier.com/food-hydrocolloids. doi:10.1016/j.foodhyd.2014.04.021.

López, O.V., García, M.A., Zaritzky, N.E., 2008. Film forming capacity of chemically modified corn starches. Carbohydr. Polym. 01448617. 73 (4), 573–581. doi:10.1016/j.carbpol.2007.12.023.

Lozano-Navarro, J.I., Díaz-Zavala, N.P., Velasco-Santos, C., Melo-Banda, J.A., Páramo-García, U., Paraguay-Delgado, F., García-Alamilla, R., Martínez-Hernández, A.L., Zapién-Castillo, S., 2018. Chitosan-starch films with natural extracts: physical, chemical, morphological and thermal properties. Materials. 19961944. 11 (1). Available from http://www.mdpi.com/1996-1944/11/1/120/pdf. doi:10.3390/ma11010120.

Marano, S., Laudadio, E., Minnelli, C., Stipa, P., 2022. Tailoring the barrier properties of PLA: a state-of-the-art review for food packaging applications. Polymers 14 (8), 1626. doi:10.3390/POLYM14081626.

Marichelvam, M.K., Jawaid, M., Asim, M., 2019. Corn and rice starch-based bio-plastics as alternative packaging materials. Fibers. 20796439. 7 (4). Available from https://res.mdpi.com/fibers/fibers-07-00032/article_deploy/fibers-07-00032-v2.pdf?filename=&attachment=1. doi:10.3390/fib7040032.

Masina, N., Choonara, Y.E., Kumar, P., du Toit, L.C., Govender, M., Indermun, S., Pillay, V., 2017. A review of the chemical modification techniques of starch. Carbohydr. Polym. 01448617. 157, 1226–1236. Available from. http://www.elsevier.com/wps/find/journaldescription.cws_home/405871/description#description. doi:10.1016/j.carbpol.2016.09.094.

Mifsud, S., Refalo, P., Rochman, A., 2023. Biodegradable polymers for cosmetic packaging: a technical and life cycle perspective. Mater. Res. Proc. 2474395X. 28, 2015–2024. www.mrforum.com/materials-research-proceedings-volumes/. doi:10.21741/9781644902479-217.

Mohamad Yazid, N.S., Abdullah, N., Muhammad, N., Matias-Peralta, H.M., 2018. Application of starch and starch-based products in food industry. J. Sci. Technol. 22298460. 10 (2). doi:10.30880/jst.2018.10.02.023.

Morel, S., Mura, G., Gallarate, M., Sapino, S., 2024. Cosmetic packaging: european regulatory aspects and sustainability. Cosmetics 11 (4), 110. doi:10.3390/COSMETICS11040110.

Mulla, M.Z., Rahman, M.R.T., Marcos, B., Tiwari, B., Pathania, S., 2021. Poly lactic acid (PLA) nanocomposites: effect of inorganic nanoparticles reinforcement on its performance and food packaging applications. Molecules 26 (7), 1967. doi:10.3390/MOLECULES26071967.

Muthuraj, R., Misra, M., Mohanty, A.K., 2017. Reactive compatibilization and performance evaluation of miscanthus biofiber reinforced poly(hydroxybutyrate-co-hydroxyvalerate) biocomposites. J. Appl. Polym. Sci. 10974628. 134 (21). Available from http://onlinelibrary.wiley.com/journal/10.1002/(ISSN)1097-4628. doi:10.1002/app.44860.

Packaging Waste Statistics—Statistics Explained—Eurostat, n.d. Available from: https://ec.europa.eu/eurostat/statistics-explained/index.php?title=Packaging_waste_statistics. (Accessed 13 October 2025).

Revenue of the cosmetics industry worldwide| statista, n.d. Available from: https://www.statista.com/forecasts/1272313/worldwide-revenue-cosmetics-market-by-segment?srsltid=AfmBOoog7DrxUTo8tGIGxXhsLdC8x9tuSijlvLYVQmgkUxT_XCGjtyDP. (Accessed 13 October 2025).

The Science and Technology of Flexible Packaging: multilayer Films from - Barry A. Morris - Βιβλία Google, n.d. Available from: https://books.google.gr/books?hl=el&lr=&id=06RXEAAAQBAJ&oi=fnd&pg=PP1&dq=Morris,+B.+A.+(2022).+The+science+and+technology+of+flexible+packaging:+multilayer+films+from+resin+and+process+to+end+use.+William+Andrew&ots=N2nDUaCI0x&sig=_-PN6LEUI5Mwb_yCD3f8KfnDWQY&redir_esc=y#v=onepage&q=Morris%2C%20B.%20A.%20(2022).%20The%20science%20and%20technology%20of%20flexible%20packaging%3A%20multilayer%20films%20from%20resin%20and%20process%20to%20end%20use.%20William%20Andrew&f=false. (Accessed 20 October 2025).

Nazir, A., Javed, S., Ahmad, A., Ahmed, S., Zahoor, A.F., 2025. Microbiological Safety and Cosmetics Sustainable Cosmeceuticals: Integrating Natural and Biotechnological Innovations. Springer Science+Business Media, Pakistan, pp. 453–478. doi:10.1007/978-3-031-86087-4_16.

Niranjana Prabhu, T., Prashantha, K., 2018. A review on present status and future challenges of starch based polymer films and their composites in food packaging applications. Polym. Compos. 15480569. 39 (7), 2499–2522. Available from http://onlinelibrary.wiley.com/journal/10.1002/(ISSN)1548-0569. doi:10.1002/pc.24236.

Oliver-Ortega, H., Vandemoortele, V., Bala, A., Julian, F., Méndez, J.A., Espinach, F.X., 2021. Nanoclay effect into the biodegradation and processability of poly(Lactic acid) nanocomposites for food packaging. Polymers. 20734360. 13 (16). Available from https://www.mdpi.com/2073-4360/13/16/2741/pdf. doi:10.3390/polym13162741.

Oluwasina, O.O., Akinyele, B.P., Olusegun, S.J., Oluwasina, O.O., Mohallem, N.D.S., 2021. Evaluation of the effects of additives on the properties of starch-based bioplastic film. SN Appl. Sci. 25233971. 3 (4). Available from https://www.springer.com/snas. doi:10.1007/s42452-021-04433-7.

Perret, J.K., Gómez Velázquez, A., Mehn, A., 2025. Green cosmetics—the effects of package design on consumers' willingness-to-pay and sustainability perceptions. Sustainability. 2071-1050. 17 (6), 2581. doi:10.3390/su17062581.

Pokhrel, S., 2015. A review on introduction and applications of starch and its biodegradable polymers. Int. J. Environ. 2091-2854. 4 (4), 114–125. doi:10.3126/ije.v4i4.14108.

Rachtanapun, P., Rachtanapun, C., Jantrawut, P., Thanakkasaranee, S., Kasi, G., Tantala, J., Panraksa, P., Chaiwarit, T., 2024. Carboxymethyl chitosan-based materials in packaging, food, pharmaceutical, and cosmetics. Adv. Polym. Sci. 292, 139–203. Available from https://www.springer.com/series/12. doi:10.1007/12_2023_158.

Resimović, L., Brozović, M., Kovačević, D., 2022. Design of sustainable packaging for natural cosmetics. J. Appl. Packag. Res. 14, 1. Available from: https://repository.rit.edu/japr/vol14/iss1/2.

Rosette, J.L., Yablonski, J., Mancuso, S., Kale, G., 2012. Packaging, Cosmetics and Pharmaceuticals Kirk-othmer Encyclopedia of Chemical Technology. Wiley, pp. 1–14. doi:10.1002/0471238961.0315191318151905.a01.pub3.

Saha, T., Hoque, M.E., Mahbub, T., 2020. Biopolymers for Sustainable Packaging in Food, Cosmetics, and Pharmaceuticals Advanced Processing, Properties, and Applications of Starch and Other Bio-based Polymers. Elsevier, Bangladesh, pp. 197–214. Available from https://www.sciencedirect.com/book/9780128196618. doi:10.1016/B978-0-12-819661-8.00013-5.

Sánchez-Safont, E.L., Arrillaga, A., Anakabe, J., Cabedo, L., Gamez-Perez, J., 2018. Toughness enhancement of PHBV/TPU/cellulose compounds with reactive additives for compostable injected parts in industrial applications. Int. J. Mol. Sci. 14220067. 19 (7). Available from http://www.mdpi.com/1422-0067/19/7/2102/pdf. doi:10.3390/ijms19072102.

Santos, F., Rodrigues, P., Vargas, P., Massano, A., Oliveira, L.M., Batista, C., Cruz, V., Mateus, A., Mitchell, G.R., Sobral, A.J.F.N., Encarnação, T., 2025. A novel fully biobased material composite for cosmetic packaging applications. Sci. Rep. 20452322. 15 (1). Available from https://www.nature.com/srep/. doi:10.1038/s41598-025-10426-y.

Sarkar, A., Biswas, D.R., Datta, S.C., Dwivedi, B.S., Bhattacharyya, R., Kumar, R., Bandyopadhyay, K.K., Saha, M., Chawla, G., Saha, J.K., Patra, A.K., 2021. Preparation of novel biodegradable starch/poly(vinyl alcohol)/bentonite grafted polymeric films for fertilizer encapsulation. Carbohydr. Polym. 01448617. 259, 117679. doi:10.1016/j.carbpol.2021.117679.

Seggiani, M., Cinelli, P., Balestri, E., Mallegni, N., Stefanelli, E., Rossi, A., Lardicci, C., Lazzeri, A., 2018. Novel sustainable composites based on poly(hydroxybutyrate-co-hydroxyvalerate) and seagrass beach-CAST fibers: performance and degradability in marine environments. Materials. 19961944. 11 (5). Available from http://www.mdpi.com/1996-1944/11/5/772/pdf. doi:10.3390/ma11050772.

Sirviö, J.A., Liimatainen, H., Niinimäki, J., Hormi, O., 2013. Sustainable packaging materials based on wood cellulose. RSC Adv. 20462069. 3 (37), 16590–16596. doi:10.1039/c3ra43264e.

Song, Z., Xiao, H., Zhao, Y., 2014. Hydrophobic-modified nano-cellulose fiber/PLA biodegradable composites for lowering water vapor transmission rate (WVTR) of paper. Carbohydr. Polym. 01448617. 111, 442–448. Available from. http://www.elsevier.com/wps/find/journaldescription.cws_home/405871/description#description. doi:10.1016/j.carbpol.2014.04.049.

Souza, V.G.L., Pires, J.R.A., Rodrigues, C., Coelhoso, I.M., Fernando, A.L., 2020. Chitosan composites in packaging industry-current trends and future challenges. Polymers. 20734360. 12 (2). Available from https://res.mdpi.com/d_attachment/polymers/polymers-12-00417/article_deploy/polymers-12-00417.pdf. doi:10.3390/polym12020417.

Su, L., Huang, J., Li, H., Pan, Y., Zhu, B., Zhao, Y., Liu, H., 2021. Chitosan-riboflavin composite film based on photodynamic inactivation technology for antibacterial food packaging. Int. J. Biol. Macromol. 18790003. 172, 231–240. Available from. www.elsevier.com/locate/ijbiomac. doi:10.1016/j.ijbiomac.2021.01.056.

Swetha, T.A., Bora, A., Mohanrasu, K., Balaji, P., Raja, R., Ponnuchamy, K., Muthusamy, G., Arun, A., 2023. A comprehensive review on polylactic acid (PLA)—synthesis, processing and application in food packaging. Int. J. Biol. Macromol. 18790003. 234. Available from https://www.sciencedirect.com/science/journal/01418130. doi:10.1016/j.ijbiomac.2023.123715.

Sylvester, O., 2024. Chapter 28: Sustainable development goal 12: Sustainable consumption and production patterns. In: Hendriks, S.L., Babu, S.C. (Eds.), Handbook on Public Policy and Food Security. Edward Elgar Publishing, pp. 289–298. doi:10.4337/9781839105449.00033.

Tabassum, Z., Mohan, A., Girdhar, M., 2024. Insight into recent trends in ZnO nanoparticle reinforced chitosan-based composite films for sustainable packaging: a critical review on its current status, challenges and perspective. Mater. Today Proc. 22147853. doi:10.1016/j.matpr.2024.05.069.

Tang, Z., Fan, F., Fan, C., Jiang, K., Qin, Y., 2020. The performance changes and migration behavior of PLA/nano-TiO_2 composite film by high-pressure treatment in ethanol solution. Polymers 12 (2), 471. doi:10.3390/POLYM12020471.

Thakur, V.K., 2014. Lignocellulosic Polymer Composites: Processing, Characterization, and Properties. Wiley, pp. 1–561. Available from: https://www.wiley.com/remtitle.cgi?isbn=1118773578. doi:10.1002/9781118773949.

Thambiliyagodage, C., Jayanetti, M., Mendis, A., Ekanayake, G., Liyanaarachchi, H., Vigneswaran, S., 2023. Recent advances in chitosan-based applications—a review. Materials. 19961944. 16 (5). Available from http://www.mdpi.com/journal/materials. doi:10.3390/ma16052073.

Tian, S., Chen, Y., Chen, Z., Yang, Y., Wang, Y., 2018. Preparation and characteristics of starch esters and its effects on dough physicochemical properties. J. Food Qual. 17454557. 2018. Available from https://www.hindawi.com/journals/jfq/. doi:10.1155/2018/1395978.

Tripathi, N., Misra, M., Mohanty, A.K., 2021. Durable polylactic acid (PLA)-based sustainable engineered blends and biocomposites: recent developments, challenges, and opportunities. ACS Eng. Au. 2694-2488. 1 (1), 7–38. doi:10.1021/acsengineeringau.1c00011.

Versino, F., Lopez, O.V., Garcia, M.A., Zaritzky, N.E., 2016. Starch-based films and food coatings: an overview. Starch/Staerke. 1521379X. 68 (11-12), 1026–1037. Available from http://onlinelibrary.wiley.com/journal/10.1002/(ISSN)1521-379X. doi:10.1002/star.201600095.

Versino, F., Ortega, F., Monroy, Y., Rivero, S., López, O.V., García, M.A., 2023. Sustainable and bio-based food packaging: a review on past and current design innovations. Foods. 23048158. 12 (5). Available from www.mdpi.com/journal/foods. doi:10.3390/foods12051057.

Vrabič-Brodnjak, U., Jestratijević, I., 2024. The future of baby cosmetics packaging and sustainable development: a look at sustainable materials and packaging innovations—a systematic review. Sustain. Dev. 10991719. 32 (3), 2208–2222. Available from http://onlinelibrary.wiley.com/journal/10.1002/(ISSN)1099-1719. doi:10.1002/sd.2775.

Wang, L., Chen, C., Wang, J., Gardner, D.J., Tajvidi, M., 2020. Cellulose nanofibrils versus cellulose nanocrystals: comparison of performance in flexible multilayer films for packaging applications. Food Packag. Shelf Life. 22142894. 23. Available from http://www.journals.elsevier.com/food-packaging-and-shelf-life/. doi:10.1016/j.fpsl.2020.100464.

Wang, S., Lu, A., Zhang, L., 2016. Recent advances in regenerated cellulose materials. Prog. Polym. Sci. 00796700. 53, 169–206. Available from. http://www.sciencedirect.com/science/journal/00796700. doi:10.1016/j.progpolymsci.2015.07.003.

Wang, W., Feng, G., Deng, Z., Zhu, Y., Zhu, J., Guo, T., Song, J., Xiao, H., 2021. Multilayer surface construction for enhancing barrier properties of cellulose-based packaging. Carbohydr. Polym. 01448617. 255, 117431. doi:10.1016/j.carbpol.2020.117431.

Wróblewska-Krepsztul, J., Rydzkowski, T., Borowski, G., Szczypiński, M., Klepka, T., Thakur, V.K., 2018. Recent progress in biodegradable polymers and nanocomposite-based packaging materials for sustainable environment. Int. J. Polym. Anal. Charact. 15635341. 23 (4), 383–395. Available from http://www.tandf.co.uk/journals/titles/1023666x.html. doi:10.1080/1023666X.2018.1455382.

Wu, C.S., 2003. Physical properties and biodegradability of maleated-polycaprolactone/starch composite. Polym. Degrad. Stab. 80 (1), 127–134. doi:10.1016/S0141-3910(02)00393-2.

Xiao, Y., Liu, Y., Kang, S., Huaide, X., 2021. Insight into the formation mechanism of soy protein isolate films improved by cellulose nanocrystals. Food Chem. 03088146. 359, 129971. doi:10.1016/j.foodchem.2021.129971.

Xu, Y.X., Kim, K.M., Hanna, M.A., Nag, D., 2005. Chitosan-starch composite film: preparation and characterization. Ind. Crops Prod. 09266690. 21 (2), 185–192. doi:10.1016/j.indcrop.2004.03.002.

Yang, J., Wang, C., Shao, K., Ding, G., Tao, Y., Zhu, J., 2015. Morphologies, mechanical properties and thermal stability of poly(lactic acid) toughened by precipitated barium sulfate. Russ. J. Phys. Chem. A. 00360244. 89 (11), 2092–2096. Available from http://springerlink.metapress.com/content/0036-0244/. doi:10.1134/S0036024415110242.

Yu, J., Chen, L.X.L., 2008. The greenhouse gas emissions and fossil energy requirement of bioplastics from cradle to gate of a biomass refinery. Environ. Sci. Technol. 0013936X. 42 (18), 6961–6966. doi:10.1021/es7032235.

Yusoff, N.H., Pal, K., Narayanan, T., de Souza, F.G., 2021. Recent trends on bioplastics synthesis and characterizations: polylactic acid (PLA) incorporated with tapioca starch for packaging applications. J. Mol. Struct. 00222860. 1232. Available from https://www.journals.elsevier.com/journal-of-molecular-structure. doi:10.1016/j.molstruc.2021.129954.

Zuo, Y., Gu, J., Tan, H., Zhang, Y., 2015. Thermoplastic starch prepared with different plasticizers: relation between degree of plasticization and properties. J. Wuhan Univ. Technol., Mater. Sci. Ed. 10002413. 30 (2), 423–428. Available from http://www.springerlink.com/content/1000-2413. doi:10.1007/s11595-015-1164-z.

Section VII

Epilogue

Chapter 28

Growth, evolution, research and development trends, and future perspectives

Maria-Parthena Lafara, Theodora Adamantidi, and Alexandros Tsoupras

Hephaestus Laboratory, School of Chemistry, Faculty of Sciences, Democritus University of Thrace, Kavala University Campus, Kavala, Greece

1 Introduction

The cosmetics industry represents one of the most dynamic and rapidly evolving sectors of the global consumer market. Over the past decades, it has experienced sustained growth, mainly driven by technological advancements, altering lifestyles, and increasing consumer awareness of cosmetic safety. Notably, the demand for cosmetics and dermatocosmetics formulated with natural ingredients and bioactive compounds has continuously increased, shaping modern market preferences and also paving the way for advances in green chemistry, formulation science, and biotechnology (Longo et al., 2022; Dwivedi et al., 2025; Liu, 2022). Globally, skincare, haircare, makeup, and fragrances constitute the main cosmetic product categories. In parallel, dermatocosmetics, as cosmeceutical counterparts, have also revealed accelerated growth, driven by consumer demand for formulations that efficiently combine esthetic benefits with enhanced biological activity. Nowadays, increasing accessibility to scientific information and social media, as well as increased consumer education and transparency initiatives, have prompted consumers to evaluate ingredient origin, manufacturing process suitability, and sustainability concerns, reinforcing a shift toward "clean beauty" and clean-label products (Dwivedi et al., 2025; Liu, 2022).

According to current cosmetic market reports, from 2021 to 2023, the European cosmetics market recorded a significant increase, with growth rates rising from 2.7% to 9.1%, showcasing the resilience and expansion potential of the cosmetics and dermatocosmetics sector. Interestingly, cosmetic consumption per capita across European countries remains significantly high, reflecting the integral role of personal care products and skincare formulations in daily life. It must be noted that on a global scale, the cosmetics and cosmeceuticals market has exhibited robust growth, supported by rising disposable income, urbanization, aging populations, and technological innovation-driven increases in skin health and preventative care awareness. Northern European countries, as presented in Fig. 28.1, as well as North America and the Asia-Pacific region, currently represent major growth drivers, with the latter demonstrating particularly rapid expansion due to a growing middle-class population, strong demand for skincare formulations, and the integration of traditional botanical knowledge with modern cosmetic science and demands (Longo et al., 2022; Turcu and Brancu, 2025; Huong et al., 2024).

According to the Cosmetics Europe Market Performance Report (2024), the European cosmetics market exceeded a total value of 96 billion euros, with skincare, haircare, makeup, and fragrances constituting the dominant product categories (Turcu and Brancu, 2025; Brancu and Turcu, 2025). Concurrently, the growing consumer preference for sustainable and naturally derived products has driven substantial expansion in the global market for natural cosmetics. This segment is projected to grow at a compound annual growth rate (CAGR) of 10.6% between 2021 and 2026, underscoring the commercial and scientific relevance of natural ingredients and bioactives in cosmetic and dermatocosmetic development (Brancu and Turcu, 2025). Fig. 28.2 illustrates the distribution of cosmetic product categories (across different countries), primarily revealing the relative contribution of each segment to the overall market (Turcu and Brancu, 2025).

Biofunctional Cosmetics for Health. https://doi.org/10.1016/B978-0-443-27500-5.00025-3

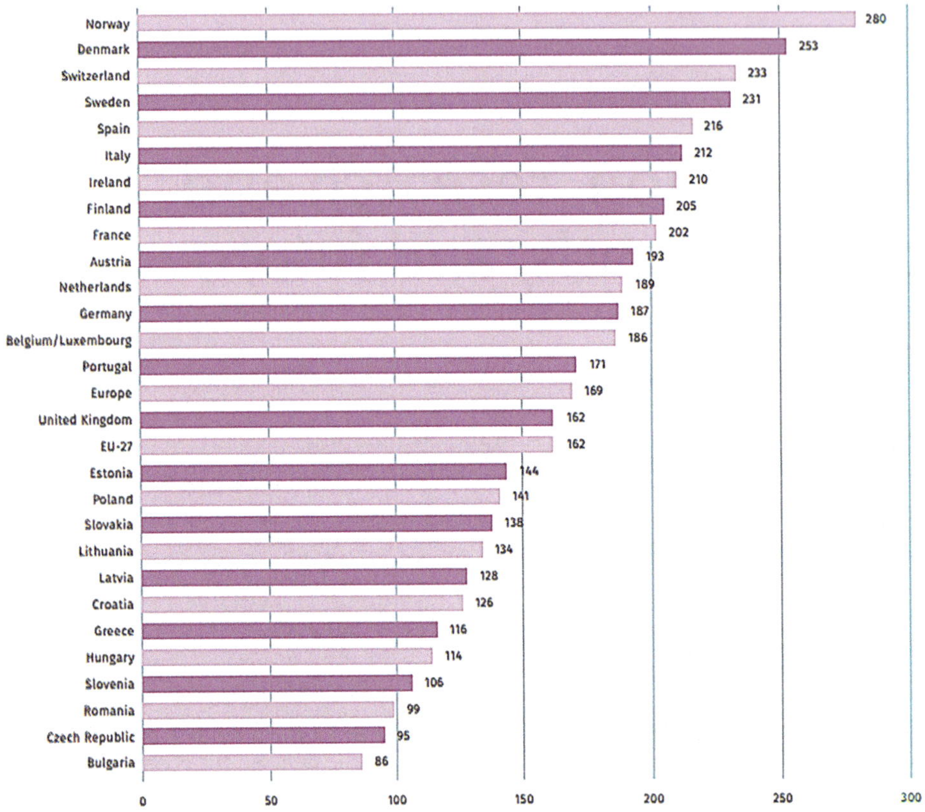

FIG. 28.1 The European cosmetics per capita consumption by country. *(Data from Turcu, O., Brancu, C., 2025. Cosmetics industry performance in the European Union: a comparative analysis. Proc. Int. Conf. Bus. Excell. 2558-9652. 19 (1), 2267–2276. doi:10.2478/picbe-2025-0175.)*

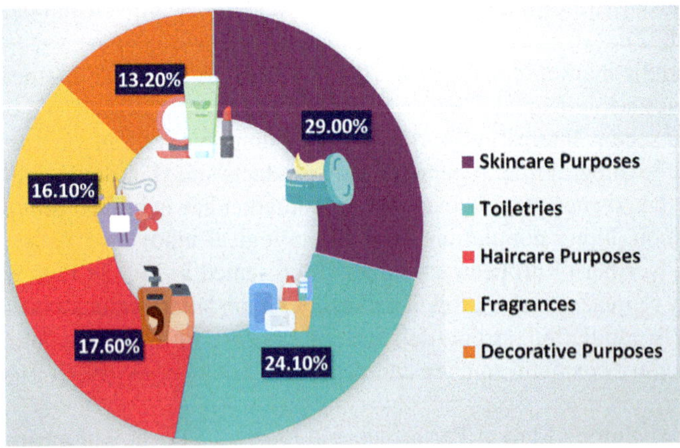

FIG. 28.2 The European cosmetics market: market changes by product category (%). *(Data from Turcu, O., Brancu, C., 2025. Cosmetics industry performance in the European Union: a comparative analysis. Proc. Int. Conf. Bus. Excell. 2558-9652. 19 (1), 2267–2276. doi:10.2478/picbe-2025-0175.)*

Cosmetics were formally described in 1945 as: "any product created to be applied, poured, sprinkled, sprayed onto, or introduced into the human body for cleansing, beautifying, promoting attractiveness, or altering appearance" (Ferreira et al., 2022; Shahanawaz et al., 2025). This definition emphasizes the external and esthetic function of cosmetic and cosmeceutical products. Subsequently, the term "cosmeceuticals" was introduced by Raymond Reed, a member of the US Society of Cosmetic Chemists, to describe products that exert specific, scientifically supported biological effects on the skin, such as antiaging, antiwrinkle, antioxidant, or skin-protective actions (Shahanawaz et al., 2025; Crespi et al., 2025; Bucur et al.,

2025). In contemporary practice, cosmetics mostly aim to enhance external appearance via topical application, including products like makeup, foundations, and mascaras. In contrast, cosmeceuticals are designed to induce measurable biological responses that result in skin improvements, such as antiaging, brightening, or firming effects, often achieved through the incorporation of bioactive ingredients, including peptides, biotics, and marine biopolymers (e.g., chitosan) in serums, creams, and oils (Baki, 2023; Badilli and Inal, 2025).

Green cosmetics, which currently represent a dominant consumer trend, refer to formulations developed using eco-friendly and sustainable manufacturing practices, with a reduced ecological footprint and an increased emphasis on ingredient traceability and biodegradability. These formulations typically incorporate naturally derived raw materials and minimize or exclude synthetic substances perceived as harmful to human health or the environment (Badilli and Inal, 2025; Dini and Laneri, 2021; Budzianowska et al., 2025; Mamta, 2025). Similarly, herbal cosmetics and cosmeceuticals constitute a related category, utilizing plant-based raw materials to confer functional properties such as antioxidant activity, moisturization, collagen-boosting, excess oil control, and antiaging effects. Their increasing popularity is often attributed to their natural origin and the perception of reduced adverse effects or allergic reactions (Shahanawaz et al., 2025; Iraqui and Das, 2022; Phatangre Piyal et al., 2023).

Recent technological advances have profoundly influenced cosmetic research, development, and effective consumer interaction. Artificial intelligence (AI) has emerged as a pivotal tool within the cosmetics industry, enabling the development of personalized skincare solutions tailored to individual consumer needs. By analyzing skin parameters, lifestyle factors, and environmental exposure, AI-driven platforms support customized product recommendations and formulation strategies (Di Guardo et al., 2025; Elder et al., 2024; Kania et al., 2024). Furthermore, augmented reality (AR) technologies have also gained prominence, particularly within e-commerce platforms, where virtual "try-on" tools allow consumers to evaluate cosmetic products digitally before purchase, enhancing user experience and decision-making processes. In addition, biotechnological innovations have enabled the formation of novel cosmetic ingredients, including bioengineered actives produced through sustainable and controlled processes, reducing reliance on nonrenewable resources and improving consistency and safety (Brancu and Turcu, 2025; Whang et al., 2021; Hemavathi et al., 2024). Interestingly, a 60% adoption of AI-related tools by cosmetic brands has been recorded, while 45% used AR digital tools, and 80% integrated e-commerce into their practices (Brancu and Turcu, 2025).

This chapter aims to provide a comprehensive overview of the growth, evolution, and current landscape of cosmetics and cosmeceuticals formulated with natural ingredients and bioactive agents. Emphasis is placed on key historical milestones, modern raw materials of natural origin, green extraction technologies, R&D strategies, regulatory frameworks, sustainability considerations, and advanced delivery systems designed to enhance stability, bioavailability, and skin performance. Furthermore, this review identifies current challenges and knowledge gaps related to standardization, safety assessment, efficacy substantiation, and consumer expectations, while efficiently pointing out future research directions and emerging technological trends.

2 Cosmetic and cosmeceutical market growth and drivers

2.1 Statistical overview of market size, CAGR, and regional trends in natural cosmetics and cosmeceuticals

As afore-mentioned, the global cosmetics and cosmeceuticals market continues to demonstrate sustained expansion, with natural and nature-inspired formulations representing one of the fastest-growing segments. Market analyses consistently indicate that natural cosmetics exhibit higher CAGR rates compared to conventional products, reflecting increasing consumer interest in safer, effective, sustainable, and ethical products, especially in the postcoronavirus disease-19 period (Shim et al., 2024; Lee and Kwon, 2022). This growth is notably evident in skincare and haircare categories, where the functional performance of natural bioactives can be directly associated with skin and scalp health benefits (Mondello et al., 2024).

From a regional perspective, Europe remains a mature, highly regulated market, characterized by strong consumer awareness, firm safety requirements, and widespread adoption of green practices. Northern European countries, in particular, show high per capita cosmetic consumption and an early adoption of natural and certified cosmetics and cosmeceuticals. The leading companies in cosmetics and beauty products are multinational corporations (e.g., L'Oréal, with revenue of USD 35 billion in 2021). However, small- and medium-sized enterprises (SMEs), which in Europe numbered 5800 in 2018, are significantly present, and in some countries, including France, they represent 80% of all cosmetic manufacturers. Moreover, at a European level, the cosmetic market is projected to register a CAGR of ~2.6% during the forecast period from 2022 to 2027, while globally it is expected to register a CAGR of ~5.5% during the 2021–2028 forecast period (Mondello et al., 2024).

North America represents another major market, driven by premium skincare demand, strong cosmeceutical positioning, and innovation-led brand strategies. In contrast, the Asia-Pacific region exhibits the most rapid growth rates, supported by growth in real incomes and wages, urbanization, demographic aging, and the merging of traditional botanical knowledge and modern cosmetic and cosmeceutical science (Nadeeshani Dilhara Gamage et al., 2022). China's cosmetics consumer market is the world's second largest, with retail sales of up to RMB 261.9 billion and a rising rate of 4.2% (2018), witnessing a boom in online sales of cosmetics of 25.3% (2018) since 2009, compared to other cosmetic market players like the United Kingdom (21.1%), the United States (10.9%), and Japan (J-beauty, 9.2%) (Akram et al., 2023). The Asia-Pacific cosmetics market was valued at USD 139.67 billion (2024) and is expected to reach USD 186.34 billion (2030) with a CAGR of 4.98% (TechSci Research, n.d.). From 2012 to 2018, the average annual growth rate of the Chinese cosmetics market was 6.52%, while the growth rate of Korean cosmetics imports in China was 14% in 2019 (Wang and Lee, 2021). Furthermore, South Korea's cosmetics market reached a value of ~USD 17.45 billion in 2024 and is projected to grow at a CAGR of 5.40% between 2025 and 2034, reaching a value of approximately USD 29.53 billion by 2034 (Expert Market Research, n.d.).

2.2 Factors driving the demand for natural cosmetics and cosmeceuticals

As technology continues to evolve, several natural alternatives are replacing synthetic ingredients used in the manufacturing of cosmetics and cosmeceuticals. Young consumers nowadays frequently prefer natural products not only for treating conditions like acne, dryness, or early aging but also for preventing their occurrence (Liu, 2022; Dini and Laneri, 2021; Mamta, 2025; Akram et al., 2023). Multiple interrelated factors contribute to the rising demand for natural cosmetics and cosmeceuticals. Heightened consumer awareness of ingredient safety and long-term health effects has encouraged scrutiny of formulation composition, particularly regarding synthetic colorants, preservatives, and fragrances (Wirtu, 2024; Alblooshi, 2025). Environmental concerns, such as climate change, biodiversity loss, and pollution, have further motivated consumers to seek sustainably sourced, eco-friendly processed, and reduced environmental footprint-related products (Wirtu, 2024; Weina and Yanling, 2022). In addition, compliance burdens and proactive sustainability strategies prompted manufacturers to reformulate existing products and shift their focus or invest in natural cosmetic alternatives (Couceiro et al., 2025).

Nowadays, digital transformation and social media platforms have amplified these trends by accelerating information distribution and dissemination, shaping consumer perception and perspectives, and promoting further transparency by using clear, certified cosmetic ingredient and agent labeling (Ngo et al., 2025). Interestingly, in an older survey conducted in ten community pharmacies in Naples, 98.5% of consumers reported that they have experienced at least one adverse cosmetic event (ACE), and 18.2% of them reported more than one event (Digiovanni et al., 2006). Recently, in a similar survey, 54.7% out of the 400 respondents used 1–2 cosmetics per day, with ~49% using them twice daily, whereas the most commonly used cosmetic products were makeup (35.9%) and personal care products (28%). A total of 132 respondents reported ACEs due to cosmetic use of ~ 33%), with the most commonly reported ACEs being itching (n = 58), redness (n = 59), and pimples (n = 42), related to skincare (~46%), haircare (~28.1%), and personal care products and formulations (17.3%) (Kumari et al., 2023).

2.3 Key market players in the natural cosmetics and cosmeceuticals sector

The natural cosmetics market is a diverse arena of competitors, where global giants and local startups exist side-by-side. This extensive mix of multinational conglomerates, including large-scale corporations, designated natural brands, independent specialist companies, SMEs, and emerging regional innovators, creates a unique balance: while the big players provide wide accessibility, smaller innovators drive the market forward with specialized, niche products (Dwivedi et al., 2025; Brancu and Turcu, 2025; Ngo et al., 2025).

Global conglomerates such as L'Oréal and Estée Lauder Companies Inc. have significantly expanded their presence in the natural cosmetic and cosmeceutical segment via brand acquisitions and dedicated product lines. For example, L'Oréal has aggressively extended its natural and botanical portfolio via luxury and mass-market extensions, while Estée Lauder's ownership, due to its strong botanical and plant-based ingredient incorporation, reflects its strategy to capture evolving consumer preferences for sustainable and naturally derived products (Eckelman et al., 2021; Martins and Marto, 2023). Furthermore, large consumer cosmetic goods firms and well-established natural/organic brands like Unilever PLC, Beiersdorf AG, Korres S.A., Laboratoires Nuxe S.A., and Yves Rocher have long operated with strong natural or botanical positioning, often supported by third-party certifications, as players that maintain high visibility, especially in Europe and North America (Eckelman et al., 2021; Martins and Marto, 2023; Lim and Kwon, 2023).

In addition to global and legacy brands, regionally focused and independent natural cosmetics companies play critical roles in shaping market niches (Huong et al., 2024; Nadeeshani Dilhara Gamage et al., 2022; Ngo et al., 2025).

Furthermore, independent and digital-native brands, along with various direct-to-consumer specialists, enhance competitiveness by mainly emphasizing transparency, ethical sourcing, and consumer engagement. Reviews indicate that the need for green and sustainable formulations, alongside ethical consciousness, transparency, and functional efficacy, is particularly prominent among younger demographics and socially engaged consumers, driving companies to adopt holistic value propositions focused on nature-based ingredients and agents and their vast incorporation in novel cosmetics and cosmeceuticals (Eckelman et al., 2021; Martins and Marto, 2023; Lim and Kwon, 2023).

3 Brief evolution of natural ingredients in cosmetics

From antiquity, natural substances derived from plants, animals, and minerals were extensively employed for beautification, skincare, and hygiene, often intertwined with medicinal and spiritual practices. Such early cosmetic rituals are deeply rooted in ethnopharmacological knowledge passed through generations via plain observation and empirical efficacy instead of regulated scientific validation. Ancient women, primarily, but men as well, used liquids, powders, or potions derived from natural sources in their daily routines for improving their appearance, cleaning their skin, masking their body odor, and toning their beauty characteristics. In ancient Egypt, women bathed in sour milk rich in lactic acid and α-hydroxy acids (AHAs), compounds currently recognized for their mild exfoliating, keratinolytic, and skin-renewing effects. Similarly, ancient Indian cosmetic rituals included the use of pumice and urine as facial scrubs. Urine, rich in urea, is well-established in dermatology for its soothing, humectant, and keratinoplastic effects (Liu, 2022; Diana Draelos, 2000; Nayak and Ligade, 2021).

Across cultures, botanicals rich in polyphenols were widely used for skin toning, pigmentation modulation, and haircare. Coffee, for instance, contains caffeic acid and caffeine, polyphenolic compounds with antioxidant, antiinflammatory, microcirculation-enhancing, and collagen-boosting properties. Currently, it is frequently incorporated into antiaging, anticellulite, and hair-growth-promoting cosmetic products (Liu, 2022; Dini and Laneri, 2021; Santos et al., 2021; Ruse et al., 2025). Other historically relevant botanicals and herbs include chamomile, aloe vera, henna, turmeric, and various essential oil-producing plants such as rosemary, which laid the groundwork for today's multifunctional cosmetic actives (Garbossa and Campos, 2016; Martínez-Burgos et al., 2022; Chen et al., 2016; Gopinath and Karthikeyan, 2017; José González-minero et al., 2020). These early applications, although empirical, laid the foundation for modern cosmetic science by identifying bioactive natural substances via repeated observation and use.

The transition toward modern cosmetic and cosmeceutical formulations represents a crucial shift in methodology. Modern cosmetic science has transformed the industry by refining traditional botanical extracts into purified active ingredients. This evolution has turned the "art" of traditional "trial-and-error" into a rigorous, evidence-based approach to beauty. This gradual shift was driven by the need for safety assurance, efficacy, reproducibility, and regulatory compliance. Advances in analytical chemistry enabled the identification of key bioactive constituents responsible for valuable cosmetic effects, such as flavonoids, phenolics, terpenes, alkaloids, and vitamins (Longo et al., 2022; Badilli and Inal, 2025; Gupta et al., 2022; Lartey, 2024; The Editors, 2022).

During the 20th century, extraction methods became increasingly refined, focusing on greener solvents and notably improving selectivity, yield, and safety (Ameer et al., 2017; Barba et al., 2016; Martins et al., 2023). The mass introduction of chromatographic and spectroscopic techniques, as well as the utilization of eco-friendly solvents and systems, allowed for structural elucidation and quantification of bioactives, improved quality control, batch-to-batch consistency, and dose-response evaluation, transforming cosmetics into industrially scalable formulations, supported by in vitro, in vivo, and clinical efficacy studies (Karageorgou et al., 2025; Alanazi, 2025). This period marked the recognition of cosmeceuticals, where natural bioactives were no longer included only for marketing appeal or beauty purposes but for their targeted antiaging, photoprotection, barrier repair, and inflammation modulation effects. This convergence of cosmetic and pharmaceutical principles established the foundation for modern dermocosmetics (Crespi et al., 2025; Badilli and Inal, 2025; Iraqui and Das, 2022; Phatangre Piyal et al., 2023; Gupta et al., 2022).

Contemporary cosmetic science has further transformed natural ingredients via the integration of pharmaceutical and biotechnological innovations. Modern delivery systems, including liposomes, microencapsulation, nanoencapsulation, nanoemulsions, lipid nanoparticles, nanofibers, polymeric matrices, or other similar carriers, have been and are currently being developed to enhance the stability, bioavailability, controlled release, and skin penetration of sensitive natural bioactives (e.g., vitamins, polyphenols, carotenoids) (Adamantidi et al., 2025; Papadopoulou et al., 2025a; Dini and Laneri, 2021). These technologies also enable dose reduction while maintaining efficacy, minimizing irritation, and improving consumer safety (Longo et al., 2022; Gupta et al., 2022). Moreover, biotechnological production and fermentation have also emerged as a sustainable alternative to traditional sourcing, enabling the production of high-purity bioactives, including hyaluronic acid, peptides, ceramides, and polysaccharides, while reducing both environmental impact and resource depletion (Dini and Laneri, 2021; Pérez-Rivero and Pablo López-gómez, 2023; Silva et al., 2025).

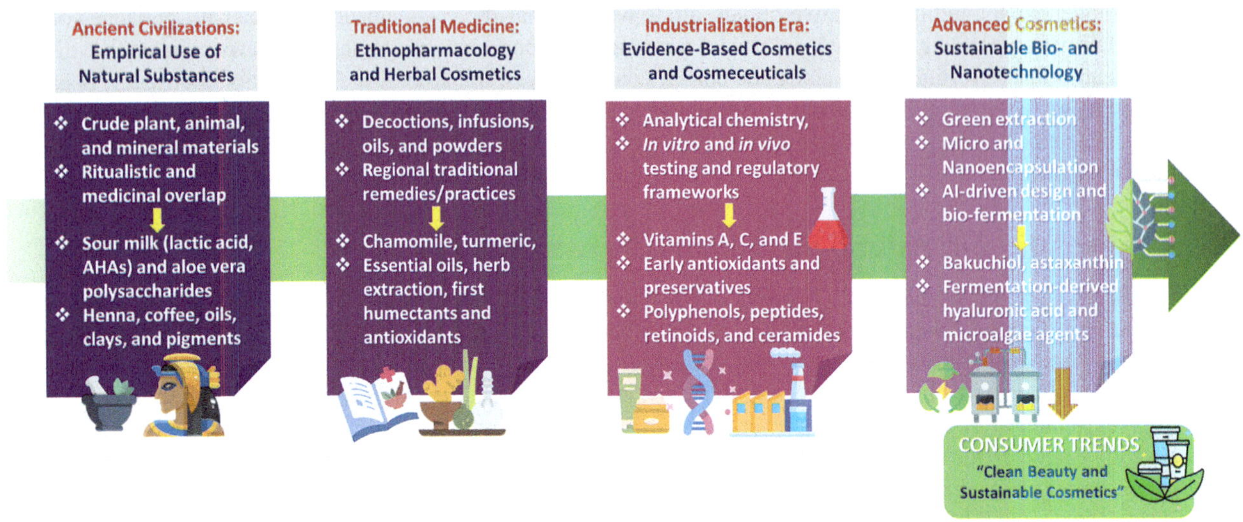

FIG. 28.3 Timeline of the evolution of natural bioactive ingredients in cosmetics. *(Parts of this figure were obtained from the open access free platform https://www.flaticon.com/ (Accessed 16 December 2025).)*

Collectively, these breakthroughs have enabled the evolution of natural cosmetics from simple, tradition-based remedies into technologically advanced, green, multifunctional, and performance-driven products aligned with modern global consumer expectations, regulatory requirements, clean-label trends, scientific validation, and sustainability goals. A timeline illustrating the evolution of natural bioactive ingredients in cosmetics, from empirical traditional practices to modern evidence-based, biotechnology-driven, and sustainable cosmetic science is presented in Fig. 28.3.

4 Natural cosmetic and cosmeceutical products: Common bioactive ingredients, agents, and indicative examples

The natural cosmetics market encompasses a broad array of product categories, reflecting the varied personal care needs of global consumers. Primary segments, mostly observed in both industry analyses and academic discussions, include skincare, haircare, makeup, fragrances, body-care, and specialized product lines such as baby-care, oral-care, and men's grooming products (Liu, 2022; Shahanawaz et al., 2025; Couceiro et al., 2025; Mondello et al., 2024).

Skincare remains the dominant category in the natural cosmetics sector, often accounting for over 50% of total product listings in global market inventories (Kumari et al., 2023). Skincare products such as soaps, creams, moisturizers, serums, toners, body lotions, makeup, nail-care products, sunscreens, and antiaging formulations often incorporate plant extracts, essential oils, antioxidants, vitamins, polyphenols, and several marine-derived agents due to their multifunctional benefits and natural efficacy claims (Adamantidi et al., 2025; de Groot and White, 2001; Amin et al., 2024; Tsoupras et al., 2024; Marra et al., 2024; Moysidou et al., 2024; Seferli et al., 2024; Tsiapali et al., 2025; Vandorou et al., 2024; Venetikidou et al., 2025; Papadopoulou et al., 2025b; Tsoupras et al., 2018; Shiels et al., 2022; Papikinou et al., 2024). Moreover, haircare follows as another major category, consisting of natural shampoos, conditioners, hair oils, scalp treatments, and styling products. These formulations often leverage botanical agents (e.g., argan oil, aloe vera, and herbal extracts) that efficiently address common concerns such as scalp sensitivity, hair breakage, and chemical avoidance, aligning with consumer demand for gentler cleansing systems and improved hair health (Pathak and Akhtar, 2019; Gubitosa et al., 2019).

Makeup and color cosmetics formulated with natural pigments, botanically derived waxes, and mineral bases have received notable attention over the past few years. While historically being less prevalent than skincare and haircare in the natural sector, botanical and mineral-based foundations, lipsticks, concealers, and eyeliners have shown increased visibility, particularly in premium and clean-label markets (Babich et al., 2025; Gălbău et al., 2024). Additional categories, such as fragrances, body-care products (e.g., scrubs, deodorants, body lotions), baby-care, oral-care, and men's grooming lines, are also integral components of the natural cosmetics portfolio (Liu, 2022; Shahanawaz et al., 2025; Babich et al., 2025; Gălbău et al., 2024).

From a chemical perspective, natural cosmetic bioactives can be classified into major groups, including polyphenols and phenolic acids, flavonoids, terpenes and terpenoids, carotenoids, peptides and proteins, vitamins, alkaloids, and polysaccharides. These natural cosmetic and cosmeceutical ingredients originate from diverse sources, including terrestrial plants, marine organisms, and microbial or biotechnological fermentation systems. Plant-derived extracts remain widely used due to their chemical diversity and consumer acceptance, while marine and microbial sources offer high-value bioactives with unique structural and functional properties, often produced through sustainable and controlled processes that still need to gain consumer acceptance (Liu, 2022; Shahanawaz et al., 2025; Shiels et al., 2022; Papikinou et al., 2024; Babich et al., 2025; Gălbău et al., 2024).

A key strategy for preventing pathological and physiological skin conditions, including acne, premature aging, and inflammation, is the control of oxidative stress. Reactive oxygen species (ROS), generated endogenously or through environmental exposure [e.g., ultraviolet (UV) radiation and pollution], disrupt the skin microbiome and compromise skin barrier integrity, ultimately triggering inflammatory responses. Antioxidants, whether synthetic or naturally derived, act as a predominant defense mechanism by neutralizing ROS, promoting cellular repair via extracellular matrix (ECM) support, and minimizing inflammation (Budzianowska et al., 2025). In addition to antioxidants, chelating agents aim to bind trace metal ions originating from water, stainless-steel processing equipment, or storage containers, thus preventing undesirable phenomena like discoloration, malodor, or final product haze. Chelators also enhance preservative efficacy by reducing metal-catalyzed oxidative reactions. Ethylenediaminetetraacetic acid (EDTA) remains the most widely used synthetic chelating agent, whereas sodium phytate and its derivatives represent effective natural alternatives increasingly adopted in green cosmetics and cosmeceuticals (Baki, 2023; Varvaresou et al., 2009). Representative examples of natural bioactives and their cosmetic functions are discussed in the following subsections. Table 28.1 represents an overview of the functional categories of natural cosmetic agents and their biological roles, while Fig. 28.4 illustrates the structures of the main representatives of each class.

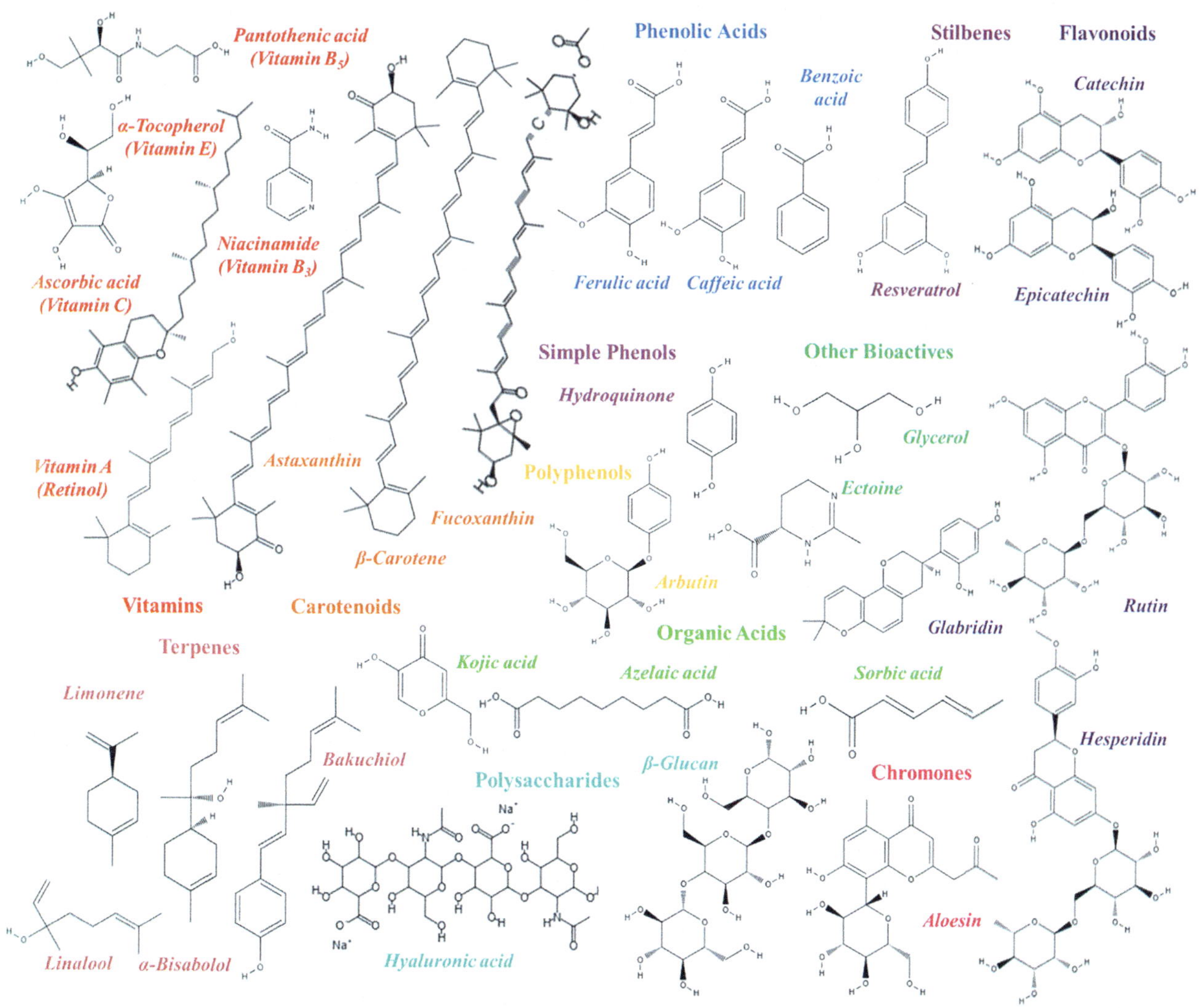

FIG. 28.4 Main representatives of each class of bioactives used in natural cosmetics and cosmeceuticals. *(Some structures were obtained from the open access free platform https://www.molview.org/ (Accessed 16 December 2025).)*

TABLE 28.1 Overview of functional categories of natural cosmetic ingredients and their biological roles.

Functional agent category	Primary biological functions	Representative natural bioactives/sources	References
Natural antioxidants and antipollution agents	Neutralization of ROS, mitigation of oxidative stress, protection against pollution-induced damage, antiinflammatory activity, and cellular repair	• Vitamins C, E, A, and B_5 • Polyphenols (ferulic acid) • Stilbenes (resveratrol) • Flavonoids (hesperidin, catechins) • Carotenoids (astaxanthin, β-carotene, fucoxanthin) • Marine antioxidants	(Dini and Laneri, 2021; Budzianowska et al., 2025; Adamantidi et al., 2025; Hoang et al., 2021; Khan et al., 2019; Chrysikopoulou et al., 2025; Al-Niaimi and Chiang, 2017; Quan, 2023; Wang et al., 2020; Lin et al., 2005; Leszczyński et al., 2025; Rodrigues and Pintado, 2024; Lee et al., 2015; Swagata Dutta and Banerjee, 2023; Arct and Mieloch, 2016; Stahl, 2012; Bakar and Setapar, 2025; Tavares et al., 2020)
Moisturizing, humectant, and barrier repair agents	Enhancement of stratum corneum hydration, lipid barrier restoration, reduction of transepidermal water loss (TEWL), and microbiome support	• Aloe vera polysaccharides • Marine polysaccharides (alginates, carrageenans) • Glycerol (natural origin) • Hyaluronic acid (biotechnologically fermented) • β-Glucans • Ceramides • Plant oils (jojoba and argan oils) • Microalgae lipids	(Liu, 2022; Silva et al., 2025; Madnani et al., 2024; Mawazi et al., 2022a; Matei et al., 2025; Çerçi et al., 2025; Zhu et al., 2025; Jabłonowska et al., 2021; Wei et al., 2024; Sousa et al., 2023; Feng et al., 2025; Schild et al., 2024; Chinjoo and Golzary, 2025; Favas et al., 2021; Gad et al., 2021; Ghannam et al., 2023; Gharby and Charrouf, 2022)
Antiaging and skin-rejuvenating agent	Stimulation of collagen and elastin synthesis, inhibition of MMPs, enhancement of epidermal renewal, and antiinflammatory protection	• Retinoids, retinol, retinal, and retinaldehyde • Bakuchiol • Niacinamide • α-Hydroxy acids • Bioactive peptides • Phytoestrogens and marine extracts	(Budzianowska et al., 2025; Adamantidi et al., 2025; Bjørklund et al., 2022; Beibei et al., 2025; Chaudhuri and Bojanowski, 2014; Iliopoulos et al., 2020; Karwal and Mukovozov, 2023; Tang et al., 2025; van Walraven et al., 2025; Amini et al., 2025; Koukouraki et al., 2020)
Skin-soothing, antiinflammatory, and sensitive skin agents	Modulation of inflammatory mediators, reduction of redness and irritation, wound healing, and barrier recovery	• Chamomile (α-bisabolol) • Calendula and *Centella asiatica* • Avenanthramides • Turmeric, green tea, apple, kiwi, avocado, grape, wine, and tomato extracts • Aloe vera-derived aloesin	(Marra et al., 2024; Moysidou et al., 2024; Tsiapali et al., 2025; Vandorou et al., 2024; Fowler et al., 2010; Batovska et al., 2025; Silva et al., 2021; Kim et al., 2023; Ejiohuo and Folami, 2024; Handayani et al., 2025; Park, 2021; Kang et al., 2018; Kim et al., 2021b; Rapti et al., 2024; Gianeti et al., 2013; Vandorou et al., 2025; Moysidou et al., 2025; Marra et al., 2025; Choleva et al., 2019; Karantonis et al., 2023; Kontaxi et al., 2024; Tsoupras et al., 2023; Abdel-Wahab et al., 2024)
Skin-brightening and pigmentation-modulating agents	Inhibition of tyrosinase activity, suppression of melanogenesis, photoprotection, and antioxidant activity	• Vitamins C derivatives • Kojic and azelaic acid • Arbutin • Licorice extract (glabridin) • Hydroquinone • Aloe vera-derived aloesin	(Liu, 2022; Chrysikopoulou et al., 2025; Al-Niaimi and Chiang, 2017; Matei et al., 2025; Abdel-Wahab et al., 2024; Couteau and Coiffard, 2016; Feng et al., 2024; Saeedi et al., 2019; Sallustio et al., 2025; Boo, 2021)
Antimicrobial, preservative, and preservative-boosting agents	Microbial growth inhibition, product stabilization, metal-ion chelation, and oxidative degradation prevention	• Essential oils (tea tree, thyme) • Organic acids (benzoic and sorbic acids) • Phenolic acids (caffeic acid) • Sodium phytate	(Herman, 2019; Hosni et al., 2013; Kairey et al., 2023; Pazyar et al., 2013; Jalil et al., 2024; Kim et al., 2025; Tang and Du, 2024; Saad et al., 2005; Bouaouz et al., 2026)
Emollients, emulsifiers, and texture-modifying agents	Sensory properties improvement, emulsion stability, spreadability, and formulation esthetics	• Plant oils and butters (shea and cocoa butter) • Beeswax and candelilla wax • Lecithin and saponins • Polysaccharides (xanthan gum)	(Cortes et al., 2024; Wongwad et al., 2025; Oliver and Kenzie, 2024)

TABLE 28.1 Overview of functional categories of natural cosmetic ingredients and their biological roles–cont'd

UV-protective and photoprotective agents	Absorption of UV radiation, reduction of photoinduced oxidative stress, and inflammation mitigation	• Polyphenols and phenolic acids (ferulic acid) • Flavonoids (rutin, catechins) • Mycosporine-like amino acids (ectoine) • Marine-derived UV-active filters • Botanical sun protection factor (SPF) extracts	(Jesus et al., 2023; Milutinov et al., 2024; Urrea-Victoria et al., 2025)
Fragrance, sensory, and consumer-experience agents	Enhancement of sensory appeal, fragrance delivery, secondary antioxidant, and antimicrobial effects	• Essential oils • Terpenes (linalool, limonene) • Natural aromatic extracts	(Rodriguez et al. (2023); Rong et al., 2025)

4.1 Natural antioxidants and antipollution agents

A fundamental strategy for preventing both pathological and natural skin conditions, such as acne, photoaging, and premature aging, is the mitigation of oxidative stress. ROS species disrupt skin barrier integrity, damage the skin microbiome, and promote inflammatory responses. Hence, antioxidants, whether synthetic or naturally derived, act as defense mechanisms by neutralizing ROS, promoting cellular repair, and combating inflammation (Hoang et al., 2021). Natural antioxidants commonly incorporated in cosmetic and cosmeceutical formulations include vitamins C, E, and A; polyphenols like ferulic acid; stilbenes like resveratrol; carotenoids such as astaxanthin (ASX) and β-carotene; flavonoids, including hesperidin or catechins; and several marine antioxidants like fucoxanthin (Hoang et al., 2021; Khan et al., 2019).

Vitamins, especially in their esterified form, are preferred due to their increased stability (Dini and Laneri, 2021). Vitamin C (ascorbic acid) and its derivatives are widely used for skin brightening, photoprotection, collagen synthesis stimulation, and prevention of hyperpigmentation. These properties are linked to their role in crossing the blood-brain barrier in oxidized form through glucose transporters, while maintaining their antioxidant capacity within the central nervous system (Dini and Laneri, 2021; Budzianowska et al., 2025; Adamantidi et al., 2025; Chrysikopoulou et al., 2025; Al-Niaimi and Chiang, 2017). Vitamin E (alpha-tocopherol) contributes to antiaging primarily by free radical scavenging (Budzianowska et al., 2025), while vitamin A (retinol) and its derivatives (retinal and retinaldehyde), the first vitamins approved by the Food and Drug Administration (FDA), exhibit well-established wrinkle-reducing and skin-smoothing effects. Topical retinol triggers glycosaminoglycan formation, enhances epidermal barrier function, increases resistance to environmental stressors, and promotes angiogenesis, leading to improved skin tone and texture (Budzianowska et al., 2025; Adamantidi et al., 2025; Quan, 2023). Vitamin B_5 (pantothenic acid), a component of coenzyme A, plays a central role in protein, lipid, and carbohydrate metabolism. In skincare, it regulates sebum production and exhibits moisturizing and antiinflammatory properties, while in haircare, it promotes hair growth, prevents split ends, enhances shine and tone, and contributes to hair detangling and smoothness manageability (Budzianowska et al., 2025; Wang et al., 2020).

Polyphenols are widely recognized for their antioxidant ability, neutralizing free radicals, and providing several neuroprotective, anticancer, antiaging, cardioprotective, and antidiabetic effects (Budzianowska et al., 2025). Phenolic acids, like ferulic acid, exert antioxidant ability through structural stabilization of free radicals, reduction of oxidative stress, and inhibition of thymidine dimer formation, thus protecting against DNA damage (Budzianowska et al., 2025; Lin et al., 2005; Leszczyński et al., 2025). Ferulic acid is frequently employed in formulations targeting acne, skin discoloration, wrinkle reduction, elasticity improvement, inflammation alleviation, and aging process downregulation, while strengthening skin barrier function against oxidative stress (Budzianowska et al., 2025; Lin et al., 2005; Leszczyński et al., 2025). Flavonoids, including hesperidin and catechins, may play critical roles in cosmetic formulations. Hesperidin, an orange-derived polyphenol, acts as a ROS scavenger and photoprotective agent, reducing epidermal thickening and modulating angiogenesis- and melanogenesis-related pathways. For example, hydrogels formulated with nanolipid carriers infused with hesperidin presented a 99% absorption of UVB radiation and 83% absorption of UVA radiation (Budzianowska et al., 2025; Rodrigues and Pintado, 2024; Lee et al., 2015).

Carotenoids such as ASX, β-carotene, and fucoxanthin provide exceptional antioxidant and photoprotective effects. ASX, naturally sourced from yeast, microalgae (mainly *Haematococcus pluvialis*), and bacteria, exhibits superior thermal and photostability and greater antioxidant activity than vitamins E and C and β-carotene. Its lipophilic nature facilitates penetration into the stratum corneum, where it reduces transepidermal water loss (TEWL), accelerates cell renewal, and promotes collagen synthesis and elastin (Budzianowska et al., 2025; Swagata Dutta and Banerjee, 2023). β-Carotene (found in fruits and vegetables) and fucoxanthin (present in several algae and seaweeds) are also potent antioxidants, capable of neutralizing singlet oxygen and decreasing UV-induced skin aging (Adamantidi et al., 2025; Arct and Mieloch, 2016; Stahl, 2012; Bakar and Setapar, 2025; Tavares et al., 2020).

4.2 Moisturizing, humectant, and barrier repair agents

Skin hydration and barrier integrity are essential determinants of skin health and appearance. Natural moisturizing agents are capable of increasing water retention in the stratum corneum, reinforcing lipid organization and the skin barrier, reducing TEWL, and providing microbiome support (Madnani et al., 2024). Widely used natural humectants and barrier-supporting agents, highly relevant in formulations targeting dry, sensitive, or compromised skin and symptoms of xerosis, inflammatory dermatoses, and aging-related barrier impairment, are aloe vera and marine polysaccharides, sorbic acid, glycerol of natural origin, hyaluronic acid produced by biotechnological fermentation, β-glucans, ceramides, and plant oils rich in essential fatty acids such as jojoba and argan oil (Liu, 2022; Madnani et al., 2024; Mawazi et al., 2022a).

Aloe vera polysaccharides and marine-derived polysaccharides (e.g., alginate from *Sargassum vulgare*, carrageenans from red seaweeds) exhibit strong humectant and film-forming properties, enabling prolonged hydration and soothing effects (Matei et al., 2025; Çerçi et al., 2025; Zhu et al., 2025). Glycerol of natural origin (e.g., *Silybum marianum*) remains a gold-standard humectant due to its ability to regulate aquaporin-3 expression, thereby facilitating water transport across epidermal layers and offering high-value antiaging effects (Jabłonowska et al., 2021). Furthermore, hyaluronic acid produced via biotechnological fermentation from, for instance, *Streptococcus,* enhances hydration at multiple molecular weights, contributing both to broad surface moisturization and deeper dermal water retention (Silva et al., 2025; Wei et al., 2024). Yeast-derived β-glucans further support barrier recovery by triggering keratinocyte proliferation and boosting innate immune defense, proving effective toward wound healing and atopic dermatitis treatment (Sousa et al., 2023; Feng et al., 2025). Moreover, ceramides (Schild et al., 2024), plant oils such as jojoba and argan oil (Gad et al., 2021; Ghannam et al., 2023; Gharby and Charrouf, 2022), and microalgae and cyanobacteria extracts (Papadopoulou et al., 2025b; Chinjoo and Golzary, 2025; Favas et al., 2021) abundant in essential fatty acids and polar lipids (e.g., polyunsaturated fatty acids like eicosapentaenoic acid and docosahexaenoic acid), restore lipid skin architecture, improve skin elasticity, and enhance resistance against environmental aggressors.

4.3 Antiaging and skin-rejuvenating agents

Antiaging remains one of the most dominant functional claims in the cosmetic and dermatocosmetic market. Natural antiaging agents act through multiple pathways, including the stimulation of collagen and elastin synthesis, the inhibition of matrix metalloproteinases (MMPs), the enhancement of cell turnover, and protection from oxidative or chronic low-grade inflammation. Representative examples include retinoids and retinol alternatives (e.g., bakuchiol), niacinamide, AHAs, peptides, phytoestrogens, and collagen-boosting botanical and marine algae extracts (Bjørklund et al., 2022).

Retinoids (Adamantidi et al., 2025) and retinol alternatives, such as bakuchiol, promote collagen synthesis while minimizing irritation, a benefit often associated with conventional retinoids. Bakuchiol, a plant meroterpene with a retinol-like activity, is capable of regulating the production of three collagen types, inhibiting melanogenesis, and improving skin photoaging, all while being more effective than retinol. Nowadays, it is widely preferred as a natural alternative to retinol in cosmeceuticals, following the trends and the need for seeking more natural, green alternatives (Budzianowska et al., 2025; Beibei et al., 2025; Chaudhuri and Bojanowski, 2014). Niacinamide (vitamin B_3) topical delivery improves barrier function, lowers hyperpigmentation occurrence, and enhances dermal ECM integrity through elevated ceramide production, offering significant antiaging benefits (Iliopoulos et al., 2020). Similarly, AHAs, such as glycolic and lactic acid, promote controlled exfoliation and stimulate epidermal renewal, providing improved skin texture and stimulating collagen synthesis and elastin preservation (Karwal and Mukovozov, 2023). In addition, bioactive peptides, particularly signal peptides (e.g., hexapeptide-12 and 10) and carrier peptides [e.g., tripeptide-1 like the glycyl-histidyl-lysine, (GHK), tripeptide-3 like the alanine-histidine-lysine (AHK)], stimulate fibroblast activity and ECM production (Tang et al., 2025; van Walraven et al., 2025). Finally, phytoestrogens (e.g., *Glycyrrhiza uralensis* extract) and collagen-boosting botanical and marine algae (e.g., *Spirulina platensis* extract) or fungi (e.g., β-glucan from *Rhodotorula* sp. DAMB1) extracts contribute to improved skin firmness, wrinkle depth reduction, and the restoration of a youthful skin appearance (Papikinou et al., 2024; Amini et al., 2025; Koukouraki et al., 2020).

4.4 Skin-soothing, antiinflammatory, and sensitive-skin agents

Natural antiinflammatory agents are essential in products designed for sensitive, irritated, or postprocedure skin. Botanical extracts such as chamomile (rich in α-bisabolol), calendula, *Centella asiatica*, oat-derived avenanthramides, turmeric extract, green tea, apple or grape extract, and aloe vera exhibit soothing, antiredness, and wound healing effects. These ingredients modulate proinflammatory mediators such as tumor necrosis factor α (TNF-α) and interleukins (e.g., IL-6) and support skin recovery while maintaining consumer preference for mild formulations (Fowler et al., 2010; Batovska et al., 2025; Silva et al., 2021; Kim et al., 2023).

Chamomile (*Matricaria chamomilla*) extract, rich in α-bisabolol, exhibits potent antiirritant, antiinflammatory, and wound healing properties (Batovska et al., 2025). Calendula (Ejiohuo and Folami, 2024) and *C. asiatica* (Handayani et al., 2025; Park, 2021) (asiaticoside-abundant) promote collagen synthesis, scar modulation, barrier support, photoaging suppression, and accelerated wound closure, making them versatile therapeutics against skin diseases and melanoma risk. Oat-derived avenanthramides, furthermore, reveal markedly strong antipruritic and antiinflammatory effects by inhibiting nuclear factor-kappa B (NF-κB) signaling, while also restoring skin barrier activity by modulating the expression of epidermal differentiation (Kim et al., 2023; Kang et al., 2018; Kim et al., 2021b). Turmeric extract (curcuminoids) (Rapti et al., 2024), green tea catechins (Gianeti et al., 2013), apple polyphenols (Vandorou et al., 2024, 2025), kiwi flavonoids (Moysidou et al., 2024, 2025), avocado phenolic acids and flavonoid derivatives (Marra et al., 2024, 2025), as well as bioactive constituents from tomato, wine, and grape pomace, further suppress proinflammatory mediators such as TNF-α and IL-6 (Tsiapali et al., 2025; Choleva et al., 2019; Karantonis et al., 2023; Kontaxi et al., 2024; Tsoupras et al., 2023). Interestingly, formulations using green tea extract exert vast moisturizing effects, reducing skin redness and roughness, while also providing antiacne and hair growth benefits as a result of epigallocatechin-3-gallate's activity (Budzianowska et al., 2025). Finally, aloe vera, containing aloesin, offers skin-lightening, soothing, and antiinflammatory properties by inhibiting melanogenesis, stimulating fibroblast proliferation, minimizing tyrosinase and 3,4-dihydroxyphenylalanine polymerase action, and supporting postinflammatory skin recovery. It also provides humectant and moisturizing benefits, decreasing TEWL and promoting water retention in the stratum corneum (Dini and Laneri, 2021; Matei et al., 2025; Abdel-Wahab et al., 2024).

4.5 Skin-brightening and pigmentation-modulating agents

Uneven skin tone and hyperpigmentation are common cosmetic and cosmeceutical concerns. Natural skin-brightening agents function primarily by inhibiting tyrosinase expression, suppressing melanin synthesis, or offering antioxidant-mediated photoprotection. Common examples include vitamin C and its derivatives, hydroquinone, kojic acid, azelaic acid, arbutin, licorice extract (glabridin), and aloesin from aloe vera (Couteau and Coiffard, 2016).

Vitamin C and its stabilized derivatives reduce melanin synthesis and promote a more uniform skin tone and texture, offering antiacne benefits (Chrysikopoulou et al., 2025; Al-Niaimi and Chiang, 2017). In addition, similar activity is expressed by azelaic acid, also used for acne, rosacea, or melasma treatment due to its inhibitory activity against tyrosinase and mitochondrial oxidoreductase, as it interferes with DNA synthesis and reduces free radical production (Liu, 2022; Feng et al., 2024). Recently, fungi-extracted kojic acid has gained vast attention, being effective at low doses and acting as a melanin suppressor, tyrosinase inhibitor, and antioxidant agent (Liu, 2022; Saeedi et al., 2019). Licorice extract, particularly glabridin, exhibits strong depigmenting and antiinflammatory benefits, whereas arbutin functions as a competitive inhibitor of melanin production (Couteau and Coiffard, 2016; Sallustio et al., 2025; Boo, 2021). In addition, hydroquinone (primarily derived from *Agaricus hondensis* mushrooms) is used in skin-bleaching products, hair dyes, and fingernail treatments due to its exceptional skin-whitening properties (Matsumoto et al., 2016). Aloesin, extracted from aloe vera, further suppresses melanogenesis through tyrosinase inhibition and cytoprotective activity, proving effective against skin discoloration and related diseases (Dini and Laneri, 2021; Matei et al., 2025; Abdel-Wahab et al., 2024).

4.6 Antimicrobial, preservative, and preservative-boosting agents

Microbial stability is critical for cosmetic product safety and shelf life. Natural antimicrobial agents, including essential oils, phenolic compounds, and organic acids, are increasingly employed as effective alternatives or even complements to conventional preservatives. Chelating agents play critical additional roles by binding metal ions originating from water, processing equipment, or packaging materials, preventing potential discoloration, malodor, haze formation, and oxidative degradation. While EDTA remains the most common synthetic chelator, natural alternatives such as sodium phytate and its derivatives are gaining attention due to their biodegradability and preservative-boosting capacity. Well-known and preferred natural antimicrobial, preservative, and preservative-boosting agents include tea tree oil and thyme (*Thymus vulgaris*) extracts, benzoic and sorbic acids, as well as a plethora of phenolic compounds like caffeic acid (Herman, 2019).

Essential oils, such as tea tree oil and wild thyme (*Thymus serpyllum* L.) extracts, exhibit broad-spectrum antimicrobial action against bacteria, yeasts, viruses, and molds by participating in membrane disruption and enzyme inhibition (Hosni et al., 2013; Kairey et al., 2023; Pazyar et al., 2013; Jalil et al., 2024). Organic acids, including benzoic and sorbic acid, function as pH-dependent antimicrobials, while phenolic compounds, such as caffeic acid, also confer antimicrobial, antioxidant, cytoprotective, and preservation-based activity (Kim et al., 2025; Tang and Du, 2024; Saad et al., 2005; Bouaouz et al., 2026).

4.7 Emollients, emulsifiers, and texture-modifying agents

Beyond biological activity, natural ingredients contribute significantly to formulation esthetics, rheology, and sensory performance. Plant oils and butters, like shea or cocoa butter, provide occlusive and emollient effects, enhancing skin softness and elasticity. Natural waxes, such as beeswax and candelilla wax, improve formulation structure and stability. Lecithin and saponins function as natural emulsifiers, while polysaccharides, like xanthan gum, act as thickeners and stabilizers. These ingredients collectively influence spreadability, absorption, and skin feel, contributing significantly to consumer acceptance and current clean-label formulation strategies (Cortes et al., 2024; Wongwad et al., 2025; Oliver and Kenzie, 2024).

4.8 UV-protective and photoprotective agents

Although organic and inorganic UV filters remain regulated, several natural compounds provide complementary phytotherapeutic and photoprotective effects. Polyphenols and phenolic acids, such as ferulic acid, enhance UV defense by scavenging free radicals generated by radiation exposure. Flavonoids like rutin and catechins absorb UV radiation and mitigate oxidative damage. Mycosporine-like amino acids, such as ectoine, and marine-derived UV filters, like oxybenzone, exhibit exceptional UV-absorbing capacity and cellular protection. Botanical extracts with high sun protection factor properties further enhance UV photoprotection by reducing photoinduced oxidative stress, inflammation, and oxidative damage (Jesus et al., 2023; Milutinov et al., 2024; Urrea-Victoria et al., 2025).

4.9 Fragrance, sensory, and consumer experience agents

Fragrance and sensory agents notably influence consumer perception and product acceptance. Essential oils, terpenes like linalool and limonene, and natural aromatic extracts offer characteristic scent profiles while simultaneously contributing antioxidant, antimicrobial, and soothing properties. However, these ingredients require careful formulation due to potential allergenicity considerations and regulatory restrictions. Modern cosmetic science increasingly focuses on balancing sensory appeal with safety, stability, and compliance, integrating fragrance agents that enhance the consumer experience without compromising skin tolerance or product integrity (; Rong et al., 2025).

5 Research and development trends regarding the use of natural bioactives in cosmetic and cosmeceutical formulations

5.1 Advances in extraction technologies of natural bioactives for cosmetic use

Extraction represents a pivotal step in the valorization of natural raw materials, as it directly determines the yield, purity, stability, and bioactivity of cosmetic and cosmeceutical bioactives. Conventional extraction methods, widely employed for cosmetic purposes, such as maceration or Soxhlet extraction, suffer from long processing times, high solvent consumption, and mass thermal degradation of thermolabile bioactives (Bisht et al., 2025; Bitwell et al., 2023; Ćujić et al., 2016; Boufetacha et al., 2025). Consequently, modern cosmetic R&D tends to adopt intensified, sustainable, and green extraction methodologies (Ameer et al., 2017; Martins et al., 2023; Dini and Laneri, 2021).

Ultrasound-assisted extraction (UAE) enhances mass transfer via acoustic cavitation, leading to cell wall disruption and improved release of intracellular compounds. UAE is particularly useful for the extraction of thermolabile constituents, including polyphenols, flavonoids, and carotenoids, while enabling reduced solvent usage and extraction duration (Armaly et al., 2022; Tiwari, 2015; Chanioti and Tzia, 2019; Dzah et al., 2020). Microwave-assisted extraction exploits dielectric heating to rapidly increase internal pressure within plant matrices, allowing for the efficient extraction of polar and moderately polar compounds with high reproducibility (Alara et al., 2021; Costa et al., 2025; da Rosa et al., 2019; Dumpler and Moraru, 2024). Moreover, enzyme-assisted extraction further improves selectivity by degrading cell wall polysaccharides, facilitating the release of bound bioactives under mild conditions, thus being especially suitable for polysaccharides, proteins, and phenolic compounds (Hosni et al., 2013; Domínguez-Rodríguez et al., 2021; Gligor et al., 2019).

Pressurized liquid extraction and supercritical fluid extraction (SFE) represent advanced solvent-based technologies offering superior extraction efficacy (Boufetacha et al., 2025; Alonso-Salces et al., 2001; Çam and Hışıl, 2010; Mantiniotou et al., 2025; Chai et al., 2020; Difonzo et al., 2021). SFE, commonly employing supercritical carbon dioxide (SFE-CO_2), is frequently preferred for the extraction of lipophilic constituents such as essential oils, terpenes, and carotenoids (e.g., ASX), while avoiding the use of toxic, nonsustainable organic solvents. SFE-CO_2, usually combined with green co-solvents such as ethanol, enables selective, less time-consuming, and high-yield extraction, while aligning with clean-label and global sustainability demands (Chai et al., 2020; Kehili et al., 2017; Kyriakoudi et al., 2024; Mihalcea et al., 2021).

One of the most promising developments is the use of natural deep eutectic solvents (NADES), composed of naturally occurring components such as organic acids, amino acids, sugars, and choline derivatives, for extraction purposes. NADES exhibit low volatility, high solvating capacity for polar and nonpolar agents, and notable biocompatibility, making them suitable as both extraction media and formulation components (Vieira et al., 2022; Bedair et al., 2024; Grozdanova et al., 2020; Szopa et al., 2024). Furthermore, adopting generally recognized as safe ingredients and biodegradable agents has become popular over the past few years. Green formulation strategies generally include solvent minimization, energy-efficient processing, renewable raw material sourcing, and the replacement of petrochemical-derived ingredients with plant-, marine-, or fermentation-based alternatives, following the principles of life-cycle assessment (LCA) (Di Guardo et al., 2025; Couceiro et al., 2025; Sasounian et al., 2024).

5.2 Encapsulation and delivery systems for natural bioactives

One of the major limitations associated with the incorporation of natural bioactives into cosmetic and cosmeceutical formulations is their intrinsic instability, low aqueous solubility, volatility, and susceptibility to oxidation, photodegradation, and hydrolysis. In addition, several natural agents exhibit limited skin penetration, primarily due to the high selectivity of the stratum corneum. To overcome these challenges, advanced encapsulation and delivery systems have gained significant attention in modern cosmetic and cosmeceutical R&D. Microencapsulation and nanoencapsulation technologies, which function by entrapping bioactive compounds with micro- and nanostructured carriers, respectively, protect sensitive compounds from oxidation, light, and thermal degradation, while enabling sustained and targeted release. Widely employed delivery systems in cosmetic and cosmeceutical applications include liposomes, niosomes, nanoemulsions, solid lipid nanoparticles (SLNs), nanostructured lipid carriers (NLCs), polymeric nanoparticles, cyclodextrin inclusion complexes, and biopolymer-based microcapsules (Mihalcea et al., 2021; Bińkowska et al., 2024; Casanova and Santos, 2016; Soh and Lee, 2019; Suganya and Anuradha, 2017; Budryn et al., 2016; Mahmoud et al., 2018; Gutiérrez-Álzate et al., 2024).

Liposomes composed of phospholipids and niosomes comprising nonionic surfactant bilayers are among the most frequently used cosmetic carriers. Due to their structural similarity to biological membranes, liposomes and niosomes facilitate enhanced skin penetration and controlled release of hydrophilic and lipophilic natural agents. Liposomal systems have been mainly studied for their efficacy in the delivery of vitamin C derivatives, polyphenols, flavonoids, and botanical extracts, demonstrating improved stability and increased deposition in the viable epidermis (Chen et al., 2017; Caddeo et al., 2008; Halevas et al., 2022; Mawazi et al., 2022b). In addition, nanoemulsions represent another versatile delivery platform that exhibits high kinetic stability, large interfacial area, and excellent sensory properties, being effective for the delivery of essential oils, carotenoids (e.g., ASX), stilbenes like resveratrol, and cosmetic agents of high applicability, such as curcumin, as enhancers of skin hydration and photoprotection (Baccarin et al., 2015; Butnariu and Giuchici, 2011; Gupta et al., 2016; Jiang et al., 2020; Rachmawati et al., 2016). Importantly, lipid-based nanocarriers like SLNs and NLCs offer additional benefits by forming occlusive films on the skin surface, thereby notably limiting TEWL, while enabling sustained release of encapsulated bioactives. These systems are particularly suitable for lipophilic agents such as retinoids, tocopherols, coenzyme Q10, phytosterols, and plant-derived oils, contributing to improved antiaging, barrier repair, photoprotective, and moisturizing effects (Gad et al., 2019; Katopodi et al., 2023; Pinna et al., 2023; Okonogi and Riangjanapatee, 2015; de Souza Guedes et al., 2021; Godase et al., 2024).

Cyclodextrins and their derivatives are increasingly applied as molecular carriers useful for the entrapment of volatile, unstable, or poorly soluble natural agents. By forming inclusion complexes, cyclodextrins enhance solubility and stability, as well as provide odor masking for compounds, including terpenes, essential oil constituents, and phenolic acids, while also enabling both sustained release and minimized skin irritation (Aksamija et al., 2016; Cid-Samamed et al., 2022; Žiemytė et al., 2023). Recently, biopolymer-based encapsulation systems like chitosan, alginate, gelatin, cellulose derivatives (e.g., carboxymethylcellulose), and protein–polysaccharide complexes have received notable attention due to their marked biodegradability, biocompatibility, and sustainability. Such systems are especially effective for the encapsulation of plant or herb extracts, peptides, probiotics, and postbiotics, supporting microbiome-friendly cosmetic concepts and prolonged skin residence time (Çerçi et al., 2025; Abdel-Wahab et al., 2024; Archana and Joydeep Dutta, 2013; Benlloch-Tinoco et al., 2025; Bayat et al., 2023; ALKaisy et al., 2023; Costa et al., 2023; Hendawy et al., 2023).

Beyond classical encapsulation, stimuli-responsive and smart delivery systems like hydrogels are emerging as next-generation cosmetic and cosmeceutical technologies. Such systems are mainly designed for releasing bioactives in response to specific external triggers, such as pH, temperature, enzymatic activity, inflammation, or oxidative stress, allowing targeted and effective agent delivery, promising for antiaging, acne, and sensitive skin formulations (Costa et al., 2025; Ahmad et al., 2022; Bustamante-Torres et al., 2021; Fan et al., 2023). An overview of the dominant encapsulation and advanced delivery systems used for the integration of natural bioactives in cosmetic and cosmeceutical formulations is illustrated in Fig. 28.5.

5.3 Omics and AI in natural ingredient discovery

The recent integration of omics technologies and AI is transforming natural ingredient discovery and cosmetic/cosmeceutical breakthroughs. Metabolomics, genomics, proteomics, and transcriptomics enable the holistic profiling of plant, microbial, and marine sources, accelerating the identification of novel bioactives, their mechanisms of action, and hidden potential (Akhter Bhat et al., 2025; de Falco et al., 2022; García-Pérez et al., 2024; Jianbiao and Jia, 2022). Moreover, robust efficacy validation remains critical, as the variability of natural raw materials complicates both standardization and reproducibility, further necessitating rapid quality control, scientifically validated analytical methods, compliance with

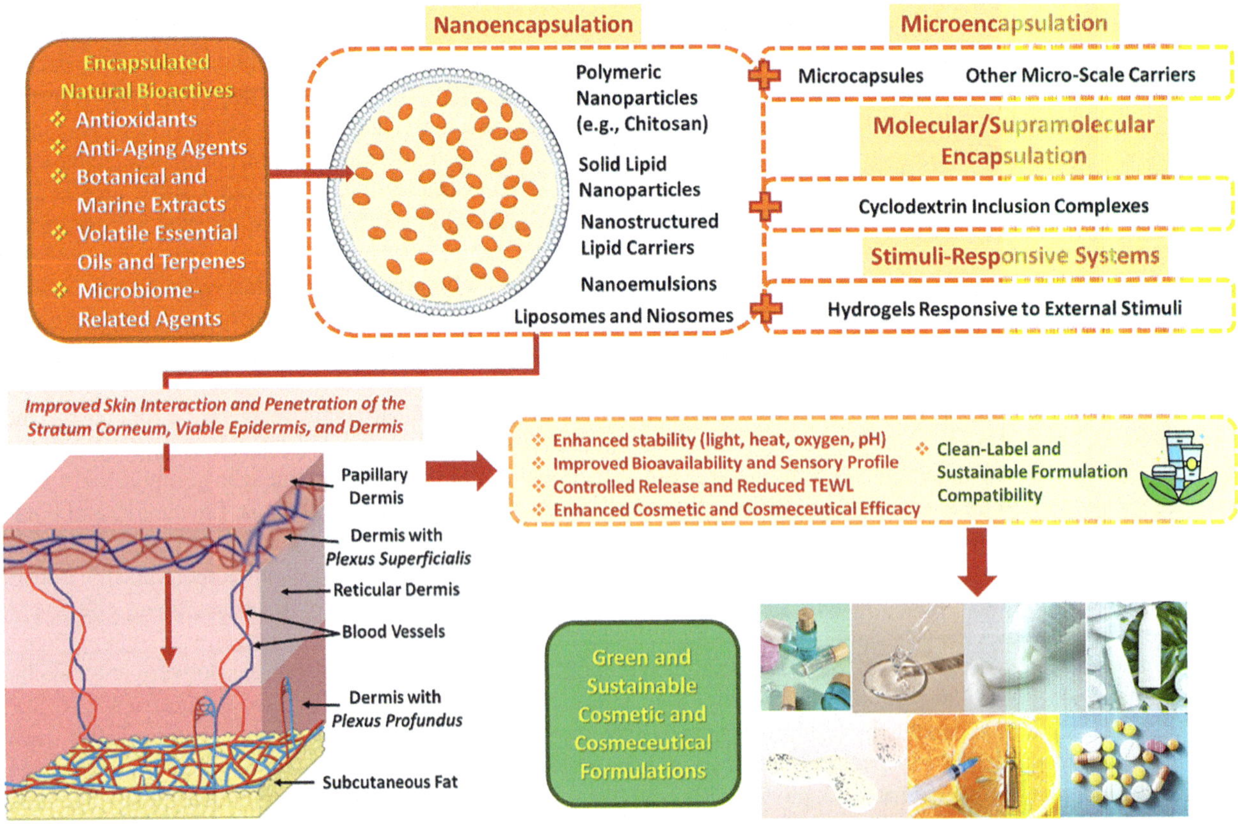

FIG. 28.5 Schematic representation of the encapsulation and delivery systems used for natural bioactives in cosmetics and cosmeceuticals. *(Parts of this figure were obtained from the open access free platform https://www.freepik.com/ (Accessed 16 December 2025).)*

regulatory frameworks, well-designed in vitro, ex vivo, and clinical studies, and data transparency (Gharby and Charrouf, 2022; García-Pérez et al., 2024; Dai et al., 2023).

6 Regulatory landscape and safety, ethical, and sustainability considerations regarding the use of natural bioactives in cosmetics and cosmeceuticals

6.1 Regulatory frameworks and categorization of cosmetic products and formulations

To ensure safety, efficacy, and compliance, cosmetics or cosmeceuticals are regulated under distinct legislative frameworks worldwide. The major markets include the European Union (EU), the United States, Canada, Brazil, China, and Japan, each applying specific regulatory approaches and competent authorities (Ferreira et al., 2022; Crespi et al., 2025; Di Guardo et al., 2025; Couceiro et al., 2025). In the EU, cosmetics are governed by Regulation (EC) No. 1223/2009, which replaced Directive 76/768/EC and established a harmonized regulatory framework across all EU Member States. This regulation introduced premarket safety assessment, mandatory Product Information Files, Cosmetic Product Safety Reports (CPSRs), responsible person designation, postmarket surveillance, and a centralized notification system through the Cosmetic Product Notification Portal. This framework ensures consumer protection and regulatory consistency, while prohibiting animal testing for cosmetic agents and finished products (Turcu and Brancu, 2025; The Editors, 2022).

In the United States, cosmetics are regulated by the FDA under the Federal Food, Drug, and Cosmetic Act (FD&C Act). Cosmetics do not require premarket approval, except for color additives. However, manufacturers are legally responsible for ensuring product safety and labeling compliance (Ferreira et al., 2022; Office of the Commissioner, 2024; Program, 2025; Wells, 2023). The Modernization of Cosmetics Regulation Act (MoCRA, 2022) notably expanded FDA authority by introducing mandatory facility registration, careful product listing, and adverse event reporting (Ferreira et al., 2022; Office of the Commissioner, 2024; Program, 2025; Wells, 2023). Meanwhile, in Canada, cosmetics are governed by the FD&C Act and Cosmetic Regulations, requiring product notification via the Cosmetic Notification Form. Canada additionally recognized Natural Health Products (NHPs) as a distinct category for cosmeceutical products (Yadav et al., 2025).

In China, cosmetic regulation was recently restructured with the introduction of the Cosmetic Supervision and Administration Regulation (CSAR) in 2021, replacing the previous Cosmetics Hygiene Supervision Regulations. Oversight is conducted by the National Medical Products Administration, as CSAR led to ingredient novelty classification (Zhe et al., 2020). Furthermore, in Japan, cosmetics are regulated under the Pharmaceuticals and Medical Devices Law by the Ministry of Health, Labor, and Welfare, where products are categorized as either cosmetics or quasi-drugs (referring to cosmeceuticals) (Ferreira et al., 2022; Rai and Rath, 2026; Inomata, 2014; bindusahithi et al., 2025). Finally, in Brazil, cosmetics are regulated by the Brazilian Health Regulatory Agency and the Hygiene, Perfume, Cosmetics, and Sanitizing Products Management, following directives such as RDC 07/2015 and 36/1999. They are classified as Grade 1 or Grade 2 products based on formulation complexity and intended use, with higher-risk products subject to registration and enhanced safety documentation (Ferreira et al., 2022; Sailaja et al., 2022).

Product categorization also differs substantially across regulatory systems. In the EU, the classification is determined by intended use and mode of action, with clear differentiation of cosmetic formulations from medicinal products, biocides, and medical devices. In the United States, under the FD&C Act, products are classified as cosmetics or drugs, with over-the-counter (OTC) drugs constituting a regulated subcategory. In Canada, products may be classified as cosmetics, OTC drugs, or NHPs, depending on claims and composition. In addition, in Japan, beauty products are categorized into cosmetics and quasi-drugs, with the latter functioning as an intermediate class, while China and Brazil apply risk-based or function-based subcategorization models. Alongside regulatory classifications, voluntary certification schemes (e.g., COSMOS, ECOCERT, NATRUE) have emerged to define "natural" and "organic" cosmetics. Nevertheless, these schemes still lack legal harmonization and regulatory compliance (Ferreira et al., 2022; The Editors, 2022; Pathak and Akhtar, 2019; Wells, 2023; Zhe et al., 2020; Rai and Rath, 2026; bindusahithi et al., 2025).

6.2 Safety assessment, packaging, labeling, claims, and greenwashing risks

Safety assessment is a core regulatory requirement for cosmetics and cosmeceuticals. In the EU, a CPSR, including ingredient toxicology, exposure assessment, safety measurements, microbiological quality, impurity profiling, and packaging compatibility, is mandatory and must be prepared by a qualified assessor before the product is available on the market (Turcu and Brancu, 2025; The Editors, 2022). It must be pointed out that animal testing is prohibited in the EU, highlighting the reliance on in vitro, in vivo, ex vivo, and clinical testing skin models for ensuring product safety and efficacy (Turcu and Brancu, 2025; The Editors, 2022). Safety evaluation and quality control, however, are notably hindered by chemical complexity, batch-to-batch variability, potential allergenicity, and the presence of heavy metals and contaminants (Turcu and Brancu, 2025; The Editors, 2022).

After addressing product safety, efficacy, and reproducibility, the final step of introducing a cosmetic or cosmeceutical product into the market is the correct and transparent packaging and labeling system. Formal packaging must ensure product stability, microbiological safety, and shelf-life compatibility, while addressing sustainability principles and consumer compliance (Regulation (EC) No. 1223/2009). Moreover, ingredient labeling across major markets follows the International Nomenclature of Cosmetic Ingredients system. Notably, claims associated with cosmetic products must be truthful and evidence-based, without misleading public concerns or implying pharmacological activity. Consumer perception has become a key driver of formulation and marketing strategies, reinforcing the need for transparent communication, scientific validation, and regulatory alignment to maintain consumer trust and market integrity (Ferreira et al., 2022; Morel et al., 2024; Schneider, 2009; Omira et al., 2025).

The growing emphasis on "natural," "green," "cruelty-free," "paraben-free," and "clean-label" cosmetics has increased the risk of greenwashing, as companies use marketing tools to make themselves or their products look more environmentally friendly than they actually are. Such marketing claims lack specific or regulatory substantiation and have prompted stricter claim governance, particularly in the EU and China, where efficacy data and documented evidence are required for functional and environmental claims before market availability (Bozza et al., 2022; Suphasomboon and Vassanadumrongdee, 2025).

6.3 Sustainability and ethical considerations

Sustainability and ethical responsibility have gained increasing attention regarding cosmetic regulation, particularly toward natural bioactive integration into cosmetics and cosmeceuticals. Regulatory authorities carefully inspect both human safety and eco- and socio-ethical implications, considering ingredient sourcing, extraction methods, processing techniques, and postconsumer fate. Sustainable sourcing of natural bioactive agents is critical to prevent biodiversity loss or ecosystem degradation due to resource depletion. Sustainable sourcing according to regulatory legislations must include renewable cultivation, controlled and sustained harvesting, biotechnological fermentation, or agricultural by-product valorization (Pérez-Rivero and Pablo López-gómez, 2023; Silva et al., 2025; Rai and Rath, 2026; Bozza et al., 2022; Rocca et al., 2022; Alviri et al., 2025). Moreover, environmental impact and biodegradability, especially concerning aquatic toxicity, persistence, and bioaccumulation risk, further imply the need for comprehensive environmental risk assessments (Wirtu, 2024; Couceiro et al., 2025; Nurkolis, 2025; Ceschin et al., 2021).

LCA is progressively adopted as a decision-support tool to evaluate the overall environmental footprint of cosmetics and cosmeceuticals, encompassing raw material extraction, processing, formulation, packaging, labeling, market distribution, shelf-life evaluation, and end-of-life disposal. Interestingly, ingredient choice, dosage, and formulation may improve the sustainability of cosmetics and cosmeceuticals (Secchi et al., 2016). Notably, ethical supply chains and fair-trade practices are particularly relevant for botanicals and marine-derived bioactives sourced from developing regions, necessitating transparent sourcing, respect for indigenous knowledge/practices, and compliance with international legislations (Nurkolis, 2025; Secchi et al., 2016; Machado et al., 2024).

7 Limitations, challenges, and future perspectives

Despite the rapid expansion of cosmetics and cosmeceuticals formulated with natural bioactives, several scientific, technological, regulatory, and market-driven limitations persist. One of the most evident challenges is market saturation, driven by the growing number of brands attempting to align with "natural," "clean," or "green" beauty trends. This intense competition often leads to limited product differentiation, exaggerated marketing claims, and difficulties in substantiating efficacy, ultimately increasing regulatory scrutiny and consumer skepticism (Brancu and Turcu, 2025; Shim et al., 2024; Bom et al., 2019).

A major scientific limitation associated with natural ingredients is their extensive variability and reduced physicochemical stability. Natural bioactive agents are often sensitive to light, oxygen, pH, and temperature fluctuations, leading to degradation, loss of activity, and shortened shelf life. Batch-to-batch variability arising from differences in plant origin, cultivation conditions, and extraction methods further complicates standardization and reproducibility (Couceiro et al., 2025; Aguilar-Toalá et al., 2019). In contrast, synthetic alternatives frequently offer high purity, stability, and cost-effectiveness, highlighting the necessity of a balanced, evidence-based, and effective integration of natural and synthetic components rather than an exclusive reliance on natural origin alone (Aguilar-Toalá et al., 2019; Bandyopadhyay et al., 2025; Ugoeze and Odeku, 2022). Another key challenge concerns the validation of efficacy and safety. While many natural bioactives demonstrate promising in vitro or preclinical activity, translation into clinically meaningful cosmetic and cosmeceutical results remains limited due to insufficient human studies and a lack of standardized protocols. The growing demand for strong claim substantiation, especially in the EU and China, necessitates more thorough clinical evaluation strategies, long-term safety data, and harmonized regulatory systems (Bozza et al., 2022; Suphasomboon and Vassanadumrongdee, 2025; Ugoeze and Odeku, 2022).

The rise of personalized skincare presents both opportunities and challenges. Advances in digital diagnostics, skin imaging, wearable sensors, and AI-driven data analysis have led to the creation of specialized formulations addressing individual skin traits, lifestyle factors, and environmental exposure (Di Guardo et al., 2025; Elder et al., 2024; Kania et al., 2024; Mantiniotou et al., 2025; Markiewicz and Idowu, 2018; Kim et al., 2021a). However, personalization significantly increases formulation complexity, production costs, data privacy concerns, and regulatory ambiguity, particularly when personalized products approach therapeutic claims (Markiewicz and Idowu, 2018; Kim et al., 2021a). From a technological standpoint, the integration of biotechnology and synthetic biology in cosmetics and cosmeceuticals was crucial. Microbial biotechnological fermentation (Pérez-Rivero and Pablo López-gómez, 2023; Silva et al., 2025), enzyme-assisted synthesis (Domínguez-Rodríguez et al., 2021; Gligor et al., 2019; Gonçalves, 2021), and genetically optimized platforms (Wei et al., 2024; Bayır et al., 2025) enable the sustainable production of high-purity agents with reduced environmental impact and improved reproducibility. Nevertheless, mass regulatory acceptance, public perception, and production scalability are still important limiting factors that must be addressed via transparent communication and regulatory guidance (Yadav et al., 2025; Rai and Rath, 2026; Machado et al., 2024; Bom et al., 2019; Markiewicz and Idowu, 2018).

Sustainability considerations further complicate product development. While consumer demand for eco-friendly yet effective formulations continuously rises, green packaging, transparent labeling, biodegradable materials, and circular economy principles increase production costs and supply chain complexity. LCAs reveal that natural ingredients do not automatically guarantee formulation safety and sustainability, reinforcing the need for a holistic evaluation of all product aspects before market availability, rather than claim-driven formulation strategies (Bucur et al., 2025; Martins and Marto, 2023; Morel et al., 2024; Omira et al., 2025; Secchi et al., 2016; Markiewicz and Idowu, 2018).

Looking forward, significant research gaps remain, particularly regarding long-term safety, environmental fate, microbiome interactions, and synergistic effects between bioactives and delivery systems. Strengthening the collaboration between academia and industry will be essential to bridge the gap between fundamental research and scalable innovation, ensuring that future cosmetic and cosmeceutical products are scientifically validated, economically viable, and eco-responsible.

8 Conclusions

The cosmetics and cosmeceuticals industry has recently undergone substantial growth and transformation, driven by increasing consumer demand for clean-label products formulated with natural ingredients and bioactive compounds. Advances in extraction technologies, green chemistry, biotechnology, encapsulation delivery systems, and digital tools have significantly expanded the functional potential of natural bioactives, enabling the development of multifunctional products targeting skin health, aging prevention, and personalized care.

However, the future success of natural bioactive-based cosmetics and cosmeceuticals relies on scientific novelty, regulatory compliance, and sustainability-driven innovation rather than plain marketing trends. Addressing challenges related to stability, standardization, efficacy validation, personalization, and environmental impact is vital for creating the next generation of cosmetic and dermatocosmetic products. By integrating R&D strategies, responsible sourcing, advanced delivery technologies, and compliance with transparent regulatory frameworks, the industry will be able to ensure the safety, efficacy, and sustainability of cosmetics and cosmeceuticals that ideally meet both global societal needs and consumer expectations.

Acknowledgments

The authors would like to thank the School of Chemistry in the Faculty of Sciences at Democritus University of Thrace for their continuous support.

Conflicts of interest

The authors declare no conflicts of interest.

Funding

This research received no external funding.

Author contributions

A.T. was involved in conceptualization, methodology, validation, supervision, and project administration. A.T., M.-P.L., and T.A. were involved in investigation, writing—review and editing, and visualization. All authors contributed to software and writing—original draft preparation and have read and agreed to the published version of the manuscript.

References

Abdel-Wahab, B.A., Haque, A., Alotaibi, H.F., Alasiri, A.S., Elnoubi, O.A.E., Ahmad, M.Z., Pathak, K., Albarqi, H.A., Walbi, I.A., Wahab, S., 2024. Eco-friendly green synthesis of silver nanoparticles utilizing olive oil waste by-product and their incorporation into a chitosan-aloe vera gel composite for enhanced wound healing in acid burn injuries. Inorg. Chem. Commun. 13877003. 165, 112587. doi:10.1016/j.inoche.2024.112587.

Adamantidi, T., Lafara, M.-P., Venetikidou, M., Likartsi, E., Toganidou, I., Tsoupras, A., 2025. Utilization and bio-efficacy of carotenoids, vitamin A and its vitaminoids in nutricosmetics, cosmeceuticals, and cosmetics' applications with skin-health promoting properties. Appl. Sci. 2076-3417. 15 (3), 1657. doi:10.3390/app15031657.

Aguilar-Toalá, J.E., Hernández-Mendoza, A., González-Córdova, A.F., Vallejo-Cordoba, B., Liceaga, A.M., 2019. Potential role of natural bioactive peptides for development of cosmeceutical skin products. Peptides. 01969781. 122, 170170. doi:10.1016/j.peptides.2019.170170.

Ahmad, Z., Salman, S., Khan, S.A., Amin, A., Rahman, Z.U., Al-Ghamdi, Y.O., Akhtar, K., Bakhsh, E.M., Khan, S.B., 2022. Versatility of hydrogels: from synthetic strategies, classification, and properties to biomedical applications. Gels. 2310-2861. 8 (3), 167. doi:10.3390/gels8030167.

Akhter Bhat, T., Rather, R.A., Bashir, S., Mishra, N.-S., John, R., 2025. Nanoparticles in plant systems: omics-based perspectives on stress adaptation and toxicological implications. Plant Nano Biol. 27731111. 13, 100181. doi:10.1016/j.plana.2025.100181.

Akram, U., Ansari, A.R., ulhaq, I., Yan, C., 2023. Cosmetics makers have always sold 'hope in a jar'! Understanding the cosmetics purchase intention in the Chinese mobile commerce environment. J. Retail. Consum. Serv. 09696989. 73, 103337. doi:10.1016/j.jretconser.2023.103337.

Aksamija, A., Polidori, A., Plasson, R., Dangles, O., Tomao, V., 2016. The inclusion complex of rosmarinic acid into beta-cyclodextrin: a thermodynamic and structural analysis by NMR and capillary electrophoresis. Food Chem. 03088146. 208, 258–263. doi:10.1016/j.foodchem.2016.04.008.

Al-Niaimi, F., Chiang, N.Y.Z., 2017. Topical Vitamin C and the skin: mechanisms of action and Clinical applications. J. Clin. Aesthet. Dermatol. 19412789. 10 (7), 14–17. Available from: http://jcadonline.epubxp.com/t/9606-journal-of-clinical-And-Aesthetic-dermatology.

Alanazi, S., 2025. Recent advances in liquid chromatography–mass spectrometry (LC–MS) applications in biological and applied sciences. Anal. Sci. Adv. 2628-5452. 6 (1). doi:10.1002/ansa.70024.

Alara, O.R., Abdurahman, N.H., Ali, H.A., Zain, N.M., 2021. Microwave-assisted extraction of phenolic compounds from Carica papaya leaves: an optimization study and LC-QTOF-MS analysis. Future Foods 26668335. 3. Available from: https://www.journals.elsevier.com/future-foods. doi:10.1016/j.fufo.2021.100035.

Alblooshi, S., 2025. The impact of perfumes and cosmetic products on human health: a narrative review. Front. Toxicol. 2673-3080. 7. doi:10.3389/ftox.2025.1646075.

ALKaisy, Q.H., Al-Saadi, J.S., AL-Rikabi, A.K.J., Altemimi, A.B., Hesarinejad, M.A., Abedelmaksoud, T.G., 2023. Exploring the health benefits and functional properties of goat milk proteins. Food Sci. Nutr. 20487177. 11 (10), 5641–5656. Available from: https://onlinelibrary.wiley.com/journal/10.1002/%28ISSN%292048-7177. doi:10.1002/fsn3.3531.

Alonso-Salces, R.M., Korta, E., Barranco, A., Berrueta, L.A., Gallo, B., Vicente, F., 2001. Pressurized liquid extraction for the determination of polyphenols in apple. J. Chromatogr. A. 00219673. 933 (1-2), 37–43. doi:10.1016/s0021-9673(01)01212-2.

Alviri, H., Lynes, J., Habib, K., 2025. Beyond green chemistry: a comprehensive review of how sustainability has been integrated into cosmetic research. Glob. Sustain. 2059-4798. 8. doi:10.1017/sus.2025.5.

Ameer, K., Shahbaz, H.M., Kwon, J.H., 2017. Green extraction methods for polyphenols from plant matrices and their byproducts: a review. Compr. Rev. Food Sci. Food Saf. 15414337. 16 (2), 295–315. Available from: http://www.interscience.wiley.com/jpages/1541-4337. doi:10.1111/1541-4337.12253.

Amin, R., Völzer, B., Genedy-Kalyoncu, M.E., Blume-Peytavi, U., Kottner, J., 2024. Skin care types, frequencies and products: a cross-sectional study in German institutional long-term care. J. Tissue Viability. 0965206X. 33 (2), 318–323. doi:10.1016/j.jtv.2024.02.005.

Amini, N., Osterlund, C., Curpen, J., Lafon-Kolb, V., Richard, T., Visdal-Johnsen, L., 2025. Phytoestrogens as natural anti-aging solutions for enhanced collagen synthesis in skin. J. Cosmet. Dermatol. 1473-2130. 24 (2). doi:10.1111/jocd.16719.

Archana, D., Joydeep Dutta, P.K.D., 2013. Evaluation of chitosan nano dressing for wound healing: characterization, in vitro and in vivo studies. Int. J. Biol. Macromol. 01418130. 57, 193–203. doi:10.1016/j.ijbiomac.2013.03.002.

Arct, J., Mieloch, M., 2016. β-carotene in skin care. Pol. J. Cosmetol. 19 (6), 206–213.

Armaly, Z., Abu-Rahme, M., Kinaneh, S., Hijazi, B., Habbasshi, N., Artul, S., 2022. An innovative ultrasound technique for early detection of kidney dysfunction: superb microvascular imaging as a reference standard. J. Clin. Med. 2077-0383. 11 (4), 925. doi:10.3390/jcm11040925.

Babich, O., Ivanova, S., Bakhtiyarova, A., Kalashnikova, O., Sukhikh, S., 2025. Medicinal plants are the basis of natural cosmetics. Process Biochem. 13595113. 154, 35–51. doi:10.1016/j.procbio.2025.04.009.

Baccarin, T., Mitjans, M., Ramos, D., Lemos-Senna, E., Vinardell, M.P., 2015. Photoprotection by *Punica granatum* seed oil nanoemulsion entrapping polyphenol-rich ethyl acetate fraction against UVB-induced DNA damage in human keratinocyte (HaCaT) cell line. J. Photochem. Photobiol. B Biol. 10111344. 153, 127–136. doi:10.1016/j.jphotobiol.2015.09.005.

Badilli, U., Inal, O., 2025. Current approaches in cosmeceuticals: peptides, biotics and marine biopolymers. Polymers. 2073-4360. 17 (6), 798. doi:10.3390/polym17060798.

Bakar, M.F.A., Setapar, S.H.M., 2025. Fucoxanthin: an emerging ingredient in cosmeceutical applications. J. Dermatol. Sci. Cosmet. Technol. 2950306X. 2 (2), 100085. doi:10.1016/j.jdsct.2025.100085.

Baki, G., 2023, Introduction to Cosmetic Formulation and Technology, second ed., John Wiley & Sons, Inc., Hoboken, NJ.

Bandyopadhyay, A., Selvan, S.A., Patial, P.K., Pal, T., 2025. Plant-based ingredients in cosmetic science: current applications, limitations, and prospects. Int. J. Cosmet. Sci. 14682494. Available from: http://onlinelibrary.wiley.com/journal/10.1111/(ISSN)1468-2494. doi:10.1111/ics.70034.

Barba, F.J., Zhu, Z., Koubaa, M., Sant'Ana, A.S., Orlien, V., 2016. Green alternative methods for the extraction of antioxidant bioactive compounds from winery wastes and by-products: a review. Trends Food Sci. Technol. 09242244. 49, 96–109. Available from: http://www.elsevier.com/wps/find/journaldescription.cws_home/601278/description#description. doi:10.1016/j.tifs.2016.01.006.

Batovska, D., Panova, N., Gerasimova, A., Tumbarski, Y., Ivanov, I., Dincheva, I., Yotkovska, I., Gentscheva, G., Nikolova, K., 2025. Chamomile matters: species- and producer-dependent variation in Bulgarian *Matricaria recutita* L. and *Chamaemelum nobile* L. essential oils and their cosmetic potential. Cosmetics. 2079-9284. 12 (3), 123. doi:10.3390/cosmetics12030123.

Bayat, G., Fallah-Darrehchi, M., Zahedi, P., Moghaddam, A.B., Ghaffari-Bohlouli, P., Jafari, H., 2023. Kiwi extract-incorporated poly(ε-caprolactone)/cellulose acetate blend nanofibers for healing acceleration of burn wounds. J. Biomater. Sci. Polym. Ed. 0920-5063. 34 (1), 72–88. doi:10.1080/09205063.2022.2110483.

Bayır, A., Saoula, S., Almansour, A., Wang, D., Bayır, M., Uzun, B.N., Turhan, S., Arslan, H., Arslan, G., 2025. CRISPR-based genetic improvement of aquaculture species. Fishes. 2410-3888. 10 (2), 84. doi:10.3390/fishes10020084.

Bedair, H.M., Samir, T.M., Mansour, F.R., 2024. Antibacterial and antifungal activities of natural deep eutectic solvents. Appl. Microbiol. Biotechnol. 14320614. 108 (1). Available from: https://www.springer.com/journal/253. doi:10.1007/s00253-024-13044-2.

Beibei, L., Wang, Z., Ying, X., Liu, Y., Ruan, B., Zhang, J., Zhang, J., Zhang, J., Zhang, T., 2025. Anti-aging and anti-inflammatory fulfilled through the delivery of supramolecular bakuchiol in ionic liquid. Supramol. Mater. 26672405. 4, 100093. doi:10.1016/j.supmat.2025.100093.

Benlloch-Tinoco, M., Gentile, P., Taylor, L., Girón-Hernández, J., 2025. Alginate edible films as delivery systems for green tea polyphenols. Food Hydrocoll. 0268005X. 158, 110518. doi:10.1016/j.foodhyd.2024.110518.

bindusahithi, L., Varadi Keerthika, V.N.L., Rajeswari, A.V.S., 2025. A comprehensive study on quasi-drugs regulations in Japan and South Korea. Int. J. Res. Publ. Rev. 25827421. 6 (8), 4051–4058. doi:10.55248/gengpi.6.0825.3106.

Bińkowska, W., Szpicer, A., Stelmasiak, A., Wojtasik-Kalinowska, I., Półtorak, A., 2024. Microencapsulation of polyphenols and their application in food technology. Appl. Sci. 2076-3417. 14 (24), 11954. doi:10.3390/app142411954.

Bisht, A., Sahu, S.C., Kumar, A., Maqsood, S., Barwant, M.M., Jaiswal, S.G., 2025. Recent advances in conventional and innovative extraction techniques for recovery of high-added value compounds for food additives and nutraceuticals. Food Phys. 29500699. 2, 100047. doi:10.1016/j.foodp.2025.100047.

Bitwell, C., Indra, S.S., Luke, C., Kakoma, M.K., 2023. A review of modern and conventional extraction techniques and their applications for extracting phytochemicals from plants. Sci. Afr. 24682276. 19, e01585. doi:10.1016/j.sciaf.2023.e01585.

Bjørklund, G., Shanaida, M., Lysiuk, R., Butnariu, M., Peana, M., Sarac, I., Strus, O., Smetanina, K., Chirumbolo, S., 2022. Natural compounds and products from an anti-aging perspective. Molecules. 1420-3049. 27 (20), 7084. doi:10.3390/molecules27207084.

Bom, S., Jorge, J., Ribeiro, H.M., Marto, J., 2019. A step forward on sustainability in the cosmetics industry: a review. J. Clean. Prod. 09596526. 225, 270–290. doi:10.1016/j.jclepro.2019.03.255.

Boo, Y.C., 2021. Arbutin as a skin depigmenting agent with antimelanogenic and antioxidant properties. Antioxidants. 2076-3921. 10 (7), 1129. doi:10.3390/antiox10071129.

Bouaouz, S., Lozano, R., Bravo, F.I., Muguerza, B., Mulero, M., Calvo, E., Ortega, P., de la Mata, F.J., 2026. Caffeic acid–functionalized silver nanoparticles for skin therapy: antioxidant, antibacterial, and anti-melanogenic properties. J. Drug Deliv. Sci. Technol. 17732247. 116, 107937. doi:10.1016/j.jddst.2025.107937.

Boufetacha, M., Gharibi, E., Benali, M., 2025. Optimising supercritical carbon dioxide extraction of rosmarinic acid from *Rosmarinus officinalis* L. and enhancing yield through soxhlet coupling. Processes. 2227-9717. 13 (3), 655. doi:10.3390/pr13030655.

Bozza, A., Campi, C., Garelli, S., Ugazio, E., Battaglia, L., 2022. Current regulatory and market frameworks in green cosmetics: the role of certification. Sustain. Chem. Pharm. 23525541. 30, 100851. doi:10.1016/j.scp.2022.100851.

Brancu, C., Turcu, O., 2025. Exploring the economic performance and market trends in the cosmetics industry: insights and analysis. Bus. Manag. Compass. 3033-0106. 69 (3), 23–32. doi:10.56065/e31nkk40.

Bucur (Popa), R.M., Stanescu, S.G., Radulescu, C., Banica, A.L., Stirbescu, R.M., 2025. Consumer habits and practices for cosmetics: a statistical approach. J. Sci. Arts. 2068-3049. 25 (2), 415–430. doi:10.46939/j.sci.arts-25.2-b03.

Budryn, G., Zaczyńska, D., Oracz, J., 2016. Effect of addition of green coffee extract and nanoencapsulated chlorogenic acids on aroma of different food products. LWT. 00236438. 73, 197–204. doi:10.1016/j.lwt.2016.06.019.

Budzianowska, A., Banaś, K., Budzianowski, J., Kikowska, M., 2025. Antioxidants to defend healthy and youthful skin—current trends and future directions in cosmetology. Appl. Sci. 2076-3417. 15 (5), 2571. doi:10.3390/app15052571.

Bustamante-Torres, M., Romero-Fierro, D., Arcentales-Vera, B., Palomino, K., Magaña, H., Bucio, E., 2021. Hydrogels classification according to the physical or chemical interactions and as stimuli-sensitive materials. Gels. 2310-2861. 7 (4), 182. doi:10.3390/gels7040182.

Butnariu, M.V., Giuchici, C.V., 2011. The use of some nanoemulsions based on aqueous propolis and lycopene extract in the skin's protective mechanisms against UVA radiation. J. Nanobiotechnol. 14773155. 9. Available from: http://www.jnanobiotechnology.com/content/9/1/3. doi:10.1186/1477-3155-9-3Romania.

Caddeo, C., Teskač, K., Sinico, C., Kristl, J., 2008. Effect of resveratrol incorporated in liposomes on proliferation and UV-B protection of cells. Int. J. Pharm. 03785173. 363 (1-2), 183–191. doi:10.1016/j.ijpharm.2008.07.024.

Çam, M., Hışıl, Y., 2010. Pressurised water extraction of polyphenols from pomegranate peels. Food Chem. 03088146. 123 (3), 878–885. doi:10.1016/j.foodchem.2010.05.011.

Casanova, F., Santos, L., 2016. Encapsulation of cosmetic active ingredients for topical application-a review. J. Microencapsul. 14645246. 33 (1), 1–17. doi:10.3109/02652048.2015.1115900.

Çerçi, N.A., Aydın, B., Naz, M., Sayın, S., Aytar, E.C., Akküçük, Ş., Kılıç, A.O., 2025. Development and evaluation of an alginate-based cream formulation from Sargassum vulgare: antimicrobial, antioxidant, and safety assessments. Algal Res. 22119264. 90, 104110. doi:10.1016/j.algal.2025.104110.

Ceschin, S., Bellini, A., Scalici, M., 2021. Aquatic plants and ecotoxicological assessment in freshwater ecosystems: a review. Environ. Sci. Pollut. Res. 0944-1344. 28 (5), 4975–4988. doi:10.1007/s11356-020-11496-3.

Chai, Y.H., Yusup, S., Ruslan, M.S.H., Chin, B.L.F., 2020. Supercritical fluid extraction and solubilization of *Carica papaya* Linn. leaves in ternary system with CO_2 + ethanol solvents. Chem. Eng. Res. Des. 02638762. 156, 31–42. Available from: http://www.elsevier.com/wps/find/journaldescription.cws_home/713871/description#description. doi:10.1016/j.cherd.2020.01.025.

Chanioti, S., Tzia, C., 2019. Evaluation of ultrasound assisted and conventional methods for production of olive pomace oil enriched in sterols and squalene. LWT. 00236438. 99, 209–216. doi:10.1016/j.lwt.2018.09.068.

Chaudhuri, R.K., Bojanowski, K., 2014. Bakuchiol: a retinol-like functional compound revealed by gene expression profiling and clinically proven to have anti-aging effects. Int. J. Cosmet. Sci. 14682494. 36 (3), 221–230. Available from: https://www.blacksci.co.uk/~cgilib/jnlpage.bin?Journal=ics&File=ics&Page=aims. doi:10.1111/ics.12117.

Chen, W., Nkosi, T.A.N., Combrinck, S., Viljoen, A.M., Cartwright-Jones, C., 2016. Rapid analysis of the skin irritant p -phenylenediamine (PPD) in henna products using atmospheric solids analysis probe mass spectrometry. J. Pharm. Biomed. Anal. 07317085. 128, 119–125. doi:10.1016/j.jpba.2016.05.020.

Chen, Y.Y., Lu, Y.H., Ma, C.H., Tao, W.W., Zhu, J.J., Zhang, X., 2017. A novel elastic liposome for skin delivery of papain and its application on hypertrophic scar. Biomed. Pharmacother. 19506007. 87, 82–91. Available from: https://www.elsevier.com/locate/biomedpharm. doi:10.1016/j.biopha.2016.12.076.

Chinjoo, N., Golzary, A., 2025. Microalgae: revolutionizing skin repair and enhancement. Biotechnol. Rep. 2215017X. 47, e00911. doi:10.1016/j.btre.2025.e00911.

Choleva, M., Boulougouri, V., Panara, A., Panagopoulou, E., Chiou, A., Thomaidis, N.S., Antonopoulou, S., Fragopoulou, E., 2019. Evaluation of anti-platelet activity of grape pomace extracts. Food Funct. 2042-6496. 10 (12), 8069–8080. doi:10.1039/c9fo02138h.

Chrysikopoulou, V., Rampaouni, A., Koutsia, E., Ofrydopoulou, A., Mittas, N., Tsoupras, A., 2025. Anti-inflammatory, antithrombotic and antioxidant efficacy and synergy of a high-dose vitamin C supplement enriched with a low dose of bioflavonoids: in vitro assessment and in vivo evaluation through a clinical study in healthy subjects. Nutrients. 2072-6643. 17 (16), 2643. doi:10.3390/nu17162643.

Cid-Samamed, A., Rakmai, J., Mejuto, J.C., Simal-Gandara, J., Astray, G., 2022. Cyclodextrins inclusion complex: preparation methods, analytical techniques and food industry applications. Food Chem. 03088146. 384, 132467. doi:10.1016/j.foodchem.2022.132467.

Cortes, N., Alves, I.A., Aragón, D.M., 2024. Innovative emulsifiers in cosmetic products: a patent review (2013–2023). ACS Omega. 2470-1343. 9 (50), 48884–48898. doi:10.1021/acsomega.4c07305.

Costa, J.M., Wang, W., Nakasu, P.Y.S., Hu, C., Forster-Carneiro, T., Hallett, J.P., 2025. Impacts of microwaves on the pectin extraction from apple pomace: technological properties in structuring of hydrogels. Food Hydrocoll. 0268005X. 160, 110766. doi:10.1016/j.foodhyd.2024.110766.

Costa, R.O.D.A., Passos, T.S., Silva, E.M.D.S., Dos Santos, N.C.S., Morais, A.H.D.A., 2023. Encapsulated peptides and proteins with an effect on satiety. Nanomaterials. 2079-4991. 13 (7), 1166. doi:10.3390/nano13071166.

Couceiro, B., Hameed, H., Vieira, A.C.F., Singh, S.K., Dua, K., Veiga, F., Pires, P.C., Ferreira, L., Paiva-Santos, A.C., 2025. Promoting health and sustainability: exploring safer alternatives in cosmetics and regulatory perspectives. Sustain. Chem. Pharm. 23525541. 43, 101901. doi:10.1016/j.scp.2024.101901.

Couteau, C., Coiffard, L., 2016. Overview of skin whitening agents: drugs and cosmetic products. Cosmetics. 2079-9284. 3 (3), 27. doi:10.3390/cosmetics3030027.

Crespi, O., Rosset, F., Pala, V., Sarda, C., Accorinti, M., Quaglino, P., Ribero, S., 2025. Cosmeceuticals for anti-aging: mechanisms, clinical evidence, and regulatory insights—a comprehensive review. Cosmetics. 2079-9284. 12 (5), 209. doi:10.3390/cosmetics12050209.

Ćujić, N., Šavikin, K., Janković, T., Pljevljakušić, D., Zdunić, G., Ibrić, S., 2016. Optimization of polyphenols extraction from dried chokeberry using maceration as traditional technique. Food Chem. 03088146. 194, 135–142. doi:10.1016/j.foodchem.2015.08.008.

da Rosa, G.S., Vanga, S.K., Gariepy, Y., Raghavan, V., 2019. Comparison of microwave, ultrasonic and conventional techniques for extraction of bioactive compounds from olive leaves (*Olea europaea* L.). Innov. Food Sci. Emerg. Technol. 14668564. 58, 102234. doi:10.1016/j.ifset.2019.102234.

Dai, Y.-L., Ying, L., Wang, Q., Niu, F.-J., Kun-Wei, L., Wang, Y.-Y., Wang, J., Zhou, C.-Z., Gao, L.-N., 2023. Chamomile: a review of its traditional uses, chemical constituents, pharmacological activities and quality control studies. Molecules. 1420-3049. 28 (1), 133. doi:10.3390/molecules28010133.

de Falco, B., Grauso, L., Fiore, A., Bonanomi, G., Lanzotti, V., 2022. Metabolomics and chemometrics of seven aromatic plants: carob, eucalyptus, laurel, mint, myrtle, rosemary and strawberry tree. Phytochem. Anal. 0958-0344. 33 (5), 696–709. doi:10.1002/pca.3121.

de Groot, A.C., White, I.R., 2001. Cosmetics and skin care products. In: Rycroft, R.J.G., Menné, T., Frosch, P.J., Lepoittevin, J.-P., Eds., Textbook of Contact Dermatitis. Springer, Berlin, Heidelberg, pp. 661–685.

de Souza Guedes, L., Martinez, R.M., Bou-Chacra, N.A., Valéria Robles Velasco, M., Rosado, C., Rolim Baby, A., 2021. An overview on topical administration of carotenoids and coenzyme Q10 loaded in lipid nanoparticles. Antioxidants. 2076-3921. 10 (7), 1034. doi:10.3390/antiox10071034.

Di Guardo, A., Trovato, F., Cantisani, C., Dattola, A., Nisticò, S.P., Pellacani, G., Paganelli, A., 2025. Artificial intelligence in cosmetic formulation: predictive modeling for safety, tolerability, and regulatory perspectives. Cosmetics. 2079-9284. 12 (4), 157. doi:10.3390/cosmetics12040157.

Diana Draelos, Z., 2000. Cosmetics and skin care products: a historical perspective. Dermatol. Clin. 07338635. 18 (4), 557–559. Available from: https://www.elsevier.com/inca/publications/store/6/2/3/3/6/3/index.htt. doi:10.1016/s0733-8635(05)70206-0.

Difonzo, G., Aresta, A., Cotugno, P., Ragni, R., Squeo, G., Summo, C., Massari, F., Pasqualone, A., Faccia, M., Zambonin, C., Caponio, F., 2021. Supercritical CO_2 extraction of phytocompounds from olive pomace subjected to different drying methods. Molecules. 1420-3049. 26 (3), 598. doi:10.3390/molecules26030598.

Digiovanni, C., Arcoraci, V., Gambardella, L., Sautebin, L., 2006. Cosmetovigilance survey: are cosmetics considered safe by consumers? Pharmacol. Res. 10436618. 53 (1), 16–21. doi:10.1016/j.phrs.2005.08.003.

Dini, I., Laneri, S., 2021. The new challenge of green cosmetics: natural food ingredients for cosmetic formulations. Molecules. 1420-3049. 26 (13), 3921. doi:10.3390/molecules26133921.

Domínguez-Rodríguez, G., Luisa Marina, M., Plaza, M., 2021. Enzyme-assisted extraction of bioactive non-extractable polyphenols from sweet cherry (*Prunus avium* L.) pomace. Food Chem. 03088146. 339, 128086. doi:10.1016/j.foodchem.2020.128086.

Dumpler, J., Moraru, C.I., 2024. Microwave vacuum drying of dairy cream: processing, reconstitution, and whipping properties of a novel dairy product. J. Dairy Sci. 00220302. 107 (2), 774–789. doi:10.3168/jds.2023-23657.

Dwivedi, S., Gupta, A., Sayal, A., 2025. Evolution of consumer perceptions and intentions in the green cosmetics market: a thematic and trend analysis. Front. Sustain. 2673-4524. 6. doi:10.3389/frsus.2025.1617779.

Dzah, C.S., Duan, Y., Zhang, H., Wen, C., Zhang, J., Chen, G., Haile, M., 2020. The effects of ultrasound assisted extraction on yield, antioxidant, anticancer and antimicrobial activity of polyphenol extracts: a review. Food Biosci. 22124292. 35, 100547. doi:10.1016/j.fbio.2020.100547.

Eckelman, M.J., Moroney, M.S., Zimmerman, J.B., Anastas, P.T., Thompson, E., Scott, P., McKeever-Alfieri, M., Cavanaugh, P.F., Daher, G., 2021. Applying green chemistry to raw material selection and product formulation at The Estée Lauder Companies. Green Chem. 14639270. 24 (6), 2397–2408. Available from: http://pubs.rsc.org/en/journals/journal/gc. doi:10.1039/d1gc03081g.

Ejiohuo, O., Folami, S., Maigoro, A.Y., 2024. Calendula in modern medicine: advancements in wound healing and drug delivery applications. Eur. J. Med. Chem. Rep. 27724174. 12, 100199. doi:10.1016/j.ejmcr.2024.100199.

Elder, A., O'donnell Cappelli, M., Ring, C., Saedi, N., 2024. Artificial intelligence in cosmetic dermatology: an update on current trends. Clin. Dermatol. 0738081X. 42 (3), 216–220. doi:10.1016/j.clindermatol.2023.12.015.

Expert Market Research, n.d. South Korea Cosmetics Market Growth Analysis - Forecast Trends and Outlook (2025-2034). Available from: https://www.marketresearch.com/Expert-Market-Research-v4220/South-Korea-Cosmetics-Growth-Forecast-42019455/ (Accessed 20 Dec 2025).

Fan, P., Zeng, Y., Zaldivar-Silva, D., Agüero, L., Wang, S., 2023. Chitosan-based hemostatic hydrogels: the concept, mechanism, application, and prospects. Molecules. 1420-3049. 28 (3), 1473. doi:10.3390/molecules28031473.

Favas, R., Morone, J., Martins, R., Vasconcelos, V., Lopes, G., 2021. Cyanobacteria and microalgae bioactive compounds in skin-ageing: potential to restore extracellular matrix filling and overcome hyperpigmentation. J. Enzyme Inhib. Med. Chem. 1475-6366. 36 (1), 1829–1838. doi:10.1080/14756366.2021.1960830.

Feng, X., Shang, J., Gu, Z., Gong, J., Chen, Y., Liu, Y., 2024. Azelaic acid: mechanisms of action and clinical applications. Clin. Cosmet. Investig. Dermatol. 11787015. 17, 2359–2371. Available from: https://www.dovepress.com/article/download/96588. doi:10.2147/CCID.S485237.

Feng, X., Shang, J., Wang, Y., Chen, Y., Liu, Y., 2025. Exploring the properties and application potential of β-glucan in skin care. Food Sci. Nutr. 2048-7177. 13 (4). doi:10.1002/fsn3.70212.

Ferreira, M., Matos, A., Couras, A., Marto, J., Ribeiro, H., 2022. Overview of cosmetic regulatory frameworks around the world. Cosmetics. 2079-9284. 9 (4), 72. doi:10.3390/cosmetics9040072.

Fowler, J.F., Woolery-Lloyd, H., Waldorf, H., Saini, R., 2010. Innovations in natural ingredients and their use in skin care. J. Drugs Dermatol. 15459616. 9 (6), s72. Available from: http://jddonline.com/articles/download_article/1257.

Gad, H.A., El-Rahman, F.A.A.A., Hamdy, G.M., 2019. Chamomile oil loaded solid lipid nanoparticles: a naturally formulated remedy to enhance the wound healing. J. Drug Deliv. Sci. Technol. 17732247. 50, 329–338. Available from: http://www.editionsdesante.fr/category.php?id_category=48. doi:10.1016/j.jddst.2019.01.008.

Gad, H.A., Roberts, A., Hamzi, S.H., Gad, H.A., Touiss, I., Altyar, A.E., Kensara, O.A., Ashour, M.L., 2021. Jojoba oil: an updated comprehensive review on chemistry, pharmaceutical uses, and toxicity. Polymers. 2073-4360. 13 (11), 1711. doi:10.3390/polym13111711.

Gălbău, C.Ş., Irimie, M., Neculau, A.E., Dima, L., da Silva, L.P., Vârciu, M., Badea, M., 2024. The potential of plant extracts used in cosmetic product applications—antioxidants delivery and mechanism of actions. Antioxidants 20763921. 13 (11). Available from: https://www.mdpi.com/journal/antioxidants. doi:10.3390/antiox13111425.

Garbossa, W.A.C., Campos, P.M.B.G.M., 2016. *Euterpe oleracea*, *Matricaria chamomilla*, and *Camellia sinensis* as promising ingredients for development of skin care formulations. Ind. Crops Prod. 09266690. 83, 1–10. Available from: https://www.elsevier.com/inca/publications/store/5/2/2/8/2/5. doi:10.1016/j.indcrop.2015.11.026.

García-Pérez, P., Becchi, P.P., Zhang, L., Rocchetti, G., Lucini, L., 2024. Metabolomics and chemometrics: the next-generation analytical toolkit for the evaluation of food quality and authenticity. Trends Food Sci. Technol. 09242244. 147, 104481. doi:10.1016/j.tifs.2024.104481.

Ghannam, M.T., Selim, M.Y.E., Thaher, A., Binamro, A., Almansoori, M., Abdallah, S., 2023. Flow characteristics of jojoba and other oil blends for skin treatment fluids. Int. J. Thermofluids. 26662027. 18, 100362. doi:10.1016/j.ijft.2023.100362.

Gharby, S., Charrouf, Z., 2022. Argan oil: chemical composition, extraction process, and quality control. Front. Nutr. 2296-861X. 8. doi:10.3389/fnut.2021.804587.

Gianeti, M.D., Mercurio, D.G., Maia Campos, P.M.B.G., 2013. The use of green tea extract in cosmetic formulations: not only an antioxidant active ingredient. Dermatol. Ther. 13960296. 26 (3), 267–271. doi:10.1111/j.1529-8019.2013.01552.x.

Gligor, O., Mocan, A., Moldovan, C., Locatelli, M., Crişan, G., Ferreira, I.C.F.R., 2019. Enzyme-assisted extractions of polyphenols – a comprehensive review. Trends Food Sci. Technol. 09242244. 88, 302–315. doi:10.1016/j.tifs.2019.03.029.

Godase, S.S., Kulkarni, N.S., Dhole, S.N., 2024. A comprehensive review on novel lipid-based nano drug delivery. Adv. Pharm. Bull. 22517308. 14 (1), 34–47. Available from: https://apb.tbzmed.ac.ir/Article/apb-37690. doi:10.34172/apb.2024.012.

Gonçalves, S., 2021. Use of enzymes in cosmetics: proposed enzymatic peel procedure. Cos ACTIVE J. https://cosmethicallyactive.com/use-of-enzymes-in-cosmetics-proposed-enzymatic-peel-procedure/ (Accessed 27 Jan 2025).

Gopinath, H., Karthikeyan, K., 2017. Turmeric: a condiment, cosmetic and cure. Indian J. Dermatol. Venereol. Leprol. 84. https://doi.org/10.4103/ijdvl.IJDVL_1143_16

Grozdanova, T., Trusheva, B., Alipieva, K., Popova, M., Dimitrova, L., Najdenski, H., Zaharieva, M.M., Ilieva, Y., Vasileva, B., Miloshev, G., Georgieva, M., Bankova, V., 2020. Extracts of medicinal plants with natural deep eutectic solvents: enhanced antimicrobial activity and low genotoxicity. BMC Chem. 2661-801X. 14 (1). doi:10.1186/s13065-020-00726-x.

Gubitosa, J., Rizzi, V., Fini, P., Cosma, P., 2019. Hair care cosmetics: from traditional shampoo to solid clay and herbal shampoo, a review. Cosmetics. 2079-9284. 6 (1), 13. doi:10.3390/cosmetics6010013.

Gupta, A., Eral, H.B., Hatton, T.A., Doyle, P.S., 2016. Nanoemulsions: formation, properties and applications. Soft Matter 17446848. 12 (11), 2826–2841. Available from: http://pubs.rsc.org/en/journals/journal/sm. doi:10.1039/c5sm02958a.

Gupta, V., Mohapatra, S., Mishra, H., Farooq, U., Kumar, K., Ansari, M., Aldawsari, M., Alalaiwe, A., Mirza, M., Iqbal, Z., 2022. Nanotechnology in cosmetics and cosmeceuticals—a review of latest advancements. Gels. 2310-2861. 8 (3), 173. doi:10.3390/gels8030173.

Gutiérrez-Álzate, K., Beltrán-Cotta, L.A., Dos Santos Rekowsky, B.S., Cavalheiro, C.P., da Costa, M.P., 2024. Micro- and Nanoencapsulation of Probiotics: exploring Their Impact on Animal-Origin Foods. ACS Food Sci. Technol. 26921944. 4 (12), 2799–2812. Available from: https://pubs.acs.org/page/afsthl/about.html. doi:10.1021/acsfoodscitech.4c00776.

Halevas, E.G., Avgoulas, D.I., Katsipis, G., Pantazaki, A.A., 2022. Flavonoid-liposomes formulations: physico-chemical characteristics, biological activities and therapeutic applications. Eur. J. Med. Chem. Rep. 27724174. 5, 100059. doi:10.1016/j.ejmcr.2022.100059.

Handayani, R., Febriyanti, R.M., Muhaimin, M., Chearunisaa, A.Y., 2025. Centella asiatica (L.) Urb. in skin health and cosmeceuticals: mechanisms, clinical evidence, and advanced delivery systems. Pharmacia 04280296. 72. Available from: https://pharmacia.pensoft.net/. doi:10.3897/pharmacia.72.e167217.

Hemavathi, M., Gnanaroy, E.R., Malar, G.S.G., 2024. A Comprehensive Analysis of the Impact of Augmented Reality on E-Commerce Cosmetics E-Commerce, Marketing, and Consumer Behavior in the AI Era. IGI Global, India, pp. 127–148. Available from: https://www.igi-global.com/book/commerce-marketing-consumer-behavior-era/340702. doi:10.4018/979-8-3693-5548-0.ch007.

Hendawy, O.M., Al-Sanea, M.M., Elbargisy, R.M., Rahman, H.U., Hassan, Y.A., Elshaarawy, R.F.M., Khedr, A.I.M., 2023. Alginate-chitosan-microencapsulated tyrosols/oleuropein-rich olive mill waste extract for lipopolysaccharide-induced skin fibroblast inflammation treatment. Int. J. Pharm. 03785173. 643, 123260. doi:10.1016/j.ijpharm.2023.123260.

Herman, A., 2019. Antimicrobial ingredients as preservative booster and components of self-preserving cosmetic products. Curr. Microbiol. 0343-8651. 76 (6), 744–754. doi:10.1007/s00284-018-1492-2.

Hoang, H.T., Moon, J.Y., Lee, Y.C., 2021. Natural antioxidants from plant extracts in skincare cosmetics: recent applications, challenges and perspectives. Cosmetics 20799284. 8 (4). Available from: https://www.mdpi.com/2079-9284/8/4/93/pdf. doi:10.3390/cosmetics8040106.

Hosni, K., Hassen, I., Chaâbane, H., Jemli, M., Dallali, S., Sebei, H., Casabianca, H., 2013. Enzyme-assisted extraction of essential oils from thyme (*Thymus capitatus* L.) and rosemary (*Rosmarinus officinalis* L.): impact on yield, chemical composition and antimicrobial activity. Ind. Crops Prod. 09266690. 47, 291–299. doi:10.1016/j.indcrop.2013.03.023.

Huong V.T.M., Hung N.P., Minh N.T.T., Thuy L.K., Duyen L.T.N., Minh T.N., 2024. Factors affecting consumers' repurchase intention toward skin care cosmetics: a cross - sectional study in Vietnam. Heliyon. 24058440. 10 (11), e32285. doi:10.1016/j.heliyon.2024.e32285.

Iliopoulos, F., Sil, B.C., Al Hossain, A.S.M.M., Moore, D.J., Lucas, R.A., Lane, M.E., 2020. Topical delivery of niacinamide: influence of neat solvents. Int. J. Pharm. 03785173. 579, 119137. doi:10.1016/j.ijpharm.2020.119137.

Inomata, S., 2014. Safety assurance of cosmetic in japan: current situation and future prospects. J. Oleo Sci. 1345-8957. 63 (1), 1–6. doi:10.5650/jos.ess13501.

Iraqui, P., Das, M.K., 2022. Herbal cosmeceuticals for beauty and skin therapy. In: Das, M.K. (Ed.), Nanocosmeceuticals. Academic Press, pp. 453–480.

Jabłonowska, M., Ciganović, P., Jablan, J., Marguí, E., Tomczyk, M., Končić, M.Z., 2021. Silybum marianum glycerol extraction for the preparation of high-value anti-ageing extracts. Ind. Crops Prod. 09266690. 168, 113613. doi:10.1016/j.indcrop.2021.113613.

Jalil, B., Pischel, I., Feistel, B., Suarez, C., Blainski, A., Spreemann, R., Roth-Ehrang, R., Heinrich, M., 2024. Wild thyme (*Thymus serpyllum* L.): a review of the current evidence of nutritional and preventive health benefits*. Front. Nutr. 2296-861X. 11. doi:10.3389/fnut.2024.1380962.

Jesus, A., Mota, S., Torres, A., Cruz, M.T., Sousa, E., Almeida, I.F., Cidade, H., 2023. Antioxidants in sunscreens: which and what for? Antioxidants. 2076-3921. 12 (1), 138. doi:10.3390/antiox12010138.

Jianbiao, H., Jia, Y., 2022. Application of omics technologies in dermatological research and skin management. J. Cosmet. Dermatol. 1473-2130. 21 (2), 451–460. doi:10.1111/jocd.14100.

Jiang, T., Liao, W., Charcosset, C., 2020. Recent advances in encapsulation of curcumin in nanoemulsions: a review of encapsulation technologies, bioaccessibility and applications. Food Res. Int. 09639969. 132, 109035. doi:10.1016/j.foodres.2020.109035.

José González-minero, F., Bravo-Díaz, L., Ayala-Gómez, A., Rosmarinus Officinalis, L., 2020. (Rosemary): an ancient plant with uses in personal healthcare and cosmetics. Cosmetics. 2079-9284. 7 (4), 77. doi:10.3390/cosmetics7040077.

Kairey, L., Agnew, T., Bowles, E.J., Barkla, B.J., Wardle, J., Lauche, R., 2023. Efficacy and safety of *Melaleuca alternifolia* (tea tree) oil for human health—a systematic review of randomized controlled trials. Front. Pharmacol. 16639812. 14. Available from: http://www.frontiersin.org/Pharmacology. doi:10.3389/fphar.2023.1116077.

Kang, C., Shin, W.S., Yeo, D., Lim, W., Ji, L.L., 2018. Anti-inflammatory effect of avenanthramides via NF-κB pathways in C2C12 skeletal muscle cells. Free Radic. Biol. Med. 18734596. 117, 30–36. Available from: https://www.elsevier.com/locate/freeradbiomed. doi:10.1016/j.freeradbiomed.2018.01.020.

Kania, B., Montecinos, K., Goldberg, D.J., 2024. Artificial intelligence in cosmetic dermatology. J. Cosmet. Dermatol. 1473-2130. 23 (10), 3305–3311. doi:10.1111/jocd.16538.

Karageorgou, E.G., Kalogiouri, N.P., Samanidou, V.F., 2025. Green approaches in high-performance liquid chromatography for sustainable food analysis: advances, challenges, and regulatory perspectives. Molecules 14203049. 30 (17). Available from: http://www.mdpi.com/journal/molecules. doi:10.3390/molecules30173573.

Karantonis, H.C., Tsoupras, A., Moran, D., Zabetakis, I., Nasopoulou, C., 2023. Olive, Apple, and Grape Pomaces with Antioxidant and Anti-inflammatory Bioactivities for Functional Foods. Elsevier BV, pp. 131–159. doi:10.1016/b978-0-12-823811-0.00007-9.

Karwal, K., Mukovozov, I., 2023. Topical AHA in dermatology: formulations, mechanisms of action, efficacy, and future perspectives. Cosmetics. 2079-9284. 10 (5), 131. doi:10.3390/cosmetics10050131.

Katopodi, A., Safari, K., Kalospyros, A., Politopoulos, K., Alexandratou, E., Detsi, A., 2023. Preparation and characterization of solid lipid nanoparticles incorporating bioactive coumarin analogues as photosensitizing agents. Colloids Surf. B Biointerfaces. 09277765. 229, 113439. doi:10.1016/j.colsurfb.2023.113439.

Kehili, M., Kammlott, M., Choura, S., Zammel, A., Zetzl, C., Smirnova, I., Allouche, N., Sayadi, S., 2017. Supercritical CO_2 extraction and antioxidant activity of lycopene and β-carotene-enriched oleoresin from tomato (*Lycopersicum esculentum* L.) peels by-product of a Tunisian industry. Food Bioprod. Process. 09603085. 102, 340–349. doi:10.1016/j.fbp.2017.02.002.

Khan, M.K., Paniwnyk, L., Hassan, S., 2019. Polyphenols as natural antioxidants: sources, extraction and applications in food, cosmetics and drugs. In: Li, Y., Chemat, F., Eds., Plant Based "Green Chemistry 2.0": Moving from Evolutionary to Revolutionary. Springer, Singapore, pp. 197–235.

Kim, H.S., Hwang, H.J., Seo, W.D., Do, S.H., 2023. Oat (*Avena sativa* L.) sprouts restore skin barrier function by modulating the expression of the epidermal differentiation complex in models of skin irritation. Int. J. Mol. Sci. 14220067. 24 (24). Available from: http://www.mdpi.com/journal/ijms. doi:10.3390/ijms242417274.

Kim, H.W., Seok, Y.S., Lee, H.G., Song, M.K., Rhee, M.S., 2021a. Consumers' lack of understanding of customized cosmetics made on the spot and implications for regulations and controls. Regul. Toxicol. Pharmacol. 02732300. 124, 104979. doi:10.1016/j.yrtph.2021.104979.

Kim, I.S., Hwang, C.W., Yang, W.S., Kim, C.H., 2021b. Multiple antioxidative and bioactive molecules of oats (*Avena sativa* L.) in human health. Antioxidants 20763921. 10 (9). Available from: https://www.mdpi.com/2076-3921/10/9/1454/pdf. doi:10.3390/antiox10091454.

Kim, K.-L., Jeon, J.-H., Kim, Y., Lim, K.-M., 2025. The antioxidant and skin-brightening effects of a novel caffeic acid derivative, caffeic acid-3,4-dihydroxyphenylpropanolester. Antioxidants. 2076-3921. 14 (7), 806. doi:10.3390/antiox14070806.

Kontaxi, N.-I., Panoutsopoulou, E., Ofrydopolou, A., Tsoupras, A., 2024. Anti-inflammatory benefits of grape pomace and tomato bioactives as ingredients in sun oils against UV radiation for skin protection. Appl. Sci. 2076-3417. 14 (14), 6236. doi:10.3390/app14146236.

Koukouraki, P., Tsoupras, A., Sotiroudis, G., Demopoulos, C.A., Sotiroudis, T.G., 2020. Antithrombotic properties of Spirulina extracts against platelet-activating factor and thrombin. Food Biosci. 22124292. 37, 100686. doi:10.1016/j.fbio.2020.100686.

Kumari, S., Pal, B., Tewari, D., Sahu, S.K., 2023. Cosmetics utilization and associated adverse events: a community based cross-sectional study. Clin. Epidemiol. Glob. Health. 22133984. 23, 101382. doi:10.1016/j.cegh.2023.101382.

Kyriakoudi, A., Mourtzinos, I., Tyśkiewicz, K., Milovanovic, S., 2024. An eco-friendly supercritical CO_2 recovery of value-added extracts from *Olea europaea* leaves. Foods. 2304-8158. 13 (12), 1836. doi:10.3390/foods13121836.

Lartey, S., 2024. The role of cosmetic products in modern beauty standards: a wealthy venture or exploitative? Future recommendations and studies. pp. 1–6. Available from: https://www.researchgate.net/publication/383862687_The_Role_of_Cosmetic_Products_in_Modern_Beauty_Standards_A_Wealthy_Venture_or_Exploitative_Future_Recommendations_and_Studies.

Lee, H.J., Lee, W.J., Chang, S.E., Lee, G.Y., 2015. Hesperidin, a popular antioxidant inhibits melanogenesis via Erk1/2 mediated MITF degradation. Int. J. Mol. Sci. 14220067. 16 (8), 18384–18395. Available from: http://www.mdpi.com/1422-0067/16/8/18384/pdf. doi:10.3390/ijms160818384.

Lee, J., Kwon, K.H., 2022. Sustainable changes in beauty market trends focused on the perspective of safety in the post-coronavirus disease-19 period. J. Cosmet. Dermatol. 1473-2130. 21 (7), 2700–2707. doi:10.1111/jocd.14493.

Leszczyński, M., Mamiński, M., Parzuchowski, P.G., 2025. Ferulic acid and polyferulic acid in polymers: synthesis, properties, and applications. Polymers 20734360. 17 (20). Available from: http://www.mdpi.com/journal/polymers. doi:10.3390/polym17202788.

Lim, H.Y., Kwon, K.H., 2023. Sustainable assessment of the environmental activities of major cosmetics and personal care companies. Sustainability. 2071-1050. 15 (18), 13286. doi:10.3390/su151813286.

Lin, F.H., Lin, J.Y., Gupta, R.D., Tournas, J.A., Burch, J.A., Selim, M.A., Monteiro-Riviere, N.A., Grichnik, J.M., Zielinski, J., Pinnell, S.R., 2005. Ferulic acid stabilizes a solution of vitamins C and E and doubles its photoprotection of skin. J. Invest. Dermatol. 15231747. 125 (4), 826–832. Available from: https://www.sciencedirect.com/science/journal/0022202X. doi:10.1111/j.0022-202X.2005.23768.x.

Liu, J.-K., 2022. Natural products in cosmetics. Nat. Prod. Bioprospect. 12, 40. doi:https://doi.org/10.1007/s13659-022-00363-y.

Longo, J.P.F., Camargo, N.S., Ferreira, G.A., Cardador, C.M., Corrêa, M.A., 2022. Nanotechnology for Cosmetics Applications—a Journey in Innovation Quantum Materials, Devices, and Applications. Elsevier, Brazil, pp. 263–278. Available from: https://www.sciencedirect.com/book/9780128205662. doi:10.1016/B978-0-12-820566-2.00010-7.

Machado, M., Silva, S., Costa, E.M., 2024. Byproducts as a sustainable source of cosmetic ingredients. Appl. Sci. 2076-3417. 14 (22), 10241. doi:10.3390/app142210241.

Madnani, N., Deo, J., Dalal, K., Benjamin, B., Murthy, V.V., Hegde, R., Shetty, T., 2024. Revitalizing the skin: exploring the role of barrier repair moisturizers. J. Cosmet. Dermatol. 1473-2130. 23 (5), 1533–1540. doi:10.1111/jocd.16171.

Mahmoud, K.F., Ali, H.S., Amin, A.A., 2018. Nanoencapsulation of bioactive compounds extracted from Egyptian prickly pear peel fruit: antioxidant and their application in guava juice. Asian J. Sci. Res. 19921454. 11 (4), 574–586. doi:10.3923/ajsr.2018.574.586.

Mamta, G.P., 2025. Publication trends and green cosmetics buying behaviour: a comprehensive bibliometric analysis. Heliyon. 24058440. 11 (2), e41513. doi:10.1016/j.heliyon.2024.e41513.

Mantiniotou, M., Athanasiadis, V., Liakos, K.G., Bozinou, E., Lalas, S.I., 2025. Artificial intelligence and extraction of bioactive compounds: the case of rosemary and pressurized liquid extraction. Processes. 2227-9717. 13 (6), 1879. doi:10.3390/pr13061879.

Markiewicz, E., Idowu, O.C., 2018. Personalized skincare: from molecular basis to clinical and commercial application. Clin. Cosmet. Investig. Dermatol. 11787015. 11, 161–171. Available from: https://www.dovepress.com/getfile.php?fileID=41479. doi:10.2147/CCID.S163799.

Marra, A., Manousakis, V., Koutis, N., Zervas, G.P., Ofrydopoulou, A., Shiels, K., Saha, S.K., Tsoupras, A., 2025. In vitro antioxidant, antithrombotic and anti-inflammatory activities of the amphiphilic bioactives extracted from avocado and its by-products. Antioxidants. 2076-3921. 14 (2), 146. doi:10.3390/antiox14020146.

Marra, A., Manousakis, V., Zervas, G.P., Koutis, N., Finos, M.A., Adamantidi, T., Panoutsopoulou, E., Ofrydopoulou, A., Tsoupras, A., 2024. Avocado and its by-products as natural sources of valuable anti-inflammatory and antioxidant bioactives for functional foods and cosmetics with health-promoting properties. Appl. Sci. 2076-3417. 14 (14), 5978. doi:10.3390/app14145978.

Martínez-Burgos, W.J., Serra, J.L., MarsigliaF, R.M., Montoya, P., Sarmiento-Vásquez, Z., Marin, O., Gallego-Cartagena, E., Paternina-Arboleda, C.D., 2022. Aloe vera: from ancient knowledge to the patent and innovation landscape – a review. S. Afr. J. Bot. 02546299. 147, 993–1006. Available from: http://www.elsevier.com. doi:10.1016/j.sajb.2022.02.034.

Martins, A.M., Marto, J.M., 2023. A sustainable life cycle for cosmetics: from design and development to post-use phase. Sustain. Chem. Pharm. 23525541. 35, 101178. doi:10.1016/j.scp.2023.101178.

Martins, R., Barbosa, A., Advinha, B., Sales, H., Pontes, R., Nunes, J., 2023. Green extraction techniques of bioactive compounds: a state-of-the-art review. Processes. 2227-9717. 11 (8), 2255. doi:10.3390/pr11082255.

Matei, C.E., Visan, A.I., Cristescu, R., 2025. Aloe Vera polysaccharides as therapeutic agents: benefits versus side effects in biomedical applications. Polysaccharides. 2673-4176. 6 (2), 36. doi:10.3390/polysaccharides6020036.

Matsumoto, M., Todo, H., Akiyama, T., Hirata-Koizumi, M., Sugibayashi, K., Ikarashi, Y., Ono, A., Hirose, A., Yokoyama, K., 2016. Risk assessment of skin lightening cosmetics containing hydroquinone. Regul. Toxicol. Pharmacol. 02732300. 81, 128–135. doi:10.1016/j.yrtph.2016.08.005.

Mawazi, S.M., Ann, J., Othman, N., Khan, J., Alolayan, S.O., thagfan, S.S.A., Kaleemullah, M., 2022a. A review of moisturizers; history, preparation, characterization and applications. Cosmetics. 2079-9284. 9 (3), 61. doi:10.3390/cosmetics9030061.

Mawazi, S.M., Ann, T.J., Widodo, R.T., 2022b. Application of niosomes in cosmetics: a systematic review. Cosmetics 20799284. 9 (6). Available from: https://www.mdpi.com/journal/cosmetics. doi:10.3390/cosmetics9060127.

Mihalcea, L., Crăciunescu, O., Gheonea (Dima), I., Prelipcean, A.-M., Enachi, E., Barbu, V., Bahrim, G.E., Râpeanu, G., Oancea, A., Stănciuc, N., 2021. Supercritical CO_2 extraction and microencapsulation of lycopene-enriched oleoresins from tomato peels: evidence on antiproliferative and cytocompatibility activities. Antioxidants. 2076-3921. 10 (2), 222. doi:10.3390/antiox10020222.

Milutinov, J., Pavlović, N., Ćirin, D., Atanacković Krstonošić, M., Krstonošić, V., 2024. The potential of natural compounds in UV protection products. Molecules. 1420-3049. 29 (22), 5409. doi:10.3390/molecules29225409.

Mondello, A., Salomone, R., Mondello, G., 2024. Exploring circular economy in the cosmetic industry: insights from a literature review. Environ. Impact Assess. Rev. 01959255. 105, 107443. doi:10.1016/j.eiar.2024.107443.

Morel, S., Mura, G., Gallarate, M., Sapino, S., 2024. Cosmetic packaging: European regulatory aspects and sustainability. Cosmetics. 2079-9284. 11 (4), 110. doi:10.3390/cosmetics11040110.

Moysidou, A.M., Cheimpeloglou, K., Koutra, S.I., Finos, M.A., Ofrydopoulou, A., Tsoupras, A., 2024. A comprehensive review on the antioxidant and anti-inflammatory bioactives of kiwi and its by-products for functional foods and cosmetics with health-promoting properties. Appl. Sci. 2076-3417. 14 (14), 5990. doi:10.3390/app14145990.

Moysidou, A.M., Cheimpeloglou, K., Koutra, S.I., Manousakis, V., Ofrydopoulou, A., Shiels, K., Saha, S.K., Tsoupras, A., 2025. In vitro antioxidant, antithrombotic and anti-inflammatory activities of bioactive metabolites extracted from kiwi and its by-products. Metabolites. 2218-1989. 15 (6), 400. doi:10.3390/metabo15060400.

Nadeeshani Dilhara Gamage, D.G., Dharmadasa, R.M., Chandana Abeysinghe, D., Saman Wijesekara, R.G., Prathapasinghe, G.A., Someya, T., 2022. Global perspective of plant-based cosmetic industry and possible contribution of Sri Lanka to the development of herbal cosmetics. Evid. Based Complement. Altern. Med. 17414288. 2022. Available from: http://www.hindawi.com/journals/ecam/contents.html. doi:10.1155/2022/9940548.

Nayak, M., Ligade, V.S., 2021. History of cosmetics in Egypt, India, and China. J. Cosmet. Sci. 15257886. 72 (4), 432–441. Available from: https://library.scconline.org/v072n041/96.

Ngo, T.T.A., Gia Khuong, A., Dao, D.K., Nguyen, N.Q.N., Phong, B.H., Nguyen, N.Y.V., Nguyen, T.B.N., 2025. Leveraging social media marketing activities (SMMAs) to enhance consumer satisfaction and purchase intention for bio-cosmetics. Acta Psychol. 00016918. 261, 105768. doi:10.1016/j.actpsy.2025.105768.

Nurkolis, F., 2025. Marine bioactives: pioneering sustainable solutions for advanced cosmetics and therapeutics. Pharmacol. Res. 10436618. 218, 107868. doi:10.1016/j.phrs.2025.107868.

Office of the Commissioner, 2024. Microbiological Safety and Cosmetics. FDA.

Okonogi, S., Riangjanapatee, P., 2015. Physicochemical characterization of lycopene-loaded nanostructured lipid carrier formulations for topical administration. Int. J. Pharm. 03785173. 478 (2), 726–735. doi:10.1016/j.ijpharm.2014.12.002.

Oliver, G., Kenzie, F., 2024. Euphorbia cerifera and candelilla wax: natural emollients with moisturizing effects and skin barrier protection in skincare products. pp. 1–9. Available from: https://www.researchgate.net/publication/384299184_Euphorbia_Cerifera_and_Candelilla_Wax_Natural_Emollients_with_Moisturizing_Effects_and_Skin_Barrier_Protection_in_Skincare_Products?channel=doi&linkId=66f3bb919e6e82486fef9a65&showFulltext=true. doi:10.13140/RG.2.2.11329.77925.

Omira, A., Grira, S., Mourad, A.H.I., Alkhedher, M., 2025. The new generation of cosmetics packaging: a paradigm shift. Glob. Transit. 25897918. 7, 223–246. Available from: https://www.sciencedirect.com/science/journal/25897918. doi:10.1016/j.glt.2025.04.004.

Papadopoulou, S.N.A., Adamantidi, T., Kranas, D., Cholidis, P., Anastasiadou, C., Tsoupras, A., 2025b. A comprehensive review on the valorization of bioactives from marine animal by-products for health-promoting, biofunctional cosmetics. Mar. Drugs. 1660-3397. 23 (8), 299. doi:10.3390/md23080299.

Papadopoulou, S.N.A., Anastasiou, E.A., Adamantidi, T., Ofrydopoulou, A., Letsiou, S., Tsoupras, A., 2025a. A comprehensive review on the beneficial roles of vitamin D in skin health as a bio-functional ingredient in nutricosmetic, cosmeceutical, and cosmetic applications. Appl. Sci. 20763417. 15 (2). Available from: https://www.mdpi.com/journal/applsci/. doi:10.3390/app15020796.

Papikinou, M.-A., Pavlidis, K., Cholidis, P., Kranas, D., Adamantidi, T., Anastasiadou, C., Tsoupras, A., 2024. Marine fungi bioactives with anti-inflammatory, antithrombotic and antioxidant health-promoting properties against inflammation-related chronic diseases. Mar. Drugs. 1660-3397. 22 (11), 520. doi:10.3390/md22110520.

Park, K.S., 2021. Pharmacological effects of *Centella asiatica* on skin diseases: evidence and possible mechanisms. Evid.-Based Complement. Altern. Med. ECAM 2021, 5462633. doi:https://doi.org/10.1155/2021/5462633.

Pathak, K., Akhtar, N., 2019. Hair care cosmetics regulation in different countries – a comparative study. Appl. Clin. Res. Clin. Trials Regul. Aff. 2213476X. 6 (1), 34–45. doi:10.2174/2213476x06666190128150054.

Pazyar, N., Yaghoobi, R., Bagherani, N., Kazerouni, A., 2013. A review of applications of tea tree oil in dermatology. Int. J. Dermatol. 00119059. 52 (7), 784–790. doi:10.1111/j.1365-4632.2012.05654.x.

Pérez-Rivero, C., Pablo López-gómez, J., 2023. Unlocking the potential of fermentation in cosmetics: a review. Fermentation. 2311-5637. 9 (5), 463. doi:10.3390/fermentation9050463.

Phatangre Piyal, L.P.P., Phatangare, T., Mani, S., 2023. An overview: herbal cosmetics and cosmeceuticals. Int. J. Pharm. Chem. Anal. 2394-2789. 10 (2), 84–90. doi:10.18231/j.ijpca.2023.017.

Pinna, N., Blasi, F., Schoubben, A., 2023. Optimization of solid lipid nanoparticles for the encapsulation of carotenoids from *Cucurbita moschata* pulp. Eng. Proc. 26734591. 37 (1). Available from: https://www.mdpi.com/journal/engproc. doi:10.3390/ECP2023-14737.

Program, H.F., 2025. BAM Chapter 23: Methods for Cosmetics, FDA.

Quan, T., 2023. Human skin aging and the anti-aging properties of retinol. Biomolecules. 2218-273X. 13 (11), 1614. doi:10.3390/biom13111614.

Rachmawati, H., Sulastri, E., Iwo, M.I., Safitri, D., Rahma, A., 2016. Bromelain encapsulated in self assembly nanoemulsion exhibits better debridement effect in animal model of burned skin. J. Nano Res. 16619897. 40, 158–166. Available from: http://www.scientific.net/1661-9897/. doi:10.4028/www.scientific.net/JNanoR.40.158.

Rai, V.K., Rath, G., 2026. Regulations in cosmetics. In: Lai, C.W., Thomas, P. (Eds.), Nanotechnology in Cosmeceuticals. Elsevier, pp. 529–540.

Rapti, E., Adamantidi, T., Efthymiopoulos, P., Kyzas, G.Z., Tsoupras, A., 2024. Potential applications of the anti-inflammatory, antithrombotic and antioxidant health-promoting properties of curcumin: a critical review. Nutraceuticals. 1661-3821. 4 (4), 562–595. doi:10.3390/nutraceuticals4040031.

Rocca, R., Acerbi, F., Fumagalli, L., Taisch, M., 2022. Sustainability paradigm in the cosmetics industry: state of the art. Cleaner Waste Syst. 27729125. 3, 100057. doi:10.1016/j.clwas.2022.100057.

Rodrigues, C.V., Pintado, M., 2024. Hesperidin from orange peel as a promising skincare bioactive: an overview. Int. J. Mol. Sci. 1422-0067. 25 (3), 1890. doi:10.3390/ijms25031890.

Rodriguez, B., Reinoso-Carvalho, F., Reyes, L.H., 2023. Sensory science in topical cosmetics: enhancing the consumer experience and emotional connection in skincare. In: 15th Pangborn Sensory Science Symposium – Meeting New Challenges in a Changing World (PSSS 2023): U10. Available from: https://ssrn.com/abstract=4550045.

Rong, Q., Chu, L., Cheng, D., 2025. Fragrance skin care: research on consumer fragrance preference and emotional value. Flavour Fragr. J. 0882-5734. 40 (4), 726–734. doi:10.1002/ffj.3858.

Ruse, G., Jîjie, A.-R., Moacă, E.-A., Pătrașcu, D., Ardelean, F., Jojic, A.-A., Ardelean, S., Tchiakpe-Antal, D.-S., 2025. *Coffea arabica*: an emerging active ingredient in dermato-cosmetic applications. Pharmaceuticals. 1424-8247. 18 (2), 171. doi:10.3390/ph18020171.

Saad, B., Bari, M.F., Saleh, M.I., Ahmad, K., Talib, M.K.M., 2005. Simultaneous determination of preservatives (benzoic acid, sorbic acid, methylparaben and propylparaben) in foodstuffs using high-performance liquid chromatography. J. Chromatogr. A. 00219673. 1073 (1-2), 393–397. doi:10.1016/j.chroma.2004.10.105.

Saeedi, M., Eslamifar, M., Khezri, K., 2019. Kojic acid applications in cosmetic and pharmaceutical preparations. Biomed. Pharmacother. 07533322. 110, 582–593. doi:10.1016/j.biopha.2018.12.006.

Sailaja, G., Bhavan, S., Snehalatha, G., Pashikanti, S., 2022. A review on regulatory requirements for approval of cosmetics in Brazil. Int. J. Nov. Res. Dev. 7 (7), 163–168.

Sallustio, V., Marto, J., Escribano-Ferrer, E., Maria Gonçalves, L., Rossi, M., Cappadone, C., Mandrone, M., Chiocchio, I., Rossello, S., Ribeiro, H., Cerchiara, T., 2025. Development and characterization of multifunctional phytonanoemulgels based on licorice extract and biocompatible polymers. Int. J. Biol. Macromol. 01418130. 319 (Pt 2), 145241. doi:10.1016/j.ijbiomac.2025.145241.

Santos, É.M.D., Macedo, L.M.D., Tundisi, L.L., Ataide, J.A., Camargo, G.A., Alves, R.C., Oliveira, M.B.P.P., Mazzola, P.G., 2021. Coffee by-products in topical formulations: a review. Trends Food Sci. Technol. 09242244. 111, 280–291. Available from: http://www.elsevier.com/wps/find/journaldescription.cws_home/601278/description#description. doi:10.1016/j.tifs.2021.02.064.

Sasounian, R., Martinez, R.M., Lopes, A.M., Giarolla, J., Rosado, C., Magalhães, W.V., Velasco, M.V.R., Baby, A.R., 2024. Innovative approaches to an eco-friendly cosmetic industry: a review of sustainable ingredients. Clean Technol. 25718797. 6 (1), 176–198. Available from: https://www.mdpi.com/journal/cleantechnol. doi:10.3390/cleantechnol6010011.

Schild, J., Kalvodová, A., Zbytovská, J., Farwick, M., Pyko, C., 2024. The role of ceramides in skin barrier function and the importance of their correct formulation for skincare applications. Int. J. Cosmet. Sci. 0142-5463. 46 (4), 526–543. doi:10.1111/ics.12972.

Schneider, S.B., 2009. Global Cosmetic Regulations? A Long Way to Go. Global Regulatory Issues for the Cosmetics Industry. Elsevier Inc, United States, pp. 189–233. Available from: http://www.sciencedirect.com/science/book/9780815515692. doi:10.1016/B978-0-8155-1569-2.50016-6.

Secchi, M., Castellani, V., Collina, E., Mirabella, N., Sala, S., 2016. Assessing eco-innovations in green chemistry: life Cycle Assessment (LCA) of a cosmetic product with a bio-based ingredient. J. Clean. Prod. 09596526. 129, 269–281. doi:10.1016/j.jclepro.2016.04.073.

Seferli, M., Kotanidou, C., Lefkaki, M., Adamantidi, T., Panoutsopoulou, E., Finos, M.A., Krey, G., Kamidis, N., Stamatis, N., Anastasiadou, C., Tsoupras, A., 2024. Bioactives of the freshwater aquatic plants, *Nelumbo nucifera* and *Lemna minor*, for functional foods, cosmetics and pharmaceutical applications, with antioxidant, anti-inflammatory and antithrombotic health-promoting properties. Appl. Sci. 2076-3417. 14 (15), 6634. doi:10.3390/app14156634.

Shahanawaz, M., Singh, K., Suvaiv, S.P.K., Kumar, A., Ahmad, S., 2025. Natural Ingredients in Pharmaceutical Technology for Cosmetics the Impact of Pharma Technology on Cosmetics: Advancements and Innovations. Bentham Science Publishers, India, pp. 128–163. Available from: https://benthambooks.com/book/9798898810726/. doi:10.2174/97988988810726125010009.

Shiels, K., Tsoupras, A., Lordan, R., Zabetakis, I., Murray, P., Saha, S.K., 2022. Anti-inflammatory and antithrombotic properties of polar lipid extracts, rich in unsaturated fatty acids, from the Irish marine cyanobacterium Spirulina subsalsa. J. Funct. Foods. 17564646. 94, 105124. doi:10.1016/j.jff.2022.105124.

Shim, J., Woo, J., Yeo, H., Kang, S., Kwon, B., Lee, E.J., Jooyoung, O., Jeong, E., Lim, J., Park, S.G., 2024. The clean beauty trend among millennial and Generation Z consumers: assessing the safety, ethicality, and sustainability attributes of cosmetic products. Sage Open. 2158-2440. 14 (2). doi:10.1177/21582440241255430.

Silva, D., Ferreira, M.S., Sousa-Lobo, J.M., Cruz, M.T., Almeida, I.F., 2021. Anti-inflammatory activity of *Calendula officinalis* L. Flower extract. Cosmetics 20799284. 8 (2). Available from: https://www.mdpi.com/2079-9284/8/2/31/pdf. doi:10.3390/cosmetics8020031.

Silva, S., Bautista-Hérnandez, I., Gomez-García, R., Costa, E.M., Machado, M., 2025. Precision fermentation as a tool for sustainable cosmetic ingredient production. Appl. Sci. 2076-3417. 15 (17), 9246. doi:10.3390/app15179246.

Soh, S.H., Lee, L.Y., 2019. Microencapsulation and nanoencapsulation using supercritical fluid (SCF) techniques. Pharmaceutics 19994923. 11 (1). Available from: https://www.mdpi.com/1999-4923/11/1/21/pdf. doi:10.3390/pharmaceutics11010021.

Sousa, P., Tavares-Valente, D., Amorim, M., Azevedo-Silva, J., Pintado, M., Fernandes, J., 2023. β-Glucan extracts as high-value multifunctional ingredients for skin health: a review. Carbohydr. Polym. 01448617. 322, 121329. doi:10.1016/j.carbpol.2023.121329.

Stahl, W., Sies, H., 2012. β-Carotene and other carotenoids in protection from sunlight. Am. J. Clin. Nutr. 00029165. 96 (5), 1179S. doi:10.3945/ajcn.112.034819.

Suganya, V., Anuradha, V., 2017. Microencapsulation and nanoencapsulation: a review. Int. J. Pharm. Clin. Res. 9. https://doi.org/10.25258/ijpcr.v9i3.8324

Suphasomboon, T., Vassanadumrongdee, S., 2025. Perceived greenwashing and its impact on consumer behavior in the cosmetic industry. Clean. Responsible Consumpt. 26667843. 100377. doi:10.1016/j.clrc.2025.100377.

Swagata Dutta, S.P.J.K., Banerjee, R., 2023. A comprehensive review on astaxanthin sources, structure, biochemistry and applications in the cosmetic industry. Algal Res. 22119264. 74, 103168. doi:10.1016/j.algal.2023.103168.

Szopa, D., Wróbel, P., Witek-Krowiak, A., 2024. Enhancing polyphenol extraction efficiency: a systematic review on the optimization strategies with natural deep eutectic solvents. J. Mol. Liq. 01677322. 404, 124902. doi:10.1016/j.molliq.2024.124902.

Tang, Y., Nie, T., Zhang, L., Liu, X., Deng, H., 2025. Peptides in cosmetics: from pharmaceutical breakthroughs to skincare innovations. Cosmetics. 2079-9284. 12 (3), 107. doi:10.3390/cosmetics12030107.

Tang, Z., Du, Q., 2024. Mechanism of action of preservatives in cosmetics. J. Dermatol. Sci. Cosmet. Technol. 1, 100054. doi:https://doi.org/10.1016/j.jdsct.2024.100054.

Tavares, R.S.N., Kawakami, C.M., Pereira, K.D.C., Amaral, G.T.D., Benevenuto, C.G., Maria-Engler, S.S., Colepicolo, P., Debonsi, H.M., Gaspar, L.R., 2020. Fucoxanthin for topical administration, a phototoxic vs. Photoprotective potential in a tiered strategy assessed by in vitro methods. Antioxidants 20763921. 9 (4). Available from: https://www.mdpi.com/2076-3921/9/4/328/pdf. doi:10.3390/antiox9040328.

TechSci Research, n.d. Asia Pacific Cosmetics Market Size, Share, and Growth Report 2030. Available from: https://www.techsciresearch.com/report/asia-pacific-cosmetics-market/28918.html. (Accessed 20 Dec 2025).

The Editors, 2022. Innovative approaches in cosmetic testing, in compliance with European regulations - June 22nd-23rd 2022. Biomed. Sci. Eng. 2531-9892 6 (s1). doi:10.4081/bse.2022.205.

Tiwari, B.K., 2015. Ultrasound: a clean, green extraction technology. TrAC Trends Anal. Chem. 01659936. 71, 100–109. doi:10.1016/j.trac.2015.04.013.

Tsiapali, O.I., Ayfantopoulou, E., Tzourouni, A., Ofrydopoulou, A., Letsiou, S., Tsoupras, A., 2025. Unveiling the utilization of grape and winery by-products in cosmetics with health-promoting properties. Appl. Sci. 2076-3417. 15 (3), 1007. doi:10.3390/app15031007.

Tsoupras, A., Lordan, R., Demuru, M., Shiels, K., Saha, S., Nasopoulou, C., Zabetakis, I., 2018. Structural elucidation of Irish organic farmed salmon (*Salmo salar*) polar lipids with antithrombotic activities. Mar. Drugs. 1660-3397. 16 (6), 176. doi:10.3390/md16060176.

Tsoupras, A., Ni, V.L.J., O'Mahony, É., Karali, M., 2023. Winemaking: "with one stone, two birds"? a holistic review of the bio-functional compounds, applications and health benefits of wine and wineries' by-products. Fermentation. 2311-5637. 9 (9), 838. doi:10.3390/fermentation9090838.

Tsoupras, A., Panagopoulou, E.A., Kyzas, G.Z., 2024. Anti-inflammatory, antithrombotic and anti-oxidant bioactives of beer and brewery by-products, as ingredients of bio-functional foods, nutraceuticals, cosmetics, cosmeceuticals and pharmaceuticals with health promoting properties. AIMS Agric. Food 24712086. 9 (2), 568–606. Available from: https://www.aimspress.com/journal/agriculture. doi:10.3934/agrfood.2024032.

Turcu, O., Brancu, C., 2025. Cosmetics industry performance in the European Union: a comparative analysis. Proc. Int. Conf. Bus. Excell. 2558-9652. 19 (1), 2267–2276. doi:10.2478/picbe-2025-0175.

Ugoeze, K.C., Odeku, O.A., 2022. Herbal bioactive–based cosmetics. In: Bakshi, I.S., Bala, R., Madaan, R., Sindhu, R.K. (Eds.), Herbal Bioactive-Based Drug Delivery Systems. Elsevier, pp. 195–226.

Urrea-Victoria, V., Casas, A.S.G., Castellanos, L., Serafini, M.R., Marcela Aragón Novoa, D., 2025. Lip photoprotection patents (2014–2024): key trends and emerging technologies. Cosmetics. 2079-9284. 12 (4), 161. doi:10.3390/cosmetics12040161.

van Walraven, N., FitzGerald, R.J., Danneel, H.-J., Amigo-Benavent, M., 2025. Bioactive peptides in cosmetic formulations: review of current in vitro and ex vivo evidence. Peptides. 01969781. 193, 171440. doi:10.1016/j.peptides.2025.171440.

Vandorou, M., Plakidis, C., Tsompanidou, I.M., Adamantidi, T., Panagopoulou, E.A., Tsoupras, A., 2024. A review on apple pomace bioactives for natural functional food and cosmetic products with therapeutic health-promoting properties. Int. J. Mol. Sci. 1422-0067. 25 (19), 10856. doi:10.3390/ijms251910856.

Vandorou, M., Plakidis, C., Tsompanidou, I.M., Ofrydopoulou, A., Shiels, K., Saha, S.K., Tsoupras, A., 2025. In vitro antioxidant, antithrombotic and anti-inflammatory properties of the amphiphilic bioactives from Greek organic Starking apple juice and its by-products (apple pomace). Appl. Sci. 2076-3417. 15 (5), 2807. doi:10.3390/app15052807.

Varvaresou, A., Papageorgiou, S., Tsirivas, E., Protopapa, E., Kintziou, H., Kefala, V., Demetzos, C., 2009. Self-preserving cosmetics. Int. J. Cosmet. Sci. 0142-5463. 31 (3), 163–175. doi:10.1111/j.1468-2494.2009.00492.x.

Venetikidou, M., Lykartsi, E., Adamantidi, T., Prokopiou, V., Ofrydopoulou, A., Letsiou, S., Tsoupras, A., 2025. Proteolytic enzyme activities of bromelain, ficin, and papain from fruit by-products and potential applications in sustainable and functional cosmetics for skincare. Appl. Sci. 2076-3417. 15 (5), 2637. doi:10.3390/app15052637.

Vieira, C., Rebocho, S., Craveiro, R., Paiva, A., Duarte, A.R.C., 2022. Selective extraction and stabilization of bioactive compounds from rosemary leaves using a biphasic NADES. Front. Chem. 2296-2646. 10. doi:10.3389/fchem.2022.954835.

Wang, L., Lee, J.H., 2021. The impact of K-beauty social media influencers, sponsorship, and product exposure on consumer acceptance of new products. Fash. Text. 21980802. 8 (1). Available from: https://www.springer.com/materials/journal/40691. doi:10.1186/s40691-020-00239-0.

Wang, Z., Nan, W., Huazhe, S., Wang, S., Zhang, H., Guangyu, L., 2020. Pantothenic acid promotes dermal papilla cell proliferation in hair follicles of American minks via inhibitor of DNA Binding 3/Notch signaling pathway. Life Sci. 00243205. 252, 117667. doi:10.1016/j.lfs.2020.117667.

Wei, M., Huang, Y., Zhu, J., Qiao, Y., Xiao, N., Jin, M., Gao, H., Huang, Y., Xiufang, H., Li, O., 2024. Advances in hyaluronic acid production: biosynthesis and genetic engineering strategies based on *Streptococcus* — a review. Int. J. Biol. Macromol. 01418130. 270 (Pt 2), 132334. doi:10.1016/j.ijbiomac.2024.132334.

Weina, A., Yanling, Y., 2022. Role of knowledge management on the sustainable environment: assessing the moderating effect of innovative culture. Front. Psychol. 1664-1078. 13. doi:10.3389/fpsyg.2022.861813.

Wells, N., 2023. FDA Regulation of Cosmetics and Personal Care Products Under the Modernization of Cosmetics Regulation Act of 2022 (MoCRA). https://www.congress.gov/crs-product/R47826 (Accessed 10 Dec 2025).

Whang, J.B., Song, J.H., Choi, B., Lee, J.H., 2021. The effect of Augmented Reality on purchase intention of beauty products: the roles of consumers' control. J. Bus. Res. 01482963. 133, 275–284. Available from: http://www.elsevier.com/locate/jbusres. doi:10.1016/j.jbusres.2021.04.057.

Wirtu, Y.D., 2024. A review of environmental and health effects of synthetic cosmetics. Front. Environ. Sci. 2296665X. 12. Available from: https://journal.frontiersin.org/journal/environmental-science. doi:10.3389/fenvs.2024.1402893.

Wongwad, E., Preedalikit, W., Rungsang, T., Srivilai, J., Aunsri, N., Mungmai, L., 2025. Evaluation of industrial crop emollients from perilla oil, cocoa butter, and wild almond butter extracts: physicochemical characterization, stability, bioactivity, and clinical efficacy of product formulations in a double-blind trial. Ind. Crops Prod. 09266690. 236, 122083. doi:10.1016/j.indcrop.2025.122083.

Yadav, S., Sinha, M., Taradia, K., Sharma, A.K., Kulshreshtha, M., 2025. Pharmacovigilance, cosmetovigilance, hemovigilance, and materiovigilance in healthcare domains. J. Med. Surg. Public Health. 2949916X. 5, 100175. doi:10.1016/j.glmedi.2024.100175.

Zhe, S., Luo, F.-Y., Pei, X.-R., Zhang, F.-L., Xing, S.-X., Wang, G.-L., 2020. Final publication of the "Regulations on the supervision and administration of cosmetics" and new perspectives of cosmetic science in China. Cosmetics. 2079-9284. 7 (4), 98. doi:10.3390/cosmetics7040098.

Zhu, C., Hong, T., Hebin, L., Chen, Y., Zheng, M., Zhipeng, L., Jiang, Z., Hui, N., Zhu, Y., 2025. κ-Carrageenan tetrasaccharide ameliorates particulate matter-induced defects in skin hydration of human keratinocytes cells and skin barrier disorders. Int. J. Biol. Macromol. 01418130. 301, 140395. doi:10.1016/j.ijbiomac.2025.140395.

Žiemytė, M., Escudero, A., Díez, P., Ferrer, M.D., Murguía, J.R., Martí-Centelles, V., Mira, A., Martínez-Máñez, R., 2023. Ficin–cyclodextrin-based docking nanoarchitectonics of self-propelled nanomotors for bacterial biofilm eradication. Chem. Mater. 0897-4756. 35 (11), 4412–4426. doi:10.1021/acs.chemmater.3c00587.

Index

Note: Page numbers followed by *f* indicate figures, *t* indicate tables.

C

D

E

H

I

K

L

M

Q

R

S

T

U

V

W

X

Y

Z

Printed and bound by CPI Group (UK) Ltd, Croydon, CR0 4YY
14/09/2026
02216388-0016